Ben Cao Gang Mu, Volume IV: Marshland Herbs, Poisonous Herbs

by Li Shizhen

The *Ben Cao Gang Mu* Series

The complete Chinese text
translated and annotated by Paul U. Unschuld

Vol. I.	Ch. 1 – 4. Introduction, History, Pharmacology, Diseases and Suitable Pharmaceutical Drugs
Vol. II.	Ch. 5 – 11. Waters, Fires, Soils, Metals, Jades, Stones, Minerals, Salts
Vol. III.	Ch. 12 – 14. Mountain Herbs, Fragrant Herbs
Vol. IV.	Ch. 15 – 17. Marshland Herbs, Poisonous Herbs
Vol. V.	Ch. 18 – 25. Creeping Herbs, Water Herbs, Herbs Growing on Stones, Mosses, Cereals
Vol. VI.	Ch. 26 – 33. Vegetables, Fruits
Vol. VII.	Ch. 34 – 37. Woods
Vol. VIII.	Ch. 38 – 46. Clothes, Utensils, Worms, Insects, Amphibians, Animals with Scales, Animals with Shells
Vol. IX.	Ch. 47 – 52. Fowls, Domestic & Wild Animals, Human Substances

Tools

The *Dictionary of the Ben Cao Gang Mu*

Vol. I.	Chinese Historical Illness Terminology
Vol. II.	Geographical and Administrative Designations
Vol. III.	Persons and Literary Sources
Vol. IV.	Substance Identification

Ben Cao Gang Mu, Volume IV: Marshland Herbs, Poisonous Herbs

by Li Shizhen

16th Century Chinese Encyclopedia of *Materia Medica* and Natural History

The complete Chinese text
translated and annotated

by

Paul U. Unschuld

UNIVERSITY OF CALIFORNIA PRESS

The generous financial support of the *Ben cao gang mu* translation project and of the publication of the resulting volumes by Mr. Rong Yumin 荣裕民 is gratefully acknowledged.

University of California Press
Oakland, California

Cataloging-in-Publication Data is on file at the Library of Congress.

Library of Congress Control Number: 2020946743

ISBN 978-0-520-38503-0 (cloth : alk. paper)
ISBN 978-0-520-38504-7 (ebook)

Manufactured in the United States of America

31 30 29 28 27 26 25 24 23 22

CONTENTS

1. Prolegomena

This book offers, together with the original Chinese text, the first complete philological and annotated English translation of chapters 15 through 17 of the *Ben cao gang mu* 本草綱目, the 16th century Chinese Encyclopedia of *Materia Medica* and Natural History by Li Shizhen 李時珍 (1518 – 1593), devoted to the natural history and pharmaceutical application of what were considered at the time "marshland herbs" and "poisonous herbs." It opens up an almost two-millennia-long panorama of wide-ranging observations and sophisticated interpretations, ingenious manipulations and practical applications of natural substances for the benefit of human health. As Prof. Zheng Jinsheng 郑金生, the pre-eminent *Ben cao gang mu* expert of present day China, has characterized it:

> "Some of the pharmaceutical substances gathered in this book have already left the platform of their clinical application. However, the data associated with them offer abundant material to study the customs of the people and the culture of the past. While he gathered data related to pharmaceutical substances, Li Shizhen never hesitated to extend his investigations and collection to all possible realms. That is, while [the *Ben cao gang mu*] appears to be a book on *materia medica*, it is in fact an encyclopedia of natural science and has become a treasure house for today's researchers of many fields of science."[1]

1.1 History of Chinese *materia medica* literature

The *Ben cao gang mu* is the culmination of a 1600-year history of Chinese *materia medica* literature. This history began at some time during the Han dynasties when, between the 2nd century BCE and the 2nd century CE, two hitherto in China undocumented genres of medical-therapeutic works appeared. Stimulated by impulses whose origin and nature remain enigmatic today, the new therapeutic approach of needling 365 "holes" spread over the human body, on the one hand; and a first detailed description of 365 individual pharmaceutical substances on the other, marked

1 Zheng Jinsheng 郑金生 and Zhang Zhibin 张志斌, *Ben cao gang mu dao du* 本草綱目导读, "Guide to Reading the *Ben cao gang mu*," Beijing, Ke xue chu ban she 科學出版社, 2016, 35.

the onset of two traditions of health care. They conceptually remained separate for one thousand years. Why the number of days in a solar year, 365 – rather unusual in the history of Chinese categorization of natural phenomena – was chosen as a starting point of both traditions is unclear.

Needling therapy, or so-called acupuncture, remained an isolated facet of Chinese medical culture until the 11th/12th century. Its seminal texts, the Yellow Thearch classics,[2] were either lost during the first millennium or survived only through a rather tenuous tradition, supported by a few members of the social elite.[3] Apparently, the Yinyang and Five Phases doctrines of systematic correspondences, which legitimated and guided needle therapy from its beginning, failed to achieve the status of a world view widely acknowledged by broad segments of the population. In contrast, pharmaceutical therapy, as evidenced by published recipe collections and works focusing on the description of individual substances, constituted the mainstay of medical practice from the first millennium to the present day.

Since the early 1970s, recipe manuscripts with data on the therapeutic properties of combinations of herbal, mineral and animal substances have been recovered from late Zhou and early Han era tombs.[4] The list of therapeutic indications and a highly developed pharmaceutical technology outlined in these texts evidence a long development of pharmaceutical therapy prior to the compilation of works with descriptions of the properties of individual substances. The earliest of these works known is the *Shen nong ben cao* 神農本草, "Shen nong's *materia medica.*" Historians agree that it was written at some time between the 1st century BCE and the 1st century CE.[5]

Even though at that time Chinese civilization recognized and documented in bibliographies and catalogues individual authorship of literary works, the authors of the seminal texts of both the needling and the pharmaceutical traditions remained anonymous. Their origins were traced to legendary culture heros, that is, Huang

2 Including the *Huang Di nei jing su wen* 黃帝內經素問, *Huang di nei jing ling shu* 黃帝內經靈樞, and a late sequel, the *Nan jing* 難經. For philological translations of these classics, see Paul U. Unschuld and Hermann Tessenow, *Huang Di Nei Jing Su Wen. An Annotated Translation of Huang Di's Inner Classic*, 2 vols. University of California Press, Berkeley and Los Angeles, 2011. Paul U. Unschuld, *Huang Di Nei Jing Ling Shu. The Ancient Classic on Needle Therapy*. University of California Press, Oakland, 2016. Paul U. Unschuld, *Nan jing. The Classic of Difficult Issues*. Oakland 2016.

3 Paul U. Unschuld, 2016, 1 – 4.

4 Donald Harper, *Early Chinese Medical Literature. The Mawangdui Medical Manuscripts*. Kegan Paul International, London and New York, 1997.

5 For details on the *Sheng non ben cao* and the subsequent history of Chinese *materia medica* literature, see Paul U. Unschuld, *Medicine in China. A History of Pharmaceutics*. Berkeley, Los Angeles, London, 1986.

Di 黃帝, the Yellow Thearch, and Shen Nong 神農, the divine husbandman. Shen Nong, also known as Yan Di 炎帝, the Fiery Thearch, was said in the *Huai nan zi* 淮南子 to have pitied the suffering of mankind. Hence he tasted all kinds of herbs and "discovered 100 with poison per day." From the very beginning, for a natural substance "to have poison" (*you du* 有毒) or "to be nonpoisonous" (*wu du* 無毒) was seen as an important criterion for assessing its acute or long-term therapeutic potential.

The *Shen nong ben cao*, closely associated with the tripartite world view of Dong Zhongshu 董仲舒 (179 – 104) and a political structure antagonistic to the hierarchy of the young empire, distinguished among three "ranks" (*pin* 品) of pharmaceutical substances. The upper rank, associated with heaven, included substances identified as *jun* 君, "rulers." These were considered nonpoisonous and capable of helping extend life. A lower rank, associated with the earth, was assigned to substances "with poison." These were given the status of *zuo* 佐and *shi* 使, that is, "helpers" and "agents," and they helped eliminate the disease. A middle rank of *chen* 臣, "officials," associated with mankind, was positioned between the upper and lower ranks. Some of these "officials" were considered "nonpoisonous," while others were known to "have poison." They acted as intermediaries between the rulers above and their helpers and agents below. The substances described, arranged according to a preface into groups of 120, 120 and 125 respectively,[6] were mostly herbal. This may be the reason behind the naming of the first *materia medica* work and henceforth the entire literature genre *ben cao* 本草, which possibly meant "based on herbs."

Tao Hongjing 陶弘景 (452-536), a Daoist naturalist, was the first author to revise and expand the "original classic," *Ben jing* 本經, as he called the *Shen nong ben cao*. In a first work, titled *Shen nong ben cao jing* 神農本草經, "Shen nong's classic on *materia medica*," he retained the original division into three chapters, but added 365 "additional records [on pharmaceutical substances recorded earlier] by renowned physicians," *ming yi bie lu* 明醫別錄. In a second work shortly thereafter, the *Shen nong ben cao jing ji zhu* 神農本草經集注, "Various annotations to Shen nong's classic on *materia medica*," Tao Hongjing significantly expanded his annotations to the 730 substances listed and divided the text into seven chapters.

Tao Hongjing initiated a "main tradition" of *ben cao* works, which would be continued by subsequent authors until the early 13th century. This tradition was characterized by an expansion of the "original classic" with ever more data on the nature, origin, therapeutic effects and pharmaceutical processing of natural and man-made

6 The *Shen nong ben cao* versions accessible today are based on reconstructions by Chinese and Japanese researchers since the 17th century. They have identified 141 substances as "upper rank," 111 substances as "middle rank," and 103 substances as "lower rank," totaling 365.

substances. This data was often adopted from an increasing number of *materia medica* works published outside of the main tradition whose authors did not feel committed to the structure and contents of the *Ben jing*. They focused on regional knowledge, their own experience, substances used as both medication and food, substances enabling survival in times of famine, pharmaceutical processing and other such special aspects of pharmaceutical lore. In the middle of the seventh century, an official named Su Jing 蘇敬 (fl. 657) suggested that the emperor support a new edition of the "original classic" to correct older data regarded since as erroneous, and include more recent knowledge of the therapeutic potential of natural substances. The result, the *Xin xiu ben cao* 新修本草, "Newly revised *materia medica*," of 659, combining 850 substance entries in 54 chapters, was the first government-sponsored and illustrated *ben cao* work in China.

The main tradition came to a halt in the 13th century for at least two reasons. The lengthy title of one of the final works of this tradition, published in 1249 and describing 1746 substances in 30 chapters, offers a clear indication of one of these reasons: *Chong xiu zheng he jing shi zheng lei bei yong ben cao* 重修正和經史證類備用本草, "Newly revised *materia medica* of the *zheng he* reign period, based on data from the classics and historical annals, based on evidence and ordered on the basis of groups, prepared for clinical application." The main tradition was stifled by the abundance of its data and the perpetuation of its claim to be merely extending the original classic. The last works were extremely unwieldy. More recent data was added to previous statements, without comments on contradictions or earlier errors. Readers were left abandoned with ever longer sequences of quotes from a wide range of sources of varying quality.

We see a second reason for the end of the main tradition in a completely new genre of *materia medica* texts initiated by Kou Zongshi's 寇宗奭 *Ben cao yan yi* 本草衍意, "Extended ideas on materia medica," in 1119 and exemplified by Wang Haogu's 王好古 *Tang ye ben cao* 湯液本草, "*Materia medica* of decoctions" in the mid 13th century. With the rise of Song Neo-Confucianism, the more than one-millennium-old schism was bridged between the therapeutic approaches of needling and pharmaceutical therapy. Needling, i.e. acupuncture, was based on the Yinyang and Five Phases doctrines of systematic correspondences. *Ben cao* literature and recipe collections were based on empirical knowledge and magic correspondences. The convergence of these two separate approaches resulted in a first pharmacology of systematic correspondences. Authors committed to this new perspective categorized each pharmaceutical substance according to its presumed association with certain kinds of flavor and qi. As these kinds of flavor and qi were associated, in turn, with certain yin and yang qualities, as well as with the Five Phases, a link appeared possible to pathologies also defined in terms of yin and yang and the Five Phases.

The main tradition was unable to integrate the ideas published by the various authors of the so-called Song-Jin-Yuan epoch of *ben cao* literature. As a result, the publication of comprehensive *materia medica* texts ended. Each of these works claimed to offer all available pharmaceutical knowledge, old and new. It was only three centuries later, in the 16th century, that two authors introduced a new structure to the contents of comprehensive *materia medica* works, leading to a brief revival of the tradition. The first result was the *Yu zhi ben cao pin hui jing yao* 御製本草品彙精要, "*Materia medica*, written on imperial order, containing essential data arranged in systematic order," in 1505. The second and more successful of these newer *ben cao* works was the *Ben cao gang mu* 本草綱目 of 1593 compiled by Li Shizhen 李時珍 (1518-1593).

1.2 Structure and contents of the *Ben cao gang mu*

It is not known whether Li Shizhen saw the *Yu zhi ben cao pin hui jing yao* before he set out to compile the *Ben cao gang mu*. In his own personal interest, Qiu Jun 邱濬 (1420 – 1495), a scholar official, had devised a scheme to overcome the unwieldy nature of the final texts of the main tradition of *ben cao* literature. By restructuring the individual substance monographs, he removed the decisive obstacle to practical use of the *ben cao* texts. He dismissed the idea that newer *ben cao* works were mere emendations of the "original classic," with whatever new knowledge had become available being added to the substance of earlier works. Qiu Jun divided each monograph in accordance with 13 characteristics of individual substances that he extracted from former texts.[7]

As a result, a reader interested in the origin, the pharmaceutical processing or the therapeutic indications of a particular substance found relevant data collected under a respective heading. To find the information they sought, users of the new text were no longer required to read through all the historical layers that had accrued among the texts of the main tradition of *ben cao* works. Qiu Jun died when he had finished writing only one chapter. After hectic intrigue and conflicts of interest, Liu Wentai 劉文泰 (fl. 1503), an official in the Imperial Medical Office, and a team of collaborators were ordered by Emperor Xiao zong 孝宗 (1470 – 1505) in 1503 "to prepare a new *ben cao* edition, to simplify the consultation of these works." They took

7 Paul U. Unschuld, 1986, 140-141

over the structural proposals of Qiu Jun but expanded the number of subheadings of each substance monograph from 13 to 24.

The new work was completed only two years later. Pleased, the emperor personally gave it the title "The Essentials of *Materia medica* with the Data on Items Arranged According to their Similar Nature, compiled on Imperial Order." Soon afterward, the emperor died. The manuscript was never published, possibly because of the exquisite color illustrations added to each entry. No technology was available in the 16th century to print such a work. Several manuscript copies were prepared and a few have ended up in libraries in Japan, Rome and Berlin. In 1701 a revised and amended version without the illustrations was prepared, by order of Emperor Kang xi 康熙. It was published by Shanghai Commercial Press in 1937.[8]

Li Shizhen chose a structure for his *Ben cao gang mu* entries similar to that of the *Yu zhi ben cao pin hui jing yao* substance monographs. However, rather than separating the data of each entry into 24 categories, he decided to limit their subheadings, where required, to the following ten:

1. *xiao zheng* 校正: Editorial Correction
2. *shi ming* 釋名: Explanation of Names
3. *ji jie* 集解: Collected Explanations
4. *xiu zhi* 脩治: Pharmaceutical Preparation
5. *bian yi* 辯疑: Discussion of Uncertain Issues
6. *zheng wu* 正誤: Correction of Errors
7. *qi wei* 氣味: Qi and Flavor
8. *zhu zhi* 主治: Therapeutic Control
9. *fa ming* 發明: Explication
10. *fu fang* 附方: Added Recipes

Li Shizhen also conceptualized a new order of the entries. The "original classic," within the three groups of "upper," "middle," and "lower rank," had listed substances following their identification as mineral, herbal, and animal-human – i.e. proceeding from dead and immobile to living and immobile, and on to living and mobile substances. A fourth and final group consisted of victuals. Later works of the main tradition omitted the "upper," "middle," and "lower rank" divisions, but retained the mineral, herbal, and animal-human classifications.

Li Shizhen introduced a different order. Based on the sequence of the Five Phases, he began, after four introductory chapters, the subsequent 48 chapters with a list of waters, followed by fires, soils, and metals, which included salts and min-

8 Ibid., 142-143

erals (chapters 5-11) and then herbal substancs (chapters 12 through 37). Separated by chapter 38, listing "fabrics and utensils," he then devoted chapters 39 through 50 to animals, ranging from "tiny" to "large," that is, from worms/bugs through fowl to four-legged creatures. Again separated by a chapter on "strange items," he eventually reached the pinnacle of his scale, human substances suitable for a medicinal application. In all, Li Shizhen wrote down ca. 1.6 million characters to describe 1892 pharmaceutical substances.

The entries in the final 48 chapters were divided into 16 sections, for 13 of which Li Shizhen identified subsections. These serve to point out related items within broader groups such as waters, herbs and worms/bugs. For example, the section on worms/bugs is subdivided into those born from eggs, those generated through transformation, and those originating from moisture. Each section is introduced by a general statement explicating the special nature of the substances grouped in it. Each individual substance is given a heading stating its earliest name documented in pharmaceutical literature and, if this was the "original classic," the upper, middle or lower rank it had been assigned to.

Where required, Li Shizhen began an entry by pointing out a formerly erroneous listing of the substance in question. Whenever he found identical substances listed in previous *ben cao* works twice under different names, he justified the combination of these names in one entry.

The length of documented Chinese pharmaceutical history, the sheer size of the country with its many regional cultures and languages, and the different kinds of sources quoted by Li Shizhen led him to list and discuss the names of the substances he described. Not infrequently, Li Shizhen saw a need to explain different names in the North and South of China assigned to an identical substance. For example, in chapter 09, he went into an extensive discussion to end an apparently millennia-old confusion concerning the substance gypsum. It was known as *shi gao* 石膏, "stone fat," *xi li shi* 細理石, "finely structured stone/mineral," and *han shui shi* 寒水石, "cold water stone/mineral." Some authors identified it as *fang jie shi* 方解石, "stone/mineral that splits into rectangular pieces," and as *chang shi* 長石, "lengthy stone/mineral." But these names had also been applied to other minerals. Li Shizhen brought all relevant quotes together and eventually offered his conclusion.

Li Shizhen titled the relevant subheading *shi ming* 釋名, "Explanation of Names," because he went beyond simply enumerating alternative names. Wherever possible he added philological explanations taking into account, for example, local dialects and the composition of characters. Substances imported from foreign countries often were given names in China transcribing the pronunciation of their original foreign pronunciation. Wherever feasible, Li Shizhen included information on the origin of such names, for example, reflecting a Sanskrit term. Furthermore, many names were written with characters possibly unfamiliar to the *Ben cao gang mu*'s readers. Hence Li Shizhen explained their pronunciation by either adducing homophones or resorting to the split-reading approach. And when he felt at his wits' end, he freely acknowledged his inability to explain a certain name.

While this explanation of names suggests an awareness of certain limits of understanding among future readers and users of the *Ben cao gang mu*, Li Shizhen rarely explained a central feature of each substance described: its therapeutic indications. The quotes on the ability of substances to "control" disease are taken from sources spanning more than 1500 years. The *Ben cao gang mu* lists more than 4500 key disease terms; by the time of Li Shizhen, perhaps most of them were still self-explanatory or could be understood by experts from their context.

In today's China, many of the disease names referred to in these quotes are no longer easily understood. Similarly, for readers of the *Ben cao gang mu* outside China, the therapeutic indications are often given with rather enigmatic disease names written in single, unfamiliar characters or using metaphors that are no longer easily grasped. The first volume of the *Dictionary of the Ben cao gang mu* traces each of the 4500 disease terms to its earliest appearance. It identifies its meaning in that early context and, where applicable, at the time of Li Shizhen.[9]

Another central feature of descriptions of pharmaceutical substances is their place of origin. From early on it was known among Chinese experts that one and the same herb was endowed with different therapeutic powers depending on where it grew in the country. The climate and the nature of the soil varied from North to South and from East to West, and so did the "qi" a plant was exposed to. Hence where considered necessary, substance entries of the *Ben cao gang mu* include related information. This is mostly comparative, that is, Li Shizhen provided a ranking of the substances from different regions in accordance with the presumed strength of their therapeutic effects. All the dynasties that followed each other during the imperial age regularly rearranged administrative structures. As a consequence, place names and the names of administrative structures were assigned new names. Hardly any location kept one and the same name throughout history. Li Shizhen regularly explained the location in his time of places mentioned in an ancient quote under a name no longer in use. Today, the current location of even more places can no longer be easily identified by their ancient names.

The second volume of the *Dictionary of the Ben cao gang mu* traces each of the place names and those of administrative structures mentioned in the *Ben cao gang*

9 See Zhang Zhibin and Paul U. Unschuld, *Dictionary of the Ben cao gang mu*. Vol. I: *Chinese Historical Illness Terminology*. University of California Press, Oakland, 2015.

mu to their current location. More importantly, the *Dictionary* offers the history of each name and each administrative structure so that a quote from a specific time period may be compared to the existence of a name and administrative structure at that time. This is of particular relevance if one identical name was given to different locations in the course of history, or if the borders of an administrative structure were moved to a degree that may have had a significant impact on the climate or nature of soil suggested by its name.[10]

No *materia medica* text prior to the *Ben cao gang mu* was based on a comparable range of literary and non-literary material. It should come as no surprise that Li Shizhen exploited the *Zheng he ben cao* 正和本草of 1249, the final work of the former main tradition of *ben cao* works, as his major source. Apparently, Li Shizhen intended to continue this tradition, but he went far beyond it. In a bibliography at the very beginning of the *Ben cao gang mu*, he listed more than 868 titles he had consulted. The number of titles quoted or mentioned in passing in the main text by far exceeds these 868 texts. Li Shizhen may not have held all of them in original editions in his hands. Many texts were quoted second- or third-hand from quotes inIn addition to drawing his data from all kinds of literary genres, Li Shizhen personally travelled to places all over the country where he expected to access data available nowhere else. This way, he also was able to record valuable data on substances not mentioned in *ben cao* literature or publicly documented elsewhere before. For example, *san qi* 三七, identified today as *Gynura segetum* (Lour.) Merr., is one of the most common herbs in Chinese medicine. Li Shizhen was the first to learn of its therapeutic potential from "locals," and introduced it with the following lines:

> "This medication was discovered for the first time only recently. The people in the South use it in their military as an important medication for wounds caused by metal objects/weapons. It is said to have an extraordinary [therapeutic] potential. It is also said: For all injuries resulting from flogging and blows, when stagnating blood is set free, it should be chewed until it is pulpy. Once this is applied [to the affected region, the bleeding] ends. Greenish swelling is dissolved. If one is to be flogged, let him ingest beforehand one or two *qian* and his blood will not rush to his heart. After a flogging it is even more advisable to ingest it. To ingest it after a birth is good, too. Generally speaking, this medication has warm qi and a sweet and slightly bitter flavor. Hence it is a medication for the blood section of the yang brilliance and ceasing yin [conduits] and can

10 See Hua Linfu, Paul D. Buell and Paul U. Unschuld, *Dictionary of the Ben cao gang mu. Vol. II: Geographical and Administrative Designations*. University of California Press, Oakland, 2017

serve to cure all kinds of blood diseases, similar to *qi lin jie* (*Daemonorops draco* Bl.) and shellac."[11]

In this manner the *Ben cao gang mu* refers to hundreds of texts and their authors, in addition to individuals (including Li Shizhen's own extended family) unassociated with any literary genre.

Many of the persons quoted or referred to as authors, patients, healers or actors in some anecdote have remained nameless to posterity. In bibliographical and biographical reference works today's readers of the *Ben cao gang mu may* easily find the more prominent book titles, authors and historical personalities encountered in the *Ben cao gang mu*. But an identification of numerous titles and many more persons requires extensive research. It is here that one wonders how many collaborators Li Shizhen may have had. Wang Shizhen, the author of a preface to the first edition of the *Ben cao gang mu*, quotes Li Shizhen verbatim with a statement that he had rewritten the entire manuscript three times.[12] A question arises here whether he had failed to notice numerous inconsistencies in the references to book titles and authors quoted. Not infrequently, one book is quoted with either its complete title or several different abbreviations. Similarly, one identical author is quoted by his full name, by his first or last name, by his style, or other possible designations. Such diversity appears plausible if one imagines a larger team around Li Shizhen supplying him with data without prior agreement on how to quote a text or refer to a person. If this diversity makes it difficult enough for readers to immediately identify a text or author quoted, the hardship is further aggravated by numerous quotes misleadingly ascribed to source texts they were never part of.

Not much later, Zhao Xuemin 趙學敏 (ca. 1730 – 1805), author of the *Ben cao gang mu shi yi* 本草綱目拾遺, suggested with the title of his book "to make up for omissions in the *Ben cao gang mu*" not only his intention to list pharmaceutically useful substances Li Shizhen had failed to include. He was also the first to point out 30 substantial errors in the description of substances recorded. In recent years, with a steep rise in *Ben cao gang mu* research, many more such errors and misleading data have been identified, as for instance in Mei Quanxi's 梅全喜(1962 -) *Ben cao gang mu bu zheng* 本草綱目補正, "Supplementing omissions and correcting errors of the *Ben cao gang mu*."[13] A comparison of numerous quotes in the *Ben cao gang mu* with their original sources often enough shows significant divergence. It is not always clear whether these are intentional modifications, perhaps adapting

---

11 *Ben cao gang mu*, chapter 09, entry 09. See also, Zheng Jinsheng 郑金生 and Zhang Zhibin 张志斌, *Ben cao gang mu dao du* 本草綱目导读, 2016, 175 - 177.

12 See below p. 27

13 Zheng Jinsheng and Zhang Zhibin, 2016, 70

an ancient wording to usages preferred at the time of Li Shizhen, or errors due to careless copying.

The third volume of the *Dictionary of the Ben cao gang mu*, devoted to "Persons and Literary Sources," offers biographical and bibliographical data on all the texts and persons encountered in Li Shizhen's encyclopedia, with a few exceptions for sources and people that appear undocumented elsewhere. This volume of the Dictionary includes the different versions of titles and names assigned by Li Shizhen or his collaborators to quotes and anecdotes. It also points out where quotes ascribed in the *Ben cao gang mu* to a specific text or author originated, in fact, elsewhere.[14]

Ever since Tao Hongjing's *Shen nong ben cao jing ji zhu* of 500 CE and throughout the history of the main tradition, authors introduced their *materia medica* works not only with at least one preface to inform readers of their motives, aims and (where relevant) the history of their texts. They also offered more general information associated with the origin, gathering, pharmaceutical processing, contra-indications, synergies and applications of pharmaceutical substances. Here, too, Li Shizhen extended the introductory sections to four voluminous chapters occupying one eighth of the entire text. In chapter one he enumerated 40 earlier *ben cao* works with brief commentaries by other authors and himself. This list is followed by another, already mentioned above, of all the literary sources he had taken into account, divided into two groups: 277 older and more recently published medical and pharmaceutical works, and 591 classics, historical annals and others. Next, Li Shizhen went into more detail informing readers of all earlier *ben cao* works he had taken drug descriptions from. Li Shizhen paid homage to the beginning of the main tradition by quoting the preliminary sections of the "original classic, " including commentaries by Tao Hongjing and others.

He eventually switched to the Song-Jin-Yuan understanding of health and pharmaceutical therapy by first quoting a passage from the *Huang Di nei jing su wen* 黃帝內經素問 concerning the influence of climatic factors on drugs. This is followed by a section on "The seven ways of compiling a recipe," with commentaries by the legendary Qi Bo 岐伯, the 8th century commentator of the *Su wen* Wang Bing 王冰, and various Song-Jin-Yuan authors. Next is a section on "The effects of the ten kinds of recipes, " with commentaries by Xu Zhicai 徐之才 (ca. 510 – 590), several Song-Jin-Yuan authors again and Li Shizhen himself. The first chapter ends with ten treatises on the medical-theoretical teachings of the Song-Jin-Yuan period.

Chapter 2 begins with an enumeration of pharmaceutical substances known by up to five alternative names. It continues with an enumeration of pharmaceutical

14 Zheng Jinsheng, Nalini Kirk, Paul D. Buell and Paul U. Unschuld, *Dictionary of the Ben cao gang mu*, Vol. III: *Persons and Literary Sources*, University of California Press, Oakland, 2018.

substances according to their reciprocal, synergistic effects when ingested together, an enumeration of foods whose consumption is forbidden during an ingestion of specific pharmaceutical substances, an enumeration of substances that must not be taken by pregnant women, and an enumeration of beverages and foods that must not be consumed together. Also in chapter 2, Li Shizhen quoted from Li Gao 李杲 (1180 – 1251), one of the main authors and theoreticians of the Song-Jin-Yuan era, whose treatise acknowledged that the treatment of certain illnesses escaped theorization. Hence he simply listed certain pathological signs and the pharmaceutical substances suitable for their treatment – without reference to the Yin-Yang and Five Phases doctrines of systematic correspondences.

Similarly, the next treatise is an "enumeration of all pharmaceutical substances that, according to Chen Cangqi 陳藏器 (8th century), are used in the treatment of depletions." From another core theoretician of the Song-Jin-Yuan era, Zhang Zihe 張子和 (1156-1228), Li Shizhen took over the treatise "The three processes of sweating, vomiting and purging." Chapter 2 ends with a section from a *Yao dui* 藥對, a work allegedly predating the "original classic," and the tables of contents of the *Ben jing* and the *Jing shi zheng lei bei ji ben cao* 經史證類備急本草 by Tang Shenwei 唐慎微 (fl.1082), one of the final works of the main tradition, written between 1080 and 1107.

Chapters 3 and 4 of the *Ben cao gang mu* include lists of all diseases, and where necessary a detailed description of their pathological conditions, with the appropriate pharmaceutical substances and information concerning their pharmacological function, preparation and administration.

Despite their prominence in chapter 2, the references to the Song-Jin-Yuan doctrines of pharmacology appear isolated. Further hints at their relevance for pharmaceutical therapy are rarely encountered in the *Ben cao gang mu*. Li Shizhen may have felt it suitable to pay lip service to a development that had lost its creative momentum prior to his lifetime. By the end of the Song-Jin-Yuan era, several authors had suggested combinations of empirical pharmaceutical knowledge with the Yinyang doctrines of systematic correspondences without reaching an agreement on one pharmacology accepted by all. Too many contradictions remained between the assessment of the properties in terms of yin and yang qualities on the one hand and their assumed and observed effects on the human body on the other. Eventually, this development found no further creative naturalists. By the time of Li Shizhen, carrying through to the very present, a status quo had emerged within which any author interested in a theoretical foundation of pharmaceutical treatment was free to pick from any of the Song-Jin-Yuan authors, whomever he felt or feels appropriate.

Li Shizhen's attitude toward a theoretical legitimation of pharmaceutical therapies may be called fragmented. Only in very few instances did he feel compelled to refer to the preference of a specific substance to enter one or more of the yin and yang conduits. Li Shizhen did not neglect magic argumentation, and he seems to have had a special inclination toward the number seven. It dominates suggestions for the length of periods and number of frequencies of ingestions as well as quantities in which pharmaceutical substances are to be taken. Categorizations of items according to their yin or yang status, or their affiliation with one of the Five Phases, are rarely seen in the *Ben cao gang mu*. Occasionally Li Shizhen resorts to a concept of *cong qi lei* 從其類, "group correspondence" to explain correspondences between items and their properties that appear to exist outside the realm of Yinyang and Five Phases correspondences. For example, in chapter 41, entry 16, "cicadas," he writes:

> Generally speaking, to cure [diseases affecting] the long-term depots and short-term repositories, the bodies of cicadas are to be used. To cure dermal sores and ulcers, wind and heat, the nymph shells of cicadas are to be used. This is always based on their group correspondences.

Similarly, in chapter 43, entry 19-02, "breficaude pit viper":

> When poisonous items are used to attack poison diseases, then this is always based on their group correspondences.

Perhaps Li Shizhen's reluctance to support his therapeutic advice with theoretical reasoning may be traced back to a perception of himself as primarily being a practitioner not interested in burdening other practitioners with a request to indulge in the complicated doctrines of systematic correspondences as a precondition of pharmaceutical therapy. If we are right to assume that a central motivation underlying Li Shizhen's compilation of the *Ben cao gang mu* was to offer a handy work to a wide public of healers, we then also grasp two more of his encyclopedia's great innovations.

Li Shizhen's *Ben cao gang mu* is the first truly inclusive encyclopedia of natural history and pharmacotherapy in China. Nothing comparable existed in the medical literature elsewhere. *Ben cao* literature had hitherto been dedicated to the description of individual substances. Li Shizhen integrated medical case histories. These are meant to illustrate, more vividly than would have been possible with theoretical statements, the therapeutic potential of certain substances. Medical case histories have been published in China ever since Sima Qian 司馬遷 included examples of treatments performed by Chunyu Yi 淳於意 (205 – 150 BCE) in the biography of this physician in his *Shi ji* 史記 of 90 BCE. Beginning with the Yuan dynasty, an increasing number of physicians chose to publish characteristic (and successful) examples of their treatments to propagate their own understanding of medicine and health care.[15] Li Shizhen included case histories from his own medical practice and others quoted from earlier collections. In this way, he certainly prevented any suspicion of promoting only his personal interpretation of generally accepted theoretical premises.

A common feature of his case histories is the emphasis on flexibility. That is, the flexibility required to sometimes abandon seemingly irrefutable principles and adapt a substance's application to the specific challenge confronting the healer. An example is his own treatment, recorded in chapter 35, of "an old woman over 60 years old" who had suffered from viscous outflow, i. e., some form of diarrhea, for an extended period of time. No established therapy had been able to end her suffering. Li Shizhen followed a recommendation by the Tang physician Wang Bing 王冰 who had traced viscous outflow to an excessive accumulation of cold. He resorted to *croton* seeds, known in China as *ba dou* 巴豆, to counteract the cold responsible for that particular patient's illness.

Since antiquity, though, *ba dou* had been described in Chinese *ben cao* literature not only as an extremely "hot" substance but also as one of the most violent purgatives. Li Shizhen had also read the Yuan era author Wang Haogu 王好古, who had pointed out, for the first time, that given an appropriate pharmaceutical processing *croton* seeds can also be applied to stop diarrhea. Hence Li Shizhen counted on the extreme heat of *croton* seeds to attack the accumulated cold in the old woman. He treated her with pills prepared with *croton* seeds and coated with beeswax, and achieved a cure.[16] Li Shizhen not only offered examples of his own reading of a patient's specific needs but also provided details of earlier physicians' creative approaches to difficult therapeutic situations. The implicit message underlying most such case histories was to promote flexibility rather than stubborn adherence to superficial principles. Hence he praised previous healers for their ingeniously individualized therapies.

Li Shizhen was also the first author in the tradition of comprehensive works to combine the genres of *ben cao* and recipe literature. With very few exceptions, he added to every substance a list of recipes with the information he may have considered essential for its application in actual clinical practice. One or more therapeutic indications, mostly down-to-earth without theoretical embellishment or legitimation, are followed by the recipe's ingredients with brief data on their raw or pro-

15 Christopher Cullen, "Yi'an (case statements): the origins of a genre of Chinese medical literature," in Elisabeth Hsü (ed.), *Innovation in Chinese Medicine.* Cambridge University Press, Cambridge, 2001, 297-323.

16 Zheng Jinsheng and Zhang Zhibin, 2016, 202 – 206.

cessed states. The recipes further include concise data on their preparation, on the external or internal mode of their application and on the number and required time span of their applications. A source is given for each recipe. For each list of recipes added to the entry of a specific substance, Li Shizhen also specifies how many of them were recorded in previous recipe collections and how many he recorded for the first time.

The perhaps most notable innovation introduced by Li Shizhen was a transition from earlier *ben cao* works that had merely propagated alleged facts as statements to an encyclopedia based on argumentation. Li Shizhen was the first to collect in a *materia medica* work the statements of earlier authors and systematically discuss them in search of what he considered as facts and truth. Earlier writers had contradicted views they failed to agree with. But Li Shizhen made this approach his basic principle. Also, simply contradicting earlier views and statements is not identical to Li Shizhen's approach of presenting several points of view. He discussed their origins and shortcomings, and eventually decided who is right and who is wrong, or presented his own dissenting perception. This is a ubiquitous principle followed throughout the *Ben cao gang mu*. It is not the least because of this feature of the *Ben cao gang mu* that Li Shizhen deserves a most prominent place in the history of Chinese natural science.

1.3 Biographical sketch of Li Shizhen (1518 – 1593)

Li Shizhen, style Dongbi 東璧, assumed name Binhu 瀕湖, was born in Qi zhou 蘄州, today's Qi chun county 蘄春縣, province Hu bei 湖北, to a family of physicians. His grandfather is known to have practiced as an itinerant healer. His father, Li Yanwen 李言聞, rose to a more respected class of physicians and was engaged for a while as medical secretary, *li mu* 吏目, in the Imperial Medical Office. For his therapeutic skills he was praised as Li xian 李仙, "immortal Li." He is remembered as author of monographs on ginseng [root] and mugwort, a plant used for moxibustion. He also wrote texts on smallpox and pulse diagnosis.

Li Shizhen was supposed to rise even higher on the social scale. He was trained to be an official and entered the sequence of government exams. At the age of 14, having studied the Confucian and other classical texts, he passed the county level exams and was granted the degree of *xiu cai* 秀才, "outstanding talent." However, even though he continued his studies for the next ten years, he failed to pass exams on the next higher level and eventually turned to the occupation of his father and grandfather.

Over time, based on experience and knowledge learned from his father and his own literate knowledge and dedication to understand the principles underlying natural processes, Li Shizhen became widely known as a competent practitioner. He was invited to noble and other high ranking families and his successful cures in 1543 eventually led to an invitation by the King of Chu 楚, Zhu Xianrong 朱顯榕, 1506 – 1545, a regional prince, to manage his palace medical office.

Details of the following years are unclear. We know that Li Shizhen was offered a position in the Imperial Medical Office but returned to his hometown after only a year. The date of this journey to Beijing and the reasons why he left so soon are not known. From the contents of the *Ben cao gang mu*, though, it is obvious that he returned from the North having accumulated much new knowledge.

In Beijing he also encountered practices he considered highly objectionable. Among the elite, a practice was widespread to "cure human ills with human substances," *yi ren bu ren* 以人補人. Based on a notion that a reverse flow of menstrual blood left the body as breast milk, practitioners advocated to knead the breasts of child girls until they released some liquid. This liquid was termed *pan tao jiu* 蟠桃酒, "flat peach wine," allegedly an elixir granting immortality. Li Shizhen recorded this practice in chapter 52, entry 15, on "human milk," clearly condemning it as "deceitful rhetoric to make a profit, aimed at those who are ignorant. It is voiced by fraudulent persons, and punished by royal law. The gentleman is to denounce it." In Beijing he also learned of the use of opium as an aphrodisiac and considered this as a therapy not to be applied by a proper healer.

Back home, in 1552, at the age of 34, Li Shizhen began to compile the *Ben cao gang mu*. 27 years later, in 1578, he concluded his manuscript. To compile a work of 1.6 million characters, based not only on extensive reading of earlier literature but also on the results of repeated short and long distance travelling, is an enormous achievement. Li Shizhen mentions family members and disciples as assistants, but the size of his team is not known. His achievement is even more astonishing given that during these 27 years he wrote and published several books. Two of these, the *Binhu mai xue* 瀕湖脈學, "[Li] Binhu's study of vessel movements," a book on pulse diagnosis, and the *Qi jing ba mai kao* 奇經八脈考, "Research of the eight extraordinary conduit vessels," survive to this day. Others, like a collection of his medical cases, *Binhu yi an* 瀕湖醫案, a "collection of [Li] Binhu's simple to use recipes," *Binhu ji jian fang* 瀕湖集簡方, and an "illustrated study of the five long-term depots," *Wu zang tu lun* 五藏圖論, have been lost as individual texts.

None of these books became as influential as the *Ben cao gang mu*. Initially, the completed manuscript of the *Ben cao gang mu* did not meet enthusiasm either. It took Li Shizhen ten years, knocking at doors here and there, until eventually Hu

Chenglong 胡承龍 in Jinling 金陵, today's Nanjing 南京, Jiangsu province, agreed to print the text. It was published in 1593 with a preface by the famous scholar Wang Shizhen 王世貞 (1526 – 1590) and supplemented by two chapters of 1109 illustrations rather hastily made by his sons Li Jianyuan 李建元 and Li Jianmu 李建木. Whether Li Shizhen ever saw this "Jinling edition" is not known. He died that same year.[17]

Today eight complete copies of the first edition and four fragments are known to exist in China, in Japan and in the USA. A second edition, supported by a local government office, was published by Xia Liangxin 夏良心 and Zhang Dingsi 张鼎思in neighboring Jiangxi 江西 province in 1603. Even though some errors crept into the text, the print and the illustrations were executed excellently. The widespread dissemination and the fame of the *Ben cao gang mu* began with this "Jiangxi edition."[18]

In 2011, the United Nations Educational, Scientific and Cultural Organization (UNESCO) certified the inscription of the *Ben cao gang mu* on the Memory of the World International Register.

2. Notes on the translation

This translation of chapters 15-17 of the *Ben cao gang mu* is based on a most remarkable critical edition of the text prepared and published by Zheng Jinsheng 郑金生and Zhang Zhibin 张志斌. Zheng Jinsheng and Zhang Zhibin have traced all quotes to their original source text. Wherever the first 1593 Jinling print of the *Ben cao gang mu* differed from the original texts because of intentional abbreviations, they have added a note with the original wording. Divergences interpreted as unintended errors, such as omissions or mistakenly written single characters, as well as erroneous ascriptions of quotes to original texts and authors, were corrected in the main text with a note added to explain such modifications. The complete text of chapters 15 - 17 presented here together with its translation includes these corrections. Readers interested in all the details, both of the errors corrected and the original wordings that were abbreviated or otherwise modified by Li Shizhen and

17 Ibid., 3 – 7.

18 Ibid. 230. For a most detailed scholarly account of Li Shizhen's life and the further history of the *Ben cao gang mu*, see Wang Jian 王剑梅全喜and Mei Quanxi 梅全喜, *Li Shizhen Ben cao gang mu, 500 nian da shi nian pu* 李时珍本草纲目500年大事年谱, "Li Shizhen's *Ben cao gang mu* – a chronicle of related major events of the past 500 years," Ren min wei sheng chu ban she 人民衛生出版社, Beijing, 2018

his collaborators, are advised to consult the text critical edition by Zheng Jinsheng and Zhang Zhibin.[19] I am most grateful to both of them for supplying me with a pre-publication version of their work. I wish to especially express my thanks to Prof. Zheng Jinsheng for helping me to understand passages and single characters my own research had been unable to clarify. Almost all philological notes accompanying my translation are based on the text edition prepared by Zheng Jinsheng and Zhang Zhibin. I have also greatly benefitted from consulting the Japanese translation of the *Ben cao gang mu* published in 1965.[20] In particular, secondary quotes within primary quotes have been marked based on the Japanese edition.

In 2003, Foreign Language Press in Beijing published a first complete English version of the *Ben cao gang mu*. The approach chosen differed significantly from the one adopted here. This is most obvious in the translation of historical Chinese illness terms. Luo Xiwen and his collaborators have attempted to identify as many diseases, ailments and signs of illness as possible encountered in the *Ben cao gang mu* in terms of modern Western medical concepts.[21]

The *Ben cao gang mu* is an encyclopedia compiled in the 16th century based on literary and non-literary data of the preceding 1800 years. It quotes authors of varying expertise and offers today's readers an incomparable view of almost two millennia of the development of pharmaceutical science and related realms of knowledge and more general aspects of culture. The translation of chapters 15 through 17 of the Chinese text honors the authors of bygone days not by telling them what they should have said if they had had the knowledge of the 20th and 21st century, but rather by illuminating as clearly as possible their thoughts and their wisdom as formed by the conceptual, social, economic and natural environment of their time. The translation offered here has resisted a temptation to make ancient views appear modern and agreeable with today's biomedical reality. Such an approach, not infrequently met in recent renderings of ancient Chinese medical texts in Western languages, is not only a sign of disrespect for the intellectual integrity of ancient experts. It is also an

19 Zheng Jinsheng 郑金生 and Zhang Zhibin 张志斌, *Ben cao gang mu yin wen ni yuan, yi*, "Tracing the quotations in the *Ben cao gang mu* to their sources." A volume of the *Ben cao gang mu yan jiu ji cheng* 本草綱目研究集成, "Collection of research on the *Ben cao gang mu*," edited by Zhang Zhibin and Zheng Jinsheng, Ke xue chu ban she 科学出版社, Beijing, 2019.

20 Kimura Kouichi 木村康 (ed.), Suzuki Shinkai 鈴木真海 (transl.), *Shinchu Koutei Kokuyaku Honzou Koumoku* 新註校定國本草綱目譯, , "A translation of the *Ben cao gang mu*. Newly annotated and checked against the original text." Shunyoudou Shoten 春陽堂書店, Tokyo 1965.

21 *Compendium of Materia Medica*. (*Bencao Gangmu*). Compiled by Li Shizhen. Translated and Annotated by Luo Xiwen.Foreign Language Press, Beijing, 2003. This edition does not include the original Chinese text.

obstacle blocking a recognition and appreciation of the never ending historical process of understanding nature and the management of human life as part of nature in China, since antiquity.

Hence I have pursued here the same approach that has guided my translations of the ancient Chinese medical classics *Huang Di nei jing su wen*, *Huang Di nei jing ling shu* and *Nan jing*. Authors from previous centuries and millennia relied on metaphors and allegories to elucidate their understandings of human physiology and pathology. Modern pathology and physiology are no different. Such fields of science need to draw on metaphors and allegories to illustrate their findings.[22] Disease names are a case in point. The *Ben cao gang mu* includes quotes with about 4500 core terms to specify all kinds of pathological conditions. Prior to the translation presented here, Prof. Zhang Zhibin and I traced them to their first appearance. Vol. I of the *Dictionary of the Ben cao gangmu* lists all of them with an explanation of their original meaning. The translation of chapters 15 through 17 provides, where appropriate, the literal meaning of disease terms. Occasionally, ancient single characters keep their meaning secret; in such cases, they are given in pinyin transcription. Notes are added to all occurrences of historical disease terms that are not self-explanatory, and readers are led to the relevant pages of Vol. I of the *Dictionary*.

The heading of each entry repeats the numbers assigned to it in the table of contents, followed by the name, in Chinese characters and pinyin, of the substance discussed and the title of the earliest work on *materia medica* identified as its FE, i. e., "first evidence." The translation of the names offers English colloquial names wherever available, a literal translation where meaningful, and scientific identifications where possible.

Place names, designations of administrative structures, names of persons and book titles appear in the translation without additional notes. Readers interested in further details should consult volumes II and III of the *Dictionary of the Ben cao gang mu*, which respectively provide information on the geographic and administrative designations and on the persons and literary sources mentioned.

A challenging feature of translating an ancient text on *materia medica* is the identification of natural substances recommended for medicinal use. European scientists have been eager to identify herbal and mineral substances they have encountered in China since the 17th century. From the beginning, this has proved to be a difficult endeavor. Different names were used for identical substances in different parts of the country; different pronunciations of an identical name in the dialects of different regions led to different writings. One and the same substance has been

22 Cynthia Taylor and Bryan M. Dewsbury, On the Problem and Promise of Metaphor Use in Science and Science Communication. J Microbiol Biol Educ. 2018; 19(1): 19.1.46.

recorded with varying names in the course of history. An herb listed in an eighth century *materia medica* text might not have been available at a later time and was substituted by another herb sold under the same name. The marketing of fakes as substitutes was sufficiently widespread at any time for Li Shizhen to caution his readers in the first chapter of the *Ben cao gang mu*. In his descriptions of individual substances he devoted much space to such issues. The fact is, despite all the many attempts published over the past three centuries, an uncertainty remains as to the true identity of quite a few of the herbs and minerals recorded in historical Chinese *materia medica* works. This translation offers – with a caveat – identifications of the substances recorded in chapters 15 through 17 of the *Ben cao gang mu* based on the most reliable reference works available today. They include:

Editing commission for *Materia Medica of China*, <Zhong hua ben cao> bian wei hui 中华本草编委会, National Chinese Medicine and Pharmacy Administration, Guo jia zhong yi yao guan li ju 国家医药管理中局, *Materia Medica of China*, *Zhong hua ben cao* 中华本草, 10 vols. Shanghai 1999.

Fèvre, Francine and Georges Métailié, *Dictionnaire RICCI des plantes de Chine*. Association Ricci – Les Éditions du Cerf, Paris 2005.

Hu Shiu-ying, *An Enumeration of Chinese Materia Medica*, The Chinese University Press, Hongkong 1980.

Needham, Joseph and Lu Gwei-Djen, *Science and Civilisation in China*, Vol 5, part 2. Cambridge University Press, Cambridge, 1972.

Read, Bernard E., *Chinese Medicinal Plants from the Pen Ts'ao Kang Mu*, 3rd edition. *Peking Natural History Bulletin* 1936, repr. Taipei 1977.

Smith, F. Porter, *Chinese Materia Medica - Vegetable Kingdom*, rev. by G. A. Stuart, Shanghai 1911. 2nd revised edition Ku T'ing Book House, Taipei 1969.

Note: Chinese names of worms/bugs/insects, animals and plants may refer to different species and substances in different geographical regions of China. Also, a species or substance indicated by a name centuries ago may no longer be the species or substance identified today. The translation offered here provides only the most likely equations. Readers interested in more detailed information are advised to consult the literature listed above. Wherever a commonly known English name was available, such as "ginger" and "ginseng [root]," it was used in the translation. All other translations refer to the Latin name of a substance. For a tentative botanical identification of herbs mentioned in recipes and elsewhere in passing, see the list at the end of this volume.

3. Wang Shizhen's preface of 1590

本草綱目原序

紀稱望龍光知古劍，覘寶氣辨明珠。故萍實商羊，非天明莫洞。厥後博物稱華，辯字稱康，析寶玉稱倚頓，亦僅僅晨星耳。楚蘄陽李君東璧，一日過予弇山園謁予，留飲數日。予窺其人，晬然貌也，癯然身也，津津然譚議也，真北斗以南一人。解其裝無長物，有《本草綱目》數十卷。謂予曰：時珍，荊楚鄙人也。幼多羸疾，質成鈍椎。長耽典籍，若啖蔗飴。遂漁獵羣書，搜羅百氏。凡子史經傳，聲韻農圃，醫卜星相，樂府諸家，稍有得處，輒著數言。古有《本草》一書，自炎、皇及漢、梁、唐、宋，下迨國朝，註解羣氏舊矣。第其中舛繆差譌遺漏，不可枚數，廼敢奮編摩之志，僭纂述之權。歲歷三十稔，書考八百餘家，稿凡三易。複者芟之，闕者緝之，譌者繩之。舊本一千五百一十八種，今增藥三百七十四種，分爲一十六部，著成五十二卷。雖非集成，亦粗大備，僭名曰《本草綱目》，願乞一言，以託不朽。予開卷細玩，每藥標正名爲綱，附釋名爲目，正始也。次以集解、辯疑、正誤，詳其土產形狀也。次以氣味、主治、附方，著其體用也。上自墳典，下及傳奇，凡有相關，靡不備採。如入金谷之園，種色奪目；如登龍君之宮，寶藏悉陳；如對冰壺玉鑑，毛髮可指數也。博而不繁，詳而有要，綜核究竟，直窺淵海。茲豈僅以醫書覯哉，實性理之精微，格物之通典，帝王之秘籙，臣民之重寶也。李君用心加惠何勤哉。噫！碔玉莫剖，朱紫相傾，弊也久矣。故辯專車之骨，必竢魯儒；博支機之石，必訪賣卜。予方著《弇州卮言》，恚博古如《丹鉛》、《卮言》後乏人也，何幸覩茲集哉。茲集也，藏之深山石室無當，盍鍥之以共天下後世味《太玄》如子雲者。

時萬曆歲庚寅春上元日，弇州山人鳳洲王世貞拜撰。

Original Preface to the *Ben cao gang mu* by Wang Shizhen.

Historical annals speak of an ancient double-edged sword that was identified for its "dragon luster," and of a shiny pearl that was discovered for its precious radiance. That is, [the delicious and auspicious nature of] the fruit *ping* [seen growing on a river by the ruler of Chu] and [the significance of the appearance in the court of the Duke of Qi of] the [one-legged bird] *shang yang* [as an omen of imminent rain] could not have been recognized [by Confucius] without an enlightenment bestowed on him by heaven. In later times, [Zhang] Hua (232-300), who was known for [compiling the encyclopedia] *Bo wu* [*zhi*], [Ji] Kang (223-262), [the poet] who is recorded to have carefully chosen the characters he wrote down, and Yi Dun (of the Warring States period), who [was wealthier than his king and] knew how to distinguish [genuine and fake] precious stones, they were as rare as stars in the morning sky. One day, Mr. Li Dongbi from Qi [zhou] in Chu came to see me in my seclusion in Shan yuan, and he stayed with me as a guest for several days. I saw a man of gentle disposition with an excessively thin body. What he said was interesting and meaningful. He truly was a unique person south of the dipper! When he opened his bag, it contained nothing valuable, but tens of volumes of the *Ben cao gang mu*. He said to me: "[I am Li] Shizhen, a man from Jing chu. In my youth I often suffered from a wasting disease. Despite a modest intelligence, I was fascinated by reading the ancient canons and various kinds of literature, as if I were eating the sweetness of sugarcane. Hence I went fishing and hunting for all kinds of books, and I collected the works of hundreds of authors. Wherever among all the experts for philosophy and history, the classics and biographies, in music and poetry, agriculture and gardening, medicine, divination, astronomy and physiognomy, and collections of tunes I found something even of only slight value, I wrote it down in many words. In ancient times there was a *ben cao* work [on materia medica]. From the times of Yan [di, i.e., Shen nong] and Huang [di] through the Han, the Liang, the Tang, and the Song [dynasty] down to our present dynasty, it has long been commented upon and provided with explanations. However, it was stained by innumerable errors, inconsistencies, contradictions and omissions. I felt encouraged to take the will to study [this field] and edit [this work], and I exceeded my legitimate limits when I engaged in a compilation based on a new narrative. For more than 30 years I have examined the books of more than 800 authors. I have rewritten the manuscript three times. Where there were repetitions, I eradicated them. Where there were omissions, I filled them up. Where there were mistakes, I corrected them. The old editions included 1518 kinds [of pharmaceutical substances]; here now 374 kinds are added. [The entries] are divided into 16 sections, written up in 52 volumes. Even though [my work] may not be complete, it is quite comprehensive and hence I dared to give it the title *Ben cao gang mu*.[23] It is my deepest desire to entrust it to you so that it will not be lost." When I opened the volumes I was pleased to see that they were written in a meticulous manner. Each pharmaceutical substance is given

23 Li Shizhen may have considered this title daring because he seemed to put his encyclopedia on a par with the *Tong jian gang mu* 通鑑綱目, which was compiled by the well-known song philosopher Zhu Xi 朱熹 (1130 – 1200)

a name as its label, that is, as its *gang*, to which are added explanations of [this and additional] names as *mu*. This is a proper beginning. Next follow "collected explanations," "discussions of ambiguities," "corrections of errors," and detailed accounts of the places of origin and physical appearances. This is followed by [data on] "qi and flavors," "control and therapy," and "added recipes," indicating the concrete usage [of the substances named]. Whether [these data] had been gathered from ancient landmark and later canonical texts above, and from legends and unusual sources below, all were relevant and nothing was chosen without thinking. [Reading these volumes] was like entering the Golden Valley Garden where all kinds of colors dazzle one's eyes. It was like entering the palace of the Dragon Sovereign where all kinds of treasures are displayed. It was like standing in front of a crystal flask and a jade mirror clearly showing each [detail like an individual] hair. [The contents] are broadly arranged but not overabundant. They are detailed with a focus on what is important. They have summed up the results of careful studies. They allow a view into the depth of the sea. How could anyone consider this as a work dedicated exclusively to medicine! In fact, it offers the essential subtleties of natural principles. It is an encyclopedia based on an investigation of things. It is a work kept secret by emperors and kings. It is a treasure highly valued by officials and the people. The diligence and the passion devoted to it by Mr. Li are extraordinary! The failure to distinguish common stones and jade, and the confusion of red and purple colors, such malpractice has lasted for long. Hence to debate the reason for the carts loaded with one bone, one had to wait for the scholar [Confucius] from Lu.[24] To recognize the stone from below the loom,[25] it was essential to enquire with a fortune teller. I myself have written the *Yan zhou zhi yan*. What a pity that in future only a few people will be able to write a broadly based works such as the ancient *Dan qian* and *Zhi yan*. So, I am all the more happy to see this collection! This collection must not be stored deep in the mountains in a stone chamber! It must be carved/printed to make it available for later generations all over the world like the work *Tai xuan* [*jing*] by Ziyun [(i. e., Yang Xiong) on the *Yi jing*].

Date: *Wan li* reign period. Year: *Geng yin*. On New Year's Day. Respectfully written by Yan zhou shan ren Wang Shizhen in Feng zhou.

24 During the Warring States period, when Wu invaded Yue, they took home from the city of Kuai ji a collection of huge bones, with one of them filling one cart. Back home they enquired with Confucius about the origin of these bones and the "scholar from Lu" explained their origin.

25 A traveller once brought back a stone he had been given by a woman he had met when he tried to reach the source of a certain river. He approached the famous fortune-teller Yan Junping who told him that this was the stone forming the foundation of the loom of a celestial fairy.

4. 本草綱目
Ben Cao Gang Mu
Chapters 15 - 17
Translation

本草綱目
Ben cao gang mu
草部目録
Section Herbs, Contents
第十五卷
Chapter 15

草之四
Herbs IV
隰草類上五十二種
Marshland Herbs Group, first, 52 kinds[26]

15-01 *Ju* 菊, *chrysanthemum*. FE *Ben jing* 本經

15-02 *Ye ju* 野菊, winter aster. FE *Shi yi* 拾遺

15-03 *Yan lü* 菴藺, Keiske *artemisia*. FE *Ben jing* 本經

15-03-A01 *Dui lu* 對廬, unidentified.

15-04 *Shi* 蓍, Siberian milfoil. FE *Ben jing* 本經

15-05 *Ai* 艾, common mugwort. FE *Bie lu* 別録

15-05-A01 *Xia tai* 夏臺, unidentified

26 This chapter consists of 53 entries. The number "52" is a mistake that was made in the original BCGM edition. It was corrected in later editions.

15-06 *Qian nian ai* 千年艾, 1000 year old common mugwort. FE *Gang mu* 綱目

15-07 *Yin chen hao* 茵蔯蒿, virgate wormwood. FE *Ben jing* 本經

15-08 *Qing hao* 青蒿, wormwood. FE *Ben jing* 本經

15-09 *Huang hua hao* 黄花蒿, yellow flower wormwood. FE *Gang mu* 綱目

15-10 *Bai hao* 白蒿, sievers wormwood. FE *Ben jing* 本經

15-11 *Jiao hao* 角蒿, Chinese *incarvillea*. FE *Tang ben* 唐本

15-12 *Lin hao* 藨蒿, *pedicularis gloriosa*. FE *Shi yi* 拾遺

15-13 *Ma xian hao* 馬先蒿, *pedicularis resupinata* L. FE *Ben jing* 本經

15-14 *Yin di jue* 陰地厥, moonwort. *Tu jing* 圖經

15-15 *Mu hao* 牡蒿, Japanese *artemisia*. FE *Bie lu* 別録

15-16 *Jiu niu cao* 九牛草, *chrysanthemum decaisneanum*. FE *Tu jing* 圖經

15-17 *Chong wei* 茺蔚, Siberian motherwort. FE *Ben jing* 本經, i. e., *yi mu cao* 益母草

15-18 *Can cai* 蔪菜, *leonurus pseudomacranthus* FE *Shi yi* 拾遺

15-19 *Mei xian* 薇蘅[27], unidentified. FE *Ben jing* 本經

15-19-A01 *Wu xin cao* 無心草, unidentified.

15-20 *Xia ku cao* 夏枯草, common selfheal herb. FE *Ben jing* 本經

15-21 *Liu ji nu cao* 劉寄奴草, Sweet wormwood. FE *Tang ben* 唐本

15-22 *Qu jie cao* 曲節草, Japanese *peristrophe*. FE *Tu jing* 圖經, i. e., *liu yue shuang* 六月霜

15-23 *Lu chun cao* 麗春草, red poppy. FE *Tu jing* 圖經

15-24 *Xuan fu hua* 旋覆花, horseheal. FE *Ben jing* 本經

15-25 *Qing xiang zi* 青葙子[28], Prince's feather. FE *Ben jing* 本經

15-25-A01 *Tao zhu shu* 陶朱術, peach-shaped red *atractylodes*.

15-25-A02 *Yan lai hong* 雁來紅, redness derived from wild geese.

15-25-A03 *Tian ling cao* 天靈草, herb of celestial magic.

15-25-A04 思蓂子, unidentified.

15-26 *Ji guan hua* 雞冠花[29], cockscomb. FE *Jia you* 嘉祐

15-27 *Hong lan hua* 紅藍花, safflower. FE *Kai bao* 開寶

15-28 *Fan hong hua* 番紅花, saffron. FE *Gang mu* 綱目

15-29 *Yan zhi* 燕脂, rouge. FE *Gang mu* 綱目

15-30 *Da ji* 大薊, *xiao ji* 小薊, *cirsium japonicum*. FE *Bie lu* 別録

15-31 *Xu duan* 續斷, Himalayan teasel [root]. FE *Ben jing* 本經

15-32 *Ku ao* 苦芺, linear leaf thistle. FE *Bie lu* 別録

---

27 Entry 15-19 writes as name *wei xian* 薇銜 instead of *wei xian* 薇蘅.

28 Entry 15-25 writes as name *qing xiang* 青葙 instead of *qing xiang zi* 青葙子.

29 Entry 15-26 writes as name *ji guan* 雞冠 instead of *ji guan hua* 雞冠花.

15-33 *Lou lu* 漏蘆[30], uniflower swisscentaury. FE *Ben jing* 本經
15-34 *Fei lian* 飛廉, welted thistle. FE *Ben jing* 本經
15-35 *Zhu ma* 苧麻, ramie plant. FE *Bie lu* 別録
15-36 *Qing ma* 茼麻, indian mallow. FE *Tang ben* 唐本, i. e., *bai ma* 白麻
15-37 *Da qing* 大青, mayflower glorybower. FE *Bie lu* 別録
15-38 *Xiao qing* 小青, coralberry. FE *Tu jing* 圖經
15-39 *Hu lu ba* 胡盧巴, fenugreek. FE *Jia you* 嘉祐
15-40 *Li shi* 蠡實, Chinese iris. FE *Ben jing* 本經, i. e., *ma lin zi* 馬藺子
15-40-A01 *Bi se le* 必似勒, unidentified.
15-41 *E shi* 惡實, great burdock. FE *Bie lu* 別録, i. e., *niu bang* 牛蒡
15-42 *Xi er* 葈耳, cocklebur. FE *Ben jing* 本經, i. e., 蒼耳
15-43 *Tian ming jing* 天名精, common *carpesium*. FE *Ben jing* 本經, i. e., *di song* 地菘, *he shi* 鶴蝨
15-44 *Xi xian* 豨薟[31], St. Paulswort. FE *Tang ben* 唐本
15-45 *Ruo* 箬, unidentified. FE *Gang mu* 綱目
15-46 *Lu* 蘆, common reed. FE *Bie lu* 別録
15-47 *Gan jiao* 甘蕉, banana. FE *Bie lu* 別録
15-48 *Rang he* 蘘荷, Japanese ginger. FE *Bie lu* 別録
15-49 *Ma huang* 麻黄, *ephedra sinica* Stopf. FE *Ben jing* 本經
15-49-A01 *Yun hua cao* 雲花草, unidentified.
15-50 *Mu zei* 木賊, winter horsetail. FE *Jia you* 嘉祐
15-50-A01 *Wen jing* 問荊, unidentified.
15-51 *Shi long chu* 石龍芻, soft rush. FE *Ben jing* 本經, i. e., *long xu cao* 龍鬚草
15-52 *Long chang cao* 龍常草, *diarrhena* herb. FE *Bie lu* 別録, i. e., *zong xin* 稯心草
15-53 *Deng xin cao* 燈心草, common rush. FE *Kai bao* 開寶

右附方舊一百四十四，新二百八十六。
Recipes added to the entries above:
144 of old. 286 newly [recorded].

30 Entry 15-33 writes as name *lou lu* 漏盧 instead of *lou lu* 漏蘆.

31 Entry 15-44 following *xi xian* 豨薟 has two appendices: *lei bi* 類鼻 and *yang niao chai* 羊尿柴.

本草綱目
Ben cao gang mu
草部
Section Herbs,
第十五卷
Chapter 15
草之四
Herbs IV
隰草類上五十三種
Marshland Herbs Group, first, 53 kinds

15-01
菊本經上品
Ju, FE *Ben jing*, upper rank.

Dendranthema morifolium* (Ramat) Tzvel. *Chrysanthemum.

【釋名】節華本經、女節别録、女華别録、女莖别録、日精别録、更生别録、傅延年别録、治蘠爾雅、金蕊綱目、陰成别録、周盈别録。【時珍曰】按陸佃埤雅云：菊，本作蘜，從鞠。鞠，窮也。月令：九月，菊有黄華。華事至此而窮盡，故謂之蘜。節華之名，亦取其應節候也。崔寔月令云：女節、女華，菊華之名也；治蘠、日精，菊根之名也。抱朴子云：仙方所謂日精、更生、周盈，皆一菊而根、莖、花、實之名異也。【頌曰】唐天寶單方圖載白菊云：原生南陽山谷及田野中。潁川人呼爲回蜂菊，汝南名荼苦蒿，上黨及建安郡、順政郡並名羊歡草，河内名地薇蒿。

Explanation of Names. *Jie hua* 節華, *Ben jing*. *Nü jie* 女節, *Bie lu*. *Nü hua* 女華, *Bie lu*. Nü jing 女莖, *Bie lu*. *Ri jing* 日精, *Bie lu*. *Geng sheng* 更生, *Bie lu*. *Fu yan nian* 傅延年, *Bie lu*. *Zhi qiang* 治蘠, *Er ya*. *Jin rui* 金蕊, *Gang mu*. *Yin cheng* 陰成, *Bie lu*. *Zhou ying* 周盈, *Bie lu*. [Li] Shizhen: According to Lu Dian in his *Pi ya*, "*ju* 菊 originally was written *ju* 蘜, based on [the character] *ju* 鞠. *Ju* 鞠 is *qiong* 窮, 'to reach an end.' *Yue ling*: In the ninth month, *ju* 菊 have yellow flowers. With them, the season of the blossoming of flowers has reached its end. Hence they are called *ju* 蘜." The name *jie hua* 節華, "seasonal blossom," too, indicates that they stick to seasonal terms, *jie hou* 節候. Cui Shi in his *Yue ling* states: "*Nü jie* 女節 and *nü hua*

女華 are names of the flowers of *ju* 菊. *Zhi qiang* 治蘠 and *ri jing* 日精 are names of the root of *ju* 菊." *Baopu zi* states: "Names such as *ri jing* 日精, *geng sheng* 更生 and *zhou ying* 周盈 found in the recipes of the hermits/immortals, they all refer to *ju* 菊, and serve to distinguish between root, stem, flower and fruit." [Su] Song: In its reference to white *ju* 菊, the Tang era *Tian bao dan fang tu* states: "Originally it grew in the mountain valleys and open country of Nan yang. The people in Ying chuan call it *hui feng ju* 回蜂菊, 'the *ju* that lets the bees return.' In Ru nan it is called *tu ku hao* 荼苦蒿, 'extremely bitter wormwood.' In Shang dang, Jian an jun and Shu zheng jun it is called *yang huan cao* 羊歡草, 'herb welcomed by sheep.' In He nei they call it *di wei hao* 地薇蒿."

【集解】【別録曰】菊花生雍州川澤及田野。正月采根，三月采葉，五月采莖，九月采花，十一月采實，皆陰乾。【弘景曰】菊有兩種。一種莖紫氣香而味甘，葉可作羹食者，爲真菊。一種青莖而大，作蒿艾氣，味苦不堪食者，名苦薏，非真菊也。華正相似，惟以甘苦别之。南陽酈縣最多，今近道處處有之，取種便得。又有白菊，莖葉都相似，惟花白，五月取之。仙經以菊爲妙用，但難多得，宜常服之。【藏器曰】白菊生平澤，五月花，紫白色。【頌曰】處處有之，以南陽菊潭者爲佳。初春布地生細苗，夏茂，秋花，冬實。然種類頗多。惟紫莖氣香，葉厚至柔者，嫩時可食。花微大，味甚甘者爲真。其莖青而大，葉細氣烈似蒿艾，花小味苦者，名苦薏，非真也。南陽菊亦有兩種。白菊葉大如艾葉，莖青根細，花白蕊黄。其黄菊葉似同蒿，花蕊都黄。今服餌家多用白者。又有一種開小花，花瓣下如小珠子，謂之珠子菊，云入藥亦佳。【宗奭曰】菊花近世有二十餘種。惟單葉花小而黄，緑葉色深小而薄，九月應候而開者是也。鄧州白菊單葉者，亦入藥。餘皆醫經不用。【瑞曰】花大而香者，爲甘菊；花小而黄者，爲黄菊；花小而氣惡者，爲野菊。【時珍曰】菊之品凡百種，宿根自生，莖葉花色，品品不同。宋人劉蒙、范致能、史正志皆有菊譜，亦不能盡收也。其莖有株蔓、紫赤、青緑之殊，其葉有大小、厚薄、尖禿之異，其花有千葉單葉、有心無心、有子無子、黄白紅紫、間色深淺、大小之别，其味有甘、苦、辛之辨。又有夏菊、秋菊、冬菊之分。大抵惟以單葉味甘者入藥。菊譜所載甘菊、鄧州黄、鄧州白者是矣。甘菊始生于山野，今則人皆栽植之。其花細碎，品不甚高。蕊如蜂窠，中有細子，亦可捺種。嫩葉及花皆可爍食。白菊花稍大，味不甚甘，亦秋月采之。菊之無子者，謂之牡菊。燒灰撒地中，能死鼃黽，説出周禮。

Collected Explanations. *Bie lu*: *Ju hua* grows in the river marshlands and open country of Yong zhou. The root is collected in the first month. The leaves are collected in the third month. The stem is collected in the fifth month. The flowers are collected in the ninth month. The fruits are collected in the eleventh month. They all are dried in the yin (i. e., shade). [Tao] Hongjing: There are two kinds of *ju*. One kind of *ju* has a violet stem, fragrant qi and a sweet flavor. The leaves can be prepared to and consumed as congee. This is the true *ju* 菊. Another kind has a greenish stem, is bigger and emits the qi of wormwood and common mugwort. It has a bitter flavor, is not edible and is called *ku yi* 苦薏, winter aster. It is not the real *ju* 菊. The flowers are truly similar, but they differ as one is sweet and the other is bitter. In Li xian of Nan yang they grow in especially large numbers. Today, they are found everywhere nearby. They can be easily obtained by gathering them [in the wild] and by planting them. There is also a white *ju* 菊. The stem and the leaves [of white *ju* and ordinary *ju*] are similar. The only difference is [that the former have] white flowers. They are gathered in the fifth month. The classics of the hermits/immortals ascribe to *ju* 菊 a wondrous usage, but it is difficult to obtain large quantities. They should be eaten continuously. [Chen] Cangqi: White *ju* grow in the marshlands of the plains. Their purple-white flowers blossom in the fifth month. [Su] Song: They are found everywhere. Those from Ju tan in Nan yang are best. At the beginning of spring they cover the ground with fine seedlings. By summer they abound. In autumn they blossom. In winter they bear fruit. But there are quite a few different kinds. Only those with a purple stem and that have fragrant qi and thick and extremely soft leaves are edible as long as they are tender. Those with flowers that are slightly larger[32] and have a very sweet flavor are true [*ju*]. Then there are those that are big with a greenish stem. The leaves are fine and the qi are quite strong, like those of wormwood and common mugwort. They have small[33] flowers, a bitter flavor and are called winter aster. They are not the real [*ju*]. The *ju* in Nan yang, too, are present in two types. The white *ju* have leaves as big as those of common mugwort. The stem is greenish and the root is fine. The flower is white and the stamens are yellow. The leaves of yellow *ju* resemble those of garden daisy. Their flowers and stamens are all yellow. Today, those who eat [such herbs as their regular] diet mostly resort to the white [*ju* variety]. Furthermore, there is one kind that opens small flowers, and it has something like small pearls underneath the petals. It is called "pearl *ju*," and it is said be an excellent medication. [Kou] Zongshi: In recent times, more than 20 kinds of *ju hua* are known. Among them, only those with single leaf, small, yellow flowers, with small, thin, deeply green leaves, and that in accordance with the season open their [flowers] in the ninth month, they are the [true *ju*]. White *ju* with a single leaf from Deng zhou can also be used as medication. All the others are not

32 Instead of *da* 大, "big," *Zheng lei* ch.6, *ju hua* 菊花, quotes the *Tu jing* as writing *xiao* 小, "small."

33 Instead of *xiao* 小, "small," *Zheng lei* ch.6, *ju hua* 菊花, quotes the *Tu jing* as writing *da* 大, "big."

[recommended for] use in the medical classics. [Wu] Rui: Those with big, fragrant flowers, they are "sweet *ju*." Those with small, yellow flowers, they are "yellow *ju*." Those with small flowers and abominable qi, they are "wild *ju*." [Li] Shizhen: There are altogether 100 *ju* kinds. They grow by themselves from a perennial root. They all differ in the color of the stem, the leaves and the flowers. Liu Meng, Fan Zhineng and Shi Zhengzhi, all these Song authors have written a "*chrysanthemum* eulogy." They are too many to list all of them here. They differ in that some stems are trunks, others are vines, and their color may be purple or red, greenish-blue or green. The leaves vary in that some are big, others are small, some are thick, others are thin, some are pointed, others are blunt. The flowers differ as they may have a thousand leaves or just one leaf. They may or may not have stamens, they may or may not have seeds, they may be yellow, white, red or purple, with mixed colors, deep colors or light colors, and they may vary in size. Their flavor may be sweet, bitter or acrid. Also, there are summer *ju*, autumn *ju* and winter *ju*. In general, only those with a one leaf flower and sweet flavor are added to medication. They are the ones referred to in the *Ju pu* as sweet *ju*, yellow ones from Deng zhou and white ones from Deng zhou. Sweet *ju* originally grew in the wild of the mountains. Nowadays all the people plant them. Their flowers are fine and fragmented. They are not very tall. Their stamens form something like a bee nest, with fine seeds in their center. They, too, can be planted by pressing them [into the ground]. Their tender leaves and the flowers can all be consumed as food. The white *ju* are a bit bigger; their flavor is not very sweet. They, too, are collected in autumn. *Ju* without seed are called *mu ju* 牡菊, "male *chrysanthemum*." By burning them and spreading the ashes on the ground one can kill frogs and toads. This is a quote from the *Zhou li*.

15-01-01
花 *Hua*
[*Ju*] flower.

葉、根、莖、實並同。

Leaves, root, stem and fruit are all identical [to the flower].

【氣味】苦，平，無毒。【别録曰】甘。【損之曰】甘者入藥，苦者不入藥。【杲曰】苦、甘，寒，可升可降，陰中微陽也。【時珍曰】本經言菊花味苦，别録言菊花味甘。諸家以甘者爲菊，苦者爲苦薏，惟取甘者入藥。謹按張華博物志言菊有兩種，苗花如一，惟味小異，苦者不中食。范致能譜序言：惟甘菊一種可食，仍入藥餌。其餘黄白二花皆味苦，雖不可餌，皆可入藥。其治頭風則白者尤良。據此二説，則是菊類自有甘苦二種，食品須用甘菊，入藥則諸菊皆可，但不得用野菊名苦薏者爾。故景煥牧豎閑談云：真菊延齡，野菊泄人。正如黃精益壽、鉤吻殺人之意。【之才曰】术及枸杞根、桑根白皮爲之使。

Qi and Flavor. Bitter, balanced, nonpoisonous. *Bie lu*: Sweet. [Yang] Sunzhi: Sweet [*ju*] specimens are added to medication; bitter specimens are not added to medication. [Li] Gao: Bitter, sweet, cold. It can rise and it can descend. It is a slight yang in yin [substance]. [Li] Shizhen: The *Ben jing* says: "The flavor of *ju* is bitter." The *Bie lu* says: "The flavor of *ju* is sweet." All experts identify sweet ones as *ju*, and bitter ones as winter aster, *ku yi* 苦薏. They only add sweet ones to medication. According to Zhang Hua's *Bo wu zhi*, "there are two kinds of *ju*. Their seedlings and flowers are identical. Only their flavors slightly differ. The bitter ones are not consumed as food." Fan Zhineng in the preface to his [*Ju*] *pu*[34] states: "Only the sweet kind is edible, and it is ingested as medication. The other two, with a yellow or white flower, cannot be eaten but can be added to medication. To cure head wind[35] the white ones are especially good." Based on these two statements, the group of *ju* comprises two kinds, one sweet and one bitter. For food sweet *ju* should be used, while all kinds can be added to medication. However, "wild *ju*", named *ku yi* 苦薏, must not be used. Hence Jing Huan in his *Mu shu xian tan* states: "True *ju* prolongs life. Wild *ju* drains humans." This is the same meaning as "solomon's seal [root] boosts longevity. *Gou wen* kills humans." [Xu] Zhicai: *Atractylodes* [rhizome] and *lycium* [herb] as well as white mulberry tree root bark serve as its guiding substances.

【主治】諸風頭眩，腫痛，目欲脱，淚出，皮膚死肌，惡風濕痺。久服利血氣，輕身耐老延年。本經。療腰痛去來陶陶，除胸中煩熱，安腸胃，利五脉，調四肢。别録。陶陶，縱緩貌。治頭目風熱，風旋倒地，腦骨疼痛，身上一切游風令消散，利血脉。並無所忌。甄權。作枕明目，葉亦明目，生熟並可食。大明。養目血，去翳膜。元素。主肝氣不足。好古。

Control. All types of wind [stroke] with a dizzy head, painful swelling, eyes about to fall out, tearflow, dying skin and muscles, blockage related to malign wind and moisture [intrusion]. Ingested over a long time it clears the passage of blood and qi, relieves the body of its weight, helps to endure aging and extends the years of life. *Ben jing*. It heals lower back pain that comes and goes endlessly, removes vexing heat from inside the chest, pacifies intestines and stomach, frees the [movement in the] five vessels, and coordinates the four limbs. *Bie lu*. >>*tao tao* 陶陶: unrestrained<< It serves to cure wind [intrusion] with heat affecting head and

34 According to the *Zhizhai shu lu jie ti* 直齋書録解題 the full title reads *Ju pu* 菊譜.

35 *Tou feng* 頭風, "head wind." Condition of wind evil attacking the head followed by pain, dizziness, itching. BCGM Dict I, 509.

eyes, and head wind[36] spin making a person fall on the ground, as well as brain-bone pain, and disperses all kinds of roaming wind on the body. [During a treatment with *ju*] there are no prohibitions to be observed. Zhen Quan. A pillowcase prepared [with *ju*] brightens the eyes. The leaves, too, serve to brighten the eyes. They can be eaten both raw and prepared with heat. Da Ming. [*Ju*] nourishes the blood in the eyes, and removes shade membranes. [Zhang] Yuansu: It controls insufficient liver qi. [Wang] Haogu.

15-01-02

白菊 *Bai ju.*

White *chrysanthemum*.

【氣味】苦、辛，平，無毒。

Qi and Flavor. Bitter, acrid, balanced, nonpoisonous.

【主治】風眩，能令頭不白。弘景。染髭髮令黑。和巨勝、茯苓蜜丸服之，去風眩，變白不老，益顏色。藏器。

Control. Dizziness caused by wind [intrusion]. It can prevent whitening of the head. [Tao] Hongjing. It serves to dye moustache and hair black. Mixed with sesame seeds and *poria*, and ingested, prepared with honey, as pills, it removes dizziness caused by wind [intrusion], changes white [hair to black hair], prevents aging and benefits complexion. [Chen] Cangqi.

【發明】【震亨曰】黄菊花屬土與金，有水與火，能補陰血，故養目。【時珍曰】菊春生夏茂，秋花冬實，備受四氣，飽經露霜，葉枯不落，花槁不零，味兼甘苦，性禀平和。昔人謂其能除風熱，益肝補陰，蓋不知其得金水之精英尤多，能益金水二臟也。補水所以制火，益金所以平木，木平則風息，火降則熱除。用治諸風頭目，其旨深微。黄者入金水陰分，白者入金水陽分，紅者行婦人血分，皆可入藥，神而明之，存乎其人。其苗可蔬，葉可啜，花可餌，根實可藥，囊之可枕，釀之可飲，自本至末，罔不有功。宜乎前賢比之君子，神農列之上品，隱士采入酒斝，騷人餐其落英。費長房言九日飲菊酒，可以辟不祥。神仙傳言康風子、朱孺子皆以服菊花成仙。荆州記言胡廣久病風羸，飲菊潭水多壽。菊之貴重如此，是豈群芳可伍哉？鍾會菊有五美贊云：圓花高懸，準天極也。純黄不雜，后土色也。早植晚發，君子德也。冒霜吐穎，象貞質也。盃中體輕，神仙食也。西京雜記言：采菊花莖葉，雜秫米釀酒，至次年九月始熟，用之。

36 *Tou feng* 頭風, "head wind." Condition of wind evil attacking the head followed by pain, dizziness, itching. BCGM Dict I, 509.

Explication. [Zhu] Zhenheng: Yellow *ju* flowers are associated with [the phases] soil and metal. They include water and fire. They are able to supplement yin blood. Hence they nourish the eyes. [Li] Shizhen: *Ju* grow in spring and are luxuriant in summer. They develop flowers in autumn and have fruit in winter. They are prepared to receive the qi of all four [seasons]. Filled with dew and frost, their leaves may wither but do not fall off. Their flowers may dry out but do not crumble. They are both sweet and bitter, and by nature balanced and harmonious. The ancients said that they are able to remove wind heat, boost the liver [qi] and supplement yin [qi]. The fact is, they did not know that [*ju* flowers] are particularly profusely endowed with the essence efflorescence of metal and water enabling them to boost [the qi of] the two long-term depots associated with [the phases] metal and water. As they supplement water, they check fire. As they boost metal, they level wood. When wood is levelled, the wind is suspended. When the fire is sent down, the heat is removed. This is the profound and subtle message underlying its application to cure all types of wind affecting head and eyes. Yellow [*ju* flowers] enter the yin section of metal and water. White ones enter the yang section of metal and water. Red ones proceed into the blood section of women. They all can be added to medication. Whether their usage is based on spirit brilliance depends on the individual [in charge of the treatment]. The seedlings can be prepared to edible vegetables. The leaves can be prepared to something sipped. The flowers can be prepared to cakes. The root and the fruit can be applied as medication. Filled in a pouch they can serve as pillow-case. Brewed they can be drunk. From the root to the top, there is no part [of *ju*] that has no potential. It was truly appropriate when former sages compared [*ju*] with a gentleman. Shen nong listed [*ju*] as upper rank. Hermits living in seclusion gathered [*ju*] to add it to wine. Poets consumed their fallen flowers. Fei Zhangfang claimed that "if *ju* wine is drunk for nine days it is able to repel the inauspicious." The *Shen xian zhuan* reports that "Kang Fengzi and Zhu Ruzi became immortals because they had ingested *ju* flowers." The *Jing zhou ji* reports that "Hu Guang suffered from wind [related] emaciation for a long time. He drank water from a *ju* pond and enjoyed a long life." This is how *ju* was valued and appreciated. Is there any other fragrant substance that could come close to it? Zhong Hui in his "Praise of the five beauties of *chrysanthemum*" states: "The round flowers hang down from above. This reflects the celestial pole. They are of pure yellow with no admixtures. This is the color of the gourgeous earth. They rise early and open themselves late. This is the virtue of the gentleman. Exposed to frost they discard their husks. This reflects their loyal nature. Given into a cup their light body [floats on the liquid]. This is the food of spirits and hermits/immortals." The *Xi jing za ji* says: "Gather *ju* flowers, stems and leaves. Mix them with glutinous millet and brew a wine. It will have matured in the ninth month of the following year, and can then be used."

【附方】舊六，新十六。

Added Recipes. Six of old. 16 newly [recorded].

服食甘菊。玉函方云：王子喬變白增年方用甘菊，三月上寅日采苗，名曰玉英；六月上寅日采葉，名曰容成；九月上寅日采花，名曰金精；十二月上寅日采根莖，名曰長生。四味並陰乾，百日取等分，以成日合擣千杵爲末，每酒服一錢匕。或以蜜丸梧子大，酒服七丸，一日三服。百日輕潤，一年髮白變黑。服之二年，齒落再生。五年，八十歲老人變爲兒童也。孟詵云：正月采葉，五月五日采莖，九月九日采花。

To ingest sweet *ju* as food. The *Yu han fang* states: "Wang Ziqiao's recipe to turn white [hair into black hair] and to add to the years [of life recommends to] use sweet *ju* [as follows]. In the third month on a first [earthly branch] *yin* 寅 day gather the seedlings; they are called *yu ying* 玉英, 'jade efflorescence.' In the sixth month on a first [earthly branch] *yin* 寅 day gather the leaves; they are called *rong cheng* 容成, 'appearance completed.' In the ninth month on a first [earthly branch] *yin* 寅 day gather the flowers; they are called *jin jing* 金精, 'gold essence.' In the twelfth month on a first [earthly branch] *yin* 寅 day gather the roots and stems; they are called *chang sheng* 長生, 'longevity.' These four items are all dried in the yin (i. e., shade). After 100 days equal amounts of them are taken up and for a whole day they are pounded together with a pestle 1000 times to generate a powder. Each time ingest with wine the amount held by a one *qian* spoon. Or form with honey pills the size of *wu* seeds. Ingest with wine seven pills. To be ingested three times a day. After 100 days, the body will be relieved of its weight and [the complexion] will be moistened.[37] After one year, black hair will have whitened. After two years, teeth that had fallen out will have grown again. After five years, an old man of 80 years will have become a young boy again." Meng Shen states: "In the first month gather the leaves. In the fifth month on the fifth day gather the stems. In the ninth month on the ninth day gather the flowers."

服食白菊。太清靈寶方引：九月九日白菊花二斤，茯苓一斤，並擣羅爲末。每服二錢，温酒調下，日三服。或以煉過松脂和丸鷄子大，每服一丸。主頭眩，久服令人好顏色不老。藏器曰：抱朴子言劉生丹法，用白菊汁、蓮花汁、地血汁、樗汁，和丹蒸服也。

37 *Qing run* 輕潤: *Zheng lei* ch. 6, *ju hua* 菊花, "*chrysanthemum* flower," quoting *Yu han fang* writes *shen qing run ze* 身輕潤澤, "the body is relieved of its weight and [the complexion] is moistened."

To ingest white *ju* as food. A quote from the *Tai qing ling bao fang*: On the ninth day of the ninth month pound two *jin* of white *ju* flowers and one *jin* of *poria* and give them through a sieve to obtain a powder. Each time ingest two *qian*, to be sent down mixed with warm wine. To be ingested three times a day. Or prepare with heat processed pine resine pills the size of chicken eggs and each time ingest one pill. This controls head dizziness. Ingested for a long time it gives one a good complexion and prevents aging. [Chen] Cangqi: The *Baopu zi* says that "Liu sheng's elixir method [is as follows]. Mix white *ju* juice, Indian lotus flower juice, *arnebia* juice and *ailanthus* juice to form an elixir,[38] steam it, and ingest it."

白菊花酒。天竇單方治丈夫婦人久患頭風眩悶，頭髮乾落，胸中痰壅，每發即頭旋眼昏，不覺欲倒者，是其候也。先灸兩風池各二七壯，并服此酒及散，永瘥。其法：春末夏初，收白菊軟苗，陰乾擣末，空腹取一方寸匕，和無灰酒服之，日再服，漸加三方寸匕。若不飲酒者，但和羹粥汁服，亦得。秋八月合花收暴乾，切取三大斤，以生絹袋盛，貯三大斗酒中，經七日服之，日三次，常令酒氣相續爲佳。蘇頌圖經。

White *ju* flower wine. The *Tian bao dan fang* [recommends to] "cure husbands and wives suffering for a long time from head wind[39] with dizziness and heart-pressure, with the hair on their head drying out and falling, and phlegm obstruction in the chest. When [the disease] effuses, it causes head spin and dizzy eyes with a tendency to become unconscious and fall down. These are its signs. First apply two times seven moxa cauterizations at the two *feng chi* [needle insertion holes, (GB-20)]. Then ingest this wine and the powder, and a healing is achieved that lasts forever. The method: At the end of spring and the beginning of summer collect tender seedlings of white *ju*, dry them in the yin (i. e., shade) and pound them into powder. Ingest on an empty stomach the amount held by a square *cun* spoon, to be ingested with ash-free wine, twice a day. Gradually increase the amount to as much as is held by three square *cun* spoons. For those who do not drink wine it is possible, too, to simply mix [the medication] with a congee juice and ingest this." In autumn, in the eighth month, collect flowers and dry them in the sun. Cut them and fill a new silk pouch with three generous *jin*. Give [the pouch] into three generous *dou* of wine, and ingest it after seven days, three times a day. It is best to continuously expose [the consumer] to the qi of this wine. Su Song, *Tu jing*.

風熱頭痛。菊花、石膏、川芎各三錢，爲末。每服一錢半，茶調下。簡便方。

38 *Dan* 丹 may be read here as both "elixir" and "[large] pill].

39 *Tou feng* 頭風, "head wind." Condition of wind evil attacking the head followed by pain, dizziness, itching. BCGM Dict I, 509.

Wind [intrusion] with heat and headache. [Grind] three *qian* each of *ju* flowers, gypsum and *ligusticum* [root] into powder. Each time ingest one and a half *qian*, to be sent down mixed with tea. *Jian bian fang*.

膝風疼痛。菊花、陳艾葉作護膝，久則自除也。吴旻扶壽方。

Painful knee wind.[40] Prepare a kneepad with *ju* flowers and long-stored common mugwort leaves. After a long time [the disease] will end as a result. Wu Min, *Fu shou fang*.

痲痘入目生瞖障。用白菊花、穀精草、緑豆皮等分，爲末。每用一錢，以乾柿餅一枚，粟米泔一盞，同煮，候泔盡，食柿，日食三枚。淺者五七日，遠者半月，見效。仁齋直指方。

Pox macules enter the eyes and generate a screen. [Grind] equal amounts of *ju* flowers, *eriocaulon* [flowers] and mung bean skin into powder. Each time use one *qian* and boil it together with one persimmon cake in one bowl of water that was used to wash millet. When all the water is consumed, eat the cake. Eat three cakes a day. If it is a case of minor severity, [continue this] for five to seven days. If it has further developed, for half a month until an effect is seen. *Ren zhai zhi zhi fang*.

病後生瞖。白菊花、蟬蜕等分，爲散。每用二三錢，入蜜少許，水煎服。大人小兒皆宜，屢驗。救急方。

A screen in the eyes in the aftermath of a disease. [Grind] equal amounts of white *ju* flowers and cicada sloughs into powder. Each time use two or three *qian*. Add a little honey, boil this in water and ingest it. It is suitable for adults and children alike, and has often proved to be effective. *Jiu ji fang*.

疔腫垂死。菊花一握，搗汁一升，入口即活，此神驗方也。冬月采根。肘後方。

Pin-illness[41] swelling bringing one close to dying. Pound a handful of *ju* flowers[42] to obtain as much as one *sheng* of juice, give it into [the patient's] mouth, and he will return to life. This is a divinely effective recipe. In winter, collect the root. *Zhou hou fang*.

---

40 *Xi feng* 膝風, "knee wind," abbreviated alternative name of *he xi feng* 鶴膝風, "crane knee wind," a condition of swelling and pain of the knee, and shrinking of the lower leg, with difficulties in bending and stretching, and a lack of strength to walk. BCGM Dict I, 214.

41 *Ding* 丁, "pin[-illness]," also *ding* 疔, "pin-illness," refers to a deep-reaching and festering hardness in a tissue, eventually rising above the skin like a pinhead. BCGM Dict I, 127-129.

42 Instead of *hua* 花, "flower," *Zheng lei* ch.6, *ju hua* 菊花 quoting *Zhou hou fang* writes *ye* 葉, "leaf."

女人陰腫。甘菊苗搗爛煎湯，先熏後洗。危氏得效方。

Swelling of a female's yin [(i. e., genital) region]. Pound sweet *ju* seedlings into a pulpy substance and boil it. First use the decoction to steam [the affected region] and then [use it to] wash it. Wei shi, *De xiao fang*.

酒醉不醒。九月九日真菊花末，飲服方寸匕。外臺秘要。

Drunk with wine, without waking up. [Grind] true *ju* [collected] on the ninth day of the ninth month into powder, and [let the person] ingest with a beverage the amount held by a square *cun* spoon. *Wai tai mi yao*.

眼目昏花。雙美丸：用甘菊花一斤，紅椒去目六兩，爲末，用新地黄汁和丸梧子大。每服五十丸，臨卧茶清下。瑞竹堂方。

Dim vision with flowers on the eye. The "double beauty pills." [Grind] one *jin* of sweet *ju* flowers and six *liang* of red Chinese pepper, with the eyes removed, into powder. Mix it with fresh Chinese foxglove [rhizome] juice to form pills the size of *wu* seeds. Each time ingest 50 pills, to be sent down with clear tea before bed. *Rui zhu tang fang*.

15-01-03
花上水 *Hua shang shui*
Water collected on [*ju*] flowers.

【主治】益色壯陽，治一切風。大明。

Control. It boosts complexion and strengthens the yang [qi (i. e., male sexuality)]. It serves to cure all types of wind [diseases]. Da Ming.

15-02
野菊拾遺
Ye ju, FE *Shi yi*

Dendranthema indicum (L.) des Moul. Winter aster.

【釋名】苦薏。【時珍曰】薏乃蓮子之心，此物味苦似之，故與之同名。

Explanation of Names. *Ku yi* 苦薏. [Li] Shizhen: *Yi* 薏 is the stamen of Indian lotus. As this item's bitter flavor is similar to that of [Indian lotus] stamens, it was given the same name.

【集解】【藏器曰】苦薏生澤畔，莖如馬蘭，花如菊。菊甘而薏苦，語曰苦如薏是也。【時珍曰】苦薏處處原野極多，與菊無異，但葉薄小而多尖，花小而蕊多，如蜂窠狀，氣味苦辛慘烈。

Collected Explanations. [Chen] Cangqi: *Ku yi* grows at the side of marshland. Its stem is similar to that of purple *chrysanthemum*. The flowers resemble *chrysanthemum* [flowers]. *Chrysanthemum* [flowers] are sweet, while those of [*ku*] *yi* are bitter. A saying is: "as bitter as [*ku*] *yi*." This is true. [Li] Shizhen: *Ku yi* is abundant all over the open country. It is not different from *chrysanthemums*. However, the leaves are thin, small and mostly pointed. The flowers are small and have many stamens, forming something like a bee nest. The qi and the bitter and acrid flavor are quite strong.

15-02-01

根、葉、莖、花 *Gen, Ye, Jing, Hua*

Root, leaf, stem, flower [of *ye ju*].

【氣味】苦、辛，温，有小毒。【震亨曰】野菊花服之大傷胃氣。

Qi and Flavor. Bitter, acrid, warm, slightly poisonous. [Zhu] Zhenheng: To ingest *ye ju* flowers massively harms stomach qi.

【主治】調中止洩，破血，婦人腹内宿血宜之。藏器。治癰腫疔毒，瘰癧眼瘜。時珍。

Control. It regulates the center, ends outflow and breaks through blood [accumulations]. It is suitable for [a treatment of] blood abiding in the abdomen of women. [Chen] Cangqi. It serves to cure swelling associated with obstruction-illness[43] and pin-illness[44] poison, scrofula pervasion-illness[45] and tumorous flesh growth in the eyes. [Li] Shizhen.

【附方】新四。

Added Recipes. Four newly [recorded].

癰疽丁腫，一切無名腫毒。孫氏集效方用野菊花連莖搗爛，酒煎熱服取汗，以渣傅之即愈。

43 *Yong* 癰, "obstruction-illness," refers to an obstruction of vessels or other ducts inside the body. Qi rushing against the obstruction may cause a local swelling and eventually break through the surface to cause an abscess. BCGM Dict I, 641.

44 *Ding* 丁, "pin[-illness]," also *ding* 疔, "pin-illness," refers to a deep-reaching and festering hardness in a tissue, eventually rising above the skin like a pinhead. BCGM Dict I, 127-129.

45 *Luo li* 瘰癧, "scrofula pervasion-illness," when two or more connected swellings of the size of plum or date kernels appear either on the neck or in the armpits, or somewhere else on the body. BCGM Dict I. 329.

Obstruction-illness, impediment-illness[46] and pin[-illness] related swelling, and all types of unspecific swelling with poison. The *Sun shi ji xiao fang* [recommends to] pound *ye ju* flowers with the stem into a pulpy substance, boil it in wine and ingest it warm to cause sweating. Then apply the dregs to [the affected region] and this results in a cure.

衛生易簡方用野菊花莖葉、蒼耳草各一握，共搗，入酒一椀，絞汁服，以渣傅之，取汗即愈。或六月六日采蒼耳葉，九月九日采野菊花，爲末，每酒服三錢，亦可。

The *Wei sheng yi jian fang* [recommends to] pound one handful each of *ye ju* flowers, stems and leaves, and cocklebur herb, give this into a bowl of wine, and squeeze it to obtain a juice that is to be ingested. The dregs are applied to [the affected region]. Once [the patient] sweats he is cured. Or, collect cocklebur leaves on the sixth day of the sixth month and *ye ju* flowers on the ninth day of the ninth month and [grind them into] powder. Each time ingest with wine three *qian*. This is possible, too.

天泡濕瘡。野菊花根、棗木，煎湯洗之。醫學集成。

Celestial blister sores[47] with moisture. Boil *ye ju* flowers and roots and date tree wood in water and use the liquid to wash [the affected region]. *Yi xue ji cheng*.

瘰癧未破。野菊花根擣爛，煎酒服，以渣傅之自消，不消亦自破也。瑞竹堂經驗方。

Scrofula pervasion-illness[48] that has not yet broken open. Pound *ye ju* flowers and roots into a pulpy substance, boil it in wine and ingest this. Apply the dregs [to the affected region and the illness] will vanish as a result. If it does not vanish it will break open. *Rui zhu tang jing yan fang*.

---

46 *Ju* 疽, "impediment-illness," refers to an obstruction of vessels or other ducts inside the body. Qi rushing against the impediment may cause a local swelling and eventually break through the surface to cause an abscess. BCGM Dict I, 277.

47 *Tian pao chuang* 天泡瘡, "celestial blister sores," a condition of sores with the appearance of blisters filled with water or pus, especially in children. BCGM Dict I, 503.

48 *Luo li* 瘰癧, "scrofula pervasion-illness," when two or more connected swellings of the size of plum or date kernels appear either on the neck or in the armpits, or somewhere else on the body. BCGM Dict I. 329.

15-03
菴藺音淹閭本經上品

Yan lü, read *yan lü*. FE *Ben jing*, upper rank.

***Artemisia keiskeana* Miq. Keiske *artemisia*.**

【釋名】覆閭。【時珍曰】菴，草屋也。閭，里門也。此草乃蒿屬，老莖可以蓋覆菴閭，故以名之。貞元廣利方謂之菴藺蒿云。又史注云：菴廬，軍行宿室也。則閭似當作廬。

Explanation of Names. *Fu lü* 覆閭. [Li] Shizhen: [*Y*]*an* 菴 is a thatched house. *Lü* 閭 is the gate to the interior. This herb belongs to the wormwood group. With its old stems one can thatch houses, [*y*]*an* 菴, and gates, *lü* 閭. Hence its name. The *Zhen yuan guang li fang* names it *yan lü hao* 菴藺蒿. Also, a comment to the *Shi* states: "[*Y*]*an lu* 菴廬 is a military barrack." Hence it may be that *lü* 閭 should be written *lu* 廬.

【集解】【別録曰】菴藺子生雍州川谷，亦生上黨及道邊，十月采實，陰乾。【弘景曰】狀如蒿艾之類，近道處處有之，仙經亦時用之，人家種此辟蛇也。【頌曰】今江淮亦有之。春生苗，葉如艾蒿，高二三尺。七月開花，八月結實，九月采實。【時珍曰】菴藺葉不似艾，似菊葉而薄，多細丫，面背皆青。高者四五尺，其莖白色，如艾莖而粗。八九月開細花，淡黄色。結細實如艾實，中有細子，極易繁衍。藝花者以之接菊。

Collected Explanations. *Bie lu*: *Yan lü* seeds grow in river valleys of Yong zhou. They also grow in Shang dang, and at the roadside. Their fruits are collected in the tenth month. They are dried in the yin (i. e., shade). [Tao] Hongjing: [The herb] is shaped like wormwood and mugwort. It can be found everywhere along the roads. The classics of the hermits/immortals, too, occasionally resort to it. The people plant it to repel snakes. [Su] Song: Today, it is also found in the Jiang Huai region. It grows a seedling in spring. The leaves are similar to those of mugwort and wormwood. They reach a height of two to three *chi*. The flowers open in the seventh month; they form fruits in the eighth month. The fruits are collected in the ninth month. [Li] Shizhen: *Yan lü* leaves are not similar to those of mugwort; they are similar to *chrysanthemum* leaves, but are thinner with many fine forks. Front and back are all greenish. Tall ones reach a height of four to five *chi*. The stem is white, similar to mugwort stems but coarser. Fine flowers open in the eighth and ninth month. They are of a light yellow color, and they form fine fruits similar to mugwort fruits. Inside of them are fine seeds, and it is very easy to profusely multiply them. Gardeners use them to graft *chrysanthemums*.

15-03-01
子 *Zi*
[*Yan lü*] seeds.

【氣味】苦、微寒，無毒。【别録曰】微温。【普曰】神農、雷公、桐君、岐伯：苦，小温，無毒。李當之：温。【權曰】辛，苦。【時珍曰】降也，陰中微陽，入足厥陰經血分。【之才曰】荆實、薏苡爲之使。

Qi and Flavor. Bitter, slightly cold, nonpoisonous. *Bie lu*: Slightly warm. [Wu] Pu: Shen nong, Lei gong, Tong jun, Qi Bo: Bitter, slightly warm, nonpoisonous. Li Dangzhi: Warm. [Zhen] Quan: Acrid, bitter. [Li] Shizhen: They sink. They are a slight yang in yin [substance]; they enter the blood section of the foot ceasing yin conduits. [Xu] Zhicai: *Schizonepeta* fruit and Job's tears serve as their guiding substance.

【主治】五臓瘀血，腹中水氣，臚脹留熱，風寒濕痺，身體諸痛。久服輕身延年不老。本經。療心下堅，隔中，寒熱周痺，婦人月水不通，消食明目。駏驉食之神仙。别録。益氣，主男子陰痿不起，治心腹脹滿。甄權。腰脚重痛，膀胱痛及骨節煩痛，不下食。大明。擂酒飲，治閃挫腰痛及婦人産後血氣痛。時珍。

Control. Stagnant blood in the five long-term depots, water qi in the abdomen with distension of the abdominal wall and abiding heat, blockage caused by wind, cold and moisture [intrusion], all types of body pain. Ingested over a long time [the seeds] relieve the body of its weight, extend the years [of life] and prevent aging. *Ben jing*. They heal hardenings below the heart, cut off center, encompassing blockage with alternating sensations of cold and heat, and blocked menstruation. [*Yan lü* seeds] dissolve food and brighten the eyes. When the *ju xu* [animal (see below Li Shizhen's explication)] ate [*yan lü* seeds] it became a spirit immortal. *Bie lu*. They boost the qi and control yin [i. e., genital member] dysfunction of males, with failure to have an erection. They serve to cure distention and a feeling of fullness in the central and abdominal region. Zhen Quan. Painful swelling of lower back and legs. Aching urinary bladder and vexing pain affecting bones and joints. Inability to eat. Da Ming. Pounded [to powder] and drunk with wine [*yan lü* seeds] serve to cure painful lower back sprain and pain related to blood and qi [disorder] of women following birth. [Li] Shizhen.

【發明】【頌曰】本經言久服輕身不老，而古方少有服食者，惟入諸雜治藥中，如胡洽治驚邪狸骨丸之類大方中用之。孫思邈千金翼、韋宙獨行方，主踠折瘀血，並單用菴蕳煮汁服，亦可末服。今人治打撲多用此法，或飲或散，其效最速。【時珍曰】吴普本草及名醫别録，並言駏驉食菴蕳神仙，此亦謂其多壽爾。駏驉乃獸名，似騾而小，前足長，後足短，不能自食，每負蟨鼠爲之齧食。

Explication. [Su] Song: The *Ben jing* says: "Ingested over a long time [*yan lü* seeds] relieve the body of its weight and prevent aging." Still, there are very few ancient recipes recommending them for ingestion as food. They are resorted to only as an addition to medication for all types of curative ends, such as Hu Qia's "pills with leopard cat bones to cure fright evil" and similar such multi-ingredient recipes. Sun Simiao in his *Qian jin yi* and Wei Zhou in his *Du xing fang* "control fractures and stagnating blood by [recommending] to solely boil *yan lü* [seeds] in water and ingest the resulting juice. It is also possible to ingest them as powder." Today people often use them to cure [injuries resulting from] blows and falls, either to be drunk or [to be ingested as] powder. The effects are very fast. [Li] Shizhen: Both the *Wu Pu ben cao* and the *Ming yi bie lu* say that "*ju xu* ate *yan lü* [seeds] and became a spirit immortal." This, too, suggests that it has a major effect on longevity. *Ju xu* is the name of an animal. It is similar to mules, but smaller. The forelegs are long; the hind legs are short. It is unable to eat itself. It always carries on its back an "alert rat/mouse]" that eats on its behalf.

【附方】舊一，新二。

Added Recipes. One of old. Two newly [recorded].

瘀血不散，變成癰腫。生菴蕳蒿擣汁一升，服之。廣利方。

Stagnating blood that does not dissipate and eventually turns into an obstruction-illness[49] with swelling. Pound fresh *yan lü hao* to obtain one *sheng* of its juice and ingest this. *Guang li fang.*

月水不通。婦人宿有風冷，留血積聚，月水不通。菴蕳子一升，桃人二升，酒浸去皮尖，研匀入瓶内，以酒二斗浸，封五日後，每飲三合，日三服。聖惠方。

Blocked menstruation. When a woman has been affected by wind and cold for some time, with abiding blood forming accumulations and collections, and the flow of menstruation blocked. Equally grind one *sheng* of *yan lü* seeds and two *sheng* of peach kernels, soaked in wine and the skin and tips removed, [to powder] and give it into a bottle to be soaked there in two *dou* of wine. Keep it sealed for five days,

49 *Yong* 癰, "obstruction-illness," refers to an obstruction of vessels or other ducts inside the body. Qi rushing against the obstruction may cause a local swelling and eventually break through the surface to cause an abscess. BCGM Dict I, 641.

and then each time [let the patient] drink three *ge*. To be ingested three times a day. *Sheng hui fang*.

產後血痛。菴藺子一兩，水一升，童子小便二盃，煎飲。頻湖集簡方。
Painful blood [disorder] following birth. Boil one *liang* of *yan lü* seeds in one *sheng* of water and two cups of boys' urine and [let the woman] drink this. *Binhu ji jian fang*.

【附録】
Appendix.

15-03-A01
對廬 *Dui lu*

Unidentified.

【别録有名未用曰】味苦，寒，無毒。主疥瘡久不瘳，生死肌，除大熱，煮汁洗之。似菴藺。八月采。
Bie lu, [section] "known by name but not in use": Flavor bitter, cold, nonpoisonous. It controls *jie*-illness[50] with sores that have not been healed for a long time. It lets dead muscles grow again, and removes massive heat. Boil it in water and wash [the affected regions] with the resulting juice. It is similar to *yan lü*. It is collected in the eighth month.

15-04
蓍音尸本經上品
Shi, read *shi*. FE *Ben jing*, upper rank.

***Achillea alpina* L. Siberian milfoil.**

【釋名】【時珍曰】按班固白虎通載：孔子云"蓍之爲言耆也"。老人歷年多，更事久，事能盡知也。陸佃埤雅云：草之多壽者，故字從耆。博物志言：蓍千歲而三百莖，其本已老，故知吉凶。
Explanation of Names. According to Ban Gu's *Bai hu tong*, "Kong zi states: '*Shi* 蓍 is to say a 'very old, *qi* 耆, [herb]'. Old people having lived many years have performed many tasks. They know all possible tasks." Lu Dian in his *Pi ya* states: "Because this herb has a long life the character [*shi* 蓍] is derived from [the character] *qi* 耆, 'very old'." *Bo wu zhi*: "When *shi* has lived for 1000 years and has 300 stems, its root is already old. Hence it [is used to] know auspicious and inauspicious events [in advance]."

50 *Jie*-illness 疥, vaguely identifiable skin ailment. BCGM Dict I, 249.

【集解】【别録曰】蓍實生少室山谷，八月、九月采實，日乾。【恭曰】此草所在有之，其莖可爲筮。陶氏誤以楮實爲之。楮實味甘，此味苦，今正之。【頌曰】今蔡州上蔡縣白龜祠旁，其生如蒿作叢，高五六尺，一本一二十莖，至多者五十莖，生便條直，所以異於衆蒿也。秋後有花，出於枝端，紅紫色，形如菊花，結實如艾實。史記龜策傳云：龜千歲乃遊於蓮葉之上。蓍百莖共一根，所生之處，獸無虎狼，蟲無毒螫。徐廣註云：劉向言龜千歲而靈，蓍百年而一本生百莖也。褚先生云：蓍滿百莖，其下必有神龜守之，其上常有青雲覆之。傳云：天下和平，王道得而蓍莖長丈，其叢生滿百莖。方今取蓍者，八十莖已上，長八尺者，即已難得。但得滿六十莖以上，長六尺者，即可用矣。今蔡州所上，皆不言如此。則此類亦神物，故不常有也。【時珍曰】蓍乃蒿屬，神草也。故易曰：蓍之德，圓而神。天子蓍長九尺，諸侯七尺，大夫五尺，士三尺。張華博物志言：以末大於本者爲主，次蒿，次荆，皆以月望浴之。然則無蓍揲卦，亦可以荆、蒿代之矣。

Collected Explanations. *Bie lu*: *Shi* fruit grow in mountain valleys of Shao shi. The fruits are collected in the eighth and ninth month. They are dried in the sun. [Su] Gong: This herb can be found everywhere. Its stem can serve to predict the future. Mr. Tao [Hongjing] wrongly assumed that these are the fruit of paper mulberry tree. Paper mulberry fruits are sweet. These [fruit here] are bitter. This is corrected now. [Su] Song: Today it grows in Cai zhou, near the Bai gui ancestral temple of Shang cai xian. It grows in clusters similar to wormwood, reaching a height of five to six *chi*. One root has ten to 20 stems, even up to as many as 50 stems. The stems rise as straight stalks, and this is different from all wormwood [plants]. They have flowers after autumn, developing at the tip of the branches. Their color is red-purple. Their shape is similar to *chrysanthemum* flowers, and they form fruits similar to mugwort fruit. The *Shi ji*, Gui ce zhuan, states: "A tortoise of 1000 years crawled on the leaves of Indian lotus. 100 stems of *shi* have one single root in common. Where [*shi*] grows, there are no wild animals such as tigers and wolves, and no bugs/worms such as poisonous scorpions." Xu Guang in his commentary states: "Liu Xiang says that a tortoise of 1000 years turns into a numinous being, while a *shi* [plant] of 100 years has one single root growing 100 stems." Mr. Chu states: "When a *shi* [plant] has fully developed 100 stems, there must be a divine tortoise underneath it to guard it, and there are always greenish clouds above to cover it. A legend states: 'When the world has harmony and peace, and the DAO of kingly [governance] is obtained, the *shi* [plants] have stems a *zhang* long. They grow in clusters of 100 stems.' The *shi* used for recipes these days should have at least 100 stems, reaching a height of eight *chi*. They already are difficult to obtain. However, those with at least 60 stems, reaching a height of six *chi*, can be used, too." The [material] submitted by Cai zhou today is not the same as was just described. It is a spiritual item. Hence it is not always available. [Li] Shizhen: *Shi* belongs to the group of wormwood. It is a spiritual herb. Hence the *Yi* says: "The virtue of *shi* is round [as heaven] and spiritual. The *shi* [employed for divination by] the Son of Heaven is nine *chi* long. That [employed for divination by] the marquises is seven *chi* long. That [employed for divination by] the senior officials is five *chi* long. That [employed for divination by] knights is three *chi* long." Zhang Hua in his *Bo wu zhi* says: "Those with an end bigger than the root are preferable. Next are wormwood, and this is followed by *schizonepeta*. They all can be resorted to to take a [ritual] bath [prior to divination] on the 15th day of a month." If no *shi* is at hand for divination, *schizonepeta* and wormwood can be used instead.

15-04-01
實 *Shi*
***Shi* [fruit].**

【氣味】苦、酸，平，無毒。

Qi and Flavor. Bitter, sour, balanced, nonpoisonous.

【主治】益氣充肌膚，明目聰慧先知。久服不饑，不老輕身。本經。

Control. They boost the qi and fill muscles and skin. They brighten the eyes, increase intelligence and enable one to know things in advance. Ingested over a long time they let one not feel hungry. They prevent aging and relieve the body of its weight. *Ben jing*.

15-04-02
葉 *Ye*
Leaf [of *shi*].

【主治】痞疾。時珍。

Control. Obstacle-illness[51] ailments. [Li] Shizhen.

【附方】新一。

Added Recipes. One newly [recorded].

腹中痞塊。蓍葉、獨蒜、穿山甲末、食鹽，同以好醋搗成餅，量痞大小貼之，兩炷香爲度。其痞化爲膿血，從大便出。劉松石保壽堂方。

Obstacle-illness lump in the abdomen. Give *shi* leaves, single clove garlic, pangolin scale powder and table salt into good vinegar, pound this to form a pie in the size of the obstacle-illness [lump] and attach it [to the affected region] for as long as it

51 *Pi* 痞, "obstacle-illness," a condition of an uncomfortable distension and fullness in the chest and abdominal region. When pressed there is no pain. BCGM Dict. I, 371.

takes two incense sticks to burn down. The obstacle-illness [lump] will transform to pus and blood and leaves [the body] with defecation. Liu Songshi, *Bao shou tang fang*.

15-05
艾別録中品
Ai, FE *Bie lu*, middle rank.

***Artemisia argyi* Lèvl. et Vant. Common mugwort [leaf].**

【釋名】冰臺爾雅、醫草別録、黄草埤雅、艾蒿。【時珍曰】王安石字説云：艾可乂疾，久而彌善，故字從乂。陸佃埤雅云：博物志言削冰令圓，舉而向日，以艾承其影則得火。則艾名冰臺，其以此乎？醫家用灸百病，故曰灸草。一灼謂之一壯，以壯人爲法也。

Explanation of Names. *Bing tai* 冰臺, "ice base," *Er ya*. *Yi cao* 醫草, "medicine herb," *Bie lu*. *Huang cao* 黄草, "yellow herb," *Pi ya*. *Ai hai* 艾蒿. [Li] Shizhen: Wang Anshi's *Zi shuo* states: "*Ai* 艾 can 'cut down', *yi* 乂, illnesses. The longer [it is stored] the better it works. Hence the character [*ai* 艾] is derived from [the character] *yi* 乂." Lu Dian in his *Pi ya* states: "The *Bo wu zhi* says: 'Cut a round piece of ice and hold it against the sun. When the *ai* underneath is met by the silhouette [of the sun] it is set afire'." Perhaps this is the origin of the name "ice base." Medical experts use it to cauterize the hundreds of diseases. Hence it is called "cauterization herb." One such scorching is called *yi zhuang* 一壯, because this is a method to "strengthen", *zhuang* 壯, one.

【集解】【別録曰】艾葉生田野，三月三日采，暴乾。【頌曰】處處有之，以複道者爲佳，云此種灸百病尤勝。初春布地生苗，莖類蒿，葉背白，以苗短者爲良。三月三日、五月五日采葉，暴乾，陳久方可用。【時珍曰】艾葉，本草不著土産，但云生田野。宋時以湯陰複道者爲佳，四明者圖形。近代惟湯陰者謂之北艾，四明者謂之海艾。自成化以來，則以蘄州者爲勝，用充方物，天下重之，謂之蘄艾。相傳他處艾灸酒壜不能透，蘄艾一灸則直透徹，爲異也。此草多生山原。二月宿根生苗成叢，其莖直生，白色，高四五尺。其葉四布，狀如蒿，分爲五尖，椏上復有小尖，面青背白，有茸而柔厚。七八月葉間出穗如車前穗，細花，結實累累盈枝，中有細子，霜後始枯。皆以五月五日連莖刈取，暴乾收葉。先君月池子諱言聞，嘗著蘄艾傳一卷。有贊云：産於山陽，采以端午。治病灸疾，功非小補。又宗懔荆楚歲時記云：五月五日雞未鳴時，采艾似人形者攬而取之，收以灸病甚驗。是日采艾爲人，懸於户上，可禳毒氣。其莖乾之，染麻油引火點灸炷，滋潤灸瘡，至愈不疼。亦可代蓍策及作燭心。

Collected Explanations. *Bie lu*: *Ai* leaves grow in the open country. They are collected on the third day of the third month. They are dried in the sun. [Su] Song: [*Ai*] can be found everywhere. Those from the roadside are excellent. It is said that this kind is especially suitable for cauterizing the hundreds of diseasses. At the beginning of spring, [*ai*] covers the ground and grows seedlings. The stems are similar to those of wormwood; the leaves are white on their back. Those are good that have short seedlings. The leaves are collected on the third day of the third month and on the fifth day of the fifth month. They are dried in the sun. After being stored for a long time they can be used according to a recipe. [Li] Shizhen: The *Ben cao* does not record a specific soil where *ai* leaves grow; it only states "open country." During the Song era, those growing in Tang yin at the roadside were considered excellent. Those from Si ming were depicted in illustrations. In recent times, only those from Tang yin were named "northern *ai*." Those from Si ming are called "sea *ai*." Since the *cheng hua* reign period (1465 – 1487) those from Qi zhou are considered superior. [*Ai* leaves from Qi] are resorted to as a local product and valued everywhere. It is called "Qi *ai*." A saying is transmitted that a cauterization with *ai* from other places is unable to penetrate a wine jug, while a cauterization with Qi *ai* passes straight through it. That is the difference. This herb often grows on plains in the mountains. Its perennial root grows seedlings forming clusters in the second month. The stem grows straight. It is white and reaches a height of four to five *chi*. The leaves spread in all four directions; they are shaped like those of wormwood. They are divided into five sections with pointed ends. These are forked again with still smaller pointed ends. The [leaves] are greenish on their front and white on their back. They have fine hair and are soft and thick. In the seventh and eighth month spikes appear between the leaves, similar to the spikes of Asiatic plantain [herbs], with fine flowers. They form a series of fruit along the twigs, and have fine seeds inside. They begin to wither after the frost. Always cut them on the fifth day of the fifth month with their stem, dry them in the sun and keep the leaves. My father [Li] Yuechi, with his surname Yanwen, once wrote a *Qi ai zhuan* in one *juan*. A praise states: "It grows on the yang (i. e., sunny) side of mountains. It is collected on the fifth day of the fifth month. It serves to cure disease and to cauterize illness. Its potential reaches beyond minor supplementation." Also, Zong Lin in his *Jing Chu sui shi ji* states: "On the fifth day of the fifth month before the cocks crow in the morning, collect *ai* shaped like a human, tie it and remove it. Keep it to cauterize diseases, and it will be very effective. On this day [people] collect *ai* and form it like humans. They suspend it above the door and this can avert poisonous qi. Dry the stem, soak it in sesame oil, light it as a moxa stick. It provides moisture to sores resulting from cauterization.

They will heal without pain. It can also be used as a substitute of yarrow-stalks/ Siberian milfoil stalks and is made to candlewicks."

15-05-01
葉 *Ye*
[*Ai*] leaf.

【脩治】【宗奭曰】艾葉乾擣，去青滓，取白，入石硫黄末少許，謂之硫黄艾，灸家用之。得米粉少許，可擣爲末，入服食藥用。【時珍曰】凡用艾葉，須用陳久者，治令細軟，謂之熟艾。若生艾灸火，則傷人肌脉。故孟子云：七年之病，求三年之艾。揀取净葉，揚去塵屑，入石臼内木杵擣熟，羅去渣滓，取白者再擣，至柔爛如綿爲度。用時焙燥，則灸火得力。入婦人丸散，須以熟艾，用醋煮乾，擣成餅子，烘乾再擣爲末用。或以糯糊和作餅及酒炒者，皆不佳。洪氏容齋隨筆云：艾難着力，若入白茯苓三五片同碾，即時可作細末。亦一異也。

Pharmaceutical Preparation. [Kou] Zongshi: Dry *ai* leaves, pound them, remove the greenish dregs and keep the white parts. Add a little sulphur powder. This is called sulphur *ai*. Cauterization specialists use it. With a little rice powder added it can be pounded into powder, and is then used by those who ingest it as food and medication. [Li] Shizhen: For all applications of *ai* leaves, it is essential to resort to those that have been stored for a long time. They are processed to generate fine, soft [pieces] that are called "prepared *ai*." If one were to use fresh *ai* for cauterization with fire, this would harm that person's skin and vessels. Hence the *Meng zi* states: "For a disease that has lasted seven years, search for *ai* that has been stored for three years." Select clean leaves and blow away dust and crumbs. Then give it into a stone mortar and pound it with a wooden pestle until it is done. Pass it through a sieve to discard the dregs. Select the white parts and pound them again until eventually something soft and pulpy is generated similar to silk floss. When it is to be used, dry it over a fire in a pan. This provides it with the strength required to cauterize with fire. For pills and powders for [treating] women, only prepared *ai* must be used. Boil it in vinegar, dry it and pound it to form a pie. Dry this by a fire and pound it again into powder that is then ready to be used. Or mix it with glutinous rice to form a pie, or fry it in wine, but all these preparations are not good. Mr. Hong [Mai] in his *Rong zhai sui bi* states: "It is difficult to develop the strength of *ai*. If it is ground together with three to five pieces of white *poria*, when the time [for an application has come] it can be prepared to a fine powder. This is a different [approach]."

【氣味】苦，微温，無毒。【恭曰】生寒，熟熱。【元素曰】苦，温，陰中之陽。【時珍曰】苦而辛，生温熟熱，可升可降，陽也。入足太陰、厥陰、少陰之經。苦酒、香附爲之使。

Qi and Flavor. Bitter, slightly warm, nonpoisonous. [Su] Gong: Fresh cold; prepared hot. [Zhang] Yuansu: Bitter, warm, a yang in yin [substance]. [Li] Shizhen: Bitter and at the same time acrid. Fresh warm; prepared hot. [The leaves] can rise and descend. They enter the foot major yin, ceasing yin and minor yin conduits. Bitter wine and nutgrass [roots] serve as their guiding [substances].

【主治】灸百病。可作煎，止吐血下痢，下部䘌瘡，婦人漏血，利陰氣，生肌肉，辟風寒，使人有子。作煎勿令見風。别録。擣汁服，止傷血，殺蚘蟲。弘景。主衄血下血，膿血痢，水煮及丸散任用。蘇恭。止崩血、腸痔血，搨金瘡，止腹痛，安胎。苦酒作煎，治癬甚良。擣汁飲，治心腹一切冷氣鬼氣。甄權。治帶下，止霍亂轉筋，痢後寒熱。大明。治帶脉爲病，腹脹滿，腰溶溶如坐水中。好古。温中逐冷除濕。時珍。

Control. They serve to cauterize the hundreds of diseases. They can be prepared as a decoction to end spitting blood and discharge with free-flux illness. [They serve to cure] sores caused by hidden worms/bugs in the lower body parts, and blood leakage of women. They free the movement of yin qi, generate skin and flesh, repel wind and cold and let one have children. When they are prepared as a decoction, they must not be exposed to wind. *Bie lu*. Pounded and the resulting juice ingested they end injuries with bleeding, and kill roundworms. [Tao] Hongjing. They control nosebleed and discharge with blood, and free-flux illness with pus and blood. They can be used, as one prefers, as an aqueous decoction, and also as pills and powder. Su Gong. They end collapsing blood[52] and bleeding intestinal piles. [In a pouch] they are applied to wounds caused by metal objects/weapons. They end abdominal pain and pacify a fetus. Prepared to a decoction with wine they are very good at curing *xuan*-illness.[53] Pounded and the resulting juice drunk, they serve to cure all types of cold qi and demon qi affecting the central and abdominal region. Zhen Quan. They end cholera with contorted sinews, and alternating sensations of cold and heat following a free-flux illness. Da Ming. They serve to cure diseases originating from the belt vessel, abdominal distension with a feeling of fullness, and a flabby lower back as if one sat in a water. [Wang] Haogu. They warm the center, drive out cold and eliminate moisture. [Li] Shizhen.

---

52 *Beng xue* 崩血, "collapsing blood," identical to [*Xue*] *beng* [血]崩, "[blood] collapse," is excessive vaginal bleeding. BCGM Dict I, 594.

53 *Xuan* 癬, "*xuan*-illness." Conditions of dermal lesions with initially erythema, papules, and itching gradually extending in all directions to form an irregular ring with clear boundaries. The skin is slightly elevated with small papules, blisters, and/or scales and scraps. The central lesion may appear to heal spontaneously, and it may reappear. Also, a designation of local lesions with itching, release of liquid and shedding of scabs. BCGM Dict I, 591.

【發明】【詵曰】春月采嫩艾作菜食，或和麵作餛飩如彈子，吞三五枚，以飯壓之，治一切鬼惡氣，長服止冷痢。又以嫩艾作乾餅子，用生薑煎服，止瀉痢及產後瀉血，甚妙。【頌曰】近世有單服艾者，或用蒸木瓜和丸，或作湯空腹飲，甚補虛羸。然亦有毒發則熱氣衝上，狂躁不能禁，至攻眼有瘡出血者，誠不可妄服也。【震亨曰】婦人無子，多由血少不能攝精。俗醫謂子宮虛冷，投以辛熱，或服艾葉。不知艾性至熱，入火灸則氣下行，入藥服則氣上行。本草止言其溫，不言其熱。世人喜溫，率多服之，久久毒發，何嘗歸咎於艾哉？予考蘇頌圖經而因默有感焉。【時珍曰】艾葉生則微苦大辛，熟則微辛大苦，生溫熟熱，純陽也。可以取太陽真火，可以回垂絕元陽。服之則走三陰，而逐一切寒濕，轉肅殺之氣爲融和。灸之則透諸經而治百種病邪，起沉痾之人爲康泰，其功亦大矣。蘇恭言其生寒，蘇頌言其有毒。一則見其能止諸血，一則見其熱氣上衝，遂謂其性寒有毒，誤矣。蓋不知血隨氣而行，氣行則血散，熱因久服致火上衝之故爾。夫藥以治病，中病則止。若素有虛寒痼.冷，婦人濕鬱帶漏之人，以艾和歸、附諸藥治其病，夫何不可？而乃妄意求嗣，服艾不輟，助以辛熱，藥性久偏，致使火躁，是誰之咎歟，於艾何尤？艾附丸治心腹少腹諸痛，調女人諸病，頗有深功。膠艾湯治虛痢乃姙娠、產後下血，尤著奇妙。老人丹田氣弱，臍腹畏冷者，以熟艾入布袋兜其臍腹，妙不可言。寒濕脚氣，亦宜以此夾入襪內。

Explication. [Meng] Shen: During spring months tender *ai* [leaves] are collected to prepare them as edible vegetables. Or they are mixed with wheat flour to make dumplings the size of bullets. To swallow three to five of them and then press them down with cooked rice, serves to cure all types of demon and malign qi. Ingested over a long time they end cold free-flux illness. Or prepare with tender *ai* [leaves] dry cakes, boil them with fresh ginger in water and ingest this to end outflow free-flux illness and outflow with blood following birth. Very wondrous. [Su] Song: In recent times, *ai* [leaves] are ingested as a single substance, or they are steamed and prepared with quince to pills, or they are boiled in water to be drunk on an empty stomach. This serves to extraordinarily supplement depletion and emaciation. However, it has also happened that [*ai* leaves] have effused poison resulting in heat rushing up [in the body] with madness and restlessness that could not be stopped, eventually attacking the eyes and causing bleeding sores. Truly, they must not be ingested without consideration. [Zhu] Zhenheng: When a woman has no children this is often so because of too little blood so that it is unable to nourish the essence [required to join with the essence/sperm of a male]. Ordinary physicians claim that there is a depletion cold in the womb, and they feed [the women] with acrid and hot [medication]. Or they let them ingest *ai* leaves. They do not know that *ai* [leaves] by their nature are very hot. If the [*ai* leaves] are applied as a fiery cauterization, their qi move downward. If they are ingested added to medication, their qi move upward. The *Ben cao* speaks of their warm [nature] only, it does not mention their heat. All the people prefer [medication of a] warm [nature]; hence they are given many [*ai* leaves] to ingest. When after a long time, they effuse poison, why should this be blamed on the *ai* [leaves]?! I have studied Su Song's *Tu jing*, and deep in my interior I am grateful [to him for making this clear to me]. [Li] Shizhen: As long as *ai* leaves are fresh/unprepared they are slightly bitter and very acrid. Once they are prepared they are slightly acrid and very bitter. Fresh they are warm; prepared they are hot. They are a pure yang [substance]. With [*ai* leaves] one can acquire the true fire of major yang and one can let the original yang return in a situation where it was close to being cut off. When they are ingested they rush into the three yin [conduits] where they expel all types of cold and moisture and transform all deadly qi to harmonious [qi]. When [*ai* leaves] are used for cauterization [their qi] penetrate all conduits and serve to cure the hundred types of disease and evil. They raise people from a state of severe sickness to one of perfect health. Their [therapeutic] potential is of such greatness. Su Gong says that when they are fresh they are cold. Su Song says that they are poisonous. One of these perspectives is based on their ability to stop all types of bleeding. The other is based on the rushing upward of their hot qi. And hence [Su Gong and Su Song] concluded that their nature is cold and that they are poisonous. Both are wrong. The fact is, they did not know that the movement of blood follows the movement of the qi. When the qi move, the blood disperses. A fire rushes upward because one has ingested something hot for a long time. That is, when pharmaceutical drugs are applied to cure a disease, once the disease is struck, the [treatment] is to end. If there are persons who because of their individual constitution have an obstinacy-illness of depletion cold, and women with pent-up moisture and leakage from [below] the belt, if their diseases are treated with *ai* [leaves], Chinese *angelica* [root] and *aconitum* [accessory tuber], why should this be impossible? If there are [women] who desperately long for offspring, who continuesly ingest *ai* [leaves] and support them with acrid and hot [medication], continuing a long-lasting one-sided exposure to the nature of such drugs, so that eventually the fire causes restlessness, who is to blame? Why should the fault lie with the *ai* [leaves]? The "pills with *ai* [leaves] and *aconitum* [accessory tuber]" serve to cure all types of pain in the central and abdominal region and in the lower abdomen. They serve to regulate all types of diseases of women. They have a far-reaching [therapeutic] potential. The "decoction with [donkey hide] glue and *ai* [leaves]" serves to cure depletion free-flux illness and blood discharge during pregnancy and after delivery. It is uniquely wondrous in all respects. When old people with a cinnabar field qi weakness and an aversion to cold in the navel and abdominal region cover the navel and abdominal region with a cloth pouch filled with prepared *ai* [leaves] the effects] are wondrous beyond words. [To cure] leg qi[54] related to cold and moisture, it is suitable to put the [*ai* leaves] into [the patient's] stockings.

【附方】舊二十四，新二十七。

Added Recipes. 24 of old. 27 newly [recorded].

傷寒時氣，温疫頭痛，壯熱脉盛。以乾艾葉三升，水一斗，煮一升，頓服取汗。肘後方。

Harm caused by cold with an affection by seasonal qi, warmth epidemics and headache, strong heat and an abundance in the vessels. Boil three *sheng* of dry *ai* leaves in one *dou* of water down to one *sheng* and ingest this in one draft to cause sweating. *Zhou hou fang*.

妊娠傷寒，壯熱，赤斑變爲黑斑，溺血。用艾葉如鷄子大，酒三升，煮二升半，分爲二服。傷寒類要。

Harm caused by cold during pregnancy, with strong heat, red macules changing to black macules and urination with blood. Boil a chicken egg size amount of *ai* leaves in three *sheng* of wine down to two and a half *sheng* and [let the woman] ingest this divided into two portions. *Shang han lei yao*.

妊娠風寒卒中，不省人事，狀如中風。用熟艾三兩，米醋炒極熱，以絹包熨臍下，良久即甦。婦人良方。

Suddenly being struck by wind and cold during pregnancy, when [the patient] recognizes neither other people nor anything else, similar to wind stroke. Fry three *liang* of prepared *ai* [leaves] in rice vinegar until they are very hot, wrap them in silk fabric and press them on the region below the abdomen. After a long time, she will regain consciousness. *Fu ren liang fang*.

中風口喎。以葦筒長五寸，一頭刺入耳内，四面以麪密封不透風，一頭以艾灸之七壯。患右灸左，患左灸右。勝金方。

Wry mouth resulting from wind stroke. Take a reed tube of five *cun* length and insert one end of it into the [patient's] ear. Tightly seal it with wheat flour on all sides so that no wind can pass through. On the other end apply *ai* cauterization seven times. If the suffering has struck the [patient's] right side, apply the cauterization on the left side. If the suffering has struck the [patient's] left side, apply the cauterization on the right side. *Sheng jin fang*.

54 *Jiao qi* 脚氣, "leg qi." Painful, weak, swollen legs. BCGM Dict I, 248.

中風口噤。熟艾灸承漿一穴，頰車二穴，各五壯。千金方。

Clenched jaw resulting from wind stroke. Apply cauterization with prepared *ai* [leaves] five times each on one *cheng jiang* [needle insertion] hole (CV-24) and on two *jia che* holes (ST-6). *Qian jin fang.*

中風掣痛，不仁不隨。並以乾艾斛許，揉團納瓦甑中，並下塞諸孔，獨留一目，以痛處着甑目，而燒艾熏之，一時即知矣。肘後方。

Wind-stroke causing painful convulsion, with numbness and paralysis. Knead about a *hu* quantity of dry *ai* [leaves] to form a ball and give this into an earthen jar. Seal all openings and leave only one eye open. Then attach this eye to the aching region and burn the *ai* [leaves] to steam it. After a while [the patient] will regain consciousness. *Zhou hou fang.*

舌縮口噤。以生艾擣傅之。乾艾浸濕亦可。聖濟録。

Contracted tongue and clenched jaw. Pound fresh *ai* [leaves] and apply [the resulting mass to the affected region]. To apply dry *ai* [leaves] soaked to moisten them is possible, too. *Sheng ji lu.*

咽喉腫痛。醫方大成用嫩艾擣汁，細嚥之。

Painful, swollen throat. The *Yi fang da cheng* [recommends to] pound tender *ai* [leaves] and to sip the resulting juice.

經驗方用青艾和莖葉一握，同醋擣爛，傅於喉上。冬月取乾艾亦得。李亞所傳方也。

The *Jing yan fang* [recommends to] pound greenish *ai* stem and leaves with vinegar into a pulpy mass and apply this to the throat. In winter dry *ai* may be used, too. A recipe handed over by Li Ya.

癲癇諸風。熟艾於陰囊下穀道正門當中間，隨年歲灸之。斗門方。

Peak-illness[55] with epilepsy and all types of wind [intrusion]. Apply cauterization, depending on the age [of the patient], between his scrotum and the anus. *Dou men fang.*

鬼擊中惡。卒然着人，如刀刺狀，胸脇腹内疞刺切痛不可按，或即吐血、鼻中出血、下血，一名鬼排。以熟艾如鷄子大三枚，水五升，煎二升，頓服。肘後方。

---

55 *Dian ji* 癲[疾], "peak ailment," a mental disturbance of depression and unhappiness, with a calm attitude and little incentive to speak. BCGM Dict I, 125.

Demon attack and being struck by the malign. When this suddenly affects a person, as if stabbed with a knife. There may be a piercing pain in chest and flanks that cannot be touched. Or [the patients] spit blood, blood leaving from their nose, and blood discharge. This is also called "demon push." Boil three pieces, the size of chicken eggs, of prepared *ai* [leaves] in five *sheng* of water down to two *sheng* and ingest this all at once. *Zhou hou fang.*

小兒臍風撮口。艾葉燒灰填臍中，以帛縛，定效。或隔蒜灸之，候口中有艾氣立愈。簡便方。

Pursed mouth of children caused by navel wind.[56] Burn *ai* leaves, place the ashes on the [child's] navel and bandage it with silk. Definitely effective. Or apply, separated by a piece of garlic, cauterization there. As soon as the *ai* qi leave from the [child's] throat and mouth it will be cured. *Jian bian fang.*

狐惑蟲𧎢。病人齒無色，舌上白，或喜睡不知痛痒處，或下痢，宜急治下部。不曉此者，但攻其上，而下部生蟲，食其肛，爛見五臟，便死也。燒艾於管中，熏下部，令烟入，或少加雄黄更妙。罌中燒烟亦可。肘後方。

Fox delusion[57] and hidden worm infestation. The patient's teeth have lost their color. The surface of the tongue is white. [The patient] may wish to sleep but feels itch and pain without knowing where. In some cases [patients suffer from] discharge with free-flux illness. It is essential to quickly apply a cure to the lower [body] part. Those who do not know this apply an attack only to the upper [body] part. But there are worms/bugs in the lower part that eat the anus so that eventually all the five long-term depots are visible and rotten, which leads to [the patient's] death. Burn *ai* [leaves] in a tube and steam the lower [body] part so that the fumes enter [the anus]. When a little realgar is added, [the effects are] even more wondrous. To burn [the *ai* leaves] in a jar to generate fumes is possible, too. *Zhou hou fang.*

頭風久痛。蘄艾揉爲丸，時時嗅之，以黄水出爲度。青囊雜纂。

Head wind[58] with long-lasting pain. Kneed Qi *ai* [leaves] to form a pill and [let the patient] repeatedly smell its [qi] until a yellow water leaves [his nose]. *Qing nan zu zuan.*

---

56 *Qi feng* 臍風, "navel wind," identical to *po shang feng* 破傷風， "wound wind," a condition brought forth by wind evil affecting the navel region of newborn children. BCGM Dict I, 382.

57 *Hu huo* 狐惑, "fox and delusion," a condition of putrid flesh and festering ulcers in the throat and private parts brought forth by moisture, heat, and bug poison. BCGM Dict I, 220.

58 *Tou feng* 頭風, "head wind." Condition of wind evil attacking the head followed by pain, dizziness, itching. BCGM Dict I, 509.

頭風面瘡，痒，出黄水。艾二兩，醋一升，砂鍋煎取汁，每薄紙上貼之，一日一兩上。御藥院方。

Head wind with facial sores, itch and yellow water leaving [from the nose]. Boil two *liang* of *ai* [leaves] in one *sheng* of vinegar in an earthenware pot to obtain a juice. Each time spread [the juice] on a piece of paper and apply this [to the affected region]. Once or twice a day. *Yu yao yuan fang.*

心腹惡氣。艾葉搗汁飲之。藥性論。

Central and abdominal region affected by malign qi. Pound *ai* leaves to obtain a juice and drink this. *Yao xing lun.*

脾胃冷痛。白艾末，沸湯服二錢。衞生易簡方。

Pain related to spleen and stomach cold. Boil white *ai* [leaf] powder in water to bubbling and ingest two *qian* [of the liquid]. *Wei sheng yi jian fang.*

蚘蟲心痛如刺，口吐清水。白熟艾一升，水三升，煮一升服，吐蟲出。或取生艾搗汁，五更食香脯一片，乃飲一升，當下蟲出。肘後方。

Roundworms causing a piercing heart pain, with clear water being spit out of the mouth. Boil one *sheng* of white, prepared *ai* [leaves] in three *sheng* of water down to one *sheng* and ingest this. The worms are spit out. Or pound fresh *ai* [leaves] to obtain a juice. In the early morning eat one slice of fragrant dried meat and then drink one *sheng* [of the juice]. This will cause a discharge of the worms. *Zhou hou fang.*

口吐清水。乾蘄艾煎湯啜之。怪證奇方。

Clear water being spit from the mouth. Boil dry Qi *ai* [leaves] in water and sip the resulting decoction. *Guai zheng qi fang.*

霍亂吐下不止。以艾一把，水三升，煮一升，頓服。外臺秘要。

Cholera with unending vomiting and discharge. Boil a handful of *ai* [leaves] in three *sheng* of water down to one *sheng* and ingest this all at once. *Wai tai mi yao.*

老小白痢。艾薑丸：用陳北艾四兩，乾薑炮三兩，爲末，醋煮倉米糊丸梧子大。每服七十丸，空心米飲下，甚有奇效。永類方。

White free-flux illness affecting old or young [persons]. The "pills with *ai* [leaves] and ginger." [Grind] four *liang* of long-stored northern *ai* [leaves] and three *liang* of dried ginger, roasted in a pan, into powder, boil it in vinegar and form with a paste made with long-stored rice pills the size of *wu* seeds. Each time ingest 70 pills, to be sent down on an empty stomach with a rice beverage. This is extraordinarily effective. *Yong lei fang.*

諸痢久下。艾葉、陳皮等分，煎湯服之，亦可爲末，酒煮，爛飯和丸，每鹽湯下二三十丸。聖濟總録。

All types of free-flux illness with a long-lasting discharge. Boil equal amounts of *ai* leaves and tangerine peels in water and drink the resulting decoction. To prepare a powder is possible, too, to form with rice, cooked until it has turned into a pulpy mass, pills. Each time send down with a salt decoction 20 to 30 pills. *Sheng ji zong lu.*

暴泄不止。陳艾一把，生薑一塊，水煎熱服。生生編。

Unending violent outflow. Boil one handful of long-stored *ai* [leaves] with one piece of fresh ginger in water and drink it hot. *Sheng sheng bian.*

糞後下血。艾葉、生薑煎濃汁，服三合。千金方。

Discharge of blood following defecation. Boil *ai* leaves and fresh ginger to obtain a thick juice and drink three *ge. Qian jin fang.*

野鷄痔病。先以槐、柳湯洗過，以艾灸上七壯，取效。郎中王及乘騾入西川，數日病痔大作，如胡瓜貫於腸頭，其熱如火，忽至僵仆，無計。有主郵者云：須灸即瘥。乃用上法灸三五壯，忽覺一道熱氣入腸中，因大轉瀉，血穢併出，瀉後遂失胡瓜所在矣。經驗方。

Piles. First wash [the affected region] with a *sophora* tree and willow tree [twig] decoction. Then apply with *ai* [leaves] seven cauterizations. This will be effective. Wang Ji of Lang zhong rode a donkey to Xi chuan. After a few days he developed a massive case of piles. As if a cucumber, as hot as fire, had passed through the end of his intestines. All of a sudden he fell to the ground and was unable to continue. A postmaster stated: "He must be cauterized; this will cure him." Then he applied the method outlined above with three to five cauterization. [The patient] suddenly felt a stream of hot qi entering his intestines and this turned into a massive outflow of blood and filth. After the outflow [the patient] no longer felt the presence of a cucumber. *Jing yan fang.*

妊娠下血。張仲景曰：婦人有漏下者，有半産後下血不絶者，有妊娠下血者，並宜膠艾湯主之。阿膠二兩，艾葉三兩，芎藭、甘草各二兩，當歸、地黄各三兩，芍藥四兩，水五升，清酒五升，煮取三升，乃納膠令消盡，每温服一升，日三服。金匱要略。

Discharge with blood during pregnancy. Zhang Zhongjing: When women have a leaking discharge, when they have incessant bleeding following a miscarriage, and when they bleed during pregnancy, all such cases can be controlled with the "decoction with [donkey hide] glue and *ai* [leaves]." [Take] two *liang* of E glue and boil three *liang* of *ai* leaves, two *liang* each of *ligusticum* [root] and *glycyrrhiza* [root], three *liang* each of Chinese *angelica* [root] and Chinese foxglove [rhizome], and four *liang* of *paeonia* [root] in five *sheng* of water and five *sheng* of clear wine down to three *sheng*. Now add the glue and let it dissolve completely. Each time [let the patient] ingest one *sheng*, to be ingested three times a day. *Jin kui yao lüe*.

妊娠胎動，或腰痛，或搶心，或下血不止，或倒產子死腹中。艾葉一鷄子大，酒四升，煮二升，分二服。肘後方。

Fetal movement during pregnancy, sometimes with lower back pain, sometimes knocking at the heart, sometimes with unending blood discharge, and for an inverted birth when the child has died in the abdomen. Boil *ai* leaves, the quantity equalling the size of a chicken egg, in four *sheng* of water down to two *sheng* and [let the woman] ingest this divided into two portions. *Zhou hou fang*

胎動迫心作痛。艾葉鷄子大，以頭醋四升，煎二升，分温服。子母秘録。

Painful fetal movement pressing against the heart. Boil *ai* leaves, the quantity equalling the size of a chicken egg, in four *sheng* of top quality vinegar down to two *sheng* and [let the woman] ingest this warm divided into several portions. *Zi mu mi lu*.

婦人崩中，連日不止。熟艾鷄子大，阿膠炒爲末半兩，乾薑一錢，水五盞，先煮艾、薑至二盞半，傾出，入膠烊化，分三服，一日服盡。初虞世古今録驗。

Collapsing center[59] of women, continuing for several days without end. Get prepared *ai* [leaves], a quantity the size of a chicken egg. Half a *liang* of E glue fried and [ground into] powder. One *qian* of dried ginger. Five cups of water. First boil the *ai* [leaves] and the ginger in the water down to two and a half cups. Pour the liquid out to remove [the leaves and the ginger]. Add the glue [to the liquid] and let it dissolve. [Let the patient] ingest this divided into three portions. All to be ingested on the same day. Chu Yushi, *Gu jin lu yan*.

產後瀉血不止。乾艾葉半兩，炙熟老生薑半兩，濃煎湯，一服止，妙。孟詵食療本草。

Unending outflow with blood following birth. Boil half a *liang* of dry *ai* leaves and half a *liang* of roasted, long-stored fresh ginger in water to obtain a thick decoction and [let the patient] ingest this to end [the outflow]. Wondrous. Meng Shen, *Shi liao ben cao*.

---

59 *Beng zhong* 崩中, "collapsing center," excessive vaginal bleeding outside of a menstruation period. BCGM Dict I, 58.

產後腹痛欲死，因感寒起者。陳蘄艾二斤，焙乾，搗鋪臍上，以絹覆住，熨斗熨之，待口中艾氣出，則痛自止矣。楊誠經驗方。

Abdominal pain following birth letting one wish to die. When this is caused by a cold affection. Bake two *jin* of long-stored Qi *ai* [leaves] over a slow fire until they are dry, pound them and apply [the mass] to the navel. Fix it with a thin, tough silk bandage and heat it with a hot iron. When the *ai* qi leave from the [patient's] mouth, the pain will end. Yang Cheng, *Jing yan fang*.

忽然吐血一二口，或心衄，或内崩。熟艾三團，水五升，煮二升服。一方：燒灰，水服二錢。千金方。

Sudden spitting of blood, one or two mouthfuls, either because of a spontaneous heart bleeding, or because of an internal [blood] collapse. Boil three balls of prepared *ai* [leaves] in five *sheng* of water down to two *sheng* and [let the patient] ingest this. Another recipe: Burn [the leaves] to ashes and [let the patient] ingest with water two *qian*. *Qian jin fang*.

鼻血不止。艾灰吹之，亦可以艾葉煎服。聖惠方。

Unending nosebleed. Blow *ai* [leaf] ashes [into the nose]. It is also possible to boil *ai* leaves and ingest [the liquid]. *Sheng hui fang*.

盜汗不止。熟艾二錢，白伏神三錢，烏梅三箇，水一鍾，煎八分，臨卧温服。通妙真人方。

Unending robber sweating.[60] Boil two *qian* of prepared *ai* [leaves], three *qian* of white *poria* and three smoked plums in one *zhong* of water down to 80% to be ingested warm when going to bed. *Tong miao zhen ren fang*.

火眼腫痛。以艾燒烟起，用盌覆之，候烟盡，盌上刮煤下，以温水調化洗眼，即瘥。更入黄連尤佳。斗門方。

Fire eye[61] with painful swelling. Boil *ai* [leaves] so that smoke rises. Cover them with a bowl until no more smoke emerges. Scrape the soot from the bowl, dissolve it in warm water and use it to wash the [affected] eyes. This will result in a cure. *Dou men fang*.

面上皯黵。艾灰、桑灰各三升，以水淋汁，再淋至三遍，以五色布納於中，同煎，令可丸時，每以少許傅之，自爛脱，甚妙。外臺秘要。

---

60 *Dao han* 盜汗, "robber sweating," (1) an illness sign of a profuse sweating during sleep that ends when one wakes up. (2) A pathological condition with robber sweating as major sign. BCGM Dict I, 122.

61 *Huo yan* 火眼, "fire eye," condition of seasonally prevalent eye diseases characterized by red and hot eyeballs that are swollen and painful. BCGM Dict I, 234.

Facial dark speckles. Let water trickle through three *sheng* each of *ai* [leaf] ashes and mulberry tree [twig] ashes to obtain a juice. Repeat this twice, altogether three times. Give "five color cloth"[62] into [the liquid] and boil this to [obtain a mass that] can be formed to pills. Each time apply a small part [to the affected region. The speckles] will soften and fall off as a result. Very wondrous. *Wai tai mi yao.*

婦人面瘡，名粉花瘡。以定粉五錢，菜子油調泥盌内，用艾一二團，燒烟熏之，候烟盡，覆地上一夜，取出調搽，永無瘢痕，亦易生肉。談埜翁試驗方。

Facial sores of women, called "cosmetic powder sores." Prepare with a mixture of five *qian* of lead carbonate and vegetable oil a paste and give this into a bowl. Then burn one or two balls of *ai* [leaves] and steam [the affected region] with the smoke. Wait until no more smoke develops. Leave [the bowl] covered on the ground for one night, remove [its contents], mix them [to generate a creme] and apply this [to the affected region]. There will never be wound scars. It is also helpful to generate [new] flesh. Tan Yeweng, *Shi yan fang.*

身面疣目。艾火炙三壯即除。聖惠方。

Warts on the body and the face. Cauterize them three times with *ai* [leaf] fire and they will be removed. *Sheng hui fang.*

鵝掌風病。蘄艾真者四五兩，水四五盌，煮五六滾，入大口瓶内盛之，用麻布二層縛之，將手心放瓶上熏之，如冷再熱，如神。陸氏積德堂方。

Goose palm wind[63] disease. Boil four to five *liang* of true Qi *ai* [leaves] in four to five cups of water five to six times to bubbling. Then fill [the liquid] into a bottle with a big mouth, cover [the opening] with a two layer hemp cloth, place the palm on the bottle [opening] and steam it. When the bottle cools off, heat it again. Divine. Lu shi, *Ji de tang fang.*

疥瘡熏法。熟蘄艾一兩，木鼈子三錢，雄黄二錢，硫黄一錢，爲末，揉入艾中，分作四條。每以一條安陰陽瓦中，置被裏烘熏，後服通聖散。醫方摘要。

Method [to cure] *jie*-illness[64] with sores by steaming. Take one *liang* of prepared Qi *ai* [leaves] and [grind] three *qian* of *momordica* seeds, two *qian* of realgar and

62 *Wu se bu* 五色布, lit.: "five color cloth," is an organic layer in many colors forming on the surface of rotten brewer's yeast.

63 *Zhang feng* 鵝掌風, "goose-palm wind," a condition of the skin of syphilis patients breaking open, festering, and desiccating on the top and soles/palms of feet and hands. BCGM Dict I, 145.

64 *Jie*-illness 疥, vaguely identifiable skin ailment. BCGM Dict I, 249.

one *qian* of sulphur into powder. Rub [the powder] with the *ai* [leaves] and form four sticks. Place each stick on a yin yang tile.[65] Place [the tiles] underneath a quilt, and heat it to generate steam. After [steaming the patient's affected region let him] ingest the "powder to communicate with sages."[66] *Yi fang zhai yao.*

小兒疳瘡。艾葉一兩，水一升，煮取四合服。備急方。

Gan-illness[67] sores of children. Boil one *liang* of *ai* leaves in one *sheng* of water down to four *ge* and [let the patient] ingest this. *Bei ji fang.*

小兒爛瘡。艾葉燒灰傅之，良。子母秘録。

Festering sores of children. Burn *ai* leaves and apply the ashes [to the affected region]. Good. *Zi mu mi lu.*

臁瘡口冷不合。熟艾燒烟熏之。經驗方。

Cold shank sore openings that fail to close. Burn prepared *ai* [leaves] and steam [the affected region] with the smoke. *Jing yan fang.*

白癩風瘡。乾艾隨多少，以浸麴釀酒如常法，日飲之，覺痺即瘥。肘後方。

White repudiation-illness (i. e., massive) wind[68] sores. Add any amount of dry *ai* [leaves] into the normal process of wine brewing with yeast and [let the patient] drink this every day. When a numbness sets in a cure is achieved.[69] *Zhou hou fang.*

疔瘡腫毒。艾蒿一擔燒灰，於竹筒中淋取汁，以一二合，和石灰如糊。先以針刺瘡至痛，乃點藥三遍，其根自拔。玉山韓光以此治人神驗。貞觀初，衢州徐使君訪得此方。予用治三十餘人，得效。孫真人千金方。

---

65 Yin yang tiles 陰陽瓦 are curved tiles layed down alternately oberlapping, one concave and one convex.

66 *Tong sheng san* 通聖散, "powder to communicate with sages," is prepared from the following ingredients: *saposhnikovia* root, *ligusticum* root, hinese *angelica* root, *paeonia* root, rhubarb root, mirabilite, *forsythia* fruit, mint, *ephedra* herb, gypsum, *platycodon* root, *scutellaria* root, *atractylodes* rhizome, *gardenia* fruit, *schizonepeta* spikes, talc, *glycyrrhiza* root and fresh ginger.

67 *Gan* 疳, "*gan*-illness," also: "sweets-illness," involves several complaints that affect children and adults, with causes and conditions too different to fall into a known disease category. BCGM Dict I, 180-188.

68 *Da feng lai* 大風癩, "massive wind [i. e.,] repudiation-illness," most likely including cases of leprosy/Aussatz. BCGM Dict I, 111, 293

69 Instead of *jue pi ji cha* 覺痺即瘥, *Zhou hou fang* ch. 5, *zhi zu de lai pi mao bian hei fang* 治卒得癩皮毛變黑方, "Recipes to cure sudden onset of repudiation-illness letting skin and hair turn black again," write *chang yin shi xun xun* 常飲使醺醺, "drunk regularly it makes one drunk."

Pin-illness[70] sores with poison swelling. Burn the load of one carrying pole, fill the ashes into a bamboo tube, let water trickle through [the tube] and mix one or two *ge* of the resulting juice with lime to make a paste. First pierce a sore with a needle until [the patient] feels a pain. Then apply the medicinal [paste to it]. After three [such applications] the root [of the pin-illness] will come out by itself. Han Guang of Yu shan used this [method] to cure people; the effects were divine. At the beginning of the *zhen guan* reign period (627 – 649), Commisioner Xu paid a visit to him and obtained this recipe. I used it myself to cure more than 30 people and it has been shown to be effective. Sun zhenren, *Qian jin fang*.

發背初起未成，及諸熱腫。以濕紙搨上，先乾處是頭，着艾灸之，不論壯數。痛者灸至不痛，不痛者灸至痛，乃止。其毒即散，不散亦免内攻，神方也。李絳兵部手集。

An effusion on the back that has only just started to rise but has not yet manifested itself. Also, all types of swelling with heat. Spread a moist paper above [the affected region]. The place where [the paper] dries first is the tip [of the effusion]. Attach *ai* [leaves] there and cauterize it, regardless of how many times. When there is pain, continue the cauterization until there is no more pain. When there is no pain, continue the cauterization until there is pain. Then stop. The poison will have dispersed. If it fails to disperse, it will not attack the interior. A divine recipe. Li Jiang, *Bing bu shou ji*.

癰疽不合，瘡口冷滯。以北艾煎湯洗後，白膠熏之。直指方。

Obstruction-illness and impediment-illness[71] [with open sores] that fail to close. Cold [qi] remain at the opening of the sores. Boil northern *ai* [leaves] in water and wash [the affected region] with the decoction. Then steam it with white [deer horn] glue. *Zhi zhi fang*.

咽喉骨哽。用生艾蒿數升，水、酒共一斗，煮四升，細細飲之，當下。外臺秘要。

Choking on a bone in the throat. Boil numerous *sheng* of fresh *ai hao* [leaves] in one *dou* of a mixture of water and wine down to four *sheng* and [let the patient] drink this in small portions. This will send [the bone] down. *Wai tai mi yao*.

70 *Ding* 丁, "pin[-illness]," also *ding* 疔, "pin-illness," refers to a deep-reaching and festering hardness in a tissue, eventually rising above the skin like a pinhead. BCGM Dict I, 127-129.

71 *Yong ju* 癰疽, "obstruction-illness, impediment-illness." refers to two vaguely distinguished obstructions/impediments of vessels or other ducts inside the body. Qi rushing against the obstruction may cause a local swelling and eventually break through the surface to cause an abscess. BCGM Dict I, 642.

誤吞銅錢。艾蒿一把，水五升，煎一升，頓服便下。錢相公篋中方。

Accidental swallowing of a copper coin. Boil one handful of *ai hao* [leaves] in five *sheng* of water down to one *sheng* and [let the patient] drink this all at once. [The coin] will be sent down. Qian xiang gong, *Qie zhong fang*.

諸蟲蛇傷。艾灸數壯，甚良。集簡方。

Harm caused by all types of worms/bugs and snakes. Cauterize [the affected region] with *ai* [leaves] several times. Very good. *Ji jian fang*.

風蟲牙痛。化蠟少許，攤紙上，鋪艾，以筯卷成筒，燒烟，隨左右熏鼻，吸烟令滿口，呵氣，即疼止腫消。靳季謙病此月餘，一試即愈。普濟方。

Toothache caused by wind [intrusion] and worms/bugs. Melt a small amount of beeswax and spread it on a piece of paper. Then spread *ai* [leaves] on it and roll it around a chopstick to form a tube. Burn it and steam with the smoke the [left or right] nostril depending on whether [the toothache] is on the left or right side. Fill the mouth with the smoke and then breathe out the qi. This will end the pain and dissolve the swelling. Jin Jiqian suffered from this disease for more a month. He tried this [method] once and was cured. *Pu ji fang*.

15-05-02

實 *Shi*

Fruit [of *ai*]

【氣味】苦、辛，暖，無毒。

Qi and Flavor. Bitter, acrid, warm, nonpoisonous.

【主治】明目，療一切鬼氣。甄權。壯陽，助水臟腰膝及暖子宮。大明。

Control. It brightens the eyes. It heals all types of [diseases related to] demon qi. Zhen Quan. It strengthens the yang [path (i. e. male sexual potency)], assists the water long-term depot (i. e., the kidneys), the lower back, and the knees, and warms the womb. Da Ming.

【發明】【詵曰】艾子和乾薑等分，爲末，蜜丸梧子大。空心每服三十丸，以飯三五匙壓之，日再服。治百惡氣，其鬼神速走出。田野之人，與此甚相宜也。

Explication. [Meng] Shen: [Grind] equal amounts of *ai zi* [leaves] and dried ginger into powder and form with honey pills the size of *wu* seeds. Each time ingest on an empty stomach 30 pills and press them down with three to five spoons of cooked rice, to be ingested twice a day. This serves to cure [diseases related to] the hundreds of malign qi and causes demon spirits to quickly rush out [of the body]. These [pills] are perfectly suited for people [who live/work] in the wild.

【附録】
Appendix

15-05-A01
夏臺 ***Xia tai***
Unidentified.

【别録有名未用曰】味甘，主百疾，濟絶氣。【弘景曰】此藥神奇乃爾，不復識用，可恨也。【時珍曰】艾名冰臺，此名夏臺，艾灸百病能回絶氣，此主百病濟絶氣，恐是一物重出也，故附於艾後。

Bie lu, [section] "known by name but not in use": Flavor sweet. It controls the hundreds of illnesses and is of assistance when the qi [flow is about to be] interrupted. [Tao] Hongjing: This is a uniquely divine pharmaceutical drug, but it is unknown and no longer in use. That is detestable! [Li] Shizhen: *Ai* [leaves] are also called *bing tai* 冰臺, "ice base." This item is called *xia tai* 夏臺, "summer base." Cauterization with *ai* [leaves is recorded] to be "able to bring back an interrupted qi [movement] associated with the hundreds of diseases." This item [is recorded to be able to] "cure the hundreds of diseases and is of assistance when the qi [flow is about to be] interrupted." Maybe this is an identical item that has been recorded twice. Therefore it is added here after the entry *ai* [leaf].

15-06
千年艾綱目
Qian nian ai, FE *Gang mu.*

1000 year old common mugwort.

【集解】【時珍曰】千年艾出武當太和山中。小莖高尺許，其根如蓬蒿，其葉長寸餘，無尖椏，面青背白。秋開黄花，如野菊而小，結實如青珠丹顆之狀。三伏日采葉，暴乾。葉不似艾，而作艾香，搓之即碎，不似艾葉成茸也。羽流以充方物。

Collected Explanations. [Li] Shizhen: 1000 year old common mugwort comes from Mount Tai he shan in Wu dang. It has a small stem of a height of a little more than a *chi*. The root is similar to that of garden daisy [herbs]. Its leaves are a bit longer than a *cun*. They are neither pointed nor forked; they are greenish on the front and white on the back. Yellow flowers open in autumn, resembling winter aster [flowers], but they are smaller. They form fruits shaped like greenish pearls/pellets. The leaves are collected during the three ten-day periods of the hot season; they are dried in the sun. The leaves are not similar to *ai* [leaves], but they have an *ai* [leaf] fragrance. When they are rubbed they turn into small pieces unlike *ai* leaves that turn into fine hair. The Daoists resort to it is a recipe ingredient.

15-06-01
葉 *Ye*
Leaf [of 1000 years old *ai*].

【氣味】辛、微苦，温，無毒。

Qi and Flavor. Acrid, slightly bitter, warm, nonpoisonous.

【主治】男子虛寒，婦人血氣諸痛，水煎服之。時珍。

Control. For depletion cold of males, and for all types of pain of women, related to blood and qi [disorders], boil [the leaves] in water and ingest this. [Li] Shizhen.

15-07
茵蔯蒿本經上品
Yin chen hao, FE *Ben jing*, upper rank.
***Artemisia scoparia* Waldst. et Kit. Virgate wormwood.**

【釋名】【藏器曰】此雖蒿類，經冬不死，更因舊苗而生，故名因陳，後加蒿字耳。【時珍曰】按張揖廣雅及吴普本草並作因塵，不知何義。

Explanation of Names. Although this [item] belongs to the wormwood, *hao* 蒿, group, it does not die throughout winter. Rather, it comes to life again "ensuing from/relying on" (*yin* 因) old seedlings. Hence it was called *yin chen* 因陳, "following from/relying on (*yin* 因) the old (*chen* 陳)." Later, the character *hao* 蒿 was added. [Li] Shizhen: According to Zhang Ji's *Guang ya* and the *Wu Pu ben cao*, it is written *yin chen* 因塵, "ensuing from dust." I have no idea what that could mean.

【集解】【别録曰】茵蔯生太山及丘陵坡岸上，五月及立秋采，陰乾。【弘景曰】今處處有之，似蓬蒿而葉緊細。秋後莖枯，經冬不死，至春又生。【韓保昇曰】葉似青蒿而背白。【大明曰】茵蔯出和州及南山嶺上，一名石茵蔯。【頌曰】近道皆有之，不及太山者佳。春初生苗，高三五寸，似蓬蒿而葉緊細，無花實，五月、七月采莖葉，陰乾，今謂之山茵蔯。江寧府一種茵蔯，葉大根粗，黄白色，至夏有花實。階州一種白蒿，亦似青蒿而背白，本土皆以爲茵蔯入藥。今南方醫人用山茵蔯，乃有數種。或著其説云：山茵蔯，汴京及北地用者，如艾蒿，葉細而背白，其氣亦如艾，味苦，乾則色黑。江南所用者，莖葉都似家茵蔯而大，高三四尺，氣極芬香，味甘辛，俗又名龍腦薄荷。吴中所用，乃石香葇也，葉至細，色黄味辛，甚香烈，性温。若誤作解脾藥服，大令人煩。以本草論之，但有茵蔯蒿，無山茵蔯。註云：葉似蓬蒿而緊細。今汴京北地所用山茵蔯是也。大體世方用山茵蔯療體痛，解傷寒發汗，行肢節滯氣，化痰利膈，治勞倦最要，詳本草正經。惟療黄疸，利小便，與世方都不應。今試取汴京所用山茵蔯爲解肌發汗藥，灼然少效。江南山茵蔯療傷寒腦痛絶勝。比見諸醫議論，謂家茵蔯亦能解肌下隔，去胸中煩。方家少用，但可研作飲服之。本草所無，自出俗方。茵蔯蒿當别是一物，主療自異，不得爲山茵蔯也。此説亦未可據。但以功較之，則江南者爲勝；以經言之，則非本草所出。醫方所用，更當考論爾。【斅曰】凡使須用葉有八角者，陰乾，去根細剉，勿令犯火。【時珍曰】茵蔯昔人多蒔爲蔬，故入藥用山茵蔯，所以别家茵蔯也，洪舜俞老圃賦云酣糟紫薑之掌，沐醯青蔯之絲是也。今淮揚人二月二日猶采野茵蔯苗，和粉麪作茵蔯餅食之。後人各據方土所傳，遂致淆亂。今山茵蔯二月生苗，其莖如艾。其葉如淡色青蒿而背白，葉歧緊細而扁整。九月開細花黄色，結實大如艾子，花實並與菴蕳花實相似，亦有無花實者。

Collected Explanations. *Bie lu*: *Yin chen* grows on Mount Tai shan and on hills and slopes of banks. It is collected in the fifth month and at Autumn Begins (7 August). It is dried in the yin (i. e., shade). [Tao] Hongjing: Today it can be found everywhere. It resembles garden daisy [herbs], but its leaves are hard and fine. After autumn, the stem withers but does not die throughout winter. By spring it comes to life again. Han Baosheng: The leaves are similar to those of wormwood, with a white back. Da Ming: *Yin chen* comes from He zhou and from the Nan shan mountain range. It is also called "rock *yin chen*," *shi yin chen* 石茵蔯. [Su] Song: Nowadays it can be found nearby, but it is not as excellent as that from Mount Tai shan. Early in spring it grows a seedling reaching a height of three to five *cun*. It is similar to that of garden daisy [herbs], but its leaves are hard and fine. It has neither flowers nor fruit. The stem and the leaves are collected in the fifth and seventh month, to be dried in the yin (i. e., shade). Today it is called "mountain *yin chen*," *shan yin chen* 山茵蔯. In Jiang ning fu is a kind of *yin chen* that has big leaves and a coarse root of yellow-white color. By summer it has flowers and fruit. In Jie zhou is a kind of "white wormwood," *bai hao* 白蒿. It, too, is similar to wormwood, but [the leaves] are white on their back. The locals regard all these kinds as *yin chen* and add them to medication. Today, the physicians in the South resort to "mountain *yin chen*," and there are several kinds of it. Some of their sayings are: "The mountain *yin chen* used in the capital and in the North is similar to *ai hao* 艾蒿, common mugwort, with fine leaves that are white on their back. Its qi, too, are similar to those of *ai* [leaves].

The flavor is bitter. When dried, the color changes to black. The kind used in Jiang nan has a stem and leaves resembling 'domestic *yin chen*.' It is three to four *chi* tall. The qi are extremely fragrant, with a sweet-acrid flavor. It has a commonly used alternative name: 'dragon brain mint.' The kind used in Wu Zhong is is Chinese *mosla* herb, *shi xiang rou* 石香葇. Its leaves are extremely fine, the color is yellow, the flavor is acrid, the fragrance is very intense and the nature is warm. If this kind is erroneously ingested as a medication to resolve spleen [disorders], it will let this person massively suffer from vexation." According to the records in the *Ben cao*, there is only a *yin chen hao* 茵蔯蒿, no "mountain *yin chen*," *shan yin chen* 山茵蔯. A comment states: "The leaves are similar to those of garden daisy [herbs], but they are hard and fine." This is the mountain *yin chen* nowadays used in the capital, in the North. In general, mountain *yin chen* is commonly used as a most important [pharmaceutical drug] to heal bodily pain, to resolve harm caused by cold by causing sweating, to stimulate the movement of sluggish qi in the limbs and joints, to transform phlegm and free the passage through the diaphragm, and to cure exhaustion and fatigue, as is described in detail in the main classics of *ben cao* literature. Only [its ability] to heal yellow *dan*-illness/jaundice and to free the passage of urine is not reflected in common recipes. A test was conducted recently using mountain *yin chen* from Bian jing as a pharmaceutical substance to dissolve muscle [disorders] and stimulate sweating. It became obvious that it had only a small effect. The mountain *yin chen* from Jiang nan has shown to be very effective in healing brain pain associated with harm caused by cold. A comparison of the discourses written by all types of physicians [of the past] is to say that "domestic *yin chen* is also able to resolve muscle [disorder], discharge [qi blocking the] diaphragm and remove vexation from within the chest. The recipe experts seldom use it; they only [say that it] can be ground to prepare a beverage for ingestion. This is not recorded in the *ben cao* literature, it has emerged from commonly used recipes. [That is,] *yin chen hao* is something else as it differs in what it controls and heals. It must not be confused with mountain *yin chen*." Such statements, too, have no basis to rely on. If one were to only compare [the various kinds of *yin chen*] in terms of [their therapeutic] potential, that from Jiang nan is superior. But in view of the classics, such [evidence] cannot be taken from the *ben cao* literature. For its application in medical recipes, further research is required. [Lei] Xiao: For all applications [of *yin chen*] use leaves with eight tips. Dry them in the yin (i. e. shade), remove the root and cut [the rest] to fine pieces. They must not be offended by fire. [Li] Shizhen: The ancients often cultivated *yin chen* as a vegetable. Hence, the mountain *yin chen* added to medication is to be distinguished from domestically cultivated *yin chen*. As Hong Shunyu aptly writes in his "Rhapsody of the Elder Gardener":

酣糟紫薑之掌
沐醯青蔯之絲
Palm-with-finger size purple ginger wrapped in distillers' grains.
Silk-thread soft greenish wormwood [leaf] sprayed with vinegar.

Today, people in Huai yang still collect wild *yin chen* seedlings on the 2nd day of the 2nd month to prepare with wheat flour *yin chen* cakes that are eaten. Later people were confused by the sayings of recipe experts. Today, mountain *yin chen* grows a seedling in the second month, with a stem resembling that of common mugwort. The leaves have a pale color like wormwood, and are white on their back. The leaves are forked, firm, fine and flat. [Mountain *yin chen*] opens fine, yellow flowers in the ninth month. They form fruits similar to common mugwort seeds. The flowers and the fruits are similar to the flowers and fruit of keiske *artemisia*. There are some that have neither flowers nor fruit.

15-07-01
莖、葉 *Jing, Ye.*
Stem, leaf [of *yin chen hao*]

【氣味】苦，平、微寒，無毒。【普曰】神農、岐伯、雷公：苦，無毒。黄帝：辛，無毒。【權曰】苦、辛，有小毒。【大明曰】石茵蔯苦，凉，無毒。伏硇砂。【張元素曰】苦、甘，陰中微陽。入足太陽經。

Qi and Flavor. Bitter, acrid, slightly cold, nonpoisonous. [Wu] Pu: Shen nong, Qi Bo, Lei gong: Bitter, nonpoisonous. Huang Di: Acrid, nonpoisonous. [Zhen] Quan: Bitter, acrid, slightly poisonous. Da Ming: Rock *yin chen* is bitter, cool, nonpoisonous. It suppresses [the effects of] sal ammoniac. Zhang Yuansu: Bitter, sweet, a slight yang in yin [substance]. It enters the foot major yang conduits.

【主治】風濕寒熱邪氣，熱結黄疸。久服輕身益氣耐老，面白悦，長年。白兔食之仙。本經。治通身發黄，小便不利，除頭熱，去伏瘕。别録。通關節，去滯熱，傷寒用之。藏器。石茵蔯，治天行時疾熱狂，頭痛頭旋，風眼疼，瘴瘧。女人癥瘕，并閃損乏絶。大明。

Control. Wind, moisture, alternating sensations of cold and heat, evil qi. Heat accumulating to yellow *dan*-illness/jaundice. Ingested over a long time they relieve the body of its weight, boost the qi and let one endure aging. The face remains white and joyful. They extend the years [of life]. White rabbits eating them turn into immortals. *Ben jing*. They serve to cure jaundice covering the entire body and blocked urination. They remove heat from the head and eliminate deeply hidden conglomeration-illness. *Bie lu*. They open the passage through the joints, remove stagnant heat, and are used for harm caused by cold. [Chen] Cangqi. Rock *yin chen* serves to cure heat and madness related to epidemic seasonal qi, headache and vertigo, wind eye[72] pain, miasmatic malaria, concretion-illness and conglomeration-illness[73] of women, and also sprains and injuries with exhaustion and fatigue. Da Ming.

【發明】【弘景曰】仙經云：白蒿，白兔食之仙。而今茵蔯乃云此，恐是誤耳。【宗奭曰】張仲景治傷寒熱甚發黄，身面悉黄者，用之極效。一僧因傷寒後發汗不徹，有留熱，面身皆黄，多熱，期年不愈。醫作食黄治不對而食不減。予與此藥，服五日病減三分之一，十日減三分之二，二十日病悉去。方用山茵蔯、山梔子各三分，秦艽、升麻各四錢，爲散。每用三錢，水四合，煎二合，去滓，食後温服，以知爲度。此藥以山茵蔯爲本，故書之。【王好古曰】張仲景茵蔯巵子大黄湯，治濕熱也。巵子蘗皮湯，治燥熱也。如苗澇則濕黄，苗旱則燥黄。濕則瀉之，燥則潤之可也。此二藥治陽黄也。韓祗和、李思訓治陰黄，用茵蔯附子湯。大抵以茵蔯爲君主，而佐以大黄、附子，各隨其寒熱也。

Explication. [Tao] Hongjing: The classics of the hermits/immortals state: "White wormwood, when white rabbits eat it they turn into immortals." If this were said of the *yin chen* available today, it might be mistaken. [Kou] Zongshi: Zhang Zhongjing uses it as an extremely effective [medication] to cure harm caused by cold with extreme heat and an effusion of yellow, with the body and the head all turning yellow. Once a monk was given [medication] to stimulate sweating in the aftermath of harm caused by cold. [The sweating] failed to penetrate [the exterior of the body] and the heat remained [in the body]. His face and body were all yellow, and there was much heat. For an entire year he was not cured. A physician considered this to be "jaundice caused by food," but his therapy was incorrect and his food was not reduced. I gave him this pharmaceutical drug. He ingested it for five days, and the disease had subsided by a third. After ten days it had subsided by two thirds. After 20 days it was all gone. My recipe [was as follows. Grind] three *fen* of mountain *yin chen* and mountain *gardenia* [fruit], with four *qian* each of large *gentiana* [root] and *cimicifuga* [rhizome] into powder. Each time boil three *qian* in four *ge* of water down to two *ge*, remove the dregs and ingest [the liquid] warm after a meal until an effect shows. This medication is based on mountain *yin chen*. Therefore it is recorded here. Wang Haogu: Zhang Zhongjing's "decoction with *yin chen*, *gardenia* [fruit] and rhubarb root" serves to cure moisture and heat. The "decoction with *gardenia*

72 *Feng yan* 風眼, "wind eye," a condition of red and festering canthi and eyelids brought about by harm caused to the eyes by heat. BCGM Dict I, 171.

73 *Zheng jia* 癥瘕, "concretion-illness and conglomeration-illness." The two terms are often used interchangeably and do not signify two distinctly different conditions. Concretion-illness and conglomeration-illness result from a disharmony of cold and warmth resulting in a failure to transform beverages and food. Nodes form when the clash with the qi of the long-term depots. BCGM Dict I, 677.

[fruit] and *phellodendron* bark" serves to cure dryness with heat. When the seedling is moist, [it is good for] moisture jaundice. When the seedling is dry, [it is good for] dryness jaundice. That is, one is able to drain in the case of moisture and the other to moisten in the case of dryness. Both these two pharmaceutical drugs serve to cure yang-type jaundice. When Han Dihe and Li Sixun cured yin-type jaundice, they used the "decoction with *yin chen* and *aconitum* [accessory tuber]." In general, *yin chen* is resorted to [in a recipe] as ruler, assisted by rhubarb root and *aconitum* [accessory tuber] – always in accordance with the respective presence of cold and heat.

【附方】舊二，新六。

Added Recipes. Two of old. Six newly [recorded].

茵陳羹。除大熱黄疸，傷寒頭痛，風熱瘴瘧，利小便。以茵陳細切，煮羹食之。生食亦宜。食醫心鏡。

Thick soup with *yin chen*. It removes yellow *dan*-illness/jaundice with massive heat, headache related to harm caused by cold, and miasmatic malaria related to wind [intrusion] and heat. It clears the passage of urine. Cut *yin chen* to fine pieces, boil them in water to a thick soup and eat it. It is also suitable to be eaten raw. *Shi yi xin jing*.

遍身風痒，生瘡疥。用茵陳煮濃汁，洗之立瘥。千金方。

The entire body is affected by wind itch, with the development of sores and *jie*-illness.[74] Boil *yin chen* in water to obtain a thick juice. Wash [the affected region] with it and [the itch] is cured immediately. *Qian jin fang*.

癧瘍風病。茵陳蒿兩握，水一斗五升，煮取七升。先以皂莢湯洗，次以此湯洗之，冷更作。隔日一洗，不然恐痛也。崔行功纂要。

Pervasion-illness with ulcer wind[75] disease. Boil two handful of *yin chen hao* in one *dou* and five *sheng* of water down to seven *sheng*. First wash [the affected region] with a *gleditsia* pod/seed decoction. Then wash it with the decoction described here. When it has become cold, make it [warm] again. Wash every other day. Otherwise there might be pain. Cui Xinggong, *Zuan yao*.

風疾攣急。茵陳蒿一斤，秫米一石，麴三斤，和匀，如常法釀酒，服之。聖濟總録。

74 *Jie*-illness 疥, vaguely identifiable skin ailment. BCGM Dict I, 249.

75 *Li yang feng* 癧瘍風, "pervasion-illness with ulcer wind." When someone has macules with interconnected dots at the sides of the neck,on the chest, and in the armpits, that appear to have come by themselves, are white and round, occasionally black, and neither itch nor ache, this is called pervasion-illness with ulcer wind."

A wind illness with contraction and tension. Mix one *jin* of *yin chen hao*, one *dan* of glutinous millet, and three *jin* of yeast and brew this to wine according to the usual method. Ingest [the wine]. *Sheng ji zong lu.*

癇黄如金，好眠吐涎。茵陳蒿、白鮮皮等分，水二鍾，煎服，日二服。三十六黄方。

Epilepsy with a yellow color similar to gold. [Patients] are sleepy and spit saliva. Boil equal amounts of *yin chen hao* and *dictamnus* [root] bark in two *zhong* of water and ingest this. To be ingested twice a day. *San shi liu huang fang.*

遍身黄疸。茵陳蒿一把，同生薑一塊，擣爛，於胸前四肢，日日擦之。

Yellow *dan*-illness/jaundice affecting the entire body. Pound a handful of *yin chen hao* together with one piece of fresh ginger to a paste and rub it on the [patient's] chest and four limbs every day.

男子酒疸。用茵陳蒿四根，梔子七箇，大田螺一箇，連殼擣爛，以百沸白酒一大盞，冲汁飲之。秘方也。

Dan-illness/jaundice of males caused by wine. Pound four *yin chen hao* roots, seven *gardenia* fruits and one large river snail, with its shell, to a paste to be boiled one hundred times to bubbling in one large bowl of white wine. Pour the juice off and drink it. A secret recipe.

眼熱赤腫。山茵陳、車前子等分，煎湯，調茶調散，服數服。直指方。

Hot, red and swollen eyes. Boil equal amounts of mountain *yin chen* and Asiatic plantain seeds in water and several times ingest [the liquid] mixed with the "powder mixed with tea."[76] *Zhi zhi fang.*

15-08
青蒿本經下品
Qing hao, FE *Ben jing*, lower rank.
Artemisia carvifolia Buch.-Ham.ex Roxb. Wormwood.

【釋名】草蒿本經、方潰本經、菣音牽去聲、犱蒿蜀本、香蒿衍義。【保昇曰】草蒿，江東人呼爲犱蒿，爲其氣臭似犱也。北人呼爲青蒿。爾雅云：蒿，菣也。孫炎注云"荆楚之間，謂蒿爲菣"，郭璞注云"今人呼青蒿，香中炙啖者爲菣"，是也。【時珍曰】晏子云：蒿，草之高者也。按

76 *Cha tiao san* 茶調散, "the powder mixed with tea," is prepared with the following ingredients: *Ligusticum* root, *saposhnikovia* root, *notopterygium* root, *glycyrrhiza* root, scouring rush, gypsum, *schizonepeta* herb, *chrysanthemum* flowers and mint.

爾雅諸蒿，獨菣得單稱爲蒿，豈以諸蒿葉背皆白，而此蒿獨青，異於諸蒿故耶？

Explanation of Names. *Cao hao* 草蒿, *Ben jing*. *Fang kui* 方潰, *Ben jing*. *Qian* 菣, read *qian* with falling tone, *xun hao* 犼蒿, *Shu ben*. *Xiang hao* 香蒿, *Yan yi*. [Han] Baosheng: *Cao hao* 草蒿 is called *xun hao* 犼蒿 by Jiang dong people because its qi are as malodorous as those of the *xun* 犼 animal.[77] The people in the North call it *qing hao* 青蒿, "greenish *hao*." The *Er ya* states: "*Hao* 蒿 is *qian* 菣." Sun Yan in his comment states: "In the Jing chu region, *hao* 蒿 is called *qian* 菣." Guo Pu in his comment states: "Today, the people call it *qing hao* 青蒿; those that are fragrant [vegetables] and are eaten after being roasted, they are *qian* 菣." That is correct. [Li] Shizhen: Master Yan [Ying] states: "*Hao* 蒿 are tall, *gao* 高, herbs, *cao* 草." According to the *Er ya*, of all the *hao* 蒿, only *qian* 菣 is simply called *hao* 蒿. As the leaves of all *hao* 蒿 have a white back, and this *hao* 蒿 is the only one with a greenish, *qing* 青, [back of leaves], maybe this is the reason why it is held to differ from all the other *hao* 蒿.

【集解】【別録曰】草蒿生華陰川澤。【弘景曰】處處有之，即今青蒿，人亦取雜香菜食之。【保昇曰】嫩時醋淹爲菹，自然香。葉似茵蔯蒿而背不白，高四尺許。四月、五月采，日乾入藥。詩云呦呦鹿鳴，食野之蒿，即此蒿也。【頌曰】青蒿春生苗，葉極細，可食。至夏高四五尺。秋後開細淡黄花，花下便結子如粟米大，八九月采子，陰乾。根、莖、子、葉並入藥用，乾者炙作飲，香尤佳。【宗奭曰】青蒿得春最早，人剔以爲蔬，根赤葉香。沈括夢溪筆談云：青蒿一類，自有二種。一種黄色，一種青色。本草謂之青蒿，亦有所别也。陝西銀綏之間，蒿叢中時有一兩窠，迥然青色者，土人謂之香蒿。莖葉與常蒿一同，但常蒿色淡青，此蒿深青，如松檜之色。至深秋餘蒿並黄，此蒿猶青，其氣芬芳。恐古人所用，以深青者爲勝。不然，諸蒿何嘗不青？【時珍曰】青蒿二月生苗，莖粗如指而肥軟，莖葉色並深青。其葉微似茵蔯而面背俱青。其根白硬。七八月開細黄花頗香。結實大如麻子，中有細子。

Collected Explanations. *Bie lu*: *Cao hao* grows in the river marshlands of Hua yin. [Tao] Hongjing: It can be found everywhere. It is today's *qing hao*. The people eat it mixed with sweet basil. [Han] Baosheng: As long as it is tender it is soaked in vinegar to prepare a pickled vegetable. It is naturally fragrant. The leaves are similar to those of *artemisia scoparia*, but their back is not white. The plant reaches a height of more than four *chi*. It is collected in the fourth and fifth month to be dried in the sun and added to medication. The *Shi* states "the sound of roaring deer; they eat the

77 *Xun* 犼, an unidentified leopard-cat like animal. BCGM 53-23: *Xun* 犼, read *xun* 迅

hao 蒿 of the wild."[78] That is the *hao* 蒿 discussed here. [Su] Song: *Qing hao* grows a seedling in spring. The leaves are extremely fine and edible. By summer it reaches a height of four to five *chi*. After autumn it opens fine flowers of a pale yellow color. Underneath the flowers fruits form the size of glutinous millet. The seeds are collected in the eighth and ninth month. They are dried in the yin (i. e., shade). The root, the stem, the seeds and the leaves alike are used added to medication. When they are dry they are roasted to be prepared for a beverage, with particularly fine fragrance. [Kou] Zongshi: When *qing hao* is obtained very early in spring, people clean it to prepare it as a vegetable. The root is red and the leaves are fragrant. Shen Gua in his *Meng xi bi tan* states: "The *qing hao* group comprises two kinds. One is of yellow color; the other is of greenish color. The *Ben cao* calls it *qing hao* to distinguish them. In the region of Yin and Sui in Shaan xi, clusters of *hao* occasionally include one or two nests of a conspicuous greenish color. The *Ben cao* names them 'greenish *hao*.' The stem and the leaves are identical to those of common *hao*, but while the color of common *hao* is pale greenish, this type of *hao* is deep greenish, similar to the color of pines and Chinese junipers. In late autumn all the other *hao* are yellow while this *hao* remains greenish with fragrant qi. Maybe the ancients considered [*hao*] of deep greenish [color] as superior. If this were not the case, why would not all types of *hao* be [considered to be] greenish?" [Li] Shizhen: *Qing hao* grows a seedling in the second month. The stem is coarse like a finger, fat and soft. Stem and leaves alike are of deep greenish [color]. The leaves are quite similar to those of *artemisia scoparia*, except that [their leaves] are greenish on the front and on the back. The root is white and hard. In the seventh and eighth month it opens fine, yellow flowers that are quite fragrant. They form fruits the size of sesame seeds with fine seeds inside.

【脩治】【斅曰】凡使，惟中爲妙，到膝即仰，到腰即俛。使子勿使葉，使根勿使莖，四件若同使，翻然成痼疾。采得葉，用七歲兒七箇溺，浸七日七夜，漉出晒乾。

Pharmaceutical Preparation: [Lei] Xiao: For all applications, only those of medium [height] are wondrous. When they reach knee [high], they look up; once they reach the lower back, they look down. If the seeds are to be used [for therapeutic purposes], do not use the leaves. If the root is to be used, do not use the stem. If all four parts are used together, they will, contrary to one's expectation, cause an obstinacy-illness ailment. When the leaves are collected, seven pees of seven year old boys are used to soak them for seven days and seven nights. Then [the liquid] is filtered off, and [the herbal drug] is dried in the sun.

78 *Shi jing*, part II, Xiao ya 小雅, Book I, Ode I: *lu ming* 鹿鳴. The original text reads 呦呦鹿鳴，食野之苹, with *ping* 苹 instead of *hao* 蒿. See below 15-10, Explication.

15-08-01
葉、莖、根、子 *Ye, Jing, Gen, Zi*
Leaf, stem, root, seed [of *qing hao*].

【氣味】苦，寒，無毒。【時珍曰】伏硫黄。

Flavor: Bitter, cold, nonpoisonous. [Li] Shizhen: They suppress the effects of sulphur.

【主治】疥瘙痂痒，惡瘡，殺蝨，治留熱在骨節間，明目。本經。鬼氣尸疰伏連，婦人血氣，腹内滿及冷熱久痢。秋冬用子，春夏用苗，並擣汁服。亦暴乾爲末，小便入酒和服。藏器。補中益氣，輕身補勞，駐顏色，長毛髮，令黑不老，兼去蒜髮，殺風毒。心痛熱黄，生擣汁服并貼之。大明。治瘧疾寒熱。時珍。生擣傅金瘡，止血止疼，良。蘇恭。燒灰隔紙淋汁，和石灰煎，治惡瘡，瘜肉黡瘢。孟詵。

Control: *Jie*-illness[79] with itch; crusts with itch. Malign sores. They kill lice. They serve to cure abiding heat in the bones and joints, and they brighten the eyes. *Ben jing*. Demon qi, corpse [qi] attachment illness,[80] hidden link.[81] Blood and qi [disorder] of women. A feeling of abdominal fullness and long-lasting free-flux illness related to cold and heat. In autumn and winter use the seeds. In spring and summer use the seedling. Pound them all alike to obtain a juice and ingest it. It is also possible to dry them in the sun, [grind them into] powder and ingest it with wine to which urine is added. [Chen] Cangqi. They supplement the center and boost the qi; they relieve the body of its weight, supplement exhaustion, maintain [a youthful] complexion, stimulate the growth of hair, keep it black and prevent aging. At the same time, they remove gray hair[82] and kill wind poison.[83] For heart pain with heat and jaundice, pound them fresh and ingest the resulting juice; it is also applied externally [to the affected region]. Da Ming. It serves to cure malaria illness with alternating cold and heat sensations. [Li] Shizhen. Pounded fresh they are applied to wounds caused by metal objects/weapons to end bleeding and to end pain. Good. Su Gong. Burn them to ashes, place [the ashes] on paper, let water trickle through [the ashes and the paper] and boil the resulting juice with lime. [The resulting liq-

79 *Jie*-illness 疥, vaguely identifiable skin ailment. BCGM Dict I, 249.

80 *Shi zhu* 尸疰, "corpse [qi] attachment-illness," a condition of a slowly developing infectious weakness. BCGM Dict I, 202.

81 *Fu lian* 伏連, "hidden link." BCGM Dict I, 175.

82 *Suan fa* 蒜髮, lit.: "garlic hair." BCGM Dict I, 481.

83 *Feng du* 風毒, "wind poison," a condition caused by *feng* 風, "wind," and *du* 毒, "poison," resulting in a pathogenic evil qi including the characteristics of both. BCGM Dict I, 160.

uid] serves to cure malign sores, tumorous flesh-growth and dermal black spots and wounds. Meng Shen.

【發明】【頌曰】青蒿治骨蒸熱勞爲最，古方單用之。【時珍曰】青蒿得春木少陽之氣最早，故所主之證，皆少陽、厥陰血分之病也。按月令通纂言：伏内庚日，采青蒿懸於門庭内，可辟邪氣。陰乾爲末，冬至、元旦各服二錢亦良。觀此，則青蒿之治鬼疰伏尸，蓋亦有所伏也。

Explication. [Su] Song: *Qing hao* is the best [pharmaceutical drug] to cure bone steaming[84] with heat and exhaustion. In ancient recipes it is used as a single substance. [Li] Shizhen: *Qing hao* is the very first in the year endowed with the minor yang qi of spring and [the phase] wood. Therefore, all the illness signs it controls are associated with diseases of the blood section of the minor yang and ceasing yin [conduits]. According to the *Yue ling tong zuan*, "to suppress [attacks of evil qi in] the interior, on every second day collect *qing hao* and hang it inside the gate to the front yard. This will repel evil qi. Dry it in the yin (i. e. shade), [grind it into] powder and on the day of Winter Solstice and the first day of the year ingest two *qian*. This is good, too." In view of this, *qing hao* not only serves to cure demon attachment-illness[85] and suppress corpse[-qi transmission].[86] The fact is, there is more that it can suppress.

【附方】舊四，新十三。

Added Recipes. Four of old. 13 newly [recorded].

男婦勞瘦。青蒿細剉，水三升，童子小便五升，同煎取一升半。去滓入器中煎成膏，丸如梧子大。每空心及卧時，温酒吞下二十丸。斗門方。

Males and women with exhaustion and emaciation. Cut *qing hao* into fine pieces and boil it in a mixture of three *sheng* of water and five *sheng* of boys's urine down to one and a half *sheng*. Remove the dregs, give [the liquid] into another vessel and boil it again until it turns into a paste, and form this to pills the size of *wu* seeds. Each time swallow on an empty stomach prior to going to bed 20 pills with warm wine. *Dou men fang*.

84 *Gu zheng* 骨蒸, "bone steaming," 1.) a condition of an infectious consumptive disease with a development of vexing heat in the afternoon. 2.) An illness sign of heat and vexation with a feeling as if this originated in the bones. BCGM Dict I, 197.

85 *Zhu* 疰, also *zhu* 注, "attachment-illness," "influx-illnesss," reflects a notion of a foreign pathogenic agent, originally of demonic nature, having attached itself to the human organism. BCGM Dict I, 688-695.

86 For the relationship between "demon attachment-illness" and "corpse-qi transmission" see BCGM Dict I, 202/203.

虛勞寒熱，肢體倦疼，不拘男婦。八九月青蒿成實時采之，去枝梗，以童子小便浸三日，晒乾爲末。每服二錢，烏梅一箇，煎湯服。靈苑方。

Depletion exhaustion with alternating feelings of cold and heat. The limbs and the body are fatigued and ache, regardless of whether this affects males or women. When in the eighth and ninth month *qing hao* forms fruit, collect [the herb], remove the branches and the stem and soak [the rest] in boys's urine for three days. Then dry it in the sun and [grind it into] powder. Each time ingest two *qian*. Boil this with one smoked plum in water and ingest the decoction. *Ling yuan fang*.

骨蒸鬼氣。童子小便五大斗澄清，青蒿五斗，八九月揀帶子者最好，細剉相和，納大釜中，以猛火煎取三大斗，去滓，溉釜令净，再以微火煎可二大斗，入豬膽十枚，同煎一大斗半，去火待冷，以瓷器盛之。每欲服時，取甘草二三兩，炙熟爲末，以煎和擣千杵爲丸。空腹粥飲下二十丸，漸增至三十丸止。崔元亮海上方。

Bone steaming[87] and demon qi. Give five generous *dou* of boys' urine, left for a while until it has become clear, and five *dou* of *qing hao*, best picked in the eighth and ninth month when it has just begun to have seeds and cut into fine pieces, into a large cauldron and boil it with a strong fire down to three generous *dou*. Remove the dregs, rinse the cauldron until it is clean and with a mild fire boil [the liquid] down to two generous *dou*. Then add ten gallbladders of pigs and boil this down to one and a half generous *dou*. Remove the fire, wait until [the liquid] has cooled and fill it into a porcelain vessel. When it is to be ingested, roast two to three *liang* of *glycyrrhiza* [roots] until done and [grind them into] powder. Mix it with [the liquid in the porcelain vessel], boil [it to a paste], pound it with a pestle a thousand times and form pills. Each time send down on an empty stomach 20 pills with a congee or with a beverage. Gradually increase the dose to 30 pills, and [the disease will] end. Cui Yuanliang, *Hai shang fang*.

骨蒸煩熱。青蒿一握，豬膽汁一枚，杏仁四十箇，去皮尖炒，以童子小便一大盞，煎五分，空心温服。十便良方。

Bone steaming[88] with vexing heat. Boil one handful of *qing hao*, the bile of one pig gallbladder and 40 almond kernels, stir fried with the skin and the tips removed, in one large cup of boys' urine down to 50%, and ingest this warm on an empty stomach. *Shi bian liang fang*.

87 *Gu zheng* 骨蒸, "bone steaming," 1.) a condition of an infectious consumptive disease with a development of vexing heat in the afternoon. 2.) An illness sign of heat and vexation with a feeling as if this originated in the bones. BCGM Dict I, 197.

88 *Gu zheng* 骨蒸, "bone steaming," 1.) a condition of an infectious consumptive disease with a development of vexing heat in the afternoon. 2.) An illness sign of heat and vexation with a feeling as if this originated in the bones. BCGM Dict I, 197.

虛勞盜汗，煩熱口乾。用青蒿一斤，取汁熬膏，入人參末、麥門冬末各一兩，熬至可丸，丸如梧子大，每食後米飲服二十丸，名青蒿煎。聖濟總録。

Depletion exhaustion with robber sweating.[89] Vexing heat and dry mouth. Press the juice out of one *jin* of *qing hao* and heat it until it has turned into a paste. Add one *liang* each of ginseng [root] and *ophiopogon* [tuber] and heat this until it can be formed to pills the size of *wu* seeds. Each time ingest after a meal 20 pills with a rice beverage. [This medication] is called "*qing hao* brew." *Sheng ji zong lu*.

瘧疾寒熱。肘後方用青蒿一握，水二升，擣汁服之。

Malaria illness with alternating sensations of cold and heat. The *Zhou hou fang* [recommends to] pound one handful of *qing hao* in two *sheng* of water and ingest the resulting juice.

仁存方用五月五日天未明時采青蒿陰乾四兩，桂心一兩，爲末。未發前，酒服二錢。

The *Ren cun fang* [recommends to] collect on the fifth day of the fifth month before dawn *qing hao*, dry it in the yin (i. e., shade) and [grind] four *liang* together with one *liang* of shaved cinnamom bark into powder. Prior to an outbreak ingest with wine two *qian*.

經驗方用端午日采青蒿葉陰乾，桂心等分，爲末。每服一錢，先寒用熱酒，先熱用冷酒，發日五更服之。切忌發物。

The *Jing yan fang* [recommends to] grind equal amounts of *qing hao* leaves, collected on the fifth day of the fifth month and dried in the yin (i. e., shade), and shaved cinnamom bark into powder. Each time ingest one *qian*. If a cold sensation comes first, [ingest it] with hot wine. If a heat sensation comes first, [ingest it] with cold wine. Ingest it on the day of an outbreak in the early morning. Avoid all [food] stimulating [qi] effusion.

温瘧痰甚，但熱不寒。用青蒿二兩，童子小便浸焙，黄丹半兩，爲末。每服二錢，白湯調下。仁存方。

Warmth malaria with extreme phlegm and a sensation of heat only, and without a sensation of cold. [Grind] two *liang* of *qing hao*, soaked in boys' urine and dried over a fire in a pan, and half a *liang* of minium into powder. Each time ingest two *qian*, to be sent down mixed with clear, boiled water. *Ren cun fang*.

---

89 *Dao han* 盜汗, "robber sweating," (1) an illness sign of a profuse sweating during sleep that ends when one wakes up. (2) A pathological condition with robber sweating as major sign. BCGM Dict I, 122.

赤白痢下。五月五日采青蒿、艾葉等分，同豆豉擣作餅，日乾，名蒿豉丹。每用一餅，以水一盞半煎服。聖濟總録。

Red and white free-flux illness discharge. On the fifth day of the fifth month collect equal amounts of *qing hao* and mugwort leaves and pound them together with fermented soy beans to prepare a cake. Dry it in the sun. It is called "[*qing*] *hao* and fermented [beans] elixir." Each time use one cake, boil it in one and a half cups of water and ingest [the liquid]. *Sheng ji zong lu.*

鼻中衄血。青蒿擣汁服之，并塞鼻中，極驗。衛生易簡方。

Nosebleed. Pound *qing hao* and ingest the resulting juice. In addition, stuff it into the nose. Extremely successful. *Wei sheng yi jian fang.*

酒痔便血。青蒿用葉不用莖，用莖不用葉，爲末。糞前冷水、糞後水酒調服。永類鈐方。

Piles caused by wine [drinking] and [defecation/urination] relief with blood. Grind *qing hao* – if the leaves are to be used, do not use the stem; if the stem is to be used, do not use the leaves – into powder. Prior to defecation ingest it mixed with cold water, after defecation mixed with water and wine. *Yong lei qian fang.*

金瘡撲損。肘後方用青蒿擣封之，血止則愈。

Wounds caused by metal objects, injuries resulting from a blow. The *Zhou hou fang* [recommends to] pound *qing hao* [to a pulp] and seal [the affected region]. Once the bleeding ends, a cure is achieved.

一方：用青蒿、麻葉、石灰等分，五月五日擣和晒乾。臨時爲末，搽之。

Another recipe. On the fifth day of the fifth month pound equal amounts of *qing hao*, hemp leaves and lime and dry them in the sun. When needed [grind them into] powder and apply it [to the affected region].

牙齒腫痛。青蒿一握，煎水漱之。濟急方。

Painful swelling of teeth. Boil a handful of *qing hao* in water and rinse [the affected region]. *Ji ji fang.*

毒蜂螫人。嚼青蒿封之即安。肘後方。

A poisonous bee/wasp has stung a person. Chew *qing hao* and seal [the affected region with the paste]. This will take care of it. *Zhou hou fang.*

耳出濃汁。青蒿末，綿裹納耳中。聖惠方。

Purulent fluid comes out of an ear. Wrap *qing hao* powder in silk and stuff it into the ear. *Sheng hui fang.*

鼻中息肉。青蒿灰、石灰等分，淋汁熬膏點之。聖濟總録。

Tumorous flesh growth in the nose. Trickle water through equal amounts of *qing hao* ashes and lime, boil the resulting juice to a paste and drip it [into the affected region]. *Sheng ji zong lu.*

15-08-02
子 ***Zi***
Seeds [of *qing hao*].

【氣味】甘，冷，無毒。

Qi and Flavor. Sweet, cold, nonpoisonous.

【主治】明目開胃，炒用。治勞瘦、壯健人小便浸用之。治惡瘡疥癬風瘮，煎水洗之。大明。治鬼氣，爲末酒服方寸匕。孟詵。功同葉。時珍。

Control. To brighten the eyes and open the stomach, use them stir fried. To cure exhaustion and emaciation and to strengthen a person, use them soaked in urine. To cure malign sores, *jie*-illness[90] and *xuan*-illness[91] and wind papules,[92] boil them in water and wash [the affected region]. Da Ming. To cure demon qi, [grind them into] powder and ingest with wine the amount held by a square *cun* spoon. Meng Shen. The [therapeutic] potential is identical to that of the leaves. [Li] Shizhen.

【附方】新一。

Added Recipes. One newly [recorded].

積熱眼澀。三月三日或五月五日，采青蒿花或子，陰乾爲末，每井華水空心服二錢。久服明目，可夜看書，名青蒿散。十便良方。

Rough eyes with accumulated heat. On the third day of the third month, or on the fifth day of the fifth month, collect *qing hao* flowers or seeds, dry them in the yin (i. e., shade) and [grind them into] powder. Each time ingest with well splendor

---

90 *Jie*-illness 疥, vaguely identifiable skin ailment. BCGM Dict I, 249.

91 *Xuan* 癬, "*xuan*-illness." Conditions of dermal lesions with initially erythema, papules, and itching gradually extending in all directions to form an irregular ring with clear boundaries. The skin is slightly elevated with small papules, blisters, and/or scales and scraps. The central lesion may appear to heal spontaneously, and it may reappear. Also, a designation of local lesions with itching, release of liquid and shedding of scabs. BCGM Dict I, 591.

92 *Feng zhen* 風瘮, "wind papules," a condition, brought forth by wind evil, of eruptive skin papules of different sizes, accompanied by unbearable itching. If scratched they rise further. BCGM Dict I, 172.

water[93] two *qian* on an empty stomach. Ingested over a long time, it brightens the eyes enabling one to read books at night. [This recipe] is called "*qing hao* powder." *Shi bian liang fang*.

15-08-03
節間蟲 *Jie jian chong*
Grubs in the nodes [of *qing hao*].

見蟲部。

See the "worms/bugs" section. (41-13)

15-09
黃花蒿綱目
Huang hua hao, FE *Gang mu*

***Artemisia annua* L. Yellow flower wormwood.**

【釋名】臭蒿。

Explanation of Names. *Chou hao* 臭蒿, "malodorous *hao*.

【集解】【大明曰】臭蒿一名草蒿。【時珍曰】香蒿、臭蒿，通可名草蒿。此蒿與青蒿相似，但此蒿色綠帶淡黃，氣辛臭不可食，人家采以罨醬黃、酒麴者是也。

Collected Explanations. Da Ming: "Malodorous *hao*" is also called *cao hao* 草蒿, "herbal *hao*." [Li] Shizhen: "Fragrant *hao*" and "malodorous *hao*" can both be named "herbal *hao*." This kind of hao is similar to "greenish hao," *qing hao* 青蒿. However, the present *hao's* green color includes some pale yellow. It qi are acrid and malodorous; it is not edible. It is collected by people to promote the growth of yellow *jiang* ferment/moulded beans,[94] and wine ferments.

15-09-01
葉 *Ye*
Leaf [of *huang hua hao*].

【氣味】辛、苦，涼，無毒。

Qi and Flavor. Acrid, bitter, cool, nonpoisonous.

---

93 *Jing hua shui* 井華水, "well splendor water," i. e., the first water drawn from a well in the morning. BCGM Vol. II, 05-15-01.

94 For details of the role of *artemisia annua* in the preparation of ferments, see Joseph Needham, *Science and Civilization in China*. Vol. 6, Biology and Biological Technology. Part V: Fermentation and Food Science, by H. T. Huang. Cambridge, 2000, 347 – 349. F. Porter Smith, *Chinese Materia Medica*. Vegetable Kingdom. Shanghai 1911, 191 – 192.

【主治】小兒風寒驚熱。時珍。

Control. Fright heat of children related to wind and cold [intrusion]. [Li] Shizhen.

15-09-02

子 *Zi*

Seeds [of *huang hua hao*].

【氣味】辛，涼，無毒。

Qi and Flavor. Acrid, cool, nonpoisonous.

【主治】治勞，下氣開胃，止盜汗及邪氣鬼毒。大明。

Control. It serves to cure exhaustion, discharges qi and opens the stomach. It ends robber sweating,[95] and [dispels] evil qi and demon poison. Da Ming.

15-10

白蒿本經上品

***Bai hao*, FE *Ben jing*, upper rank.**

***Artemisia sieversiana* Ehrhart ex Willd. Sievers wormwood.**[96]

【釋名】蘩爾雅、由胡爾雅、蔞蒿食療、蔏音商。【時珍曰】白蒿有水陸二種，爾雅通謂之蘩，以其易蘩衍也。曰蘩，皤蒿，即今陸生艾蒿也，辛薰不美。曰蘩，由胡，即今水生蔞蒿也，辛香而美。曰蘩之醜，秋爲蒿，則通指水陸二種而言，謂其春時各有種名，至秋老則皆呼爲蒿矣。曰籟，曰蕭，曰萩，皆老蒿之通名，象秋氣肅賴之氣。

Explanation of Names. *Fan* 蘩, *Er ya*. *You hu* 由胡, *Er ya*. *Lou hao* 蔞蒿, *Shi liao*. *Shang* 蔏, read *shang* 商. [Li] Shizhen: There are two kinds of *bai hao*. One "water" [*bai hao*] and one "land" [*bai hao*]. The *Er ya* calls both of them *fan* 蘩, because they multiply, *fan yan* 蘩衍, easily. When it is said "*fan* 蘩 is *po hao* 皤蒿," then this is today's *ai hao* 艾蒿, common mugwort, growing on land. It is acrid and has a bad smell. When it is said "*Fan* 蘩 is *you hu* 由胡," then this is today's *lou hao* 蔞蒿, growing in waters. It is acrid and has a nice fragrance. When it is said "The unsightly kind of *fan* 蘩 turning into *hao* 蒿 in autumn," then this is a reference to both the water and the land kinds. That is, in spring they have individually descriptive names, and by autumn, when they turn old, they all alike are called *hao* 蒿. *Lai* 籟, *xiao* 蕭 and *qiu* 萩 are designations of old *hao* 蒿. They reflect the solemn, *su* 肅, and trustworthy, *lai* 賴, qi of autumn, *qiu* 秋.

95 *Dao han* 盜汗, "robber sweating," (1) an illness sign of a profuse sweating during sleep that ends when one wakes up. (2) A pathological condition with robber sweating as major sign. BCGM Dict I, 122.

96 *Bai hao* 白蒿, lit.: "white *hao*."

【集解】【别録曰】白蒿生中山川澤，二月采。【弘景曰】蒿類甚多，而俗中不聞呼白蒿者。方藥家既不用，皆無復識之。【恭曰】爾雅皤蒿，即白蒿也，所在有之。葉頗似細艾，上有白毛錯澀，粗於青蒿。從初生至秋，白於衆蒿。【禹錫曰】蓬蒿可以爲茹。故詩箋云，以豆薦蘩菹也。陸機詩疏云：凡艾白色爲皤蒿。今白蒿先諸草發生，香美可食，生蒸皆宜。【頌曰】此草古人以爲菹。今人但食蔞蒿，不復食此。或疑白蒿即蔞蒿，而孟詵食療又別著蔞蒿條，所說不同，明是二物，乃知古今食品之異也。又今階州以白蒿爲茵蔯，其苗葉亦相似，然以入藥，恐不可用也。【時珍曰】白蒿處處有之，有水陸二種。本草所用，蓋取水生者，故曰生中山川澤，不曰山谷平地也。二種形狀相似，但陸生辛薰，不及水生者香美爾。詩云：呦呦鹿鳴，食野之苹。苹即陸生皤蒿，俗呼艾蒿是矣。鹿食九種解毒之草，白蒿其一也。詩云："于以采蘩，于沼于沚。"左傳云：蘋蘩蘊藻之菜，可以薦於鬼神，羞於王公。並指水生白蒿而言，則本草白蒿之爲蔞蒿無疑矣。鄭樵通志謂苹爲蔞蒿，非矣。鹿乃山獸，蔞乃水蒿。陸機詩疏謂苹爲牛尾蒿，亦非矣。牛尾蒿色青不白，細葉直上，狀如牛尾也。蔞蒿生陂澤中，二月發苗，葉似嫩艾而歧細，面青背白。其莖或赤或白，其根白脆。采其根莖，生熟菹曝皆可食，蓋嘉蔬也。景差大招云：吴酸蒿蔞不沾薄。謂吴人善調酸，瀹蔞蒿爲齏，不沾不薄而甘美，此正指水生者也。

Collected Explanations. *Bie lu*: *Bai hao* grows in the river marshlands of Mount Zhong shan. It is collected in the second month. [Tao] Hongjing: There are very many kinds of *hao* 蒿. But *bai hao* is not commonly spoken of. The experts of pharmaceutical recipes do not use it; they all do not know it. [Su] Gong. The *po hao* 皤蒿, "white [hair] *hao*," of the *Er ya* is *bai hao* 白蒿, "white *hao*." It can be found everywhere. The leaves are quite similar to those of fine common mugwort. Their upper side is covered with white hair and rough. They are coarser than those of *qing hao* wormwood. From the very beginning of their growth until autumn, they are whiter than those of all the other *hao* 蒿. [Zhang] Yuxi: Garden daisy can be prepared as an edible vegetable. Hence the *Shi jian* states: "Soybean fodder and *fan* 蘩 [can be made to] pickled vegetables." Lu Ji in his *Shi shu* states: "All mugwort of white color is *po hao* 皤蒿, "white [hair] wormwood." Today, *bai hao* develops [in a year] earlier than all other herbs; it is fragrant, delicious and edible. It is suitable for consumption both fresh and steamed. [Su] Song: This herb was considered by the ancients to be a vegetable. Today, people only eat *lou hao* 蔞蒿; they no longer eat this [*bai hao*]. Some wonder whether *bai hao* is not the same as *lou hao*, but Meng Shen in his *Shi liao* treats *lou hao* in a separate entry. Even though the statements differ, it is clear that these are two different items and from this one knows that the food of ancient times and today is not the same. Also, in current Jie zhou, *bai hao* is *yin chen* 茵蔯, virgate wormwood. Their seedlings and leaves are similar. But [*bai hao*] may not be suitable for therapeutic use. [Li] Shizhen: *Bai hao* can be found everywhere. There are two kinds, one water [*bai hao*] and one land [*bai hao*]. The *Ben cao* accepts for [therapeutic use] only that which grows in water. Hence it says "grows in river marshlands of Mount Zhong shan." It does not say "mountain valleys and flatlands." The two kinds resemble each other in their physical shape, but the land [kind of *bai hao*] has an acrid fragrance that is not as nice a fragrance as that of the water [kind of *bai hao*]. A poem states "the sound of roaring deer; they eat the *ping* 苹 of the wild."[97] *Ping* 苹 is the *po hao*, white [hair] *hao*, growing on land. It is commonly called *ai hao* 艾蒿. Deer eat nine kinds of herbs that serve to resolve poison. *Bai hao* is one of them. Another poem states: "Where they collect *fan* 蘩, in ponds and on islets." The *Zuo zhuan* states: "Vegetables prepared from *ping* 蘋, *fan* 蘩, *yun* 蘊 (green algae) and *zao* 藻 (brown algae) can be recommended to demons and spirits; they disgrace kings and dukes." Both [these poems] refer to the *bai hao* growing in waters. That is, the *bai hao* mentioned in the *Ben cao* undoubtedly is *lou hao*. When Zheng Qiao in his *Tong zhi* says: "*Ping* 苹 is *lou hao* 蔞蒿," he is wrong. Deer are animals of the mountains. *Lou* [*hao*] 蔞[蒿] is a water *hao* 蒿. When Lu Ji in his *Shi shu* says: "Ping 苹 is *niu wei hao* 牛尾蒿, 'oxtail *hao*'," he, too, is wrong. Oxtail *hao* is greenish, not white. Its fine leaves reach straight upward, shaped like an oxtail. *Lou hao* grows on slopes and in marshland. It develops a seedling in the second month. The leaves resemble tender mugwort [leaves], but are forked and finer. The front is greenish and the back is white. The stems may be red or white. The root is white and brittle. Collect the root stem; it is edible fresh or prepared, preserved and dried. The fact is, it is a good vegetable. Jing Chai in his *Da zhao* states: "In Wu they add sour [flavor] to *hao* 蒿 and *lou* 蔞; neither too much, nor too little." That is to say, in Wu the people love to mix [food] with sour [flavor]. They boil *lou hao* to become a spice, and they add neither too much nor too little to achieve a sweet and delicious [flavor]. This is certainly a reference to the [*hao*] growing in waters.

15-10-01

苗、根 *Miao, Gen.*

Seedling, root [of *bai hao*].

【氣味】甘，平，無毒。【思邈曰】辛，平。【時珍曰】發瘡疥。

Qi and Flavor. Sweet, balanced, nonpoisonous. [Sun] Simiao. Acrid, balanced. [Li] Shizhen: It stimulates outbreaks of sores and *jie*-illness.[98]

---

97 *Shi jing*, part II, Xiao ya 小雅, Book I, Ode I: *lu ming* 鹿鳴.

98 *Jie*-illness 疥, vaguely identifiable skin ailment. BCGM Dict I, 249.

【主治】五臟邪氣，風寒濕痺，補中益氣，長毛髮令黑，療心懸，少食常饑。久服輕身，耳目聰明不老。本經。生挼，醋淹爲菹食，甚益人。擣汁服，去熱黃及心痛。曝爲末，米飲空心服一匙，治夏月暴水痢。燒灰淋汁煎，治淋瀝疾。孟詵。利膈開胃，殺河豚魚毒。時珍。

Control. Evil qi affecting the five long-term depots. Blockage related to the presence of wind, cold and moisture. They supplement the center and boost the qi. They stimulate the growth of hair and let them remain black. They heal heart suspension.[99] When people eat little and are permanently hungry. Ingested over a long time, they relieve the body of its weight. They clear and brighten ears and eyes and prevent aging. *Ben jing*. Collected fresh and consumed prepared with vinegar to a vegetable, they greatly benefit one. Pounded to obtain a juice, its ingestion removes heat jaundice and heart pain. Dried in the sun, [ground into] powder and the amount held by a spoon drunk with a rice beverage on an empty stomach they serve to cure in summer sudden watery free-flux illness. Burned to ashes, and the juice obtained by trickling water [through the ashes] boiled, they serve to cure dripping [urine] illnesses. Meng Shen. They free the passage through the diaphragm and open the stomach. They kill the poison of globefish.

【發明】【弘景曰】服食家七禽散云，白兔食白蒿仙，與菴蔄同法耳。【時珍曰】本經列白蒿於上品，有功無毒，而古今方家不知用，豈不得服之之訣與？

Explication. [Tao] Hongjing: The "seven fowl powder" of the experts who ingest [medicinal substances] for food states: "White hares/rabbits eat *bai hao* and become immortals." The method is the same as that of preparing keiske *artemisia*. [Li] Shizhen: The *Ben jing* lists *bai hao* as "upper rank." It has a [therapeutic] potential and is nonpoisonous. But the recipe masters of ancient times did not know how to use it. Is this so because nobody instructed them on how to ingest it?

【附方】舊一。

Added Recipes. One of old.

惡瘡癩疾。但是惡疾遍體，面目有瘡者，皆可服之。用白艾蒿十束如升大，煮取汁，以麴及米一如釀酒法，候熟，稍稍飲之。梅師方。

99 *Xin xuan* 心懸, "heart suspension," a condition with a feeling of the "heart," i. e., the stomach, not being firmly fixed and dangling in a hollow space. BCGM Dict I, 581.

Malign sores and repudiation-illness[100] ailments. When a malign illness affects the entire body, with sores covering face and eyes, in all these cases they can be ingested. Boil ten bundles of *bai ai hao*, the size of a *sheng*, in water and prepare the resulting juice with yeast and rice in the same way as one brews wine. Wait until it is done and drink [the liquid] in small quantities. *Mei shi fang*.

15-10-02
子 *Zi*
Seeds [of *bai hao*].

【氣味】缺。

Qi and Flavor. Missing.

【主治】鬼氣。爲末，酒服之，良。孟詵。

Control. Demon qi. [Grind them into] powder and ingest it with wine. Good. Meng Shen.

15-11
角蒿唐本草
Jiao hao, FE *Tang ben cao.*

***Incarvillea sinensis* Lam. Chinese *incarvillea*.**[101]

【集解】【恭曰】角蒿葉似白蒿，花如瞿麥，紅赤可愛，子似王不留行，黑色作角，七月、八月采。【保昇曰】葉似蛇牀、青蒿，子角似蔓菁，實黑而細，秋熟，所在皆有之。【宗奭曰】莖葉如青蒿，開淡紅紫花，大約徑三四分。花罷結角，長二寸許，微彎。【斅曰】凡使，勿用紅蒿并邪蒿，二味真似角蒿，只是此香而角短爾。采得，於槐砧上細剉用之。

Collected Explanations. [Su] Gong: *Jiao hao* leaves are similar to those of Sievers wormwood. The flowers are like those of fringed pink. They are of a lovely red. The seeds resemble those of cowherbs. They are black and have protuberances. They are collected in the seventh and eighth month. [Han] Baosheng: The leaves resemble those of *cnidium* [herbs] and greenish wormwood. The seeds have protuberances similar to those of rape turnips. They are black and fine, and they ripen in autumn. They are found everywhere. [Kou] Zongshi: The stem and the leaves are similar to those of greenish wormwood. They open flowers of a pale red-purple color with a diameter of about three to four *fen*. When the flowers decay the protuberances are formed; they are about two *cun* long and a little bent. [Lei] Xiao: For all applications

100 *Lai* 癩, "repudiation-illness," most likely referring to leprosy, "Aussatz." BCGM Dict I, 111, and 293-294.

101 *Jiao hao* 角蒿, lit.: "wormwood with protuberances."

do not resort to *hong hao*, red wormwood, and to *xie hao*, *libanotis* [herb]. Both these substance are very similar to *jiao hao*. The only [difference is that *jiao hao*] is fragrant and has short protuberances. When [the herb] is collected, cut it on a *sophora* wood block to fine pieces and then use them.

【氣味】辛、苦，有小毒。
Qi and Flavor. Acrid, bitter, slightly poisonous.

【主治】乾濕䘌諸惡瘡有蟲者。唐本。治口齒瘡絶勝。宗奭。
Control. All malign sores with worms/bugs, with the hidden worms/bugs related to either dryness or moisture. *Tang ben*. It serves to cure dental sores and is very effective. [Kou] Zongshi.

【附方】舊二，新一。
Added Recipes. Two of old. One newly [recorded].

齒齦宣露。多是疳也。角蒿燒灰，夜塗上。切忌油膩、沙糖、乾棗。外臺秘要。
Cases of teeth and gums exposure are mostly *gan*-illness.[102] Burn *jiao hao* and apply the ashes [to the gums] overnight. Fat items, sugar and dry dates are to be avoided. *Wai tai mi yao.*

口瘡不瘥，入胸中並生者。不拘大人小兒，以角蒿灰塗之，有汁吐去，一宿效。千金方。
Oral sores that fail to heal and have entered the chest to develop there, too. Regardless of whether adults or children are concerned, apply *jiao hao* ashes [to the affected region]. When a juice [collects in the mouth, the patient is to] spit it out. Effective after one night. *Qian jin fang.*

月蝕耳瘡。用蒿灰摻之良。集簡方。
Lunar eclipse[103] ear sores. Apply wormwood ashes [to the affected region]. Good. *Ji jian fang.*

102 *Gan* 疳, "*gan*-illness," also: "sweets-illness," involves several complaints that affect children and adults, with causes and conditions too different to fall into a known disease category. BCGM Dict I, 180-188.

103 *Yue shi* 月蝕, "lunar eclipse," a condition of *chuang* 瘡, "sores" developing on the ears, nose, face, and to the side of the orifices in the anal and genital region. BCGM Dict I, 65.

15-12
藨蒿拾遺
Lin hao. FE *Shi yi*.

***Pedicularis gloriosa* Biss.**

【釋名】莪蒿爾雅、蘿蒿同上、抱娘蒿。【時珍曰】陸農師云：藨之爲言高也。莪，亦峨也。莪科高也。可以覆蠶，故謂之蘿。抱根叢生，故曰抱娘。

Explanation of Names. *E hao* 莪蒿, *Er ya*. *Luo hao* 蘿蒿, same source as previous. *Bao nang hao* 抱娘蒿. [Li] Shizhen: Lu Nongshi states: "*Lin* 藨 is to say *gao* 高, 'tall.' *E* 莪, too, is *e* 峨, 'high'." The class of *e* 莪 comprises tall [items]. It can serve to cover silkworms. Hence it is called *luo* 蘿. As it grows in clusters "embracing," *bao* 抱, the root, *gen* 根, it is called *bao nang* 抱娘, "embracing the mother."

【集解】【時珍曰】藨蒿生高崗，似小薊，宿根先於百草。爾雅云"莪，蘿"是也。詩小雅云：菁菁者莪。陸機注云：即莪蒿也。生澤國漸洳處，葉似斜蒿而細科，二月生。莖、葉可食，又可蒸，香美。頗似蔞蒿。但味帶麻，不似蔞蒿甘香。

Collected Explanations. [Li] Shizhen: *Lin hao* grows on high hills; it is similar to cat thistles. The perennial root [develops a seedling early in the year] prior to all other herbs. The *Er ya* states: "*E* 莪 is *luo* 蘿." That is correct. The *Shi*, Xiao ya, states: "Those growing luxuriantly are *e* 莪." Lu Ji in a comment states: "This is *e hao* 莪蒿. It grows in marshland countries and increasingly damp places. The leaves resemble those of common *seseli*, but are finer. They grow in the second month. Stem and leaves are edible. Also, they can be [consumed] steamed. They are fragrant and delicious." They are quite similar to those of Sievers wormwood but their flavor has some numbing effects. It is not as sweet and fragrant as that of Sievers wormwood.

【氣味】辛，温，無毒。

Qi and Flavor. Acrid, warm, nonpoisonous.

【主治】破血下氣，煮食之。藏器。

Control. To break through blood [accumulation] and to discharge qi, boil it [in water] and eat it. [Chen] Cangqi.

15-13
馬先蒿本經中品
Ma xian hao, FE *Ben jing*, middle rank.

***Pedicularis resupinata* L.**

【釋名】馬新蒿唐本、馬矢蒿本經、練石草別録、爛石草同上、虎麻。【時珍曰】蒿氣如馬矢，故名。馬先，乃馬矢字訛也。馬新，又馬先之訛也。【弘景曰】練石草，一名爛石草，即馬矢蒿。公方藥不復用之。

Explanation of Names. *Ma xin hao* 馬新蒿, *Tang ben*. *Ma shi hao* 馬矢蒿, *Ben jing*. *Lian shi cao* 練石草, *Bie lu*. *Lan shi cao* 爛石草, source identical to the previous. *Hu ma* 虎麻. [Li] Shizhen: The qi of this kind of *hao* resembles [the smell of] horse dung, *ma shi* 馬矢, hence the name. *Ma xian* 馬先 is an erroneous writing of *ma shi* 馬矢. *Ma xin* 馬新, in turn, is an erroneous writing of *ma xian* 馬先. [Tao] Hongjing: *Lian shi cao* 練石草, "white silk stone herb," alternatively named *lan shi cao* 爛石草, "rotten stone herb," is [a less offensive writing of] *ma shi cao* 馬矢蒿, "horse dung *hao*." In commonly[104] resorted to pharmaceutical recipes it is no longer used.

【集解】【別録曰】馬先蒿、練石草，並生南陽川澤。【恭曰】葉大如茺蔚，花紅白色。二月、八月采莖葉，陰乾用。八月、九月實熟，俗謂之虎麻是也。一名馬新蒿，所在有之。茺蔚苗短小，其子夏中熟。二物初生極相似也。【禹錫曰】按爾雅云：蔚，牡菣。註云，即蒿之無子者。詩云：匪莪伊蔚。陸機云：牡蒿也。二月始生，七月花，花似胡麻花而紫赤，八月生角，似小豆角，銳而長，一名馬新蒿是也。【頌曰】郭璞以牡菣爲無子，而陸機云有子，二説小異。今當用有子者爲正。【時珍曰】別録牡蒿、馬先蒿，原是二條。陸機所謂有子者，乃馬先蒿，而復引無子之牡蒿釋之，誤矣。牡蒿詳見本條。

Collected Explanations. *Bie lu*: *Ma xian hao* and *lian shi cao* grow in river marshlands of Nan yang. [Su] Gong: The leaves are as big as those of Siberian motherwort. The flowers are of red-white color. Stem and leaves are collected in the second and eighth month to be dried in the yin (i. e., shade) before they are used. The fruit ripen in the eighth and ninth month. They are the ones commonly called *hu ma* 虎麻, "tiger sesame." [Zhang] Yuxi: According to the *Er ya*, "wei 蔚 is male *qian* 菣." As a comment explains: "These are childless kinds of wormwood." The *Shi* states: "[I] am] not the outstanding [item (*e* 莪)] my parents had looked forward to. I am] only of mediocre [talent (*wei* 蔚)]."[105] Lu Ji states: "This is a reference to male (i. e., infertile) wormwood." It begins to grow in the second month and has flowers in the

104 *Zheng lei* ch. 9, *ma xian hao* 馬先蒿, does not have the character *gong* 公. It may be an erroneous writing of the similar character *jin* 今, "today."

105 *Shi jing*, part II, Xiao ya 小雅, Book V, Ode VIII: *lu e* 蓼莪.

seventh month. The flowers resemble *hu ma* flowers, but are purple-red. They develop protuberances in the eighth month, resembling small bean protuberances. They are pointed and lengthy. This is [the item] called *ma xin hao* 馬新蒿 with an alternative name. [Su] Song: Guo Pu considers *mu qian* 牡菣, "male *qian*," to be without seeds, while Lu Ji states that it has seeds. Their two statements are slightly different. Today it is appropriate to use those with seeds. [Li] Shizhen: In the *Bie lu*, *mu hao* 牡蒿 and *ma xian hao* 馬先蒿 originally were treated in two entries. [The herb] said by Lu Ji to have seeds is *ma xian hao*. When this in turn is identified as *mu hao* 牡蒿, then this is wrong. For details on *mu hao* 牡蒿 see the respective entry (15-15).

【氣味】苦，平，無毒。別録曰：練石草，寒。

Qi and Flavor. Bitter, balanced, nonpoisonous. *Bie lu*: *Lian shi cao*, cold.

【主治】寒熱鬼疰，中風濕痺，女子帶下病，無子。本經。練石草，治五癃，破石淋、膀胱中結氣，利水道小便。別録。惡瘡。弘景。

Control. Demon attachment-illness[106] with alternating sensations of cold and heat. Blockage related to wind stroke and moisture. Diseases of women below the belt. Childlessness. *Ben jing*. *Lian shi cao* serves to cure the five types of protuberance-illness,[107] breaks through urinary stone dripping and bound qi[108] in the urinary bladder. It clears the passage of urine through the passageways of water. *Bie lu*. Malign sores. [Tao] Hongjing.

【附方】舊一。

Added Recipes. One of old.

大風癩疾。骨肉疽敗，眉鬚墮落，身體痒痛。以馬先蒿，一名馬矢蒿，一名爛石草，炒，擣末。每服方寸匕，食前温酒下，一日三服，一年都瘥。肘後方。

106 *Zhu* 疰, also *zhu* 注, "attachment-illness," "influx-illnesss," reflects a notion of a foreign pathogenic agent, originally of demonic nature, having attached itself to the human organism. BCGM Dict I, 688-695.

107 *Wu long* 五癃, "five kinds of protuberance-illness." Reference to various, not clearly distinguished *long* 癃, "protuberance-illnesses," associated with a passing of urine in small amounts, or a completely blocked passage. BCGM Dict I, 323, 541.

108 *Jie qi* 結氣, "bound qi," are pathological qi halting and congealing at any place in the body. BCGM Dict I, 240.

For massive wind,[109] [i. e.,] repudiation-illness,[110] ailments. Bones and flesh are decayed with impediment-illness.[111] Eyebrows and hair have fallen off. The entire body itches and is in pain. Stir-fry *ma xian hao*, also named *ma shi hao* and also named *lan shi cao*, and pound it into powder. Each time ingest the amount held by a square *cun* spoon. To be sent down prior to meals with warm wine. To be ingested three times a day. A complete healing will be achieved within one year. *Zhou hou fang*.

15-14
陰地厥宋圖經
Yin di jue, FE Song, *Tu jing*.

Scerpteridium ternatum (Thunb.) Lyon. Moonwort.

【集解】【頌曰】生鄧州順陽縣内鄉山谷。葉似青蒿，莖青紫色，花作小穗，微黄，根似細辛。七月采根用。【時珍曰】江浙亦有之。外家采制丹砂、硫黄。

Collected Explanations. [Su] Song: It grows in the rural areas and mountain valleys of Shun yang in Deng zhou. The leaves are similar to those of greenish wormwood. The stems are greenish-purple. The flowers form small spikes; they are slightly yellow. The root resembles that of *asarum heteropoides*. The root is collected for use in the seventh month. [Li] Shizhen: It is also found in Jiang and Zhe. Specialists of external [medical therapy] collect it to check [the effects] of cinnabar and sulphur.

15-14-01
根、苗 *Gen, Miao*
Root, seedling [of *yin di jue*].

【氣味】甘、苦，微寒，無毒。

Qi and Flavor. Sweet, bitter, slightly cold, nonpoisonous.

【主治】腫毒風熱。蘇頌。

Control. Wind and heat [intrusion] with poison swelling. Su Song.

---

109 *Da feng* 大風, "massive wind," may refer to sores caused by a massive intrusion of wind evil and also to conditions of leprosy. BCGM Dict I, 111.

110 *Lai* 癩, "*lai*-illness," "repudiation-illness," including cases of leprosy/Aussatz." BCGM Dict I, 293.

111 *Ju* 疽, "impediment-illness," refers to an obstruction of vessels or other ducts inside the body. Qi rushing against the impediment may cause a local swelling and eventually break through the surface to cause an abscess. BCGM Dict I, 277.

【附方】新一。

Added Recipes. One newly [recorded].

男婦吐血後，胸膈虛熱。陰地厥、紫河車、貫衆、甘草各半兩。每服三錢，水煎服。聖濟總録。

Males and women with depletion heat in chest and diaphragm following an episode of blood spitting. Each time ingest three *qian* of [a mixture of] half a *liang* each of *yin di jue*, human placenta, *dryopteris* [root] and *glycyrrhiza* [root]. To be ingested boiled in water. *Sheng ji zong lu.*

15-15
牡蒿別録下品

Mu hao, FE *Bie lu*, lower rank.

***Artemisia japonica* Thunb. Japanese *artemisia*.**

【釋名】齊頭蒿。【時珍曰】爾雅：蔚，牡菣。蒿之無子者。則牡之名以此也。諸蒿葉皆尖，此蒿葉獨奓而秃，故有齊頭之名。

Explanation of Names. *Qi tou hao* 齊頭蒿. [Li] Shizhen: *Er ya*: "*Wei* 蔚 is *mu qian* 牡菣. These are *hao* 蒿 without seeds." This explains the name *mu* 牡, "male," (i. e. childless, *wu zi* 無子). The leaves of all kinds of *hao* 蒿 are pointed. The leaves of the present *hao* 蒿 are the only ones that are broad and blunt. Hence the name *qi tou* 齊頭.

【集解】【别録曰】牡蒿生田野，五月、八月采。【弘景曰】方藥不復用。【恭曰】齊頭蒿也，所在有之。葉似防風，細薄而無光澤。【時珍曰】齊頭蒿三四月生苗，其葉扁而本狹，末奓有秃岐。嫩時可茹。鹿食九草，此其一也。秋開細黄花，結實大如車前實，而内子微細不可見，故人以爲無子也。

Collected Explanations. *Bie lu*: *Mu hao* grows in the open country. It is collected in the fifth and eighth month. [Tao] Hongjing: It is no longer used in pharmaceutical recipes. [Su] Gong: *Qi tou hao* can be found everywhere. The leaves resemble those of *saposhnikovia* [herbs]. They are fine, thin and lack glossiness. [Li] Shizhen: *Qi tou hao* grows a seedling in the third to fourth month. The leaves are flat and narrow at their origin. They are broad at the end with a blunt tip. As long as they are tender, they can be eaten. The deer eat nine herbs [that resolve poison]. This is one of them. [*Mu hao*] opens fine, yellow flowers in autumn, and forms fruit as big as Asiatic plantain fruit. The seeds inside are too fine to be visible. Hence, people assume [*mu hao*] has no seeds.

15-15-01
苗 *Miao*
Seedling [of *mu hao*].

【氣味】苦、微甘，温，無毒。

Qi and Flavor. Bitter, slightly sweet, warm, nonpoisonous.

【主治】充臟膚，益氣，令人暴肥。不可久服，血脉滿盛。别録。擂汁服，治陰腫。時珍。

Control. It fills muscles and skin, boosts the qi and lets one quickly become fat. It should not be ingested for a long time, so that it does not fill the blood vessels excessively. *Bie lu*. Pound it and ingest the resulting juice. This serves to cure swelling of the yin [(i. e., genital) region]. [Li] Shizhen.

【附方】新一。
Added Recipes. One newly [recorded].

瘧疾寒熱。齊頭蒿根、滴滴金根各一把，擂生酒一鍾，未發前服。以渣傅寸口，男左女右。二日便止。海上名方。

Malaria illness with alternating sensations of cold and heat. Ingest prior to an outbreak one *zhong* of fresh wine in which were pounded a handful each of *qi tou hao* root and horseheal root. Apply the dregs to the inch opening [on the wrist]; for males on the left and for females on the right [wrist]. Within two days [the outbreak] will end. *Hai shang ming fang*.

15-16
九牛草宋圖經
***Jiu niu cao*. FE Song, *Tu jing*.**
***Chrysanthemum decaisneanum* Matsum.**

【集解】【頌曰】生筠州山岡上。二月生苗，獨莖，高一尺。葉似艾葉，圓而長，背有白毛，面青。五月采苗用。【時珍曰】陳嘉謨本草蒙筌以此爲蕲艾，謬矣。

Collected Explanations. [Su] Song: It grows on mountains and hills of Yun zhou. It grows a seedling in the second month. A single stem reaches a height of one *chi*. The leaves resemble mugwort leaves. They are round and lengthy, and on their back they have white hair. The front side is greenish. The seedling is collected in the fifth month for [therapeutic] use. [Li] Shizhen: Chen Jiamo in his *Ben cao meng quan* identifies it as Qi *ai*. That is wrong.

15-16-01
苗 *Miao*
Seedling [of *jiu niu cao*].

【氣味】微苦，有小毒。

Qi and Flavor. Slightly bitter. Slightly poisonous.

【主治】解風勞，治身體痛。與甘草同煎服，不入衆藥用。蘇頌。

Control. It resolves exhaustion related to wind [intrusion] and serves to cure body pains. Boil it together with *glycyrrhiza* [root] and ingest this. It is not used added to any [other] medication. Su Song.

15-17
茺蔚本經上品

Chong wei. FE *Ben jing*, upper rank.

***Leonurus japonicus* Houtt. Siberian motherwort.**

【釋名】益母本經、益明本經、貞蔚別録、蓷爾雅音推、野天麻會編、豬麻綱目、火杴本經、鬱臭草圖經、苦低草圖經、夏枯草外臺、土質汗綱目。【時珍曰】此草及子皆充盛密蔚，故名茺蔚。其功宜於婦人及明目益精，故有益母之稱。其莖方類麻，故謂之野天麻。俗呼爲豬麻，豬喜食之也。夏至後即枯，故亦有夏枯之名。近效方謂之土質汗。林億云：質汗出西番，乃熱血合諸藥煎成，治金瘡折傷。益母亦可作煎治折傷，故名爲土質汗也。【禹錫曰】爾雅：萑，蓷。注云：今茺蔚也，又名益母。劉歆云：蓷，臭穢也。臭穢，即茺蔚也。機云：蓷，益母也。故曾子見之感思。

Explanation of Names. *Yi mu* 益母, *Ben jing*. *Yi ming* 益明, *Ben jing*. *Zhen wei* 貞蔚, *Bie lu*. *Tui* 蓷, according to the *Er ya* read *tui* 推. *Ye tian ma* 野天麻, *Hui bian*. *Zhu ma* 豬麻, *Gang mu*. *Huo xian* 火杴, "fire shovel," *Ben jing*. *Yu chou cao* 鬱臭草, "pent-up stench herb," *Tu jing*. *Ku di cao* 苦低草, "bitter drooping herb," *Tu jing*. *Xia ku cao* 夏枯草, *Wai tai*. *Tu zhi han* 土質汗, *Gang mu*. [Li] Shizhen: This herb and its seeds flourish in dense and luxurious growth, *chong* ... *wei* 充 ... 蔚. Hence it is called *chong wei* 茺蔚. Its [therapeutic] potential is suitable for women; it brightens the eyes and boosts, *yi* 益, the essence/sperm. Hence its designation as "good for mothers," *yi mu* 益母. Its stem is square like that of hemp, *ma* 麻, hence it is called "wild heavenly hemp," *ye tian ma* 野天麻. A common name is *zhu ma* 豬麻, "pig's hemp," as pigs love to eat it. After Summer Solstice it withers. Hence it is also called "withers in summer," *xia ku* 夏枯. The *Jin xiao fang* calls it *tu zhi han* 土質汗, "local *zhi han*." Lin Yi states: "*Zhi han* comes from foreign lands in the West. It is prepared by boiling a mixture of hot blood and all types of medication, and serves to cure wounds caused by metal objects/weapons with fracture damage. *Yi mu*, too, can be prepared to a decoction to cure fracture damage. Hence it is called 'local *zhi han*', *tu zhi han* 土質汗." [Zhang] Yuxi: *Er ya*: "*Tui* 萑 is *tui* 蓷." A commentary states: "This is today's *chong wei* 茺蔚. It is also called *yi mu* 益母." Liu Xin states: "*Tui* 蓷 is malodorous and filthy, *chou hui* 臭穢. *Chou hui* 臭穢 is *chong wei* 茺蔚." Lu Ji: "*Tui* 蓷 is *yi mu* 益母. This is why Zeng Zi when he saw it was moved to think [of his mother]."

【集解】【别録曰】茺蔚生海濱池澤，五月采。【弘景曰】今處處有之。葉如荏，方莖，子形細長，有三稜。方用亦稀。【頌曰】今園圃及田野極多。郭璞註爾雅云：葉似荏，方莖白華，華生節間，節節生花。實似鷄冠子，黑色。莖作四方稜，五月采。又云：九月采實，醫方稀有用實者。【宗奭曰】茺蔚初春生時，亦可浸洗，淘去苦水，煮作菜食。淩冬不凋悴也。【時珍曰】茺蔚，近水濕處甚繁。春初生苗如嫩蒿，入夏長三四尺，莖方如黄麻莖。其葉如艾葉而背青，一梗三葉，葉有尖歧。寸許一節，節節生穗，叢簇抱莖。四五月間，穗内開小花，紅紫色，亦有微白色者。每萼内有細子四粒，粒大如茼蒿子，有三稜，褐色，藥肆往往以作巨勝子貨之。其草生時有臭氣，夏至後即枯，其根白色。蘇頌圖經謂其葉似荏，其子黑色，似鷄冠子，九月采實，寇宗奭衍義謂其淩冬不凋者，皆誤傳也。此草有白花、紫花二種，莖、葉、子、穗皆一樣。但白者能入氣分，紅者能入血分，别而用之可也。按閨閣事宜云：白花者爲益母，紫花者爲野天麻。返魂丹註云：紫花者爲益母，白花者不是。陳藏器本草云：茺蔚生田野間，人呼爲鬱臭草。天麻生平澤，似馬鞭草，節節生紫花，花中有子，如青葙子。孫思邈千金方云：天麻草，莖如火麻，冬生苗，夏着赤花，如鼠尾花。此皆似以茺蔚、天麻爲二物，蓋不知其是一物二種。凡物花皆有赤白，如牡丹、芍藥、菊花之類是矣。又按郭璞爾雅註云：蓷，音推，即茺蔚，又名益母。葉似荏，白華，華生節間。又云：蓷，音推，方莖，葉長而鋭，有穗，穗間有花紫縹色，可以爲飲，江東呼爲牛蘈。據此則是蓷、蘈名本相同，但以花色分别之，其爲一物無疑矣。宋人重修本草，以天麻草誤註天麻，尤爲謬失。陳藏器本草又有鏨菜，云生江南陰地，似益母，方莖對節白花，主産後血病。此即茺蔚之白花者，故其功主血病亦相同。

Collected Explanations. *Bie lu*: *Chong wei* grows in ponds and marshlands at the seaside. It is collected in the fifth month. [Tao] Hongjing: Today it can be found everywhere. The leaves are similar to those of *perilla*. The stem is square. The seeds are fine and lengthy, with three edges. [*Chong wei*], too, is seldom used in pharmaceutical recipes. [Su] Song: Today it can be found very often in gardens and in the open country. Guo Pu in his comment on the *Er ya* states: "The leaves are similar to *perilla* [leaves]. The stem is square and has white flowers. The flowers grow from between the nodes. Every two nodes grow a flower. The fruits are similar to cockscomb seeds; they are black. The stem is rectangular with four edges. It is collected in the fifth month." It is also said: "Collect the fruit in the ninth month." Physicians seldom use the fruits. [Kou] Zongshi: When *chong wei* grows in early spring, it can be soaked and washed. It is washed in a pan and its bitter [flavor] is discarded with the water. Then it is boiled and eaten as a vegetable. It does not wither in winter. [Li] Shizhen: *Chong wei* grows very strongly in waters and moist locations nearby. In early spring a seedling grows similar to tender wormwood. By summer, it reaches a height of three to four *chi*. The stem is square like a yellow hemp stem. The leaves resemble mugwort leaves with a greenish back. One stalk has three leaves, and the leaves have pointed ends. The nodes are situated in a distance of about one *cun*. Spikes develop between two nodes, forming clusters embracing the stem. In the fourth and fifth month, small flowers open in the spikes; they are of red-purple color. There are also some of a pale white color. Each calyx includes four fine seed kernels. These kernels have the size of garden daisy seeds. They have three edges and are brown. Apothecary's shops often substitute them with sesame seeds. When the herb grows it emits malodorous qi. After Summer Solstice it withers and the root is white. When Su Song in the *Tu jing* says: "Its leaves are similar to *perilla* [leaves], its seeds are black, similar to cockscomb seeds. The fruits are collected in the ninth month," and when Kou Zongshi in his *Yan yi* says: "They do not wither in winter," they are both wrong. This herb has two kinds of flowers, white flowers and purple flowers. Stem, leaves, seeds and spike are the same. However, the white ones can enter the qi section, while the red ones enter the blood section, and their application should differ accordingly. According to the *Gui ge shi yi*, "those with white flowers are *yi mu* 益母; those with red flowers are *ye tian ma* 野天麻." A commentary to the [*Zhi zhi fang* recipe of] the "elixir to let the *hun*-soul return" states: "Those with purple flowers are *yi mu* 益母; those with white flowers are not." Chen Cangqi in his *Ben cao* states: "*Chong wei* grows in the open country. People call it 'pent-up malodorous stench herb.' *Tian ma* 天麻 grows in the plains, in marshlands. It resembles vervain. Always between two nodes purple flowers grow, and in these flowers are seeds, similar to *celosia* [herb] seeds." Sun Simiao in his *Qian jin fang* states: "*Tian ma cao* 天麻草 has a stem like hemp [herbs]. It grows a seedling in winter and develops red flowers in summer, similar to the flowers of Japanese *salvia*." Apparently, all these statements suggest that *chong wei* and *tian ma* are two items. The fact is, they do not know that these are two kinds of one item. Many items have red and white flowers, such as [tree] *paeonia*, *paeonia* and *chrysanthemum* flowers. Also, as Guo Pu in his commentary on the *Er ya* states: "*Tui* 萑, read *tui* 推, is *chong wei*

茺蔚, alternative name: *yi mu* 益母. The leaves are similar to *perilla* [leaves]. It has white flowers. The flowers grow between the nodes." It is also stated: "*Tui* 蓷, read 推, has a square stem. The leaves are long and pointed. It has spikes. Flowers are situated between the spikes; they are of a purple, indistinct color. They can be prepared to a beverage. In Jiang dong it is called *niu tui* 牛蘈." That is, the names *tui* 蓷 and *tui* 蓷 are basically identical; the [plants] differ only in terms of the color of their flowers. Hence it is without doubt that they are one and the same item. In the *Ben cao* newly revised by Song people, *tian ma cao* 天麻草 is erroneously commented upon as *tian ma* 天麻. This is a particularly gross mistake. The *Chen Cangqi ben cao* also mentions a *zan cai* 鏨菜, stating that "it grows at yin (i. e., shady) places in Jiang nan and is similar to *yi mu* 益母. It has a square stem and white flowers growing facing each other at the nodes, and controls blood diseases following birth." These are the *chong wei* 茺蔚 with white flowers. Hence they have the same [therapeutic] potential of controlling blood disease.

15-17-01
子 *Zi*
Seeds [of *chong wei*].

【修治】【時珍曰】凡用，微炒香，亦或蒸熟，烈日曝燥，舂簸去殼，取仁用。

Pharmaceutical Preparation. [Li] Shizhen: For all uses, slightly stir-fry them until they develop a fragrance; it is also possible to steam them until done, and to dry them in the hot sun. [Crush them in a] mortar, and winnow away the shells. Remove the kernels for [therapeutic] use.

【氣味】辛、甘，微温，無毒。【別録曰】甘，微寒。【時珍曰】甘、辛，温。灰制硫黄。

Qi and Flavor. Acrid, sweet, slightly warm, nonpoisonous. *Bie lu*: Sweet, slightly cold. [Li] Shizhen: Sweet, acrid, warm. The ashes serve to check the effects of sulphur.

【主治】明目益精，除水氣，久服輕身。本經。療血逆大熱，頭痛心煩。別録。産後血脹。大明。舂仁生食，補中益氣，通血脉，填精髓，止渴潤肺。吴瑞。治風解熱，順氣活血，養肝益心，安魂定魄，調女人經脉，崩中帶下，産後胎前諸病。久服令人有子。時珍。

Control. They brighten the eyes. boost the essence/sperm and remove water qi. Ingested over a long time they relieve the body of its weight. *Ben jing*. They heal blood countermovement with massive heat, headache and heart vexation. *Bie lu*. Distention related to blood following birth. Da Ming. The kernels [obtained after crushing the seeds in a] mortar and eaten fresh supplement the center and boost the qi. They penetrate the blood vessels and fill essence and marrow. They end thirst and moisten the lung. Wu Rui. They serve to cure wind [intrusion] and resolve heat. They correct the [flow of] qi and quicken the blood. They nourish the liver and boost the heart. They pacify the *hun*-soul and stabilize the *po*-soul. They bring in order the [movement in the] conduit-vessels of women and [serve to cure] collapsing center[112] and [further ailments] below the belt, as well as all diseases after delivery and prior to birth. Ingested over a long time, they let one have children. [Li] Shizhen.

【發明】【震亨曰】茺蔚子活血行氣，有補陰之功，故名益母。凡胎前產後所恃者，血氣也。胎前無滯，產後無虛，以其行中有補也。【時珍曰】茺蔚子味甘微辛，氣温，陰中之陽，手、足厥陰經藥也。白花者入氣分，紫花者入血分。治婦女經脉不調，胎產一切血氣諸病妙品也，而醫方鮮知用。時珍常以之同四物、香附諸藥治人，獲效甚多。蓋包絡生血，肝藏血。此物能活血補陰，故能明目益精，調經，治女人諸病也。東垣李氏言：瞳子散大者，禁用茺蔚子，爲其辛温主散，能助火也。當歸雖辛温，而兼苦甘，能和血，故不禁之。愚謂目得血而能視，茺蔚行血甚捷，瞳子散大，血不足也，故禁之，非助火也。血滯病目則宜之，故曰明目。

Explication. [Zhu] Zhenheng. *Chong wei* seeds quicken the blood and stimulate qi movement; they have a potential of supplementing yin [qi]. Hence they are named "good for mothers." All vital processes prior to birth and following delivery depend on [the condition of] blood and qi. Prior to birth there should be no sluggishness [of blood and qi]. After delivery there should be no depletion. This is achieved [with *chong wei* as in addition to stimulating movement it has a supplementing function. [Li] Shizhen: *Chong wei* seeds are sweet and slightly acrid. Their qi are warm. They are a yang in yin [substance]. They are a pharmaceutical drug for the hand and foot ceasing yin conduits. Those [of *chong wei* herbs] with white flowers enter the qi section. Those [of *chong wei* herbs] with purple flowers enter the blood section. They serve to cure irregular [movements] in the conduit vessels of females, and they occupy a wondrous rank for all types of diseases related to blood and qi [disorder] prior to birth. Still, they are rarely acknowledged and resorted to in medicinal recipes. [I, myself, Li] Shizhen have continuously used them together with all the pharmaceutical drugs of the "[decoction with] four items"[113] and nutgrass [root] to cure people, and they have often shown to be effective. The fact is, the [heart] enclosing network generates blood and the liver stores blood. This item [*chong wei*]

112 *Beng zhong* 崩中, "collapsing center," excessive vaginal bleeding outside of a menstruation period. BCGM Dict I, 58.

113 Ingredients include *paeonia* root, Chinese foxglove rhizome, Chinese *angelica* root and *ligusticum* root.

can quicken the blood and supplement yin [qi]. Hence it is able to brighten the eyes and boost the essence/sperm, to regulate [movement in the conduits] and to cure all diseases of females. Mr. Li Dongyuan says: "For an extension of the eye's pupils one must not use *chong wei* seeds because its acrid [flavor] and warm [nature] control dispersion and can assist fire. Chinese *angelica* [root] is acrid and warm, but at the same time it is bitter and sweet and can harmonize blood. Therefore it is not forbidden [treat pupil extension]." I say, when the eyes are supplied with blood they can see. *Chong wei* lets the blood move very fast. In the case of an extension of the pupils, the blood is insufficient. This is why it is forbidden [to use *chong wei*]; not because it assists fire. It is suitable for eye diseases related to sluggish blood. Hence it is said "to brighten the eyes."

15-17-02
莖 *Jing*
Stem [of *chong wei*].

【大明曰】苗、葉、根同功。

Da Ming: The seedling, the leaves and the root have the same [therapeutic] potential.

【氣味】【藏器曰】寒。【時珍曰】莖、葉：味辛、微苦。花：味微苦、甘。根：味甘。並無毒。【鏡源曰】制硫黄、雌黄、砒石。

Qi and Flavor. [Chen] Cangqi: Cold. [Li] Shizhen: Stem and leaves: Flavor acrid, slightly bitter. Flowers: Flavor slightly bitter, sweet. Root: Flavor sweet. All nonpoisonous. *Jing yuan*: It checks [the effects of] sulphur, realgar and arsenic.

【主治】癮瘮，可作浴湯。本經。擣汁服，主浮腫，下水，消惡毒丁腫、乳癰、丹遊等毒，并傅之。又服汁，主子死腹中及產後血脹悶。滴汁入耳中，主聤耳。擣傅蛇虺毒。蘇恭。入面藥，令人光澤，治粉刺。藏器。活血破血，調經解毒，治胎漏產難，胎衣不下，血運血風血痛，崩中漏下，尿血瀉血，疳痢痔疾，打撲内損瘀血，大便小便不通。時珍。

Control. For hidden papules[114] it can be used to prepare a hot bath. *Ben jing*. Pounded and the resulting juice ingested it controls surface swelling, discharges water and dissolves all the poison associated with pin[-illness][115] swelling with malign

114 *Yin zhen* 癮疹, "dormant papules," identical to *feng zhen* 風疹, "wind papules," a condition brought forth by wind evil, of eruptive skin papules of different sizes, accompanied by unbearable itching. If scratched they rise further. BCGM Dict. I, 172.

115 *Ding* 丁, "pin[-illness]," also *ding* 疔, "pin-illness," refers to a deep-reaching and festering hardness in a tissue, eventually rising above the skin like a pinhead. BCGM Dict I, 127-129.

poison, breast obstruction-illness[116] and roaming cinnabar [poison].[117] For all these it is to be applied [externally to the affected region]. Also, the juice ingested serves to control a child that has died in the abdomen, and blood related distension and heart-pressure after delivery. The juice dripped into the ears controls festering ears. Pounded [to a pulp] it is applied [to regions affected by] the poison of snakes and venomous vipers. Su Gong. Added to facial medication, it lets one regain glossiness and serves to cure acne. [Chen] Cangqi. It quickens the blood and breaks through blood [accumulation]. It regulates the [movement in the] conduits and resolves poison. It serves to cure fetal leakage and difficult birth, when the placenta fails to be discharged, blood[-induced brain] movement,[118] blood wind[119] and blood [disorder] pain, collapsing center[120] and leakage discharge, urination with blood and outflow with blood, *gan*-illness,[121] free-flux illness and piles ailment, stagnating blood resulting from blows, falls and internal injury, as well as blocked defecation and urination. [Li] Shizhen.

【發明】【時珍曰】益母草之根、莖、花、葉、實，並皆入藥，可同用。若治手、足厥陰血分風熱，明目益精，調女人經脉，則單用茺蔚子爲良。若治腫毒瘡瘍，消水行血，婦人胎產諸病，則宜並用爲良。蓋其根莖花葉專于行，而子則行中有補故也。

Explication. [Li] Shizhen: Root, stem, flowers, leaves and fruit of *yi mu cao* are all added to medication. Their possible usages are identical. If it is required to cure wind and heat affecting the blood section of the hand and foot ceasing yin [conduits], to brighten the eyes, to boost the essence/sperm, and to regulate [the movement]

---

116 *Ru yong* 乳癰, "breast obstruction-illness," a condition of acute putrefication of a woman's breast. Often encountered if a woman, following delivery, experiences *chui nai* 吹奶, "inflated breast," or *du ru* 妒乳, "jealousy breast." BCGM Dict I, 412.

117 *Dan you* 丹游, "roaming cinnabar [poison]," identical to *Chi you dan du* 赤游丹毒," red roaming cinnabar poison," a condition of *dan du* 丹毒, "cinnabar poison," with rashes that seem to be hiding. They move here and there and have no permanent location. BCGM Dict I, 89.

118 *Xue yun* 血運, "blood[-induced brain] movements;" a condition of sudden vertigo brought forth by sudden and violent depletion of qi and blood following parturition. [Patients] pant and vomit. In severe cases this includes a clouded mind. BCGM Dict I, 602.

119 *Xue feng* 血風, "blood wind," a condition brought about by an intrusion of wind evil qi into an unbalanced state of qi and blood, mostly in women. BCGM Dict I, 594.

120 *Beng zhong* 崩中, "collapsing center," excessive vaginal bleeding outside of a menstruation period. BCGM Dict I, 58.

121 *Gan* 疳, "*gan*-illness," also: "sweets-illness," involves several complaints that affect children and adults, with causes and conditions too different to fall into a known disease category. BCGM Dict I, 180–188.

in the conduit vessels of women, then it is good to resort to *chong wei* seeds only. If it is intended to cure sores and ulcers with swelling and poison, to disperse water, quicken the blood and [to treat] all types of diseases of women related to pregnancy and birth, then it is good to use all of them together. The fact is, root, stem, flowers and leaves especially serve to stimulate movement, while the seeds in addition to stimulating movement have a supplementing function.

【附方】舊十四，新七。

Added Recipes. 14 of old. Seven newly [recorded].

濟陰返魂丹。昝殷產寶曰：此方，乃吉安文江高師禹備禮求于名醫所得者，其效神妙，活人甚多，能治婦人胎前產後諸疾危證。用野天麻，又名益母，又名火杴，又名負擔，即茺蔚子也。葉似艾葉，莖類火麻，方梗凹面，四五六月節節開花，紅紫色如蓼花，南北隨處皆有，白花者不是。于端午、小暑，或六月六日花正開時，連根收采，陰乾，用葉及花、子。忌鐵器，以石器碾爲細末，煉蜜丸如彈子大，隨證嚼服，用湯使。其根燒存性爲末，酒服，功與黑神散不相上下。其藥不限丸數，以病愈爲度。或丸如梧子大，每服五七十丸。又可搗汁濾净，熬膏服之。

The "elixir to support yin [qi] and let the *hun*-soul return." Zan Yin, *Chan bao*: This recipe was obtained by Gao Shiyu of Wen jiang in Ji an after he had supported his request by showing his respect to a famous physician. Its effects are divinely wondrous. It has kept many people alive and is able to cure critical conditions associated with all types of diseases of women prior to and after birth. It is based on *ye tian ma* 野天麻, also named *yi mu* 益母, *huo xian* 火杴 and *fu dan* 負擔, which are *chong wei* 茺蔚 seeds. The leaves are similar to common mugwort leaves; the stem resembles that of hemp. It has a square stalk and an indented surface. During the fourth, fifth and sixth month always two nodes open flowers. They are of a red-purple color similar to those of knotweed. They are found everywhere, in the North and in the South. Those with white flowers are not the ones discussed here. On the fifth day of the fifth month, at the solar term Minor Heat (July 7) and on the sixth day of the sixth month, when the flowers are truly open, collect [the herb] with the root and dry it in the yin (i. e., shade). When using the leaves, the flowers and the seeds, avoid iron utensils and pound them in a stoneware utensil to fine powder to be formed with heat refined honey to pills the size of bullets. Chew and ingest them as required by the individual illness condition [as listed below], and send them down with hot, boiled water. Burn the root with its nature retained and [grind it into] powder. It is to be ingested with wine. Its [therapeutic] potential is not better or worse than that of the "black spirit powder."[122] The quantity of pills resorted to as medication is not limited [to any definite number]. The healing of the diseases determines the limit. If the pills are prepared the size of *wu* seeds, each time ingest 50 to 70 pills. It is also possible to pound [the substances] to obtain a juice. This is strained to obtain a clear liquid that is then heated to generate a paste for ingestion. [The recipe is applied for the following conditions as indicated.]

胎前臍腹痛，或作聲者，米飲下。

Pain prior to birth in the navel and abdominal region, sometimes with sounds. Send it down with a rice beverage.

胎前產後，臍腹刺痛，胎動不安，下血不止，當歸湯下。

A piercing pain in the navel and abdominal region prior to and after birth, a fetus movement that does not calm down, a discharge of blood that does not end. Send it down with a Chinese *angelica* decoction.

產後，以童子小便化下一丸，能安魂定魄，血氣自然調順，諸病不生。又能破血痛，養脉息，調經絡，並溫酒下。

After delivery, one pill dissolved in boys' urine can pacify a *hun*-soul and stabilize the *po*-soul. Blood and qi will return to order by themselves and no disease will develop. It is also able to break through painful blood [accumulation], nourish the pulsating [movements in the] vessels, and regulate the [movement in the] conduits and network [vessels]. For all these send it down with warm wine.

胎衣不下及横生不順，死胎不下，經日脹滿，心悶心痛，並用炒鹽湯下。

When the placenta fails to be discharged, when [a child] is born in a not agreeable transverse position, when a dead fetus fails to be discharged, for distension and a sensation of fullness during menstruation, as well as for heart-pressure and heart pain, for all these send it down with a decoction of stir-fried salt.

產後血運，眼黑血熱，口渴煩悶，如見鬼神，狂言不省人事，以童子小便和酒化下。

Blood[-induced brain] movement[123] following birth, blackened eyes related to blood heat, thirst and vexing heart-pressure, if one sees demon-spirits, talks mad-

122 The ingredients of the "black spirit powder," *hei shen san* 黑神散, include: Black soybeans, Chinese foxglove rhizome, Chinese *angelica* root, unscraped bark of cinnamom tree, prepared ginger, prepared *glycyrrhiza* root, paeonia root and cattail pollen.

123 *Xue yun* 血運, "blood[-induced brain] movements;" a condition of sudden vertigo brought forth by sudden and violent depletion of qi and blood following parturition. [Patients] pant and vomit. In severe cases this includes a clouded mind. BCGM Dict I, 602.

ly and does not know other persons or anything else, send it down dissolved in a mixture of boys' urine and wine.

產後結成血塊，臍腹奔痛，時發寒熱，有冷汗，或面垢顏赤，五心煩熱，並用童子小便、酒下，或薄荷自然汁下。

Bound [qi] causing blood clots after birth, with a running pain in the navel and abdominal region, recurring outbreaks of cold and heat, cold sweat, a dirty complexion and red face, as well as the five types of heart vexation with heat. For all these send it down with boys' urine and wine. Or send it down with the natural juice of mint.

產後惡露不盡，結滯刺痛，上衝心胸滿悶，童子小便、酒下。

Unending malign lochia after birth, with bound, sluggish [qi] causing a piercing pain, and rushing upward to the heart and chest causing a sensation of fullness and heart-pressure. Send it down with boys' urine and wine.

產後瀉血水，以棗湯下。

Outflow with blood and water after birth. Send it down with a Chinese date decoction.

產後痢疾，米湯下。

Free-flux illness after birth. Send it down with a rice decoction.

產後血崩漏下，糯米湯下。

Blood collapse[124] and leakage discharge after birth. Send it down with a glutinous rice decoction.

產後赤白帶下，煎膠艾湯下。

Red and white [outflow from] below the belt after birth. Send it down with the "decoction with [donkey hide] glue and mugwort [leaves]."

月水不調，温酒下。

Irregular menstruation. Send it down with warm wine.

產後中風，牙關緊急，半身不遂，失音不語，童便、酒下。

Being struck by wind after birth, clenched jaws, one half of the body paralyzed, and an inability to speak. Send it down with boys' urine and wine.

---

124 *Xue beng* 血崩, blood collapse. Excessive vaginal bleeding, identical to *beng zhong* 崩中, collapsing center. BCGM Dict I, 594; 58.

產後氣喘欬嗽，胸膈不利，惡心吐酸水，面目浮腫，兩脇疼痛，舉動失力，温酒下。

Panting and cough after birth, with the movement through chest and diaphragm blocked, nausea, spitting of sour water, face and eyes with surface swelling, the two flanks aching and no strength left to rise and move. Send it down with warm wine.

產後月内欬嗽，自汗發熱，久則變爲骨蒸，童便、酒下。

Cough within the first month after birth, with spontaneous sweating and heat effusion, which after a long time changes to bone steaming.[125] Send it down with boys' urine and wine.

產後鼻衄，舌黑口乾，童便、酒下。

Nosebleed following birth, with a black tongue and a dry mouth. Send it down with boys' urine and wine.

產後兩太陽穴痛，呵欠心忪，氣短羸瘦，不思飲食，血風身熱，手足頑麻，百節疼痛，並米飲化下。

When following birth the two major yang [needle insertion] holes (i. e., the temples) ache, [patients] breathe out, yawn and are agitated, with shortness of [breath] qi and emaciation, no desire to drink and eat, body heat with blood wind,[126] numbness of hands and feet and all the hundred joints aching, for all these send it down dissolved in a rice beverage.

產後大小便不通，煩躁口苦者，薄荷湯下。

Blocked major [defecation] and minor [urination] relief after birth, with vexing restlessness and a bitter taste in the mouth. Send it down with a mint decoction.

婦人久無子息，温酒下。

A woman that does not have a child for a long time. Send it down with warm wine.

益母膏。近效方治產婦諸疾及折傷内損有瘀血，每天陰則痛，神方也。三月采益母草，一名負擔，一名夏枯草，連根、葉、莖、花洗擇令净，於箔上攤暴水乾，以竹刀切長五寸，勿用鐵刀，置於大鍋中，以水浸過二三寸，煎煮，候草爛水減三之二，漉去草，取汁約五六斗，入盆中澄半日，以綿濾去濁滓，以清汁入釜中，慢火煎取一斗，如稀餳狀，瓷瓶封收。每

125 *Gu zheng* 骨蒸, "bone steaming," 1.) a condition of an infectious consumptive disease with a development of vexing heat in the afternoon. 2.) An illness sign of heat and vexation with a feeling as if this originated in the bones. BCGM Dict I, 197.

126 *Xue feng* 血風, "blood wind," a condition brought about by an intrusion of wind evil qi into an unbalanced state of qi and blood, mostly in women. BCGM Dict I, 594.

取梨大，暖酒和服，日再服。或和羹粥亦可。如遠行，即更煉至可丸收之。服至七日，則疼漸平復也。產婦惡露不盡及血運，一二服便瘥。其藥無忌。又能治風，益心力。外臺秘要。

Yi mu paste. A divine recipe [recommended by the] *Jin xiao fang* to cure all types of illnesses of women giving birth as well as stagnating blood related to fracture damage and internal injury that are painful whenever a day is yin (i. e., cloudy, without sunshine). In the third month collect *yi mu cao* 益母草, also called *fu dan* 負擔 and *xia ku cao* 夏枯草, together with root, leaves, stem and flowers, and wash them clean. Spread them on bamboo trays to dry them in the sun. With a bamboo knife cut them into five *cun* long pieces; do not use iron knives. Then place them into a large pot, soak them in water exceeding them by two or three *cun*. Boil this until the herbs have become pulpy and the water has decreased by two thirds. Then strain off the herbs and pour about five to six *dou* of the juice into another pot where it is left to become clear for half a day. With silk strain [the liquid off] to remove the dregs and fill the clear juice into a cauldron. Boil it with a slow fire down to one *dou*, with a consistency similar to that of watery malt sugar. Keep it sealed in a porcelain jar. For each [application] take as much as the size of a pear and ingest it mixed with warm wine. To be ingested twice a day. It may also be [ingested] mixed with a congee. If one is to go on a long journey, it can be processed further with heat to prepare pills that can be taken along. Ingested for up to seven days, it diminishes pain and restores health. Women with malign lochia that fails to end and also those with blood[-induced brain] movement,[127] will be healed after ingesting it once or twice. This medication is not tied to any prohibitions. It is also able to cure wind [intrusion] and it boosts the strength of the heart. *Wai tai mi yao.*

女人難產。益母草搗汁七大合，煎減半，頓服立止。無新者，以乾者一大握，水七合，煎服。韋宙獨行方。

Women with difficult birth. Pound *yi mu cao* to obtain seven generous *ge* of juice, boil it down to one half and [let the patient] ingest it all at once. This will end [the pain] immediately. If no new/fresh [*yi mu cao*] is available, boil one large handful in seven *ge* of water and let her ingest this. Wei Zhou, *Du xing fang.*

胎死腹中。益母草搗熟，以暖水少許，和絞取汁，頓服之。韋宙獨行方。

127 *Xue yun* 血運, "blood[-induced brain] movements" a condition of sudden vertigo brought forth by sudden and violent depletion of qi and blood following parturition. [Patients] pant and vomit. In severe cases this includes a clouded mind. BCGM Dict I, 602.

A fetus has died in the abdomen. Pound *yi mu cao* to a pulp and wring it with a small amount of warm water to obtain a juice. [Let the woman] ingest it all at once. Wei Zhou, *Du xing fang*.

產後血運，心氣欲絶。益母草研汁，服一盞，絶妙。子母秘録。

Blood[-induced brain] movement[128] following birth, with the [movement of] heart qi about to be interrupted. Grind *yi mu cao* to obtain a juice and [let the woman] ingest one cup. Definitely wondrous. *Zi mu mi lu*.

產後血閉不下者。益母草汁一小盞，入酒一合，温服。聖惠方。

Blocked blood following birth that fails to be discharged. One small cup of *yi mu zhi* juice is added to one *ge* of wine. [Let the woman] ingest this warm. *Sheng hui fang*.

帶下赤白。益母草花開時采，搗爲末。每服二錢，食前温湯下。集驗方。

Red and white [outflow] from below the belt. Collect *yi mu cao* when its flowers have opened and pound it into powder. Each time [let the woman] ingest two *qian*, to be sent down prior to a meal with warm, boiled water. *Ji yan fang*.

小便尿血。益母草搗汁，服一升立差。此蘇澄方也。外臺秘要。

Urination with blood. Pound *yi mu cao* to obtain a juice and ingest one *sheng*. Immediately effective. This is a recipe of Su Cheng. *Wai tai mi yao*.

赤白雜痢困重者。益母草日乾，陳鹽梅燒存性，等分爲末。每服三錢，白痢乾薑湯、赤痢甘草湯下。名二靈散。衞生家寶方。

Mixed red and white free-flux illness with considerable hardship. [Grind] equal amounts of dried *yi mu cao* and long-stored salted plums, burned with their nature retained, into powder. Each time ingest three *qian*. In the case of white free-flux illness to be sent down with a dried ginger decoction. In the case of red free-flux illness to be sent down with a *glycyrrhiza* [root] decoction. This [recipe] is called the "powder with the two magic [ingredients]." *Wei sheng jia bao fang*.

小兒疳痢垂死者。益母草嫩葉，同米煮粥食之，取足，以瘥爲度，甚佳。飲汁亦可。廣利方。

Gan-illness[129] and free-flux illness of children bringing them close to death. Boil tender *yi mu cao* leaves with rice to prepare a congee and [let the patient] eat it.

128 *Xue yun* 血運, "blood[-induced brain] movements" a condition of sudden vertigo brought forth by sudden and violent depletion of qi and blood following parturition. [Patients] pant and vomit. In severe cases this includes a clouded mind. BCGM Dict I, 602.

129 *Gan* 疳, "*gan*-illness," also: "sweets-illness," involves several complaints that affect children and adults, with causes and conditions too different to fall into a known disease

Prepare a sufficient quantity to [feed the child] until a cure is achieved. Very fine. It may also drink the juice. *Guang li fang*.

痔疾下血。益母草葉，擣汁飲之。食醫心鏡。

Piles with blood discharge. Pound *yi mu cao* leaves and drink the juice. *Shi yi xin jing*.

一切癰瘡。婦人妬乳乳癰，小兒頭瘡及浸淫黄爛熱瘡，疥疽陰蝕。並用天麻草切五升，以水一斗半，煮一斗，分數次洗之以殺痒。千金方。

All types of obstruction-illness sores.[130] Jealousy breast[131] and breast obstruction-illness[132] of women. Head sores of children and heat sores sodden with yellow [liquid], *jie*-illness,[133] impediment-illness[134] and yin (i. e., vaginal) erosion. For all these cut *tian ma cao* into pieces and boil five *sheng* in one and a half *dou* of water down to one *dou*. Divide [the liquid] into several portions to wash [the affected region]. This will kill the itch. *Qian jin fang*.

急慢疔瘡。聖惠方用益母草搗封之，仍絞五合服，即消。

Acute or chronic pin-illness[135] sores. The *Sheng hui fang* [recommends to] pound *yi mu cao* [to a pulp] and use it to seal [the affected region]. Also, wring it [to obtain] five *ge* [of juice] and ingest it. This will dissolve [the pin].

醫方大成用益母草四月連花采之，燒存性。先以小尖刀十字劃開疔根，令血出。次遶根開破，捻出血，拭乾。以稻草心蘸藥撚入瘡口，令到底。良久，當有紫血出，捻令血净，再撚藥入，見紅血乃止。一日夜撚藥三五

---

category. BCGM Dict I, 180-188.

130 *Yong* 癰, "obstruction-illness," refers to an obstruction of vessels or other ducts inside the body. Qi rushing against the obstruction may cause a local swelling and eventually break through the surface to cause an abscess. BCGM Dict I, 641.

131 *Du ru* 妒(妬)乳, "jealousy breast," a condition with milk blocked after delivery and the breasts turning red and swelling, being hot and painful, accompanied by fever. BCGM Dict I, 135.

132 *Ru yong* 乳癰, "breast obstruction-illness," a condition of acute putrefication of a woman's breast. Often encountered if a woman, following delivery, experiences *chui nai* 吹奶, "inflated breast," or *du ru* 妒乳, "jealousy breast." BCGM Dict I, 412.

133 *Jie*-illness 疥, vaguely identifiable skin ailment. BCGM Dict I, 249.

134 *Ju* 疽, "impediment-illness," refers to an obstruction of vessels or other ducts inside the body. Qi rushing against the impediment may cause a local swelling and eventually break through the surface to cause an abscess. BCGM Dict I, 277.

135 *Ding* 丁, "pin[-illness]," also *ding* 疔, "pin-illness," refers to a deep-reaching and festering hardness in a tissue, eventually rising above the skin like a pinhead. BCGM Dict I, 127-129.

度。重者二日根爛出，輕者一日出。有瘡根脹起，即是根出，以針挑之。出後仍傅藥，生肌易愈。忌風寒、房室、酒肉、一切毒物。

The *Yi fang da cheng* [recommends to] collect *yi mu cao* with flowers in the fourth month and burn it with its nature retained. First cut a cross with a small, sharp knife to lay free the root of the pin-illness and cause a bleeding. Then cut around the root, sever it and squeeze it until no more blood appears. Twist the [burned *yi mu cao*] drug with the fingers and insert it [into the wound]. Stop when red blood appears. On one day and one night insert the twisted drug three to five times. In severe cases, the root is softened and will come out the second day. In mild cases it comes out within one day. When the root of the sore swells and rises, this is a sign that the root comes out. Now pick it with a needle. Once it is removed apply the drug [to the open wound]. This will generate muscles and an easy cure is achieved. [During the treatment] wind and cold, sex, wine and meat and all poisonous items are forbidden.

癤毒已破。益母草搗敷甚妙。斗門方。

Pimples with poison that have broken open. Pound *yi mu cao* and apply it [to the affected region]. Very wondrous. *Dou men fang*.

勒乳成癰。益母爲末，水調塗乳上，一宿自瘥。生擣亦得。聖惠方。

A tightly strapped breast develops an obstruction-illness.[136] [Grind] *yi mu cao* into powder, mix it with water and apply it to the breast. A cure will be achieved within one night. It is also possible to pound fresh [*yi mu cao* for an application to the breast]. *Sheng hui fang*.

喉閉腫痛。益母草擣爛，新汲水一盌，絞濃汁頓飲，隨吐愈。冬月用根。衛生易簡方。

Throat blockage with painful swelling. Pound *yi mu cao* to a pulp and squeeze it with one bowl of newly drawn water to obtain a thick juice. Drink it all at once. This will cause vomiting, and this results in a cure. In winter, use the root. *Wei sheng yi jian fang*.

聤耳出汁。茺蔚莖葉汁滴之。聖惠方。

Festering ears emitting a juice. [Pound] *chong wei* stems and leaves to obtain a juice and drip this [into the affected ears]. *Sheng hui fang*.

---

136 *Yong* 癰, "obstruction-illness," refers to an obstruction of vessels or other ducts inside the body. Qi rushing against the obstruction may cause a local swelling and eventually break through the surface to cause an abscess. BCGM Dict I, 641.

粉刺黑斑。閨閣事宜云：五月五日收帶根天麻紫花者，晒乾燒灰。以商陸根搗自然汁，加酸醋和，搜灰作餅，炭火煅過收之。半年方用入面藥，甚能潤肌。

Acne with black dermal spots. The *Gui ge shi yi* states: "On the fifth day of the fifth month collect purple flower *tian ma* with its root, dry it in the sun and burn it to ashes. Pound Indian pokeweed roots to obtain its natural juice, add sour vinegar and mix this with the ashes to prepare a cake. Calcine [the cake] with a charcoal fire and keep it. Half a year later add it to facial medication. It is very much able to moisten the muscles."

蘇頌曰：唐天后鍊益母草澤面法，五月五日采根苗具者，勿令着土，暴乾搗羅，以麪水和成團，如鷄子大，再暴乾。仍作一爐，四旁開竅，上下置火，安藥中央。大火燒一炊久，即去大火，留小火養之，勿令火絶。經一伏時出之，瓷器中研，治篩，再研，三日收用，如澡豆法，日用。

Su Song: The method applied by the Tang Empress to provide glossiness to her face with refined *yi mu cao*. On the fifth day of the fifth month collect the root with the seedling attached, and make sure that they are not stained with soil. Dry them in the sun, pound them [to powder and pass it] through a screen, mix this with wheat flour and water and form a ball, the size of a chicken egg. Then dry this again in the sun. Now build a stove with openings on all four sides. Add fire above and below and place the medication into the middle. Light a big fire for as long as it takes to have a meal, and remove the big fire. Then nourish a small fire and do not let it go out. Remove [the medication] after a full day and night, grind it in a porcelain utensil, pass it through a sieve and grind it again. Store it for three days before using it. Apply it daily, just like bathing beans.[137]

一方：每十兩，加滑石一兩，臙脂一錢。

Another recipe. To each 10 *liang* add one *liang* of talc and one *qian* of rouge.

馬咬成瘡。苦低草，切細，和醋炒塗之。孫真人方。

Sores/wounds resulting from a horse bite. Cut *ku di cao* (i. e., *chong wei*) to fine pieces, mix them with vinegar, stir-fry this and apply this [to the affected region]. A recipe of Sun zhenren.

新生小兒。益母草五兩，煎水浴之，不生瘡疥。簡要濟衆。

137 *Zao dou* 澡豆, "bathing beans," an ancient detergent prepared from pig pancreas and bean powder.

For newborns. Boil five *liang* of *yi mu cao* in water and wash [the child]. It will never develop sores with *jie*-illness.[138] *Jian yao ji chong*.

15-18
鏨菜音慙拾遺
Can cai, read *can*. FE *Shi yi*.

***Leonurus pseudomacranthus* Kitag.**

【集解】【藏器曰】鏨菜生江南陰地，似益母，方莖對節，白花。【時珍曰】此即益母之白花者，乃爾雅所謂"蓷"是也。其紫花者，爾雅所謂蓷是也。蓷、蓷皆同一音，乃一物二種。故此條亦主血病，與益母功同。郭璞獨指白花者爲益母，昝殷又謂白花者非益母，皆欠詳審。嫩苗可食，故謂之菜。寇宗奭言茺蔚嫩苗可煮食，正合此也。

Collected Explanations. [Chen] Cangqi: *Can cai* grows in yin [(i. e., shady) locations] of Jiang nan. It is similar to Siberian motherwort. It has a square stem, with white flowers growing facing each other at the nodes. Those with purple flowers are the ones called *tui* 蓷 in the *Er ya*. *Tui* 蓷 and *tui* 蓷 are read alike. These are two kinds of one item. Hence the [item discussed in] the present entry also serves to control blood diseases, identical to Siberian motherwort. Guo Pu identifies only those with white flowers as Siberian motherwort, while Zan Yin says that those with white flowers are not Siberian motherwort. Both failed to examine them carefully. [*Can cai*] has tender seedlings that are edible. Hence it is called *cai* 菜, "vegetable." Kou Zongshi says: "The tender seedlings of Siberian motherwort can be boiled to be eaten." This is exactly identical to the [item discussed] here.

15-18-01
苗 *Miao*

Seedling [of *can cai*].

【氣味】辛，平，無毒。

Qi and Flavor. Acrid, balanced, nonpoisonous.

【主治】破血，產後腹痛，煮汁服。藏器。

Control. It breaks through blood [accumulation]. Abdominal pain after delivery. Boil it and ingest the juice. [Chen] Cangqi.

---

138 *Jie*-illness 疥, vaguely identifiable skin ailment. BCGM Dict I, 249.

15-19
薇銜薇音眉本經上品
Mei xian, 薇 read *mei*. FE *Ben jing*, upper rank.

Unidentified.

【釋名】麋銜本經、鹿銜唐本、吴風草唐本、無心吴普、無顛吴普、承膏別録、承膱吴普。【恭曰】南人謂之吴風草。一名鹿銜草，言鹿有疾，銜此草即瘥也。【時珍曰】據蘇説，則薇銜、麋銜當作鹿銜也。鹿、麋一類也。按酈道元水經註云：魏興錫山多生薇銜草，有風不偃，無風獨摇。則吴風亦當作無風，乃通。【藏器曰】一名無心草，非草之無心者，方藥少用。

Explanation of Names. *Mi xian* 麋銜, "Pére David's deer bit," *Ben jing*. *Lu xian* 鹿銜, "deer bit," *Tang ben*. *Wu feng cao* 吴風草, *Tang ben*. *Wu xin* 無心, Wu Pu. *Wu dian* 無顛, Wu Pu. *Cheng gao* 承膏, *Bie lu*. *Cheng ji* 承膱, Wu Pu. [Su] Gong: The people in the South call it *wu feng cao* 吴風草, and also *lu xian cao* 鹿銜草. That is to say, when deer, *lu* 鹿, have an illness they use this herb as a bit, *xian* 銜, and it will be healed. [Li] Shizhen: According to Su [Gong], *mei xian* 薇銜 and *mi xian* 麋銜 should be written *lu xian* 鹿銜. Deer, *lu* 鹿, and *mi* 麋, Pére David's deer, belong to the same group. According to Li Daoyuan in his *Shui jing zhu*, "plenty of *wei xian cao* grows on Mount Xi shan in Wei xing. When wind blows it does not lie down. When there is no wind, *wu feng* 無風, it sways by itself." Hence *wu feng* 吴風 should be written *wu feng* 無風, "in the absence of wind." That makes sense. [Chen] Cangqi: It is also called *wu xin cao* 無心草, "herb without 'heart'." But this is not an herb "without heart." It is seldem resorted to in medicinal recipes.

【集解】【别録曰】薇銜生漢中川澤及寃句、邯鄲。七月采莖葉，陰乾。【恭曰】此草叢生，似茺蔚及白頭翁，其葉有毛，赤莖。又有大小二種，楚人謂大者爲大吴風草，小者爲小吴風草。【保昇曰】葉似茺蔚，叢生有毛，其花黄色，其根赤黑色。

Collected Explanations. *Bie lu*: *Wei xian* grows in rivers and marshlands of Han zhong, and also in Yuan ju and Han dan. The stem and the leaves are collected in the seventh month. They are dried in the yin (i. e., shade). [Su] Gong: This herb grows in clusters. It is similar to Siberian motherwort and *pulsatilla* [herb]. Its leaves have hair; the stem is red. There are two kinds; one large, one small. The people in Chu call the large ones *da wu feng cao* 大吴風草, "large *wu feng* herb," and the small ones *xiao wu feng cao* 小吴風草, "small *wu feng* herb." [Han] Baosheng: The leaves are similar to those of Siberian motherwort; they grow as clusters and have hair. The flowers are yellow. The root is red-black.

15-19-01
莖、葉 ***Jing, Ye***
Stem, leaves [of *wei xian*].

【氣味】苦，平，無毒。【别録曰】微寒。【之才曰】得秦皮良。

Qi and Flavor. Bitter, acrid, nonpoisonous. *Bie lu*: Slightly cold. [Xu] Zhicai: Combined with *fraxinus* bark, [their therapeutic effects are] good.

【主治】風濕痺，歷節痛，驚癇吐舌，悸氣賊風，鼠瘻癰腫。本經。暴癥，逐水，療痿蹷。久服輕身明目。别録。婦人服之，絶産無子。藏器。煎水，洗瘰疽、甲疽、惡瘡。時珍。出外科精義。

Control. Blockage related to wind and moisture [intrusion]. Painful pervading joints [wind].[139] Fright epilepsy with tongue protrusion, palpitating qi,[140] robber wind,[141] mouse fistula[142] and obstruction-illness[143] swelling. *Ben jing*. Sudden concretion-illness. They eliminate water and heal dysfunction with an inability to walk. Ingested for long, they relieve the body of its weight and brighten the eyes. *Bie lu*. When women eat them, they will become infertile and have no children. [Chen] Cangqi. An aqueous decoction serves to wash [regions affected by] flaming-heat-illness and impediment-illness,[144] nails with impediment-illness and malign sores. [Li] Shizhen, quoted from *Wai ke jing yi*.

【發明】【時珍曰】麋銜乃素問所用治風病自汗藥，而後世不知用之，誠缺略也。素問：黄帝曰：有病身熱懈惰，汗出如浴，惡風少氣，此爲何病？岐伯曰：病名酒風。治之以澤瀉、术各三五分，麋銜五分，合以三指撮爲後飯。後飯者，先服藥也。

139 *Li jie [feng]* 歷節[風], pervading joints [wind], a condition of *tong feng* 痛風, "pain wind," characterized by spontaneous sweating, shortness of qi/breath, aching joints, and difficulties in bending and stretching. BCGM Dict I, 314.

140 *Ji qi* 悸氣, "palpitating qi," a condition with fright, fear and heart palpitation. BCGM Dict I, 240.

141 *Zei feng* 賊風, "robber wind," a condition caused by qi that appear in a season they do not belong to. More at BCGM Dict I, 667.

142 *Shu lou* 鼠瘻, "mouse fistula," BCGM Dict I, 466, identical to *luo li* 瘰癧, "scrofula pervasion-illnes."

143 *Yong* 癰, "obstruction-illness,"refers to an obstruction of vessels or other ducts inside the body. Qi rushing against the obstruction may cause a local swelling and eventually break through the surface to cause an abscess. BCGM Dict I, 641.

144 *Ju* 疽, "impediment-illness," refers to an obstruction of vessels or other ducts inside the body. Qi rushing against the impediment may cause a local swelling and eventually break through the surface to cause an abscess. BCGM Dict I, 277.

Explication. [Li] Shizhen: *Mi xian* is a pharmaceutical drug [recommended] in the *Su wen* for curing wind diseases and spontaneous sweating. But in later times nobody knew how to use it. What a loss! *Su wen*: "Huang Di: Someone suffers from [the following]: His body is hot and sluggish. Sweat leaves [his body] as if he had taken a bath. He has an aversion to wind and is short of [breath] qi. Which disease is that? Qi Bo: The disease is called 'wine wind.'[145] To cure it take three to five *fen* each of *alisma* [root] and *atractylodes* [rhizome], and five *fen* of *mi xian*. Mix them and take before meals as much as can be taken up with three fingers." *Hou fan* 後飯, "before meals," is to say: ingest the medication before [having a meal].

【附方】新二。

Added Recipes. Two newly [recorded].

年深惡瘡。無心草根、釣苓根、狼毒、白丁香各五錢，麝香一字，爲末摻之。

Malign sores lasting for years. [Grind] five *qian* each of *wu xin cao* root, *diao qin* root,[146] wolfsbane and male sparrow feces, and one *zi* of musk into powder and apply this [to the affected region].

又方：無心草根、乾薑各二錢，釣苓根三錢，爲末摻之。並外科精義。

Another recipe. [Grind] two *qian* each of *wu xin cao* root and dried ginger and three *qian* of *diao qin* root into powder and apply this [to the affected region]. Both: *Wai ke jing yi*.

小兒破傷風病，拘急口噤。没心草[147]半兩，白附子炮二錢半，爲末。每服一字，薄荷酒灌下。聖濟録。

Wound wind[148] disease of children, with cramps, tension and clenched jaw. [Grind] half a *liang* of *mei xin cao* and two and a half *qian* of white *aconitum* [accessory tuber] into powder. Each time [let the child] ingest one *zi*, to be sent down, force-fed, with mint wine. *Sheng ji lu*.

145 *Jiu feng* 酒風, "wine wind," a condition of a hot and sluggish body with heavy perspiration, an aversion to wind and short breath, brought forth by excessive consumption of alcoholic beverages. BCGM Dict I, 271. *Su wen* ch. 46. Paul U. Unschuld and Hermann Tessenow, *Huang Di Nei Jing Su Wen. An Annotated Translation of Huang Di's Inner Classic*, 2 vols. University of California Press, Berkeley and Los Angeles, 2011. Vol. 1, 685.

146 *Diao qin* 釣苓, Unidentified herb

147 *Mei xin cao* 没心草, "herb without heart," alternative writing of *wu xin cao* 無心草.

148 *Po shang feng* 破傷風, "wound wind," a condition of lockjaw, arched back rigidity and convulsions, resulting from wounds struck by wind. BCGM Dict I, 379.

【附録】
Appendix.

15-19-A01

無心草宋圖經 ***Wu xin cao*,** FE Song, *Tu jing*

Unidentified.

【頌曰】生秦州及商州，鳳翔各縣皆出之。三月開花，五月結實，六七月采根苗，陰乾用。性温，無毒。主積血，逐氣塊，益筋節，補虛損，潤顏色，療澼洩腹痛。【時珍曰】麋銜一名無心草，此草功用與之相近，其圖形亦相近，恐即一物也，故附之俟訪攷焉。鼠耳草亦名無心，與此不同。

[Su] Song: It grows in Qin zhou and Shang zhou, and comes from all the counties in Feng xiang. It opens flowers in the third month, and forms fruit in the fifth month. Root and seedling are collected in the sixth and seventh month. They are dried in the yin (i. e., shade) and then used [for therapeutic purposes]. Nature: Warm; nonpoisonous. They control accumulated blood, eliminate qi lumps, benefit sinews and joints, supplement depletion injury, moisten one's complexion and heal [intestinal] flush outflow with abdominal pain. [Li] Shizhen: *Mi xian* is also named *wu xin cao*. Their [therapeutic] potential and usages are quite similar, and so are their physical images. Presumably, they are one and the same item. Hence [*wu xin cao*] is added here pending further studies. Cudweed, too, is named *wu xin* 無心. It is different from [the item discussed] here.

15-20

夏枯草本經下品

***Xia ku cao*, FE *Ben jing*, lower rank.**

***Prunella vulgaris* L. Common selfheal herb.**

【釋名】夕句本經、乃東本經、燕面別録、鐵色草。【震亨曰】此草夏至後即枯。蓋禀純陽之氣，得陰氣則枯，故有是名。

Explanation of Names. *Xi ju* 夕句, *Ben jing*. *Nai dong* 乃東, *Ben jing*. *Yan mian* 燕面, "sparrow face," *Bie lu*. *Tie se cao* 鐵色草, "iron color herb." [Zhu] Zhenheng: This herbs withers in the aftermath of Summer Solstice. The fact is, it is endowed with pure yang qi. Once it is affected by yin qi it withers. Hence this name.

【集解】【別録曰】夏枯草生蜀郡川谷，四月采。【恭曰】處處有之，生平澤。【頌曰】冬至後生，葉似旋復。三月、四月開花作穗紫白色，似丹參花，結子亦作穗。五月便枯，四月采之。【時珍曰】原野間甚多，苗高一二尺許，其莖微方。葉對節生，似旋復葉而長大，有細齒，背白多故。

莖端作穗，長一二寸，穗中開淡紫小花，一穗有細子四粒。丹溪云無子，亦欠察矣。嫩苗瀹過，浸去苦味，油鹽拌之可食。

Collected Explanations. *Bie lu*: *Xia ku cao* grows in the river valleys of Shu jun. It is collected in the fourth month. [Su] Gong: It can be found everywhere. It grows in marshlands in the plains. [Su] Song: It grows after Winter Solstice. The leaves are similar to those of horseheal. It opens flowers in the third and fourth month forming purple-white spikes, similar to the flowers of Chinese sage. The seeds, too, form spikes. It begins to wither in the fifth month; it is collected in the fourth month. [Li] Shizhen: Originally, plenty of it grew in the open country. Its seedlings reach a height of more than one or two *chi*. The stems are almost square. The leaves grow in pairs facing each other at the nodes, similar to the leaves of horseheal, but longer and bigger, with fine teeth. They are white on the back with many lines.[149] Spikes form at the end of the stem, with a length of one to two *cun*. Inside the spikes small flowers open of a pale purple color. Each spike has four fine seed kernels. [Zhu] Danxi states: "It has no seeds." He did not examine it carefully. The tender seedlings are cleansed and soaked [in water] to eliminate their bitter flavor. Mixed with oil and salt they can be eaten.

【正誤】【宗奭曰】今謂之鬱臭。自秋便生，經冬不悴，春開白花，夏結子。【震亨曰】鬱臭草有臭味，即茺蔚是也。夏枯草無臭味，明是兩物。俱生於春。夏枯先枯而無子，鬱臭後枯而結子。

Correction of Errors. [Kou] Zongshi: Today it is called *yu chou* 鬱臭, "pent-up malodorous [qi]." It begins to grow in autumn and does not deteriorate throughout winter. In spring it opens white flowers. In summer it forms seeds. [Zhu] Zhenheng: The *yu chou* herb that has a malodorous flavor is *chong wei* 茺蔚, common motherwort. *Xia ku cao* has no malodorous flavor. Obviously, these are two different items. Both grow in spring. *Xia ku* is the first to wither and has no seeds. *Yu chou* withers later and forms seeds.

***Jing* 莖, *ye* 葉。**

Stem, leaf [of *xia ku*].

【氣味】苦、辛，寒，無毒。【之才曰】土瓜爲之使。伏汞砂。

Qi and Flavor. Bitter, acrid, cold, nonpoisonous. [Xu] Zhicai: Japanese snake gourd serves as their guiding [substance]. [Xia ku cao] suppresses the effects of mercury and cinnabar.

149 Instead of *gu* 故, the Zhang edition writes *wen* 紋. This makes sense and is adopted here.

【主治】寒熱，瘰癧鼠瘻，頭瘡，破癥，散癭結氣，脚腫濕痺，輕身。本經。

Control. Alternating sensations of cold and heat. Scrofula pervasion-illness,[150] mouse fistula,[151] head sores. [*Xia ku cao*] breaks through concretion-illness, dispels goiter with bound qi,[152] [cures] swollen legs and blockage related to [the presence of] moisture. It relieves the body of its weight. *Ben jing*.

【發明】【震亨曰】本草言夏枯草大治瘰癧，散結氣。有補養厥陰血脉之功，而不言及。觀其退寒熱，虚者可使。若實者以行散之藥佐之，外以艾灸，亦漸取效。【時珍曰】黎居士簡易方：夏枯草治目疼，用沙糖水浸一夜用，取其能解内熱、緩肝火也。樓全善云：夏枯草治目珠疼至夜則甚者，神效。或用苦寒藥點之反甚者，亦神效。蓋目珠連目本，即係也，屬厥陰之經。夜甚及點苦寒藥反甚者，夜與寒亦陰故也。夏枯禀純陽之氣，補厥陰血脉，故治此如神，以陽治陰也。一男子至夜目珠疼，連眉稜骨及頭半邊腫痛。用黄連膏點之反甚，諸藥不效。灸厥陰、少陽，疼隨止，半日又作，月餘。以夏枯草二兩，香附二兩，甘草四錢，爲末。每服一錢半，清茶調服。下咽則疼减半，至四五服良愈矣。

Explication. [Zhu] Zhenheng: The *Ben cao* says that *xia ku cao* is very capable of curing scrofula pervasion-illness and of dispersing bound qi.[153] Its potential of supplementing and nourishing the ceasing yin blood vessels is not recorded [in the *Ben cao*]. In view of its ability to push back cold and heat, it can be resorted to [to supplement] depletion. In the case of repletion, it should be assisted by pharmaceutical drugs that stimulate movement and disperse [evil qi]. If this is supported from the outside by cauterization with common mugwort [leaves], a gradual effect will be achieved. [Li] Shizhen: Li Jushi, *Jian yi fang*: "*Xia ku cao* serves to cure pain in the eyeballs. After soaking it in sugar water for one night one can use its ability to resolve internal heat and to calm down liver fire." Lou Quanshan states: "*Xia ku cao* serves to cure, with divine effects, pain in the eyeballs that increases in severity by night. When [pain in the eyeballs] is treated by dripping bitter and cold medication [into the eyes] with the adverse [effect that the pain] further increases in severity, [an application of *xia ku cao*] will be divinely effective, too. The fact is, the eyeballs

150 *Luo li* 瘰癧, "scrofula pervasion-illness," when two or more connected swellings of the size of plum or date kernels appear either on the neck or in the armpits, or somewhere else on the body. BCGM Dict I. 329.

151 *Shu lou* 鼠瘻, "mouse fistula," BCGM Dict I, 466, identical to *luo li* 瘰癧, "scrofula pervasion-illnes."

152 *Jie qi* 結氣, "bound qi," are pathological qi halting and congealing at any place in the body. BCGM Dict I, 240.

153 *Jie qi* 結氣, "bound qi," are pathological qi halting and congealing at any place in the body. BCGM Dict I, 240.

are tied to the base of the eyes by means of the '[eye] ribbons.'[154] They are linked to the ceasing yin conduits. When [the pain] is severe at night and one drips bitter and cold medication [into the eyes] and contrary [to one's intention, the pain] increases in severity, this is so because night and cold are both yin. *Xia ku cao* has pure yang qi. It supplements [qi in] the ceasing yin blood vessels. It is therefore divinely suitable to cure this, simply because this is to cure a yin condition with yang [qi]. There was a male who suffered from eyeball pain once the night began, reaching to the bone ridge behind the eyebrows and causing a swelling of one half of his head. When a *coptis* [rhizome] paste was applied [the pain] only increased in severity. All types of medication remained without effect. When the ceasing yin and minor yang [conduits] were cauterized, the pain ended but came back half a day later. This lasted for more than a month. [I suggested the following treatment]. [Grind] two *liang* of *xia ku cao*, two *liang* of *aconitum* [accessory tuber] and four *qian* of *glycyrrhiza* [root] into powder. Each time ingest one and a half *qian*. To be ingested mixed with clear tea. When this was sent down the throat, the pain subsided by one half. After four or five ingestions it was well healed."

【附方】舊一，新六。

Added Recipes. One of old. Six newly [recorded].

明目補肝。肝虛目睛痛，冷淚不止，筋脉痛，羞明怕日。夏枯草半兩，香附子一兩，爲末。每服一錢，臘茶湯調下。簡要濟衆。

To brighten they eyes by supplementing liver [qi]. When the liver [qi] are depleted and the eyes ache, with unending cold tearflow, painful sinews and vessels, fear of light and fear of sunlight. [Grind] half a *liang* of *xia ku cao* and one *liang* of nutgrass [root] into powder. Each time ingest one *qian*, to be sent down mixed with a *la* tea[155] decoction. *Jian yao ji chong*.

赤白帶下。夏枯草，花開時采，陰乾爲末。每服二錢，米飲下，食前。徐氏家傳方。

---

154 Instead of *ji* 即, the Zhang edition writes *gan* 肝, "liver." However, *Ling shu*, ch. 21, Han re bing 寒熱病, "Cold and Heat Disease, states *zu tai yang you tong xiang ru yu nao zhe zheng shu mu ben ming yue yan xi* 正屬足太陽有通項入于腦者正屬目本名曰眼系, "the foot major yang [conduit] passing through the neck to the brain is connected to the base of the eyes. This is named the 'eye ribbon,". That is, *ji* 即 may be an erroneous writing of *yan* 眼, "eye."

155 *La* tea, *la cha* 臘茶, lit: "tea of the 12th month," mentioned by Ouyang Xiu and Shen Kua during the Song era. As it is colored like melted wax it is also called *la cha* 蠟茶, "wax tea."

Red and white discharge from below the belt. Dry *xia ku cai*, collected after its flowers have opened, in the yin (i. e., shade) and [grind it into] powder. Each time ingest two *qian*. To be sent down with a rice beverage. Prior to meals. *Xu shi jia chuan fang*.

血崩不止。夏枯草爲末，每服方寸匕，米飲調下。聖惠方。

Unending blood collapse.[156] [Grind] *xia ku cao* into powder. Each time ingest the amount held by a square cun spoon. To be sent down mixed with a rice beverage. *Sheng hui fang*.

產後血運，心氣欲絶者。夏枯草擣絞汁，服一琖，大妙。徐氏家傳方。

Blood[-induced brain] movement[157] after birth, with the [movement of] heart qi about to be interrupted. Pound *xia ku cai*, and wring [the pulp] to obtain a juice. Ingest one small cup. Highly wondrous. *Xu shi jia chuan fang*.

撲傷金瘡。夏枯草口嚼爛，署上即愈。衛生易簡方。

Harm caused by a blow, wounds caused by metal objects/weapons. Chew *xia ku cao* to obtain a pulpy substance and place it on [the affected region]. This will result in a cure. *Wei sheng yi jian fang*.

汗斑白點。夏枯草煎濃汁，日日洗之。乾坤生意。

Sweat macules with white spots. Boil *xia ku cao* to obtain a thick juice and wash the [affected region] every day. *Qian kun sheng yi*.

瘰癧馬刀。不問已潰未潰，或日久成漏。用夏枯草六兩，水二鍾，煎七分，食遠温服。虛甚者則煎汁熬膏服。并塗患處，兼以十全大補湯加香附、貝母、遠志尤善。此物生血，乃治瘰癧之聖藥也。其草易得，其功甚多。薛己外科經驗方。

Saber shaped scrofula pervasion-illness,[158] regardless of whether is has begun to fester or not. Also for those that after several days have developed a leakage. Boil six *liang* of *xia ku cao* in two *zhong* of water down to 70% and ingest this between meals. In the case of an extreme depletion, boil it to obtain a juice, heat it to generate a paste and ingest it. At the same time, apply it [to the affected region]. Also, to resort

156 *Xue beng* 血崩, blood collapse. Excessive vaginal bleeding, identical to *beng zhong* 崩中, collapsing center. BCGM Dict I, 594; 58.

157 *Xue yun* 血運, "blood[-induced brain] movements;" a condition of sudden vertigo brought forth by sudden and violent depletion of qi and blood following parturition. [Patients] pant and vomit. In severe cases this includes a clouded mind. BCGM Dict I, 602.

158 *Ma dao* 馬刀, "saber," a condition of saber-shaped, hard *luo li* 瘰癧, scrofula with pervasion-illness, developing in the armpits. BCGM Dict I, 331.

to the "decoction that massively supplements [qi] with 100% success,"[159] to which are added *aconitum* [accessory tuber], *fritillaria* [root] and *polygala* [root], will yield particularly good results. This item generates blood. Hence it is a sage-like pharmaceutical drug to cure scrofula pervasion-illness. The herb is easily obtainable and its [therapeutic] potentials are many. Xue Ji, *Wai ke jing yan fang*.

15-21
劉寄奴草唐本草
Liu ji nu cao, FE *Tang ben cao.*

***Artemisia anomala* S.Moore. Sweet wormwood.**

【釋名】金寄奴大明、烏藤菜綱目。【時珍曰】按李延壽南史云：宋高祖劉裕，小字寄奴。微時伐荻新洲，遇一大蛇，射之。明日往，聞杵臼聲。尋之，見童子數人皆青衣，於榛林中搗藥。問其故。荅曰：我主爲劉寄奴所射，今合藥傅之。裕曰：神何不殺之？曰：寄奴王者，不可殺也。裕叱之，童子皆散，乃收藥而反。每遇金瘡傅之即愈。人因稱此草爲劉寄奴草。鄭樵通志云：江南人因漢時謂劉爲卯金刀，乃呼劉爲金，是以又有金寄奴之名。江東人謂之烏藤菜云。

Explanation of Names. *Jin ji nu* 金寄奴, Da Ming. *Wu teng cai* 烏藤菜, "black cane vegetable," *Gang mu*. [Li] Shizhen: According to Li Yanshou's *Nan shi*, "Song [Emperor] Gao zu, Liu Yu, with childhood name Jinu, prior to his ascending the throne was on a military mission against the Northern Barbarians in Xin zhou when he encountered a huge snake and shot it. The next day when he went there again he heard the sound of pestles pounding in a mortar. He searched for it and saw several boys, all wearing greenish clothes, in a hazel wood pounding medicinal substances. He asked them why they did so and they answered: Our master was shot by Liu Jinu. Today we compose a medication to apply [to his wounds]. [Liu] Yu asked: He is a spirit, why didn't he kill [Liu Yu]? They said: Jinu is a king; he must not be killed. [Liu] You shouted at them, and they all dispersed. He then took the medication and returned. After this, whenever he was confronted with a wound caused by a weapon, he applied it and [the victim] was cured. This is why the people call this herb Li Jinu herb." Zheng Qiao in his *Tong zhi* states: "In Jiang nan during the Han era, because people said the name Liu [comprises the three components] *mao* 卯, *jin* 金 and *dao* 刀, they called him Liu Weijin 劉爲金. Therefore [he and the item discussed here] also had the name Jin Jinu 金寄奴, 'metal sent out to make slaves'." The people in Jiang dong call it *wu teng cai* 烏藤菜, "black vine vegetable."

---

159 Ingredients of *shi quan da bu tang* 十全大補湯 include: Ginseng root, *cassia* bark, *ligusticum* root, Chinese foxglove rhizome, *poria*, *atractylodes* rhizome, prepared *glycyrrhiza* root, *astragalus* root, white paeonia root, fresh ginger and Chinese dates.

【集解】【恭曰】劉寄奴草生江南。莖似艾蒿，長三四尺，葉似山蘭草而尖長，一莖直上有穗，葉互生，其子似稗而細。【保昇曰】今出越州，蒿之類也。高四五尺，葉似菊，其花白色，其實黃白色作穗，夏月收苗，日乾之。【頌曰】今河中府、孟州、漢中、滁州亦有之。春生苗，莖似艾蒿，上有四稜，高二三尺以來。葉青似柳，四月開碎小黃白花，形如瓦松，七月結實似黍而細，根淡紫色似萵苣。六月、七月采苗及花子，通用。【時珍曰】劉寄奴一莖直上。葉似蒼朮，尖長糙澀，而深背淡。九月莖端分開數枝，一枝攢簇十朵小花，白瓣黃蕊，如小菊花狀。花罷有白絮，如苦蕒花之絮。其子細長，亦如苦蕒子。所云實如黍、稗者，似與此不同，其葉亦非蒿類。

Collected Explanations. [Su] Gong: *Liu ji nu cao* grows in Jiang nan. The stem is similar to that of common mugwort. It is three to four *chi* long. The leaves are similar to those of *shan lan cao*,[160] but are pointed and longer. One stem rises upward and has spikes. The leaves grow in pairs. The seeds are similar to those of barnyard grass, but finer. [Han] Baosheng. Today it comes from Yue zhou. It belongs to the group of *hao* 蒿, wormwood. During the summer months the seedling is collected; it is dried in the sun. [Su] Song: Today it is also found in He zhong fu, Meng zhou, Han zhong and Chu zhou. In spring it grows a seedling with a stem similar to that of common mugwort. Above it has four edges; it reaches a height of about two to three *chi*. The leaves are greenish and are similar to willow [leaves]. In the fourth month it opens fragmentated, small, yellow-white flowers, shaped like roof pine [flowers]. In the seventh month it forms fruit similar to those of millet, but finer. The root is of pale purple color, similar to that of garden lettuce. Stem, flowers and seeds are collected in the sixth and seventh month; they are all used [for therapeutic purposes]. [Li] Shizhen: *liu ji nu* has one stem that rises straight up. The leaves are similar to those of *atractylodes* [herbs], but they are pointed, lengthy and rough; their front[161] is deeply [colored]; the back is pale. In the ninth month, the tip of the stem divides into several forks, with one such fork holding a cluster of ten small flowers with white petals and yellow anther bearing filaments, shaped similar to small *chrysanthemum* flowers. When the flowers decay a white wadding appears, similar to the wadding of *sow thistle* flowers. The seeds are fine and lengthy. They, too, are similar to those of *sow thistle*. When it is said that the fruits resemble those of millet and barnyard grass, this is different from the [item discussed] here. The leaves, too, are not those typical of *hao* 蒿, wormwood.

---

160 *Shan lan cao* 山蘭草, lit.: "mountain orchid herb." Unidentified.

161 The usual phrasing of such descriptions and the meaning of the present phrase suggest that *er* 而 is a writing error for *mian* 面, "face," "front side."

15-21-01
子 *Zi*
Seeds [of *liu ji nu cao*]

苗同。

Identical to the seedling.

【修治】【斅曰】凡采得，去莖葉，只用實。以布拭去薄殼令净，拌酒蒸，從巳至申，暴乾用。【時珍曰】莖、葉、花、子皆可用。

Pharmaceutical Preparation. [Lei] Xiao: When [the herb] is collected, remove the stem and the leaves, and use only the fruit. Rub them with a cloth to remove the thin shell and clean them. Then steam them mixed with wine, from *si* 巳 hours (9 – 11) to *shen* 申 hours (15 – 17), and dry them in the sun. [Li] Shizhen: The stem, the leaves, the flowers and the seeds can all be used.

【氣味】苦，温，無毒。

Qi and Flavor. Bitter, warm, nonpoisonous.

【主治】破血下脹。多服令人下痢。蘇恭。下血止痛，治産後餘疾，止金瘡血，極效。别本。心腹痛，下氣，水脹血氣，通婦人經脉癥結，止霍亂水瀉。大明。小便尿血，新者研末服。時珍。

Control. It breaks through blood [accumulation] and discharges [qi causing a] distension. Eaten in large quantities it causes discharge with free-flux illness. Su Gong. It discharges [sluggish] blood and ends pain. It serves to cure ailments in the aftermath of a dbirth. It very effectively ends bleeding of wounds caused by metal objects/weapons. *Bie ben*. Painful central and abdominal region. It discharges qi, water causing distension and [ends] blood and qi [disorder]. It passes through concretion-illness nodes blocking the conduit vessels of women. It ends cholera with watery outflow. Da Ming. For urination with blood, grind fresh [*liu ji nu cao*] into powder and ingest it. [Li] Shizhen.

【附方】舊一，新七。

Added Recipes. One of old. Seven newly [recorded].

大小便血。劉寄奴爲末，茶調空心服二錢，即止。集簡方。

Major (defecation) and minor (urination) relief with blood. [Grind] *liu ji nu into powder*, mix it with tea and ingest on an empty stomach two *qian*. This will end [the disease]. *Ji jian fang*.

折傷瘀血在腹内者。劉寄奴、骨碎補、延胡索各一兩，水二升，煎七合，入酒及童子小便各一合，頓温服之。千金方。

Stagnant blood in the abdomen related to fracture harm. Boil one *liang* each of *liu ji nu*, polypody and *corydalis* [tuber] in two *sheng* of water down to seven *ge*, add one *ge* each of wine and boys' urine and ingest this warm all at once. *Qian jin fang.*

血氣脹滿。劉寄奴穗實爲末，每服三錢，酒煎服。不可過多，令人吐利。此破血之仙藥也。衛生易簡方。

Blood and qi [disorder causing] distension and a sensation of fullness. [Grind] *liu ji nu* spikes with their fruit into powder. Each time ingest three *qian*. To be ingested boiled in wine. It must not be ingested excessively lest it cause vomiting and free flow. This is an hermit/immortal's drug to break through blood [accumulation]. *Wei sheng yi jian fang.*

霍亂成痢。劉寄奴草煎汁飲。聖濟總録。

Cholera resulting in free-flux illness. Boil *liu ji nu* herb in water and drink the juice. *Sheng ji zong lu.*

湯火傷灼。劉寄奴擣末，先以糯米漿鷄翎掃上，後乃摻末。並不痛，亦無痕，大驗之方。凡湯火傷，先以鹽末摻之，護肉不壞，後乃摻藥爲妙。本事方。

Scalding from hot water and burning from fire. Pound *liu ji nu* into powder. First spread with a chicken feather a thick glutinous rice soup on [the affected region]. Then apply the powder to it. There will be no pain and there will be no scars. A recipe based on massive success. For all types of harm caused by hot water and fire, apply salt powder first to protect the flesh from rotting. Then apply the medication. This is wondrous. *Ben shi fang.*

風入瘡口腫痛。劉寄奴爲末，摻之即止。聖惠方。

Wind has entered a wound causing painful swelling. [Grind] *liu ji nu* into powder and apply it [to the affected region]. This will end [the painful swelling]. *Sheng hui fang.*

小兒夜啼。劉寄奴半兩，地龍炒一分，甘草一寸，水煎，灌少許。聖濟總録。

Wailing of children at night. Boil half a *liang* of *liu ji nu*, one *fen* of stir-fried earthworms and a one *cun* long piece of *glycyrrhiza* [root] in water and force-feed this in small amounts [to the child]. *Sheng ji zong lu.*

赤白下痢。陰陽交滯，不問赤白。劉寄奴、烏梅、白薑等分，水煎服。赤加梅，白加薑。艾元英如宜方。

Red and white discharge with free-flux illness. Yin (i. e., the cold causing free-flux illness with pus) and yang (i. e., the heat causing free-flux illness with blood) block each other. There is no point in trying to distinguish red from white [discharge]. Boil equal amounts of *liu ji nu*, smoked plums and white/dried ginger in water and ingest this. If [the discharge] is red, add plums; if it is white, add ginger. Ai Yuan-ying, *Ru yi fang*.

15-22
曲節草宋圖經
Qu jie cao, FE Song, *Tu jing*.

***Peristrophe japonica* (Thunb.) Bremek. Japanese *peristrophe*.**[162]

【釋名】六月凌音令圖經、六月霜綱目、緑豆青圖經、蛇藍。【時珍曰】此草性寒，故有凌、霜、緑豆之名。

Explanation of Names. *Liu yue ling* 六月凌, "sixth month's ice," read *ling* 令, *Tu jing*. *Liu yue shuang* 六月霜, "sixth month's frost," *Gang mu*. *Lü dou qing* 緑豆青, *Tu jing*. *She lan* 蛇藍. [Li] Shizhen: This herb is of cold nature. It was therefore named *ling* 凌, "ice," *shuang* 霜, "frost," and *lü dou* 緑豆, (lit.:) "green bean."

【集解】【頌曰】曲節草生筠州。四月生苗，莖方色青有節，葉似劉寄奴而青軟，七八月着花似薄荷，結子無用。五月、六月采莖葉，陰乾。

Collected Explanations. [Su] Song: *Qu jie cao* grows in Yun zhou. It grows a seedling in the fourth month. The stem is square, of greenish color and has nodes. The leaves are similar to those of sweet wormwood, but are greenish and soft. In the seventh and eighth month it has flowers similar to those of mint. It forms seeds of no use. Stem and leaves are collected in the fifth and sixth month. They are dried in the yin (i. e., shade).

15-22-01
莖、葉 *Jing, Ye*
Stem, leaf [of *qu jie cao*].

【氣味】甘，平，無毒。

Qi and Flavor. Sweet, balanced, nonpoisonous.

【主治】發背瘡，消癰腫，拔毒。同甘草作末，米汁調服。蘇頌。

162 *Qu jie cao* 曲節草, lit.: "bent nodes herb."

Control. Effusion-of-the-back sores.[163] They dissolve swelling related to an obstruction-illness and serve to pull out the poison. [Grind] them together with *glycyrrhiza* [root] into powder and ingest this mixed with rice juice. Su Song.

15-23
麗春草宋圖經
Li chun cao, FE Song, *Tu jing*.

***Papaver rhoeas* L. Red poppy.**[164]

【釋名】仙女蒿圖經、定參草。【頌曰】麗春草生檀嵎山川谷，檀嵎山在高密界。河南淮陽郡、潁川及譙郡、汝南郡等，並呼爲龍芊草。河北近山、鄴郡、汲郡，並名叢蘭艾。上黨紫團山亦有，名定參草，又名仙女蒿。今所在有之。甚療瘾黄，人莫能知。【時珍曰】此草有殊功，而不著其形狀。今罌粟亦名麗春草，九仙子亦名仙女嬌，與此同名，恐非一物也。當俟博訪。

Explanation of Names. *Xian nü hao* 仙女蒿, "immortal girl's wormwood," *Tu jing*. *Ding shen cao* 定參草. [Su] Song: *Li chun cao* 麗春草 grows in the river valleys of Mount Tan yu shan. Mount Tan yu shan is located at the border of Gao mi. In He nan's Huai yang jun and Ying chuan, and in Qiao jun and Ru nan jun, everywhere it is called *long qian cao* 龍芊草. In He bei, adjacent to the mountains, in Ye jun and Ji jun, everywhere it is called *cong lan ai* 叢蘭艾. On Mount Zi tuan in Shang dang it can be found, too. There it is called *ding shen cao* 定參草, and also *xian nü hao* 仙女蒿. Today it can be found everywhere. It is very much able to heal hidden-illness jaundice that people [even if they are affected] cannot know about. [Li] Shizhen: This herb has an outstanding [therapeutic] potential, but its physical appearance is not recorded [in *materia medica* literature]. Today, opium poppy (23-17), too, is named *li chun cao* 麗春草, and *jiu xian zi* 九仙子 (unidentified, 18-34) is also named *xian nü qiao* 仙女嬌. These are the same names as those given to the [item has that is discussed] here. Presumably they are not one and the same item. Further investigations are required.

163 *Fa bei* 發背, "effusion of the back," a condition of *yong* 癰, "obstruction-illnesses," and *ju* 疽, "impediment-illnesses," developing on one's back. As it was believed that the transporter holes of the five long-term depots and six short-term repositories are located on the back, conditions of obstruction-illnesses and impediment-illnesses there, often apparent as abscesses, were considered threatening. BCGM Dict I, 148.

164 *Li chun cao* 麗春草, lit.: "gorgeous spring herb."

15-23-01
花及根 ***Hua ji gen***
Flower and root [of *li chun cao*].

【氣味】缺。

Qi and Flavor. Missing.[165]

【主治】癃黄黄疸。蘇頌。

Control. Hidden-illness jaundice, yellow *dan*-illness/jaundice. Su Song.

【發明】【頌曰】唐天寶中，潁川郡楊正進方，名醫皆用有效。其方云：麗春草療因時患傷熱，變成癃黄，遍身壯熱，小便黄赤，眼如金色，面又青黑，心頭氣痛，遶心如刺，頭旋欲倒，兼脇下有瘕氣，及黄疸等，經用有驗。其藥春三月采花，陰乾一升，擣散。每平明空腹取三方寸匕，和生麻油一盞頓服，日一服，隔五日再進，以知爲度。其根療黄疸，擣汁一盞，空腹頓服，須臾即利三兩行，其疾立已。一劑不能全愈，隔七日更一劑，永瘥。忌酒、麪、豬、魚、蒜、粉酪等。

Explication. [Su] Song: During the Tang era, in the reign period *tian bao* (742- 755) Yang Zheng of Ying chuan jun submitted a recipe. All famous physicians used it with success. The recipe states: "*Li chun cao* heals suffering from harm caused by heat related to seasonal [qi] that may change to hidden-illness jaundice. The entire body is very hot. Urine is yellow-red. The eyes assume a golden color. The face is greenish-black. The top of the stomach aches, and this winds around the heart as if it were pierced. Vertigo with a tendency to fall to the ground, together with conglomeration-illness qi below the flanks, as well as yellow *dan*-illness/jaundice. For all this, [this recipe] has shown to be effective. In spring, in the third month, collect the flowers. Dry one *sheng* in the yin (i. e., shade) and pound it into powder. Each time at dawn take on an empty stomach the amount held by three square *cun* spoons, mix this with fresh sesame oil and ingest this all at once, once a day. Five days later take it again, and so on until an effect shows. The root heals yellow *dan*-illness/jaundice. Pound it to obtain one cup of juice and ingest it on an empty stomach all at once. After a short time this will result in two or three free flow episodes, and this ends the illness. If one dose is unable to bring abaout a complete cure, take another dose seven days later, and this will result in an everlasting cure. [During this treatment] wine, wheat flour, pork, fish, garlic and junket are to be avoided."

165 *Zheng lei* ch. 30, *li chun cao* 麗春草, quoting the *Tu jing* writes: *wei gan wei wen wu du* 味甘，微温，無毒, "flavor sweet, slightly warm, nonpoisonous."

15-24
旋覆花本經下品

Xuan fu hua, FE *Ben jing*, lower rank.

***Inula japonica* Thunb. Horseheal.**

【釋名】金沸草本經、金錢花綱目、滴滴金綱目、盜庚爾雅、夏菊綱目、戴椹別録。【宗奭曰】花緣繁茂，圓而覆下，故曰旋覆。【時珍曰】諸名皆因花狀而命也。爾雅云：䕰，盜庚也。蓋庚者金也，謂其夏開黄花，盜竊金氣也。酉陽雜俎云：金錢花一名毘尸沙，自梁武帝時始進入中國。

Explanation of Names. *Jin fei cao* 金沸草, "boiled gold herb," *Ben jing*. *Jin qian hua* 金錢花, "gold coin flowers," *Gang mu*. *Di di jin* 滴滴金, "Dripping gold," *Gang mu*. *Dao geng* 盜庚, "Robber of *geng* (i. e., metal)," *Er ya*. *Xia ju* 夏菊, "summer *chrysanthemum*," *Gang mu*. *Dai shen* 戴椹, *Bie lu*. [Kou] Zongshi: Because its flowers are luxuriant, round and being overturned cover, *fu* 覆, what is below, [the herb] is called *xuan fu* [*hua*] 旋覆[花], "[flowers] circling and overturned covering." [Li] Shizhen: All the names refer to the shape of the flowers. The *Er ya* states: "*Fu* 䕰 is *dao geng* 盜庚." The fact is, *geng* 庚 is [associated with the phase] *jin* 金, "metal." That is to say, in summer [this herb] opens yellow flowers because it has stolen[166] the qi of metal/gold. The *You yang za zu* states: "*Jin qian hua* 金錢花 is also called *pi shi sha* 毘尸沙. It has been brought to China ever since the times of Emperor Liang Wu di (420 – 589)."

【集解】【別録曰】旋覆生平澤川谷。五月采花，日乾，二十日成。【弘景曰】出近道下濕地，似菊花而大。別有旋葍根，出河南，北國亦有，形似芎藭，惟合旋葍膏用之，餘無所用，非此旋覆花根也。【保昇曰】葉似水蘇，花黄如菊，六月至九月采花。【頌曰】今所在皆有。二月以後生苗，多近水旁，大似紅藍而無刺，長一二尺以來，葉如柳，莖細。六月開花如菊花，小銅錢大，深黄色。上黨田野人呼爲金錢花，七八月采花。今近道人家園圃所蒔金錢花，花葉並同，極易繁盛，恐即旋覆也。【宗奭曰】旋覆葉如大菊，又如艾蒿。秋開花大如梧桐子，花淡黄色，其香過於菊。別有旋花，乃鼓子花，非此花也。見本條。【時珍曰】花狀如金錢菊。水澤邊生者，花小瓣單。人家栽者，花大蕊簇，蓋壤瘠使然。其根細白。俗傳露水滴下即生，故易繁，蓋亦不然。

Collected Explanation. *Bie lu*: *Xuan fu* grows in the marshlands of the plains and in river valleys. Its flowers are collected in the fifth month. They are dried in the sun. [This process of drying] is completed after 20 days. [Tao] Hongjing: [*Xuan fu*] comes from low-lying marshlands nearby. It is similar to *chrysanthemum* flowers, but

166 Since it blooms in the summer it would have been legitimate to only adopt the qi of the phase fire. Contrary to the laws of nature, it acquired the qi of metal, that is, the qi of autumn. Hence it is said to have "stolen" the qi of metal.

is bigger. There is also a *xuan fu* root, *xuan fu gen* 旋葍根, it comes from He nan and is also found in the Northern countries. Its physical shape is similar to *ligusticum* root. It is used only to prepare the *xuan fu* paste; it is not used for anything else. It is not the root of *xuan fu hua* discussed here. [Han] Baosheng: The leaves are similar to those of camphor mint. The flowers are yellow like those of chrysanthemums. The flowers are collected from the sixth month to the ninth month. [Su] Song: Today [*xuan fu*] can be found everywhere. It grows a seedling beginning with the second month, mostly close to waters. Its size is similar to that of safflower, but it has no thorns. It reaches a length of one to two *chi*. The leaves are similar to willow [leaves]. The stem is fine. In the sixth month it opens flowers similar to *chrysanthemum* flowers. They have the size of small copper coins and are of a deep yellow color. The people in the open country of Shang dang call them "gold coin flowers." They collect the flowers in the seventh and eighth month. The "gold coin flowers" that are now planted by nearby households in their gardens have the same flowers and leaves, and they grow easily and luxuriantly. Presumably, these are *xuan fu* [plants]. [Kou] Zongshi: The leaves of *xuan fu* are similar to those of big chrysanthemums, and they also resemble those of common mugwort. In autumn [*xuan fu*] opens flowers as big as those of Chinese parasol trees. The flowers are of a pale yellow color and their fragrance exceeds that of chrysanthemums. There is also a *xuan hua* 旋花, also [called] *gu zi hua* 鼓子花, but this is not the flower [discussed] here. See the respective entry (18-14). [Li] Shizhen: The flowers are shaped like gold coin chrysanthemums. Those growing near waters and marshland have small flowers with only one petal. Those cultivated by households have flowers with big stamen clusters. The fact is, [such differences] result from the good or bad quality of the soil [they grow on]. The root is fine and white. A common tradition is that [this herb] grows where dew has dropped down and that it is therefore that it grows easily and luxuriantly. The fact is, this, too, is not so.

15-24-01
花 *Hua*
Flower [of *xuan fu hua*].

【修治】【斅曰】采得花，去蕊并殼皮及蒂子，蒸之，從巳至午，曬乾用。

Pharmaceutical Preparation. [Lei] Xiao: Collect the flowers, remove the stamens, the shells with the skin, the fruit base and seeds. Steam [the rest] from the *si* hours (9 – 11) to the *wu* hours (11 – 13), dry it in the sun and then use it.

【氣味】鹹，温，有小毒。【别録曰】甘，微温，冷利。【權曰】甘，無毒。【大明曰】無毒。【宗奭曰】苦、甘、辛。

Qi and Flavor. Salty, warm, slightly poisonous. *Bie lu*: Sweet, slightly warm. It has cold [qi] causing free flow. [Zhen] Quan: Sweet, nonpoisonous. Da Ming: Nonpoisonous. [Kou] Zongshi: Bitter, sweet, acrid.

【主治】結氣脇下滿，驚悸，除水，去五臟間寒熱，補中下氣。本經。消胸上痰結，唾如膠漆，心胸痰水，膀胱留飲，風氣濕痺，皮間死肉，目中眵䁾，利大腸，通血脉，益色澤。别録。主水腫，逐大腹，開胃，止嘔逆不下食。甄權。行痰水，去頭目風。宗奭。消堅軟痞，治噫氣。好古。

Control. Bound qi[167] causing a sensation of fullness below the flanks. Fright palpitation. It removes water, eliminates cold and heat from among the five long-term depots, supplements [qi in] the center and discharges qi. *Ben jing*. It dissolves phlegm nodes that have risen in the chest, saliva similar to sticky lacquer, phlegm water in the central region and the chest,[168] beverages abiding in the urinary bladder, blockage related to the presence of wind, [evil] qi and moisture, dead flesh in the skin, and tearflow with sticky secretion in the eyes. It clears the passage through the large intestine, penetrates the blood vessels and boosts complexion and luster. *Bie lu*. It controls water swelling, ends an enlarged abdomen, opens the stomach, and stops vomiting of counterflow food that fails to move down. Zhen Quan. It stimulates the passage of phlegm and water, and removes wind from head and eyes. [Kou] Zongshi: If dissolves hardenings and softens obstacle-illness.[169] It serves to cure hiccup qi. [Wang] Haogu.

【發明】【頌曰】張仲景治傷寒汗下後，心下痞堅，噫氣不除，有七物旋覆代赭湯。雜治婦人，有三物旋覆湯。胡洽居士治痰飲在兩脇脹滿，有旋覆花丸，用之尤多。成無己曰：鞕則氣堅，旋覆之鹹，以軟痞堅也。【震亨曰】寇宗奭言其行痰水去頭目風，亦走散之藥。病人涉虛者，不宜多服，冷利大腸，宜戒之。【時珍曰】旋覆乃手太陰肺、手陽明大腸藥也。所治諸病，其功只在行水下氣通血脉爾。李衛公言嗅其花能損目，唐慎微本草誤以旋花根方收附此下，今改正之。

Explication. [Su] Song: To cure obstacle-illness hardening and hiccup-qi that fail to end following a treatment of harm caused by cold by means of [a therapy stimulating] sweating and discharge, Zhang Zhongjing uses the "decoction with - seven

167 *Jie qi* 結氣, "bound qi," are pathological qi halting and congealing at any place in the body. BCGM Dict I, 240.

168 Instead of *xiong* 胸, "chest," *Zheng lei* ch. 10, *xuan fu hua* 旋覆花, write *xie* 脇, "flanks."

169 *Pi* 痞, "obstacle-illness," a condition of an uncomfortable distension and fullness in the chest and abdominal region. When pressed there is no pain. BCGM Dict I. 371.

items including - *xuan fu* and hematite."[170] For curing various [ailments of] women, he uses the "decoction with - three items including - *xuan fu*."[171] Hu Qia jushi especially often resorts to "*xuan hua* pills" to cure distension and a sensation of fullness in the two flanks related to phlegm rheum. Cheng Wuji: Flogging/lashing causes qi hardening. The salty [qi] of *xuan fu* soften obstacle-illness[172] hardening. [Zhu] Zhenheng: [Kou] Zongshi refers to its ability to stimulate the passage of phlegm and water, and to remove wind from head and eyes. That is, it is also a pharmaceutical drug that [stimulates qi] to rush and disperse. Patients with a condition of depletion must not ingest much of it lest it cause free flow in the large intestine. They use it moderately. [Li] Shizhen: *Xuan fu* is a pharmaceutical drug for the hand major yin lung and hand yang brilliance large intestine [conduits]. In the treatment of all types of diseases, its potential is focused on stimulating the movement of water, discharging qi and penetrating the blood vessels. Li Weigong says: "Smelling the flowers hurts the eyes." Tang Shenwei's *Ben cao* erroneously adds *xuan hua* root, hedge bindweed (18-14), as an attachment to the present item. This is corrected now.

【附方】舊一，新三。

Added Recipes. One of old. Three newly [recorded].

中風壅滯。旋覆花，洗净焙研，煉蜜丸梧子大。夜卧以茶湯下五丸至七丸、十丸。經驗後方。

Struck by wind, with obstructed and sluggish [qi flow]. Wash *xuan fu hua* clean, dry it over a fire in a pan, grind it [to powder] and with heat refined honey form pills the size of *wu* seeds. At night, when going to sleep, send down with a tea decoction five to seven pills, or even ten pills. *Jing yan hou fang*.

半產漏下。虚寒相搏，其脉弦芤。旋覆花湯：用旋覆花三兩，葱十四莖，新絳少許，水三升，煮一升，頓服。金匱要略。

Dribbling discharge related to miscarriage. Cold has availed itself of the depletion, with a thread-like, hollow [movement in the] vessels. The "decoction with *xuan fu*": Boil three *liang* of *xuan fu hua*, 14 onion stalks and a small piece of newly dyed red

170 Ingredients of the *xuan fu dai he tang* 旋覆代赭湯, "decoction with *xuan fu* and hematite," include *xuan fu hua*, hematite, ginseng root, *glycyrrhiza* root, *pinellia* tuber, fresh ginger and Chinese dates.

171 Ingredients of the *xuan fu tang* 旋覆湯, "decoction with *xuan fu*," include *xuan fu*, onion and red silk fabric, newly dyed with madder, safflower juice or similar sources of red color. See below, Added Recipes.

172 *Pi* 痞, "obstacle-illness," a condition of an uncomfortable distension and fullness in the chest and abdominal region. When pressed there is no pain. BCGM Dict I. 371.

[silk fabric] in three *sheng* of water down to one *sheng* and ingest this all at once. *Jin kui yao lüe*.

月蝕耳瘡。旋覆花燒研，羊脂和塗之。集簡方。

Lunar eclipse[173] ear sores. Burn *xuan fu hua*, grind [the residue into powder], mix it with sheep fat and apply this [to the affected region]. *Ji jian fang*.

小兒眉癬。小兒眉毛眼睫因癬退不生。用野油花即旋覆花、赤箭即天麻苗、防風等分，爲末。洗净，以油調塗之。總微論。

Xuan-illness[174] affecting the eyebrows of children. When eyebrows and eyelashes of a child fail to grow once a *xuan*-illness has receded. [Grind] equal amounts of *ye you hua*, that is, *xuan fu hua*, of *chi jian*, that is *gastrodia* seedling, and of *saposhnikovia* [root] into powder. Wash [the affected region] clean and apply [the powder] with oil there. *Zong wei lun*.

15-24-02

葉 *Ye*

Leaf [of *xuan fu hua*].

【主治】傅金瘡，止血。大明。治疔瘡腫毒。時珍。

Control. Applied to wounds caused by metal objects/weapons, it stops bleeding. Da Ming. It serves to cure poison swelling related to pin-illness[175] sores. [Li] Shizhen.

15-24-03

根 *Gen*

Root [of *xuan fu hua*].

【主治】風濕。别録。

Control. Wind and moisture [intrusion]. *Bie lu*.

---

173 *Yue shi* 月蝕, "lunar eclipse," a condition of *chuang* 瘡, "sores" developing on the ears, nose, face, and to the side of the orifices in the anal and genital region. BCGM Dict I, 65.

174 *Xuan* 癬, "*xuan*-illness." Conditions of dermal lesions with initially erythema, papules, and itching gradually extending in all directions to form an irregular ring with clear boundaries. The skin is slightly elevated with small papules, blisters, and/or scales and scraps. The central lesion may appear to heal spontaneously, and it may reappear. Also, a designation of local lesions with itching, release of liquid and shedding of scabs. BCGM Dict I, 591.

175 *Ding* 丁, "pin[-illness]," also *ding* 疔, "pin-illness," refers to a deep-reaching and festering hardness in a tissue, eventually rising above the skin like a pinhead. BCGM Dict I, 127-129.

15-25
青葙本經下品

Qing xiang, FE *Ben jing*, lower rank.

***Celosia argentea* L. Prince's feather.**

【釋名】草蒿本經、萋蒿本經、崑崙草唐本、野鷄冠綱目、鷄冠莧綱目。子名草决明本經。【時珍曰】青葙名義未詳。胡麻葉亦名青蘘，此草又多生于胡麻地中，與之同名，豈以其相似而然耶？青蒿亦名草蒿，其功相似，而名亦相同，何哉？其子明目，與决明子同功，故有草决明之名。其花葉似鷄冠，嫩苗似莧，故謂之鷄冠莧。鄭樵通志言俗名牛尾蒿者，誤矣。

Explanation of Names. *Cao gao* 草蒿, "herbal wormwood," *Ben jing* . *Qi hao* 萋蒿, "luxuriant wormwood," *Ben jing*. *Kun lun cao* 崑崙草, "Kun lun herb," *Tang ben*. *Ye ji guan* 野鷄冠, "wild cockscomb," *Gang mu*. *Ji guan xian* 鷄冠莧, cockscomb amaranth," *Gang mu*. The seeds are named *cao jue ming* 草决明, "herbal fetid *cassia*," *Ben jing*. [Li] Shizhen: The meaning of *qing xiang* 青葙 is not clear. Sesame leaves, too, are called *qing xiang* 青蘘. This herb often grows on the ground together with sesame. Could it be, they have the same name because they are so similar? The seeds [of the item discussed here] brighten the eyes. This potential is identical to that of fetid *cassia* seeds. Hence [*qing xiang*] is also called "herbal fetid *cassia*." The flowers and leaves are similar to those of cockscomb, and the tender seedling resembles that of *amaranth*. Hence an alternative name [of *qing xiang*] is cockscomb *amaranth*. Zheng Qiao in his *Tong zhi* mentions "oxtail wormwood," *niu wei hao* 牛尾蒿 as its commonly used name. That is wrong.

【集解】【別録曰】青葙生平谷道旁。三月采莖葉，陰乾。五月、六月采子。【弘景曰】處處有之。似麥柵花，其子甚細。别有草蒿，或作草藁，主療殊相類，形名又相似可疑，而實兩種也。【恭曰】此草苗高尺餘，葉細軟，花紫白色，實作角，子黑而扁光，似莧實而大，生下濕地，四月、五月采，荆襄人名爲崑崙草。【頌曰】今江淮州郡近道亦有之。二月生青苗，長三四尺。葉闊似柳而軟。莖似蒿，青紅色。六月、七月内生花，上紅下白。子黑光而扁，似莨菪。根亦似蒿根而白，直下獨莖生根。六月、八月采子。【時珍曰】青葙生田野間，嫩苗似莧可食，長則高三四尺。苗葉花實與鷄冠花一樣無别。但鷄冠花穗或有大而扁或團者，此則稍間出花穗，尖長四五寸，狀如兔尾，水紅色，亦有黄白色者。子在穗中，與鷄冠子及莧子一樣，難辨。蘇恭言其結角，誤矣。蕭炳言黄花者名陶珠術，與陳藏器所説不同。又有天靈草，亦此類也，並附於下。

Collected Explanations. *Bie lu*: *Qing xiang* grows on the sides of the roads in Ping gu. Stem and leaves are collected in the third month, to be dried in the yin (i. e., shade). The seeds are collected in the fifth and sixth month. [Tao] Hongjing: It can be found everywhere. It is similar to *mai zha hua* 麥柵花.[176] Its seeds are very fine. There is also a *cao hao* 草蒿, sometimes written *cao gao* 草藁, with a rather similar therapeutic potential. The physical appearance and the nature of this [herb] and the item discussed here are suspiciously similar. And yet, they are two different kinds. [Su] Gong: The seedling of this herb reaches a height of more than a *chi*. The leaves are fine and soft. The flowers are purple-white. The fruits form protuberances with black, flat and shiny seeds, similar to the fruit of amaranth, but they are bigger. [*Qing xiang*] grows in low-lying marshlands. It is collected in the fourth and fifth month. The people in Jing and Xiang call it Kun lun herb. [Su] Song: Today it is also found nearby in the *zhou* and prefectures of the Jiang Huai region. It grows a greenish seedling in the second month, *three* to four *chi* long. The leaves are broad, similar to those of willows, but soft. The stem is similar to that of wormwood; it has a greenish-red color. [*Qing xiang*] grows flowers in the sixth and seventh month. They are red above and white below. The seeds are black, shiny and flat. They are similar to those of henbane. The root, too, is similar to wormwood roots, but is white. It is a single stem going straight down as a root. The seeds are collected in the sixth and eighth month. [Li] Shizhen: *Qing xiang* grows in the open country. Its tender seedlings are similar to those of amaranth, and can be eaten. They grow to be three to four *chi* tall. Seedling, leaves, flowers and fruits are identical to those of cockscomb; there is no difference. However, the flower spikes of cockscomb may be large and flat or round. The present [*qing xiang*'s] flower spikes emerge from the end; they are pointed and extend to a length of four to five *cun*. They are shaped like a hare/rabbit's tail. They are of a watery red color; some are of a yellow-white color. The seeds in the spikes are identical to cockscomb seeds and amaranth seeds. They are difficult to distinguish. Su Gong says: "They form protuberances." That is wrong. Xiao Bing says: "Those with yellow flowers are called *tao zhu zhu* 陶珠術, 'pottery bead *atractylodes*'." This is different from what Chen Cangqi says. There is also a *tian ling cao* 天靈草, "heavenly numinous/magic herb." It, too, belongs to the same group. They are attached below.

176 *Mai zha hua* 麥柵花, unidentified plant.

【附録】
Appendix.

15-25-A01
桃朱術 *Tao zhu shu*
Peach-shaped red atractylodes.

【炳曰】青葙一種花黄者名陶朱術，苗相似。【藏器曰】桃朱術生園中，細如芹，花紫，子作角。以鏡向旁敲之，則子自發。五月五日乃收子，帶之令婦人爲夫所愛。

[Xiao] Bing: A *qing xiang* variety with yellow flowers is called *tao zhu*[177] *zhu*; the seedlings are similar. [Chen] Cangqi: *Tao zhu zhu* grows in gardens. It is as fine as Chinese celery. The flowers are purple; the seeds form protuberances. When the protuberances are struck with a mirror from the side, the seeds will be emitted. The seeds are gathered on the fifth day of the fifth month. Worn on her clothes they will seduce a male to make love with that woman.

15-25-A02
雁來紅 *Yan lai hong*
Redness derived from wild geese.[178]

【時珍曰】莖、葉、穗、子並與鷄冠同。其葉九月鮮紅，望之如花，故名。吴人呼爲老少年。一種六月葉紅者，名十樣錦。

[Li] Shizhen: Stem, leaves, spikes and seeds are all identical to those of cockscomb. The leaves are bright red in the ninth month. Seen from a distance they look like flowers. Hence the name. The people in Wu call them *lao shao nian* 老少年, "old and young age." There is one kind with leaves turning red in the sixth month. It is called *shi yang jin* 十樣錦, the "ten variations brocade."

15-25-A03
天靈草 *Tian ling cao*
Herb of celestial magic.

【時珍曰】按土宿真君本草云：狀如鷄冠花，葉亦如之，折之有液如乳，生江、湖、荆南陂地間。五月取汁，可制雄、硫，煮雌煉砂。

[Li] Shizhen: According to the *Tu su zhen jun ben cao*, "it is shaped like cockscomb. When broken, it shows a milk-like fluid. It grows in the region of Jiang, Hu and

177 Instead of *zhu* 朱, *Zheng lei* ch. 10, *xuan fu hua* 旋覆花, quoting Xiao Bing writes *zhu* 珠. The *Tu jing*, quoting this in turn, also writes *zhu* 珠. The *Shi yi* writes zhu 朱. Li Shizhen followed the *Shi yi*.

178 Wild geese were known to arrive in the ninth month. The leaves turn red with the arrival of wild geese.

Jing nan. Collect the juice in the fifth month. It can check [the effects of] realgar and sulphur. It is boiled with orpiment, and heat processed with cinnabar."

15-25-A04

思莫子 *Si mi zi*

Unidentified.

【斅曰】思蓂子、鼠細子，二件真似青葙子，只是味不同。思蓂子味跙，煎之有涎。

[Lei] Xiao: *Si mi* seeds and *shu xi* seeds, these two items are truly similar to *qiang xiang* seeds. Only their flavors differ. *Si mi* seeds have a bad flavor; when they are boiled in water, a saliva[-like fluid] is generated.

15-25-01

莖、葉 *Jing, Ye*

Stem, leaf [of *qing xiang*].

【修治】【斅曰】凡用先燒鐵杵臼，乃擣用之。

Pharmaceutical Preparation. [Lei] Xiao: First heat an iron pestle and mortar, then pound [stem and leaves of *qing xiang*] for later use.

【氣味】苦，微寒，無毒。

Qi and Flavor. Bitter, slightly cold, nonpoisonous.

【主治】邪氣，皮膚中熱，風瘙身癢，殺三蟲。本經。惡瘡，疥蝨，痔蝕，下部䘌瘡。别録。擣汁服，大療温癘。蘇恭。止金瘡血。大明。

Control. Evil qi. Heat in the skin. Wind itch; body itch. They kill the three worms/bugs. *Ben jing*. Malign sores. *Jie*-illness[179] and lice. Piles erosion. Sores with hidden worms/bugs in the lower body section. *Bie lu*. To pound them and ingest the resulting juice serves to massively heal warmth epidemics. Su Gong. It ends the bleeding of wounds caused by metal objects/weapons. Da Ming.

15-25-02

子 *Zi*

Seeds [of *qing xiang*].

【氣味】苦，微寒，無毒。【權曰】苦，平。

Qi and Flavor. Bitter, slightly cold, nonpoisonous. [Zhen] Quan. Bitter, balanced.

---

179 *Jie*-illness 疥, vaguely identifiable skin ailment. BCGM Dict I, 249.

【主治】脣口青。本經。治五臟邪氣，益腦髓，鎮肝，明耳目，堅筋骨，去風寒濕痺。大明。治肝臟熱毒衝眼，赤障青盲，翳腫，惡瘡，疥瘡。甄權。

Control: Greenish lips and mouth. *Ben jing*. They serve to cure the five long-term depots affected by evil qi. They boost brain marrow, ease the liver [qi], brighten ears and eyes, harden sinews and bones, and remove blockage related to [the presence of] wind, cold and moisture. Da Ming. They serve to cure heat poison of the liver long-term conduit rushing against the eyes, with a red screen, green-blindness, and a shade [in the eyes] with swelling, malign sores, and *jie*-illness sores. Zhen Quan.

【發明】【炳曰】理眼，有青葙子丸。【宗奭曰】青葙子，經中不言治眼，惟藥性論、日華子始言治肝明目。今人多用治眼，殊與經意不相當。【時珍曰】青葙子治眼，與決明子、莧實同功。本經雖不言治眼，而云一名草決明，主脣口青，則其明目之功可知矣。目者肝之竅，脣口青者足厥陰經之證，古方除熱亦多用之，青葙子之爲厥陰藥，又可知矣。況用之治目，往往有驗，尤可徵。據魏略云：初平中有青牛先生，常服青葙子丸，年百餘歲，如五六十者。

Explication. [Xiao] Bing: To cure the eyes, the "pills with *qing xiang* seeds" are available. [Kou] Zongshi: There is no record in the classics of a potential of *qing xiang* seeds to cure the eyes. The *Yao xing lun* and *Rihua zi* were the first to mention their ability to cure the liver and brighten the eyes. Today, people often use them to cure the eyes. This is certainly not in agreement with the meaning conveyed by the classics. [Li] Shizhen: The potential of *qing xiang* seeds to cure the eyes is identical to that of fetid *cassia* seeds and amaranth fruit. The *Ben jing* may not explicitly mention their potential to cure the eyes, but it states: "Alternative name herbal fetid *cassia*, controls greenish lips." From this it is obvious that they have the potential to brighten the eyes. The eyes are the orifice of the liver. When the lips are greenish, this is an illness sign related to the foot ceasing yin conduits. Ancient recipes often resorted to them to remove heat [from these conduits]. It is clear, therefore, that *qing xiang* seeds are a pharmaceutical drug for the ceasing yin [conduits]. Also, when they are used to cure [ailments affecting] the eyes, they have proved to be effective again and again. This is particularly valid evidence. According to the *Wei lüe*, during the *chu ping* reign period (190 – 193), "Gentleman Black Ox regularly ingested the 'pills with *qing xiang* seeds.' Even at the age of over a hundred, he looked like someone in his fifties or sixties."

【附方】舊一。
Added Recipes. One of old.

鼻衄不止，眩冒欲死。青葙子汁三合，灌入鼻中。貞元廣利方。

Unending nosebleed. Veiled eye dizziness[180] bringing [a patient] close to dying. Force-feed three *ge* of *qing xiang* seeds into the [patient's] nose. *Zhen yuan guang li fang*.

15-26
鷄冠宋嘉祐
Ji guan. FE *Jia you*.

***Celosia cristata* L. Cockscomb.**

【釋名】【時珍曰】以花狀命名。

Explanation of Names. [Li] Shizhen: The name [*ji guan* 鷄冠, "cockscomb"] reflects the shape of the flowers.

【集解】【時珍曰】鷄冠處處有之。三月生苗，入夏高者五六尺，矬者纔數寸。其葉青柔，頗似白莧菜而窄，[角肖]有赤脉。其莖赤色，或圓或扁，有筋起。六七月稍間開花，有紅、白、黄三色。其穗圓長而尖者，儼如青葙之穗；扁卷而平者，儼如雄鷄之冠。花大有圍一二尺者，層層卷出可愛。子在穗中，黑細光滑，與莧實一様。其穗如秕麥狀。花最耐久，霜後始蔫。

Collected Explanations. [Li] Shizhen: Cockscomb can be found everywhere. It grows a seedling in the third month; by summer it reaches a height of five to six *chi*. Short ones are only a few *cun* long. The leaves are greenish and soft. They are quite similar to those of white amaranth, but are narrower. They are pointed and have red veins. The stems are red. They may be round or flat, and they have protruding sinews. In the sixth and seventh month, flowers open at the tip [of the stem]. They may be of any of the three colors red, white, and yellow. Their spikes are round, lengthy and pointed, and they are as majestic as the spikes of prince's feather. Big flowers have a circumference of one or two *chi*. They appear curled up layer upon layer in an amiable manner. The seeds in the spikes are black, fine and shiny with a smooth surface, identical to the fruit of amaranth. The spikes are shaped like those of wheat that have not yet developed fruit. The flowers last very long. They begin to wither only after the begin of frost.

180 *Xuan mao* 眩冒, "veiled eyes dizziness," an illness sign of *xuan yun* 眩運, "vertigo," with severe cases resulting in a clouding. BCGM Dict I, 592-

15-26-01
苗 *Miao*
Seedling [of *ji guan*].

【氣味】甘，涼，無毒。

Qi and Flavor. Sweet, cool, nonpoisonous.

【主治】瘡痔及血病。時珍。

Control. Sores, piles and blood diseases. [Li] Shizhen.

15-26-02
子 *Zi*
Seeds [of *ji guan*].

【氣味】甘，涼，無毒。

Qi and Flavor. Sweet, cool, nonpoisonous.

【主治】止腸風瀉血，赤白痢。藏器。崩中帶下，入藥炒用。大明。

Control. They end intestinal wind and outflow with blood. Red and white free-flux illness. [Chen] Cangqi. Collapsing center[181] and [further diseases] below the belt. They are to be stir-fried to be added to medication. Da Ming.

15-26-03
花 *Hua*
Flower [of *ji guan*].

【氣味】同上。

Qi and Flavor. Identical to those listed above.

【主治】痔漏下血，赤白下痢，崩中，赤白帶下，分赤白用。時珍。

Control. Piles with a dribbling discharge of blood. Red and white discharge with free-flux illness. Collapsing center. Red and white [outflow] from below the belt. [The flowers] are applied in accordance with the red and white color [of the outflow]. [Li] Shizhen.

【附方】新十。

Added Recipes. Ten newly [recorded].

吐血不止。白鷄冠花，醋浸煮七次，爲末。每服二錢，熱酒下。經驗方。

181 *Beng zhong* 崩中, "collapsing center," excessive vaginal bleeding outside of a menstruation period. BCGM Dict I, 58.

Unending spitting of blood. Soak white *ji guan* flowers in vinegar, boil them seven times and [grind them into] powder. Each time ingest two *qian*, to be sent down with hot wine. *Jing yan fang*.

結陰便血。鷄冠花、椿根白皮等分，爲末，煉蜜丸梧子大。每服三十丸，黄芪湯下，日二服。聖濟總録。

Bound yin [qi] with [major/defecation and minor/urination] relief with blood. [Grind] equal amounts of *ji guan* flowers and white skin of *ailanthus* trees into powder and form with heat refined honey pills the size of *wu* seeds. Each time ingest 30 pills, to be sent down with an *astragalus* [root] decoction. To be ingested twice a day. *Sheng ji zong lu*.

糞後下血。白鷄冠花并子炒，煎服。聖惠方。

Blood discharge following defecation. Stir-fry white *ji guan* flowers with their seeds, then boil them [in water] and ingest this. *Sheng hui fang*.

五痔肛腫，久不愈，變成瘻瘡。用鷄冠花、鳳眼草各一兩，水二盌，煎湯頻洗。衛生寶鑑。

The five types of piles with anal swelling that has not been healed for a long time and eventually has turned into scrofula sores. Boil one *liang* each of *ji guan* flowers and *ailanthus* herb in two bowls of water and repeatedly wash [the affected region] with the decoction. *Wei sheng bao jian*.

下血脱肛。白鷄冠花、防風等分，爲末，糊丸梧子大，空心米飲每服七十丸。

Anal prolapse related to a discharge with blood. [Grind] equal amounts of white *ji guan* flowers and *saposhnikovia* [root] into powder and form with [wheat flour] paste pills the size of *wu* seeds. Each time ingest with a rice beverage 70 pills on an empty stomach.

一方：白鷄冠花炒、椶櫚灰、羌活各一兩，爲末。每服二錢，米飲下。永類鈐方。

Another recipe. [Grind] one *liang* each of stir-fried white *ji guan* flowers, *trachycarpus* [palm] ashes and *notopterygium* [root] into powder. Each time ingest two *qian*, to be sent down with a rice beverage. *Yong lei qian fang*.

經水不止。紅鷄冠花一味，晒乾爲末。每服二錢，空心酒調下。忌魚腥、猪肉。孫氏集效方。

Unending menstruation. Dry red *ji guan* flowers as an individual substance in the sun and [grind them into] powder. Each time [let the patient] ingest two *qian*, to be sent down mixed with wine on an empty stomach. [During the treatment] fish, items with the smell of fish and pork are to be avoided. Sun shi, *Ji xiao fang*.

產後血痛。白鷄冠花，酒煎服之。李樓奇方。

Painful bleeding following birth. Boil white *ji guan* flowers in wine and [let the woman] ingest this. *Li Lou qi fang*.

婦人白帶。白鷄冠花晒乾爲末，每旦空心酒服三錢。赤帶用紅者。孫氏集效方。

White [outflow from below the] belt of women. Dry white *ji guan* flowers in the sun and [grind them into] powder. Every morning [let the patient] ingest with wine three *qian* on an empty stomach. In the case of red [outflow from below the] belt, use red [flowers]. Sun shi, *Ji xiao fang*.

白帶沙淋。白鷄冠花、苦壺蘆等分，燒存性，空心火酒服之。摘玄方。

White [outflow from below the] belt with [urinary] sand dripping. Burn equal amounts of white *ji guan* flowers and calabashs with their nature retained and [let the patient] ingest this with brandy on an empty stomach. *Zhai xuan fang*.

赤白下痢。鷄冠花煎酒服。赤用紅，白用白。集簡方。

Red and white discharge with free-flux illness. Boil *ji guan* flowers in wine and ingest this. For red [discharge] use red [flowers]. For white [discharge] use white [flowers]. *Ji jian fang*.

15-27
紅藍花宋開寶
Hong lan hua, FE Song, *Kai bao*.

***Carthamus tinctorius* L. Safflower.**

【釋名】紅花開寶、黄藍。【頌曰】其花紅色，葉頗似藍，故有藍名。

Explanation of Names. *Hong hua* 紅花, "red flowers," *Kai bao*. *Huang lan* 黄藍. [Su] Song: The flowers, *hua* 花, are of red, *hong* 紅, color; the leaves are similar to those of indigo plants, *lan* 藍. Hence the name *lan* 藍.

【集解】【志曰】紅藍花即紅花也，生梁漢及西域。博物志云：張騫得種於西域。今魏地亦種之。【頌曰】今處處有之。人家場圃所種，冬月布子於熟地，至春生苗，夏乃有花。花下作梂彙多刺，花出梂上。圃人乘露采之，采已復出，至盡而罷。梂中結實，白顆如小豆大。其花暴乾，以染真紅，又作臙脂。【時珍曰】紅花二月、八月、十二月皆可以下種，雨後布子，如種麻法。初生嫩葉、苗亦可食。其葉如小薊葉。至五月開花，如大薊花而紅色。侵晨采花搗熟，以水淘，布袋絞去黄汁又搗，以酸粟米泔清又淘，又絞袋去汁，以青蒿覆一宿，晒乾，或捏，成薄餅，陰乾收之。入藥搓碎用。其子五月收采，淘浄搗碎煎汁，入醋拌蔬食，極肥美。又可爲車脂及燭。

Collected Explanations. [Ma] Zhi: *Hong lan hua* 紅藍花 is *hong hua* 紅花. It grows in Liang and Han and in the western regions. The *Bo wu zhi* states: "Zhang Qian obtained the seeds in the western regions." Nowadays it is also planted in Wei. [Su] Song: Today it can be found everywhere. Households plant it in gardens. The seeds are spread on fertile ground in winter; by the time of spring a seedling grows and in summer flowers appear. Below the flowers a ball-shaped cluster is formed with many thorns. The flowers emerge from above this ball. The gardeners collect them when they are covered with dew. When they are removed, new [flowers] appear. This is repeated until they are exhausted and decay. The fruits are formed inside the balls. These are white seeds the size of rice beans. The flowers are dried in the sun; they serve as a red dye. Also, they are made to rouge. [Li] Shizhen: *Hong hua* seeds can be planted in the second, eighth and twelfth month. The seeds are sown after a rain, the same way as hemp/sesame is sown. The tender leaves that grow first and also the seedling are edible. The leaves are similar to small cat thistle leaves. The flowers open in the fifth month. They are similar to the flowers of Japanese thistles, but are red. Collect the flowers in the early morning, pound them and wash them with water in a pan or basket. Put them into a cloth pouch, squeeze them to remove their yellow juice and pound them again. Rinse them with water in which millet has been washed and squeeze them again in a pouch to remove the juice. Then cover them with greenish wormwood for one night and dry them in the sun. Or knead them with your fingers to prepare a thin cake, dry it in the yin (i. e., shade) and store it. For medicinal application, rub it with your hands into small pieces. The seeds are collected in the fifth month. They are washed clean, ground to small pieces and boiled to obtain a juice. This is mixed with vinegar to be eaten with vegetables. A very fat and delicious item. It can also be used as cart grease and to prepare candles.

15-27-01
花 *Hua*
Flower [of *hong hua*].

【氣味】辛，温，無毒。【元素曰】入心養血，謂其苦温，陰中之陽，故入心。佐當歸，生新血。【好古曰】辛而甘苦，温，肝經血分藥也。入酒良。

Qi and Flavor. Acrid, warm, nonpoisonous. [Zhang] Yuansu: It enters the heart and nourishes blood. It is said that it enters the heart because of its being bitter and warm, a yang in yin [quality]. Assisted by Chinese *angelica*, it generates new blood. [Wang] Haogu: Acrid and at the same time sweet and bitter, warm. It is a pharmaceutical drug for the blood section of the liver conduits. Added to wine it yields good [results].

【主治】產後血運口噤，腹内惡血不盡絞痛，胎死腹中，並酒煮服。亦主蠱毒。開寶。多用破留血，少用養血。震亨。活血，潤燥，止痛，散腫，通經。時珍。

Control. Blood [induced brain] movement and lockjaw following delivery, a contracting pain in the abdomen caused by malign blood that does not completely come out, and when a fetus has died in the abdomen, for all these ingest [*hong hua* flowers] in wine. They also control *gu* poison.[182] *Kai bao*. Used often/in larger amounts they break through abiding blood. Used seldom/in small amounts they nourish blood. [Zhu] Zhenheng. They quicken the blood, moisturize dryness, end pain, disperse [qi causing a] swelling and penetrate the conduits. [Li] Shizhen.

【發明】【時珍曰】血生於心包，藏於肝，屬於衝任。紅花汁與之同類，故能行男子血脈，通女子經水。多則行血，少則養血。按養痾漫筆云：新昌徐氏婦，病産運已死，但胸膈微熱。有名醫陸氏曰：血悶也。得紅花數十斤，乃可活。遂亟購得，以大鍋煮湯，盛三桶於窗格之下，舁婦寢其上熏之，湯冷再加。有頃指動，半日乃蘇。按此亦得唐許胤宗以黄芪湯熏柳太后風病之法也。

Explication: [Li] Shizhen: The blood is generated in the heart enclosing [network]. It is stored in the liver and it is associated with the throughway and controller [vessels]. *Hong hua* juice belongs to the same group [as blood]. Hence it is able to pass through the blood vessels of males and to open the flow of menstruation of females. Large amounts stimulate the movement of blood. Small amounts nourish blood. According to the *Yang ke man bi*, "the wife of Mr. Xu in Xin chang had died of the disease [blood induced brain] movement following delivery. Still, there was some heat left in her chest and diaphragm. The famous physician Mr. Lu said: 'This is blood[-related] heart-pressure. With tens of *jin* of *hong hua* she can be brought back to live.' Hence, a large quantity was purchased and boiled in a huge cauldron. The resulting decoction was filled into three buckets that were then placed underneath the window. The woman was lifted and placed on [the buckets] to be steamed [by the vapors of the hot decoction]. When the decoction cooled, [hot liquid] was added again. After a short while her fingers began to move. After half a day she

182 *Gu du* 蠱毒, "*gu*-poison[ing]." (1) A poison emitted by certain worms/snakes with an ability to cause varying pathological changes in a person who has taken it in by means of wine or food. (2) Abdominal fullness, in some cases with blood spitting, and blood in the stool and urine. BCGM Dict I, 192 - 193. See BCGM 42-22.

awoke." Now, this was an application of the same method used during the Tang era by Xu Yinzong to treat the wind disease of the empress dowager Liu tai hou by steaming her with an *astragalus* [root decoction].[183]

【附方】舊五，新三。

Added Recipes. Five of old. Three newly [recorded].

六十二種風。張仲景治六十二種風，兼腹内血氣刺痛。用紅花一大兩，分爲四分，以酒一大升，煎鍾半，頓服之。不止再服。圖經本草。

The 62 kinds of [diseases related to] wind [intrusion]. This is Zhang Zhongjing's treatment of 62 kinds of [diseases related to] wind [intrusion], accompanied by a piercing pain caused by blood and qi [disorder] in the abdomen. Divide one generous *liang* of *hong hua* into four portions and boil [each of] them in one generous *sheng* of wine down to half a *sheng* to be ingested all at once. If [the disease] does not end, ingest this again. *Tu jing ben cao.*

一切腫疾。紅花熟搗取汁服，不過三服便瘥。外臺秘要。

All types of illnesses with a swelling. Pound heat prepared *hong hua* to obtain its juice and ingest it. A cure is achieved after not more than three ingestions. *Wai tai mi yao.*

喉痺壅塞不通者。紅藍花搗，絞取汁一小升服之，以瘥爲度。如冬月無生花，以乾者浸濕絞汁煎服，極驗。廣利方。

Blocked, impassable throat. Pound *hong lan hua*, squeeze [the resulting mass] to obtain a small *sheng* of its juice and ingest it until a cure is achieved. If in winter no fresh flowers are available, moisturize dry [flowers] by soaking them and then squeeze them. Boil the resulting juice and ingest [the liquid]. Extremely effective. *Guang li fang.*

熱病胎死。紅花酒煮汁，飲二三盞。熊氏補遺。

Death of a fetus related to a heat disease. Boil *hong hua* in wine and [let the woman] drink two or three cups of the resulting juice. Xiong shi, *Bu yi.*

胎衣不下。方同上。楊氏產乳。

Failure to discharge the placenta. Recipe identical to the one above. Yang shi, *Chan ru.*

183 See BCGM 12-02-01, *huang qi* root, "Explication," for a more detailed account of this treatment.

產後血運，心悶氣絶。紅花一兩，爲末，分作二服，酒二盞，煎一盞，連服。如口噤，斡開灌之。或入小便尤妙。子母秘録。

Blood[-induced brain] movement following birth, with heart-pressure and interrupted qi [flow]. [Grind] one *liang* of *hong hua* into powder and divide it for ingestion into two portions. Boil [each of] them in two cups of wine down to one cup, and ingest [both portions] one after another. In the case of clenched jaws, break open [the woman's teeth] to force-feed her. The addition of urine leads to even better results. *Zi mu mi lu.*

聤耳出水。紅藍花三錢半，枯礬五錢，爲末，以綿杖繳净吹之。無花則用枝葉。一方去礬。聖惠方。

Festering ears releasing water. [Grind] three and a half *qian* of *hong lan hua* and five *qian* of processed alum into powder. Wrap silk floss around a wooden stick, wipe [the interior of the affected ear] clean and blow the [powder into it]. If no flowers are available, use twigs and leaves. Another recipe omits the alum. *Sheng hui fang.*

噎膈拒食。端午采頭次紅花，無灰酒拌，焙乾，血竭瓜子樣者，等分爲末，無灰酒一盞，隔湯頓熱，徐嚥。初服二分，次日四分，三日五分。楊起簡便方。

Choking with food rejected at the diaphragm. On the fifth day of the fifth month collect the very first blossoming *hong hua* flowers, mix them with ash-free wine, dry them over a fire in a pan, mix them with an equal amount of melon seed-sized pieces of dragon's blood and [grind this into] powder. Give it into one cup of ash-free wine and heat [the cup] in a water-bath of boiling water. This is then slowly drunk [by the patient]. He is to first ingest two *fen*, the next day four *fen*, and on the third day five *fen*. Yang Qi, *Jian bian fang.*

15-27-02
子 *Zi*
Seeds [of *hong hua*].

【主治】天行瘡痘，水呑數顆。開寶。功與花同。蘇頌。

Control. For epidemic smallpox, swallow with water several seeds. *Kai bao.* The [therapeutic] potential [of *hong hua* seeds] is identical to that of the flowers. Su Song.

【附方】舊二，新一。

Added Recipes. Two of old. One newly [recorded].

血氣刺痛。紅藍子一升，擣碎，以無灰酒一大升拌子，暴乾，重擣篩，蜜丸梧子大，空心酒下四十丸。張仲景方。

Piercing pain related to blood and qi [disorder]. Pound one *sheng* of *hong hua* seeds to small pieces. Mix the seeds with one generous *sheng* of ash-free wine and dry this in the sun. Pound this again, pass it through a sieve and with honey form pills the size of *wu* seeds. Send 40 pills down with wine on an empty stomach. A recipe of Zhang Zhongjing.

瘡疽不出。紅花子、紫草茸各半兩，蟬蛻二錢半，水酒鍾半，煎減半，量大小加減服。龐安常傷寒論。

Sores and impediment-illness that fail to release [liquid]. Boil half a *liang* each of *hong hua* seeds and fine *arnebia* herbs and two and a half *qian* of cicada sloughs in one and a half *zhong* of a water and wine mixture down to one half, and [let the patient] ingest an amount depending on his age. Pang Anchang, *Shan han lun.*

女子中風，血熱煩渴。以紅藍子五合，熬擣，旦日取半大匙，以水一升，煎取七合，去滓細細嚥之。貞元廣利方。

Females struck by wind, with blood heat and vexing thirst. Heat five *ge* of *hong lan* seeds and pound them. At dawn boil half a big spoonful in one *sheng* of water down to seven *ge*. Remove the dregs and [let the patient] cautiously sip [the liquid]. *Zhen yuan guang li fang.*

15-27-03
苗 ***Miao***
Seedling [of *hong hua*].

【主治】生擣，塗遊腫。開寶。

Control. Pound fresh [seedlings] and apply [the resulting mass] on a roaming swelling. *Kai bao.*

15-28
番紅花綱目
Fan hong hua, FE *Gang mu*

***Crocus sativus* L. Saffron.**[184]

【釋名】洎夫藍綱目、撒法即。

184 *Fan hong hua* 番紅花, lit.: "foreign *hong hua*/safflower,"

Explanation of Names. *Ji fu lan* 洎[185]夫藍, *Gang mu*. *Safaji* 撒法即[186].

【集解】【時珍曰】番紅花出西番、回回地面及天方國，即彼地紅藍花也。元時以入食饌用。按張華博物志言，張騫得紅藍花種於西域，則此即一種，或方域地氣稍有異耳。

Collected Explanations. [Li] Shizhen: *Fan hong hua* comes from foreign lands in the West, from Muslim territories and from Tian fang guo. It is the safflower of these regions. During the Yuan era it was introduced to China as a delicacy. According to Zhang Hua's *Bo wu zhi*, "Zhang Qian obtained safflower and planted it in the Western regions." But this is a kind different from the one discussed here. The qi of the region [where a plant grows] causes a little difference.

【氣味】甘，平，無毒。

Qi and Flavor. Sweet, balanced, nonpoisonous.

【主治】心憂鬱積，氣悶不散，活血。久服令人心喜。又治驚悸。時珍。

Control. A worried mind with pent-up and accumulated [heat qi] pressing against the heart and failing to disperse. It quickens the blood. Ingested over a long time it lets one by happy. Also, it serves to cure fright palpitation. [Li] Shizhen.

【附方】新一。

Added Recipes. One newly [recorded].

傷寒發狂，驚怖恍惚。用撒法即二分，水一盞，浸一夕服之。天方國人所傳。王璽醫林集要。

Harm caused by cold with eruptions of madness, horror and absent-mindedness. Soak two *fen* of *safaji* in one cup of water for one night and ingest this. Transmitted by people from Tian fang guo. Wang Xi, *Yi lin ji yao*.

185 *Ji* 洎 is most likely an erroneous writing of *zan* 咱. Yin shan zheng yao ch. 3, Liao wu xing wei 料物性味, "Nature and flavor of victuals," writes *zan fu lan* 咱夫蘭. The alternative names of *fan hong hua*, such as *zan fu lan* 咱夫藍 and *sa fa lang* 撒法郎 are transcriptions [of the foreign name saffron]. A writing *ji* 洎 appears inappropriate.

186 *Ji* 即 is most likely an erroneous writing of *lang* 郎, for the same reason as outlined above. This mistake started with Wang Xi's Yi lin ji yao.

15-29
燕脂綱目
Yan zhi, FE *Gang mu*

Rouge.[187]

【釋名】赮赦。【時珍曰】按伏侯中華古今注云：燕脂起自紂，以紅藍花汁凝作之。調脂飾女面，產於燕地，故曰燕脂。或作赮赦。匈奴人名妻爲閼氏，音同燕脂，謂其顏色可愛如燕脂也。俗作臙肢、胭支者，並謬也。

Explanation of Names. *Yan she* 赮赦. [Li] Shizhen: According to Fu Hou's *Zhong hua gu jin zhu*, "*yan zhi* 燕脂 came up during [the reign of the Shang ruler] Zhou. It is produced by mixing the coagulated juice of safflower with fat to decorate the face of women. As it is produced in Yan 燕 it is called 'Yan fat,' *yan zhi* 燕脂. It is also written *yan she* 赮赦. The Xiong nu people call their wives *yan zhi* 閼氏, with a pronunciation identical to that of *yan zhi* 燕脂, stating that the complexion [of their wives] is as amiable as that of *yan zhi* 燕脂." Commonly used designations such as *yan zhi* 臙肢 and *yan zhi* 胭支 are all wrong.

【集解】【時珍曰】燕脂有四種：一種以紅藍花汁染胡粉而成，乃蘇鶚演義所謂燕脂葉似薊，花似蒲，出西方，中國謂之紅藍，以染粉爲婦人面色者也。一種以山燕脂花汁染粉而成，乃段公路北户録所謂端州山間有花叢生，葉類藍，正月開花似蓼，土人采含苞者爲燕脂粉，亦可染帛，如紅藍者也。一種以山榴花汁作成者，鄭虔胡本草中載之。一種以紫[金丱]染綿而成者，謂之胡燕脂，李珣南海藥譜載之。今南人多用紫[金丱]燕脂，俗呼紫梗是也。大抵皆可入血病藥用。又落葵子亦可取汁和粉飾面，亦謂之胡燕脂，見菜部。

Collected Explanations. There are four kinds of *yan zhi*. One kind is made by mixing safflower juice with lead carbonate. This is the one referred to in the Su E *yan yi*: "*Yan zhi* leaves are similar to those of Japanese thistles. The flowers resemble those of dandelion. [*Yan zhi*] comes from the West. In China it is called *hong lan* 紅藍 (15-27). It is used to color a cosmetic face powder for women." Another kind is made by mixing a powder with the juice of mountain *yan zhi* flowers. This is the one referred to by Duan Gonglu in his *Bei hu lu*: "In Duan zhou in the mountains clusters of flowers grow with leaves similar to those of *eupatorium* herbs. The flowers open in the first month and are similar to those of knotweed. The locals collect them as flower buds and prepare a *yan zhi* powder. It can also be used to dye silks. This is similar to *hong lan* 紅藍 (15-27)." Another kind is made with mountain pomegranade juice. Zheng Qian lists it in his *Hu ben cao*. Another kind is made by dying silk fabric with shellac. It is called *hu yan zhi* 胡燕脂. Li Xun lists it in his *Nan hai yao*

187 *Yan zhi* 燕脂, lit.: "a swallow's fat."

pu. Today, people in the South often use shellac *yan zhi*; it is the commonly called *zi geng* 紫梗. "purple stick." In general, all [the kinds mentioned above] can be added to medication for blood diseases. Furthermore, the juice of Malabar nightshade can also be mixed with powder to prepare facial cosmetics. This, too, is called *hu yan zhi*. See the section "vegetables." (27-21)

【氣味】甘，平，無毒。

Qi and Flavor. Sweet, balanced, nonpoisonous.

【主治】小兒聤耳，浸汁滴之。開寶。活血，解痘毒。時珍。

Control. For festering ears of children, soak it to obtain a juice and drip it [into the affected ears]. *Kai bao*. It quickens blood and dissolves smallpox poison. [Li] Shizhen.

【附方】新五。

Added Recipes. Five newly [recorded].

乳頭裂破。燕脂、蛤粉爲末，傅之。危氏得效方。

Chapped breast nipples. [Grind] *yan zhi* and clam shell powder into powder and apply it [to the affected region]. *Wei shi de xiao fang*.

嬰孩鵝口，白厚如紙。用坯子燕脂，以乳汁調塗之，一宿效。男用女乳，女用男乳。集簡方。

Goose mouth of children[188] with a thick, white layer resembling paper. Mix semi-finished *yan zhi* with the nursing mother's milk and apply this [to the affected region]. An effect will show after one night. For baby boys use the milk for a baby girl. For baby girls use the milk for a baby boy. *Ji jian fang*.

漏瘡腫痛：豬膽七箇，綿燕脂十個，洗水和勻，搽七次即可。救急方。

Dripping sores with painful swelling. Wash seven pig gallbladders and ten pieces of *yan zhi* made from [dyed] silk in water and mix them evenly. Apply this seven times [to the affected region] and [a cure] can be achieved. *Jiu ji fang*.

防痘入目。臙脂嚼汁點之。集簡方。

To prevent smallpox from entering the eyes. Chew *yan zhi* to obtain a juice and drip it into [the eyes]. *Ji jian fang*.

---

188 *E kou* 鵝口, "goose mouth," refers to a white layer covering the mucous membranes and top of the tongue in a child's mouth making it resemble a goose-mouth. BCGM Dict I, 141.

痘瘡倒陷。乾臙脂三錢，胡桃燒存性一箇，研末，用胡荽煎酒服一錢，再服取效。救急方。

Inverted smallpox sores. Grind three *qian* of dried *yan zhi* and walnuts, heated with their nature retained, into powder. Boil it with coriander seeds and ingest one *qian* of this with wine. After repeated ingestions an effect will be achieved. *Jiu ji fang*.

15-30
大薊小薊別録中品

***Da ji, xiao ji*.** FE *Bie lu*, middle rank.

***Cirsium japonicum* DC. Japanese thistle.**

【釋名】虎薊弘景、馬薊范汪、貓薊弘景、刺薊日華、山牛蒡日華、鷄項草圖經、千針草圖經、野紅花綱目。【弘景曰】大薊是虎薊，小薊是貓薊，葉並多刺，相似。田野甚多，方藥少用。【時珍曰】薊猶髻也，其花如髻也。曰虎、曰貓，因其苗狀狰獰也。曰馬者，大也。牛蒡，因其根似牛蒡根也。鷄項，因其莖似鷄之項也。千針、紅花，皆其花狀也。鄭樵通志謂爾雅之蘩曰狗毒者即此，未知是否？【藏器曰】薊門以多薊得名，當以北方者爲勝也。

Explanation of Names. *Hu ji* 虎薊, "tiger thistle," [Tao] Hongjing. *Ma ji* 馬薊, "horse thistle," Fan Wang. *Mao ji* 貓薊, "cat thistle," [Tao] Hongjing. *Ci ji* 刺薊, "thorny thistle," Rihua. *Shan niu bang* 山牛蒡, "mountain burdock," Rihua. *Ji xiang cao* 鷄項草, "chicken nape herb," *Tu jing*. *Qian zhen cao* 千針草, "thousand needles herb," *Tu jing*. *Ye hong hua* 野紅花, "wild safflower," *Gang mu*. [Tao] Hongjing: *Da ji* 大薊, "large thistle," is *hu ji* 虎薊, "tiger thistle." *Xiao ji* 小薊, "small thistle," is *mao ji* 貓薊, "cat thistle." The leaves of both have many thorns and are similar. Many of them are found in the open country. They are seldom resorted to as recipe drugs. [Li] Shizhen: *Ji* 薊 is equal to *ji* 髻, "coiled hair." The flowers resemble coiled hair. *Da ji* and *xiao ji* are named after tigers and cats because of the ferocious shape of the seedlings. They are named "horse *ji*" because they are big. [They are named "mountain] burdock", [*shan*] *niu bang* [山]牛蒡, because their root resembles the root of "great burdock," *niu bang* 牛蒡. [They are named] "chicken nape" because their stem resembles the nape of chicken. "Thousand needles" and "red flower/safflower", *hong hua* 紅花, are references to their flowers. Zheng Qiao in his *Tong zhi* says: "The *Er ya* has *ji* 蘩, also called 'dog poison,' *gou du* 狗毒. This is the [substance discussed here]." It is not known yet whether this is so indeed. [Chen] Cangqi: Ji men 薊門 (today's Bei jing) is named so because of the many burdocks, *ji* 薊, found there. Those from the North must be the best.

【集解】【别録曰】大小薊，五月采。【恭曰】大小薊葉[雖相似，功力有殊。大薊生山谷，根療癰腫。小薊生平澤，不能消腫，而俱能破血。【頌曰】小薊處處有之，俗名青刺薊。二月生苗，二三寸時，併根作菜，茹食甚美。四月高尺餘，多刺，心中出花，頭如紅藍花而青紫色，北人呼爲千針草。四月采苗，九月采根，並陰乾用。大薊苗根與此相似，但肥大爾。【宗奭曰】大小薊皆相似，花如髻。但大薊高三四尺，葉皺；小薊高一尺許，葉不皺，以此爲異。作菜雖有微芒，不害人。

Collected Explanations. *Bie lu*: *Da* [*ji*] and *xiao ji* are collected in the fifth month. [Su] Gong: The leaves of *da* [*ji*] and *xiao ji* are similar but their [therapeutic] potentials differ. *Da ji* grows in mountain valleys. The root serves to cure swelling related to obstruction-illness.[189] *Xiao ji* grows in the plains, in marshlands. It is unable to dissolve swelling. But both can break through blood [accumulation]. [Su] Song: *Xiao ji* can be found everywhere. It is commonly called "greenish thorny thistle." It grows a seedling in the second month. When it has reached a length of two or three *cun*, together with the root it can serve as a very tasty vegetable. By the fourth month [*xiao ji*] has reached a height of more than one *chi*, with many thorns. Flowers come out of the center. Their top is similar to that of safflower flowers, with a greenish-purple color. People in the North call it "thousand needle herb." The seedling is collected in the fourth month; the root is collected in the ninth month. Both [seedling and root] are dried in the yin (i. e., shade) before they are made use of. The seedling and the root of *Da ji* are similar to those [of *xiao ji*]; they are just fatter and bigger. [Kou] Zongshi: *Da* [*ji*] and *xiao ji* are similar to each other in all respects. Their flowers resemble coiled hair. However, *da ji* reaches a height of three to four *chi*, and the leaves are wrinkled. *Xiao ji* is more than one *chi* tall; the leaves are not wrinkled. That is the difference. When they are prepared as vegetable they have some fine awns, but this is not harmful to humans.

15-30-01
大薊根 *Da ji gen*
Root of *da ji*.

葉同。

Identical with the leaves.

【氣味】甘，温，無毒。【弘景曰】有毒。【權曰】苦，平。【大明曰】葉涼。

189 *Yong* 癰, "obstruction-illness,"refers to an obstruction of vessels or other ducts inside the body. Qi rushing against the obstruction may cause a local swelling and eventually break through the surface to cause an abscess. BCGM Dict I, 641.

Qi and Flavor. Sweet, warm, nonpoisonous. [Tao] Hongjing: Poisonous. [Zhen] Quan: Bitter, balanced. Da Ming: The leaves are cool.

【主治】女子赤白沃，安胎，止吐血鼻衄，令人肥健。别録。擣根絞汁服半升，主崩中血下立瘥。甄權。葉：治腸癰，腹臟瘀血作運，撲損，生研，酒并小便任服。又惡瘡疥癬，同鹽研署之。大明。

Control. Red and white [discharge of] foam by females. It calms a fetus and ends blood spitting and nosebleed. It lets one become fat and strong. *Bie lu*. Pound the root and squeeze [the resulting pulp] to obtain a juice and ingest half a *sheng*. This controls collapsing center[190] with blood discharge and has an immediate effect. Zhen Quan. The leaves: To cure intestinal obstruction-illness, [brain] movement caused by blood stagnating in the abdomen and the long-term depots, and injuries resulting from a blow, grind them fresh and eat, mixed with wine and urine, as much as seems preferable. Also, for malign sores, *jie*-illness[191] and *xuan*-illness,[192] grind them with salt and apply this [to the affected region]. Da Ming.

15-30-02
小薊根 *Xiao ji gen*
Root of *xiao ji*.

苗同。

Identical with the seedling.

【氣味】甘，温，無毒。【大明曰】涼。

Qi and Flavor. Sweet, warm, nonpoisonous. Da Ming: Cool.

【主治】養精保血。别録。破宿血，生新血，暴下血血崩，金瘡出血，嘔血等，絞取汁温服。作煎和糖，合金瘡及蜘蛛蛇蠍毒，服之亦佳。藏器。治熱毒風，並胸膈煩悶，開胃下食，退熱，補虚損。苗：去煩熱，生研汁服。並大明。作菜食，除風熱。夏月熱煩不止，擣汁半升服，立瘥。孟詵。

Control. It nourishes the essence/sperm and guards the blood. *Bie lu*. It breaks through abiding blood and generates new blood. [To cure] sudden blood discharge

190 *Beng zhong* 崩中, "collapsing center," excessive vaginal bleeding outside of a menstruation period. BCGM Dict I, 58.

191 *Jie*-illness 疥, vaguely identifiable skin ailment. BCGM Dict I, 249.

192 *Xuan* 癬, "*xuan*-illness." Conditions of dermal lesions with initially erythema, papules, and itching gradually extending in all directions to form an irregular ring with clear boundaries. The skin is slightly elevated with small papules, blisters, and/or scales and scraps. The central lesion may appear to heal spontaneously, and it may reappear. Also, a designation of local lesions with itching, release of liquid and shedding of scabs. BCGM Dict I, 591.

and blood collapse,[193] bleeding wounds caused by metal objects/weapons, and vomiting of blood, squeeze it to obtain a juice and ingest it warm. Boiled and the decoction ingested mixed with sugar, it is also an excellent [medication] for wounds caused by metal objects/weapons and [to resolve] the poison of spiders, snakes and skorpions. [Chen] Cangqi. It serves to cure heat poison associated with wind [intrusion], and also vexing heart-pressure affecting chest and diaphragm. It opens the stomach and allows food to pass down. It repels heat and supplements [qi] in the case of depletion injury. The seedling: To remove vexing heat, grind fresh [seedlings] and ingest the juice. All this from Da Ming. Prepared as vegetable and eaten it eliminates heat related to wind [intrusion]. [To cure] unending vexation related to summer month heat, pound it and ingest half a *sheng* of the resulting juice. Immediately effective. Meng Shen.

【發明】【大明曰】小薊力微，只可退熱，不似大薊能健養下氣也。【恭曰】大小薊皆能破血。但大薊兼療癰腫，而小薊專主血，不能消腫也。

Explication. Da Ming: The [therapeutic] potential of *xiao ji* is mild. It can only be used to repel heat. This is not like the ability of *Da ji* to strengthen, nourish and discharge qi. [Su] Gong: Both *da* [*ji*] and *xiao ji* are able to break through blood [accumulation]. However, *da ji* also heals swelling related to obstruction-illness,[194] while *xiao ji* in particular controls blood [disorder]. It is unable to dissolve swelling.

【附方】舊五，新九。

Added Recipes. Five of old. Nine newly [recorded].

心熱吐血，口乾。用刺薊葉及根，搗絞取汁，每頓服二小盞。聖惠方。

Heart heat with blood spitting; dry mouth. Pound the leaves and root of *ci ji* and squeeze [the resulting mass] to obtain a juice. Each time ingest a quantity of two small cups. *Sheng hui fang.*

舌硬出血不止。刺薊搗汁，和酒服。乾者爲末，冷水服。普濟方。

Unending bleeding of a hardened tongue. Pound *ci ji* to obtain a juice, mix it with wine and ingest it. Dry [*ci ji* is ground into] powder to be ingested with cold water. *Pu ji fang.*

---

193 *Xue beng* 血崩, blood collapse. Excessive vaginal bleeding, identical to *beng zhong* 崩中, collapsing center. BCGM Dict I, 594; 58.

194 *Yong* 癰, "obstruction-illness,"refers to an obstruction of vessels or other ducts inside the body. Qi rushing against the obstruction may cause a local swelling and eventually break through the surface to cause an abscess. BCGM Dict I, 641.

九竅出血。方同上。簡要濟衆。

Bleeding from the nine orifices. Recipe identical to the one above. *Jian yao ji zhong*.

卒瀉鮮血。小薊葉搗汁，温服一升。梅師方。

Sudden outflow of fresh blood. Pound *xiao ji* leaves to obtain a juice and ingest one *sheng* warm. *Mei shi fang*.

崩中下血。大小薊根一升，酒一斗，漬五宿，任飲。亦可酒煎服，或生搗汁温服。

Collapsing center[195] with a discharge of blood. Soak one *sheng* of *da* [*ji*] and *xiao ji* in one *dou* of water for five days and nights and drink this at will.

又方：小薊莖葉洗切，研汁一盞，入生地黄汁一盞，白朮半兩，煎減半，温服。千金方。

Another recipe: Wash stem and leaves of *xiao ji* and cut them into small pieces. Grind them to obtain a small cup of juice. Add one small cup of fresh Chinese foxglove [rhizome] juice and half a *liang* of *atractylodes macrocephala* [rhizome]. Boil this down to one half and ingest it warm. *Qian jin fang*.

墮胎下血。小薊根葉、益母草五兩，水三大盌，煮汁一盌，再煎至一盞，分二服，一日服盡。聖濟總録。

Discharge of blood related to abortion/miscarriage. Boil five *liang* [each] of root and leaves of *xiao ji* and of Siberian motherwort herb in three large bowls of water down to obtain a juice of one bowl. Boil it again down to one small cup and [let the patient] ingest this divided into two portions. To be ingested completely within one day. *Sheng ji zong lu*.

金瘡出血不止。小薊苗擣爛塗之。孟詵食療本草。

Unending bleeding from wounds caused by metal objects/weapons. Pound *xiao ji* seedlings and apply the resulting pulp [to the wounds]. Meng Shen, *Shi liao ben cao*.

小便熱淋。馬薊根搗汁服。聖惠方。

Dripping hot urine. Pound *ma ci* roots and ingest the resulting juice. *Sheng hui fang*.

鼻塞不通。小薊一把，水二升，煮取一升，分服。外臺秘要方。

Blocked nose. Boil one handful of *xiao ji* in two *sheng* of water down to one *sheng* and ingest it in several portions. A *Wai tai mi yao* recipe.

---

195 *Beng zhong* 崩中, "collapsing center," excessive vaginal bleeding outside of a menstruation period. BCGM Dict I, 58.

小兒浸淫瘡，痛不可忍，發寒熱者。刺薊葉新水調傅瘡上，乾即易之。簡要濟衆方。

Drenched sores of children, with unbearable pain and alternating sensations of cold and heat. Mix *ci ji* leaves with fresh water and apply this to the sores. When they are dry change them. *Jian yao ji zhong fang.*

癬瘡作痒。刺薊葉擣汁服之。千金方。

Xuan-illness[196] sores with itch. Pound *ci ji* leaves and ingest the resulting juice. *Qian jin fang.*

婦人陰痒。小薊煮湯，日洗三次。普濟方。

Itching yin [(i. e., genital) region] of women. Boil *xiao ji* [in water] and use the decoction to wash [the affected region] three times a day. *Pu ji fang.*

諸瘻不合。虎薊根、貓薊根、酸棗根、枳根、杜衡各一把，班蝥三分，炒，爲末，蜜丸棗大，日一服。并以小丸納瘡中。肘後方。

All types of fistula that fail to close. [Grind] one handful each of *hu ji* root, *mao ji* root, jujube root, bitter orange root and *asarum caulescens* [root], with three *fen* of stir-fried blister beetles into powder and form with honey pills the size of dates. Ingest one [pill] per day. Also, insert a small pill into the sores. *Zhou hou fang.*

丁瘡惡腫。千針草四兩，乳香一兩，明礬五錢，爲末。酒服二錢，出汗爲度。普濟方。

Pin[-illness] sores with a malign swelling. [Grind four *liang* of *qian zhen cao*, one *liang* of frankincense and five *qian* of alum into powder and ingest with wine two *qian* until sweat leaves [the body]. *Pu ji fang.*

15-31
續斷本經上品

Xu duan, FE *Ben jing*, upper rank.

***Dipsacus asperoides* C. Y. Cheng et T. M. Ai. Himalayan teasel [root].**[197]

【釋名】屬折本經、接骨别録、龍豆别録、南草。【時珍曰】續斷、屬折、接骨，皆以功命名也。

---

196 *Xuan* 癬, "*xuan*-illness." Conditions of dermal lesions with initially erythema, papules, and itching gradually extending in all directions to form an irregular ring with clear boundaries. The skin is slightly elevated with small papules, blisters, and/or scales and scraps. The central lesion may appear to heal spontaneously, and it may reappear. Also, a designation of local lesions with itching, release of liquid and shedding of scabs. BCGM Dict I, 591.

197 *Xu duan* 續斷, lit.: "to join what has broken off."

Explanation of Names. *Zhu she* 屬折, "reconnecting fractures," *Ben jing*. *Jie gu* 接骨, "joining bones," *Bie lu*. *Long dou* 龍豆, "dragon bean," *Bie lu*. *Nan cao* 南草, "southern herb." [Li] Shizhen: *Xu duan* 續斷, *Zhu she* 屬折 and *jie gu* 接骨, all these are names referring to the [therapeutic] potential [of this herb].

【集解】【别録曰】續斷生常山山谷，七月、八月采，陰乾。【普曰】出梁州，七月七日采。【弘景曰】按桐君藥録云：續斷生蔓延，葉細莖如荏，大根本，黄白有汁，七月、八月采根。今皆用莖葉節節斷，皮黄皺，狀如鷄脚者，又呼爲桑上寄生。時人又有接骨樹，高丈餘許，葉似蒴藋，皮主金瘡。廣州又有續斷藤，一名諾藤，斷其莖，以器承取汁飲，療虛損絶傷，用沐頭，長髮，折枝插地即生。恐皆非真。李當之云是虎薊，與此大乖，但虎薊亦療血。【恭曰】所在山谷皆有。今俗用者，葉似苧而莖方，根如大薊，黄白色。陶説非也。【頌曰】今陝西、河中、興元、舒、越、晉、絳諸州亦有之。三月以後生苗，幹四稜，似苧麻，葉兩兩相對而生。四月開花紅白色，似益母花。根如大薊，赤黄色。謹按范汪方云：續斷即是馬薊，與小薊葉相似，但大於小薊爾。葉似旁翁菜而小厚，兩邊有刺，刺人。其花紫色，與今越州所圖者相類。而市之貨者亦有數種，少能辨其粗良。醫人但以節節斷、皮黄皺者爲真。【斅曰】凡使，勿用草茅根，緣真相似，若誤服令人筋軟。【時珍曰】續斷之説不一。桐君言是蔓生，葉似荏。李當之、范汪並言是虎薊。日華子言是大薊，一名山牛蒡。蘇恭、蘇頌皆言葉似苧麻，根似大薊。而名醫别録復出大小薊條，頗難依據。但自漢以來，皆以大薊爲續斷，相承久矣。究其實，則二蘇所云似與桐君相符，當以爲正。今人所用，以州中來，色赤而瘦，折之有烟塵起者爲良焉。鄭樵通志謂范汪所説者乃南續斷，不知何據？蓋以别川續斷耳。

Collected Explanations. *Bie lu*: *Xu duan* grows in the mountain valleys of Mount Chang shan. It is collected in the seventh and eighth month. It is dried in the yin (i. e., shade). [Wu] Pu: It comes from Liang zhou. It is collected in the seventh month on the seventh day. [Tao] Hongjing: According to Tong jun's *Yao lu*, "*xu duan* grows as an extending creeper, with fine leaves and a stem similar to that of *perilla* [herbs]. It has a large, yellow-white root base with juice. The root is collected in the seventh and eighth month." Today, everyone uses the stem and the leaves of those specimens that are divided into sections from knot to knot, with a yellow, wrinkled bark, shaped like a chicken leg. They are also called "parasites on mulberry trees." Occasionally, people come up with a *jie gu* tree more than one *zhang* tall and with leaves similar to those of Chinese elder. Its bark serves to control wounds caused by metal objects/weapons. Furthermore, in Guang zhou is a *xu duan* vine, also called *nuo teng* 諾藤, "*nuo* vine." It has a juice that is caught in a bowl and then drunk. It serves to heal depletion injury and harm related to cut offs. It is used to wash the head to stimulate hair growth. Break a twig off and insert it into the ground, and [a new plant] will grow. I guess, all this does not agree with the facts. Li Dangzhi's statement concerns tiger thistle; this is something very different from the item discussed here. Still, tiger thistle, too, heals blood [disorders]. [Su] Gong: It can be found everywhere in mountain valleys. Those commonly used today have leaves similar to ramie plants with a square stem. The root is similar to that of Japanese thistles. What Tao [Hongjing] has said is wrong. [Su] Song: Today it can be found in Shaanxi, He zhong, Xing yuan, and all the *zhou* of Shu, Yue, Jin and Jiang. Beginning with the third month it grows a seedling. This is a stalk with four edges, similar to that of ramie plants. The leaves grow two and two facing each other. In the fourth month flowers of red-white color open. They are similar to Siberian motherwort flowers. The root is similar to that of Japanese thistle; it is of red-yellow color. According to the *Fan Wang fang*, "*xu duan* is horse thistle. Its leaves resemble those of Japanese thistle, but are larger than those of Japanese thistle. The leaves are similar to those of *pang weng cai*,[198] but they are smaller and thicker. They have thorns on both sides that pierce humans. The flowers are purple." They resemble those on illustrations [of this herb] from Yue zhou. On the markets many kinds are offered and there is hardly a possibility to distinguish between coarse and good quality. The physicians consider only those as genuine that can be broken from section to section and have a yellow, wrinkled bark. [Lei] Xiao: For all applications do not use those of Japanese buttercup. The reason is, they really are very similar, but if [Japanese buttercup] is mistakenly ingested it softens one's sinews. [Li] Shizhen. The descriptions of *xu duan* differ. Tong jun says: "It grows as a creeper, with leaves similar to those of *perilla* [herbs]." Both Li Dangzhi and Fan Wang say that [*xu duan*] is tiger thistle. The *Rihua zi* says it is Japanese thistle, also named *shan niu bang* 山牛蒡. Both Su Gong and Su Song say that the leaves are similar to those of ramie plants, and the root resembles that of Japanese thistle. And the *Ming yi bie lu* treats the *da ji* and *xiao ji* [variations of Japanese thistle] in separate entries. All these [statements] are difficult to rely on. However, since the Han era everyone identified *da ji*/Japanese thistle as *xu duan*, and this has been transmitted for a long time. Considering the facts, it seems that what the two Su [Song and Su Gong] say agrees with Tong jun, and should be accepted as correct. Of those used by people today, those are good that come from Zhou[199] zhong, that are red and slim and when broken release a smoke of dust. Zheng Qiao in his *Tong zhi* says that "the [item] described by Fan

198 *Pang weng cai* 旁翁菜, an unidentified herb mentioned only once in the BCGM.

199 Instead of *zhou* 州, the Zhang edition writes *chuan* 川. In view of Li Shizhen's reference to a *chuan xu duan* 川續斷, "xu duan from [Si] chuan," below, *zhou zhong* 州中 as a place name may be a mistaken writing of *chuan zhong* 川中

Wang is a 'southern *xu duan*'." I do not know what this could rely on. The fact is, he meant to distinguish *xu duan* from [Si] chuan.

15-31-01
根 *Gen*
Root [of *xu duan*].

【修治】【斆曰】凡采得根，横切剉之，又去向裏硬筋，以酒浸一伏時，焙乾，入藥用。

Pharmaceutical Preparation. [Lei] Xiao: Always collect the roots, cut them transversely into segments and file them. Also, remove the hard sinews extending toward the interior. Soak [the pieces] in wine for one full day and dry them over a fire in a pan. Then they may be added to medication for [therapeutic] applications.

【氣味】苦，微温，無毒。【別録曰】辛。【普曰】神農、雷公、黄帝、李當之：苦，無毒。扁鵲：辛，無毒。【之才曰】地黄爲之使，惡雷丸。

Qi and Flavor. Bitter, slightly warm, nonpoisonous. *Bie lu*: Acrid. [Wu] Pu: Shen nong, Lei gong, Huang Di, Li Dangzhi: Bitter, nonpoisonous. Bian Que: Acrid, nonpoisonous. [Xu] Zhicai: Chinese foxglove [rhizome] serves as its guiding [substance]. [Ingested together,] it abhors thunderball fungus.

【主治】傷寒，補不足，金瘡，癰傷，折跌，續筋骨，婦人乳難。久服益氣力。本經。婦人崩中漏血，金瘡血内漏，止痛，生肌肉，及踠傷，惡血腰痛，關節緩急。別録。去諸温毒，通宣血脉。甄權。助氣，補五勞七傷，破癥結瘀血，消腫毒，腸風，痔瘻，乳癰，瘰癧，婦人産前後一切病，胎漏，子宫冷，面黄虚腫，縮小便，止泄精尿血。大明。

Control. Harm caused by cold. It supplements insufficient [qi]. Wounds caused by metal objects/weapons. Harm related to obstruction-illness.[200] Fractures resulting from a fall. It reconnects sinews and bones. [It serves to cure] women with difficulties in letting down milk. Ingested for a long time it boosts the qi and one's strength. *Ben jing*. Collapsing center[201] and dripping bleeding of women. Wounds caused by metal objects/weapons with internal dripping of blood. It ends pain and generates muscles and flesh. Also, [it serves to cure] physical fracture harm, malign blood with lower back pain, and cramped joints. *Bie lu*. It removes all types of warmth [epidemic] poison. It opens the passage through the blood vessels. Zhen Quan. It supports the qi, supplements [qi depletion related to] the five types of exhaustion and sev-

200 *Yong* 癰, "obstruction-illness," refers to an obstruction of vessels or other ducts inside the body. Qi rushing against the obstruction may cause a local swelling and eventually break through the surface to cause an abscess. BCGM Dict I, 641.

201 *Beng zhong* 崩中, "collapsing center," excessive vaginal bleeding outside of a menstruation period. BCGM Dict I, 58.

en types of harm, breaks through concretion-illness nodes and stagnating blood, dissolves swelling with poison, [cures] intestinal wind, piles fistula, female breast obstruction-illness, scrofula pervasion-illness,[202] all the diseases affecting women prior to or following delivery, fetal dripping, womb cold, and yellow face with hollow swelling. It restrains [involuntary] urination and ends outflow of sperm and urination with blood. Da Ming.

【發明】【時珍曰】宋張叔潜秘書，知劍州時，其閣下病血痢。一醫用平胃散一兩，入川續斷末二錢半，每服二錢，水煎服即愈。紹熙壬子，會稽時行痢疾。叔潜之子以方傳人，往往有驗。小兒痢服之皆效。

Explication. [Li] Shizhen: During the Song era, secretary Zhang Shuqian was stationed in Jian zhou when his Excellency[203] suffered from bleeding free-flux illness. One physician resorted to one *liang* of the "powder to balance the stomach" and added two and a half *qian* of [Si] chuan *xu duan*. [The patient was asked to] ingest two *qian* per dose. [The items were] boiled in water and after ingesting them [the patient] was cured. In the *ren zi* year of the *shao xi* reign period (1192) an epidemic of free-flux illness ailments occurred in Kuai ji. [Zhang] Shuqian's son gave this recipe to others, and it was often effective. When it was given to children suffering from free-flux illness it was always effective.

【附方】舊二，新二。

Added Recipes. Two of old. Two newly [recorded].

小便淋瀝。生續斷搗絞汁服，即馬薊根也。初虞世古今録驗。

Dribbling free-flux illness of children. Pound fresh *xu duan*, squeeze [the resulting mass] to obtain a juice and ingest it. This is the root of horse thistle. Chu Yushi, *Gu jin lu yan*.

妊娠胎動。兩三月墮，預宜服此。川續斷酒浸，杜仲薑汁炒去絲，各二兩，爲末，棗肉煮爛杵和丸梧子大。每服三十丸，米飲下。

---

202 *Luo li* 瘰癧, "scrofula pervasion-illness," when two or more connected swellings of the size of plum or date kernels appear either on the neck or in the armpits, or somewhere else on the body. BCGM Dict I. 329.

203 Instead of *ge xia* 閣下, "excellency," *Bai yi xuan fang* ch. 6, *zhi xue li* 止血痢, "to cure bleeding free-flux illness," writes *ge zhong* 閣中. *Pu ji fang* 普濟方, *Si ku quan shu* 四庫全書 edition, ch. 220, *xue li* 血痢, "bleeding free-flux illness," writes *kun xia* 閫下. *Ge zhong* 閣中 and *kun xia* 閫下 both refer to a member of one's household. This appears to make more sense here than *ge xia* 閣下, "excellency."

Fetal movement during pregnancy with a possibility of a miscarriage in the second or third month. To prevent this it is advisable to ingest the following [medication]. [Grind] two *liang* each of [Si] chuan *xu duan*, soaked in wine, and *eucommia* [bark], fried in ginger juice, into powder. Boil Chinese date meat to obtain a pulp and mix it [with the powder] to form pills the size of *wu* seeds. Each time ingest 30 pills, to be sent down with a rice beverage.

產後諸疾。血運，心悶煩熱，厭厭氣欲絶，心頭硬，乍寒乍熱。續斷皮一握，水三升，煎二升，分三服。如人行一里，再服。無所忌。此藥救産後垂死。子母秘録。

All illnesses following delivery. Blood [caused brain] movement, heart-pressure with vexing heat. [When the woman] is depressed to a degree that the flow of qi may be interrupted, the top section of the stomach hardens, and an alternating sensation of cold and heat sets in, boil one handful of *xu duan* in three *sheng* of water down to two *sheng* and let her ingest this divided into three portions. After a time it takes one to walk three miles, she is to ingest it again. There are no prohibitions to be observed. This medication rescues [women] close to dying after delivery. *Zi mu mi lu*.

打撲傷損，閃肭骨節。用接骨草葉搗爛罨之，立效。衛生易簡方。

Injury damage from a blow or fall, with a sprain of the bone joints. Pound the leaves of *jie gu cao* and apply the pulpy mass [to the affected region]. Immediately successful. *Wei sheng yi jian fang*.

15-32
苦芙音襖別録下品
Ku ao read *ao*, FE *Bie lu*, lower rank.

Cirsium chinense Gardn. et Champ. Linear leaf thistle.

【釋名】鉤芙爾雅、苦板。【時珍曰】凡物穉曰芙，此物嫩時可食，故以名之。

Explanation of Names. *Gou ao* 鉤芙, *Er ya*. *Ku ban* 苦板. [Li] Shizhen: All items that are tender shoots are called *ao* 芙. The present item is edible as long as it is tender. Hence this name.

【集解】【弘景曰】苦芙處處有之，傖人取莖生食之。【保昇曰】所在下濕地有之，莖圓無刺，可生噉，子若猫薊。五月五日采苗，暴乾。【恭曰】今人以爲漏蘆，非也。【時珍曰】爾雅鉤芙即此苦芙也。芙大如拇指，中空，莖頭有蔓似薊，初生可食。許慎説文言：江南人食之下氣。

今浙東人清明節采其嫩苗食之，云一年不生瘡疥。亦搗汁和米爲食，其色清，久留不敗。造化指南云：苦板大者名苦藉，葉如地黄，味苦，初生有白毛，入夏抽莖有毛，開白花甚繁，結細實。其無花實者，名地膽草，汁苦如膽也。處處濕地有之。入爐火家用。

Collected Explanations. [Tao] Hongjing: *Ku ao* can be found everywhere. Uncivilized people collect the stems and eat them raw. [Han] Baosheng: They are found everywhere in low-lying marshlands. The stem is round and has no thorns. It can be eaten raw. The seeds are similar to those of cat thistle. The seedling is collected on the fifth day of the fifth month; it is dried in the sun. [Su] Gong: Today's people identify it as *stemmacantha* herb. That is wrong. [Li] Shizhen: The *gou ao* 鉤芺 mentioned in the *Er ya* is the present *ku ao* 苦芺. [*Ku*] *ao* is as big as a thumb, and hollow inside. At the top of the stem is a calyx resembling that of thistles. When it has just begun to grow it can be eaten. Xu Shen in his *Shuo wen* says: "The people in Jiang nan eat it to discharge qi." Today the people in Zhe dong on the day of the *qing ming* festival collect the tender seedlings and eat them. They say this will prevent the generation of sores and *jie*-illness[204] for an entire year. They also pound [the seedlings], mix the resulting juice with rice and eat it. The color is distinct and it can be kept for a long time without turning bad. The *Zao hua zhi nan* states: "Large specimens of *ku ban* are called *ku ji* 苦藉. The leaves are similar to those of Chinese foxglove, with a bitter flavor. When they have just begun to grow they have white hair. In early summer, a stem with hair rises and opens white flowers in great abundance. They form fine fruit. Those without flowers and fruits are call *di dan cao* 地膽草, 'ground bile herb.' Their juice is bitter like bile. They are found everywhere in marshlands. Experts of furnace [preparation of elixirs] use them."

15-32-01
苗 *Miao*
Seedling [of *ku ao*].

【氣味】苦，微寒，無毒。

Qi and Flavor. Bitter, slightly cold, nonpoisonous.

【主治】面目通身漆瘡，燒灰傅之。亦可生食。别録。燒灰療金瘡，甚驗。弘景。治丹毒。大明。煎湯洗痔，甚驗。汪穎。下氣解熱。時珍。

Control. Lacquer sores[205] covering the face, the eyes and the entire body. Burn [the seedlings] to ashes and apply them [to the affected region]. They can also be eaten raw. *Bie lu*. Burned to ashes they very effectively heal wounds caused by metal

204 *Jie*-illness 疥, vaguely identifiable skin ailment. BCGM Dict I, 249.

205 *Qi chuang* 漆瘡, "lacquer sores," are conditions developing as an allergic reaction to having been affected by the qi of lacquer. After the naked skin has come into contact with

object/weapons. [Tao] Hongjing. They serve to cure cinnabar poison.[206] Da Ming. They are boiled in water and the decoction serves to wash piles. Very effective. Wang Ying. They discharge qi and resolve heat. [Li] Shizhen.

15-33
漏盧本經上品
Lou lu, FE *Ben jing*, upper rank.

***Stemmacantha uniflorum* (L.) Dittrich. Uniflower swisscentaury.**

【釋名】野蘭本經、莢蒿蘇恭、鬼油麻日華。【時珍曰】屋之西北黑處謂之漏。凡物黑色謂之盧。此草秋後即黑，異於衆草，故有漏盧之稱。唐韻作蔏。其莢如麻，故俗呼爲鬼油麻云。

Explanation of Names. *Ye lan* 野蘭, "wild orchid," *Ben jing*. *Jia hao* 莢蒿, Su Gong. *Gui you ma* 鬼油麻, "demon sesame," *Rihua*. [Li] Shizhen: The black/darkest corner in the North-West of a house is called *lou* 漏. All black items are called *lu* 盧. This herb turns black after autumn. This is different from all other herbs. Hence the designation *lou lu* 漏盧. The *Tang yun* writes [the character *lou*] as 蔏. The pod/fruits are similar to sesame [seeds], *ma* 麻. Hence [the plant] is commonly called "demon sesame," *gui you ma* 鬼油麻.

【集解】【別録曰】漏盧生喬山山谷，八月采根，陰乾。【弘景曰】喬山應是黄帝所葬處，乃在上郡。今出近道。市人取苗用之。俗中取根名鹿驪根，苦酒摩以療瘡疥。【恭曰】此藥俗名莢蒿，莖葉似白蒿，花黄，生莢，長似細麻之莢，大如筯許，有四五瓣，七八月後皆黑，異於衆草，蒿之類也。常用其莖葉及子，未見用根。其鹿驪，山南謂之木黎蘆，有毒，非漏盧也。今人以馬薊似苦芙者爲漏盧，亦非也。【志曰】別本言漏盧莖大如筯，高四五尺，子房似油麻房而小。江東人取其苗用，勝於根。江寧及上黨者佳。陶云鹿驪，蘇云木黎蘆，皆非也。漏盧自別。【藏器曰】南人用苗，北土用根，乃樹生，如茱萸，樹高二三尺，有毒，殺蟲，山人以洗瘡疥。【保昇曰】葉似角蒿，今曹、兖州下濕處最多。六月、七月采莖，日乾，黑於衆草。【大明曰】花苗並可用。形并氣味似乾牛蒡，頭上有白花子。【頌曰】今汴東州郡及秦、海州皆有之。舊説莖葉似白蒿，花黄有莢，莖若筯大，房類油麻而小。今諸郡所圖上，惟單州者差相類。沂州者花葉頗似牡丹。秦州者花似單葉寒菊，紫色，五七枝同一幹。海州者花紫碧，如單葉蓮花，花萼下及根旁有白茸裹之，根如蔓菁而細，又類葱本，黑色，淮甸人呼爲老翁花。三州所生花雖別，而葉頗相類，但秦、海

lacquer qi it suddenly turns red, is inflamed and itches. Small streaks or blisters emerge. If scratched they open to fester and emit liquid. BCGM Dict I, 382.

206 *Dan du* 丹毒, "cinnabar poison," a skin ailment with red rashes. BCGM Dict I, 118

州者葉更作鋸齒狀。一物而殊類如此，醫家何所適從？當依舊説，以單州出者爲勝。又本草飛廉一名漏盧，云與苦芙相類，其根生則肉白皮黑，乾則黑如玄參，七八月采花，陰乾用。所説與秦州、海州所圖漏盧花葉及根頗相近，然彼人但名漏盧，不曰飛廉也。【斆曰】一種真似漏盧，只是味苦酸，誤服令人吐不止。【時珍曰】按沈存中筆談云：今方家所用漏盧乃飛廉也。飛廉一名漏盧，苗似苦芙，根如牛蒡，綿頭者是也。采時用根。今閩中所謂漏盧，莖如油麻，高六七寸，秋深枯黑如漆，采時用苗，乃真漏盧也。餘見"飛廉"下。

Collected Explanations. *Bie lu*: *Lou lu* grows in the mountain valleys of Mount Qiao shan. The root is collected in the eighth month. It is dried in the yin (i. e., shade). [Tao] Hongjing: Mount Qiao shan should be the place where the Yellow Thearch was buried. It is located in Shang jun. Today [*lou lu*] comes from nearby. The market merchants collect the seedlings [and offer them for therapeutic] use. The common people collect the roots, called *lu li gen* 鹿驪根 ("deer and black horse root"). They grind them with vinegar to heal sores and *jie*-illness.[207] [Su] Gong: This pharmaceutical drug is commonly called *jia hao* 莢蒿. Its stem and leaves are similar to those of Sievers wormwood, *bai hao* 白蒿. The flowers are yellow; they generate pods/fruit with a length similar to the pods/fruit of fine sesame, and a size like chopsticks. They have four or five petals, all of them turn black from the seventh and eighth month on. This is different from all other herbs. They belong to the group of *hao* 蒿/wormwood plants. Their stem, leaves and seeds are in frequent use; the use of the root has not been observed. The [root named] *lu li* 鹿驪 is called *mu li lu* 木黎蘆 in Shan nan. It is poisonous; it is not *lou lu* 漏盧. Today, people consider horse thistle that is similar to linear leaf thistle to be *lou lu*. That is wrong, too. [Ma] Zhi: Another copy [of the *Ben cao*] says that the stems of *lou lu* have the size of chopsticks, reaching a height of four to five *chi*. The seed chambers are similar to sesame seed chambers, but they are smaller. The people in Jiang dong gather the stems for [pharmaceutical] use. They are superior to the roots. Those from Jiang ning and Shang dang are excellent. What Tao [Hongjing] says about *lu li* 鹿驪 and what Su [Gong] says about *mu li lu* 木黎蘆, is all wrong. These [items] differ from *lou li*. [Chen] Cangqi: The Southerners use the seedling; in the North they use the roots. Now, [*lou lu*] grows as trees, similar to *evodia*. The trees reach a height of two to three *chi*. [*Lou lu*] is poisonous; it kills *gu* [poison][208]. The people in the mountains use it to wash sores and *jie*-illness. [Han] Baosheng: The leaves are similar to those

207 *Jie*-illness 疥, vaguely identifiable skin ailment. BCGM Dict I, 249.

208 *Gu du* 蠱毒, "*gu*-poison[ing]." (1) A poison emitted by certain worms/snakes with an ability to cause varying pathological changes in a person who has taken it in by means of wine or food. (2) Abdominal fullness, in some cases with blood spitting, and blood in the stool and urine. BCGM Dict I, 192 - 193. See BCGM 42-22.

of Chinese *incarvillea*. Nowadays, very many [*lou lu*] are found in Cao [zhou] und Yan zhou. The stem is collected in the sixth and seventh month. It is dried in the sun. It is darker in color than that of all other herbs. Da Ming: Flower and stem can all be used. From their physical appearance and their qi and flavor they are similar to those of dried great burdock. On the top [of the stem] are a white flower and the seeds. [Su] Song: Today, [*lou lu*] can be found in the *zhou* and prefectures of Bian dong and also in Qin and Hai zhou. Formerly it was said that the stem and the leaves are similar to those of Sievers wormwood, that the flowers are yellow and have pods, that the stem has the size of a chopstick and that the [fruit] chambers are like those of sesame, but smaller. Today, judged from illustrations coming from all the prefectures, only those from Shan zhou are quite similar [to the descriptions quoted above]. The flower and leaves of those from Yi zhou are quite similar to those of *paeonia suffruticosa*. The flower and leaves of those from Qin zhou are similar to single leaf *han ju* 寒菊.[209] They are of purple color with five to seven branches on one stem. Those from Haizhou have flowers of a purple-jade green color, similar to the single leaf lotus flowers. The parts below the calyx and to the side of the root are covered by fine white hair. The root is similar to that of rape turnips, but finer. It also looks like an onion, but it is black. The people in Huai dian call [*lou lu*] *lao weng hua* 老翁花, "greybeard flower." The flowers growing in these three *zhou* may differ, but the leaves are quite similar. Still, the leaves [of *lou lu*] from Qin and Hai zhou have more serrated edges. With one item having such different variations, what should physicians orientate themselves to? Following the old records, those from Shan zhou are superior. Furthermore, the welted thistle, *fei lian* 飛廉, mentioned in the *Ben cao* is also named *lou lu* 漏盧. It says that it is related to linear leaf thistle, *ku ao* 苦芺. As long as the root is fresh, its flesh is white and the skin is black. When it is dried, it turns black like a *scrophularia* root. The flowers are collected in the seventh and eighth month; they are dried in the yin (i. e., shade) and are then used [for therapeutic purposes]. It is said that the [*fei lian* 飛廉, welted thistle, mentioned above] is similar to the flowers and leaves of *lou lu* depicted on illustrations from Qin zhou and Hai zhou. But the people there only know the name *lou lu*; they do not say *fei lian* 飛廉. [Lei] Xiao: There is a kind that is truly similar to *lou lu*, except for its bitter and sour flavor. When it is mistakenly ingested it causes endless vomiting. [Li] Shizhen: According to Shen Cunzhong's *Bi tan*, "the *lou lu* used by today's recipe experts is *fei lian* 飛廉, welted thistle. An alternative name of *fei lian* is *lou lu*. The seedling is similar to that of linear leaf thistle. The root is similar to that of great burdock. They have a silk floss (i. e., hairy) top. The root is collected for [therapeutic] use." The so-called *lou lu* of Min zhong today has a stem similar to that of

209 *Han ju* 寒菊, lit.: "cold chrysanthemum," an unidentified herb.

sesame [herbs], reaching a height of six to seven *cun*. In autumn when it withers it takes on a deep black color, similar to [black] lacquer. The seedling is collected for [therapeutic] use. This is the genuine *lou lu*. For more, see under *fei lian* 飛廉 (15-34).

15-33-01

根、苗 *Gen, Miao*

Root, seedling [of *lou lu*].

【修治】【斅曰】凡采得漏盧，細剉，以生甘草相對拌蒸之，從巳至申，揀出晒乾用。

Pharmaceutical Preparation. [Lei] Xiao: Whenever *lou lu* is collected, it is cut into fine pieces. These are mixed with an equal amount of *glycyrrhiza* [root] and then steamed from *si* [hours (9 – 11)] to *shen* [hours (15-17)]. Pick out [the *lou lu* pieces] and dry them in the sun. Then they can be used [for therapeutic purposes].

【氣味】鹹，寒，無毒。【別録曰】大寒。【藏器曰】有毒。【杲曰】無毒。足陽明本經藥也。【日華曰】連翹爲之使。

Qi and Flavor. Salty, cold, nonpoisonous. *Bie lu*: Very cold. [Chen] Cangqi: Poisonous. [Li] Gao: Nonpoisonous. This is a pharmaceutical drug for the foot yang brilliance conduits. *Rihua*: *Forsythia* [fruit] serves as its guiding [substances].

【主治】皮膚熱毒，惡瘡疽痔，濕痺，下乳汁。久服輕身益氣，耳目聰明，不老延年。本經。止遺溺。熱氣瘡痒如麻豆，可作浴湯。別録。通小腸，泄精，尿血，腸風，風赤眼，小兒壯熱，撲損，續筋骨，乳癰，瘰癧，金瘡，止血排膿，補血長肉，通經脉。大明。

Control. Heat poison in the skin. Malign sores, impediment-illness,[210] piles. Blockage related to the presence of moisture. It stimulates [women] to let down milk sap. Ingested over a long time, it relieves the body of its weight and boosts the qi. It clears the ears and brightens the eyes. It prevents aging and extends the years [of life]. *Ben jing*. It ends uncontrolled loss [of sperm] and urination, itching sores with heat qi similar to smallpox. Its decoction can be used for bathing. *Bie lu*. It penetrates the small intestine and [serves to cure] outflow of sperm, urination with blood, intestinal wind, red eyes caused by wind, strong heat of children, and injuries caused by an attack. It reconnects sinews and bones It [serves to cure] breast

210 *Ju* 疽, "impediment-illness," refers to an obstruction of vessels or other ducts inside the body. Qi rushing against the impediment may cause a local swelling and eventually break through the surface to cause an abscess. BCGM Dict I, 277.

obstruction-illness,[211] scrofula pervasion-illness,[212] wounds caused by metal objects/weapons, and ends bleeding and festering. It supplements blood and stimulates the growth of flesh. It penetrates the conduit-vessels. Da Ming.

【發明】【弘景曰】此藥久服甚益人，而服食方罕見用之。近道出者，惟療瘻疥耳。市人皆取苗用。【時珍曰】漏盧下乳汁，消熱毒，排膿止血，生肌殺蟲。故東垣以爲手足陽明藥，而古方治癰疽發背，以漏盧湯爲首稱也。龐安常傷寒論治癰疽及預解時行痘疹熱，用漏盧葉，云無則以山巵子代之。亦取其寒能解熱，蓋不知其能入陽明之故也。

Explication. [Tao] Hongjing: When this pharmaceutical drug is ingested over a long time, it very much boosts one's [qi]. But it is rarely seen to be resorted to in recipes of [pharmaceutical drugs] ingested as food. [*Lou lu*] from nearby is only used to heal fistula and *jie*-illness.[213] The market merchants always supply the seedling for [therapeutic] use. [Li] Shizhen: *Lou lu* stimulates the let down [reflex] for milk juice. It dissolves heat poison, eliminates pus and ends bleeding. It stimulates the growth of muscles and kills worms/bugs. Therefore, [Li] Dongyuan identifies it as a pharmaceutical drug for the hand and foot yang brilliance [conduits], and when ancient recipes were designed to cure obstruction-illness and impediment-illness[214] with an effusion on the back, a *lou lu* decoction was named first. Pan Anchang in his *Shang han lun* cured obstruction-illness and impediment-illness and prevented epidemic smallpox and macula heat with *lou lu* leaves, and he stated that "if [such leaves] were not available, mountain *gardenia* fruit could be used instead." This way, the cold [of *gardenia* fruit] is used to resolve the heat. The fact is, he did not know that [it is effective] because it enters the yang brilliance [conduits].

【附方】舊二，新六。

Added Recipes. Two of old. Six newly [recorded].

腹中蚘蟲。漏盧爲末，以餅臛和方寸匕，服之。外臺秘要。

211 *Yong* 癰, "obstruction-illness,"refers to an obstruction of vessels or other ducts inside the body. Qi rushing against the obstruction may cause a local swelling and eventually break through the surface to cause an abscess. BCGM Dict I, 641.

212 *Luo li* 瘰癧, "scrofula pervasion-illness," when two or more connected swellings of the size of plum or date kernels appear either on the neck or in the armpits, or somewhere else on the body. BCGM Dict I. 329.

213 *Jie*-illness 疥, vaguely identifiable skin ailment. BCGM Dict I, 249.

214 *Yong ju* 癰疽, "obstruction-illness, impediment-illness." refers to two vaguely distinguished obstructions/impediments of vessels or other ducts inside the body. Qi rushing against the obstruction may cause a local swelling and eventually break through the surface to cause an abscess. BCGM Dict I, 642.

Roundworms in the abdomen. [Grind] *lou lu* into powder. Mix it with the amount of cake and meat gruel held by a square *cun* spoon and ingest this. *Wai tai mi yao.*

小兒無辜疳，病肚脹，或時泄痢，冷熱不調。以漏盧一兩，杵爲散。每服一錢，以豬肝一兩，入鹽少許，同煮熟，空心頓食之。聖惠方。

Innocence[215] *gan*-illness[216] of children. [Patients] suffer from an abdominal distension and occasional outflow and free-flux illness, with irregular feelings of cold and heat. Pound one *liang* of *lou lu* into powder and each time [let the child] ingest one *qian*. Boil this until done together with one *liang* of pig liver and a little salt added and [let the child] ingest this all at once on an empty stomach. *Sheng hui fang.*

冷勞泄痢。漏盧一兩，艾葉炒四兩，爲末。米醋三升，入藥末一半，同熬成膏，入後末和丸梧子大，每温水下三十丸。聖濟總録。

Cold exhaustion[217] with outflow and free-flux illness. [Grind] one *liang* of *lou lu* and four *liang* of common mugwort leaves, fried, into powder. Add half of the drug powder to three *sheng* of rice vinegar and boil this to obtain a paste. Then add the remaining powder to form pills the size of *wu* seeds. Each time ingest with warm water 30 pills. *Sheng ji zong lu.*

產後帶下。方同上。

[Diseases of women] below the belt following delivery. Recipe identical to the one above.

乳汁不下。乃氣脉壅塞也。又治經絡凝滯，乳内脹痛，邪畜成癰，服之自然内消。漏盧二兩半，蛇退十條炙焦，瓜蔞十箇燒存性，爲末。每服二錢，温酒調下，良久以熱之，以通爲度。和劑方。

Failure to let down milk. This is an obstruction of qi vessels. This also serves to cure coagulation and sluggishness in the conduits and network [vessels] with painful distention in the breast and an accumulation of evil [qi] generating an obstruction-illness.[218] When this is ingested, [the obstruction] will dissolve internally as a

215 *Wu gu* 無辜, "innocence," a type of *gan*-illness accompanied by scrofula affecting the head and neck. BCGM Dict I, 537.

216 *Gan* 疳, "*gan*-illness," also: "sweets-illness," involves several complaints that affect children and adults, with causes and conditions too different to fall into a known disease category. BCGM Dict I, 180-188.

217 *Leng lao* 冷勞, "cold exhaustion," a condition of *xu lao* 勞, "depletion exhaustion," with yang qi depletion and internal cold. BCGM Dict I, 306.

218 *Yong* 癰, "obstruction-illness,"refers to an obstruction of vessels or other ducts inside the body. Qi rushing against the obstruction may cause a local swelling and eventually break

result. [Grind] two and a half *liang* of *lou lu*, ten snake slough strings, roasted and scorched, and ten Japanese snake gourd [fruit], burned with their nature retained, into powder. Each time [let the woman] ingest two *qian*, to be sent down mixed with warm wine. After quite some time [let the woman] consume a hot soup in addition. This is continued until [the passage through the vessels] is open. *He ji fang*.

歷節風痛，筋脉拘攣。古聖散：用漏盧麸炒半兩，地龍去土炒半兩，爲末。生薑二兩取汁，入蜜三兩，同煎三五沸，入好酒五合，盛之。每以三盃，調末一錢，温服。聖濟總録。

Painful pervading joints wind.[219] Sinews and vessels are cramped and contracted. The "powder of the ancient sages." [Grind] half a *liang* of *lou lu*, fried with wheat bran, and half a *liang* of earthworms, fried, with the soil removed, into powder. Also, boil three to five times to bubbling the juice obtained from two *liang* of fresh ginger and three *liang* of honey. Then add five *ge* of good wine and keep this. Each time mix one *qian* of the powder with three cups [of the liquid] and ingest this warm. *Sheng ji zong lu*.

一切癰疽。發背初發二日，但有熱證，便宜服漏盧湯，退毒下膿，乃是宣熱拔毒之劑，熱退即住服。漏盧用有白茸者、連翹、生黄耆、沉香各一兩，生粉草半兩，大黃微炒一兩，爲細末。每服二錢，薑、棗湯調下。李迅癰疽集驗方。

All types of obstruction-illness and impediment-illness.[220] When an effusion on the back has lasted for two days and there are only signs of heat, then it is advisable to ingest the "decoction with *lou lu*" to repel the poison and discharge the pus. This is a preparation to lead off the heat and to pull out the poison. Once the heat is repelled, stop ingesting [this medication]. [Grind] one *liang* each of *lou lu* with white hair, *forsythia* [fruit], fresh *astragalus* [root] and aloes wood, half a *liang* of fresh *glycyrrhiza* [root] powder, and one *liang* of rhubarb root, slightly fried, into powder. Each time ingest two *qian*, to be sent down mixed with a ginger and Chinese dates decoction. Li Xun, *Yong ju ji yan fang*.

白秃頭瘡。五月收漏盧草，燒灰，豬膏和塗之。聖濟總録。

---

through the surface to cause an abscess. BCGM Dict I, 641.

219 *Li jie feng* 歷節風, "pervading joints wind." A condition characterized by spontaneous sweating, shortness of breath/qi, and difficulties in bending and stretching. BCGM Dict I, 318.

220 *Yong ju* 癰疽, "obstruction-illness, impediment-illness." refers to two vaguely distinguished obstructions/impediments of vessels or other ducts inside the body. Qi rushing against the obstruction may cause a local swelling and eventually break through the surface to cause an abscess. BCGM Dict I, 642.

Baldness with head sores. Gather *lou lu* in the fifth month, burn it to ashes, mix them with lard and apply this [to the affected region]. *Sheng ji zong lu.*

15-34
飛廉本經上品

Fei lian. FE *Ben jing*, upper rank.

***Carduus crispus* L. Welted thistle.**

【釋名】漏蘆別録、木禾別録、飛雉同上、飛輕同、伏兔同、伏豬同、天薺同。【時珍曰】飛廉，神禽之名也。其狀鹿身豹文，雀頭蛇尾，有角，能致風氣。此草附莖有皮如箭羽，復療風邪，故有飛廉、飛雉、飛輕諸名。

Explanation of Names. *Lou lu* 漏蘆, *Bie lu. Mu he* 木禾, "tree/wooden grain," *Bie lu. Fei zhi* 飛雉, same as before. *Fei qing* 飛輕, same. *Fu tu* 伏兔, "crouching hare/rabbit," same. *Fu zhu* 伏豬, "crouching pig," same. *Tian qi* 天薺, "heaven's apricot-leaved *adenophora* [root]," same. [Li] Shizhen: *Fei lian* 飛廉 is the name of a divine fowl. Its shape includes a deer body and a leopard line design, the head of a sparrow and the tail of a snake. It has horns and can arouse wind qi. The herb has a skin similar to arrow feathers attached to its stem, and it serves to heal wind evil [intrusion]. Therefore it has names such as *fei lian* 飛廉, "flying integrity," *fei zhi* 飛雉, "flying pheasant," and *fei qing* 飛輕, "flying light weight."

【集解】【別録曰】飛廉生河內川澤，正月采根，七月、八月采花，陰乾。【弘景曰】處處有之。極似苦芺，惟葉多刻缺，葉下附莖，輕有皮起似箭羽，其花紫色。俗方殆無用，而道家服其枝莖，可得長生，又入神枕方。今既別有漏蘆，則此漏蘆乃別名爾。【恭曰】此有兩種：一種生平澤中，是陶氏所説者。一種生山岡上者，葉頗相似，而無刻缺，且多毛，其莖亦無羽，其根直下，更無旁枝，生則肉白皮黑，中有黑脉，日乾則黑如玄參。用莖葉及根，療疳蝕殺蟲，與平澤者俱有驗。今俗以馬薊、以苦芺者爲漏蘆，並非是也。【保昇曰】葉似苦芺，莖似軟羽，花紫色，子毛白。所在平澤皆有，五月、六月采，日乾。【斅曰】凡使勿用赤脂蔓，與飛廉形狀相似，只赤脂蔓見酒則色便如血，以此可表識之。【頌曰】今秦州所圖漏蘆，花似單葉寒菊，紫色，五七枝同一幹。海州所圖漏盧，花紫碧色，如單葉蓮花，花蕚下及根旁有白茸裹之，根黑色，如蔓菁而細，又類葱本。與陶、蘇所説飛廉相近，然彼但謂之漏蘆。今醫家罕有用飛廉者，不能的識。【時珍曰】飛廉亦蒿類也。蘇頌圖經疑海州所圖之漏蘆是飛廉。沈存中筆談亦言飛廉根如牛蒡而綿頭。古方漏蘆散下云"用有白茸者"，則是有白茸者乃飛廉無疑矣。今考二物氣味功用俱不相遠，似可通用。豈或一類有數種，而古今名稱各處不同乎？

Collected Explanations. *Bie lu*: *Fei lian* grows in river marshlands of He nei. The root is collected in the first month; the flowers are collected in the seventh and eighth month. They are dried in the yin (i. e., shade). [Tao] Hongjing: It can be found everywhere and it is extremely similar to linear leaf thistle. The only [difference is:] the leaves have many indentations, below the leaves attached to the stem is a light skin similar to arrow feathers and the flowers are purple. In common recipes it is hardly ever used, but Daoists ingest its branches and stems because they let them enjoy a long life. It is also an ingredient of the "divine pillow" recipe. Today, there is a separate [item called] *lou lu*. The present item has *lou lu* as an alternative name. [Su] Gong: Of this there are two kinds. One kind grows in the marshlands of the plains. It is the one referred to by Mr. Tao [Hongjing]. Another kind grows on mountains. Its leaves are similar, but have no indentations and they are very hairy. Also, the stem has no [arrow] feathers. The root reaches straight down and has no branches to the side. As long as it is fresh/unprepared it has white meat and a black skin. Inside are black vessels. When it is dried in the sun, it turns as black as *scrophularia* [root]. The stem, the leaves and the root are used to heal *gan*-illness[221] erosion and to kill worms/bugs. They are as effective as those from the marshlands in the plains. Today, horse thistle and linear leaf thistle are commonly held to be *lou lu*. Both assumptions are wrong. [Han] Baosheng: The leaves are similar to those of linear leaf thistle. The stem resembles soft feathers. The flowers are purple, and the seeds have white hair. They are found everywhere in the marshlands in the plains. They are collected in the fifth and sixth month, and dried in the sun. [Lei] Xiao: Whenever [*fei lian*] is to be applied, do not use *chi zhi man* 赤脂蔓.[222] It is shaped similar to *fei lian*, but when *chi zhi man* comes into contact with wine, the [wine] assumes the color of blood. This way it can be identified. [Su] Song: The *lou lu* depicted on illustrations from Qin zhou has flowers similar to those of the single leaf *han ju* 寒菊.[223] The region below the calyx and to the side of the root is covered by soft hair. The root is black, similar to that of rape turnips, but it is finer. Also, it is of the kind of onions. This comes close to the descriptions of *fei lian* by Tao [Hongjing] and Su [Gong], but they have spoken only of *lou lu*. Today's medical experts seldom resort to *fei lian*. Therefore it is unknown. [Li] Shizhen: *Fei lian* is another member of the wormwood, *hao* 蒿, group. Su Song in his *Tu jing* wonders whether the illustration of *lou lu* does not in fact show *fei lian*. Shen Cunzhong in his *Bi tan* also says that "the root of *fei lian* is similar to that of great burdock with a silk floss

221 *Gan* 疳, "*gan*-illness," also: "sweets-illness," involves several complaints that affect children and adults, with causes and conditions too different to fall into a known disease category. BCGM Dict I, 180-188.

222 *Chi zhi man* 赤脂蔓, lit.: "red, fat vine." An unidentified herb.

223 *Han ju* 寒菊, lit.: "cold chrysanthemum," an unidentified herb.

(i. e., hairy) top." Below the ancient recipes for a "powder with *lou lu*" it says "use that with white, soft hair." That is, that with white, soft hair undoubtedly is *fei lian*. Today's examination of the two items shows that their qi, flavor and [medicinal] usage are not very different; apparently both can be used. How can this be that there are several kinds within one group that are given different names in all the places where they are found?!

15-34-01
及、花 *Gen, Hua*
Root and Flower [of *fei lian*]

【修治】【斆曰】凡用根，先刮去粗皮，杵細，以苦酒拌，一夜，漉出，日乾細杵用。

Pharmaceutical Preparation. [Lei] Xiao: For all usages of the root, first scrape off the coarse skin, pound [the rest] to fine [powder] and mix this with bitter wine for one night. Then filter [the liquid] to take [out the drug]. Dry it in the sun, pound it to obtain a fine [powder] and this is then used [for therapeutic purposes].

【氣味】苦，平，無毒。【權曰】苦、鹹，有毒。【之才曰】得烏頭良，惡麻黄。

Qi and Flavor. Bitter, acrid, nonpoisonous. [Zhen] Quan: Bitter, salty, poisonous. [Xu] Zhicai: Combined with *aconitum* [main tuber] it achieves good results. [Ingested together,] it abhors *ephedra* herb.

【主治】骨節熱，脛重酸疼。久服令人身輕。本經。頭眩頂重，皮間邪風，如蜂螫針刺，魚子細起，熱瘡癰疽，痔，濕痺，止風邪欬嗽，下乳汁。久服益氣明目不老，可煮可乾用。别録。主留血。甄權。療疳蝕，殺蟲。蘇恭。小兒疳痢，爲散，水漿服，大效。蕭炳。治頭風旋運。時珍。

Control. Bone join heat. A feeling of heaviness in the shinbone with soreness. Ingested over a long time it relieves one's body of its weight. *Ben jing*. Dizziness in the head and a feeling of heaviness at the top. Evil wind in the skin with a piercing pain as if stung by a bee. Fine [pimples similar to] fish roe rise. Heat obstruction-illness and impediment-illness.[224] Piles. Blockage related to the presence of moisture. It ends cough caused by wind evil [intrusion]. It stimulates the let down reflex for milk. Ingested over a long time it boosts the qi, brightens the eyes and prevents aging. It can be used boiled in water and also dried. *Bie lu*. It controls abiding

224 *Yong ju* 癰疽, "obstruction-illness, impediment-illness." refers to two vaguely distinguished obstructions/impediments of vessels or other ducts inside the body. Qi rushing against the obstruction may cause a local swelling and eventually break through the surface to cause an abscess. BCGM Dict I, 642.

blood. Zhen Quan. It heals *gan*-illness[225] erosion and kills worms/bugs. Su Gong. For *gan*-illness and free-flux illness of children, prepare it into a powder and [let the children] ingest it with fermented water of foxtail millet. Very effective. Xiao Bing. It serves to cure head wind,[226] dizziness and vertigo. [Li] Shizhen.

【發明】【時珍曰】葛洪抱朴子書言：飛廉單服，可輕身延壽。又言：服飛廉煎，可遠涉疾行，力數倍於常。本經、别録所列亦是良藥，而後人不知用，何哉？

Explication. [Li] Shizhen: Ge Hong in his *Baopu zi* says: "*Fei lian* ingested alone can relieve the body of its weight and extends the years of life." He also says: "Ingesting a watery decoction of Fei Lian will allow you to go far and fast and multiply your strength many times more than normal." The *Ben jing* and the *Bie lu*, too, list it as a good pharmaceutical drug, but people in later times no longer knew how to use it. Why?

【附方】舊一。

Added Recipes. One of old.

疳䘌蝕口及下部。用飛廉蒿燒灰擣篩，以兩錢匕着痛處。甚痛，則忍之。若不痛，非疳也。下部蟲如馬尾大，相纏出無數。十日瘥，二十日平復。千金翼方。

Sweets-illness with hidden worms/bugs[227] and erosions in the mouth and the lower [body] part. Burn *fei lian* wormwood ínto ashes, pound them and give them through a sieve to apply the amount held by two one-*qian* spoons to the location of the pain. If this causes an extreme pain, it must be endured. If [the treatment] fails to cause pain, it is not a sweets-illness. Countless worms/bugs emerge from the lower body parts; they are interwoven in the size of a horse tail. After ten days a cure is achieved. After 20 days a complete recovery is achieved. *Qian jin yi fang*.

---

225 *Gan* 疳, "*gan*-illness," also: "sweets-illness," involves several complaints that affect children and adults, with causes and conditions too different to fall into a known disease category. BCGM Dict I, 180-188.

226 *Tou feng* 頭風, "head wind." Condition of wind evil attacking the head followed by pain, dizziness, itching. BCGM Dict I, 509.

227 *Gan ni* 疳䘌, "sweets-illness with hidden worms," a disease brought forth by frequent consumption of sweet items, with the teeth turning black and rotting, or ulcers developing in the anal and genital areas, and festering with stench. BCGM Dict I, 184.

15-35
苧麻別録下品
Zhu ma, FE *Bie lu*, lower rank.

Boehmeria nivea (L.) Gaud. Ramie plant.

【釋名】【時珍曰】苧麻作紵，可以績紵，故謂之紵。凡麻絲之細者爲絟，粗者爲紵。陶弘景云：苧即今績苧麻是也。麻字從广，從林，音派，象屋下林麻之形。广音掩。

Explanation of Names. [Li] Shizhen: [The first character *zhu* 苧 of] *zhu ma* 苧麻 is also written *zhu* 紵, because [*zhu ma*] can be used to weave "sack cloth," *zhu* 紵. Hence [this herb] is called *zhu* [*ma*] 紵[麻], "sack cloth [bast fibers]. All fine fibers and silk threads are *quan* 絟, "fine cloth." Coarse ones are *zhu* 紵, "sack cloth." Tao Hongjing: "*Zhu* 苧 is the ramie, *zhu ma* 苧麻, used for weaving today." The character *ma* 麻 is a combination of *yan* 广, "thatched hut," and 林, read *pai* 派. It is to reflect the fitting underneath a roof by means of bamboo shingles, *lin* 林, and bast fibers, *ma* 麻.[228] 广 is read *yan* 掩.

【集解】【頌曰】苧麻舊不著所出州土，今閩、蜀、江、浙多有之。剥其皮可以績布。苗高七八尺。葉如楮葉而無叉，面青背白，有短毛。夏秋間着細穗青花。其根黄白而輕虚，二月、八月采。按陸機草木疏云：苧一科數十莖，宿根在土中，至春自生，不須栽種。荆、揚間歲三刈，諸園種之歲再刈，便剥取其皮，以竹刮其表，厚處自脱，得裏如筋者煮之，用緝布。今江、浙、閩中尚復如此。【宗奭曰】苧如蕁麻，花如白楊而長成穗，每一朶凡數十穗，青白色。【時珍曰】苧，家苧也。又有山苧，野苧也。有紫苧葉面紫，白苧葉面青，其背皆白。可刮洗煮食救荒，味甘美。其子茶褐色，九月收之，二月可種。宿根亦自生。

Collected Explanations. [Su] Song: Formerly, the *zhou* where *zhu ma* came from were not mentioned in the literature. Today, much of it can be found in Min, Shu, Jiang and Zhe. When its skin/bark is scraped off, it can be used to weave fabrics. The seedling is seven to eight *chi* tall. The leaves are similar to those of the paper mulberry tree, but they are not forked. They are greenish on their front side and white on the back; they have short hair. During summer and autum fine spikes form with greenish flowers. The root is yellow-white, and light and hollow. It is collected in the second and eighth month. According to Lu Ji's *Cao mu shu*, "[the plant] *zhu* 苧 forms clusters of several stems. The perennial root in the soil grows [new seedlings]

---

228 The original version of this statement is recorded in the *Shuo wen*, which Li Shizhen fails to point out here. The *Shuo wen* states: *ma yu lin tong, ren suo zhi, zai wu xia. cong yan cong lin* 麻与林同,人之所治,在屋下,從广從林, "*Ma* ("bast fibers") is identical to *lin*. People use them to construe the ceiling under the roof. [The character *ma* 麻] is built from *yan* 广 ("thatched hut") and *lin* 林].

by itself in spring. It does not have to be replanted. In Jing and Yang it is cut three times in a year; in all the gardens where it is planted it is cut twice a year. The skin/bark is peeled first. Then the exterior is scraped with a bamboo knife and the thicker parts fall off. The interior parts, with something resembling vessels, is boiled in water and can then be used for weaving fabrics." This is still practiced today in Jiang, Zhe and Min. *Zhu* [*ma*] 苧[麻] is similar to *qian ma* 蕁麻, "nettle." Its flowers are similar to those of poplars, but they are lengthy and grow spikes. These are clusters of several tens of greenish-white spikes. [Li] Shizhen: *Zhu* 苧 is domestic *zhu* 苧. There are also "mountain *zhu*," *shan zhu* 山苧, and "wild *zhu*," *ye zhu* 野苧. Then there are "purple *zhu*," *zi zhu* 紫苧, with leaves that are purple on their front side, and "white *zhu*," *bai zhu* 白苧, with leaves that are greenish on their front and all white on their back. When [the skin/bark] is scraped off and they are washed and boiled [in water], they can be eaten in times of famine. Their flavor is sweet-delicious. The seeds are tea-brown. They are collected in the ninth month; they can be planted in the second month. The perennial root grows [new plants] also by itself.

15-35-01
根 *Gen*
Root [of *zhu ma*].

【氣味】甘，寒，無毒。【權曰】甘，平。【大明曰】甘、滑，冷，無毒。

Qi and Flavor. Sweet, cold, nonpoisonous. [Zhen] Quan: Sweet, balanced. Da Ming: Sweet, oily, cold, nonpoisonous.

【主治】安胎，貼熱丹毒。別録。治心膈熱，漏胎下血，産前後心煩，天行熱疾，大渴大狂，服金石藥人心熱，罯毒箭蛇蟲咬。大明。漚苧汁，止消渴。別録。

Control. It calms a fetus. It is applied to cinnabar poison[229] with heat. *Bie lu*. It serves to cure heat affecting heart and diaphragm, leaking fetus[230] with discharge of blood, heart vexation prior to and following delivery, epidemic heat illness with great thirst and madness, and heart heat of persons ingesting metal and mineral medication. Apply it to [regions affected by] poisoned arrows and bites by snakes and worms/bugs. Da Ming. The juice obtained by soaking *zhu* ends melting with thirst.[231] *Bie lu*.

229 *Dan du* 丹毒, "cinnabar poison," a skin ailment with red rashes. BCGM Dict I, 118

230 *Lou tai* 漏胎, "leaking fetus," is vaginal bleeding during pregnancy. BCGM Dict I, 327.

231 *Xiao ke* 消渴, "melting with thirst," most likely including cases of diabetes. BCGM Dict Vol I, 567.

【發明】【震亨曰】苧根大能補陰而行滯血，方藥或惡其賤，似未曾用也。【藏器曰】苧性破血，將苧麻與產婦枕之，止血運。產後腹痛，以苧安腹上即止也。又蠶咬人毒入肉，取苧汁飲之。今人以苧近蠶種，則蠶不生是矣。

Explication. [Zhu] Zhenheng: The root of *zhu* is very much able to supplement yin [qi] and to stimulate the movement of sluggish blood. [Specialists of] recipe medication abhor it because it is so cheap; this may be the reason why they do not use it. [Chen] Cangqi: *Zhu* by its nature breaks through blood [accumulation]. When *zhu ma* is placed as a pillow underneath the head of a woman who has just given birth it ends blood [induced brain] movement. For pain following delivery, place *zhu* on the [patient's] abdomen and [the pain] ends. Also, when someone was bitten by silkworms, with the poison entering the flesh, [let that person] drink *zhu* juice. Today, people plant *zhu* close to silkworm [eggs]. This has the effect that the silkworms cannot develop.

【附方】舊四，新七。

Added Recipes. Four of old. Seven newly [recorded].

痰哮欬嗽。苧根煅存性，爲末，生豆腐蘸三五錢食，即效。未全可以肥豬肉二三片蘸食，甚妙。醫學正傳。

Phlegm roaring[232] and cough. [Grind] *zhu ma*, calcined with its nature retained, into powder and eat this together with three to five *qian* of fresh bean curd. This is effective. If no complete recovery is achieved, dip two or three slices of fat pork [into the powder] and eat them. Very wondrous. *Yi xue zheng chuan*.

小便不通。聖惠方用麻根、蛤粉各半兩，爲末。每服二錢，空心新汲水下。

Blocked urination. The *Sheng hui fang* [recommeds to] grind half a *liang* each of [*zhu*] *ma* root and clam shell powder into powder. Each time ingest two *qian*, to be sent down on an empty stomach with freshly drawn water.

摘玄方用苧根洗研，攤絹上，貼少腹連陰際，須臾即通。

The *Zhai xuan fang* [recommends to] wash a *zhu* [*ma*] root, grind it [to powder], spread it out on tough silk and attach it to the lower abdomen including the yin [(i.e., genital) region]. After a short while [the passage of urine] will be open.

小便血淋。苧根煎湯頻服，大妙。亦治諸淋。聖惠方。

232 *Tan xiao* 痰哮, "phlegm roaring," is a condition of *xiao chuan* 哮喘, "roaring panting," brought forth by phlegm and saliva congestion. BCGM Dict I, 497.

Dripping urine with blood. Boil *zhu* [*ma*] root [in water] and repeatedly ingest the resulting decoction. Very wondrous. This also serves to cure all other types of dripping. *Sheng hui fang*.

五種淋疾。苧麻根兩莖，打碎，以水一盌半，煎半盌，頓服即通，大妙。斗門方。

The five kinds of dripping [urine] illness. Pound two *zhu ma* root stems to small pieces and boil them in one bowl of water down to half a bowl. Ingest this all at once and [the passage of urine] will be open. Very wondrous. *Dou men fang*.

妊娠胎動，忽下黄汁如膠，或如小豆汁，腹痛不可忍者。苧根去黑皮切二升，銀一斤，水九升，煎四升。每服以水一升，入酒半升，煎一升，分作二服。一方不用銀。梅師方。

Fetal movement during pregancy with a sudden discharge of a yellow, glue-like juice, or of a rice bean juice, with an unbearable abdominal pain. Remove the black skin/bark from two *sheng* of *zhu* [*ma*] root, cut them into pieces and boil them together with one *jin* of silver in nine *sheng* of water down to four *sheng*. For each dose add half a *sheng* of wine to one *sheng* of the water, boil this down to one *sheng* and [let the woman] ingest it divided into two portions. Another recipe does not use the silver. *Mei shi fang*.

肛門腫痛。生苧根搗爛，坐之良。瀕湖集簡方。

Painful swelling of the anus. Pound fresh *zhu* [*ma*] root to obtain a pulpy mass and sit on it. Good. *Binhu ji jian fang*.

脱肛不收。苧根搗爛，煎湯熏洗之。聖惠方。

Anal prolapse with [the colon] drawn in again. Pound *zhu* [*ma*] root to obtain a pulpy mass, boil it [in water] and use the resulting decoction to steam and wash [the affected region]. *Sheng hui fang*.

癰疽發背，初起未成者。苧根熟搗傅上，日夜數易，腫消則瘥。圖經本草。

Obstruction-illness and impediment-illness[233] with an effusion on the back that has just begun to rise but has not broken open yet. Pound *zhu* [*ma*] root, [boiled until] done, [into a pulpy mass] and apply this [to the affected region]. Change [the application] several times during day and night. Once the swelling dissolves a cure is achieved. *Tu jing ben cao*.

233 *Yong ju* 癰疽, "obstruction-illness, impediment-illness." refers to two vaguely distinguished obstructions/impediments of vessels or other ducts inside the body. Qi rushing against the obstruction may cause a local swelling and eventually break through the surface to cause an abscess. BCGM Dict I, 642.

五色丹毒。苧根煮濃汁，日三浴之。外臺秘要。

Multi-colored cinnabar poison.[234] Boil *zhu* [*ma*] root to obtain a thick juice and bathe [the affected region] three times a day. *Wai tai mi yao.*

鷄魚骨哽。談野翁試驗方用苧麻根擣汁，以匙挑灌之，立效。

Choking on a chicken or fish bone. Tan Yeweng in his *Shi yan fang* [recommends to] pound *zhu ma* root to obtain a juice and force-feed it [to the patient] by pushing the spoon [into his throat]. Immediately effective.

醫方大成用野苧麻根擣碎，丸如龍眼大，魚骨魚湯下，鷄骨鷄湯下。

The *Yi fang da cheng* [recommends to] pound wild *zhu ma* root to small pieces to form pills the size of dragon eyes/longan seeds. In the case of [a choking on] a fish bone, send them down with a fish soup. In the case of [a choking on] a chicken bone, send them down with a chicken soup.

15-35-02
葉 *Ye*
Leaf [of *zhu ma*].

【氣味】同根。

Qi and Flavor. Identical to the root.

【主治】金瘡傷折，血出瘀血。時珍。

Control. Wounds caused by metal objects/weapons and fracture harm, with bleeding and stagnating blood. [Li] Shizhen.

【發明】【時珍曰】苧麻葉甚散血，五月五日收取，和石灰擣作團，晒乾收貯。遇有金瘡折損者，研末傅之，即時血止，且易痂也。按李仲南永類方云：凡諸傷瘀血不散者，五六月收野苧葉、蘇葉，擂爛，傅金瘡上。如瘀血在腹内，順流水絞汁服即通，血皆化水。以生豬血試之，可驗也。秋冬用乾葉亦可。

Explication. [Li] Shizhen: *Zhu ma* leaves are very much able to disperse blood. Collect them on the fifth day of the fifth month, mix them with lime and pound them to [a pulpy mass to] form a ball. Dry it in the sun and store it [for later use]. In the case of a wound caused by a metal object/weapon or any other injury, grind [the ball] into powder and apply it [to the affected region]. This stops the bleeding and a scar is easily formed. According to Li Zhongnan's *Yong lei fang*, "for all types of harm with stagnating blood that fails to disperse, in the fifth and sixth month gather wild *zhu* [*ma*] leaves and *perilla* leaves, pound them to obtain a pulpy mass

234 *Dan du* 丹毒, "cinnabar poison," a skin ailment with red rashes. BCGM Dict I, 118

and apply this to the wound. If the blood stagnates in the abdomen, soak [the leaves] in water running its due course, squeeze them to obtain a juice and ingest it. This will open the passage [of the blood], and all the blood will be transformed to water. Perform a test with fresh pig blood and it will be successful. In autumn and winter dried leaves may be used, too."

【附方】新三。

Added Recipes. Three newly [recorded].

驟然水瀉，日夜不止，欲死，不拘男婦。用五月五日采麻葉，陰乾爲末。每服二錢，冷水調下。勿喫熱物，令人悶倒。只喫冷物。小兒半錢。楊子建護命方。

Sudden watery outflow that does not end for days and nights, letting one wish to die – regardless of whether [the patient] is a man or a woman. Collect [*zhu*] *ma* leaves on the fifth day of the fifth month, dry them in the yin (i. e., shade) and [grind them into] powder. Each time ingest two *qian*, to be sent down mixed with cold water. [During the treatment] do not consume anything hot, this would cause heart-pressure and a fall to the ground. Only eat cold items. Children are to ingest half a *qian*. Yang Zitian, *Hu ming fang*.

冷痢白凍。方同上。

Cold free-flux illness with a white jelly [discharge]. Recipe identical to the one above.

蛇虺咬傷。青麻嫩頭擣汁，和酒等分，服三盞。以渣傅之，毒從竅中出，以渣棄水中即不發。看傷處有竅是雄蛇，無竅是雌蛇，以針挑破傷處成竅，傅藥。摘玄方。

Harm caused by snake and venomous viper bites. Pound the tender tip of greenish [*zhu*] *ma* [leaves] to obtain a juice, mix it with an equal amount of wine and ingest three cups. Apply the dregs [to the affected region]. The poison will leave [the body with the dregs] through an opening. Discard the dregs into some water, and [the poison] will not effuse [in the body]. Take a look at the affected location. If there is an opening, it was a male snake. If there is no opening, it was a female snake. Poke the affected location with a needle to open a hole and apply the medication there. *Zhai xuan fang*.

15-36
苘麻苘音頃唐本草

Qing ma, 苘 is read *qing* 頃. FE *Tang ben cao*.

Abutilon theophrasti **Medic. Indian mallow.**

【釋名】白麻。【時珍曰】苘一作藚，又作檾。種必連頃，故謂之藚也。

Explanation of Names. *Bai ma* 白麻, "white hemp." [Li] Shizhen: *Qing* 苘 is also written *qing* 藚 and *qing* 檾. [To obtain a harvest of highest quality,] plant it in a field that covers many neighboring hectars. Therefore it is named *qing* 藚.

【集解】【恭曰】苘即藚麻也。今人取皮作布及索者。實似大麻子，九月、十月采，陰乾。【頌曰】處處有之。北人種以績布及打繩索。苗高四五尺或六七尺，葉似苧而薄，花黄，實殼如蜀葵，其中子黑色。【時珍曰】苘麻，今之白麻也。多生卑濕處，人亦種之。葉大似桐葉，團而有尖。六七月開黄花。結實如半磨形，有齒，嫩青老黑。中子扁黑，狀如黄葵子。其莖輕虛潔白。北人取皮作麻。以莖蘸硫黄作焠燈，引火甚速。其嫩子小兒亦食之。

Collected Explanations. [Su] Gong: *Qing* 苘 is *qing ma* 藚麻. Today, people take the bark to prepare cloths and large ropes. The fruit is similar to hemp seeds. It is collected in the ninth and tenth month and dried in the yin (i. e., shade). [Su] Song: It can be found everywhere. The Northerners plant it to weave fabric and to prepare ropes. The seedling reaches a height of four to five *chi* or six to seven *chi*. The leaves are similar to those of ramie, but they are thinner. The flowers are yellow. The fruit capsule is similar to that of common hollyhock. The seeds inside are black. [Li] Shizhen: *Qing ma* is today's *bai ma* 白麻. It often grows at low, moist places. People also plant it. The leaves are big and resemble dragon tree leaves. They are round and pointed. Yellow flowers open in the sixth and seventh month. They form fruits similar to the size of half a grindstone with teeth. As long as they are tender, they are greenish. When they are old, they are black. The seeds are flat and black, and they are shaped like yellow Chinese malva seeds. The stem is light, hollow and pure white. The Northerners use the bark to prepare fibers. They dip the stem into sulphur to light the lanterns. [*Qing ma*] guides fire very quickly. The tender seeds are also eaten by children.

15-36-01
實 *Shi*
Fruit [of Indian mallow].

【氣味】苦，平，無毒。

Qi and Flavor. Bitter, balanced, nonpoisonous.

【主治】赤白冷熱痢，炒研爲末，每蜜湯服一錢。癰腫無頭者吞一枚。蘇恭。主眼翳瘀肉，起倒睫拳毛。時珍。

Control. Red and white free-flux illness related to cold and heat. Fry *qing ma* and grind it into powder. Each time ingest with hot honey water one *qian*. In the case of an obstruction-illness[235] with a swelling without a tip [filled with pus], swallow one root. Su Gong. It controls eyes with shades and excessive flesh, and lifts inverted eyelashes. [Li] Shizhen.

15-36-02
根 *Gen*
Root [of *qing ma*].

【主治】亦治痢。古方用之。蘇頌。

Control. It, too, serves to cure free-flux illness. It is [recommended for] use in ancient recipes. Su Song.

【附方】新二。
Added Recipes. Two newly [recorded].

一切眼疾。茼麻子一升，爲末。以豶豬肝批片，蘸末炙熟，再蘸再炙，末盡，乃爲末。每服一字，陳米飲下，日三服。聖濟總録。

All types of illnesses of the eyes. [Grind] one *sheng* of *qing ma* seeds into powder. Cut the liver of a castrated pig into slices. Dip them into the powder and roast them until done. Dip them again [into the powder] and roast them again until all the powder is used up. Then [grind them into] powder. Each time ingest one *zi*, to be sent down with a beverage made of long-stored rice. To be ingested three times a day. *Sheng ji zong lu*.

目生翳膜久不愈者。用檾實，以柳木作磑，磨去殼，馬尾篩取黄肉去焦殼，每十兩可得四兩，非此法不能去殼也。用豬肝薄切，滚藥慢炙熟，爲末，醋和丸梧子大。每服三十丸，白湯下。一方：以檾實内袋中蒸熟，暴爲末，蜜丸，温水下。聖濟總録。

The eyes grow shades and membranes that are not cured for a long time. Break *qing* [*ma*] fruit with an implement made of willow wood, and rub them to discard the shells. With a horse tail sieve take out the yellow flesh [of the fruit] and discard the charred shells. Out of every ten *liang* [of *qing ma* fruit] four *liang* [of the flesh] remain. There is no other way to get rid of the shells. Cut pig liver into thin slices,

235 *Yong* 癰, "obstruction-illness," refers to an obstruction of vessels or other ducts inside the body. Qi rushing against the obstruction may cause a local swelling and eventually break through the surface to cause an abscess. BCGM Dict I, 641.

Roll them in the medicinal [powder] and roast them until done. Then [grind them into] powder. Mix it with vinegar and form pills the size of *wu* seeds. Each time ingest 30 pills, to be sent down with clear, boiled water. Another recipe: Fill *qing* [*ma*] fruit into a pouch and steam them until they are done. Dry them in the sun and [grind them into] powder. With honey form pills and send them down with warm water. *Sheng ji zong lu.*

15-37
大青別録中品
Da qing, FE *Bie lu*, middle rank.

***Clerodendrum cyrtophyllum* Turcz. Mayflower glorybower.**

【釋名】【時珍曰】其莖葉皆深青，故名。

Explanation of Names. [Li] Shizhen: Its stem and leaves are all deep greenish, *qing* 青. Hence the name.

【集解】【别録曰】大青，三四月采莖，陰乾。【弘景曰】今出東境及近道，紫莖長尺許，莖葉皆用。【頌曰】今江東州郡及荆南、眉、蜀、濠、淄諸州皆有之。春生青紫莖，似石竹苗葉，花紅紫色，似馬蓼，亦似芫花，根黄，三月、四月采莖葉，陰乾用。【時珍曰】處處有之。高二三尺，莖圓。葉長三四寸，面青背淡，對節而生。八月開小花，紅色成簇。結青實大如椒顆，九月色赤。

Collected Explanations. *Bie lu*: *Da qing*, the stem is collected in the third and fourth month; it is dried in the yin (i. e., shade). [Tao] Hongjing: Today it comes from Dong jing and nearby regions. The purple stem is more than a *chi* long. Stem and leaves are all used. [Su] Song: Today it can be found in the *zhou* and prefectures of Jiang dong, as well as in all the *zhou* of Jing nan, Mei, Shu, Hao and Zi. In spring it grows a greenish-purple seedling, similar to the seedling and the leaves of fringed pink. The flowers are of a red-purple color, similar to those of *ma liao* 馬蓼 (16-49) and also to daphne flowers. The root is yellow. Stem and leaves are collected in the third and fourth month. They are dried in the yin (i. e., shade) and can then be used. [Li] Shizhen: It can be found everywhere. It is two to three *chi* tall; the stem is round. The leaves are three to four *cun* long. They are greenish on their front side and pale on their back. They grow facing each other in segments. Small flowers of red color open in the eighth month in clusters. They form greenish fruits the size of Chinese pepper kernels. They turn red in the ninth month.

莖、葉 *Jing, Ye*

Stem, leaves [of *da qing*].

【氣味】苦，大寒，無毒。【權曰】甘。【時珍曰】甘、微鹹，不苦。

Qi and Flavor. Bitter, very cold, nonpoisonous. [Zhen] Quan: Sweet. [Li] Shizhen: Sweet, slightly salty, not bitter.

【主治】時氣頭痛，大熱口瘡。别録。除時行熱毒，甚良。弘景。治温疫寒熱。甄權。治熱毒風，心煩悶，渴疾口乾，小兒身熱疾，風瘮，及金石藥毒。塗署腫毒。大明。主熱毒痢，黄疸，喉痺，丹毒。時珍。

Control. Headache caused by seasonal qi. Oral sores with great heat. *Bie lu*. It removes heat poison related to seasonal epidemic [qi]. Very good. [Tao] Hongjing: It serves to cure warmth epidemics with alternating sensations of cold and heat. Zhen Quan. It serves to cure heat poison associated with wind [intrusion], heart vexation with heart-pressure, thirst illness and dry mouth, body heat illnesses of children, wind papules[236] and the poison of metal and stone/mineral drugs. Apply it to a swelling with poison. Da Ming. It controls free-flux illness related to heat poison, yellow *dan*-illness/jaundice, throat closure, and cinnabar poison.[237] [Li] Shizhen.

【發明】【頌曰】古方治傷寒黄汗、黄疸等，有大青湯。又治傷寒頭身强、腰脊痛，葛根湯内亦用大青。大抵時疾多用之。【時珍曰】大青氣寒，味微苦鹹，能解心胃熱毒，不特治傷寒也。朱肱活人書治傷寒發赤斑煩痛，有犀角大青湯、大青四物湯。故李象先指掌賦云：陽毒則狂斑煩亂，以大青、升麻，可回困篤。

Explication. [Su] Song: Ancient recipes included a "decoction with *da qing*"[238] to cure harm caused by cold with yellow sweat, and yellow *dan*-illness/jaundice. It also serves to cure a stiff head and body related to harm caused by cold, and lower back and back pain. The "decoction with *pueraria* root," too, includes *da qing*. In general, many [recipes] for seasonal qi resort to it. [Li] Shizhen: The qi of *da qing* are cold. Its flavor is slightly bitter and salty. It is able to resolve heat poison affecting the heart and the stomach. It does not only serve to cure harm caused by cold. Zhu Gong in his *Huo ren shu* cures red macules and vexing pain related to harm caused by cold with a "decoction with rhinoceros horn and *da qing*"[239] and also with the

236 *Feng zhen* 風瘮, "wind papules," a condition, brought forth by wind evil, of eruptive skin papules of different sizes, accompanied by unbearable itching. If scratched they rise further. BCGM Dict I, 172.

237 *Dan du* 丹毒, "cinnabar poison," a skin ailment with red rashes. BCGM Dict I, 118

238 For details, see below under "Added Recipes."

239 For details, see below under "Added Recipes."

"decoction with four items and *da qing*."[240] Hence Li Xiangxian in his *Zhi zhang fu* states: "When yang poison causes a chaotic situation of madness, macules and vexation, a recovery can be achieved with *da qing* and *cimicifuga* [rhizome]."

【附方】新五。
Added Recipes. Five newly [recorded].

喉風喉痺。大青葉搗汁灌之，取效止。衛生易簡方。

Throat wind,[241] throat closure. Pound *da qing* leaves to obtain a juice and force-feed it [to the patient]. When an effect shows, stop [the treatment]. *Wei sheng yi jian fang.*

小兒口瘡。大青十八銖，黄連十二銖，水三升，煮一升服。一日二服，以瘥爲度。千金方。

Oral sores of children. Boil 18 *zhu* of *da qing* and 12 *zhu* of *coptis* [rhizome] down to one *sheng* and [let the child] ingest it. To be ingested twice per day until a cure is achieved. *Qian jin fang.*

熱病下痢困篤者。大青湯：用大青四兩，甘草、赤石脂各三兩，膠二兩，豉八合，水一斗，煮三升，分三服，不過二劑瘥。肘後方。

Heat disease and discharge with a severe free-flux illness. The "decoction with *da qing*." Boil four *liang* of *da qing*, three *liang* each of *glycyrrhiza* [root] and red halloysite, two *liang* of [donkey-hide] glue, and eight *ge* of [soybean] relish in one *dou* of water down to three *sheng* and ingest this divided into three portions. A cure is achieved after ingesting no more than two such preparations. *Zhou hou fang.*

熱病發斑，赤色煩痛。大青四物湯：用大青一兩，阿膠、甘草各二錢半，豉二合，分三服。每用水一盞半，煎一盞，入膠烊化服。

Heat disease with an eruption of red macules and a vexing pain. The "decoction with four items and *da qing*." One *liang* of *da qing*, two and a half *qian* of E glue and *glycyrrhiza* [root] and two *ge* of [soybean] relish are ingested divided into three portions. Each time boil them in one and a half cup of water down to one cup, let the glue melt in it and ingest this.

又犀角大青湯：用大青七錢半，犀角二錢半，巵子十枚，豉二撮，分二服。每服水一盞半，煎八分，温服。南陽活人書。

240 For details, see below under "Added Recipes."

241 *Hou feng* 喉風, "throat wind," various conditions with mouth, tongue, and throat swelling and pain. BCGM Dict I, 217.

Also, the "decoction with rhinoceros horn and *da qing*." Seven and a half *qian* of *da qing*, two and a half *qian* of rhinoceros horn, ten *gardenia* fruit and two pinches of [soybean] relish are ingested divided into two portions. Each time boil them in one and a half cup of water down to 80% and ingest this warm. *Nan yang huo ren shu.*

肚皮青黑。小兒卒然肚皮青黑，乃血氣失養，風寒乘之，危惡之候也。大青爲末，納口中，以酒送下。保幼大全方。

Greenish-black colored abdominal skin. When a child's abdominal skin suddenly assumes a greenish-black color, this is because blood and qi are insufficiently nourished and wind and cold have availed themselves of the [resulting depletion]. This is a critical, bad sign. [Grind] *da qing* into powder, stuff it into [the child's] mouth and send it down with wine. *Bao you da quan fang.*

15-38
小青宋圖經
Xiao qing, FE Song, *Tu jing*.

***Ardisia pusilla* A. DC. Coralberry.**

【集解】【頌曰】小青生福州，三月生花，彼土人當月采葉用之。

Collected Explanations. [Su] Song: *Xiao qing* grows in Fu zhou. It develops flowers in the third month. The local people collect the leaves in the same month and make use of them.

15-38-01
葉 *Ye*
Leaf [of *xiao qing*].

【氣味】缺。

Qi and Flavor. Missing.

【主治】生擣，傅癰腫瘡癤，甚效。蘇頌。治血痢腹痛，研汁服，解蛇毒。時珍。

Control. Pound the fresh [leaves] and apply [the resulting mass] to a swelling related to obstruction-illness,[242] sores, and pimples. Very effective. Su Song. They serve to cure free-flux illness with abdominal pain. Grind them to obtain a juice and ingest it to resolve snake poison. [Li] Shizhen.

---

242 *Yong* 癰, "obstruction-illness,"refers to an obstruction of vessels or other ducts inside the body. Qi rushing against the obstruction may cause a local swelling and eventually break through the surface to cause an abscess. BCGM Dict I, 641.

【附方】新二。

Added Recipes. Two newly [recorded].

蛇虺螫傷。衛生易簡方用小青一握，細研，入香白芷半兩，酒調服。手挼患處，候黄水出爲效。

Harm caused by snake and venomous viper bites. The *Wei sheng yi jian fang* [recommends to] grind a handful of *xiao qing* to fine powder, add half a *liang* of fragrant *angelica dahurica* [root] and ingest this mixed with wine. Squeeze the affected location until a yellow water is released. This shows the effect.

摘玄方用小青、大青、牛膝葉同搗汁，和酒服，以渣傅之。

The *Zhai xuan fang* [recommends to] pound *xiao qing*, *da qing*/mayflower glorybower and *achyranthes* leaves to obtain a juice and ingest it mixed with wine. Apply the dregs [to the affected region].

中暑發昏。小青葉井水浸去泥，控乾，入沙糖擂汁，急灌之。壽域方。

Confusion caused by summer heat stroke. Soak *xiao qing* leaves in well water and remove the mud. Hang it up so the liquid can drip out. Add sugar and pound it to obtain a juice. Quickly force-feed it [to the patient]. *Shou yu fang*.

15-39
胡盧巴宋嘉祐

Hu lu ba, FE Song, *Jia you*.

***Trigonella foenum-graecum* L. Fenugreek.**[243]

【釋名】苦豆。

Explanation of Names. *Ku dou* 苦豆, "bitter bean."

【集解】【禹錫曰】胡盧巴出廣州并黔州。春生苗，夏結子，子作細莢，至秋采。今人多用嶺南者。或云是番蘿蔔子，未審的否。【頌曰】今出廣州。或云種出海南諸番，蓋其國蘆菔子也。舶客將種蒔於嶺外亦生，然不及番中來者真好。今醫家治元臟虛冷爲要藥，而唐已前方不見用，本草不著，蓋是近出也。

Collected Explanations. [Zhang] Yuxi: *Hu lu ba* comes from Guang zhou and Qian zhou. It grows a seedling in spring and forms seeds in summer. The seeds have small

243 The Chinese name *hu lu ba* 胡盧巴 is a tranliteration of the Arabic term *hulba*, known in Persia as *hulbat*. For this and further examples of transliterations with Chinese characters of foreign plant and food terms, see Herbert Franke, Additional Notes on Non-Chinese Terms in the Yüan-Imperial Dietary Compendium *Yin-shan cheng-yao*" in *Zentralasiatische Studien des Seminars für Sprach- und Kulturwissenschaft Zentralasiens der Universität Bonn*, 4, Wiesbaden 1970.

pods that are collected in autumn. Today's people often use those from Ling nan. Some say [*hu lu ba*] is the seed of "foreign radish," *fan luo bo* 番蘿蔔, but there are no studies on whether this the case or not. [Su] Song: Today it comes from Guang zhou. Some say it is planted and comes from Hai nan where all the foreigners are. The fact is, these are the seeds of that country's *lu fu* 蘆菔. Passengers have brought it on ships to plant it in Ling wai and it grows there, too. But it is not really as good as that coming here from foreign lands. Today's physicians consider it an important pharmaceutical drug to cure depletion cold of the original long-term depot (i. e., the kidneys), but in recipes devised prior to the Tang era its application is not seen. The *Ben cao* does not list it. The fact is, it is a recent arrival.

【修治】【時珍曰】凡入藥，淘净，以酒浸一宿，晒乾，蒸熟或炒過用。

Pharmaceutical Preparation. [Li] Shizhen: Whenever [*hu lu ba* seeds] are added to a medication, wash them clean in a pan or basket and soak them in wine for one night. Then dry them in the sun and steam them until done, or fry them. Then they can be used.

【氣味】苦，大温，無毒。【杲曰】純陽。

Qi and Flavor. Bitter, very warm, nonpoisonous. [Li] Gao: Pure yang.

【主治】元臟虛冷氣。得附子、硫黄，治腎虛冷，腹脇脹滿，面色青黑。得蘹香子、桃仁，治膀胱氣，甚效。嘉祐。治冷氣疝瘕，寒濕脚氣，益右腎，暖丹田。時珍。

Control. Depletion of original [qi in the kidney] long-term depot with the presence of cold qi. Together with *aconitum* [accessory tuber] and sulphur, [*hu lu ba* seeds] serve to cure kidney depletion cold, with a distension of and a feeling of fullness in the abdomen and the flanks, and a greenish-black complexion. Together with fennel seeds and peach seeds they serve to cure urinary bladder qi [disorder], and are very effective. *Jia you*. They serve to cure elevation-illness with conglomeration-illness[244] related to cold qi [presence], and leg qi[245] related to [the presence of] cold and moisture. They boost [the qi of] the right kidney, and warm the cinnabar field. [Li] Shizhen.

【發明】【宗奭曰】膀胱氣，用此合桃仁麸炒，等分爲末。半爲散，半以酒糊和丸梧子大。每服五七十丸，空心鹽酒下。其散以熱米湯下，與丸子相間，空心服。日各一二服。【時珍曰】胡盧巴，右腎命門藥也。元陽不足，冷氣潛伏，不能歸元者，宜之。宋惠民和劑局方有胡盧巴丸，治大

244 *Shan jia* 疝瘕, "elevation-illness with conglomeration-illness." A lump-like swelling in the abdomen that alternately collects and then dissolves again. BCGM Dict I, 418.

245 *Jiao qi* 脚氣, "leg qi." Painful, weak, swollen legs. BCGM Dict I, 248.

人、小兒小腸奔豚偏墜及小腹有形如卵，上下走痛，不可忍者。用胡盧巴八錢，茴香六錢，巴戟去心、川烏頭炮去皮各二錢，楝實去核四錢，吴茱萸五錢，並炒爲末，酒糊丸梧子大。每服十五丸，小兒五丸，鹽酒下。太醫薛己云：一人病寒疝，陰囊腫痛，服五苓諸藥不效，與此而平也。又張子和儒門事親云：有人病目不覩，思食苦豆，即胡盧巴，頻頻不缺。不周歲而目中微痛，如蟲行入眦，漸明而愈。按此亦因其益命門之功，所謂益火之原，以消陰翳是也。

Explication. [Kou] Zongshi: For urinary bladder qi [disorders, grind] equal amounts of these [*hu lu ba* seeds] and peach kernels, fried together with wheat bran, into powder. Leave one half as a powder, and mix the other half with wine and [wheat flour] paste to form pills the size of *wu* seeds. Each time ingest 50 to 70 pills, to be sent down on an empty stomach with salted wine. The powder is to be sent down with a hot rice decoction, at an interval after the pills, on an empty stomach. Both [the pills and the powder] are to be ingested once or twice a day. [Li] Shizhen: *Hu lu ba* is a pharmaceutical drug for the right kidney, (i. e.) the Gate of Life. It is suitable to be resorted to when the original yang [qi] are insufficient because cold qi lies hidden and [the yang qi] are unable to return to their origin. The Song era *Hui min he ji ju fang* lists "pills with *hu lu ba*" to cure, regardless of whether adult males or children are concerned, small intestinal running piglet[246] and unilateral collapse of testes, and a mass shaped like an egg in the lower abdomen, with unbearable pain rushing up and down. Fry together and [grind into] powder eight *qian* of *hu lu ba*, six *qian* of fennel, two *qian* each of *morinda* [root], its heart removed, and Si chuan *aconitum* [main tuber], roasted with the skin removed, four *qian* of Persian lilac fruit, with the kernels removed, and five *qian* of *evodia* [fruit], and with wine and wheat flour form pills the size of *wu* seeds. Each time ingest 15 pills, children five pills, to be sent down with salted wine. The imperial physician Xue Ji states: "Someone suffered from cold elevation-illness.[247] His scrotum was painfully swollen. He ingested the 'powder with five [ingredients including *zhu*] *ling* [猪]苓,'[248] and other medication, but all remained without effect. Then he was given this preparation and his health was restored." Also, Zhang Zihe in his *Ru men shi qin* states: "Someone

246 *Ben tun* 賁豚, "running piglet," a condition of an accumulation in the kidneys assuming the shape of a piglet moving up and down at irregular intervals. BCGM Dict I, 57.

247 *Shan qi* 疝氣, "elevation-illness qi," a pathological condition of (1) an item having entered the scrotum, with pain, sometimes ascending, sometimes descending, (2) a condition affecting the scrotum or a testicle, (3) of violent abdominal pain, in some cases associated with constipation and anuria. BCGM Dict I, 419, 417.

248 *Wu ling san* 五苓散, the "powder with five [ingredients including *zhu*] *ling* [猪]苓," a recipe first recorded in the *Shang han lun*. Ingredients include: *Polyporus* sclerotium, *alisma* root, *atractylodes macrocephala* rhizome, *poria*, and *cassia* twigs. Several other powders of the same name were designed in later times.

suffered from a loss of his eyesight and he thought of eating 'bitter beans', *ku dou* 苦豆, which are *hu lu ba* [seeds]. He took them again and again and within less than a year he felt a slight pain in his eyes as if worms/bugs were moving into the canthi. Gradually his eyes turned clear again and he was cured." Now, this result was achieved because of the potential [of *hu lu ba*] to boost the [qi of the] Gate of Life. This is [in conformity with] the so-called "boost the source of the fire to dissolve the shades [generated by] yin [qi]."

【附方】新六。

Added Recipes. Six newly [recorded].

小腸氣痛。胡盧巴炒，研末，每服二錢，茴香酒下。直指方。

Painful qi [disorder] in the lower abdomen. Fry *hu lu ba* [seeds] and grind them into powder. Each time ingest two *qian*, to be sent down with fennel wine. *Zhi zhi fang*.

腎臟虚冷，腹脇脹滿。胡盧巴炒二兩，熟附子、硫黄各七錢五分，爲末，酒煮麴糊丸梧桐子大，每鹽湯下三四十丸。聖濟總録。

Kidney long-term depot depletion cold, with distension of abdomen and flanks and a sensation of fullness. [Grind] two *liang* of *hu lu ba* [seeds], roasted, seven *qian* and five *fen* each of heat prepared *aconitum* [accessory tuber] and sulphur into powder. Boil it wine and with brewer's yeast and [wheat flour] paste form pills the size of *wu tong* seeds. Each time send down with a salt decoction 30 to 40 pills. *Sheng ji zong lu*.

冷氣疝瘕。胡盧巴酒浸晒乾，蕎麥炒研麪，各四兩，小茴香一兩，爲末，酒糊丸梧子大。每服五十丸，空心鹽湯或鹽酒下。服至兩月，大便出白膿則除根。方廣心法附餘。

Elevation-illness and conglomeration-illness[249] related to [the presence of] cold qi. [Grind] four *liang* each of *hu lu ba* [seeds], soaked in wine and then dried in the sun, and buckwheat [rhizome], fried and ground to flour, and one *liang* of fennel into powder and form with wine and [wheat flour] paste pills the size of *wu* seeds. Each time ingest 50 pills, to be sent down on an empty stomach with an aqueous salt decoction or salted wine. After ingesting this for two months, white pus is emitted with defecation, and this way the root [of the diseases] is eliminated. Fang Guang, *Xin fa fu yu*.

249 *Shan jia* 疝瘕, "elevation-illness with conglomeration-illness." A lump-like swelling in the abdomen that alternately collects and then dissolves again. BCGM Dict I, 418.

陰㿉腫痛偏墜，或小腸疝氣，下元虛冷，久不愈者，沉香内消丸主之。沉香、木香各半兩，胡盧巴酒浸炒，小茴香炒，各二兩，爲末，酒糊丸梧子大。每服五七十丸，鹽酒下。

Yin breakdown-illness, painful swelling, unilateral collaps of testicles, or small intestinal elevation-illness,[250] with depletion cold in the lower [long-term depot of] original [qi (i. e., the kidneys)], that have not been cured for a long time, are controlled by the "pills with aloes wood for internal dissolving." [Grind] half a *liang* each of aloes wood and *costus* [root], two *liang* each of *hu lu ba* [seeds], soaked in wine and roasted, and fennel, roasted, into powder and form with wine and [wheat flour] paste pills the size of *wu* seeds. Each time ingest 50 to 70 pills, to be sent down with salted wine.

氣攻頭痛。胡盧巴炒，三稜酒浸焙，各半兩，乾薑炮二錢半，爲末，薑湯或温酒每服二錢。濟生方。

Headache following a qi attack. [Grind] half a *liang* each of *hu lu ba* [seeds], roasted, and *sparganium* [root], soaked in wine and dried over a fire in a pan, and two and a half *qian* of dried ginger, roasted, into powder. Each time ingest, with a ginger decoction or with warm wine, two *qian*. *Ji sheng fang*.

寒濕脚氣。腿膝疼痛，行步無力。胡盧巴酒浸一宿焙，破故紙炒香，各四兩，爲末。以木瓜切頂去瓤，安藥在内令滿，用頂合住簽定，爛蒸，搗丸梧子大。每服七十丸，空心温酒下。楊氏家藏方。

Leg qi[251] related to cold and moisture. Painful leg and knee, with not enough strength to walk. [Grind] four *liang* each of *hu lu ba* [seeds], soaked in wine for one night and dried over a fire in a pan, and scurfy peas, roasted until they emit fragrance, into powder. Then cut off the top of a quince, remove the pulp and fill it completely with the medicinal [powder]. Close the opening again with the top and fix it. Then steam this until it has become pulpy, pound it and form pills the size of *wu* seeds. Each time ingest 70 pills, to be sent down on an empty stomach with warm wine. *Yang shi jia cang fang*.

250 *Shan qi* 疝氣, "elevation-illness qi," a pathological condition of (1) an item having entered the scrotum, with pain, sometimes ascending, sometimes descending, (2) a condition affecting the scrotum or a testicle, (3) of violent abdominal pain, in some cases associated with constipation and anuria. BCGM Dict I, 419, 417.

251 *Jiao qi* 脚氣, "leg qi." Painful, weak, swollen legs. BCGM Dict I, 248.

15-40
蠡實本經中品
Li shi, FE *Ben jing*, middle rank.

***Iris lactea* Pall. var. *chinensis* (Fisch.) Koidz. Chinese iris.**

【釋名】荔實別録、馬藺子唐本、馬楝子圖經、馬薤禮記注、馬帚爾雅、鐵掃帚救荒、劇草本經、旱蒲禮記、豕首本經、三堅。【弘景曰】方藥不用，俗無識者。惟天名精亦名豕首。【恭曰】此即馬藺子也。月令：仲冬荔挺出。鄭玄注云：荔，馬薤也。通俗文云：一名馬藺。本草謂之荔實。【頌曰】馬藺子，北人訛爲馬楝子。廣雅云：馬薤，荔也。高誘云：荔挺出，荔草挺出也。講禮者不識，呼爲荔挺，又作馬莧，並誤矣。馬莧亦名豚耳，即馬齒也。【時珍曰】爾雅云：荓，音瓶，馬帚也。此即荔草，謂其可爲馬刷，故名。今河南北人呼爲鐵掃帚，是矣。

Explanation of Names. *Li shi* 荔實, *Bie lu*. *Ma lin zi* 馬藺子, *Tang ben*. *Ma lian zi* 馬楝子, *Tu jing*. *Ma xie* 馬薤, "horse chives," *Li ji zhu*, *Ma zhou* 馬帚, "horse brush," *Er ya*. *Tie sao zhou* 鐵掃帚, "iron brush," *Jiu huang*. *Ju cao* 劇草, "intense herb," *Ben jing*. *Han pu* 旱蒲, "dryland cattail," *Li ji*. *Shi shou* 豕首, "pig head," *Ben jing*. *San jian* 三堅, "triple strength." [Tao] Hongjing: It is not used as a recipe drug; it is widely unknown. It is just that *carpesium abrotanoides* is also called *shi shou* 豕首. [Su] Gong: This is *ma lin zi* 馬藺子. *Yue ling*: "In the middle period of winter, *li* 荔 [seedlings] rise out of [the ground]." Zheng Xuan in a commentary states: "*Li* 荔 is *ma xie* 馬薤. The *Tong su wen* states: 'Another name is *ma lin* 馬藺.' The *Ben cao* calls it *li shi* 荔實, '*li* fruit'." Su] Song: *Ma lin zi* 馬藺子 is mistakenly called *ma lian zi* 馬楝子 in the North. The *Guang ya* states: "*Ma xie* 馬薤 is *li* 荔." Gao You states: "'*Li* 荔 [seedlings] rise, *ting* 挺, out of [the ground]' is: '*Li* 荔 herbs, *cao* 草, rise out of [the ground]'." Those who know the *Li* [*ji*], they do not know [this herb]. They call it *li ting* 荔挺, and they write [the name] *ma xian* 馬莧. Both are wrong. *Ma xian* 馬莧 is also called *tun er* 豚耳, "piglet ear," and this is *ma chi* 馬齒, "horse tooth," purslane. [Li] Shizhen: The *Er ya* states: "*Ping* 荓, read *ping* 瓶, is *ma zhou* 馬帚." This is *li cao* 荔草. [*Ma zhou* 馬帚] is to say: It can be made to horse brushes. Hence the name. It is the *tie sao zhou* 鐵掃帚, "iron broom," called by the people in He nan bei today.

【集解】【別録曰】蠡實生河東川谷，五月采實，陰乾。【頌曰】今陝西諸郡及鼎、澧州亦有之，近汴尤多。葉似薤而長厚，三月開紫碧花，五月結實作角子，如麻大而赤色有稜，根細長，通黄色，人取以爲刷。三月開花，五月采實，並陰乾用。許慎説文云：荔似蒲而小，根可爲刷。高誘云：河北平澤率生之。江東頗多，種於階庭，但呼爲旱蒲，不知即馬薤也。【時珍曰】蠡草生荒野中，就地叢生，一本二三十莖，苗高三四尺，葉中抽莖，開花結實。

Collected Explanations. *Bie lu*: *Li shi* grows in the river valleys of He dong. The fruits are collected in the fifth month. They are dried in the yin (i. e., shade). [Su] Song: Today it can be found in all the prefectures of Shaan xi and also in Ding and Li zhou. It is especially abundant near Bian. The leaves are similar to those of Chinese chives, but they are long and thick. [*Li shi*] opens purple-jade blue flowers in the third month. In the fifth month they generate fruits forming [protuberances like] horns with seeds. They are as big as sesame [seeds], red and have edges. The root is small and lengthy; it is of yellow color throughout. The people gather [the roots] to make brushes. The flowers open in the third month; the fruits are collected in the fifth month. All are dried in the yin (i. e., shade) and can then be used. Xu Shen in his *Shuo wen* states: "*Li* is similar to *pu* 蒲, cattail, but is smaller. The root can be used to make brushes." Gao You states: "Much of it grows in the flat land, in the marshlands of He bei." There are especially many in He dong. They are planted in terrace gardens, but [people there] call them *han pu* 旱蒲, "dryland cattail," because they are unaware that these are *ma xie* 馬薤, "horse chives." [Li] Shizhen: *Li cao* grow in the wilds. They form clusters on the ground. One root has 20 to 30 stems; the seedlings reach a height of three to four *chi*. The stem rises from the middle of the leaves. It opens flowers and forms fruit.

【正誤】【宗奭曰】蠡實，陶隱居言方藥不用，俗無識者。本草諸家所注不相應。若果是馬藺，則日華子本草不當更言可爲蔬菜。蓋馬藺葉出土已硬，又無味，馬牛皆不食，豈堪人食。今不敢以蠡實爲馬藺，更俟博識。【時珍曰】别録蠡實亦名荔實，則蠡乃荔字之訛也。張揖廣雅云"荔又名馬藺"，其説已明。又按周憲[252]王救荒本草言其嫩苗味苦，煠熟換水浸去苦味，油鹽調食，則馬藺亦可作菜矣。寇氏但據陶説疑之，欠考矣。陶氏不識之藥多矣。今正其誤。

Correction of Errors. [Kou] Zongshi: *Li shi*, Tao Yinju says: "It is not used as a recipe drug. Therefore it is unknown." The comments written by all the *Ben cao* experts do not agree. If it were actually *ma lin* 馬藺, then the *Rihu zi ben cao* should not say that it can be prepared as a vegetable. The fact is, when *ma lin* leaves come out of the ground, they are already hard, and they have no flavor. Neither horses nor oxen eat them, how could humans endure them as food? For the time being, [I] do not dare to identify *li shi* 蠡實 as *ma lin* 馬藺. Further studies are required to improve knowledge. [Li] Shizhen: The *Bie lu* lists *li shi* 荔實 as an alternative name of *li shi* 蠡實. That is, *li* 蠡 is a mistaken writing of the character *li* 荔. Zhang Ji in

252 According to *Ming shi*, Zhou Ding wang xiao zhuan 周定王橚傳, *Xian* 憲 should be Ding 定.

his *Guang ya* states: "*Li* 荔 is also called *ma lin* 馬藺." This should be clear enough! Also, according to Zhou Xian wang's *Jiu huang ben cao*, "its tender seedlings have a bitter flavor. Heat them until done, change the water, soak them to remove the bitter flavor and eat them mixed with vinegar and salt." This way, *ma lin*, too, can be prepared as a vegetable. Mr. Kou [Zongshi] bases his doubts on nothing but the sayings of Tao [Hongjing]. He failed to examine them. Mr. Tao was not familiar with many pharmaceutical drugs. Here now this error is corrected.

15-40-01
實 *Shi*
Fruit [of *li shi*]

【修治】【時珍曰】凡入藥炒過用，治疝則以醋拌炒之。

Pharmaceutical Preparation. [Li] Shizhen: When this is added to medication it is to be used fried. To cure elevation-illness[253] [qi] fry it mixed with vinegar.

【氣味】甘，平，無毒。【保昇曰】寒。【頌曰】山人服之，云大溫，甚有奇效。

Qi and Flavor. Sweet, balanced, nonpoisonous. [Han] Baosheng: Cold. [Su] Song: Mountain people ingest them. They claim them to be very warm, and extraordinarily effective.

【主治】皮膚寒熱，胃中熱氣，風寒濕痺，堅筋骨，令人嗜食。久服輕身。本經。止心煩滿，利大小便，長肌膚，肥大。別録。療金瘡血内流，癰腫，有效。蘇恭。婦人血氣煩悶，產後血運，并經脉不止，崩中帶下。消一切瘡癤，止鼻衄吐血，通小腸，消酒毒，治黄病，殺蕈毒，傅蛇蟲咬。大明。治小腹疝痛，腹内冷積，水痢諸病。時珍。

Control. Cold and heat affecting the skin. Heat qi in the stomach. Blockage related to [the presence of] wind, cold and moisture. They harden sinews and bones and let one long for food. Ingested for a long time, they relieve the body of its weight. *Ben jing*. They end heart vexation and a sensation of fullness. They free the passage of major (i. e., defecation) and major (i. e., urination) relief, stimulate the growth of muscles and skin and let one become fat and big. *Bie lu*. They effectively heal wounds caused by metal objects/weapons with an internal flow of blood, and swelling related to obstruction-illness.[254] Su Gong. Vexing heart-pressure related to

253 *Shan qi* 疝氣, "elevation-illness qi," a pathological condition of (1) an item having entered the scrotum, with pain, sometimes ascending, sometimes descending, (2) a condition affecting the scrotum or a testicle, (3) of violent abdominal pain, in some cases associated with constipation and anuria. BCGM Dict I, 419, 417.

254 *Yong* 癰, "obstruction-illness," refers to an obstruction of vessels or other ducts inside the body. Qi rushing against the obstruction may cause a local swelling and eventually break

blood and qi [disorders] of women, blood [induced brain] movement following delivery, unending menstruation, collapsing center[255] [and further diseases] below the belt. They dissolve all types of sores and pimples, end nosebleed and blood spitting, penetrate the small intestine, dissolve the poison of wine, serve to cure jaundice, and kill the poison of fungi. They are applied to bites of snakes and worms/bugs. Da Ming. They serve to cure painful elevation-illness [qi][256] of children, cold [qi] accumulation in the abdomen and all types of watery free-flux illness. [Li] Shizhen.

【附方】舊二，新六。

Added Recipes. Two of old. Six newly [recorded].

諸冷極病，醫所不治者。馬藺子九升洗净，空腹服一合，酒下，日三服。千金方。

All diseases related to extreme cold that cannot be cured by medicine. Wash nine *sheng* of *ma lin zi* clean and ingest on an empty stomach one *ge*, to be sent down with wine. To be ingested three times a day. *Qian jin fang*.

寒疝諸疾。寒疝不能食及腹内一切諸疾，消食肥肌。馬藺子一升，每日取一把，以麪拌煮吞之，服盡愈。姚僧坦集驗方。

All illnesses of cold [qi] elevation-illness. All illnesses related to cold [qi] elevation-illness making it impossible to eat. [This medication] dissolves food and fattens muscles. From one *sheng* of *ma lin zi* every day take one handful, boil them mixed with wheat flour and eat this. When [the entire *sheng*] is ingested, a cure is achieved. Yao Sengtan, *Ji yan fang*.

喉痺腫痛。衛生易簡方用蠡實一合，升麻五分，水一升，煎三合，入少蜜攪匀，細呷，大驗。

Throat closure and painful swelling. The *Wei sheng yi jian fang* [recommends to] boil one *ge* of *li* fruit and five *fen* of *cimicifuga* [rhizome] down to three *ge*, add a little honey, stir this to generate an even mixture and sip this in small amounts. Very effective.

聖惠方用馬藺子二升，升麻一兩，爲末，蜜丸，水服一錢。

through the surface to cause an abscess. BCGM Dict I, 641.

255 *Beng zhong* 崩中, "collapsing center," excessive vaginal bleeding outside of a menstruation period. BCGM Dict I, 58.

256 *Shan qi* 疝氣, "elevation-illness qi," a pathological condition of (1) an item having entered the scrotum, with pain, sometimes ascending, sometimes descending, (2) a condition affecting the scrotum or a testicle, (3) of violent abdominal pain, in some cases associated with constipation and anuria. BCGM Dict I, 419, 417.

The *Sheng hui fang* [recommends to grind] two *sheng* of *ma lin zi* and one *liang* of *cimicifuga* [rhizome] into powder and form with honey pills. Ingest with water one *qian*.

又方：馬藺子八錢，牛蒡子六錢，爲末，空心温水服方寸匕。
Another recipe. [Grind] eight *qian* of *ma lin zi* and six *qian* of great burdock seeds into powder, and ingest on an empty stomach with warm water the amount held by a square *cun* spoon.

水痢百病。張文仲備急方用馬藺子，以六月六日麪熬，各等分，爲末，空心米飲服方寸匕。如無六月六日麪，常麪亦可，牛骨灰亦可。
The hundred diseases related to watery free-flux illness. Zhang Wenzhong in his *Bei ji fang* [recommends to grind] equal amounts of *ma lin zi* with roasted wheat flour from the sixth day of the sixth month into powder and ingest on an empty stomach with a rice beverage the amount held by a one square *cun* spoon. If no wheat flour of the sixth day of the sixth month is at hand, normal wheat flour will do, too. The ashes of the bones of oxen can be used, too.

又方：馬藺子、乾薑、黄連各等分，爲散，熟湯服二方寸匕，入腹即斷也。冷熱皆治，常用神效，不得輕之。忌豬肉、冷水。
Another recipe. [Grind] equal amounts of *ma lin zi*, dried ginger and *coptis* [rhizome] into powder. Boil it until done and ingest of the decoction the amount held by two square *cun* spoons. Once it enters the abdomen, [the disease] ends. [Diseases related to] cold and heat are all cured; a regular application yields divine effects. [This recipe] must not be considered unimportant. Pork and cold water are to be avoided [during such a treatment].

腸風下血。有疙瘩瘡，破者不治。馬藺子一斤，研破酒浸，夏三、冬七日，晒乾，何首烏半斤，雄黄、雌黄各四兩，爲末，以浸藥酒打糊丸梧子大。每服三十丸，温酒下，日三服，見效。普濟方。
Intestinal wind with a discharge of blood. When pimples have broken open, this can no longer be cured. Grind and break into pieces one *jin* of *ma lin zi* and soak them in wine, in summer for three and in winter for seven days. Then dry them in the sun and [grind] them with half a *jin* of *polygonum multiflorum* [root] and four *liang* each of realgar and orpiment into powder. With the wine in which the [*ma lin zi*] drug was soaked prepare a paste to form pills the size of *wu* seeds. Each time ingest 30 pills, to be sent down with warm wine. To be ingested three times a day. An effect will show. *Pu ji fang*.

花、在[257] 根、葉 *Hua, Gen, Ye*

Flowers, root and leaves [of *li*].

【主治】去白蟲本經。療喉痺，多服令人溏洩。別録。主癰疽惡瘡。時珍。

Control. They remove white worms and heal throat closure. Ingested in large amounts they cause semi-liquid outflow. *Bie lu.* They control malign sores related to obstruction-illness and impediment-illness.[258] [Li] Shizhen.

【發明】【頌曰】蠡草花實皆入藥。列仙傳云寇先生宋人，好種荔，食其葩實"，是矣。【時珍曰】按葉水東日記云：北方田野人患胸腹飽脹者，取馬楝花擂凉水服，即泄數行而愈。據此則多服令人泄之説有驗，而蠡實之爲馬藺更無疑矣。

Explication. [Su] Song: Flowers and fruit of *li* herbs are all added to medication. The *Lie xian zhuan* states: "Mr. Kou was a person of the Song era. He loved to plant *li* and ate the flowers and the fruit." This is [the item discussed here]. [Li] Shizhen: According to the *Ye shui dong ri ji*, "when people in the open country in the North suffer from bloated chest and abdomen after eating to repletion, they resort to *ma lian* flowers, pound them in cold water and ingest this. Then they have several outflows and are cured." Judging from these records, the saying that ingesting them in large amounts causes outflow is based on experience, and there is even less doubt that *li shi* 蠡實, "*li* fruit," are identical to *ma lin* 馬藺 [seeds].

【附方】舊三，新六。

Added Recipes. Three of old. Six newly [recorded].

睡死不寤。蠡實根一握，杵爛，以水絞汁，稍稍灌之。外臺秘要。

[A person] sleeping [like] dead who cannot be awoken. Pound a handful of *li shi* to obtain a pulpy mass, squeeze it with water to obtain a juice and force-feed it in small amounts [to the patient]. *Wai tai mi yao.*

---

257 The Jiang xi edition has the character *zai* 在 here, too. All later edition have replaced it with the characters *shi* 實, "fruit," or *jing* 莖, "stem." However, the fruits are treated individually above, and this item has no "stem." Therefore, this changes are all wrong. The character *zai* 在 may have been an erroneous insertion from the beginning.

258 *Yong ju* 癰疽, "obstruction-illness, impediment-illness." refers to two vaguely distinguished obstructions/impediments of vessels or other ducts inside the body. Qi rushing against the obstruction may cause a local swelling and eventually break through the surface to cause an abscess. BCGM Dict I, 642.

喉痺口噤。馬藺花二兩，蔓荆子一兩，爲末，温水服一錢。

Throat closure and lockjaw. [Grind] two *liang* of *ma lin zi* and one *liang* of simpleleaf chastetree seeds into powder and [let the patient] ingest with warm water one *qian*.

喉痺腫痛，喘息欲死者。外臺秘要用馬藺根葉二兩，水一升半，煮一盞，細飲之，立瘥。

Throat closure with painful swelling, with a wheezing breath bringing one close to dying. The *Wai tai mi yao* [recommends to] boil two *liang* of *ma lin* root and leaves in one and a half *sheng* of water down to one cup and drink this in small amounts. A cure is achieved immediately.

聖惠方用根擣汁三合，蜜一合，慢火熬成，徐徐嚥之，日五七度。

The *Sheng hui fang* [recommends to] pound the root to obtain three *ge* of its juice and heat it with one *ge* of honey over a slow fire until it is ready [for ingestion. Let the patient] swallow it in small amounts, five to seven times a day.

一方：單汁飲之，口噤者灌下。無生者，以刷煎汁。

Another recipe. [Let the patient] drink only the juice. In the case of lockjaw, force-feed it to him. If no fresh [*li* stem, root and leaves] are at hand, boil a brush [made of them] to obtain the juice.

沙石熱淋。馬藺花七枚燒，故筆頭二七枚燒，粟米一合炒，爲末。每服三錢，酒下，日二服。名通神散。

Urinary dripping of sand and stones related to heat. [Grind] seven *ma lin* flowers, burned [to ashes], two times seven old writing brush tips, burned [to ashes], and one *ge* of millet, fried, into powder. Each time ingest three *qian*, to be sent down with wine. To be ingested twice a day. This [medication] is called "powder based on communication with spirits."

小便不通。馬藺花炒，茴香炒，葶藶炒[259]，爲末，每酒服二錢。十便良方。

Blocked urination. [Grind] *ma lin* flowers, fried, fennel, fried, and wood whitlow grass, fried, into powder. Each time ingest with wine two *qian*. *Shi bian liang fang*.

259 The *Shi bian liang fang* extent today does not list this recipe. However, *Pu ji fang*, ch. 216, *Xiao bian lin mi* 小便淋秘, "dripping and closed urination," has it, writing here: *ting li chao ge den fen* 葶藶炒各等分, "three *fen* each of .. and wood whitlow grass, fried."

一切癰疽：發背惡瘡。用鐵掃帚，同松毛、牛膝，以水煎服。乾坤生意。

All types of obstruction-illness and impediment-illness[260] with an effusion of malign sores on the back. Boil *tie sao zhou* together with pine hair (i. e., leaves) and *achyranthes* [leaves] in water and ingest this. *Qian kun sheng yi.*

面上瘢黶。取鐵掃帚地上自落葉并子，煎湯頻洗，數次自消。壽域神方。

Facial scars and moles. Boil in water the leaves and the seeds that have fallen by themselves to the ground from *tie sao chou* and repeatedly wash [the affected region] with the resulting decoction. After several times [the scars and moles] will dissolve as a result. *Shou yu shen fang.*

面皰鼻皶。馬藺子花，杵傅之佳。肘後方。

Facial blisters and nose sediments. Pound *ma lin zi* flowers and apply this to [the affected region]. Excellent. *Zhou hou fang.*

【附録】

Appendix

15-40-A01

必似勒拾遺 *Bi si le*, FE *Shi yi*

Unidentified.

【藏器曰】辛，温，無毒。主冷氣，胃閉不消食，心腹脹滿。生崑崙，狀似馬藺子也。

[Chen] Cangqi: Acrid, warm, nonpoisouns. It controls cold qi and a stomach closure with a failure to dissolve food, with distention and a sensation of fullness in the central and abdominal region. It grows in Kun lun and is shaped like *ma lin zi.*

15-41

惡實別録中品

***E shi*, FE *Bie lu*, middle rank.**

***Arctium lappa* L. Great burdock.**

【釋名】鼠粘別録、牛蒡別録、大力子綱目、蒡翁菜綱目、便牽牛綱目、蝙蝠刺。【時珍曰】其實狀惡而多刺鉤，故名。其根葉皆可食，人呼爲牛

260 *Yong ju* 癰疽, "obstruction-illness, impediment-illness." refers to two vaguely distinguished obstructions/impediments of vessels or other ducts inside the body. Qi rushing against the obstruction may cause a local swelling and eventually break through the surface to cause an abscess. BCGM Dict I, 642.

菜，術人隱之，呼爲大力也。俚人謂之便牽牛。河南人呼爲夜叉頭。【頌曰】實殼多刺，鼠過之則綴惹不可脱，故謂之鼠粘子，亦如羊負來之比。

Explication of Names. *Shu nian* 鼠粘, "clinging to rats/mice,", *Bie lu*. *Niu bang* 牛蒡, "oxen burdock," *Bie lu*. *Da li zi* 大力子, "great strength seeds," *Gang mu*. *Bang weng cai* 蒡翁菜, "father burdock vegetable," *Gang mu*. *Bian qian niu* 便牽牛, "conveniently pulling oxen," *Gang mu*. *Bian fu ci* 蝙蝠刺, "bat thorns." [Li] Shizhen: These fruit have an abominable shape with many thorns. Hence the name ["abominable fruit," *e shi* 實] The root and the leaves are edible. People call them "oxen vegetable," *niu cai* 牛菜. Persons practicing the arts [of longevity] conceal [this name] and call it *da li* 大力, "great strength." Ordinary people call it *bian qian niu* 便牽牛, "conveniently pulling oxen." People in Hen nan call it *ye cha tou* 夜叉頭, "nightly fork tip." [Su] Song: The fruit shell has many thorns. When mice/rats pass by it, [the fruit] cling to them and cannot be thrown off. Hence they are called "seeds clinging to rats/mice," *shu nian zi* 鼠粘子. This is similar to cocklebur [fruit], named *yang fu lai* 羊負來, "they come carried by sheep."

【集解】【别録曰】惡實生魯山平澤。【恭曰】魯山在鄧州東北。此草葉大如芋，子殻似栗狀，實細長如茺蔚子。【頌曰】惡實即牛蒡子也，處處有之。葉大如芋葉而長。實似葡萄核而褐色，外殻似栗梂而小如指頭，多刺。根有極大者，作菜茹益人。秋後采子入藥。【時珍曰】牛蒡古人種子，以肥壤栽之。剪苗汋淘爲蔬，取根煮曝爲脯，云甚益人，今人亦罕食之。三月生苗，起莖高者三四尺。四月開花成叢，淡紫色。結實如楓梂而小，萼上細刺百十攢簇之，一梂有子數十顆。其根大者如臂，長者近尺，其色灰黪。七月采子，十月采根。

Collected Explanations. *Bie lu*: *E shi* grows in the marshlands of the plains of Mount Lu shan. [Su] Gong: Mount Lu shan lies in the North-East of Deng zhou. The leaves of this herb as as big as those of Chinese chestnuts. The seed shells resemble the shape of millet. The fruits are fine and long, similar to those of Siberian motherwort [herbs]. Su] Song: *E shi* is *niu bang zi*. It can be found everywhere. Its leaves are as big as those of taro, but they are longer. The fruits are similar to grape kernels, but they are of brown color. Their outer shell is similar to that of Chinese chestnuts, but they are as small as a finger tip and have many thorns. The root may be extremely big; prepared as vegetable it is good for humans. The seeds are collected from autumn on to be added to medication. [Li] Shizhen: When the ancients planted the seeds of *niu bang*, they inserted them into fat soil. They cut the seedlings into small slices and washed them under running water to prepare them as a vegetable. They boiled the roots, dried them in the sun and stored them as preserved foot, claiming that they greatly benefit humans. Today, people seldom eat them. [*E shi*] grows a seedling in the third month. A stem rises to reach a height of three to four *chi*. In the fourth month, the flowers open, forming clusters. They are of a pale purple color. They form fruits similar to the [resin] balls of Chinese sweet gum, but they are smaller. Tens to hundreds of fine thorns form a cluster on the calyx. In one [fruit] ball are tens of seeds. The root is as big as a [human] arm, reaching a length of almost one *chi*, and it is ash-grey-black. The seeds are collected in the seventh month. The root is collected in the tenth month.

15-41-01
子 *Zi*
Seeds [of *e shi*].

【修治】【斅曰】凡用揀净，以酒拌蒸，待有白霜重出，以布拭去，焙乾擣粉用。

Pharmaceutical Preparation. [Lei] Xiao: For all usages, pick out the clean [seeds], mix them with wine and steam them until they release a white frost. Wipe off [the frost] with a cloth and dry [the seeds] over a fire in a pan. Then pound them into powder, and this can be used.

【氣味】辛，平，無毒。【藏器曰】苦。【元素曰】辛，温，陽中之陰，升也。【杲曰】辛，平，陽也，降也。

Qi and Flavor. Acrid, balanced, nonpoisonous. [Chen] Cangqi: Bitter. [Zhang] Yuansu: Acrid, warm, a yin in yang [substance]; it rises. [Li] Gao: Acrid, balanced, a yang [substance]. It descends.

【主治】明目補中，除風傷。别録。風毒腫，諸瘻。藏器。研末浸酒，每日服三二盞，除諸風，去丹石毒，利腰脚。又食前熟挼三枚吞之，散諸結節、筋骨煩、熱毒。甄權。吞一枚，出癰疽頭。蘇恭。炒研煎飲，通利小便。孟詵。潤肺散氣，利咽膈，去皮膚風，通十二經。元素。消斑疹毒。時珍。

Control. They clear the eyes and supplement the center. They eliminate harm caused by wind [intrusion]. *Bie lu*. Swelling related to the presence of wind poison. All types of fistula. [Chen] Cangqi. Grind [them into] powder, soak them in wine and ingest three small cups a day. This will eliminate all types of wind [intrusion], removes the poison of elixirs and mineral [drugs] and frees [the movement of/through] lower back and legs. Also, prior to meals rub three ripe [seeds] between your hands and swallow them. This will disperse all types of nodes [blocking the] joints, with sinew and bone irritation, and heat poison. Zhen Quan. To swallow one piece opens the tip of obstruction-illness and impediment illness.[261] Su Gong. Fry [the seeds], grind [them into powder], boil [them in water] and drink [the liquid]

261 *Yong ju* 癰疽, "obstruction-illness, impediment-illness." refers to two vaguely distinguished obstructions/impediments of vessels or other ducts inside the body. Qi rushing

to free the passage of urine. Meng Shen. They moisten the lung, disperse qi, free [the passage through] the throat and the diaphragm, and penetrate the 12 conduits. [Zhang] Yuansu. They dissolve the poison of macules and papules. [Li] Shizhen.

【發明】【杲曰】鼠粘子其用有四：治風濕癮疹，咽喉風熱，散諸腫瘡瘍之毒，利凝滯腰膝之氣，是也。

Explication. [Li] Gao. *Shu nian zi* have four usages. They serve to cure dormant papules related to wind and moisture, and wind and heat affecting the throat. They disperse all types of poison related to swelling, sores and ulcers. They free the passage of coagulated and sluggish qi in the lower back and knees.

【附方】舊五，新十一。

Added Recipes. Five of old; 11 newly [recorded].

風水身腫欲裂。鼠粘子二兩，炒研爲末。每温水服二錢，日三服。聖惠方。

Wind and water,[262] with the body swollen and threatening to crack open. Fry two *liang* of *shu nian zi*, and grind them into powder. Each time ingest with warm water two *qian*. To be ingested three times a day. *Sheng hui fang*.

風熱浮腫，咽喉閉塞。牛蒡子一合，半生半熟，爲末，熱酒服一寸匕。經驗方。

Wind heat with a surface swelling and throat closure. [Grind] one *ge* of *niu bang zi*, one half fresh, one half prepared with heat, into powder. Ingest with hot wine the amount held by a one square *cun* spoon. *Jing yan fang*.

痰厥頭痛。牛蒡子炒、旋覆花等分，爲末。臘茶清服一錢，日二服。聖惠方。

Phlegm recession[263] with headache. [Grind] equal amounts of *niu ban zi*, fried, and horseheal flowers into powder and ingest with clear *la*-tea[264] one *qian*. To be ingested twice a day. *Sheng hui fang*.

against the obstruction may cause a local swelling and eventually break through the surface to cause an abscess. BCGM Dict I, 642.

262 *Feng shui* 風水, "wind and water," a condition of *shui zhong* 水腫, "edemata," brought forth by wind that harms a body while it is sweating. It is often accompanied by aching joints and an aversion to wind. BCGM Dict I, 168.

263 *Tan jue* 痰厥, "phlegm recession." 1.) Etiological agent of blocked phlegm and closed-in qi causing headaches. 2.) Pathological condition of recession cold affecting the four limbs, brought forth by an abundance of phlegm and closed-in qi. In severe cases this may include the pathological condition of black-out with loss of consciousness, and an inability to recognize things and persons. BCGM Dict I, 493.

264 *La* tea, *la cha* 臘茶, lit: "tea of the 12th month," mentioned by Ouyang Xiu and Shen Kua during the Song era. As it is colored like melted wax it is also called *la cha* 蠟茶, "wax tea."

頭痛連睛。鼠粘子、石膏等分，爲末，茶清調服。醫方摘要。

Headache involving the eyes. [Grind] equal amounts of *shu nian zi* and gypsum into powder and ingest it mixed with clear tea. *Yi fang zhai yao.*

咽膈不利。疏風壅涎唾多，牛蒡子微炒、荆芥穗各一兩，炙甘草半兩，爲末。食後湯服二錢，當緩緩取效。寇氏本草衍義。

[The passage through] the throat and diaphragm is blocked. To disperse wind causing obstruction, and massive salivation, [grind] one *liang* each of *niu bang zi*, slightly fried, and *schizonepeta* spikes with half a *liang* of roasted *glycyrrhiza* [root] into powder and ingest, after meals, two *qian* with boiled water. Slow by slow this will show an effect. Kou shi, *Ben cao yan yi.*

懸癰喉痛。風熱上搏也。惡實炒、甘草生，等分，水煎含嚥，名啓關散。普濟方。

Suspended obstruction-illness[265] and painful throat, with wind and heat rising to attach themselves above. Boil equal amounts of fried *e shi* and fresh *glycyrrhiza* [root] in water, hold [the liquid] in the mouth and swallow it. This is called the "powder that opens a gate." *Pu ji fang.*

喉痺腫痛。牛蒡子六分，馬藺子六分，爲散。每空心温水服方寸匕，日再服。仍以牛蒡子三兩，鹽二兩，研勻，炒熱包熨喉外。廣濟方。

Throat blockage with a painful swelling. [Grind] six *fen* of *niu bang zi* and six *fen* of Chinese iris into powder. Each time ingest on an empty stomach with warm water the amount held by a square *cun* spoon. To be ingested twice a day. In addition evenly grind three *liang* of *niu bang zi* and two *liang* of salt [to powder], fry it, wrap it, and attach it as a hot compress from the outside to the throat. *Guang ji fang.*

咽喉痘疹。牛蒡子二錢，桔梗一錢半，粉甘草節七分，水煎服。痘疹要訣。

Smallpox with papules on the throat. Boil in water two *qian* of *niu bang zi*, one and a half *qian* of *platycodon* [root] and seven *fen* of *glycyrrhiza* [root] node powder, and [let the patient] ingest this. *Dou zhen yao jue.*

風熱癮疹。牛蒡子炒、浮萍等分，以薄荷湯服二錢，日二服。初虞世古今録驗。

Dormant papules related to wind and heat. Ingest with a mint decoction equal amounts of fried *niu bang zi* and ducksmeat. To be ingested twice a day. Chu Yushi, *Gu jin lu yan.*

---

265 *Xuan yong* 懸癰, "suspended obstruction-illness," a condition developing either in the perineum or in the bend between the jaws and pharynx. BCGM Dict I, 593.

風齲牙痛。鼠粘子炒，煎水含，冷吐之。延年方。

Painful decayed teeth, related to wind [intrusion]. Boil fried *shu nian zi* in water and hold [the liquid] in the mouth. Spit it out when it is cold. *Yan nian fang.*

小兒痘瘡。時出不快，壯熱狂躁，咽膈壅塞，大便秘澀。小兒咽喉腫不利。若大便利者，勿服。牛蒡子炒一錢二分，荆芥穗二分，甘草節四分，水一盞，同煎至七分，温服。已出亦可服。名必勝散。和劑局方。

Smallpox of children with a slow release of sores, strong heat, madness and restlessness, as well as blocked throat and constipated or rough defecation, Impassable, swollen throat of children. If the bowel movement is free, do not ingest [the following medication]. Boil one *qian* and two *fen* of *niu bang zi*, two *fen* of *schizonepeta* spikes, and four *fen* of *glycyrrhiza* [root] nodes in water down to 70% and [let the child] ingest this warm. This may also be ingested when [the sores] have been released. The name [of this medication] is: the "powder that must win."[266] *He ji ju fang.*

婦人吹乳。鼠粘二錢，麝香少許，温酒細吞下。袖珍方。

Inflated breast[267] of women. Mix two *qian* of *shu nian* [*zi*] with a small amount of musk and [let the woman] swallow this with warm wine in small quantities. *Xiu zhen fang.*

便癰腫痛。鼠粘子二錢炒，研末，入蜜一匙，朴硝一匙，空心温酒服。袖珍方。

Painful swelling associated with an obstruction-illness[268] [blocking defecation/urination] relief. Grind two *qian* of fried *shu nian zi* into powder, add one spoon of honey and one spoon of mirabilite and ingest this on an empty stomach with warm wine. *Xiu zhen fang.*

蛇蝎蠱毒。大力子煮汁服。衛生易簡方。

Snake, scorpion and *gu* poison.[269] Boil *da li zi* and ingest the juice. *Wei sheng yi jian fang.*

---

266 Instead of *bi sheng san* 必勝散, "powder that must win," *Ju fang* ch. 10, *zhi xiao er zhu ji* 治小兒諸疾, "to cure all illnesses of children," writes *xiao du san* 消毒散, "powder to dissolve poison."

267 *Chui ru* 吹乳, "inflated breast." Identical to *chui nai* 吹奶, "inflated breast." A condition with milk blocked after delivery and the breasts turning red and swelling. BCGM Dict I, 101.

268 *Yong* 癰, "obstruction-illness,"refers to an obstruction of vessels or other ducts inside the body. Qi rushing against the obstruction may cause a local swelling and eventually break through the surface to cause an abscess. BCGM Dict I, 641.

269 *Gu du* 蠱毒, "*gu*-poison[ing]." (1) A poison emitted by certain worms/snakes with an ability to cause varying pathological changes in a person who has taken it in by means of

水蠱腹大。惡實微炒一兩，爲末，麪糊丸梧子大，每米飲下十丸。張文仲方。

Enlarged abdomen caused by water *gu* [poison].[270] [Grind] one *liang* of *e shi*, slightly fried, into powder and form with a wheat flour paste pills the size of *wu* seeds. Each time send down with a rice beverage ten pills. *Zhang Wenzhong fang*.

歷節腫痛。風熱攻手指，赤腫麻木，甚則攻肩背兩膝，遇暑熱則大便秘。牛蒡子三兩，新豆豉炒、羌活各一兩，爲末。每服二錢，白湯下。本事方。

Painful swelling related to pervading joints [wind].[271] Wind heat attacks the fingers, with redness, swelling and numbness. In severe cases, [wind heat] attacks shoulders, back and both knees, and in the heat of summer months defecation is blocked. *Ben shi fang*.

15-41-02
根、莖 *Gen, Jing*
Root, stem [of *e shi*].

【氣味】苦，寒，無毒。【權曰】甘，平。【藏器曰】根須蒸熟暴乾用。不爾，令人欲吐。

Qi and Flavor. Bitter, cold, nonpoisonous. [Zhen] Quan: Sweet, balanced. [Chen] Cangqi: To use the root it must be steamed until done. Then it is dried in the sun. Otherwise it lets one develop an urge to vomit.

【主治】傷寒寒熱汗出，中風面腫，消渴熱中，逐水。久服輕身耐老。別録。根主牙齒痛，勞瘧諸風，脚緩弱風毒，癰疽，欬嗽傷肺，肺壅，疝瘕，冷氣積血。蘇恭。根浸酒服，去風及惡瘡。和葉搗碎，傅杖瘡、金瘡，永不畏風。藏器。主面目煩悶，四肢不健，通十二經脉，洗五臟惡氣。可常作菜食，令人身輕。甄權。切根如豆，拌麪作飯食，消脹壅。莖葉煮汁作浴湯，去皮間習習如蟲行。又入鹽花生搗，搨一切腫毒。孟詵。

Control. Harm caused by cold, with alternating sensations of cold and heat, and sweating. Wind stroke with facial swelling. Melting with thirst[272] with central heat.

wine or food. (2) Abdominal fullness, in some cases with blood spitting, and blood in the stool and urine. BCGM Dict I, 192 - 193. See BCGM 42-22.

270 *Shui gu* 水蠱, "water *gu*[-distension," identical to *gu zhang* 鼓脹, "drum[-like] distension." A condition of an abdominal distension and big upswell brought forth by stagnant water qi accumulating in the abdomen. BCGM Dict 409, 196.

271 *Li jie feng* 歷節風, "pervading joints wind," a condition of *tong feng* 痛風, "pain wind," characterized by spontaneous sweating, shortness of qi/breath, aching joints, and difficulties in bending and stretching. BCGM Dict I, 314.

272 *Xiao ke* 消渴, "melting with thirst," most likely including cases of diabetes. BCGM Dict Vol I, 567.

It eliminates water. Ingested over a long time, it relieves the body of its weight and helps to endure aging. *Bie lu*. The root controls toothache, exhaustion, malaria and all types of wind [intrusion], weakness of legs with wind poison, obstruction-illness and impediment-illness,[273] cough related to harmed lung, lung obstruction,[274] elevation-illness and conglomeration-illness[275] with cold qi and accumulated blood. Su Gong. To soak the root in wine and ingest it eliminates wind and malign sores, Pounded together with the leaves and applied to wounds caused by flogging and wounds caused by metal objects/weapons one does not have to fear that they could be struck by wind. [Chen] Cangqi. It controls irritation affecting face and eyes, and heart-pressure, with the four limbs losing their strength. It penetrates the 12 conduit vessels and cleans the five long-term depots of malign qi. It can be prepared as vegetable for continuous consumption to relieve one from the weight of his body. Zhen Quan. Cut the root into bean-size pieces, mix them with wheat flour and prepare a meal for consumption. This will dissolve swelling related to an obstruction. The stem and the leaves boiled and the juice prepared to a hot bathing liquid removes an itching in the skin as if there were bugs/worms moving. Also, pound the fresh [stem and leaves] with crystallized salt and rub this on all types of swelling with poison. Meng Shen.

【發明】【頌曰】根作脯食甚良。莖葉宜煮汁釀酒服。冬月采根，蒸暴入藥。劉禹錫傳信方：療暴中風，用緊細牛蒡根，取時避風，以竹刀或荆刀刮去土，生布拭了，搗絞取汁一大升，和好蜜四大合，温分兩服，得汗出便瘥。此方得之岳鄂鄭中丞。鄭因食熱肉一頓，便中暴風。外甥盧氏爲潁陽令，有此方。服，當時便瘥。

Explication. [Su] Song: The root prepared to and consumed as preserved food is very good. The stem and the leaves are boiled in water and this is used to brew wine to be ingested. Collect the root during the winter months, steam it, dry it in the sun and add it to medication. Liu Yuxin, *Chuan xin fang*: "For sudden wind stroke use a solid, fine *niu bang* [*zi*] root to remove the wind as soon as possible. Remove the soil with a bamboo knife or with a knife made from simpleleaf chastetree wood, wipe [the root] with a piece of cloth, pound it and squeeze [the resulting pulp] to

273 *Yong ju* 癰疽, "obstruction-illness, impediment-illness." refers to two vaguely distinguished obstructions/impediments of vessels or other ducts inside the body. Qi rushing against the obstruction may cause a local swelling and eventually break through the surface to cause an abscess. BCGM Dict I, 642.

274 *Fei yong* 肺癰, "lung obstruction-illness," also: *fei yong* 肺壅, "lung obstruction," a condition of abscesses in the lung, with fever, chest pain, and vomiting of bad-smelling pus and blood. BCGM Dict I, 156.

275 *Shan jia* 疝瘕, "elevation-illness with conglomeration-illness." A lump-like swelling in the abdomen that alternately collects and then dissolves again. BCGM Dict I, 418.

obtain one generous *sheng* of the juice. Mix it with four *ge* of good honey and ingest this warm divided into two portions. When sweating begins healing is achieved. This recipe was obtained from Vice Censor-in-Chief Zheng from Yue e. Zheng once suffered from a sudden wind stroke after he had eaten hot meat. His nephew. Mr. Lu, governor of Ying yang, had this recipe. [Zheng] ingested it and was cured in due time."

【附方】舊五，新一十六。

Added Recipes. Five of old. 16 newly [recorded].

時氣餘熱不退，煩燥發渴，四肢無力，不能飲食。用牛蒡根搗汁，服一小盞，效。聖惠方。

Heat that remains following seasonal qi affection, with vexing dryness causing thirst. The four limbs have lost their strength, and [patients] can neither drink nor eat. Pound *niu ban zi* and ingest one small cup of the resulting juice. Effective. *Sheng hui fang*.

天行時疾。生牛蒡根搗汁五合，空腹分爲二服。服訖，取桑葉一把，炙黄，以水一升，煮取五合，頓服取汗，無葉用枝。孫真人食忌。

Epidemic illness. Pound fresh *niu bang* root to obtain five *ge* of juice and on an empty stomach ingest it divided into two portions. After ingesting them roast a handful of mulberry tree leaves until they turn yellow, boil them in one *sheng* of water down to five *ge* and ingest this to stimulate sweating. If no [mulberry tree] leaves are available, the twigs will do. *Sun zhenren shi ji*.

熱攻心煩，恍惚。以牛蒡根搗汁一升，食後分爲二服。食醫心鏡。

Vexation caused by heat attacking the heart, with absent-mindedness. Pound *niu bang* root to obtain one *sheng* of juice and after meals ingest it divided into two portions. *Shi yi xin jing*.

傷寒搐搦。汗後覆蓋不密，致腰背手足搐搦者，牛蒡根散主之。牛蒡根十條，麻黄、牛膝、天南星各六錢，剉，於盆内研細，好酒一升同研，以新布絞取汁。以炭火半秤燒一地坑令赤，掃净，傾藥汁入坑内，再燒令黑色，取出於乳鉢内細研。每服一錢，温酒下，日三服。朱肱活人書。

Convulsions related to harm caused by cold. If someone is not covered tightly after sweating and suffers from convulsions affecting his lower back, back, hands and feet, this will be controlled by the "powder with *niu bang* [*zi*] root." File ten *niu bang* [*zi*] roots and six *qian* each of *ephedra* [herb], *achyranthes* [leaves] and Indian turnip [root] and grind them in a basin to fine [powder]. Add one *sheng* of good wine and grind this. Squeeze [the pulp] with a new piece of cloth to obtain a juice. Heat a pit in the ground with a fire lit by half a *cheng* of charcoal until it is red. Sweep it clean, pour the medicinal juice into the pit and heat it again to let [the juice] turn into a black [mass]. Remove [the black mass] and grind it to fine [powder]. Each time ingest one *qian*, to be sent down with warm wine. To be ingested three times a day. Zhu Gong, *Huo ren shu*.

一切風疾，十年、二十年者。牛蒡根一升，生地黄、枸杞子、牛膝各三升，用袋盛藥，浸無灰酒三升内，每任意飲之。外臺秘要。

All types of wind illnesses. They may have lasted for ten or 20 years. Fill a pouch with one *sheng* of *niu bang* [*zi*] roots, and three *sheng* each of fresh Chinese foxglove [rhizomes], *lycium* seeds, and *achyranthes* [roots]. Soak [the pouch] in three *sheng* of ash-free wine and each time drink as much as you wish. *Wai tai mi yao*.

老人中風。口目瞤動，煩悶不安。牛蒡根切一升，去皮晒乾，杵爲麪，白米四合淘净，和作餺飥，豉汁中煮，加葱、椒、五味，空心食之。恒服極效。壽親養老書。

Old persons struck by wind. Mouth and eyes making involuntary, uncontrolled movements. With vexing heart-pressure and restlessness. Cut one *sheng* of *niu bang* [*zi*] root, remove the skin and dry [the rest] in the sun. Pound it to flour. Rinse four *ge* of white rice, mix it with [the dried *niu ban zi* root] and prepare cakes. Boil them in the juice of [soybean] relish. Add onions, pepper, and the five flavor [spices] and eat this on an empty stomach. When this is ingested permanently it is very effective. *Shou qin yang lao shu*.

老人風濕久痺，筋攣骨痛。服此壯腎，潤皮毛，益氣力。牛蒡根一升切，生地黄一升切，大豆二升炒，以絹袋盛，浸一斗酒中五六日，任性空心温服二三盞，日二服。集驗方。

Old persons with blocked [joints] related to wind and moisture [intrusion], with sinew contraction and aching bones. To ingest this will strengthen the kidneys, moisten skin and hair and boost the strength of qi. Fill one *sheng* of *niu bang* [*zi*] root, cut [to pieces], one *sheng* of fresh Chinese foxglove [rhizome], cut [to pieces], and two *sheng* of soybeans, fried, into a silk pouch and soak it in one *dou* of wine for five to six days. Drink at will on an empty stomach two or three cups. To be ingested twice a day. *Ji yan fang*.

頭面忽腫。熱毒風氣内攻，或連手足赤腫，觸着痛者。牛蒡子根，一名蝙蝠刺，洗净研爛，酒煎成膏，絹攤貼腫處。仍以熱酒服一二匙，腫消痛減。斗門方。

Sudden swelling of head and face. When heat poison and wind qi have attacked internally, in some cases associated with redness and swelling of hands and feet, and pain felt when they are touched. Wash clean a *niu bang zi* root, also called "bat thorns," and grind it into a pulpy mass. Boil it in wine to obtain a paste. Spread [the paste] on a piece of silk and apply this to the location of the swelling. Also, ingest with hot wine the amount held by one or two spoons. This will dissolve the swelling and reduce the pain. *Dou men fang*.

頭風掣痛不可禁者，摩膏主之。取牛蒡莖葉，搗取濃汁二升，無灰酒一升，鹽花一匙頭，煻火煎稠成膏，以摩痛處，風毒自散。摩時，須極力令熱乃效。冬月用根。篋中方。

Head wind[276] and unstoppable convulsion pain.[277] This is controlled by rubbing the paste [described below on the affected region]. Pound stem and leaves of *niu bang* [*zi*] to obtain two *sheng* of a thick juice. Add an amount of crystallized salt held by the tip of a spoon and boil this over a warming fire to generate a thick paste. When this is rubbed on the aching region the wind poison will disperse as a result. The rubbing must be carried out with utmost strength to generate heat, and this will result in an effect. During the winter months use the root [instead of stem and leaves]. *Jia zhong fang*.

頭風白屑。牛蒡葉搗汁，熬稠塗之。至明，皂莢水洗去。聖惠方。

Head wind with white dandruff. Pound *niu bang* [*zi*] leaves to obtain a juice. Boil it to generate a thick [paste] and apply this [to the affected region]. The next morning wash it with *gleditsia* pod/seed water to remove [the paste]. *Sheng hui fang*.

喉中熱腫。鼠粘根一升，水五升，煎一升，分三服。延年方。

Swollen throat with heat. Boil one *sheng* of *shu nian* [*zi*] root in five *sheng* of water down to one *sheng* and ingest this divided into three portions. *Yan nian fang*.

小兒咽腫。牛蒡根搗汁，細嚥之。普濟方。

Swollen throat of children. Pound *niu bang* [*zi*] root to obtain a juice and [let the child] swallow small quantities. *Pu ji fang*.

熱毒牙痛。熱毒風攻頭面，齒齦腫痛不可忍。牛蒡根一斤搗汁，入鹽花一錢，銀器中熬成膏。每用塗齒齦下，重者不過三度瘥。聖惠方。

---

276 *Tou feng* 頭風, "head wind." Condition of wind evil attacking the head followed by pain, dizziness, itching. BCGM Dict I, 509.

277 *Zhi tong* 掣痛, "convulsion pain," an illness sign of pain accompanied by a twitching sensation. BCGM Dict I, 681.

Toothache related to heat poison. Wind related to heat poison attacks head and face, letting the gums swell with an unbearable pain. Pound *niu bang* [*zi*] roots to obtain a juice. Add one *qian* of crystallized salt and heat this in a silver vessel to generate a paste. Each time apply it to below the [affected] gum. Even serious cases will be healed after no more than three applications. *Sheng hui fang.*

項下癭疾。鼠粘子根一升，水三升，煮取一升半，分三服。或爲末，蜜丸常服之。救急方。

Goiter illness below the neck. Boil one *sheng* of *shu nian zi* root in three *sheng* of water down to one and a half *sheng* and ingest this divided into three portions. Or prepare a powder, form it with honey to pills, and ingest them continuously. *Jiu ji fang.*

耳卒腫痛。牛蒡根切，絞汁二升，銀鍋内熬膏塗之。聖濟總録。

Sudden painful swelling of an ear. Cut *niu bang* [*zi*] roots [to pieces] and squeeze them to obtain two *sheng* of a juice. Heat it in a silver pot to generate a paste and apply this [to the affected region]. *Sheng ji zong lu.*

小便不通，臍腹急痛。牛蒡葉汁、生地黄汁二合，和匀，入蜜二合。每服一合，入水半盞，煎三五沸，調滑石末一錢服。聖濟總録。

Blocked urination, with an acute pain in the navel and abdominal region. Evenly mix two ge of *niu bang* [*zi*] leaf juice and fresh Chinese foxglove [rhizome] juice, and add two *ge* of honey. Each time ingest one *ge*. Give it into half a cup of water, boil it three to five times to bubbling, mix it with one *qian* of talcum powder, and ingest this. *Sheng ji zong lu.*

癤子腫毒。鼠粘子葉貼之。千金方。

Pimples with swelling and poison. Attach *shu nian zi* leaves [to the affected region]. *Qian jin fang.*

石瘻出膿，堅實寒熱。鼠粘子葉爲末，和鷄子白封之。外臺秘要。

Stone fistula emitting pus. Hard and solid [fistula] with alternating sensations of cold and heat. [Grind] *shu nian zi* leaves into powder, [mix it] with egg white and use this to cover [the fistula]. *Wai tai mi yao.*

諸瘡腫毒。牛蒡根三莖洗，煮爛搗汁，入米煮粥，食一椀，甚良。普濟方。

All types of sores with swelling and poison. Wash three *niu bang* [*zi*] root stems, boil them to generate a pulpy mass and pound this to obtain a juice. Add rice and boil this to generate a congee. Eat one bowl. Very good. *Pu ji fang.*

積年惡瘡、反花瘡、漏瘡不瘥者。牛蒡根擣，和臘月猪脂，日日封之。千金方。

Malign sores lasting for several years. Reversed-blossom sores.[278] Leaking sores that have not been healed. Pound *niu bang* [*zi*], mix [the resulting pulp] with lard of the 12th month and seal [the affected region] with it every day. *Qian jin fang*.

月水不通，結成癥塊，腹肋脹大欲死。牛蒡根二斤剉，蒸三遍，以生絹袋盛之，以酒二斗浸五日，每食前温服一盞。普濟方

Blocked menstruation, with a formation of concretion lumps and a distension of abdomen and flanks bringing one close to dying. File two *jin* of *niu bang* [*zi*] root [to pieces], steam them three times and fill them into a new silk pouch. Soak [the pouch] in two *dou* of wine for five days. Each time ingest prior to a meal one cup of the warm [wine]. *Pu ji fang*.

15-42
葈耳本經中品
Xi er, FE *Ben jing*, middle rank.

***Xanthium sibiricum* Patrin ex Widder. Cocklebur.**

【釋名】胡葈本經、常思弘景、蒼耳爾雅、卷耳詩經、爵耳詩疏、豬耳綱目、耳璫詩疏、地葵本經、葹音施、羊負來弘景、道人頭圖經、進賢菜記事珠、喝起草綱目、野茄綱目、縑絲草。【頌曰】詩人謂之卷耳，爾雅謂之蒼耳，廣雅謂之葈耳，皆以實得名也。陸機詩疏云：其實正如婦人耳璫，今或謂之耳璫草。鄭康成謂是白胡葈，幽州人呼爲爵耳。博物志云：洛中有人驅羊入蜀，胡葈子多刺，粘綴羊毛，遂至中土，故名羊負來。俗呼爲道人頭。【弘景曰】傖人皆食之，謂之常思菜，以葉覆麥作黄衣者。方用甚稀。【時珍曰】其葉形如葈麻，又如茄，故有葈耳及野茄諸名。其味滑如葵，故名地葵，與地膚同名。詩人思夫賦卷耳之章，故名常思菜。張揖廣雅作常葈，亦通。

Hu xi 胡葈, "hemp of the Hu," *Ben jing*. *Chang si* 常思, "continously longed for," [Tao] Hongjing. *Cang er* 蒼耳, "dark green ear," *Er ya*. *Juan er* 卷耳, "curled up ear," *Shi jing*. *Jue er* 爵耳, *Shi shu*. *Zhu er* 豬耳, "pig ear," *Gang mu*. *Er dang* 耳璫, "earring," *Shi shu*. *Di kui* 地葵, "ground mallow," *Ben jing*. *Shi* 葹, read *shi* 施, [and] *yang fu lai* 羊負來, "those that come carried by sheep," [Tao] Hongjing. *Dao ren tou* 道人頭, "Daoist's head," *Tu jing*. *Jin xian cai* 進賢菜, "vegetable presented to the virtuous," *Ji shi zhu*. *He qi cao* 喝起草, "herb to let one rise and shout loudly," *Gang mu*. *Ye jia* 野茄, "wild eggplant," *Gang mu*. *Jian si cao* 縑絲草, "fine silk threads

278 *Fan hua chuang* 反花瘡, "reversed-blossoms sores," a condition with a festering ulcer generating a fleshgrowth assuming the shape of a flower. BCGM Dict I, 149.

herb." [Su] Song: A poet has called it *juan er* 卷耳. The *Er ya* calls it *cang er* 蒼耳. The *Guang ya* calls it *xi er* 葈耳. All these names refer to [the shape of] the fruit. Lu Ji in his *Shi shu* states: "Its fruits are really similar to the earrings of women. Today it is sometimes called 'earring herb'." Zheng Kangcheng says: "It is *bai hu xi* 白胡葈. People in You zhou call it *Jue er* 爵耳." The *Bo wu zhi* states: "In Lu zhong people drive sheep to Shu. The seeds of *hu xi* 胡葈 have many thorns. They cling to the fur of the sheep and are brought to Zhong tu. Hence they are named 'those that come carried by sheep'," *yang fu lai* 羊負來." A common designation [of these burdocks] is "Daoist's head," *dao ren tou* 道人頭. [Tao] Hongjing: All the poor people eat [this herb]. They call it "the vegetable of continuous longing," *chang si cai* 常思菜. They use the leaves [of *xi er*] to cover wheat and give it a yellow coating. They are rarely used in recipes. [Li] Shizhen: The leaves are shaped like those of hemp, *xi ma* 葈麻, and also like those of eggplants, *qie* 茄. Hence [the plant] was given names such as *xi er* 葈耳, "hemp ears," and *ye qie* 野茄, "wild eggplant." Its flavor is as oily as that of mallows, *kui* 葵, hence it is called *di kui* 地葵, "ground mallow," which is also the name of the broomplant, *di fu* 地膚, "ground skin." A poet has written a piece *Si fu fu* 思夫賦, "Verses on longing for the husband," [with a reference to a plant named] "curled up ear," *juan er* 卷耳. Hence it is named "vegetable of continuous longing," *chang si cai* 常思菜. Zhang Qi in his *Guang ya* writes [the name] *chang xi* 常葈. This makes sense, too.

【集解】【別録曰】葈耳生安陸川谷及六安田野，實熟時采。【頌曰】今處處有之。陸氏詩疏云：其葉青白似胡荽，白華細莖，蔓生，可煮爲茹，滑而少味。四月中生子，正如婦人耳璫。郭璞云：形如鼠耳，叢生如盤。今之所有皆類此，但不作蔓生。【時珍曰】按周憲王救荒本草云：蒼耳葉青白，類粘糊菜葉。秋間結實，比桑椹短小而多刺。嫩苗煠熟，水浸淘拌食，可救飢。其子炒，去皮，研爲麪，可作燒餅食，亦可熬油點燈。

Collected Explanations. *Bie lu*: *Xi er* grows in the river valleys of An lu and in the open country of Liu an. The fruits are collected when they are ripe. [Su] Song: Today it can be found everywhere. Mr. Lu [Ji] in his *Shi shu* states: "Its leaves are greenish-white similar to those of coriander. It has white flowers and fine stems. It grows as a creeper and can be cooked as food. It is oily and has little flavor. It grows seeds in the middle of the fourth month that really resemble the earrings of women." Guo Pu: "They are shaped like the ears of rats/mice. They form clusters shaped like trays." All those found today are of this type, but they do not grow as creepers. [Li] Shizhen: According to Zhou xian wang's *Jiu huang ben cao*, "the leaves of *cang er* are greenish-white, of the same type as the leaves of St. Paulswort. Fruits form in autumn. They are comparable to those of mulberry trees, but they are shorter, smaller and have many thorns. The tender seeds are fried in fat/oil until done. When they are soaked and washed in a pan and mixed with food, they can rescue one during a famine. The seeds are fried, the skin is discarded, and they are ground to flour. This can be used to cook cakes. They can also be boiled to prepare an oil that serves to light lamps."

15-42-01
實 *Shi*
Fruit [of *xi er*].

【修治】【大明曰】入藥炒熟，搗去刺用，或酒拌蒸過用。

Pharmaceutical Preparation. Da Ming: For adding them to medication, fry them until done, pound them, remove the thorns and then use them. Or use them after steaming them mixed with oil.

【氣味】甘，温，有小毒。【别録曰】苦。【權曰】甘，無毒。【恭曰】忌豬肉、馬肉、米泔，害人。

Qi and Flavor. Sweet, warm, slightly poisonous. *Bie lu*: Bitter. [Zhen] Quan: Sweet, nonpoisonous. [Su] Gong: [During a treatment with them] pork, horse meat, and slop from rinsing rise are to be avoided; they would be harmful.

【主治】風頭寒痛，風濕周痺，四肢拘攣痛，惡肉死肌，膝痛。久服益氣。藏器。治肝熱，明目。甄權。治一切風氣，填髓，暖腰脚，治瘰癧、疥瘡及瘙癢。大明。炒香浸酒服，去風補益。時珍。

Control. Painful wind head[279] with cold. Blockage [of joints] throughout [the body] related to the presence of wind and moisture. Painful contraction of the four limbs. Malign flesh [growth] and dead muscles. Aching knees. Ingested for a long time they boost the qi. [Chen] Cangqi.[280] They serve to cure liver heat; they clear the eyes. Zhen Quan. They serve to cure all types of wind qi [intrusion], fill the marrow, warm the lower back and the legs, and serve to cure scrofula pervasion-illness,[281] *jie*-illness[282] sores and itching. Da Ming.

279 *Feng tou* 風頭, "wind head," a condition wind evil attacking the head followed by pain, or dizziness, or itching. BCGM Dict I, 509.

280 藏器：此前引文乃出證類卷八葈耳實所載本經、别録。

281 *Luo li* 瘰癧, "scrofula pervasion-illness," when two or more connected swellings of the size of plum or date kernels appear either on the neck or in the armpits, or somewhere else on the body. BCGM Dict I. 329.

282 *Jie*-illness 疥, vaguely identifiable skin ailment. BCGM Dict I, 249.

【附方】舊三，新四。

Added Recipes. Three of old; four newly [recorded].

久瘧不瘥。蒼耳子，或根莖亦可，焙，研末，酒糊丸梧子大。每酒服三十丸，日二服。生者擣汁服亦可。朱氏集驗方。

Long-lasting malaria that has not been cured. Dry *cang er* seeds – the root and the stem will do, too – over a fire in a pan and grind them into powder. With wine and [wheat flour] prepare a paste to form pills the size of *wu* seeds. Each time ingest with wine 30 pills. To be ingested twice a day. When they are fresh it is also possible to pound them and ingest the resulting juice. *Zhu shi ji yan fang.*

大腹水腫，小便不利。蒼耳子灰、葶藶末等分。每服二錢，水下，日二服。千金方。

Enlarged abdomen with a water swelling. Blocked urination. Each time ingest, to be sent down with water, two *qian* of equal amounts of *cang er* seed ashes and wood whitlow grass powder. To be ingested twice a day. *Qian jin fang.*

風濕攣痺，一切風氣。蒼耳子三兩，炒，爲末，以水一升半，煎取七合，去滓呷之。食醫心鏡。

Contraction and blockage [of joints] related to the presence of wind and moisture. All types of wind [intrusion] illnesses. Fry three *liang* of *cang er* seeds and [grind them into] powder. Boil them in one and a half *sheng* of water down to seven *ge*. Discard the dregs and sip [the liquid]. *Shi yi xin jing.*

牙齒痛腫。蒼耳子五升，水一斗，煮取五升，熱含之。冷即吐去，吐後復含，不過一劑瘥。莖葉亦可，或入鹽少許。孫真人千金翼。

Toothache with a swelling. Boil five *sheng* of *cang er* seeds in one *dou* of water down to five *sheng* and hold [a first portion of] the hot [liquid] in the mouth. Spit it out when it is cold. After spitting [the cold liquid] out, once again hold [hot liquid] in the mouth. After no more than one preparation [is ingested] a cure is achieved. Stem and leaves will do, too. A small amount of salt may be added. Sun zhenren, *Qian jin yi.*

鼻淵流涕。倉耳子，即縑絲草子，炒，研爲末，每白湯點服一二錢。證治要訣。

Nasal deep source outflow[283] of snivel. Fry *cang er* seeds, these are the seeds of *jian si cao*, and grind them into powder. Each time ingest, with clear, boiled water, one or two *qian*. *Zheng zhi yao jue.*

283 *Bi yuan* 鼻淵, "nasal deep-source [outflow]," a condition with much snivel that is malodorous, dirty and turbid, or resembles yellow liquid. BCGM Dict I, 64.

眼目昏暗。菒耳實一升，爲末，白米半升作粥，日食之。普濟方。

Clouding of the eyes with dim vision. [Grind] one *sheng* of *cang er* fruits into powder and with half a *sheng* of white rice prepare a congee. Eat this every day. *Pu ji fang*.

嗜酒不已。氈中蒼耳子七枚，燒灰投酒中飲之，即不嗜。陳藏器本草。

Endless addiction to wine. Burn seven *cang er* seeds found in felt to ashes, give them into wine and drink it. There will be no more addiction. *Chen Cangqi ben cao*.

15-42-02

莖、葉 *Jing, Ye*

Stem, leaf [of *xi er*].

【修治】【斅曰】凡采得去心，取黄精，以竹刀細切，拌之蒸，從巳至亥時出，去黄精，陰乾用。

Pharmaceutical Preparation. [Lei] Xiao: Whenever they are collected, remove the heart. With a bamboo knife cut [the *xi er* stems and leaves together with] solomon's seal [root] into fine pieces, mix them and steam them from the *si* hours (9 – 11) to the *hai* hours (21- 23). Then remove the Solomon's seal [root]. Dry [the *xi er* pieces] in the yin (i. e., shade) and use them.

【氣味】苦，辛，微寒，有小毒。【恭曰】忌豬肉、馬肉、米泔。伏硇砂。

Qi and Flavor. Bitter, acrid, slightly cold, slightly poisonous. [Su] Gong: [During a treatment] pork, horse meat and slop from rinsing rice are to be avoided. They suppress [the effects of] sal ammoniac.

【主治】溪毒。别録。中風傷寒頭痛。孟詵。大風癲癇，頭風濕痺，毒在骨髓，腰膝風毒。夏月采曝，爲末，水服一二匕，冬月酒服。或爲丸，每服二三十丸，日三服，滿百日，病出如瘑疥，或癢，汁出，或斑駁甲錯皮起，皮落則膿如凝脂。令人省睡，除諸毒螫，殺蟲疳濕䘌。久服益氣，耳目聰明，輕身强志。蘇恭。挼葉安舌下，出涎，去目黄好睡。燒灰和臘豬脂，封丁腫出根。煮酒服，主狂犬咬毒。藏器。

Control. Rivulet poison.[284] *Bie lu*. Massive wind[285] and peak-illness[286] epilepsy. Head wind[287] and blockage [of joints] related to the presence of moisture. Poison in bones and marrow. Wind poison affecting lower back and knees. Collect [stem and leaves] during the summer months and [grind them into] powder. Ingest with water a spoon or two. In winter ingest it with wine. Or prepare pills and each time ingest 20 to 30 pills. To be ingested three times a day. After 100 days the disease will be released similar to a lair-illness[288] or *jie*-illness.[289] It may be accompanied by itch and the release of a juice. The skin may show streak variegation with a flaky, risen surface. Once the skin has fallen off, the muscles will appear like congealed lard. [This treatment] will let one want to sleep less, and it removes all types of poison resulting from stings. It kills worms/bugs causing *gan*-illness[290] and hidden worms/bugs related to the presence of moisture. Ingested for a long time, it boosts the qi, clears the ears and the eyes, relieves the body of its weight and strengthens the mind. Su Gong. Pick the leaves and place them under the tongue to stimulate salivation. This serves to remove yellow color from the eyes and [to end] an inclination to sleep. Burned and the ashes mixed with lard from the 12th month it is used to seal a swelling associated with a pin[-illness][291] and lets the root come out. Ingested boiled with wine it controls the poison of rabid dog bites. [Chen] Cangqi.

【發明】【時珍曰】蒼耳藥久服去風熱有效，最忌豬肉及風邪，犯之則遍身發出赤丹也。按蘇沈良方云：菓耳根、苗、葉、實，皆洗濯陰乾，燒灰湯淋，取濃汁，泥連兩竈煉之。灰汁耗，即旋取傍釜中熱灰湯益之。一日

284 *Xi du* 溪毒, "rivulet poison," 1.) A tiny bug assumed to live in bodies of water and supposedly capable of striking humans when they enter the water, thereby causing disease. 2.) A condition resulting from being struck by rivulet poison. BCGM Dict I, 548.

285 *Da feng* 大風, "massive wind," may refer to sores caused by a massive intrusion of wind evil and also to conditions of leprosy. BCGM Dict I, 111.

286 *Dian ji* 癲[疾], "peak ailment," a mental disturbance of depression and unhappiness, with a calm attitude and little incentive to speak. BCGM Dict I, 125.

287 *Tou feng* 頭風, "head wind." Condition of wind evil attacking the head followed by pain, dizziness, itching. BCGM Dict I, 509.

288 *Guo chuang* 瘑瘡, "lair-illness sores," a vaguely defined skin ailment associated with pain, itch and a gradual extension. BCGM Dict I, 203-204.

289 *Jie*-illness 疥, vaguely identifiable skin ailment. BCGM Dict I, 249.

290 *Gan* 疳, "*gan*-illness," also: "sweets-illness," involves several complaints that affect children and adults, with causes and conditions too different to fall into a known disease category. BCGM Dict I, 180-188.

291 *Ding* 丁, "pin[-illness]," also *ding* 疔, "pin-illness," refers to a deep-reaching and festering hardness in a tissue, eventually rising above the skin like a pinhead. BCGM Dict I, 127-129.

夜不絶火，乃旋得霜，乾瓷瓶收之。每日早晚酒服二錢，補煖去風駐顔，尤治皮膚風，令人膚革清净。每澡沐入少許尤佳。宜州文學昌從諫，服此十餘年，至七八十，紅潤輕健，皆此藥力也。斗門方云：婦人血風攻腦，頭旋悶絶，忽死倒地，不知人事者，用喝起草嫩心陰乾爲末，以酒服一大錢，其功甚效，此物善通頂門連腦。蓋即蒼耳也。

Explication: [Li] Shizhen: Long-term ingestion of *cang er* drugs[292] effectively eliminates wind heat. [During such a treatment] pork and [exposure to] wind evil are to be strictly avoided lest the entire body release red cinnabar.[293] According to the *Su Shen liang fang*, "wash the root, seedling, leaves and fruits of *xi er* and dry them in the yin (i. e., shade). Burn them and pour hot water on the ashes to obtain a thick juice. Process it with heat on two stoves connected with clay. When the ash juice is used up (on one of the stoves), add hot ash liquid from the cauldron [on the other stove] next to it. For one day and night the fire must not be interrupted. Eventually a frost forms that is then stored in a dry porcelain jar. Ingest two *qian* a day in the morning and in the evening. This supplements warmth, eliminates wind and maintains [a youthful] complexion. In particular, it serves to cure wind [intrusion] in the skin and lets one's skin remain clear and clean. If a small amount is given into the bathing water, this is especially good. Chang Congjian, a scholar from Yi zhou, ingested this for more than ten years. When he turned 80, he was still rosy. [His body was] light and strong. All these are signs of the strength of this medication." The *Dou men fang* states: "When in a woman the wind in the blood attacks the brain,[294] resulting in vertigo, heart-pressure and an interruption [of qi movement], with sudden death letting her fall to the ground, unable to recognize persons or anything else, dry the tender heart of *he qi cao* in the yin (i. e., shade) and [grind it into] powder. Let her ingest with wine one generous *qian*. Its therapeutic potential is very effective as this item tends to penetrate the neck gate and tie up with the brain." The fact is, this is *cang er*.

292 The character *yao* 藥, "pharmaceutical drug," may be a writing error here for *ye* 葉, "leaves."

293 *Chi dan* 赤丹, "red cinnabar," a condition of *dan du* 丹毒, "cinnabar poison," with massive heat poison and red skin rash. BCGM Dict I, 85.

294 *Xue feng* 血風, "blood wind," a condition brought about by an intrusion of wind evil qi into an unbalanced state of qi and blood, mostly in women. BCGM Dict I, 594.

【附方】舊十二，新十七。

Added Recipes. 12 of old. 17 newly [recorded].

萬應膏。治一切癰疽發背，無頭惡瘡，腫毒疔癤，一切風癢，臁瘡杖瘡，牙疼喉痺。五月五日采蒼耳根葉數擔，洗净晒萎細剉，以大鍋五口，入水煮爛，以篩濾去粗滓，布絹再濾。復入净鍋，武火煎滚，文火熬稠，攪成膏，以新罐貯封，每以敷貼即愈。牙疼即敷牙上，喉痺敷舌上或噙化，二三次即效。每日用酒服一匙，極有效。集簡方。

The "ointment with a myriad [positive] responses." It serves to cure all types of effusion on the back related to obstruction-illness and impediment-illness,[295] malign sores without a tip [filled with pus], swelling with poison related to pin-illness and pimples,[296] all types of wind itch, calf sores and sores caused by flogging, toothache and throat closure. On the fifth day of the fifth month collect several *dan* of *cang er* roots and leaves. Dry them in the sun so that they wither and file them to fine pieces. Give them into five large cauldrons, add water and boil them to generate a pulpy [mass]. Pass it through a sieve to discard the rough dregs, and strain [the rest] through a silk cloth. Give it again into a clean cauldron and boil it with a strong fire first and then with a mild fire to generate a thick mass. Stir it to obtain a paste. This is stored in a tightly sealed new jar. Each time apply [the paste to the affected region] and a cure is achieved. For toothache apply it to the teeth. For throat closure apply it to the surface of the tongue or hold it in the mouth to let it transform. Do this twice or three times and an effect will show. To ingest one spoon with wine every day is extremely effective. *Ji jian fang.*

一切風毒。并殺三蟲腸痔，能進食。若病胃脹滿，心悶發熱，即宜服之。五月五日午時附地刈取葈耳葉，洗暴燥，搗下篩。每服方寸匕，酒或漿水下，日二、夜三。若覺吐逆，則以蜜丸服，準計方寸匕數也。風輕者，日二服。若身體作粟或麻豆出，此爲風毒出也。可以針刺，潰去黄汁乃止。七月七、九月九，亦可采用。

All types of wind poison. [The following medication] also kills the three [types of] worms/bugs in the intestines and those related to piles. It stimulates eating. If someone suffers from stomach distension and [a feeling of] fullness, heart-pressure and effusion of heat, it is suitable to ingest it. Cut down and gather *xi er* leaves

295 *Yong ju* 癰疽, "obstruction-illness, impediment-illness." refers to two vaguely distinguished obstructions/impediments of vessels or other ducts inside the body. Qi rushing against the obstruction may cause a local swelling and eventually break through the surface to cause an abscess. BCGM Dict I, 642.

296 *Ding* 丁, "pin[-illness]," also *ding* 疔, "pin-illness," refers to a deep-reaching and festering hardness in a tissue, eventually rising above the skin like a pinhead. BCGM Dict I, 127-129.

at noon on the fifth day of the fifth month. Wash them and dry them in the sun. Pound them and pass [the powder] through a sieve. Each time ingest the amount held by a square *cun* spoon, to be sent down with wine or formented water of foxtail millet. Twice each day, three times during the night. If [the patient] feels nausea and countermovement [of qi/food], ingest it as pills prepared with honey, with their number calculated in accordance with [the amount of powder held by] a square *cun* spoon. If it is a light case of wind [intrusion], ingest it twice a day. If the body releases something like millet or hemp seeds, this is the release of the wind poison. They can be pierced with a needle. This way a yellow juice flows out and [the disease] ends. [The leaves] can also be collected for such usage on the seventh [day] of the seventh month and on the ninth [day] of the ninth month.

一切風氣。蒼耳嫩葉一石切，和麥糵五升作塊，於蒿艾中署二十日成麴。取米一斗，炊作飯，看冷暖，入麴三升釀之，封二七日成熟。每空心暖服，神驗。封此酒可兩重布，不得令密，密則溢出。忌馬肉、豬肉。孟詵食療本草。

All types of wind qi [intrusion]. Cut one *dan* of tender *cang er* leaves [to pieces] add five *sheng* of fermenting grain and form lumps. Place them amidst wormwood and mugwort for 20 days to generate yeast. Get one *dou* of rice, cook it and watching the change of temperature add three *sheng* of the yeast to initiate a brewing process. Keep it sealed for two times seven days until [the distillation] is done. Each time ingest [the resulting wine] warm on an empty stomach. Divinely effective. This wine should be sealed with two layers of fabric. The sealing must not be tight. If it is tight, [the contents] will spill over. [During such a treatment] horse meat and pork at to be avoided. Meng Shen, *Shi liao ben cao.*

諸風頭運。蒼耳葉晒乾爲末，每服一錢，酒調下，日三服。若吐，則以蜜丸梧子大，每服二十丸。十日全好矣。楊氏經驗方。

All types of vertigo related to wind [intrusion]. Dry *cang er* leaves in the sun and [grind them into] powder. Each time ingest one *qian*, to be sent down mixed with wine. To be ingested three times a day. If this leads to vomiting, resort to pills prepared with honey the size of *wu* seeds and each time ingest 20 pills. Within ten days a complete restoration is achieved. *Yang shi jing yan fang.*

血風腦運。方見發明下。

Blood and wind brain movements.[297] For a recipe, see under "Explication."

---

297 *Xue feng nao yun* 血風腦運, "blood and wind brain-movements," a condition identical to *xue yun* 血運, "blood[-induced brain] movements." BCGM Dict I, 595, 602.

毒攻手足，腫痛欲斷。蒼耳搗汁漬之，并以滓傅之，立效。春用心，冬用子。千金翼。

Poison attacking hands and feet, with a painful swelling as if they were about to be cut off. Pound *cang er* to obtain a juice and soak [the affected parts] in it. In addition, apply the dregs to them. Immediately effective. In spring use the heart [of the stems]; in winter use the seeds. *Qian jin yi.*

卒中水毒。初覺頭目微痛，惡寒，骨節强急，旦醒暮劇，手足逆冷，三日則蟲蝕下部，六七日膿潰，食至五臟，殺人也。搗常思草，絞汁服一二升，并以綿染，導其下部。肘後方。

Suddenly being struck by water poison.[298] This begins with a feeling of a slight pain in the head and the eyes, an aversion to cold and a stiffening of bone joints. When [the patient] wakes up in the morning it is more serious. Hands and feet are cold because of [qi] countermovement. On the third day erosions caused by worms/bugs appear in the lower [body] part, festering on the sixth and seventh day when they start to eat on the five long-term depots. Eventually they kill that person. Pound *chang si cao* and squeeze the [resulting pulp]. Ingest one to two *sheng* of the resulting juice. Also, stain a piece of cloth [with the juice] and insert it into the lover [body] part. *Zhou hou fang.*

毒蛇溪毒、沙虱、射工等所傷，口噤眼黑，手足强直，毒攻腹内成塊，逡巡不救。蒼耳嫩苗一握，取汁和酒，温灌之，以滓厚傅傷處。勝金方。

Harm caused by poisonous snakes, rivulet poison,[299] sand lice[300] and the archer,[301] with clenched jaw, blackened eyes, and stiffened hands and feet. When the poison attacks inside the abdomen and forms lumps, this is an irreversible condition without possibility to rescue [the victim]. [Squeeze] a handful of tender *cang er* leaves to obtain a juice. Mix it with wine and force-feed it [to the patient]. Also, use the dregs to place a thick cover on the location of the initial harm. *Sheng jin fang.*

---

298 *Shui du* 水毒, "water poison," an etiological agent identical to *xi du* 溪毒, "rivulet poison." BCGM Dict I, 468, 548.

299 *Xi du* 溪毒, "rivulet poison," 1.) A tiny bug assumed to live in bodies of water and supposedly capable of striking humans when they enter the water, thereby causing disease. 2.) A condition resulting from being struck by rivulet poison. BCGM Dict I, 548.

300 *Sha shi* 沙虱, "sand lice," small bugs, in former times assumed to live in waters or at the banks of waters and being able of penetrating the skin of people and cause disease.

301 *She gong* 射工, "archer," (1) a small bug in ancient times believed to live in water and be capable of "shooting" poison from its mouth at people, thereby causing disease; (2) a condition caused by the archer's poison. BCGM Dict. I, 432. See 42-15.

疫病不染。五月五日午時多采蒼耳嫩葉，陰乾收之。臨時爲末，冷水服二錢，或水煎，舉家皆服，能辟邪惡。千金方。

To prevent being infected by epidemic disease. On the fifth day of the fifth month collect many tender *cang er* leaves. Dry them in the yin (i. e., shade) and store them. When the time has come [grind them into] powder and ingest with cold water two *qian*, or boil them in water. When all members of a family ingest this, they can ward off evil and malign [epidemic qi]. *Qian jin fang*.

風瘙癮疹，身痒不止。用蒼耳莖、葉、子等分，爲末。每服二錢，豆淋酒調下。聖惠方。

Wind itching[302] and dormant papules. Endless itch affecting the entire body. [Grind] equal amounts of *cang er* stems, leaves and seeds into powder. Each time ingest two *qian*, to be sent down with wine prepared with black soybeans. *Sheng hui fang*.

面上黑斑。蒼耳葉焙爲末，食後米飲調服一錢，一月愈。摘玄方。

Black spots on the face. Dry *cang er* leaves over a fire in a pan and [grind them into] powder. After a meal ingest mixed with a rice beverage one *qian*. A cure will be achieved within one month. *Zhai xuan fang*.

赤白汗斑。蒼耳嫩葉尖，和青鹽擂爛，五六月間擦之五七次，效。摘玄方。

Red and white sweat macules.[303] Pound the tips of tender *cang er* leaves together with greenish salt/halite into a pulpy mass and in the fifth and sixth month apply it five to seven times [to the affected region]. Effective. *Zhai xuan fang*.

大風癘疾。袖珍方用嫩蒼耳、荷葉等分，爲末。每服二錢，温酒下，日二服。

Massive wind[304] epidemic. The *Xiu zhen fang* [recommends to grind] equal amounts of tender *cang er* and lotus leaves into powder. Each time ingest two *qian*, to be sent down with warm wine. To be ingested twice a day.

302 *Feng sao* 風瘙, "wind itching," a condition of wind evil or wind cold entering the skin, with the skin itching, or the emergence of skin papules, as major signs. BCGM Dict I, 167.

303 *Han ban* 汗斑, "sweat macule," a condition identical to *li yang feng* 癧瘍風, "pervasion-illness with ulcers wind," with white macules and dots appearing on the skin in the neck, on the chest,and below the armpits, without itching or pain. BCGM Dict I, 205, 315.

304 *Da feng* 大風, "massive wind," may refer to sores caused by a massive intrusion of wind evil and also to conditions of leprosy. BCGM Dict I, 111.

乾坤生意用蒼耳葉爲末，以大楓子油和丸梧子大。每服三四十丸，以茶湯下，日二服。

The *Qian kun sheng yi* [recommends to grind] *cang er* leaves into powder, mix it with chaulmoogra oil and prepare pills the size of *wu* seeds. Each time ingest 30 to 40 pills, to be sent down with a tea decoction. To be ingested twice a day.

又方：五月五日或六月六日，五更帶露采蒼耳草，搗取汁，熬作錠子。取半斤鱧魚一尾，剖開不去肚腸，入藥一錠，線縫，以酒二盌，慢火煮熟令喫，不過三五箇魚即愈也。忌鹽一百日。

Another recipe. On the fifth day of the fifth month or on the sixth day of the sixth month in the early morning collect *cang er* herbs with the dew on them, pound them to obtain a juice and heat it to form ingots. Take half a *jin* of the tail of snake-head fish, cut it open without discarding the stomach and the intestines and insert the medicinal ingots. Then sew it up with a thread and boil it in two bowls of wine over a mild fire until done. Let [the patient] eat this. No more than three to five fish are required to achieve a cure. Salt is to be avoided for 100 days.

卒得惡瘡。蒼耳、桃皮作屑，納瘡中。百一方。

Sudden suffering from malign sores. [Grind] *cang er* and peach bark to crumbs and insert them into the sores. *Bai yi fang*.

反花惡瘡。有肉如飯粒，破之血出，隨生反出。用蒼耳葉搗汁，服三合，并塗之，日二上。聖濟總録。

Reversed-blossom malign sores.[305] With flesh resembling rice grains. When they are pierced they release blood. Then they grow again and [blood] is released again. Pound *cang er* leaves to obtain a juice. Ingest three *ge* and also apply it [to the affected region]. Twice a day. *Sheng ji zong lu*.

一切丁腫。詵曰：危困者，用蒼耳根葉搗，和小兒尿絞汁，冷服一升，日三服，拔根甚驗。

All types of swelling associated with pin[-illness].[306] [Meng] Shen: In critical situations pound root and leaves of *cang er*, mix them with the urine of a child and squeeze this to obtain a juice. Ingest one *sheng* cold. To be ingested three times a day. This is a very successful method to pull out the root.

---

305 *Fan hua chuang* 反花瘡, "reversed-blossoms sores," a condition with a festering ulcer generating a fleshgrowth assuming the shape of a flower. BCGM Dict I, 149.

306 *Ding* 丁, "pin[-illness]," also *ding* 疔, "pin-illness," refers to a deep-reaching and festering hardness in a tissue, eventually rising above the skin like a pinhead. BCGM Dict I, 127-129.

養生方用蒼耳根苗燒灰，和醋淀塗之，乾再上。不十次，即拔根出。

The *Yang sheng fang* [recommends to] burn *cang er* root and seedling to ashes, mix them with vinegar sediments and apply this [to the affected region]. When it has dried apply it again. After no more than ten applications the root will be pulled out.

邵真人方：蒼耳根三兩半，烏梅肉五箇，連鬚葱三根，酒二鍾，煎一鍾，熱服取汗。

Shao zhenren fang: Boil three and a half liang of *cang er* roots, the meat of five plums and three onions with the "beard" in two handleless cups of wine down to one cup and ingest this hot to stimulate sweating.

齒風動痛。蒼耳一握，以漿水煮，入鹽含漱。外臺秘要。

Tooth wind[307] with moving pain. Boil one handful of *cang er* with fermented water of foxtail millet, add salt and hold it in the mouth to rinse [the affected teeth]. *Wai tai mi yao.*

纏喉風病。蒼耳根一把，老薑一塊，研汁，入酒服。聖濟總録。

Throat constricting wind[308] disease. Grind one handful of *cang er* roots and one piece of old ginger to obtain a juice. Add it to wine and ingest this. *Sheng ji zong lu.*

赤目生瘡，作痛。道人頭末二兩，乳香一錢，每用一錢，燒烟嗃鼻。聖濟總録。

Red eyes with a generation of painful sores. Mix two *liang* of *dao ren tou* powder and one *qian* of frankincense. Each time burn one *qian* [of this mixture] and inhale the fumes with the nose. *Sheng ji zong lu.*

鼻衄不止。蒼耳莖葉搗汁一小盞服。聖惠方。

Unending nosebleed. Pound *cang er* stems and leaves and ingest one small cup of the resulting juice. *Sheng hui fang.*

五痔下血。五月五日采蒼耳莖葉爲末，水服方寸匕，甚效。千金翼。

The five types of piles with blood discharge. On the fifth day of the fifth month collect *cang er* stems and leaves and [grind them into] powder. Ingest with water the amount held by a square *cun* spoon. Very effective. *Qian jin fang.*

---

307 *Chi feng* 齒風, "tooth wind," a condition of toothache and exposure of tooth roots brought about by *feng xie* 風邪, "wind evil." BCGM Dict I, 171

308 *Chan hou feng* 纏喉風, "throat-constricting wind," a condition of throat blockage, with a rapid onset, a swelling of throat and cheeks, and a closure of the throat that makes it impossible to ingest even a liquid. BCGM Dict I, 74.

赤白下痢。蒼耳草不拘多少洗净，用水煮爛，去渣，入蜜，用武火熬成膏。每服一二匙，白湯下。醫方摘玄。

Red and white discharge with free-flux illness. Wash clean any quantity of *cang er* herb and boil it with water to generate a pulpy [mass. Press it through a sieve,] remove the dregs, add honey [to the liquid], and heat this with a strong fire to generate a paste. Each time ingest one or two spoons, to be sent down with clear, boiled water. *Yi fang zhai xuan*.

產後諸痢。蒼耳葉擣絞汁，温服半中盞，日三四服。聖惠方。

All types of free-flux illness following delivery. Pound *cang er* leaves, squeeze [the pulp to obtain a] juice and ingest the amount filling half a medium size cup warm. To be ingested three to four times a day. *Sheng hui fang*.

誤吞銅錢。蒼耳頭一把，以水一升，浸水中十餘度，飲水，愈。肘後方。

Mistakenly having swallowed a copper coin. Soak one handful of *cang er* tips in one *sheng* of water and repeat this ten times or more. Drink the water. This results in a cure. *Zhou hou fang*.

花蜘蛛毒。咬人，與毒蛇無異。用野縑絲，即道人頭，擣汁一盞服，仍以渣傅之。摘玄方。

The poison of a versicolor spider. When it bites a human this is not different from [the bite of] a venomous snake. Pound *jian si cao*, this is *dao ren tou*, and ingest one cup of the resulting juice. In addition, apply the dregs to [the affected region]. *Zhai xuan fang*.

15-42-03
花 *Hua*
Flower [of *xi er*].

【主治】白癩頑癢。時珍。

Control. White repudiation-illness[309] with persistent itch. [Li] Shizhen.

309 *Lai* 癩, "*lai*-illness," "repudiation-illness," including cases of leprosy/Aussatz." BCGM Dict I, 293.

15-43
天名精本經上品

Tian ming jing, FE *Ben jing*, upper rank.

***Carpesium abrotanoides* L. Common *carpesium*.**

【校正】【時珍曰】據蘇、沈二說，併入唐本鶴虱、開寶地菘、別録有名未用埊松。

Editorial Correction. [Li] Shizhen: Based on Su [Shi's] and Shen [Gua's book, the items *he shi* 鶴虱 from the *Tang ben*, *di song* 地菘 from the *Kai bao* and *di song* 埊松 from the section "known by name but not in use" of the *Bie lu* are included here.

【釋名】天蔓菁別録、天門精別録、地菘唐本、埊松別録埊與地同、玉門精別録、麥句薑本經、蟾蜍蘭別録、蝦蟆藍本經、蚵蚾草綱目、豕首本經、彘顱別録、活鹿草異苑、劉愭草愭音胡革反、皺面草綱目、母豬芥綱目。實名鶴虱，根名杜牛膝。【恭曰】天名精，即活鹿草也。別録一名天蔓菁，南人名爲地菘。葉與蔓菁、菘菜相類，故有此名。其味甘辛，故有薑稱。狀如藍，而蝦蟆好居其下，故名蝦蟆藍。香氣似蘭，故又名蟾蜍蘭。【時珍曰】天名精乃天蔓菁之訛也。其氣如豕彘，故有豕首、彘顱之名。昔人謂之活鹿草，俗人因其氣臊，訛爲狐狸臊者是也。爾雅云：菵甄，豕首也。郭璞注云：江東呼爲豨首，可以熓蠶蛹食。【藏器曰】郭璞注爾雅蘧麥，云"即麥句薑"者，非也。陶公注"釣樟"條云：有一草似狼牙，氣辛臭，名爲地菘，人呼爲劉愭草，主金瘡。按異苑云：宋元嘉中，青州劉愭射一麞，剖五臟以此草塞之，蹶然而起。愭怪而拔草，便倒，如此三度。愭因密録此草，種之，主折傷，愈多人，因以名之。既有活鹿之名，雅與麞事相合。陶、蘇俱說是地菘，定非二物。

Explanation of Names. *Tian man jing* 天蔓菁, *Bie lu*. *Tian men jing* 天門精, *Bie lu*. *Di song* 地菘, *Tang ben*. *Di song* 埊松, *Bie lu*. *Di* 埊 is identical to *di* 地. *Yu men jing* 玉門精, *Bie lu*. *Mai ju jiang* 麥句薑, *Ben jing*. *Chan chu lan* 蟾蜍蘭, *Bie lu*. *Ha mo lan* 蝦蟆藍, *Ben jing*. *He bo cao* 蚵蚾草, *Gang mu*. *Shi shou* 豕首, *Ben jing*. *Zhi lu* 彘顱, *Bie lu*. *Huo lu cao* 活鹿草, *Yi yuan*. *Liu Huai cao* 劉愭草, with 愭 read *hu* 胡革反, and *zou mian cao* 皺面草, *Gang mu*. *Mu zhu jie* 母豬芥, *Gang mu*. The fruit is called *he shi* 鶴虱, "a crane's lice;" the root is called *du niu xi* 杜牛膝. [Su] Gong: *Tian ming jing* 天名精 is *huo lu cao* 活鹿草. The *Bie lu* has *tian man jing* 天蔓菁 as an alternative name. The Southerners call it *di song* 地菘. The leaves are similar to those of turnips, *man jing* 蔓菁, and pak choi, *song cai* 菘菜. Therefore these names. The flavor is sweet-acrid; hence it is named "ginger," *jiang* 薑. It is shaped like *eupatorium* herb, *lan* 藍, and toads, *ha mo* 蝦蟆, love to rest underneath it. Therefore the name *ha mo lan* 蝦蟆藍. Its fragrant qi are similar to those of orchids, *lan* 蘭. Hence it is also called *chan chu lan* 蟾蜍蘭. [Li] Shizhen: *Tian ming jing* 天名精 is a writing error of *tian man jing* 天蔓菁. Its qi are similar to those of pigs, *shi zhu* 豕彘 Hence the names "pig head," *shi shou* 豕首, and "pig skull," *zhu lu* 彘顱. The ancients named it "herb that brings deer back to life," *huo lu cao* 活鹿草. As its qi are foul, *sao* 臊, the common people have miswritten this as *hu li sao* 狐狸臊, "foul fox stench." The *Er ya* states: "*Lie zeng* 茢甄 is *shi shou* 豕首." Guo Pu comments: "In Jiang dong they write *xi shou* 豨首. It can be used to fry silkworm pupae that are then eaten." [Chen] Cangqi: When Guo Pu in his comment on *qu mai* 蘧麥 in the *Er ya* states: "This is *mai ju jiang* 麥句薑," he is wrong. Mr. Tao [Hongjing] commenting on the silky spike bush entry, *diao zhang* 釣樟 (34-17), states: "There is an herb similar to *agrimonia* herb, *lang ya* 狼牙. Its qi are acrid and malodorous. It is named *di song* 地菘. People call it *Liu Huai cao* 劉憓草. It controls wounds caused by metal objects/weapons. According to the *Yi yuan*, "during the *yuan jia* reign period (424 -452) of the Song dynasty, in Qing zhou Liu Huai shot a roebuck. He cut out the five long-term depots and filled [the animal's abdomen] with this herb. Thereupon it suddenly jumped up. [Liu] Huai found this strange. He pulled the herb out again whereupon [the roebuck] fell to the ground. This continued three times. [Liu] Huai made notes of this herb and planted it. It controls harm associated with fractures. He cured many people with it and gave it this name." The name "[herb that] brings deer back to life," *huo lu* 活鹿, agrees with the roebuck [record in the *Er*] *ya*. Both Tao [Hongjing] and Su [Gong] say that it is *di song* 地菘. So, these are definitely not two different items

【正誤】【弘景曰】天名精即今之豨薟，亦名豨首。夏月杵汁服之，除熱病。味至苦而云甘，或非是也。【恭曰】豨首苦而臭，名精辛而香，全不相類也。【禹錫曰】蘇恭云：天名精南人名地菘。陳藏器本草解紛，亦言天名精爲地菘。開寶本草不當重出地菘條，例宜刊削。【時珍曰】按沈括筆談云：世人既不識天名精，又妄認地菘爲火杴，本草又出鶴虱一條，都成紛亂。不知地菘即天名精，其葉似菘，又似蔓菁，故有二名，鶴虱即其實也。又別録有名未用埊松，即此地菘，亦係誤出，今並正之，合而爲一。
Correction of Errors. [Tao] Hongjing: *Tian ming jing* 天名精 is today's St. Paulswort, *xi xian* 豨薟. It is also called "pig head," *xi shou* 豨首. During summer months it is pounded and the resulting juice is ingested to eliminate heat disease. It has an extremely bitter flavor, but [some texts] state that it is sweet. This is definitely wrong. [Su] Gong: *Xi shou* 豨首 is bitter and malodorous. [*Tian*] *ming jing* is acrid and fragrant. [These two items] are completely unrelated. [Zhang] Yuxi: Su Gong states: "The Southerners call *tian ming jing* 天名精 *di song* 地菘." Chen Cangqi in his *Ben cao* resolved the confusion. He, too, says: "*Tian ming jing* is *di song*." The *Kai bao ben cao* did no longer devote a separate entry to *di song*. It should be deleted. [Li]

Shizhen: According to Shen Gua's *Bi tan*, "common people do not know *tian ming jing*. They mistakenly identifiy *di song* as *huo xian* 火杴, and the *Ben cao* devotes an entry to *he shi* 鶴虱, this way contributing to utter confusion. They are unaware that *di song* is *tian ming jing*. The leaves are similar to those of pak choi, *song* [*cai*] 菘[菜], and they also resemble those of turnips, *man jing* 蔓菁. Therefore [this herb] has two names. *He shi* 鶴虱, "crane lice," are its fruit." Also, the *Bie lu* in its section "known by name but not in use" lists a *di song* 埊松 as *di song* 地菘. This, too, is a mistake. Here now all this is corrected and [*tian ming jing* 天名精 and *di song* 地菘] are combined in one [entry].

【集解】【别録曰】天名精生平原川澤，五月采。【保昇曰】地菘也。小品方名天蔓菁，又名天蕪菁。葉似山南菘菜，夏秋抽條，頗似薄荷，花紫白色，味辛而香。【志曰】地菘所在皆有，生人家及路旁陰處，高二三寸，葉似菘葉而小。又曰：鶴虱，出波斯者爲勝。今上黨亦有，力勢薄於波斯者。【恭曰】鶴虱生西戎，子似蓬蒿子而細，合莖葉用之。【頌曰】天名精，江湖間皆有之，狀如韓保昇所説。又曰：鶴虱，江、淮、衡、湘皆有之。春生苗，葉皺似紫蘇，大而尖長，不光。莖高二尺許。七月生黄白花，似菊。八月結實，子極尖細，乾即黄黑色。南人呼其葉爲火杴。按火杴即豨薟，雖花實相類，而别是一物，不可雜用。【時珍曰】天名精嫩苗緑色，似皺葉菘芥，微有狐氣。淘浸煠之，亦可食。長則起莖，開小黄花，如小野菊花。結實如同蒿，子亦相似，最粘人衣，狐氣尤甚。炒熟則香，故諸家皆云辛而香，亦巴人食負蠜，南人食山柰之意爾。其根白色，如短牛膝。此物最賤，而唐本草言鶴虱"出西戎"，宋本草言"出波斯"者何哉？蓋當時人不知用之，惟西戎、波斯始知入藥，且土産所宜故爾。亦苜蓿云出西域，而不知中國飼馬者即是也。詳見"豨薟"下。

Collected Explanations: *Bie lu*: *Tian ming jing* 天名精 grows in river marshlands of the plains. It is collected in the fifth month. [Han] Baosheng: *Di song* 地菘, the *Xiao pin fang* names it *tian man jing* 天蔓菁; it also names it *tian wu jing* 天蕪菁. The leaves are similar to those of pak choi, *song cai* 菘菜. A bough rises in summer and autumn, quite similar to that of mint. The flowers are of purple-white color. The flavor is acrid and fragrant. [Ma] Zhi: *Di song* can be found everywhere. It grows in private [gardens] and in yin (i. e., shady) places at the roadside, reaching a height of two to three *cun*. The leaves are similar to those of pak choi, but they are smaller. It is also said: *He shi* 鶴虱 from Po si/Persia is best. Today it is also found in Shang dang. But its strength is weaker than that [of *he shi*] from Po si. [Su] Gong: *He shi* grows in Xi rong. The seeds are similar to garden daisy seeds, but they are finer. They are used together with the stem and the leaves. [Su] Song: *Tian ming jing* is present everywhere at rivers and lakes. It is shaped as is said by Han Baosheng.

It is also said: *He shi* is present in Jiang, He, Heng and Xiang. In spring it grows a seedling. The leaves are creased similar to those of *perilla*. They are big, pointed and long, without shine. The stem is more than two *chi* tall. In the seventh month it grows yellow-white flowers, similar to *chrysanthemum* [flowers]. Fruits are formed in the eighth month. The seeds are extremely fine and pointed. When they are dried they assume a yellow-black color. The Southerners call the leaves *huo xian* 火枕. Now, *huo xian* 火枕 is *xi xian* 豨薟. Although flowers and fruits are similar, these are two different items. They must not be used interchangeably. [Li] Shizhen: The green, tender seedling of *tian ming jing* resembles that of creased leaf pak choi and black mustard. It has a slight fox qi [odor]. Washed in a pan, soaked and heated it is edible. When it grows, a stem rises and opens small yellow flowers similar to the flowers of small winter asters. They form fruits resembling those of garden daisy. Their seeds resemble each other, too. They easily cling to the garments of humans. Their fox qi [odor] is particularly strong. When they are fried they assume a fragrant odor. Hence all experts state that they are acrid and fragrant. When people in Ba eat ground beetles, *fu fan* 負蠜 (41-26), and Southerners eat galgant, this is based on the same idea. The root is white, similar to short *achyranthes* [root]. This item is very cheap, and how can it be that the *Tang ben cao* says "*he shi* comes from Xi rong," while the Song era *Ben cao* says "it comes from Po si"? The fact is, the people of those times did not know how to use it. In the beginning, only [people in] Xi rong and Po si knew that it can be added to medication, simply because it is a local product there. Alfalfa, too, is said to come from Xi rong, and [those who say so] are unaware that it is something used in China to feed horses. For details see under "*xi xian* 豨薟" (15-44).

15-43-01

葉、根同 *Ye, Gen*

Leaf, root [of *tian ming jing*], identical.

【氣味】甘，寒，無毒。【别録曰】埊松：辛，無毒。【時珍曰】微辛，甘，有小毒。生汁吐人。【之才曰】垣衣、地黄爲之使。

Qi and Flavor. Sweet, cold, nonpoisonous. *Bie lu*: *Di song* 埊松: Acrid, nonpoisonous. [Li] Shizhen: Slightly acrid, sweet, slightly poisonous. The fresh juice lets one vomit. [Xu] Zhicai: Wall moss and Chinese foxglove [rhizome] serve as guiding [substances].

【主治】瘀血血瘕欲死，下血止血，利小便。久服輕身耐老。本經。除小蟲，去痺，除胸中結熱，止煩渴，逐水，大吐下。别録。破血，生肌，止鼻衄，殺三蟲，除諸毒腫丁瘡，瘻痔，金瘡内射，身癢癮疹不止者，揩之立已。唐本。地菘：主金瘡，止血，解惡蟲蛇螫毒，挼以傅之。開寶。吐痰止瘧，治牙痛，口緊，喉痺。時珍。埊松：主眩痺。別録有名未用。

Control. Stagnating blood, blood conglomeration-illness,[310] bringing one close to dying. Blood discharge. It stops bleeding and clears the passage of urine. Ingested for a long time, it relieves the body of its weight and helps to endure aging. *Ben jing*. It eliminates small worms/bugs. It removes blockages and discards heat nodes in the chest. It ends vexing thirst, drives out water and stimulates massive vomiting and discharge. *Bie lu*. It breaks through blood [accumulations], stimulates the growth of muscles, ends nosebleed, kills the three types of worms/bugs, and removes all types of poison swelling, pin[-illness][311] sores, fistula and, piles, wounds caused by metal objects/weapons with the [poison] remaining stuck inside,[312] and unending body itch with dormant papules. For all these, wipe [the affected regions with *tian ming jing* leaves] and [the ailments] end immediately. *Tang ben*. *Di song* 地菘: It controls wounds caused by metal objects/weapons. It ends bleeding. It resolves the poison of malign worms/bugs and snake bites. Rub [the herb] and apply [the resulting mass]. *Kai bao*. It induces vomiting of phlegm and ends malaria. It serves to cure toothache, lockjaw, and throat closure. [Li] Shizhen. *Di song* 埊松: It controls dizziness and blockage [of joints]/numbness. *Bie lu*, [section] "known by name but not in use."

【發明】【時珍曰】天名精，併根苗而言也。地菘、埊松，皆言其苗葉也。鶴虱，言其子也。其功大抵只是吐痰止血，殺蟲解毒，故擂汁服之能止痰瘧，漱之止牙疼，挼之傅蛇咬，亦治豬瘟病也。按孫天仁集效方云：凡男婦乳蛾，喉嚨腫痛，及小兒急慢驚風，牙關緊急，不省人事者，以鶴虱草，一名鰍面草，一名母豬芥，一名杜牛膝，取根洗凈搗爛，入好酒絞汁灌之，良久即甦。仍以渣傅項下，或醋調搽亦妙。朱端章集驗方云：余被檄任淮西幕府時，牙疼大作。一刀鑷人以草藥一捻，湯泡少時，以手蘸湯挹痛處即定。因求其方，用之治人多效，乃鰍面地菘草也，俗人訛爲地

310 *Xue jia* 血瘕, "blood conglomeration-illness," a condition which has formed from stagnant blood and fails to dissolve. Such a condition mostly develops in women with irregular menstruation or out of stagnant blood present in the body following delivery. BCGM Dict I, 596.

311 *Ding* 丁, "pin[-illness]," also *ding* 疔, "pin-illness," refers to a deep-reaching and festering hardness in a tissue, eventually rising above the skin like a pinhead. BCGM Dict I, 127-129.

312 *Jin chuang nei she* 金瘡内射 is attested nowhere else in medical literature. *Nei she* 内射, "internal shooting/spouting," appears only in the works of Sun Simiao, but in a different context. *Jin chuang nei she* 金瘡内射 may be an erroneous writing of *jin chuang nei se* 金瘡内塞, a common phrase referring to poison in a wound caused by a knife or other weapon that remains stuck inside. A translation of "wounds caused by metal objects/weapons with the poison shooting into the body's interior" is possible, too.

葱。沈存中筆談專辯地菘，其子名鶴虱，正此物也。錢季誠方：用鶴虱一枚，擢置齒中。高監方：以鶴虱煎米醋漱口，或用防風、鶴虱煎水噙漱，仍研草塞痛處，皆有效也。

Explication. [Li] Shizhen: *Tian ming jing* 天名精 refers to both the root and the seedling. Both *di song* 地菘 and *di song* 埊松 refer to seedling and leaves. *He shi* 鶴虱 refers to the seeds. Their therapeutic] potential is basically limited to letting one vomit phlegm and to end bleeding, to kill worms/bugs and to resolve poison. Hence to pound them and ingest the juice can end phlegm malaria. To rinse [the mouth] ends toothache. Rub them and apply [the resulting mass] on the location of snake bites. It also serves to cure warmth diseases of pigs. According to Sun Tianren's *Ji xiao fang*, "for all cases of nipple moths,[313] regardless of wether [a patient is] male or a women, with painful throat swelling, and also for acute or chronic fright wind of children with clenched jaw and an inability to recognize persons or anything else, take the root of *he shi* herb, also called *zou mian* 皺面 herb, also called *mu zhu jie* 母豬芥, also called *du niu xi* 杜牛膝, wash it clean, pound it into a pulpy [mass], add good wine, squeeze this to obtain a juice and force-feed it [to the patient]. After some considerable time, he will regain his consciousness. In addition, apply the dregs below the neck, or apply them mixed with vinegar. This, too, is wondrous." Zhu Duanzhang in his *Ji yan fang*[314] states: "When I was appointed Tent Secretary in Huai xi, I suffered from massive toothache. A person selling knives and forceps let a pinch of an herbal drug soak in hot water for a short while. Then he dipped his finger into the hot water and rubbed the aching location. This ended [the pain]. Hence I asked him for the recipe and when I used it to cure people it was often effective. This was the *zou mian di song* 皺面地菘 herb. Common people mistakenly change [the name] to *di cong* 地葱, 'ground onion.' Shen Cunzhong in his *Bi tan* specifically deals with *di song* 地菘, naming the seeds *he shi* 鶴虱. This is the item [discussed] here." Qian Jicheng's recipe: "Place one *he shi* 鶴虱 into the [aching] teeth." Gao Jian's recipe: "Boil *he shi* in rive vinegar and rinse the mouth [with the liquid]. Or boil *saposhnikovia* [root] and *he shi* in water and hold it in the mouth to rinse [the affected teeth]. Also, grind the herb and stuff [the resulting mass] into the aching location. All these are effective [treatments]."

313 *Ru e* 乳蛾, "nipple moth," acute tonsillitis. A condition with red swelling and pain on both sides of the throat, in severe cases including the generation of pus forming white dots, as a major sign. BCGM Dict I, 410.

314 This recipe is copied here not from a *Ji yan fang* by a Zhu Duanzhang, but from the *Bai yi xuan fang* ch. 8, *zhi feng re shang gong chi tong* 治風熱上攻齒痛, "to cure toothache caused by an attack of rising heat." Also, the author of the *Ji yan fang* is Zhu Zuo 朱佐, not Zhu Duanzhang 朱端章.

【附方】舊二，新九。

Added Recipes. Two of old. Nine newly [recorded].

男女吐血。皺面草即地菘，晒乾爲末。每服一二錢，以茅花泡湯調服，日二次。衛生易簡。

Males and females spitting blood. *Zou mian cao*, i. e., *di song*, is dried in the sun and [ground into] powder. Each time ingest one or two *qian*, to be ingested mixed with a floss grass macerated in hot water. Twice a day. *Wei sheng yi jian.*

咽喉腫塞。傷寒蘊要治痰涎壅滯，喉腫水不可下者，地菘，一名鶴虱草，連根葉搗汁，鵝翎掃入，去痰最妙。

Swollen, blocked throat. A cure [recommended] by the *Shang han yun yao* for sluggish phlegm and saliva blocking [the throat] and throat swelling so that water cannot be sent down. Pound *di song*, also called *he shi cao*, with root and leaves to obtain a juice and sweep it down the [patient's] throat with a goose feather. Very wondrous [method] to remove phlegm.

聖濟總録用杜牛膝、鼓鎚草，同搗汁灌之。不得下者，灌鼻，得吐爲妙。

The *Sheng ji zong lu* [recommends to] pound *du niu xi* together with *gu chui cao*[315] to obtain a juice and force-feed it [to the patient]. If it cannot be sent down [through the mouth], force-feed it through the nose. A wondrous [method] to induce spitting/vomiting.

又方：土牛膝，春夏用莖，秋冬用根，一把，青礬半兩，同研，點患處，令吐膿血痰沫，即愈。

Another recipe. Grind one handful of *du niu xi* – in spring and summer use the stem, in autumn and winter use the root – with half a *liang* of melanterite and apply [the resulting pulp] to the affected location. This will cause [the patient] to spit bloody pus and phlegm foam, and this is the cure.

纏喉風腫。蚵蚾草，即皺面草，細研，以生蜜和丸彈子大，每噙一二丸即愈。乾者爲末，蜜丸亦可。名救生丸。經效濟世方。

Throat constricting wind[316] swelling. Grind *he bo cao*, this is *zou mian cao*, to a fine [powder], and form with fresh honey pills the size of a bullet. Each time hold in the mouth one or two pills, and this results in a cure. If only dried [*he bo cao*] is at hand,

315 *Gu chui cao* 鼓鎚草, lit.: "drumstick herb," an unidentified herb.

316 *Chan hou feng* 纏喉風, "throat-constricting wind," a condition of throat blockage, with a rapid onset, a swelling of throat and cheeks, and a closure of the throat that makes it impossible to ingest even a liquid. BCGM Dict I, 74.

[grind it into] powder and with honey form pills. This is possible, too. [The recipe] is called "life saving pills." *Jing xiao ji shi fang.*

諸骨哽咽。地菘、馬鞭草各一握，去根，白梅肉一箇，白礬一錢，搗作彈丸，綿裹含嚥，其骨自軟而下也。普濟方。

All types of choking on a bone. Pound one handful each of *di song* and vervain, with the roots removed, one salted plum and one *qian* of alum, and form pills the size of a bullet. Wrap them in silk fabric, hold them in the mouth and swallow [the resulting liquid]. The bone will soften and move down. *Pu ji fang.*

風毒瘰癧，赤腫。地菘搗傅，乾即易之。聖惠方。

Scrofula pervasion-illness[317] related to wind poison, with a red swelling. Pound *di song* and apply [the moist pulp to the affected region]. When it has dried, replace it [with moist pulp]. *Sheng hui fang.*

疔瘡腫毒。鶴虱草葉，浮酒糟，同搗傅之，立效。孫氏集效方。

Pin-illness[318] sore swelling with poison. Pound *he shi* herb leaves with floating distillers' grains [to a pulp] and apply this [to the affected region]. Immediately effective. Sun shi, *Ji xiao fang.*

發背初起。地菘杵汁一升，日再服，瘥乃止。傷寒類要。

An effusion on the back[319] that has just begun to rise. Pound *di song* to obtain one *sheng* of juice and ingest it twice a day. Once a cure is achieved, stop [ingesting the juice]. *Shang han lei yao.*

惡瘡腫毒。地菘搗汁，日服三四次。外臺秘要。

Malign sores with swelling and poison. Pound *di song* to obtain a juice and ingest it three to four times a day. *Wai tai mi yao.*

---

317 *Luo li* 瘰癧, "scrofula pervasion-illness," when two or more connected swellings of the size of plum or date kernels appear either on the neck or in the armpits, or somewhere else on the body. BCGM Dict I. 329.

318 *Ding* 丁, "pin[-illness]," also *ding* 疔, "pin-illness," refers to a deep-reaching and festering hardness in a tissue, eventually rising above the skin like a pinhead. BCGM Dict I, 127-129.

319 *Fa bei* 發背, "effusion on/of the back," a condition of *yong* 癰, "obstruction-illnesses," and *ju* 疽, "impediment-illnesses," developing on one's back. As it was believed that the transporter holes of the five depots and six palaces are located on the back, conditions of obstruction-illnesses and impediment-illnesses there, often apparent as abscesses, were considered threatening. BCGM Dict I, 148.

惡蛇咬傷。地菘擣傅之。易簡方。

Harm caused by malign snake bites. Pound *di song* [to a pulp] and apply it [to the site of the bite]. *Yi jian fang.*

15-43-02

鶴虱唐本草 *He shi* FE *Tang ben cao*

Fruit [of *tian ming jing*].

【氣味】苦，辛，有小毒。【大明曰】凉，無毒。

Qi and Flavor. Bitter, acrid, slightly poisonous. Da Ming: Cool. Nonpoisonous.

【主治】蚘、蟯蟲，爲散，以肥肉臛汁服方寸匕，亦入丸散用。唐本。蟲心痛，以淡醋和半匕服，立瘥。開寶。殺五臟蟲，止瘧，傅惡瘡。大明。

Control. Roundworm and pinworms. Prepare a powder and ingest with a fat meat souce the amount held by a square *cun* spoon. It can also be used added to pills and powders. *Tang ben.* Heart/stomach pain caused by worms/bugs. Mix the amount held by half a spoon with bland vinegar and ingest this. Immediately effective. *Kai bao.* It kills the five long-term depot worms/bugs. It ends malaria. Apply it to malign sores. Da Ming.

【發明】【頌曰】鶴虱，殺蟲方中爲最要藥。初虞世古今録驗方：療蚘咬心痛，取鶴虱十兩，擣篩，蜜丸梧子大，以蜜湯空腹吞四五十丸。忌酒肉。韋雲患心痛十年不瘥，於雜方内見，合服之便愈。李絳兵部手集方，治小兒蚘蟲嚙心腹痛，亦單用鶴虱研末，以肥豬肉汁下之。五歲一服二分，蟲出即止也。

Explication. [Su] Song: *He shi* is the most important drug in recipes designed to kill worms/bugs. Chu Yushi, in his *Gu jin lu yan fang*, [recommends the following recipe]. "To cure heart/stomach pain caused by roundworm bites pound ten *liang* of *he shi*, pass it through a sieve and with honey form pills the size of *wu* seeds. Swallow on an empty stomach 40 to 50 pills with a honey decoction. [During such a treatment] wine and meat are to be avoided. Wei Yun suffered from heart/stomach pain for ten years without being cured. He discovered [this recipe] in a list of various recipes. He prepared it, ingested it and was cured." A recipe in Li Jiang's *Bing bu shou ji*: To cure children with pain in the teeth and the central and abdominal region caused by roundworms, grind *he shi* as a single item into powder and [let them] send it down with a fat pork soup. If they are five years old they ingest two *fen* once. When the worms are emitted, [the therapy] ends.

【附方】新一。

Added Recipes. One newly [recorded].

大腸蟲出不斷，斷之復生，行坐不得。鶴虱末，水調半兩服，自愈。怪疾奇方。

Unending release of worms from the large intestine. When this is ended, they develop again. [Patients] are unable to walk or sit. Ingest half a *liang* of *he shi* powder mixed with water. This results in a cure. *Guai ji qi fang*.

15-44

豨薟音喜枕唐本

Xi xian, read *xi xian*. FE *Tang ben*.

***Siegesbeckia orientalis* L. St. Paulswort.**

【校正】併入唐本豬膏莓。

Editorial Correction. *Zhu gao mei*, recorded [separately] in the *Tang ben*, is included here.

【釋名】希仙綱目、火枕草唐本、豬膏莓唐本、虎膏唐本、狗膏唐本、粘糊菜救荒。【時珍曰】韻書楚人呼豬爲豨，呼草之氣味辛毒爲薟。此草氣臭如豬而味薟螫，故謂之豨薟。豬膏、虎膏、狗膏，皆因其氣似，及治虎狗傷也。火枕當作虎薟，俗音訛爾，近人復訛豨薟爲希仙矣。救荒本草言其嫩苗煠熟，浸去苦味，油鹽調食，故俗謂之粘糊菜。

Explanation of Names. *Xi xian* 希仙, *Gang mu*. *Huo xian cao* 火枕草, *Tang ben*. *Zhu gao mei* 豬膏莓, *Tang ben*. *Hu gao* 虎膏, *Tang ben*. *Gou gao* 狗膏, *Tang ben*. *Nian hu cai* 粘糊菜, *Jiu huang*. [Li] Shizhen: According to rhyme books, in Chu people call *zhu* 豬, "pigs," *xi* 豨, and they refer to the acrid and poisonous qi of herbs as *xian* 薟. This herb has malodorous qi similar to pigs and the flavor is poisonous and stinging, *xian shi* 薟螫. Hence it is called *xi xian* 豨薟. "Pig paste," *zhu gao* 豬膏, "tiger paste," *hu gao* 虎膏 and "dog paste," *gou gao* 狗膏, are all based on the similarities of their qi. Also, [this herb] serves to cure harm caused by tigers and dogs. *Huo xian* 火枕 should be *hu xian* 虎薟: This is a common mispronunciation. In recent times, people have mistakenly converted *xi xian* 豨薟 to *xi xian* 希仙, "invisible hermit/immortal." The *Jiu huang ben cao* says: "Heat its tender leaves until done and soak them to eliminate the bitter flavor. Then eat them mixed with oil and salt. Hence it is commonly said to be a 'vegetable sticky like a paste,' *nian hu cai* 粘糊菜."

【集解】【恭曰】豨薟，田野皆識之，一名火杴。葉似酸漿而狹長，花黄白色。三月、四月采苗葉，暴乾。又曰：豬膏苺生平澤下濕地，所在皆有。一名虎膏，一名狗膏。葉似蒼耳，莖圓有毛。【頌曰】豨薟處處有之。春生苗，葉似芥葉而狹長，文粗。莖高二三尺。秋初有花如菊。秋末結實，頗似鶴虱。夏采葉，暴乾用。【藏器曰】豬膏草葉似荏有毛。【保昇曰】豬膏葉似蒼耳，兩枝相對，莖葉俱有毛黄白色，五月、六月采苗，日乾。【時珍曰】按蘇恭唐本草謂，豨薟似酸漿，豬膏苺似蒼耳，列爲二種。而成訥進豨薟丸表言此藥與本草所述相異，多生沃壤，高三尺許，節葉相對。張詠豨薟丸表言此草金稜銀線，素莖紫荄，對節而生，蜀號火杴，莖葉頗同蒼耳。又按沈括筆談云：世人妄認地菘爲火杴。有單服火杴法者，乃是地菘，不當用火杴。火杴乃本草名豬膏苺者，後人不識，重複出條也。按此數説各異，而今人風痺多用豨薟丸，將何適從耶？時珍常聚諸草訂視，則豬膏草素莖有直稜，兼有斑點，葉似蒼耳而微長，似地菘而稍薄，對節而生，莖葉皆有細毛。肥壤一株分枝數十。八九月開小花，深黄色，中有長子如同蒿子，外萼有細刺粘人。地菘則青莖，圓而無稜，無斑無毛，葉皺似菘、芥，亦不對節。觀此則似與成、張二氏所説相合。今河南陳州采豨薟充方物，其狀亦是豬膏草，則沈氏謂豨薟即豬膏苺者，其説無疑矣。蘇恭所謂似酸漿者，乃龍葵，非豨薟，蓋誤認爾。但沈氏言世間單服火杴，乃是地菘，不當用豬膏苺，似與成、張之説相反。今按豨薟、豬膏苺條，並無治風之説。惟本經地菘條，有去痺除熱，久服輕身耐老之語，則治風似當用地菘。然成、張進御之方，必無虛謬之理。或者二草皆有治風之功乎？而今服豬膏苺之豨薟者，復往往有效。其地菘不見有服之者。則豨薟之爲豬膏，尤不必疑矣。

Collected Explanations. [Su] Gong: *Xi xian* is known to everybody in the open country. Another name is *huo xian* 火杴. The leaves are similar to those of Chinese lantern plants, but they are narrower and longer. The flowers are yellow-white. Seedling and leaves are collected in the third and fourth month. They are dried in the sun. It is also said: *Zhu gao mei* grows in the plains in marshlands, on low-lying, moist ground. It can be found everywhere. Another name is "tiger paste," and yet another name is "dog paste." The leaves are similar to those of cocklebur. The stem is round and has hair. [Su] Song: *Xi xian* can be found everywhere. It grows a seedling in spring. The leaves resemble black mustard leaves, but are narrower and longer, with a coarse line design. The stem is two to three *chi* tall. At the beginning of autumn flowers similar to *chrysanthemum* [flowers] appear. At the end of autumn they form fruits, quite similar to those of *carpesium* [herbs]. The leaves are collected in summer. They are dried in the sun before they are used. [Chen] Cangqi: The leaves of *zhu gao cao* are similar to those of *perilla* herbs, but they have hair. [Han] Baosheng: The leaves of *zhu gao* [*cao*] resemble those of *carpesium* herbs. Always two branches grow facing each other. Stem and leaves have yellow-white hair. The seedling is collected in the fifth and sixth month. It is dried in the sun. [Li] Shizhen: According to Su Gong's *Tang ben cao*, *xi xian* is similar to Chinese lantern plant, while *zhu gao mei* is similar to cocklebur herbs. So, these are two different kinds. Cheng Na submitted a "*Xi xian* pill memorandum," saying that "this drug differs from the description in the *Ben cao*. It often grows on fertile land and is more than three *chi* tall. The leaves at the nodes grow facing each other." Zhang Yong in his "*Xi xian* pill memorandum" says: "This herb has gold edges and silver threads, a plain stem and a purple root. [The leaves] grow facing each other at the nodes. In Shu it is called *huo xian* 火杴. Stem and leaves are similar to those of cocklebur." Also, according to Shen Gua's *Bi tan*, "the common people erroneously identify *carpesium* herb as *huo xian*. There exists a [therapeutic] method of ingesting *huo xian* as a single substance, but this refers to *carpesium* herb; it is not suitable to resort to *huo xian*. *Huo xian* is named *zhu gao mei* in the *Ben cao*, but this was unknown to people of later times and they established a separate entry." Now, all these many statements differ, and when today people with wind blockage [of joints] often use *xi xian* pills, which of them should they follow? [I, Li] Shizhen have gathered all types of [these] herbs and have studied them. Now, *zhu gao cao* has a plain stem with a straight edge, covered with many dots. The leaves are similar to those of cocklebur, but they are a little longer. They resemble those of *carpesium* but are a little thinner. They grow facing each other at the nodes. Stem and leaves have fine hair. On fertile land one stem develops several tens of branches. In the eighth and ninth month small flowers open; they are of a deep yellow color. In their midst they have lengthy seeds similar to garden daisy seeds. On the outside of the calyx are many fine thorns that let them cling to humans. *Di song* 地菘, *carpesium* herb, has a greenish stem. It is round and has no edges, no dots and no hair. The leaves are wrinkled like those of pak choi and black mustard, and they do not grow facing each other at nodes. This view [on these two items] is in agreement with the statements by Cheng [Na] and Zhang [Yong]. Today, in Chen zhou of He nan *xi xian* is collected and then served as a local item. It is shaped like *zhu gao cao*, and when Mr. Shen [Gua] states that *xi xian* is in fact *zhu gao mei*, this is not to be doubted. That which Su Gong says is similar to Chinese lantern plant is common nightshade. It is not *xi xian*. The fact is, his identification is wrong. However, when Mr. Shen [Gua] says that "*huo xian* is commonly ingested as a single substance and that this is *carpesium*, and that [it must not be substituted by] *zhu gao mei*," then this contradicts the statements of Cheng [Na] and Zhang [Yong]. According to the [*Ben cao*] entries on *xi xian* and *zhu gao mei*, none of them serves to cure wind [intrusion]. Only the *Ben jing*, in its *di song* 地菘, *carpesium*, entry, says: "It removes blockage [of joints] and eliminates heat. Ingested over a long time it relieves the body of its weight and helps to endure aging." That is, to cure wind [intrusion] it seems as if one had to resort to *di song*. Still, the recipes submitted to the Emperor by Cheng [Na] and Zhang [Yong] are definitely not based on a principle of omission and error. But maybe the two substances have a potential of curing wind [intrusion] nevertheless? Today, the application of *xi xian* as *zhu gao mei* regularly yields good effects, but such [effects] are not observed when *di song* is ingested. Hence it is without doubt that *xi xian* is *zhu gao mei*.

豨薟。【氣味】苦，寒，有小毒。又曰：豬膏莓，辛、苦，平，無毒。【藏器曰】有小毒。蘇恭曰豬膏無毒，誤矣。

Xi xian. Qi and Flavor. Bitter, cold, slightly poisonous. It is also said: *Zhu gao mei*: Acrid, bitter, balanced, nonpoisonous. [Chen] Cangqi: Slightly poisonous. When Su Gong says: "*Zhu gao mei* is nonpoisonous," this is wrong.

【主治】豨薟治熱䘌煩滿不能食。生擣汁三合服，多則令人吐。又曰：豬膏莓主金瘡止痛，斷血生肉，除諸惡瘡，消浮腫。搗封之，湯漬、散傅並良。蘇恭。主久瘧痰[疒陰]，搗汁服，取吐。搗傅虎傷、狗咬、蜘蛛咬、蠶咬、蠼螋溺瘡。藏器。治肝腎風氣，四肢麻痺，骨痛膝弱，風濕諸瘡。時珍。

Control: *Xi xian* serves to cure heat with hidden worms/bugs letting one feel a vexing fullness and making it impossible to eat. Pound fresh [*xi xian*] and ingest three *ge* of the juice. [To ingest] more lets one vomit. It is also said: *Zhu gao mei* controls wounds caused by metal objects/weapons and ends pain, it stops bleeding and stimulates the growth of flesh, it eliminates all types of malign sores and dissolves surface swelling. Pound it and cover [the affected region with the resulting pulp]. To steep [the affected region] in a [*xi xian*] decoction or to apply a [*xi xian*] powder, all this yields good results. Su Gong. To control long-lasting malaria and phlegm rheum,[320] pound it and ingest the juice to stimulate vomiting. Pound it and apply [the resulting pulp] to harm caused by tigers, dog bites, spider bites, silkworm bites and sores caused by the urine of earwigs. [Chen] Cangqi. It serves to cure wind qi affecting liver and kidneys, numbness of the four limbs, aching bones, weakness of knees and all types of sores related to the presence of wind and moisture. [Li] Shizhen.

【發明】【頌曰】蜀人單服豨薟法：五月五日、六月六日、九月九日，采葉，去根、莖、花、實，净洗暴乾。入甑中，層層洒酒與蜜蒸之，又暴。如此九過，則氣味極香美。熬搗篩末，蜜丸服之。云甚益元氣，治肝

320 *Tan yin* 痰[疒陰] is similar to *tan yin* 痰飲, "phlegm rheum," an accumulation of water and phlegm in the chest and diaphragm region.

腎風氣，四肢麻痺，骨間冷，腰膝無力者，亦能行大腸氣。諸州所説，皆云性寒有小毒，與唐本同。惟文州及高郵軍云：性熱無毒，服之補益，安五臟，生毛髮，兼主風濕瘡，肌肉頑痺。婦人久冷尤宜用。須去粗莖，留枝、葉、花、實蒸暴。兩説不同。豈單用葉則寒而有毒，并枝、花、實則熱而無毒乎？抑土地所産不同而然歟？【時珍曰】生搗汁服則令人吐，故云有小毒。九蒸九暴則補人去痺，故云無毒。生則性寒，熟則性温，云熱者非也。【慎微曰】按江陵府節度使成訥進豨薟丸方表略云：臣有弟訮[321]，年二十一中風，伏枕五年，百醫不瘥。有道人鍾針因覩此患，曰：可餌豨薟丸，必愈。其草多生沃壤，高三尺許，節葉相對。當夏五月以來收之，每去地五寸剪刈，以温水洗去泥土，摘葉及枝頭。凡九蒸九暴，不必太燥，但以取足爲度。仍熬搗爲末，煉蜜丸如梧子大，空心温酒或米飲下二三十丸。服至二千丸，所患忽加，不得憂慮，是藥攻之力。服至四千丸，必得復故。至五千丸，當復丁壯。臣依法修合，令訮服之，果如其言。服後須喫飯三五匙壓之。五月五日采者佳。奉勑宣付醫院詳録。又知益州張詠進豨薟丸表略云：切以餐石飲水，可作充腸之饌；餌松含栢，亦成救病之功。是以療飢者不在於羞珍，愈病者何煩於異術？倘獲濟時之藥，輒陳鄙物之形。不耻管窺，輒干天聽。臣因換龍興觀，掘得一碑，内説修養氣術，并藥方二件。依方差人訪問采覓，其草頗有異，金稜銀線，素莖紫荄，對節而生。蜀號火枚，莖葉頗同蒼耳。不費登高歷險，每常求少獲多。急采非難，廣收甚易。倘勤久服，旋見神功。誰知至賤之中，乃有殊常之效。臣自喫至百服，眼目清明。即至千服，髭鬚烏黑，筋力輕健，效驗多端。臣本州有都押衙羅守一，曾因中風墜馬，失音不語。臣與十服，其病立瘥。又和尚智嚴，年七十，忽患偏風，口眼喎斜，時時吐涎。臣與十服，亦便得痊。今合一百劑，差職員史元奏進。

Explication. [Su] Song: The method of people in Shu to ingest *xi xian* as a single substance. Collect the leaves on the fifth day of the fifth month, the sixth day of the sixth month and the ninth day of the ninth month. Discard the root, the stem, the flowers and the fruit and wash [the leaves] clean. Then dry them in the sun and give them into a jar. Place them in layers with each layer sprinkled with wine and honey, and steam this. Then dry them again in the sun. Do this nine times. This will result in extremely fragrant qi and a delicious flavor. Heat them, pound them and pass them through a sieve to obtain a powder to be formed with honey to pills. To ingest them, they say, very much boosts the original qi, cures liver and kidneys affected by wind qi, numbness of the four limbs, cold in the bones and lack of strength in the lower back

321 *Zheng lei* ch. 11, *xi xian* 豨薟 has changed *yan* 訮 to *xin* 訢. However, *Yi shuo* ch. 3, *xi xian wan* 豨薟丸, "*xi xian* pills," and *Ben shi fang* ch. 7, *za bing* 雜病, "various diseases, both write *yan* 訮. According to the *Shuo wen*, *xin* 訢 is *xi* 喜, "to enjoy," *yan* 訮 is to speak freely; *na* 訥 is to stutter. Yan 訮 and his brother's name Na 訥 form a pair." Therefore, *yan* 訮 makes sense here.

and knees. They also stimulate the passage of qi through the large intestine. In all the *zhou* it is said that their nature is cold and that they are slightly poisonous. This is in agreement with the *Tang ben*. Only in Wen zhou and Gao you jun they state: "Their nature is hot and nonpoisonous. To ingest them is supplementing and boosting. They calm the five long-term depots, stimulate the growth of hair, and also control sores related to the presence of wind and moisture, as well as stubborn blockage/numbness of muscles and flesh. When women are affected by cold for a long time, [to ingest the leaves] is suitable, too. One must discard the coarse stem, and leave the twigs, leaves, flowers and fruit. They are steamed and then dried in the sun." These two statements do not agree. How can it be that the leaves, when used alone, are cold and poisonous, while when [they are used] together with the twigs, the flowers and the fruit, they are hot and nonpoisonous? Is this related to differences in the soil where they grow? [Li] Shizhen: When [this herb] is pounded as long as it is fresh and the resulting juice is ingested, this lets one vomit. Hence it is said: "Slightly poisonous." When it is steamed nine times and dried in the sun nine times, then it supplements one's [qi] and eliminates blockages/numbness. Hence it is said: "Poisonous." When it is fresh, its nature is cold. When it is prepared with heat, its nature is warm. To state that it is hot, is wrong. [Tang] Shenwei: The "*Xi xian* pill recipe memorandum" submitted to the Emperor by Cheng Na, stationed in Jiang ling fu as Military Commissioner, reads: "I, your subject, have a younger brother, Yan, who at the age of 21 years was struck by wind. He stayed in bed for five years. A hundred physicians were unable to cure him. Then a Daoist named Zhong Zhen saw his suffering and said: 'He can take *xi xian* pills, and he will definitely be cured. Much of this herb grows on fertile land. It is more than three *chi* tall. Leaves grow facing each other at the nodes. It must be gathered in summer beginning with the fifth month. Each time cut it five *cun* above the ground. Wash it clean with warm water to remove muddy soil and select the leaves and the tips of the twigs. Always steam them nine times and dry them in the sun nine times. They must not become too dry, though. Stop when there is sufficient [moisture] left. Then heat it, pound it and form the powder with heat prepared honey to pills the size of *wu* seeds. Send down on an empty stomach with warm wine or a rice beverage 20 to 30 pills. Ingest up to 2000 pills. When the suffering increases, do not worry. This is a sign of the strength of the medication. When 4000 pills are ingested, a restoration of health will be achieved. By the time 5000 pills are ingested, [the patient] will be very strong.' I, your subject, prepared [the medication] as prescribed and let [my younger brother] Yan ingest it. The result was as [the Daoist had] predicted. After ingesting this medication one must eat three to five spoons of cooked rice to press it down. [The herb] collected on the fifth day of the fifth month is excellent." On request of the Emperor, the memorandum was submitted to the Medical Office for detailed recording. Also, a "Memorandum on *xi xian* pills submitted" by Zhang Yong, governor of Yi zhou, states: "I[322] have eaten stones and drunk water and got delicacies filling the stomach. I have eaten pines and held cypresses in my mouth to realize their potential to rescue me from disease. That is, those who heal hunger will not shy away from the unusual, and those who cure disease, why should they be irritated by procedures that are different?! If a drug is acquired that helps in times of seasonal [epidemics], then it should be propagated even if it is of a vulgar shape. One must not look at it narrow-mindedly, but propagate it to everybody. I, your subject, during the restoration of the Rising Dragon Monastery excavated a stele on which was written a procedure to nourish one's qi, accompanied by two recipes. Based on these recipes, I sent people out to make enquiries and gather [information]. The herb [mentioned on the stele] is quite unique. It has golden edges and a silver thread, a plain stalk and purple roots. [The leaves] grow opposite at the nodes. In Shu, they call it *huo xian* 火枕. Stem and leaves are quite similar to those of cocklebur. There is no need to waste efforts to climb on high mountains and to pass through dangerous terrain, and each time obtain only a small amount [of this herb]. It is quickly collected without any difficulty, and large quantities are collected most easily. When it is ingested regularly and for a long time, its divine potential will be obvious. Who could imagine that in such an extremely cheap item such extraordinary effects are contained?! When I, your subject, had ingested it a 100 times, my eyes were cleared. When I had ingested it a 1000 times, my hair and beard had turned black. My sinews felt light and my strength had returned. So many effects and [therapeutic] successes. In my, your subject's, *zhou* a Chief Lackey Luo Shouyi was struck by wind and fell from his horse. He lost his voice and could no longer speak. I, your subject, gave him [this herb] to ingest it ten times and his disease was cured. Also, the monk Zhi Yan, at the age of 70 years, suddenly suffered from a hemilateral wind [stroke]. His mouth and eyes were slanted and again and again he spat saliva. I, your subject, gave him, too, [this herb] to ingest it ten times and his health also was fully restored. Now I have put together 100 preparations and send the official Shi Yuan to submit it to Your Majesty."

【附方】新五。

Added Recipes. Five newly [recorded].

風寒泄瀉。火枕丸：治風氣行於腸胃，泄瀉。火枕草爲末，醋糊丸梧子大。每三十丸，白湯下。聖濟總録。

Outflow related to wind [intrusion and] cold. The "*huo xian* pills." They serve to cure intestines and stomach invaded by wind qi, with outflow. [Grind] *huo xian* into

322 The character *qie* 切 most likely stands here for *qie* 窃, "myself."

powder and form with a vinegar [wheat flour] paste pills the size of *wu* seeds. Each time ingest 30 pills, to be sent down with clear, boiled water. *Sheng ji zong lu.*

癰疽腫毒，一切惡瘡。豨薟草端午采者一兩，乳香一兩，白礬燒半兩，爲末。每服二錢，熱酒調下。毒重者連進三服，得汗妙。乾坤秘韞。

Swelling with poison related to obstruction-illness and impediment-illness.[323] All types of malign sores. [Grind] one *liang* of *xi xian* herb, collected on the fifth day of the fifth month, one *liang* of frankincense and half a *liang* of alum, burned, into powder. Each time ingest two *qian*, to be sent down mixed with hot wine. In the case of a severe affect by poison ingest [the dose] three times one after another. This will stimulate sweating with a wondrous [effect]. *Qian kun mi yun.*

發背丁瘡。豨薟草、五葉草即五爪龍、野紅花即小薊、大蒜等分，擂爛，入熱酒一盌，絞汁服，得汗立效。乾坤生意。

Effusion on the back[324] of pin[-illness][325] sores. Pound equal amounts of *xi xian* herb, five-leaves herb, that is "five claws dragon" [herb], and "wild red flowers," that is cat thistle, and garlic into a pulpy [mass]. Give this into a bowl of hot wine, and squeeze it to obtain a juice. Ingest it to stimulate sweating. Immediately effective. *Qian kun sheng yi.*

丁瘡腫毒。端午采豨薟草，日乾爲末。每服半兩，熱酒調下。汗出即愈，極有效驗。集簡方。

Pin[-illness] with poison swelling. Collect *xi xian* herb on the fifth day of the fifth month, dry it in the sun and [grind it into] powder. Send it down mixed with hot wine. When sweating begins a cure is achieved. Extremely effective. *Ji jian fang.*

反胃吐食。火杴草焙爲末，蜜丸梧子大，每沸湯下五十丸。百一選方。

Turned over stomach and vomiting of food. Dry *huo xian* herb over a fire in a pan and [grind it into] powder. With honey form pills the size of *wu* seeds. Each time send down 50 pills with boiled water heated to bubbling. *Bai yi xuan fang.*

---

323 *Yong ju* 癰疽, "obstruction-illness, impediment-illness." refers to two vaguely distinguished obstructions/impediments of vessels or other ducts inside the body. Qi rushing against the obstruction may cause a local swelling and eventually break through the surface to cause an abscess. BCGM Dict I, 642.

324 *Fa bei* 發背, "effusion on/of the back," a condition of *yong* 癰, "obstruction-illnesses," and *ju* 疽, "impediment-illnesses," developing on one's back. As it was believed that the transporter holes of the five depots and six palaces are located on the back, conditions of obstruction-illnesses and impediment-illnesses there, often apparent as abscesses, were considered threatening. BCGM Dict I, 148.

325 *Ding* 丁, "pin[-illness]," also *ding* 疔, "pin-illness," refers to a deep-reaching and festering hardness in a tissue, eventually rising above the skin like a pinhead. BCGM Dict I, 127-129.

【附録】
Appendix.

15-44-A01
類鼻 *Lei bi*

【別録有名未用曰】味酸，温，無毒。主痿痺。生田中高地。葉如天名精，美根，五月采。【時珍曰】此似豬膏草也。古今名謂或不同，故附於此。

Bie lu, section "known by name but not in use." Flavor sour, warm, nonpoisonous. Cures dysfunction and blockage/numbness. It grows on elevated locations in the fields. The leaves are similar to those of *carpesium*, with a beautiful root. It is collected in the fifth month. [Li] Shizhen: This herb is similar to *zhu gao* [*mei*] herb. Its ancient and the contemporary names may differ. Therefore it is attached here.

15-44-A02
羊尿柴 *Yang niu chai*

Sheep urine firewood.

【時珍曰】按乾坤生意云：一名牛屎柴。生山野中。葉類鶴虱，四月開白花。其葉主癰疽發背，搗傅之。冬月用根。可以毒魚。

[Li] Shizhen: According to the *Qian kun sheng yi*, "it has another name, *niu shi chai* 牛屎柴, "ox dung firewood."[326] It grows in the wild of mountains. The leaves are similar to those of *carpesium*. It opens white flowers in the fourth month. The leaves control obstruction-illness and impediment-illness[327] with an effusion on the back.[328] Pound [the leaves] and apply them [to the affected region]. In winter use the root. It can serve to poison fish."

326 The *Qian kun mi yun*, section *zhu chuan* 諸瘡, "all types of sores," only writes *yang niao chai* 羊尿柴. It does not mention an alternative name.

327 *Yong ju* 癰疽, "obstruction-illness, impediment-illness." refers to two vaguely distinguished obstructions/impediments of vessels or other ducts inside the body. Qi rushing against the obstruction may cause a local swelling and eventually break through the surface to cause an abscess. BCGM Dict I, 642.

328 *Fa bei* 發背, "effusion on/of the back," a condition of *yong* 癰, "obstruction-illnesses," and *ju* 疽, "impediment-illnesses," developing on one's back. As it was believed that the transporter holes of the five depots and six palaces are located on the back, conditions of obstruction-illnesses and impediment-illnesses there, often apparent as abscesses, were considered threatening. BCGM Dict I, 148.

15-45
箬綱目
Ruo, FE *Gang mu*.

Unidentified.

【釋名】篛與箬同、蓼葉。【時珍曰】箬若竹而弱，故名。其生疏遼，故又謂之遼。

Explanation of Names. *Ruo* 篛 is identical to *ruo* 箬, "skin of bamboo." *Liao ye* 蓼葉, "*liao* leaves." [Li] Shizhen: *Ruo* 箬 is similar to bamboo, but it is weaker, *ruo* 弱. Hence the name. It grows sparsely distributed, *liao* 遼. Hence it is also called *liao* 遼.[329]

【集解】【時珍曰】箬生南方平澤。其根與莖皆似小竹，其節籜與葉皆似蘆荻，而葉之面青背淡，柔而韌，新舊相代，四時常青。南人取葉作笠及裹茶、鹽，包米糉，女人以襯鞵底。

Collected Explanations. [Li] Shizhen: *Ruo* grows in marshlands of the planis in the South. Its root and stem resemble those of small bamboo. The joints, the sheaths of its shoots and its leaves all resemble those of common reed, while its leaves are greenish on their front and pale on their back. They are soft but strong and pliable. Old and new [leaves] follow each other; [*ruo*] is greenish throughout the four seasons. The Southerners use the leaves to make large bamboo hats and to wrap tea, salt and dumplings. Women use them to make shoe soles.

15-45-01
葉 *Ye*
Leaf [of *ruo*].

【氣味】甘，寒，無毒。

Qi and Flavor. Sweet, cold, nonpoisonous.

【主治】男女吐血、衄血、嘔血、咯血、下血。並燒存性，溫湯服一錢匕。又通小便，利肺氣喉痺，消癰腫。時珍。

Control. Blood spitting of males and females, nosebleed, vomiting of blood, coughing up of blood, blood discharge. For all these burn them with their nature retained and ingest with warm, boiled water the amount held by a one *qian* spoon. Also, they free the passage of urine. They free the passage of lung qi and open throat blockage. They dissolve swelling related to obstruction-illness.[330]

---

329 This may be an error and based on the name listed before should be *liao* 蓼.

330 *Yong* 癰, "obstruction-illness,"refers to an obstruction of vessels or other ducts inside the body. Qi rushing against the obstruction may cause a local swelling and eventually break through the surface to cause an abscess. BCGM Dict I, 641.

【附方】新一十二。

Added Recipes. 12 newly [recorded].

一切眼疾。籠篛燒灰，淋汁洗之，久之自效。經驗方。

All types of eye illnesses. Burn *ruo* that had been used to prepare a basket to ashes, pour water through them and wash [the affected eyes with the liquid]. Continue this for some time and an effect will show. *Jing yan fang.*

咽喉閉痛。蓼葉、燈心草燒灰等分，吹之，甚妙。集簡方。

Painful throat closure. Burn equal amounts of *liao* leaves and common rush to ashes and blow them [into the patient's throat]. Very wondrous. *Ji jian fang.*

耳忽作痛，或紅腫内脹。將經霜青箬露在外將朽者燒存性，爲末。傅入耳中，其疼即止。楊起簡便方。

Sudden pain in the ears, possibly with a red swelling extending internally. Take a rotten piece of green *ruo* that was exposed to frost outside and burn it with its nature retained. [Grind] it into powder and insert it into the [affected] ear. The pain will end. Yang Qi, *Jian bian fang.*

肺壅鼻衄。箬葉燒灰、白麪三錢，研勻，井花水服二錢。聖濟總録。

Lung obstruction[331] and nosebleed. Burn *ruo* leaves to ashes and evenly grind them with three *qian* of white wheat flour. Ingest two *qian* of this with the first water drawn from a well. *Sheng ji zong lu.*

經血不止。箬葉灰、蠶紙灰等分，爲末。每服二錢，米飲下。聖濟總録。

Unending menstruation. [Grind] equal amounts of *ruo* leaf ashes and egg shells of mulberry silkworms to ashes. Each time ingest two *qian*, to be sent down with a rice beverage. *Sheng ji zong lu.*

腸風便血。茶簍内箬葉，燒存性。每服三匙，空心糯米湯下。或入麝香少許。王璆百一選方。

Intestinal wind and [urination/defecation] relief with blood. Burn, with their nature retained, *ruo* leaves that had been used to prepare a tea basket. Each time ingest the amount held by three spoons, to be sent down on an empty stomach with a glutinous rice decoction. Or add a small amount of musk. Wang Qiu, *Bai yi xuan fang.*

331 *Fei yong* 肺癰, "lung obstruction-illness," also: *fei yong* 肺壅, "lung obstruction," a condition of abscesses in the lung, with fever, chest pain, and vomiting of bad-smelling pus and blood. BCGM Dict I, 156.

男婦血淋。亦治五淋。多年煮酒瓶頭箬葉，三五年至十年者尤佳。每用七箇，燒存性，入麝香少許，陳米飲下，日三服。有人患此，二服愈。福建煮過夏月酒多有之。百一選方。

Dripping [urination] with blood of men and women. It also serves to cure the five types of [urinary] dripping. Each time use seven *ruo* leaves from the top of a flask that was used for many years to boil wine – those from [flasks] three to five years, or even up to ten years old are especially excellent – and boil them with their nature retained. Add a little musk and send them down with a beverage made from long-stored rice. To be ingested three times a day. Someone suffered from this and was cured after ingesting [this medication] twice. In Fu jian it is often contained in wine boiled during summer months. *Bai yi xuan fang.*

尿血如注，小腹氣痛。茶籠内箬葉燒存性，入麝香少許，米飲下。經驗方。

Urination with blood as if it where pouring. Painful qi [disorder] in the lower abdomen. Burn, with their nature retained, *ruo* leaves that had been used to prepare a tea basket, add a little musk and send this down with a rice beverage. *Jing yan fang.*

小便澀滯不通。乾箬葉一兩燒灰，滑石半兩，爲末，每米飲服三錢。普濟方。

Rough urination that cannot flow freely. Burn one *liang* of dry *ruo* leaves to ashes and grind them with half a *liang* of talcum into powder. Each time ingest with a rice beverage three *qian*. *Pu ji fang.*

男婦轉脬。方同上。

Contorted bladder[332] of men and women. Recipe identical to the one above.

吹奶乳癰。五月五日糉箬燒灰，酒服二錢即散，累效。濟急仙方。

Inflated breast,[333] and breast obstruction-illness.[334] On the fifth day of the fifth month burn *ruo* leaves that had been used to wrap rice dumplings. Ingest with wine two *qian* to disperse [the qi responsible for the obstruction]. Repeatedly effective. *Ji ji xian fang.*

---

332 *Zhuan pao* 轉脬, "contorted bladder," a condition of a distended, tight and painful urinary bladder because of a blockage of the 'bladder connection' (*bao xi* 胞系, i.e. the urethra) and resulting inhibition of the flow of urine. BCGM Dict I, 697.

333 *Chui ru* 吹乳, "inflated breast." Identical to *chui nai* 吹奶, "inflated breast." A condition with milk blocked after delivery and the breasts turning red and swelling. BCGM Dict I, 101.

334 *Yong* 癰, "obstruction-illness," refers to an obstruction of vessels or other ducts inside the body. Qi rushing against the obstruction may cause a local swelling and eventually break through the surface to cause an abscess. BCGM Dict I, 641.

痘瘡倒靨。箬葉灰一錢，麝香少許，酒服。張德恭痘疹便覽方。

Smallpox sores with inverted moles. Burn *ruo* leaves to obtain one *qian* of ashes. Add a little musk and ingest this with wine. Zhang Degong, *Dou zhen bian lan fang*.

15-46
蘆別録下品
Lu, FE *Bie lu*, lower rank.

Phragmites communis **Trin. Common reed.**

【校正】併入拾遺江中采出蘆。

Editorial correction. Included here is "reed collected from the middle of a river," [formerly listed separately] in the *Shi yi*.

【釋名】葦音偉、葭音加。花名蓬蕽唐本。笋名虇音拳。【時珍曰】按毛萇詩疏云：葦之初生曰葭，未秀曰蘆，長成曰葦。葦者，偉大也。蘆者，色盧黑也。葭者，嘉美也。

Explanation of Names. *Wei* 葦, read *wei* 偉; *jia* 葭, read *jia* 加. The flowers are called *peng nong* 蓬蕽, *Tang ben*. The shoots are called *quan* 虇, read *quan* 拳. [Li] Shizhen: According to Mao Chang's *Shi shu*, when *wei* 葦 has just begun to grow it is called *jia* 葭. Before its flowers blossom it is *lu* 蘆. When it has matured it is called *wei* 葦. *Wei* 葦 is "great," *wei da* 偉大. *Lu* 蘆 is *lu hei* 盧黑, "soot-black." *Jia* 葭 is *jia mei* 嘉美, "beautiful."

【集解】【恭曰】蘆根生下濕地。莖葉似竹，花若荻花，名蓬蕽。二月、八月采根，日乾用。【頌曰】今在處有之，生下濕陂澤中。其狀都似竹，而葉抱莖生，無枝。花白作穗若茅花。根亦若竹根而節疏。其根取水底味甘辛者。其露出及浮水中者，並不堪用。按郭璞注爾雅云：葭即蘆也，葦即蘆之成者。菼、薍，似葦而小，中實，江東呼爲烏蓲，音丘。或謂之藡，即荻也。至秋堅成，即謂之萑，音桓。蒹似萑而細長，高數尺，江東謂之蒹。其花皆名芀，音調。其萌皆名虇，堪食如竹笋。若然，則蘆、葦通爲一物也。所謂蒹，乃今作簾者是也。所謂菼者，今以當薪者是也。而人罕能別蒹、菼與蘆。葦也。又北人以葦與蘆爲二物。水旁下濕所生者皆名葦，其細不及指大。人家池圃所植者皆名蘆，其幹差大。深碧色者，亦難得。然則蘆、葦皆可通用矣。【時珍曰】蘆有數種。其長丈許，中空皮薄色白者，葭也，蘆也，葦也。短小於葦而中空皮厚色青蒼者，菼也，薍也，荻也，萑也。其最短小而中實者，蒹也，薕也。皆以初生、已成得名。其身皆如竹，其葉皆長如箬葉，其根入藥，性味皆同。其未解葉者，古謂之紫籜。【斆曰】蘆根須要逆水生，並黃泡肥厚者，去鬚節並赤黃皮用。

Collected Explanations. [Su] Gong: The root of *lu* grows in low-lying, moist areas. The stem and the leaves are similar to those of bamboo. The leaves resemble those of *di* 荻 flowers. They are named *peng nong* 蓬蕽. The root is collected in the second and eighth month. [Su] Song: Today it can be found everywhere. It grows in low-lying moist reservoirs and marshlands. Its shape in every respect is similar to bamboo, but the leaves grow enclosing the stem. It has no branches. The flowers are white and form spikes similar to floss grass. Even the root is similar to bamboo roots, but the nodes are more distant to each other. The root gathered from the ground of waters has a sweet-acrid flavor. Those that have [left the water/ground and have] come to the open, and those floating on waters, they are not suitable for [medicinal] use. According to Guo Pu's comment on the *Er ya*, *jia* 葭 is *lu* 蘆. *Wei* 葦 is matured *lu* 蘆. *Tan* 菼 and *wan* 薍 are similar to *wei* 葦, but they are smaller and they are solid inside. In Jiang dong they are called *wu qiu* 烏蓲, read *qiu* 丘, and some call them *di* 薍. This is *di* 荻. In autumn it hardens and matures and is then called *huan* 萑, *read huan* 桓. *Jian* 蒹 resembles *huan* 萑, but is finer and lengthy. It reaches a height of several *chi*. In Jiang dong they call it *jian* 蒹.[335] Its flower is called *diao* 艻, read *diao* 調. The buds are called *quan* 虇; they are edible, just like bamboo sprouts. In view of all this, *lu* 蘆 and *wei* 葦 are one identical item. The [reed] called *jian* 蒹 is used today to make screens, *lian* 簾. The [reed] called *tan* 菼 serves as firewood today. Now, people are rarely able to distinguish *jian* 蒹 and *tan* 菼 from *lu* 蘆, which is *wei* 葦. Also, the Northerners identify *wei* 葦 and *lu* 蘆 as two different items. They name those [reeds] that grow near waters and in low-lying, moist areas *wei* 葦. They are fine and do not even reach the size of a finger. Those planted by people in ponds and gardens are always called *lu* 蘆. The trunk is much bigger. Those of a deep jade-blue color are difficult to obtain. So, *lu* 蘆 and *wei* 葦 can be used interchangeably. [Li] Shizhen: There are several kinds of *lu* 蘆. That wich is longer than a *zhang*, is hollow inside and has a thin, white bark is *jia* 葭, is *lu* 蘆 and is *wei* 葦. That which is shorter and smaller than *wei* 葦, hollow inside and has a thick bark of greenish-dark green color is *tan* 菼, is *wan* 薍, is *di* 荻 and is *huan* 萑. The shortest and smallest kind that is solid inside, is *jian* 蒹, is *lian* 蒹. All of them are named this way from the beginning of their growth to their maturity. The body of all of them is similar to bamboo. The leaves are all long, similar to *ruo* leaves (15-45). The root is added to medication. They all have an identical nature and flavor. The leaves were never explained before. In ancient times they were called "purple sheaths," *zi tuo* 紫籜. [Lei] Xiao: The roots of *lu* must be those growing in water flowing against their normal current. Of those that are yellow, fluffy, fat and thick, remove the hair, the nodes and the red-yellow bark before making use of them

335 *Er ya, shi cao* 釋草, "Explaining herbs," Guo Pu writes *jian* 蒹 instead of *Jian* 蒹.

15-46-02
根 *Gen*
Root [of *lu*]

【氣味】甘，寒，無毒。

Qi and Flavor. Sweet, cold, nonpoisonous.

【主治】消渴客熱，止小便利。別録。療反胃嘔逆不下食，胃中熱，傷寒内熱，彌良。蘇恭。解大熱，開胃，治噎噦不止。甄權。寒熱時疾，煩悶，瀉痢人渴，孕婦心熱。大明。

Control. Melting with thirst[336] with visitor heat.[337] It stops free flow of urine. *Bie lu.* It heals turned over stomach with vomiting and food unable to move down. It is good at [healing] heat in the stomach and Harm caused by cold with internal heat. Su Gong. It resolves massive heat, opens the stomach and serves to cure unending gullet occlusion and retching. Zhen Quan. Alternating sensations of cold and heat associated with seasonal [epidemic] illnesses. Vexing heart-pressure. Outflow with free-flux illness letting one be thirsty. Heart/stomach heat of pregnant women. Da Ming.

15-46-02
笋 *Sun*
Sprout [of *lu*].

【氣味】小苦，冷，無毒。【寗原曰】忌巴豆。

Qi and Flavor. Slightly bitter, cold, nonpoisonous. Ning Yuan: [During a treatment with this drug] avoid *croton* seeds.

【主治】膈間客熱，止渴，利小便，解河豚及諸魚蟹毒。寗原。解諸肉毒。時珍。

Control. Visitor heat[338] in the diaphragm region. It ends thirst and frees the flow of urine. It resolves the poison of globefish and all types of fish and crabs. Mi Yuan. It resolves the poison of all types of meat. [Li] Shizhen.

---

336 *Xiao ke* 消渴, "melting with thirst," most likely including cases of diabetes. BCGM Dict Vol I, 567.

337 *Ke re* 客熱, "visitor heat," 1.) an etiological agent identified as heat evil intruding into the human organism from outside. 2.) A condition identical to *re* 熱, "heat." BCGM Dict I, 282.

338 *Ke re* 客熱, "visitor heat," 1.) an etiological agent identified as heat evil intruding into the human organism from outside. 2.) A condition identical to *re* 熱, "heat." BCGM Dict I, 282.

【發明】【時珍曰】按雷公炮炙論序云：益食加觴，須煎蘆、朴。注云：用逆水蘆根并厚朴二味等分，煎湯服。蓋蘆根甘能益胃，寒能降火故也。

Explication. According to the preface of the *Lei gong pao zhi lun*, "To increase [a person's]eating and drinking, it is essential to boil *lu* and *magnolia* bark." The comment states: "Boil equal amounts of the two items *lu* root out of a water that flows against its usual current and *magnolia* bark, and ingest the decoction." The fact is, *lu* root is sweet and can boost stomach [qi] because its cold can cause the fire to descend.

【附方】舊六，新六。

Added Recipes. Six of old. Six newly [recorded].

骨蒸肺痿不能食者，蘇遊蘆根飲主之。蘆根、麥門冬、地骨皮、生薑各十兩，橘皮、茯苓各五兩，水二斗，煮八升，去滓，分五服，取汗乃瘥。外臺秘要。

Bone steaming,[339] lung dysfunction and inability to eat. This is controlled by Su You's "*lu* root beverage." Boil in two *dou* of water down to eight *sheng* ten *liang* each of *lu* root, *ophiopogon* [tuber], *lycium* root bark and fresh ginger, together with five *liang* each of tangerine peels and *poria*. Remove the dregs and ingest [the decoction] divided into five portions. When a sweating begins, the cure is achieved. *Wai tai mi yao.*

勞復食復，欲死。並以蘆根煮濃汁飲。肘後方。

Relapse [of a disease] because of exhaustion and relapse because of food, bringing one close to dying. For both boil *lu* root to obtain a thick juice and drink it. *Zhou hou fang.*

嘔噦不止厥逆者。蘆根三斤切，水煮濃汁，頻飲二升，必效。若以童子小便煮服，不過三服愈。肘後方。

Unending vomiting and retching with [yang qi] recession and [qi] countermovement. Cut three *jin* of *lu* roots and frequently drink up to two *sheng*. This will be effective. If this is ingested boiled with boys' urine, a cure is achieved after no more than three ingestions. *Zhou hou fang.*

五噎吐逆，心膈氣滯，煩悶不下食。蘆根五兩剉，以水三大盞，煮取二盞，去滓溫服。金匱玉函方。

339 *Gu zheng* 骨蒸, "bone steaming," 1.) a condition of an infectious consumptive disease with a development of vexing heat in the afternoon. 2.) An illness sign of heat and vexation with a feeling as if this originated in the bones. BCGM Dict I, 197.

The five types of gullet occlusion[340] with vomiting and [qi] countermovement, sluggish qi in the heart and diaphragm, vexing heart-pressure and failure to move down food. Cut five *liang* of *lu* root and boil them in three large cups of water down to two small cups. Remove the dregs and ingest the warm [liquid]. *Jin kui yu han fang.*

反胃上氣。蘆根、茅根各二兩，水四升，煮二升，分服。千金方。

Turned over stomach with rising qi. Boil two *liang* each of *lu* root and floss grass root in four *sheng* of water down to two *sheng* and ingest this in several portions. *Qian jin fang.*

霍亂煩悶。蘆根三錢，麥門冬一錢，水煎服。千金方。

Cholera with vexing heart-pressure. Boil in water three *qian* of *lu* root and one *qian* of *ophiopogon* [tuber] and ingest [the decoction]. *Qian jin fang.*

霍亂脹痛。蘆根一升，生薑一升，橘皮五兩，水八升，煎三升，分服。太平聖惠方。

Cholera with painful [abdominal] distension. Boil one *sheng* of *lu* root, one *sheng* of fresh ginger and five *liang* of tangerine peels in three *sheng* of water and ingest this in several portions. *Tai ping sheng hui fang.*

食狗肉毒。心下堅，或腹脹口乾，忽發熱妄語，蘆根煮汁服。梅師方。

Poisoning after eating dog meat. With a hardening below the heart, and possibly an abdominal distention with a dry mouth, sudden effusion of heat and mad talking. Boil *lu* root and ingest the resulting juice. *Mei shi fang.*

中馬肉毒。方同上。聖惠。

Poisoning by horse meat. Recipe identical to the one above. *Sheng hui.*

鯸鮧魚毒。方同上。千金。

Poisoning by globefish. Recipe identical to the one above. *Qian jin.*

食蟹中毒。方同上。千金。

Poisoning after eating crabs. Recipe identical to the one above. *Qian jin.*

中藥箭毒。方同上。千金。

Struck by the poison of a medicated arrow. Recipe identical to the one above. *Qian jin.*

340 For a detailed list of the five types of gullet occlusion by qi, anxiety, food, exhaustion, and pondering, see BCGM Dict I, 545.

15-46-03
莖、葉 *Jing, Ye*
Stem, leaf [of *lu*]

【氣味】甘，寒，無毒。

Qi and Flavor. Sweet, cold, nonpoisonous.

【主治】霍亂嘔逆，肺癰煩熱，癰疽。燒灰淋汁，煎膏，蝕惡肉，去黑子。時珍。

Control. Cholera with vomiting and [qi] countermovement. Lung obstruction-illness[341] with vexing heat, obstruction-illness and impediment-illness.[342] Burn them to ashes and drip water through them to obtain a juice. Boil it to generate a paste [and apply this to] eat away malign flesh and to remove black [skin] spots. [Li] Shizhen.

15-46-04
蘀 *Tuo*
Leaves fallen from *lu*.

治金瘡，生肉滅瘢。徐之才。

They serve to cure wounds caused by metal objects/weapons. They stimulate the growth of flesh and they minimize scars. Xu Zhicai.

15-46-05
江中采出蘆 *Jiang zhong cai chu lu*
***Lu* collected from amidst a river.**

令夫婦和同，用之有法。藏器。

It lets husband and wife form a harmonious union. The application follows a specific method. [Chen] Cangqi.

【發明】【時珍曰】古方煎藥多用勞水及陳蘆火，取其水不强，火不盛也。蘆中空虛，故能入心肺，治上焦虛熱。

Explication. [Li] Shizhen: Ancient recipes often [recommended] to use exhausted water (05-14) and fire made of long-stored *lu*/reed to boil pharmaceutical drugs.

341 *Fei yong* 肺癰, "lung obstruction-illness," also: *fei yong* 肺壅, "lung obstruction," a condition of abscesses in the lung, with fever, chest pain, and vomiting of bad-smelling pus and blood. BCGM Dict I, 156.

342 *Yong ju* 癰疽, "obstruction-illness, impediment-illness." refers to two vaguely distinguished obstructions/impediments of vessels or other ducts inside the body. Qi rushing against the obstruction may cause a local swelling and eventually break through the surface to cause an abscess. BCGM Dict I, 642.

This way they were sure that the water was not strong and the fire was not violent. *Lu* is hollow. Hence it can enter heart and lung and serve to cure depletion heat in the upper [section of the Triple] Burner.

【附方】新六。

Added Recipes. Six newly [recorded].

霍亂煩渴，腹脹。蘆葉一握，水煎服。

Cholera with vexing thirst and abdominal distension. Boil a handful of *lu* leaves in water and ingest [the decoction].

又方：蘆葉五錢，糯米二錢半，竹茹一錢，水煎，入薑汁、蜜各半合，煎兩沸，時時呷之。聖惠方。

Another recipe. Boil in water five *qian* of *lu* leaves, two and a half *qian* of glutinous rice and one *qian* of bamboo shavings. Add half a *ge* each of ginger juice and honey, boil this to bubbling twice and frequently sip the [liquid]. *Sheng hui fang.*

吐血不止。蘆荻外皮燒灰，勿令白，爲末，入蚌粉少許，研勻，麥門冬湯服一二錢。三服可救一人。聖惠方。

Unending blood spitting. Burn the external bark of *lu*, [that is,] *di*, to ashes, but do not let them turn white. [Grind them into] powder, add a little freshwater mussel powder and grind this to an evenly mixed powder. Ingest with an *ophiopogon* [tuber] decoction one to two *qian*. Three ingestions can rescue one. *Sheng hui fang.*

肺癰欬嗽，煩滿微熱，心胸甲錯。葦莖湯：用葦莖切二升，水二斗，煮汁五升。入桃仁五十枚，薏苡仁、瓜瓣各半升，煮取二升，服。當吐出膿血而愈。張仲景金匱玉函方。

Lung obstruction-illness[343] with cough. A vexing [sensation of] fullness with a little heat, and a flaky skin in the heart and chest region. The "decoction with *wei* stems." Cut two *sheng* of *wei* stems [into small pieces] and boil them in two *dou* of water to obtain a juice of five *sheng*. Add 50 peach kernels and half a *sheng* each of Job's tears and wax gourd petals. Boil this down to two *sheng* and ingest it. This will cause vomiting pus and blood, and [the patient] is cured. Zhang Zhongjing, *Jin kui yu han fang.*

343 *Fei yong* 肺癰, "lung obstruction-illness," also: *fei yong* 肺壅, "lung obstruction," a condition of abscesses in the lung, with fever, chest pain, and vomiting of bad-smelling pus and blood. BCGM Dict I, 156.

發背潰爛。陳蘆葉爲末，以葱椒湯洗净，傅之神效。乾坤秘韞。

Effusion on the back[344] with festering of a pulpy mass. [Grind] long-stored *lu* leaves into powder. Wash [the affected region] clean with a decoction of onions and pepper. Then apply the [powder]. Divinely effective. *Qian kun mi yun.*

癰疽惡肉。白炭灰、白荻灰等分，煎膏塗之，蝕盡惡肉，以生肉膏貼之。亦去黑子。此藥只可留十日，久則不效。葛洪肘後方。

Obstruction-illness and impediment-illness,[345] with malign flesh growth. Boil equal amounts of white charcoal ashes and white *di* ashes [in water] to a paste and apply it [to the affected region]. It will eat away all the malign flesh. Then apply a paste that stimulates the growth of new flesh. It also serves to remove black [dermal] spots. This medication can be stored for ten days only. After a long time it is no longer effective. Ge Hong, *Zhou hou fang.*

小兒禿瘡。以鹽湯洗净，蒲葦灰傅之。聖濟總録。

Baldness sores of children. Wash [the affected region] clean with a salt decoction and apply the ashes of *acorus* and *wei* to it. *Sheng ji zong lu.*

15-46-06
蓬蕽 *Peng nong*
Flower [of *lu*].

【氣味】甘，寒，無毒。

Qi and Flavor. Sweet, cold, nonpoisonous.

【主治】霍亂。水煮濃汁服，大驗。蘇恭。煮汁服，解中魚蟹毒。蘇頌。燒灰吹鼻，止衄血，亦入崩中藥。時珍。

Control. Cholera. Boil [*lu* flowers] in water to obtain a thick juice and ingest it. Very effective. Su Gong. Boil it and ingest the juice. This resolves poisoning [after eating] fish and crabs. Su Song. Burned to ashes and blown into the nose it ends nosebleed. It is also added to medication for collapsing center.[346] [Li] Shizhen.

344 *Fa bei* 發背, "effusion on/of the back," a condition of *yong* 癰, "obstruction-illnesses," and *ju* 疽, "impediment-illnesses," developing on one's back. As it was believed that the transporter holes of the five depots and six palaces are located on the back, conditions of obstruction-illnesses and impediment-illnesses there, often apparent as abscesses, were considered threatening. BCGM Dict I, 148.

345 *Yong ju* 癰疽, "obstruction-illness, impediment-illness." refers to two vaguely distinguished obstructions/impediments of vessels or other ducts inside the body. Qi rushing against the obstruction may cause a local swelling and eventually break through the surface to cause an abscess. BCGM Dict I, 642.

346 *Beng zhong* 崩中, "collapsing center," excessive vaginal bleeding outside of a menstruation period. BCGM Dict I, 58.

【附方】新二。

Added Recipes. Two newly [recorded].

乾霍亂病，心腹脹痛。蘆蓬茸一把，水煮濃汁，頓服二升。小品方。

Dry cholera disease, with a painful distension of the central and abdominal region. Boil one handful of soft *lu* flowers in water to obtain a thick juice and ingest two *sheng* at a time. *Xiao pin fang*.

諸般血病。水蘆花、紅花、槐花、白鷄冠花、茅花等分，水二鍾，煎一鍾服。萬表積善堂方。

All types of blood disease. Boil equal amounts of water *lu* flowers, safflower, *sophora* flowers, white cockscomb flowers and floss grass flowers in two *zhong* of water down to one *zhong* and ingest this. Wan Biao, *Ji shan tang fang*.

15-47
甘蕉別録下品

Gan jiao, FE *Bie lu*, lower rank.

***Musa sapientum* L. Banana.**

【釋名】芭蕉衍義、天苴史記注、芭苴。【時珍曰】按陸佃埤雅云：蕉不落葉，一葉舒則一葉焦，故謂之蕉。俗謂乾物爲巴，巴亦蕉意也。稽聖賦云：竹布實而根苦，蕉舒花而株稿。芭苴乃蕉之音轉也。蜀人謂之天苴。曹叔雅異物志云：芭蕉結實，其皮赤如火，其肉甜如蜜，四五枚可飽人，而滋味常在牙齒間，故名甘蕉。

Explanation of Names. *Ba jiao* 芭蕉, *Yan yi*. *Tian ju* 天苴, *Shi ji* commentary. *Ba ju* 芭苴. [Li] Shizhen: According to Lu Dian's *Pi ya*, "the leaves of *jiao* do not fall off. When a [new] leaf unfolds, an [old] leaf is 'scorched,' *jiao* 焦. Therefore [the plant] is called *jiao* 蕉. Dry items are commonly called *ba* 巴. *Ba* 巴, too, has the meaning of *jiao* 蕉, 'scorched plant'." The *Ji sheng fu* states: "When bamboo displays fruits, the root turns bitter. When *jiao* 蕉 unfolds flowers, its stem withers." *Ba ju* 芭苴 is a modified reading [of *ba jiao*]. In Shu, people call it *tian ju* 天苴. Cao Shuya in his *Yi wu zhi* states: "The fruits formed by *ba jiao* have a skin as red as fire and the flesh is sweet like honey. Four or five can fill a person. Its flavor remains between the teeth for a long time. Hence it is called 'sweet *jiao*,' *gan jiao* 甘蕉."

【集解】【弘景曰】甘蕉本出廣州。今江東並有，根葉無異，惟子不堪食耳。【恭曰】甘蕉出嶺南者，子大味甘；北間者但有花無實。【頌曰】今二廣、閩中、川蜀皆有，而閩、廣者實極甘美可啖，他處雖多，而作花者亦少，近時中州種之甚盛，皆芭蕉也。其類亦多。有子者名甘蕉，卷心中抽幹作花。初生大萼，似倒垂菡萏，有十數層，層皆作瓣，漸大則花出瓣中，極繁盛。紅者如火炬，謂之紅蕉。白者如蠟色，謂之水蕉。其花大類象牙，故謂之牙蕉。其實亦有青黄之别，品類亦多，最甘美，曝乾可寄遠，北土得之以爲珍果。其莖解散如絲，閩人以灰湯練治，紡績爲布，謂之蕉葛。【宗奭曰】芭蕉三年已上即有花，自心中抽出，一莖止一花，全如蓮花，瓣亦相似，但色微黄緑，中心無蕊，悉是花葉也。花頭常下垂，每一朵自中夏開，直至中秋後方盡，凡三葉開則三葉脱落也。【時珍曰】按萬震南州異物志云：甘蕉即芭蕉，乃草類也。望之如樹，株大者一圍餘。葉長丈許，廣尺餘至二尺。其莖虚軟如芋，皆重皮相裹。根如芋魁，青色，大者如車轂。花着莖末，大如酒杯，形色如蓮花。子各爲房，實隨花長，每花一闔，各有六子，先後相次，子不俱生，花不俱落也。蕉子凡三種，未熟時皆苦澀，熟時皆甜而脆，味如葡萄，可以療饑。一種子大如拇指，長六七寸，鋭似羊角，兩兩相抱者，名羊角蕉，剥其皮黄白色，味最甘美。一種子大如鷄卵，有類牛乳者，名牛乳蕉，味微減。一種子大如蓮子，長四五寸，形正方者，味最弱也。並可蜜藏爲果。又顧玠海槎録云：海南芭蕉常年開花結實，有二種。板蕉大而味淡，佛手蕉小而味甜，通呼爲蕉子。不似江南者，花而不實。又范成大虞衡志云：南中芭蕉有數種。極大者凌冬不凋，中抽一條，長數尺，節節有花，花褪葉根有實，去皮取肉，軟爛如緑柹，味極甘冷，四季恒實。土人以飼小兒，云去客熱，謂之蕉子，又名牛蕉子。以梅汁漬，曝，壓扁，味甘酸，有微霜，名芭蕉乾。一種鷄蕉子，小於牛蕉，亦四季實。一種牙蕉子，小於鷄蕉，尤香嫩甘美，惟秋初結子。一種紅蕉，葉瘦，類蘆箬，花色正紅，如榴花，日拆一兩葉，其端有一點鮮緑可愛，春開至秋盡猶芳，俗名美人蕉。一種膽瓶蕉，根出土時肥飽，狀如膽瓶也。又費信星槎勝覽云：南番阿魯諸國，無米穀，惟種芭蕉、椰子，取實代粮也。

Collected Explanations. [Tao] Hongjing. *Gan jiao* originally came from Guang zhou. Today it is also found in Jiang dong. The roots and the leaves [of *gan jiao* from Jiang dong] are not different [from those grown in Guang zhou]; only their fruits are not edible. [Su] Gong: The fruits of *gan jiao* from Ling nan are big and sweet. [*Gan jiao*] from Bei jian has flowers only, without fruit. [Su] Song: Today it can be found in Er guang, Min zhong and Chuan shu, with the fruit of [*gan jiao*] from Min and Guang being extremely sweet and delicious; they can be eaten with great pleasure. At other places there may be many [*gan jiao*], too, but very few of them produce flowers. In recent times they have been planted abundantly in the central *zhou*. These are all *ba jiao* 芭蕉. There are many kinds. Those with seeds are called *gan jiao* 甘蕉. A stem rises from the curled bud and produces flowers. At the beginning, a large calyx appears, resembling lotus flowers hanging upside down. It has many layers, and each layer has petals. When they have grown large, flowers come out of the petals. They are extremely lush. Red ones resemble a torch made of bundled reeds. They are called *hong jiao* 紅蕉, "red banana." White ones have a color like wax; they are called *shui jiao* 水蕉, "water banana." The flowers are similar to ivory; hence they are called *ya jiao* 牙蕉, "tooth/ivory banana." Their fruit, too, vary from greenish to yellow and there are many different types. They are very sweet and delicious, dried in the sun they can be sent to distant places. When the northerners get them, they consider them a precious fruit. The stem can be split into threads. The people in Min process them with an ash decoction to [threads] suitable for weaving fabrics. They call them *jiao ge* 蕉葛, "banana fibers." [Kou] Zongshi: *Ba jiao* of three years or more have a flower that rises straight out of the heart [of the stem]. One stem has only one flower. It is in all respects similar to Indian lotus flowers. The petals, too, resemble each other. Only the color is slightly yellow-green, and in its center [the flower] lacks anther bearing filaments. These are all flower-leaves/petals. The tip of the flower always hangs down. Each flower begins to open in mid-summer and this ends after mid-autumn. When a total of three [flower] leaves/petals open, then these three leaves/petals eventually fall off. [Li] Shizhen: According to Wan Zhen's *Nan zhou yi wu zhi*, "*gan jiao* 甘蕉 is *ba jiao* 芭蕉, and belongs to the group of herbs. From a distance it looks like a tree. Trunks may be more than a double-handspan big. The leaves reach a length of about one *zhang*, and they are more than one *chi* up to two *chi* wide. The stem is hollow and soft like that of taro. It is covered by a bark of several layers, one wrapping around the other. The root is similar to taro tubers. It is of greenish color. Large ones resemble the hub of a wheel. The flower is attached to the end of the stem. It is as big as a wine cup. Its shape and color are similar to Indian lotus flowers. Each seed has a chamber; the fruit grow in accordance with the growth of the flower. Each flower has one capsule of six seeds. They follow each other [in their development]; the seeds do not grow together; the flowers do not fall off together. There are three types of *jiao* 蕉 fruit in total. Before they have ripened, they are all bitter and rough. When they are ripe, they are all sweet and crisp. They have a flavor similar to grapes and can serve to heal hunger. One kind of fruit is as big as a thumb, with a length of six to seven *cun*. They are pointed like the horns of sheep, with always two clinging to each other. They are called 'sheep horn banana.' When their skin is peeled, [the interior] is of a yellow-white color. The flavor is very sweet and delicious. Another type is as big as a chicken egg. There are also some resembling the teat of a cow. They are called 'cow teat banana.' Their flavor is weaker. Another type is of the size of Indian lotus seeds, with a length of four to five *cun*. They are exactly square shaped, and their flavor is very weak. All [the variations mentioned] can be prepared with honey to be stored as fruit." Also, Gu Jie in his *Hai chuo lu* states: "In Hai nan, *ba jiao* open flowers and form fruit all year long.

There are two kinds. 'Board banana' is big and has a bland flavor. 'Buddha's hand banana' is small and has a sweet flavor. All of them are called 'banana fruit.' They differ from those in Jiang nan that have flowers without fruit." Also, Fan Chengda in his *Yu heng zhi* states: "The *ba jiao* of Nan zhong has many kinds. The largest ones do not wither even in cold winter. In their center a stem rises, reaching a length of several *chi*, with flowers at all the nodes. When the flowers vanish, fruit develop at the base of the leaves. The skin is discarded, and the meat is kept. It is soft and pulpy like that of green persimmons, with an extremely sweet and cold flavor. It has fruit throughout the four seasons. The locals use them to feed children, claiming that they eliminate visitor heat.[347] They call them 'bananas,' and also 'ox bananas.' When they soak them in plum juice, dry them in the sun and press them flat, they have a sweet-sour flavor, with some frost on it. This is called 'dried banana.' Yet another kind are the 'chicken bananas.' They are smaller than the 'ox bananas.' They, too, bear fruit throughout the four seasons. Then there are the 'tooth/ivory bananas.' They are smaller than the chicken bananas. They are particularly fragrant and tender, sweet and delicious. They form seeds only at the beginning of autumn. There is also a 'red banana.' It has thin leaves, resembling those of reed, and the flower is exactly red, similar to a pomegranate flower. Per day it unfolds two leaves with an amiable dot of fresh green color at their tips. They remain open from spring on throughout autumn with a permanent fragrance. They are commonly called 'beauty banana.' Yet another kind is the 'bile vase banana.' When the root leaves the soil it is fat, similar to a vase used for storing bile." Also, Fei Xin in his *Xing cha sheng lan* states: "In all the countries of E lu in the southern foreign regions, there is no rice or other grain. They only plant *ba jiao* and coconut trees, resorting to their fruit as food."

【氣味】甘，大寒，無毒。【恭曰】性冷，不益人。多食動冷氣。

Qi and Flavor. Sweet, very cold, nonpoisonous. [Su] Gong: Its nature is cold; it does not boost human [qi]. Eaten in large quantities it excites one's cold qi.

【主治】生食，止渴潤肺。蒸熟晒裂，舂取仁食，通血脉，填骨髓。孟詵。生食，破血，合金瘡，解酒毒。乾者，解騰熱煩渴。吴瑞。除小兒客熱，壓丹石毒。時珍。

Control. Eaten fresh, it ends thirst and moistens the lung. Steamed until done and exposed to the sun it cracks. [Pound it in a] mortar, take out the kernels and eat them. They will penetrate the blood vessels and fill the bones with marrow. Meng Shen. Eaten fresh, they break through blood [accumulation], close wounds caused

347 *Ke re* 客熱, "visitor heat," 1.) an etiological agent identified as heat evil intruding into the human organism from outside. 2.) A condition identical to *re* 熱, "heat." BCGM Dict I, 282.

by metal objects/weapons and resolve the poison of wine. Dried, they resolve muscle heat with vexing thirst. Wu Rui. They eliminate visitor heat[348] of children and suppress the poison of elixirs and minerals. [Li] Shizhen.

15-47-01
根 *Gen*
Root [of *gan jiao*].

【氣味】甘，大寒，無毒。【恭曰】寒。【頌曰】甘蕉、芭蕉，性相同也。

Qi and Flavor. Sweet, very cold, nonpoisonous. [Su] Gong: Cold. [Su] Song: *Gan jiao* and *ba jiao* are of identical nature.

【主治】癰腫結熱。别録。擣爛傅腫，去熱毒。擣汁服，治産後血脹悶。蘇恭。主黄疸。孟詵。治天行熱狂，煩悶消渴，患癰毒，并金石發動，躁熱口乾，并絞汁服之。又治頭風遊風。大明。

Control. Obstruction-illness[349] swelling with heat nodes. *Bie lu*. When it is pounded into a pulpy [mass] and applied to a swelling it removes heat poison. Pounded and the resulting juice ingested, it serves to cure distensions and heart-pressure related to blood [disorder] after birth. Su Gong. It controls yellow *dan*-illness/jaundice. Meng Shen. It serves to cure epidemic heat causing madness, vexing heart-pressure, melting with thirst[350] and suffering from obstruction-illness poison. Also, excitement [of qi] caused by [an ingestion of] metals and minerals, with restlessness, heat and a dry mouth. For all these, squeeze them to obtain a juice and ingest it. It also serves to cure head wind[351] and roaming wind.[352] Da Ming.

【附方】舊四，新六。

Added Recipes. Four of old. Six newly [recorded].

發背欲死。芭蕉根擣爛塗之。肘後方。

---

348 *Ke re* 客熱, "visitor heat," 1.) an etiological agent identified as heat evil intruding into the human organism from outside. 2.) A condition identical to *re* 熱, "heat." BCGM Dict I, 282.

349 *Yong* 癰, "obstruction-illness,"refers to an obstruction of vessels or other ducts inside the body. Qi rushing against the obstruction may cause a local swelling and eventually break through the surface to cause an abscess. BCGM Dict I, 641.

350 *Xiao ke* 消渴, "melting with thirst," most likely including cases of diabetes. BCGM Dict Vol I, 567.

351 *Tou feng* 頭風, "head wind." Condition of wind evil attacking the head followed by pain, dizziness, itching. BCGM Dict I, 509.

352 *You feng* 游風, "roaming wind," a condition of roaming and sudden pain and itching brought about by *feng xie* 風邪, "wind evil." BCGM Dict I, 645.

Effusion on the back[353] bringing one close to dying. Pound *ba jiao* root into a pulpy [mass] and apply it [to the affected region]. *Zhou hou fang*.

一切腫毒。方同上。

All types of swelling with poison. Recipe identical to the one above.

赤遊風瘮。方同上。

Red roaming wind papules.[354] Recipe identical to the one above.

風熱頭痛。方同上。

Headache related to wind [intrusion] and heat. Recipe identical to the one above.

風蟲牙痛。芭蕉自然汁一椀，煎熱含漱。普濟。

Toothache related to wind [intrusion and the presence of] worms/bugs. Boil one bowl of the natural juice of *ba jiao* to obtain a juice and hold it hot in the mouth to rinse [the affected teeth]. *Pu ji*.

天行熱狂。芭蕉根擣汁飲之。日華子本草。

Epidemic heat causing madness. Pound *ba jiao* root to obtain a juice and [let the patient] drink it. *Rihua zi ben cao*.

消渴飲水，骨節煩熱。用生芭蕉根擣汁，時飲一二合。聖惠方。

Melting with thirst[355] and [an urge to] drink water, with a vexing heat in the bone joints. Pound fresh *ba jiao* to obtain a juice and regularly drink one to two *ge*. *Sheng hui fang*.

353 *Fa bei* 發背, "effusion on/of the back," a condition of *yong* 癰, "obstruction-illnesses," and *ju* 疽, "impediment-illnesses," developing on one's back. As it was believed that the transporter holes of the five depots and six palaces are located on the back, conditions of obstruction-illnesses and impediment-illnesses there, often apparent as abscesses, were considered threatening. BCGM Dict I, 148.

354 *Feng zhen* 風疹, "wind papules," a condition, brought forth by wind evil, of eruptive skin papules of different sizes, accompanied by unbearable itching. If scratched they rise further. BCGM Dict I, 172.

355 *Xiao ke* 消渴, "melting with thirst," most likely including cases of diabetes. BCGM Dict Vol I, 567.

血淋澀痛。芭蕉根、旱蓮草各等分，水煎服，日二。聖惠方。

[Urinary] painful, rough dripping with blood. Boil equal amounts of *ba jiao* root and ink plant in water and ingest it. Twice a day. *Sheng hui fang*.

產後血脹。擣芭蕉根絞汁，溫服二三合。

Distension related to blood [disorder] following birth. Pound *ba jiao* root [to a pulp], squeeze it to obtain a juice, and [let the woman] ingest two to three *ge*.

瘡口不合。芭蕉根取汁，抹之良。直指方。

When a wound opening fails to close. Obtain the juice of *ba jiao* root and apply it [to the wound]. Good. *Zhi zhi fang*.

15-47-02
蕉油 *Jiao you*
Oil of [*ba*] *jiao*.

以竹筒插入皮中，取出，瓶盛之。

Insert a bamboo tube through the skin into the center [of a *ba jiao* fruit] and let [the oil] come out to fill a bottle.

【氣味】甘，冷，無毒。

Qi and Flavor. Sweet, cold, nonpoisonous.

【主治】頭風熱，止煩渴及湯火傷。梳頭，止女人髮落，令長而黑。大明。暗風癇病，涎作運悶欲倒者，飲之取吐，極有奇效。蘇頌。

Control. Head wind[356] with heat. It ends vexing thirst and harm caused by scalding and fire. Used for combing the head it ends hair loss of women, and lets [their hair] grow long and remain/turn black. Da Ming. Dim-vision wind[357] and epileptic disease, with salivation causing [brain] movement, heart-pressure and a tendency to fall to the ground. Drink [the oil] to stimulate vomiting. Excellent, with an extraordinary effect. Su Song.

---

356 *Tou feng* 頭風, "head wind." Condition of wind evil attacking the head followed by pain, dizziness, itching. BCGM Dict I, 509.

357 *An feng* 暗風, "dim-vision wind," a condition of sudden dizziness or transient unconsciousness. BCGM Dict I, 43.

【附方】新一。

Added Recipes. One newly [recorded].

小兒截驚。以芭蕉汁、薄荷汁煎勻，塗頭項，留顖門，塗四肢，留手足心勿塗，甚效。鄧筆峰雜興。

To cut fright in children. Boil equal amount of *ba jiao* juice and mint juice and apply this to the crown of the head, leaving the fontanel free, and apply it to the four limbs, leaving the palms of the hands and the soles of the feet free; do not apply it there!. Very effective. Deng Bifeng, *Za xing*.

【主治】腫毒初發，研末，和生薑汁塗之。時珍。聖惠方。

Control. Swelling with poison that has just begun to effuse. [Grind it into] powder, mix it with fresh ginger juice and apply this [to the affected region]. [Li] Shizhen. *Sheng hui fang*.

15-47-03
葉 *Ye*
Leaf [of *gan jiao*]

【附方】新一。

Added Recipes. One newly [recorded].

岐毒初起。芭蕉葉，熨斗内燒存性，入輕粉，麻油調塗，一日三上，或消或破，皆無痕也。仁齋直指方。

Scrofula poison swelling[358] that has just begun to rise. Burn *ba jiao* leaves in an iron vessel with their nature retained. Add calomel and apply this mixed with sesame oil. To be applied three times a day. [The poison swelling] will be either dissolved or broken open, and there will never be a scar left. *Renzhai zhi zhi fang*.

15-47-04
花 *Hua*
Flower [of *gan jiao*].

【主治】心痺痛。燒存性研，鹽湯點服二錢。日華。

Control. Painful blockage of heart [qi]. Burn [*gan jiao* flowers] with their nature retained and grind [the residue into powder]. Drip two *qian* [of the powder] into a salt decoction and ingest this. *Rihua*.

358 *Qi du* 岐毒 is a mistaken writing of [疾-失+其]毒, a kind of *luo li* 瘰癧, "scrofula pervasion-illness," whereby two or three connected swellings of the size of plum or date kernels appear either in the female breast or in the loins.

15-48
蘘荷別録中品
Rang he, FE *Bie lu*, Middle rank.

***Zingiber mioga* (Thunb.) Rosc. Japanese ginger.**

【校正】自菜部移入此，併入有名未用蘘草爲一。

Editorial Correction. Moved here from the section "vegetables." *Rang cao* 蘘草, formerly listed in the section "known by name but not in use" [of the *Bie lu*], is also included here.

【釋名】覆葅別録、蘘草別録、猼苴音博、蒚苴説文、嘉草。【弘景曰】本草白蘘荷，而今人呼赤者爲蘘荷，白者爲覆苴。蓋食以赤者爲勝，入藥以白者爲良，葉同一種爾。【時珍曰】覆苴，許氏説文作蒚苴，司馬相如上林賦作猼苴，與芭蕉音相近。離騷大招云：醢豚苦狗膾苴蓴。王逸注云：苴蓴，音愽，蘘荷也，見本草。而今之本草無之，則脱漏亦多矣。

Explanation of Names. *Fu ju* 覆葅, *Bie lu*. *Rang cao* 蘘草, *Bie lu*. *Bo ju* 猼苴, read *bo* 博, *Fu ju* 蒚苴, *Shuo wen*. *Jia cao* 嘉草. [Tao] Hongjing: The *Ben cao* lists a white/*bai rang he* 白蘘荷, and today's people call red specimens *rang he* 蘘荷, and white ones *fu ju* 覆苴. The fact is, for eating, the red ones are superior. For adding them to medication, the white ones are good. The leaves of both kinds are identical. [Li] Shizhen: *Fu ju* 覆苴 is written *fu ju* 蒚苴 in Mr. Xu [Shen's] *Shuo wen*. Sima Xiangru in his *Shang lin fu* writes *bo ju* 猼苴, a name read similar to *ba jiao* 芭蕉. *Li sao*, *Da zhao*, states: "Pickled pork is as bitter tasting as dog [meat] prepared with *ju bo* 苴蓴." Wang Yi in his comment states: "*Ju bo* 苴蓴, read *bo* 愽, is *rang he* 蘘荷. See the *Ben cao*." But the *Ben cao* available today does not list it. Many former listings are lost.

【集解】【別録曰】蘘草生淮南山谷。【頌曰】蘘荷，荆、襄江湖間多種之，北地亦有。春初生，葉似甘蕉，根似薑芽而肥，其葉冬枯，根堪爲葅。其性好陰，在木下生者尤美。潘岳閑居賦云蘘荷依陰，時藿向陽，是也。宗懔荆楚歲時記云：仲冬以鹽藏蘘荷，用備冬儲，又以防蟲。史游急就篇云：蘘荷冬日藏，其來遠矣。然有赤白二種，白者入藥，赤者堪噉，及作梅果多用之。【宗奭曰】蘘荷八九月間淹貯，以備冬月作蔬果。治病止用白者。【時珍曰】蘇頌圖經言"荆、襄江湖多種"，今訪之無復識者。惟楊慎丹鉛録云：急就章註蘘荷即今甘露。考之本草形性相同，甘露即芭蕉也。崔豹古今注云：蘘荷似芭蕉而白色，其子花生根中，花未敗時可食，久則消爛矣。根似薑。宜陰翳地，依蔭而生。又按王旻山居録云：蘘荷宜樹陰下，二月種之。一種永生，不須鋤耘，但加糞耳。八月初踏其苗令死，則根滋茂。九月初取其傍生根爲葅，亦可醬藏。十月中以糠覆其根下，則過冬不凍死也。

Collected Explanations. *Bie lu*: *Rang cao* grows in the mountain valleys of Huai nan. [Su] Song: *Rang he* is often planted in the region of rivers and lakes in Jing and Xiang. It is also found in the North. In spring it begins to grow. The leaves are similar to those of bananas. The root resembles that of ginger and taro, but is fatter. The leaves wither in winter. The root is suitable for a preparation as preserved vegetable. By its nature it prefers yin [(i. e., shady) locations] and [the roots of *rang he*] that grow under trees are especially delicious. When Pan Yue in his *Xian ju fu* states "*rang he* is inclined to yin; *agastache* [herbs] lean toward the yang," he is correct. Zong Lin in his *Jing Chu sui shi ji* states: "By mid-winter *rang he* preserved with salt is used as a winter provision. Also, it serves to keep away worms/bugs." When Shi You in his *Ji jiu pian* states: "*Rang he* is stored in winter," this has an origin long ago. There are two kinds, one red, one white. White ones are added to medication. Red ones are suitable for eating, and they are often used for preserving plums [and other] fruit. [Kou] Zongshi: *Rang he* is steeped and stored in the eighth and ninth month to be prepared for consumption in the winter months as vegetable or fruit. To cure diseases, only white ones are used. [Li] Shizhen: Su Song in his *Tu jing* says that "[*rang he*] is often planted in the region of the rivers and lakes of Jing and Xiang." According to a recent inquiry, [*rang he*] is no longer known there. Only Yang Shen in his *Dan qian lu* states: "A comment to the *Ji jiu zhang* says: '*Rang he* is today's *gan lu* 甘露, 'sweet dew'." Based on the *Ben cao*, *gan lu* are identical to bananas, as their physical appearance and nature are described as being the same. Cui Bao in his *Gu jin zhu* states: "*Rang he* resemble bananas, but they are white. Their seeds/fruit and flowers grow from inside the roots. They can be eaten as long as the flowers have not deteriorated. After a long time, they dissolve and turn pulpy. The root is similar to that of ginger. It needs a yin (i. e., shady) and concealed ground. It relies on a shady place to grow." Also, as Wang Min in his *Shan ju lu* states: "For *rang he* the yin (i. e., shady area) underneath trees is suitable. It is planted in the second month. There is no need to remove weeds with a hoe. Just add some manure [as fertilizer]. In the eighth month, trample on the seedlings to kill them. This will stimulate a profuse growth of the roots. In the ninth month gather the side roots and prepare them for [storage as] a preserved vegetable. They can also be stored in soy sauce. In the tenth month cover the ground underneath the roots with chaff. This way they will not freeze to death throughout winter."

【修治】【斅曰】凡使勿用革牛草，真相似，其革牛草腥澀。凡使白蘘荷，以銅刀刮去粗皮一重，細切，入砂盆中研如膏，取自然汁鍊作煎，新器攤冷，如乾膠狀，刮取用之。

Pharmaceutical Preparation. [Lei] Xiao: For all applications be sure not to use *ge niu cao*.[359] They are truly similar, but *ge niu cao* has a fishy smell and is astringent. For all applications of white *rang he*, use a copper knife to remove one layer of the coarse bark. Cut [the remaing item] into fine pieces, give them into a pottery basin and grind them to generate a paste. [Squeeze it] to get its natural juice and boil it. Give it then into a new vessel to let it turn cold. When it has reached the appearance of dry glue, scrape it off and remove it for later use.

15-48-01

根 *Gen*

Root [of *rang he*].

【氣味】辛，温，有小毒。【思邈曰】辛，微温，濇，無毒。

Qi and Flavor. Acrid, warm, slightly poisonous. [Sun] Simiao: Acrid, slightly warm, astringent, nonpoisonous.

【主治】中蠱及瘧，擣汁服。别録。溪毒，沙蝨，蛇毒。弘景。諸惡瘡。根心：主稻麥芒入目中不出，以汁注目即出。蘇恭。赤眼澀痛，擣汁點之。時珍。

Control. For being struck by *gu*,[360] and malaria, pound it to obtain a juice and ingest it. *Bie lu*. Rivulet poison.[361] Sand lice[362] Snake poison. [Tao] Hongjing. All types of malign sores. The core of the root [serves to] control the intrusion of rice and wheat awns into the eyes. Drip the juice into the [affected eyes] and they will come out. Su Gong. Red eyes with painful roughness. Pound [the root] and drip the [resulting] juice [into the affected eyes]. [Li] Shizhen.

15-48-02

蘘草 *Rang cao*

The herb of *rang* [*he*].

【氣味】苦、甘，寒，無毒。【大明曰】平。

Qi and Flavor. Bitter, sweet, cold, nonpoisonous. Da Ming: Balanced.

---

359 *Ge niu cao* 革牛草, lit: "herb depriving oxen of their skin," an unidentified herb.

360 *Gu du* 蠱毒, "*gu*-poison[ing]." (1) A poison emitted by certain worms/snakes with an ability to cause varying pathological changes in a person who has taken it in by means of wine or food. (2) Abdominal fullness, in some cases with blood spitting, and blood in the stool and urine. BCGM Dict I, 192 - 193. See BCGM 42-22.

361 *Xi du* 溪毒, "rivulet poison," 1.) A tiny bug assumed to live in bodies of water and supposedly capable of striking humans when they enter the water, thereby causing disease. 2.) A condition resulting from being struck by rivulet poison. BCGM Dict I, 548.

362 *Sha shi* 沙虱, "sand lice," small bugs, in former times assumed to live in waters or at the banks of waters and being able of penetrating the skin of people and cause disease.

【主治】温瘧寒熱，酸嘶邪氣，辟不祥。别録。

Control. Warmth malaria, with alternating sensations of cold and heat. Distress[363] related to the presence of evil qi. It wards off the inauspicious. *Bie lu*.

【發明】【弘景曰】中蠱者服蘘荷汁，并卧其葉，即呼蠱主姓名。多食損藥力，又不利脚。人家種之，亦云辟蛇。【頌曰】按干寳搜神記云：外姊夫蔣士先得疾下血，言中蠱。其家密以蘘荷置於席下，忽大笑曰：蠱我者，張小小也。乃收小小，小小亡走。自此解蠱藥多用之，往往驗也。周禮庶氏以嘉草除蠱毒，宗懔謂嘉草即蘘荷，是也。陳藏器云“蘘荷、茜根爲主蠱之最”，謂此。【時珍曰】别録菜部蘘荷，謂根也；草部蘘草，謂葉也。其主治亦頗相近，今併爲一云。

Explication. [Tao] Hongjing: Let a person struck by *gu* [poison][364] ingest *rang he* [herb] juice. Then he is to lie on [*rang he*] leaves and he will call the name of the person in control of the *gu*. Eaten in large quantities, it decreases the strength of medication [taken simultaneously], and it is not beneficial for leg [movement]. People plant it; they also claim that it keeps snakes away. [Su] Song: According to Gan Bao in his *Sou shen ji*, "Jiang Shixian, husband of his elder sister, fell ill with blood discharge. It was said that he was struck by *gu*. His family secretly placed *rang he* under his mat. Suddenly he laughed and shouted with a loud voice: 'The one who has plagued me with *gu* [poison] is Zhang Xiaoxiao.' [They went to] get [Zhang] Xiaoxiao, but [Zhang] Xiaoxiao had already disappeared; he had run away. Since then [*rang he* juice and leaves] are often used as medication to resolve *gu* [poison], and this has been successful again and again." According to the *Zhou li*, "Mr. Shu used *jia cao* 嘉草 to remove *gu* poison," and Zong Lin said: "*Jia cao* is *rang he*." This is correct. Chen Cangqi states: "*Rang he* and madder root are the very best [items] to control *gu* [poison]." [Li] Shizhen: The *rang he* listed in the *Bie lu* in the section "vegetables" is the root, while the *rang cao* listed in the section "herbs" refers to the leaves. Their potentials of therapeutic control are quite similar. Here now they are discussed in one entry.

363 *Suan si* 酸嘶, identical to *suan xi* 酸㾷, "distress." BCGM Dict I, 481/482.

364 *Gu du* 蠱毒, "*gu*-poison[ing]." (1) A poison emitted by certain worms/snakes with an ability to cause varying pathological changes in a person who has taken it in by means of wine or food. (2) Abdominal fullness, in some cases with blood spitting, and blood in the stool and urine. BCGM Dict I, 192 - 193. See BCGM 42-22.

【附方】舊八，新一。

Added Recipes. Eight of old. One newly [recorded].

卒中蠱毒，下血如鷄肝，晝夜不絶，臟腑敗壞待死者。以蘘荷葉密置病人席下，勿令知之，必自呼蠱主姓名也。梅師方。

Suddenly being struck by *gu* poison,[365] with a discharge of blood looking like chicken liver, ending neither during the day nor at night. When the long-term depots and short-term repositories have decayed, [victims] are bound to die. Secretly place *rang he* leaves under the patient's mat. He must not be informed of this. He will automatically shout out the name of the person controlling the *gu* [poison]. *Mei shi fang*.

喉中似物，吞吐不出，腹脹羸瘦。取白蘘荷根擣汁服，蠱立出也。梅師方。

A sensation in the throat as if an item were present there that cannot be made to come out either by swallowing it or by vomiting it, resulting in an abdominal distension and emaciation. Pound a *rang he* root and ingest the juice. The *gu* will come out immediately. *Mei shi fang*.

喉舌瘡爛。酒漬蘘荷根半日，含漱其汁，瘥乃止。外臺秘要。

Sores and pulpy deterioration of throat and tongue. Soak a *rang he* root in wine for half a day. Then hold the juice in the mouth and rinse [the affected region]. Stop [the treatment] when a cure is achieved. *Wai tai mi yao*.

吐血痔血。向東蘘荷根一把，擣汁三升服之。肘後方。

Blood spitting; bleeding piles. Pound a handful of *rang he* roots that have grown toward the East and ingest three *sheng* of their juice. *Zhou hou fang*.

婦人腰痛。方同上。

Painful lower back of women. Recipe identical to the one above.

月信澀滯。蘘荷根細切，水煎取二升，空心入酒和服。經驗方。

Rough and sluggish menstruation. Cut *rang he* roots into fine pieces and boil them in water to obtain two *sheng*. Add wine and ingest this on an empty stomach. *Jing yan fang*.

---

365 *Gu du* 蠱毒, "*gu*-poison[ing]." (1) A poison emitted by certain worms/snakes with an ability to cause varying pathological changes in a person who has taken it in by means of wine or food. (2) Abdominal fullness, in some cases with blood spitting, and blood in the stool and urine. BCGM Dict I, 192 - 193. See BCGM 42-22.

風冷失聲，咽喉不利。蘘荷根二兩，擣絞汁，入酒一大盞，和匀，細細服，取瘥。肘後方。

Loss of voice related to wind [intrusion] and [the presence of] cold, with a blocked throat passage. Pound two *liang* of *rang he* roots and squeeze [the pulp] to obtain a juice. Add one large cup of wine and mix it evenly. Ingest this in small quantities until a cure is achieved. *Zhou hou fang*.

傷寒時氣，温病初得，頭痛壯熱，脉盛者。用生蘘荷根葉合擣，絞汁服三四升。肘後。

Harm caused by cold related to [epidemic] seasonal qi. The beginning of an affliction by warmth disease, with headache and massive heat. Pound *rang he* root and leaves together, squeeze [the resulting pulp] to obtain a juice and ingest three to four *sheng*. *Zhou hou*.

雜物入目。白蘘荷根取心擣，絞取汁，滴入目中，立出。普濟方。

Various items have entered the eyes. Remove the core from a white *rang he* root and pound it. Squeeze [the pulp] to obtain a juice and drip it into the [affected] eyes. [The foreign item] will come out immediately. *Pu ji fang*.

15-49
麻黄本經中品
Ma huang. FE *Ben jing*, middle rank.

***Ephedra sinica* Stopf.**

【釋名】龍沙本經、卑相別録、卑鹽別録。【時珍曰】諸名殊不可解。或云其味麻，其色黄，未審然否？張揖廣雅云：龍沙，麻黄也。狗骨，麻黄根也。不知何以分別如此？

Explanation of Names. *Long sha* 龍沙, "dragon sand/droppings," *Ben jing*. *Bei xiang* 卑相, *Bie lu*. *Bei yan* 卑鹽, *Bie lu*. [Li] Shizhen: These names cannot be explained. Some say, the flavor [of *ma huang*] is "numbing," *ma* 麻, and its color is "yellow," *huang* 黄. Could this be so? Zhang Qi in his *Guang ya* states: "*Long sha* 龍沙 is *ma huang* 麻黄; *gou gu* 狗骨, 'dog bone,' is the root of *ma huang* 麻黄." It is not clear how these [names] can serve to distinguish these [items from others].

【集解】【別録曰】麻黄生晉地及河東，立秋采莖，陰乾令青。【弘景曰】今出青州、彭城、滎陽、中牟者爲勝，色青而多沫。蜀中亦有，不好。【恭曰】鄭州鹿臺及關中沙苑河旁沙州上最多，同州沙苑亦多。其青、徐者亦不復用。【禹錫曰】按段成式酉陽雜俎云：麻黄莖頭開花，花小而黄，叢生。子如覆盆子，可食。【頌曰】今近汴京多有之，以滎陽、中牟者爲勝。春生苗，至夏五月則長及一尺以來。梢上有黄花，結實如百合瓣而小，又似皂莢子，味甜，微有麻黄氣，外皮紅，裹仁子黑。根紫赤色。俗説有雌雄二種。雌者於三月、四月内開花，六月結子。雄者無花，不結子。至立秋後收莖，陰乾。【時珍曰】其根皮色黄赤，長者近尺。

Collected Explanations. *Bie lu*: *Ma huang* grows in Jin and in He dong. The stem is collected at Autumn Begins (August 7). It is dried in the yin (i. e., shade) and this lets it turn green. [Tao] Hongjing: Today, [*ma huang*] from Qing zhou, Peng cheng, Xing yang and Zhong mou is superior. Its color is greenish, and it contains much foam. It is also found in Shu, but not of good quality. [Su] Gong: The largest quantities grow in Lu tai of Zheng zhou and Sha yuan of Guang zhong, at river banks on sandy grounds. Much of it is also found in Sha yuan of Tong zhou. That from Qing and Xu is no longer in use. [Zhang] Yuxi: According to Duan Chengshi's *You yang za zu*, "the flowers of *ma huang* open at the top of the stem. The flowers are small and yellow; they grow in clusters. The seeds are similar to *rubus* seeds; they are edible." [Su] Song: Today it can be found in large quantities near Bian jing. Those from Xin yang and Zhong mou are superior. In spring [*ma huang*] grows a seedling. By summer, in the fifth month, it has reached a height of one *chi*. On its tip is a yellow flower. It forms fruits similar to those of Brown's lily, but they are smaller. Also, they resemble *gleditsia* pods/seeds. They have a sweet flavor and slightly emit *ma huang* qi. The outer bark is red; the kernels inside are black. The root is of a purple-red color. It is commonly said that there are two kinds: female and male. The females open flowers in the third and fourth month; they form seeds in the sixth month. The males have no flower, and they do not form seeds. After Autumn Begins (August 7) the stems are gathered; they are dried in the yin (i. e., shade). [Li] Shizhen: The bark of the root is yellow-red. Long ones reach a length of close to one *chi*.

【附録】
Appendix.

15-49-A01
雲花子 *Yun hua zi*
Unidentified.

【時珍曰】按葛洪肘後方治馬疥，有雲花草，云狀如麻黄而中堅實也。

[Li] Shizhen: According to Ge Hong's *Zhou hou fang*, to cure horse *jie*-illness,[366] *yun hua cao* is available. It states: "It is shaped like *ma huang*, but its center is solid."

366 *Ma jie* 馬疥, "horse *jie*-illness," a condition of *jie chuang* 疥瘡, "*jie*-illness sores," whereby the skin forms scales and scraps, while its base is rough and thick. It itches and if scratched one does not feel any pain. BCGM Dict I, 332.

莖 *Jing*
Stem [of *ma huang*].

【修治】【弘景曰】用之折去節根，水煮十餘沸，以竹片掠去上沫。沫令人煩，根節能止汗故也。

Pharmaceutical Preparation. [Tao] Hongjing: To use it [for therapeutic purposes], break it and remove the nodes and the root. Boil [the rest] in water at least ten times to bubbling. With a piece of bamboo remove the foam floating on the surface. The reason is, when the foam is cold it lets one experience vexation, and the root and the nodes can stop sweating.

【氣味】苦，温，無毒。【別録曰】微温。【普曰】神農、雷公：苦，無毒。扁鵲：酸。李當之：平。【權曰】甘，平。【元素曰】性温，味苦而甘辛，氣味俱薄，輕清而浮，陽也，升也。手太陰之藥，入足太陽經，兼走手少陰、陽明。【時珍曰】麻黄微苦而辛，性熱而輕揚。僧繼洪云：中牟有麻黄之地，冬不積雪，爲泄内陽也，故過用則洩真氣。觀此，則性熱可知矣。服麻黄自汗不止者，以冷水浸頭髮，仍用撲法即止。凡服麻黄藥，須避風一日，不爾病復作也。凡用須佐以黄芩，則無赤眼之患。【之才曰】厚朴、白微爲之使。惡辛夷、石韋。

Qi and Flavor. Bitter, warm, nonpoisonous. *Bie lu*: Slightly warm. [Wu] Pu: Shen nong, Lei gong: Bitter, nonpoisonous. Bian Que: Sour. Li Dangzhi: Balanced. [Zhen] Quan: Sweet, balanced. [Zhang] Yuansu: Its nature is warm; its flavor is bitter and sweet-acrid. Qi and flavor are all weakly pronounced. It is light and clear, and it floats. It is a yang [item]. It rises. It is a pharmaceutical drug for the hand major yin [conduits]. It enters the foot major yang conduits, and also rushes toward the hand minor yin and yang brilliance [conduits]. [Li] Shizhen: *Ma huang* is slightly bitter and acrid. Its nature is hot, and it is light and raising. Monk Ji Hong states: "In Zhong mou is an area where *ma huang* grows. No snow accumulates there in winter because of an outflow of the internal yang [qi of *ma huang*]. Hence its excessive application results in an outflow of true qi." In view of this, it is clear that its nature is hot. When an ingestion of *ma huang* results in unending sweating, [that person] should submerge the hair on his head in cold water. He needs to apply the method of bending over [into cold water] and [the sweating] ends. When a *ma huang* medication is ingested, wind is to be avoided for an entire day, lest the disease become active again. All applications [of *ma huang*] should be assisted by *scutellaria* [root]. This prevents suffering from red eyes. [Xu] Zhicai: *Magnolia* bark and *cynanchum atratum* [root] serve as guiding [substances]. [If ingested together,] it abhors *magnolia* flower buds and *pyrrosia* [leaves].

【主治】中風傷寒頭痛，温瘧，發表出汗，去邪熱氣，止欬逆上氣，除寒熱，破癥堅積聚。本經。五臟邪氣緩急，風脅痛，字乳餘疾，止好唾，通腠理，解肌，洩邪惡氣，消赤黑斑毒。不可多服，令人虛。别録。治身上毒風㿏痺，皮肉不仁，主壯熱温疫，山嵐瘴氣。甄權。通九竅，調血脉，開毛孔皮膚。大明。去營中寒邪，泄衛中風熱。元素。散赤目腫痛，水腫風腫，産後血滯。時珍。

Control. Headache related to wind stroke and harm caused by cold. Warmth malaria. It effuses [qi from] the exterior, stimulates sweating, removes evil heat qi, ends cough with qi rising in countermovement, ends alternating sensations of cold and heat and breaks through concretion-illness hardenings, accumulations and collections. *Ben jing*. Alternating episodes of slackening and tension related to the presence of evil qi in the five long-term depots, pain in the flanks because of wind [intrusion]. Ailments in the aftermath of delivery. It ends sleepiness, opens the passage through the interstitial structures, resolves [evil qi affecting] the muscles, drains evil and malign qi, and dissolves the poison in red and black macules. It must not be ingested in large amounts, lest it cause depletion. *Bie lu*. It serves to cure wind papules[367] and blockage related to rising poison, with numbness of the skin, and it controls strong heat and warmth epidemics, and hazy miasma qi in the mountains. Zhen Quan. It penetrates the nine orifices, regulates the blood vessels, and opens the hair pores in the skin. Da Ming. It removes cold evil from within the camp [qi, (i. e. blood)] and drains wind and heat from within the guardian [sector (i. e., qi)]. [Zhang] Yuansu. It disperses painful swelling of red eyes, water swelling and wind swelling, and sluggish blood following delivery. [Li] Shizhen.

【發明】【弘景曰】麻黄療傷寒，解肌第一藥。【頌曰】張仲景治傷寒，有麻黄湯及葛根湯、大小青龍湯，皆用麻黄。治肺痿上氣，有射干麻黄湯、厚朴麻黄湯，皆大方也。【杲曰】輕可去實，麻黄、葛根之屬是也。六淫有餘之邪，客於陽分皮毛之間，腠理閉拒，營衛氣血不行，故謂之實。二藥輕清成象，故可去之。麻黄微苦，其形中空，陰中之陽，入足太陽寒水之經。其經循背下行，本寒而又受外寒，故宜發汗，去皮毛氣分寒邪，以泄表實。若過發則汗多亡陽，或飲食勞倦及雜病自汗表虚之證用之，則脱人元氣，不可不禁。【好古曰】麻黄治衛實之藥，桂枝治衛虚之藥，二物雖爲太陽證藥，其實營衛藥也。心主營爲血，肺主衛爲氣。故麻黄爲手太陰肺之劑，桂枝爲手少陰心之劑。傷寒傷風而欬嗽，用麻黄、桂枝，即湯液之源也。【時珍曰】麻黄乃肺經專藥，故治肺病多用之。張仲景治傷寒無汗用麻黄，有汗用桂枝。歷代明醫解釋，皆隨文傅

367 *Feng zhen* 風疹, "wind papules," a condition, brought forth by wind evil, of eruptive skin papules of different sizes, accompanied by unbearable itching. If scratched they rise further. BCGM Dict I, 172.

會，未有究其精微者。時珍常釋思之，似有一得，與昔人所解不同云。津液爲汗，汗即血也。在營則爲血，在衛則爲汗。夫寒傷營，營血内濇，不能外通於衛，衛氣閉固，津液不行，故無汗發熱而憎寒。夫風傷衛，衛氣外泄，不能内護於營，營氣虚弱，津液不固，故有汗發熱而惡風。然風寒之邪，皆由皮毛而入。皮毛者，肺之合也。肺主衛氣，包羅一身，天之象也。是證雖屬乎太陽，而肺實受邪氣。其證時兼面赤怫鬱，欬嗽有痰，喘而胸滿諸證者，非肺病乎？蓋皮毛外閉，則邪熱内攻，而肺氣膹鬱。故用麻黄、甘草同桂枝，引出營分之邪，達之肌表，佐以杏仁泄肺而利氣。汗後無大熱而喘者，加以石膏。朱肱活人書，夏至後加石膏、知母，皆是泄肺火之藥。是則麻黄湯雖太陽發汗重劑，實爲發散肺經火鬱之藥也。腠理不密，則津液外泄，而肺氣自虚。虚則補其母。故用桂枝同甘草，外散風邪以救表，内伐肝木以防脾。佐以芍藥，泄木而固脾，泄東所以補西也。使以薑、棗，行脾之津液而和營衛也。下後微喘者加厚朴、杏仁，以利肺氣也。汗後脉沉遲者加人參，以益肺氣也。朱肱加黄芩爲陽旦湯，以瀉肺熱也。皆是脾肺之藥。是則桂枝雖太陽解肌輕劑，實爲理脾救肺之藥也。此千古未發之秘旨，愚因表而出之。又少陰病發熱脉沉，有麻黄附子細辛湯、麻黄附子甘草湯。少陰與太陽爲表裏，乃趙嗣真所謂熟附配麻黄，補中有發也。一錦衣夏月飲酒達旦，病水泄，數日不止，水穀直出，服分利、消導、升提諸藥則反劇。時珍診之，脉浮而緩，大腸下弩，復發痔血。此因肉食、生冷、茶水過雜，抑遏陽氣在下，木盛土衰，素問所謂久風成飧泄也。法當升之揚之。遂以小續命湯投之，一服而愈。昔仲景治傷寒六七日，大下後，脉沉遲，手足厥逆，咽喉不利，唾膿血，泄利不止者，用麻黄湯平其肝肺，兼升發之，即斯理也。神而明之，此類是矣。

Explication. [Tao] Hongjing: *Ma huang* is the number one pharmaceutical drug to heal harm caused by cold and to resolve [evil qi affecting] the muscles. [Su] Song: Zhang Zhongjing [in his recipes] to cure harm caused by cold resorted to the "decoction with *ma huang*"[368] and the "decoction with *pueraria* [root],"[369] as well as the major and minor "greenish dragon decoctions."[370] They all include *ma huang*, and they all are important recipes to cure lung dysfunction with rising qi. Then there are

368 *Ma huang tang* 麻黄湯及葛根湯, "decoction with ma huang," with the following ingredients: *Ma huang*, *cassia* twig, *glycyrrhiza* root, apricot seed.

369 *Ge gen tang* 葛根湯, "decoction with *pueraria* root," with the following ingredients: *Pueraria* root, *ma huang*, *cassia* twig, white *paeonia* root, *glycyrrhiza* root, fresh ginger, Chinese date.

370 *Da qing long tang* 大青龍湯, "major greenish dragon decoction," with the following ingredients: *Ma huang*, *cassia* twig, *glycyrrhiza* root, apricot seed, fresh ginger, Chinese date, gypsum. *Xiao qing long tang* 小青龍湯, "minor greenish dragon decoction," with the ingredients *ma huang*, *paeonia* root, *asarum heteropoides* herb, dried ginger, *glycyrrhiza* root, *cassia* twig, *schisandra* seed, and *pinellia* tuber.

the "decoction with blackberry lily [root]"[371] and the "decoction with *magnolia* bark and *ma huang*."[372] Both are great recipes. [Li] Gao: "Light [substances] can eliminate repletion. *Ma huang* and *pueraria* root belong to this group." When evil [qi] of excessively pronounced six types of licentiousness have settled in the region of skin and hair of the yang section, with a closure of the intersticial structures and a blocked passage of camp and guardian [qi, (i. e.,)] blood and qi, this is called repletion. The two pharmaceutical drugs [*ma huang* and *pueraria* root] exemplify lightness and purity. It is therefore that they can eliminate such [repletion]. *Ma huang* is slightly bitter. Its physical form is hollow inside; it is a yang in yin [item]. It enters the foot major yang conduit of cold water. This conduit passes downward along the spine. Its basic [nature] is cold, and it also accepts cold from outside. Hence it is advisable to stimulate sweating to remove cold evil from the qi section of skin and hair, in order to drain a repletion in the [body's] outer region. If such stimulation of sweating is excessive, with much sweating, yang [qi, too,] are lost. Or, if it is applied in the case of illness signs of a depletion in the [body's] outer region, as may be the result of drinking and eating, or physical overexertion, then this leads to a loss of that person's original qi. This must be avoided! [Wang] Haogu: *Ma huang* is a pharmaceutical drug to cure guardian [qi] repletion. *Cassia* twig is a pharmaceutical drug to cure guardian [qi] depletion. Although these two items are drugs for major yang signs, they are in fact drugs for the camp and guardian [qi]. The heart controls the camp [qi, (i. e.,)] the blood. The lung controls the guardian [qi, (i. e.,)] qi. Therefore, *ma huang* is a preparation for the hand major yang [conduits of the] lung. *Cassia* twigs are a preparation for the hand minor yin [conduits of the] heart. When for harm caused by cold and harm caused by wind with cough *ma huang* and *cassia* twigs are resorted to, then they constitute the very source of the respective decoctions. [Li] Shizhen: *Ma huang* is a pharmaceutical drug especially for the lung conduits. Hence it is often used to cure lung diseases. When Zhang Zhongjing cured harm caused by cold without sweating, he used *ma huang*. For [harm caused by cold] with sweating, he used *cassia* twigs. In the course of history, when famous physicians explained [their therapeutic approach] they followed him, clinging to his texts without further consideration. There has never been an investigation of the seminal essentials [underlying Zhang Zhongjing's treatments]. [I, Li] Shizhen have always thought about an explanation. When eventually [I] arrived at it, it differed

---

371 *She gan ma huan tang* 射干麻黄湯, "decoction with blackberry lily and *ma huang*,"with the following ingredients: Blackberry lily root, *ma huang*, fresh ginger, *asarum heteropoides* herb, winter aster root, coltsfoot, *schisandra* seed, *pinellia* root and Chinese date.

372 *Hou po ma huang tang* 厚朴麻黄湯, "decoction with *magnolia* bark and *ma huang*," with the following ingredients: *Magnolia* bark, gypsum, *pinellia* root, *schisandra* seed, dried ginger, *asarum heteropoides* herb, and wheat.

from the explanations offered by persons of former times, as follows. Body liquids form the sweat, and sweat is blood. In terms of camp [qi] it is blood; in terms of guardian [qi] it is sweat. Now, cold harms the camp [qi]. When the camp [qi] are locked down in the interior, they are unable to communicate with the guardian [qi] in the exterior. When the guardian [qi] are blocked and shut in, the body liquids fail to pass. Hence there is no sweating. Heat effusion and an aversion to cold result. Now, when wind harms the guardian [qi], the guardian [qi] flow off toward the outside and are unable to offer protection to the camp [qi] inside. When the camp qi are depleted and weak, the body liquids are unstable. This then results in sweating, an effusion of heat and an aversion to wind. As it is, the evil [qi] of wind and cold always enter [the body] via skin and hair. Skin and hair form a union with the lung. The lung controls the guardian qi; enclosing the entire body like a net. This is the image of heaven. Although the [illness] signs [listed above] belong to major yang, it is a lung repletion resulting from its having received evil qi. The [illness] signs may include a red face with anger and depression, cough with phlegm, panting and a feeling of fullness in the chest. When all such signs appear – is this not a lung disease? The fact is, when skin and hair are closed on the outside, evil heat attacks internally and the lung qi are pent up. Therefore, one resorts to *ma huang* and *glycyrrhica* [root] joined by *cassia* twigs to lead away the evil [qi] in the camp [qi] section, guiding them to the exterior [section] of the muscles. This is assisted by apricot seeds to drain the lung and free the flow of its qi. If following sweating no great heat effuses, with [the patient] panting, one adds gypsum. Zhu Gong in his *Huo ren shu* [recommends to] "add gypsum and *anemarrhena* [root] after Summer Solstice (June 21)." Both are drugs draining lung fire. That is, even though the "decoction with *ma huang*" is an important preparation stimulating sweating in the major yang [region], it is truly a pharmaceutical drug serving to effuse and disperse pent-up fire in the lung conduits. When the intersticial structures are not closed, the body liquids flow off toward the outside and the lung qi will be depleted as a result. "In the case of such a depletion, one supplements [qi in] the [long-term depot lung's] mother [i. e., the long-term depot spleen]." Hence *cassia* twigs and *glycyrrhiza* [root] are used to disperse the evil [qi] of wind and safeguard the exterior [body section] in the outer [region] and to fell the liver [associated with the phase] wood in the interior to protect the spleen [associated with the phase soil, the mother phase of metal, associated with the lung]. This is assisted by *paeonia* [root] medication, serving to drain wood [i. e., liver qi] and to stabilize the spleen. That is, one drains in the East to supplement in the West. Ginger and Chinese dates serve as guiding [substances] to stimulate the passage of the body liquids of the spleen and to harmonize [the communication of] camp and guardian [qi]. If following [such a therapy patients] suffer from slight panting, add *magnolia* bark and apricot seeds to free the passage of lung qi. If after the sweating the [movement in the] vessels is in the depth, add ginseng [root] to boost the lung qi. Zhu Gong adds *scutellaria* [root] to create the "decoction for a daybreak of yang [qi]," to drain lung heat. All these are medications for the spleen and the lung. That is, although *cassia* twigs are a light preparation to resolve muscle [qi] in the major yang section, they are really a pharmaceutical drug to order spleen [qi] in order to safeguard the lung. This is a secret aim that has never been disclosed since a thousand [years] before. Hence I have published it here. Also, for a minor yin disease with heat effusion and a deep [movement in the] vessels, the "decoction with *ma huang*, *aconitum* [accessory tuber] and *asarum heteropoides* [root]" and the "decoction with *ma huang*, *aconitum* [accessory tuber] and *glycyrrhiza* [root]" are available. A minor yin and major yang constitute outside and inside. This corresponds to what Zhao Sizhen has said to require a combination of *aconitum* [accessory tuber] with *ma huang*, that is an effusion within supplementation. An embroidered-uniform guard once in a summer month drank wine until daybreak and then suffered from a watery outflow that lasted for several days. Water and grain [consumed] left [the body] right away. He ingested all types of medication to rearrange the flow [of liquid and solid food], to dissolve and lead off [evil qi], and to raise [the qi responsible for unending discharge], but contrary [to expectations, the disease only] increased in severity. [I, Li] Shizhen diagnosed his [condition]. The [movement in the] vessels was in the depth and slowed. His large intestine had descended to generate a tumorous flesh growth, repeatedly developing bleeding piles. This had resulted from an excessive mixture of meat, raw and cold items, tea and water, repressing and holding back yang qi below. The wood [i. e., the liver qi] flourished, while the soil [i. e., the spleen qi] was weakened. This was a case termed in the *Su wen* "outflow of undigested food caused by wind."[373] The [appropriate therapeutic] approach requires "to raise, to lift." Hence [I] prescribed the "minor decoction to prolong life."[374] One single ingestion resulted in a cure. Formerly, when [Zhang] Zhongjing cured harm caused by cold lasting six, seven days, after stimulating massive discharge, the [movement in the] vessels was in the depth and slowed down. Hands and feet experienced a [yang qi] recession and countermovement. The throat was blocked. [Patients] spat pus and blood and expe-

373 Worded *jiu feng wei sun xie* 久風為飧泄 in *Su wen*, ch. 17. Paul U. Unschuld and Hermann Tessenow, *Huang Di Nei Jing Su Wen. An Annotated Translation of Huang Di's Inner Classic*, 2 vols. University of California Press, Berkeley and Los Angeles, 2011. Vol. 1, 293

374 *Xiao xu ming tang* 小續命湯, the "minor decoction to prolong life," includes the following ingredients: *Ma huang*, *stephania tetandra* root, ginseng root, *scutellaria* root, shaved cinnamom bark, *glycyrrhiza* root, *paeonia* root, *ligusticum* root, apricot seed, *aconitum* accessory tuber, *saposhnikovia* root and fresh ginger.

rienced unending outflow with free flow. In such a situation, [Zhang Zhongjing] used the "decoction with *ma huang*" to balance liver and lung [qi], and to simultaneously raise and effuse [qi]. This was based on the principle outlined above. It belongs to those [principles] that reflect a divine understanding.

【附方】舊五，新七。

Added Recipes. Five of old. Seven newly [recorded].

天行熱病，初起一二日者。麻黄一大兩去節，以水四升煮，去沫，取二升，去滓，着米一匙及豉爲稀粥。先以湯浴後，乃食粥，厚覆取汗，即愈。孟詵必效方。

Epidemic heat disease that has just begun one or two days before. Boil one generous *liang* of *ma huang*, with its nodes removed, in four *sheng* of water, continuously removing the foam, down to two *sheng*. Remove the dregs. Add one spoon of rice and some [soybean] relish and prepare a congee. [Let the patient] first bathe in hot water and then eat the congee. Cover him thickly so that he sweats, and this results in a cure. Meng Shen, *Bi xiao fang*.

傷寒雪煎。麻黄十斤去節，杏仁四升去皮熬，大黄一斤十二兩。先以雪水五碩四斗，漬麻黄於東向竈釜中。三宿後，納大黄攪匀，桑薪煮至二石，去滓。納杏仁同煮至六七斗，絞去滓，置銅器中。更以雪水三斗合煎，令得二斗四升，藥成，丸如彈子大。有病者以沸白湯五合，研一丸服之，立汗出。不愈，再服一丸。封藥勿令洩氣。千金方。

Harm caused by cold, [medication] boiled with snow [water]. [Prepare the following items.] Ten *jin* of *ma huang*, with the nodes removed. Four *jin* of apricot kernels, with the skin removed and then simmered. One *jin* and 12 *liang* of rhubarb root. First soak the *ma huang* in five *dan* and four *dou* of snow water in a cauldron on a stove facing East. After three days add the rhubarb root and mix it evenly. Boil this over a mulberry twig fire down to two *dan*, remove the dregs, add the apricot seeds and boil this down to six, seven *dou*. Squeeze this to discard the dregs, and place [the juice] into a copper vessel. Add further three *dou* of snow water and and boil this down to two *dou* and four *sheng*. Now the medication is ready; it is prepared to pills the size of a bullet. In the case of a disease, grind one pill in five *ge* of bubbling hot water and ingest it. This will stimulate an immediate sweating. If no cure results, ingest one more pill. Keep the medication tightly sealed so that its qi do not drain away. *Qian jin fang*.

傷寒黄疸。表熱者，麻黄醇酒湯主之。麻黄一把，去節綿裹，美酒五升，煮取半升，頓服取小汗。春月用水煮。千金方。

Harm caused by cold with yellow *dan*-illness/jaundice and effusion of heat is controlled by the "decoction with *ma huang* and pure wine." Remove the nodes from one handful of *ma huang*, wrap it in silk floss and boil this in five *sheng* of delicious wine down to half a *sheng*. Ingest it all at once to stimulate a slight sweating. During spring months boil it in water. *Qian jin fang*.

裹水黄腫。張仲景云：一身面目黄腫，其脉沉，小便不利，甘草麻黄湯主之。麻黄四兩，水五升，煮去沫，入甘草二兩，煮取三升。每服一升，重覆汗出。不汗再服。慎風寒。千金云：有患氣急久不瘥，變成水病，從腰以上腫者，宜此發其汗。

Yellow swelling[375] with water inside [the body]. Zhang Zhongjing: "When the entire body, the face and the eyes are yellow and swollen, with a deep [movement in the] vessels, and blocked urination, this is controlled by the "decoction with *glycyrrhiza* [root] and *ma huang*." Boil four *liang* of *ma huang* in five *sheng* of water and remove the foam. Add two *liang* of *glycyrrhiza* [root] and boil this down to three *sheng*. Each time [let the patient] ingest one *sheng* and cover him warmly to stimulate sweating. If he fails to sweat, let him ingest [the liquid] again. Keep him away from wind and cold." The *Qian jin* states: "If someone suffers from acute qi [disorder] that is not cured for a long time, this may change into a water disease. In the case of a swelling extending from the lower back upward, this [medication] is suitable for stimulating sweating."

水腫脉沉。屬少陰。其脉浮者爲風，虚脹者爲氣，皆非水也。麻黄附子湯汗之。麻黄三兩，水七升，煮去沫，入甘草二兩，附子炮一枚，煮取二升半。每服八分，日三服，取汗。張仲景金匱要略。

A water swelling with a deep [movement in the] vessels is associated with the minor yin. When the [movement in the] vessels is floating, this is a sign of wind. In the case of a depletion swelling, it is a qi [disorder]. All these are not water [swellings]. Induce sweating with the "decoction with *ma huang* and *aconitum* [accessory tuber]." Boil three *liang* of *ma huang* in seven *sheng* of water and remove the foam. Add two *liang* of *glycyrrhiza* [root] and one *aconitum* [accessory tuber], roasted in a pan, and boil this down to two and a half *sheng*. Each time ingest eight *fen*, to be ingested three times a day, to stimulate sweating. Zhang Zhongjing, *Jin kui yao lüe*.

375 *Huang zhong* 黄腫, "yellow swelling," an illness sign of a *shui zhong* 水腫, "water swelling," an edematose disease with a swelling covering the entire body and the skin assuming a yellow complexion. BCGM Dict I, 227.

風痺冷痛。麻黄去根五兩，桂心二兩，爲末，酒二升，慢火熬如餳。每服一匙，熱酒調下，至汗出爲度。避風。聖惠方。

Painful closure/numbness related to the presence of wind and cold. [Grind] five *liang* of *ma huang*, with the root removed, and two *liang* of shaved cinnamom bark into powder and boil this in two *sheng* of wine over a slow fire until it has taken on a consistency of malt-sugar. Each time ingest the amount held by one spoon, to be sent down mixed with hot wine until a sweating results. [During this treatment] avoid an exposure to wind. *Sheng hui fang.*

小兒慢脾風，因吐泄後而成。麻黄長五寸十箇去節，白术指面大二塊，全蠍二箇，生薄荷葉包煨，爲末。二歲以下一字，三歲以上半錢，薄荷湯下。聖惠方。

Slow spleen wind[376] of children following an episode of spitting/vomiting and outflow. [Grind] ten *ma huang* [stems] of a lengh of five *cun*, with the nodes removed, two *atractylodes macrocephala* [rhizomes], the size of a thumb, and two complete scorpions, wrapped in fresh mint leaves, into powder. Let [children] up to the age of two years ingest one *zi* , and [children] aged three years or older half a *qian*, to be sent down mixed with a mint decoction. *Sheng hui fang.*

尸咽痛痺，語聲不出。麻黄以青布裹，燒烟筒中熏之。聖惠方。

Corpse [bugs/worms] throat[377] with a painful closure and an inability to speak. Wrap *ma huang* in a greenish piece of cloth, burn this and steam [the affected region] with the fumes passing through a tube. *Sheng hui fang.*

産後腹痛，及血下不盡。麻黄去節，爲末，酒服方寸匕，一日二三服，血下盡即止。子母秘録。

Abdominal pain after delivery, with an unending discharge of blood. [Grind] *ma huang*, with the nodes removed, into powder and ingest with wine the amount held by a square *cun* spoon. To be ingested two or three times a day. End [the treatment] when the bleeding ends. *Zi mu mi lu.*

心下悸病。半夏麻黄丸：用半夏、麻黄等分，末之，煉蜜丸小豆大。每飲服三丸，日三服。金匱要略。

Palpitation disease below the heart. The "pills with *pinellia* [root] and *ma huang.*" Grind equal amounts of *pinellia* [root] and *ma huang* and form with heat refined

376 *Man pi feng* 慢脾風, "slow spleen wind," a condition of a *jing feng* 驚風, "fright wind," characterized by recurrent cramps in the presence or absence of fever. The cramps are slow and not very forceful. BCGM Dict I, 334.

377 *Shi yan* 屍咽, "corpse [bugs/worms] throat," a condition of a disease affecting the throat with pain and itching and loss of voice. BCGM Dict I, 458.

honey pills the size of mung beans. Each time ingest with a beverage three pills, to be ingested three times a day. *Jin kui yao lüe.*

痘瘡倒黶。寇宗奭曰：鄭州麻黄去節半兩，以蜜一匙同炒良久，以水半升煎數沸，去沫，再煎去三分之一，去滓，乘熱服之。避風，其瘡復出也。

Smallpox sores with inverse moles. Kou Zongshi: Fry half a *liang* of *ma huang* from Zhen zhou, with the nodes removed, in one spoonful of honey for an extended period of time. Then boil this with half a *sheng* of water several times to bubbling. Remove the foam and again boil [the liquid], this time down by one third. Remove the dregs and ingest [the liquid] hot. [During the treatment, exposure to] wind is to be avoided, lest the sores break out again.

一法：用無灰酒煎，其效更速。仙源縣筆工李用之子病斑瘡，風寒倒黶已困，用此一服便出，如神。

Another method. Boil [the *ma huang*] in ash-free wine and the effects will be even faster. The son of Li Yong, a maker of writing brushs in Xian yuan xian, suffered from [smallpox] macule sores. The presence of wind and cold had caused inverse moles, and his condition was critical. He ingested one dose of this and [the moles] came out. Divine.

中風諸病。麻黄一秤去根，以王相日、乙卯日，取東流水三石三斗，以净鐺盛五七斗，先煮五沸，掠去沫，逐旋添水，盡至三五斗，漉去麻黄，澄定，濾去滓，取清再熬至一斗，再澄再濾，取汁再熬，至升半爲度，密封收之，一二年不妨。每服一二匙，熱湯化下取汗。熬時要勤攪，勿令着底，恐焦了。仍忌鷄犬陰人見之。此劉守真秘方也。宣明方。

All types of wind stroke diseases. On *wang xiang*[378] and *yi mao* days[379] acquire three *dan* and three *dou* of water flowing toward the East. Fill five to seven *dou* into a clean flat pan and boil it first [with the *ma huang*] five times to bubbling. Remove the foam, and alternately add water, up to three to five *dou*. Then seep it through a filter to remove the *ma huang* and wait for the dregs to settle. Filter [the liquid] to remove the dregs. Boil the clear liquid down to one *dou*, and alternately let [the dregs] settle, filter [the liquid] and heat the juice again until one and a half *sheng*

378 *Wang xiang ri* 王相日, lit.: "sovereign and prime minister days," refer to auspicious "sovereign days," *wang ri* 王日, and "prime minister days," *xiang ri* 相日, in the course of the four seaons. "Sovereign days" are *yan* 寅 days in spring, *si* 巳 days in summer, *shen* 申 in autumn, and *hai* 亥 days in winter. "Prime minister days" are *si* 巳 days in spring, *shen* 申 days in summer, *hai* 亥 days in autumn, and *yan* 寅 days in winter.

379 *Yi mao ri* 乙卯日, auspicious days identified as days associated with *yi* 乙, the second of the celestial stems, *tian gan* 天干, and *mao* 卯, the fourth of the earth branches, *di zhi* 地支.

are left. Store this tightly sealed and do not touch it for one or two years. Each time ingest one or two spoons, to be sent down dissolved in hot water to stimulate sweating. While [the liquid] is being heated, stir it continuously. Do not let it attach itself to the bottom for too long, as it might be scorched. Also, see to it that no chickens, dogs or yin (i. e., female] persons come in view. This is a secret recipe of Liu Shouzhen. *Xuan ming fang*.

15-49-01
根節 *Gen jie*
Root and nodes [of *ma huang*].

【氣味】甘，平，無毒。

Qi and Flavor. Sweet, balanced, nonpoisonous.

【主治】止汗，夏月雜粉撲之。弘景。

Control. To end sweating, mix them with a powder and apply this. [Tao] Hongjing.

【發明】【權曰】麻黄根節止汗，以故竹扇杵末同撲之。又牡蠣粉、粟粉并麻黄根等分，爲末，生絹袋盛貯。盜汗出，即撲，手摩之。【時珍曰】麻黄發汗之氣駃不能禦，而根節止汗效如影響，物理之妙，不可測度如此。自汗有風濕、傷風、風温、氣虚、血虚、脾虚、陰虚、胃熱、痰飲、中暑、亡陽、柔痓諸證，皆可隨證加而用之。當歸六黄湯加麻黄根，治盜汗尤捷。蓋其性能行周身肌表，故能引諸藥外至衛分而固腠理也。本草但知撲之之法，而不知服餌之功尤良也。

Explication. [Zhen] Quan: To end sweating with *ma huang* root and nodes grind them together with an old bamboo fan into powder and apply it [to the patient's skin]. Also, [grind] oyster shell powder and millet powder with *ma huang* root into powder and keep this filled in a pouch made of new tough silk. In the case of robber sweating,[380] apply it [to the skin] by rubbing it with the hand. [Li] Shizhen: The qi of *ma huang* that stimulate sweating can hardly be controlled, and the potential of its root and nodes to end sweating is tied to them like a shadow or an echo. These are the wondrous principles underlying the items. Nobody can imagine them. Spontaneous sweating may be associated with the following conditions: Wind and moisture [intrusion], harm caused by wind, wind and warmth [intrusion], qi depletion, blood depletion, spleen [qi] depletion, yin [qi] depletion, stomach heat, phlegm rheum, struck by summer heat, loss of yang [qi] and soft spasms.[381] For all these

380 *Dao han* 盜汗, "robber sweating," (1) an illness sign of a profuse sweating during sleep that ends when one wakes up. (2) A pathological condition with robber sweating as major sign. BCGM Dict I, 122.

381 *Rou si* 柔痓, identical to *rou jing* 柔痙, "soft spasms," a condition of *jing bing* 痙病, "spasms disease," with the special characteristic of feverish sweating without an aversion

cases [of spontaneous sweating] decide about adding [the respective pharmaceutical drugs] in accordance with the presence of any of these conditions. When *ma huang* root is added to the "decoction with Chinese *angelica* [root] and the six [items bearing in their names the character] *huang*,"[382] this serves to cure robber sweating especially fast. The fact is, its nature can pass through all the muscles in the outer sphere of the entire body. Therefore it is capable of pulling all types of drugs toward the outside into the guardian [qi] section and to stabilize the membrane/intersticial structures.[383] The *Ben cao* knows only the method of applying it [to the skin]; it does not know that ingesting it has an especially good [therapeutic] potential.

【附方】新八。
Added Recipes. Eight newly [recorded].

盗汗陰汗。麻黄根、牡蠣粉爲末，撲之。

Robber sweating, yin sweating.[384] [Grind] *ma huang* root and oyster shell powder into powder and apply it [to the affected region].

盗汗不止。麻黄根、椒目等分，爲末。每服一錢，無灰酒下。外以麻黄根、故蒲扇爲末，撲之。奇效良方。

Unending robber sweating. [Grind] equal amounts of *ma huang* root and Chinese pepper into powder. Each time ingest one *qian*, to be sent down with ash-free wine. For external [use, grind] *ma huang* root and an old cattail leaf fan into powder and apply this [to the affected region]. *Qi xiao liang fang*.

小兒盗汗。麻黄根三分，故蒲扇灰一分，爲末，以乳服三分，日三服。仍以乾蕫三分同爲末，三分撲之。古今録驗。

Robber sweating[385] of children. [Grind] three fen of *ma huang* root and one fen of an old cattail leaf fan into powder and ingest three *fen* of this with a nursing mother's

to cold. BCGM Dict I, 409.

382 *Dang gui liu huang tang* 當歸六黄湯, "decoction with Chinese *angelica* [root] and the six [items bearing in their names the character] *huang*," has the following ingredients: Chinese *angelica* root, Chinese foxglove rhizome, prepared Chinese foxglove rhizome, *coptis* rhizome, *scutellaria* root, *phellodendron* bark, *astragalus* root.

383 Instead of *mo li* 膜理, "membrane structure," the Zhang edition writes *cou li* 腠理

384 *Yin han* 陰汗, "yin sweating," an illness sign of sweating in the frontal 'yin region', at the scrotum and at the perineum. Also, a condition with sweating in the yin (i. e., genital) region as a major sign. BCGM Dict I, 634.

385 *Dao han* 盗汗, "robber sweating," (1) an illness sign of a profuse sweating during sleep that ends when one wakes up. (2) A pathological condition with robber sweating as major sign. BCGM Dict I, 122.

milk. To be ingested three times a day. Also, grind three *fen* [of the powder] together with dried ginger into powder, and apply three *fen* [to the affected region]. *Gu jin lu yan.*

諸虛自汗：夜卧即甚，久則枯瘦。黄芪、麻黄根各一兩，牡蠣米泔浸洗煅過一兩，爲散。每服五錢，水二盞，小麥百粒，煎服。和劑局方。

All types of spontaneous sweating associated with a depletion, reaching an extreme at nighttime during one's sleep. If this continues for a long time, [the patient's body] is withered and emaciated. [Grind] one *liang* each of *astragalus* [root] and *ma huang* root with one *liang* of oysters, steeped in water that was used to wash rice first and then calcined, into powder. Each time ingest five *qian*. Boil this in two cups of water to which are added 100 grains of wheat, and ingest [the resulting decoction]. *He ji ju fang.*

虛汗無度。麻黄根、黄芪等分，爲末，飛麪糊作丸梧子大。每用浮麥湯下百丸，以止爲度。談埜翁試驗方。

Boundless sweating associated with a depletion. [Grind] equal amounts of *ma huang* root and *astragalus* [root] into powder and form, with wheat flour, pills the size of *wu* seeds. Each time send down 100 pills with a wheat bran decoction until [the sweating] ends. Tan Yeweng, *Shi yan fang.*

産後虛汗。黄芪、當歸各一兩，麻黄根二兩。每服一兩，煎湯下。

Depletion sweating following delivery. Each time ingest one *liang* each of *astragalus* [root] and Chinese *angelica* [root], and three *liang* of *ma huang* root, to be sent down as a decoction.

陰囊濕瘡，腎有勞熱。麻黄根、石硫黄各一兩，米粉一合，爲末，傅之。千金方。

Moist scrotum sores, with exhaustion heat[386] in the kidneys. [Grind] one *liang* each of *ma huang* root and sulphur, and one *ge* of rice powder into powder and apply this [to the affected region]. *Qian jin fang.*

内外障翳。麻黄根一兩，當歸身一錢，同炒黑色，入麝香少許，爲末。嗃鼻，頻用。此南京相國寺東黑孩兒方也。普濟。

Internal and external obstructive shade [in the eyes]. Fry one *liang* of *ma huang* root together with one *qian* of Chinese *angelica* [root] body until they have assumed a black color. Add a little musk and [grind this] into powder. Inhale this through the

386 *Lao re* 勞熱, "exhaustion heat," a condition of depletion heat brought forth by yin [qi] depletion. BCGM Dict I, 299.

nose and use it repeatedly. This is a Black Child[387] recipe from the eastern part of the Prime Minister monastery in Nan jing. *Pu ji.*

15-50
木賊宋嘉祐
Mu zei, FE *Jia you.*

***Hippochaete hyemale* (L.) Borher. Winter horsetail.**

【釋名】【時珍曰】此草有節，面糙澀。治木骨者，用之磋擦則光净，猶云木之賊也。

Explanation of Names. [Li] Shizhen: This herb has nodes, and its surface is rough. It is used to process *acanthopanax* [root bark/stem], *mu gu* 木骨 (lit.: "wooden bone"), by rubbing it so that it becomes clean and shiny. This may be the reason why it is called "the robber of wood," *mu zhi zei* 木之賊.

【集解】【禹錫曰】木賊出秦、隴、華、成諸郡近水地。苗長尺許，叢生。每根一幹，無花葉，寸寸有節，色青，凌冬不凋。四月采之。【頌曰】所在近水地有之，采無時，今用甚多。【時珍曰】叢叢直上，長者二三尺，狀似鳧茈苗及粽心草而中空有節，又似麻黄莖而稍粗，無枝葉。

Collected Explanations. [Zhang] Yuxi: *Mu zei* comes from all the prefectures of Qin, Long, Hua and Cheng that lie close to waters. The seedlings are more than one *chi* long; they grow as clusters. Each root develops one stalk; they have neither flowers nor leaves. They have nodes *cun* after *cun*. They are greenish and even in cold winter they do not wither. They are collected in the fourth month. [Su] Song: [*Mu zei*] can be found on grounds near a water. It can be collected any time. Today it is used very often. [Li] Shizhen: Clusters of it rise straight upward. They may reach a length of two or three *chi*. They resemble *eleocharis* seedlings and *diarrhena* herb, but they are hollow and have nodes. They also resemble *ephedra* herb stems, but are a little rougher. They have no branches and leaves.

15-50-01
莖 *Jing*
Stem [of *mu zei*]

【氣味】甘，微苦，無毒。【時珍曰】温。

Qi and Flavor: Sweet, slightly bitter, nonpoisonous. [Li] Shizhen: Warm.

387 For *hei hai er* 黑孩兒, "black child," see BCGM Dict III, 180.

【主治】目疾，退翳膜，消積塊，益肝膽，療腸風，止痢，及婦人月水不斷，崩中赤白。嘉祐。解肌，止淚止血，去風濕，疝痛，大腸脱肛。時珍。

Control. Eye afflictions. It pushes back shades and membranes. It dissolves accumulation lumps, boosts liver and gallbladder [qi], heals intestinal wind, and ends free-flux illness, also unending menstruation and red and white collapsing center[388] of women. *Jia you.* It resolves muscles, ends tearflow and bleeding, eliminates wind and moisture, painful elevation-illness[389] and anal prolapse of the great intestine. [Li] Shizhen.

【發明】【禹錫曰】木賊得牛角腮、麝香，治休息久痢。得禹餘粮、當歸、芎藭，治崩中赤白。得槐蛾、桑耳，治腸風下血。得槐子、枳實，治痔疾出血。【震亨曰】木賊去節烘過，發汗至易，本草不曾言及。【時珍曰】木賊氣温，味微甘苦，中空而輕，陽中之陰，升也，浮也。與麻黄同形同性，故亦能發汗解肌，升散火鬱風濕，治眼目諸血疾也。

Explication. [Zhang] Yuxi: *Mu zei* supported by ox horn bone pith and musk serves to cure long-lasting free-flux illness with some periods of dormancy. Supported by limonite, Chinese *angelica* [root] and *ligusticum* [root] it serves to cure collapsing center with red and white [discharge]. Supported by moths from a *sophora japonica* tree and jelly ear from a mulberry tree, it serves to cure intestinal wind with blood discharge. Supported by *sophora japonica* seeds and bitter orange fruit it serves to cure bleeding piles illnesses. [Zhu] Zhenheng: *Mu zei*, with the nodes removed and dried by the fire, easily induces sweating, but this is not recorded in the *Ben cao*. [Li] Shizhen: *Mu zei* has warm qi and a slightly sweet and bitter flavor. It is hollow and light. It is a yin in yang substance; it rises and it floats. It has the same appearance and the same nature as *ephedra* herb. Therefore, it, too, induces sweating and resolves [evil qi in the] muscles. It rises to disperse pent-up fire and wind and moisture. It serves to cure ailments of the eyes and all types of blood illnesses.

【附方】舊三，新九。

Added Recipes. Three of old. Nine newly [recorded].

目昏多淚。木賊去節，蒼朮泔浸，各一兩，爲末。每服二錢，茶調下。或蜜丸亦可。

388 *Beng zhong* 崩中, "collapsing center," excessive vaginal bleeding outside of a menstruation period. BCGM Dict I, 58.

389 *Shan* [*qi*] 疝[氣], "elevation-illness [qi]," a pathological condition of (1) an item having entered the scrotum, with pain, sometimes ascending, sometimes descending, (2) a condition affecting the scrotum or a testicle, (3) of violent abdominal pain, in some cases associated with constipation and anuria. BCGM Dict I, 419, 417.

Dim vision and profuse tearflow. [Grind] one *liang* each of *mu zei*, with the nodes discarded, and *atractylodes* [rhizome] into powder. Each time ingest two *qian*, to be sent down mixed with tea. It is also possible to form [the powder] with honey to pills.

急喉痺塞。木賊以牛糞火燒存性，每冷水服一錢，血出即安也。聖惠方。
Acute throat numbness/blockage. Burn *mu zei* with an ox manure fire with its nature retained. Each time ingest with cold water one *qian*. When a bleeding begins, this is the cure. *Sheng hui fang*.

舌硬出血。木賊煎水漱之，即止。聖惠方。
Hardening of the tongue with bleeding. Boil *mu zei* in water and rinse [the tongue with the decoction]. This ends [the hardening and the bleeding]. *Sheng hui fang*.

血痢不止：木賊五錢，水煎温服，一日一服。聖惠方。
Unending free-flux illness with blood. Boil five *qian* of *mu zei* in water and ingest the warm [decoction]. To be ingested once a day. *Sheng hui fang*.

瀉血不止。方同上，日二服。廣利方。
Unending outflow with blood. Recipe identical to the one above. To be ingested twice a day. *Guang li fang*.

腸痔下血，多年不止。用木賊、枳殻各二兩，乾薑一兩，大黄二錢半，並於銚内炒黑存性，爲末。每粟米飲服二錢，甚效也。蘇頌圖經本草。
Intestinal piles with a bloody discharge that has not ended for many years. Give two *liang* each of *mu zei* and bitter orange fruit, one *liang* of dried ginger and two and a half *qian* of rhubarb root into a kettle, fry them until they have turned black, still retaining their nature, and [grind this into] powder. Each time ingest with a millet beverage two *qian*. Very effective. Su Song, *Tu jing ben cao*.

大腸脱肛。木賊燒存性，爲末摻之，按入即止。一加龍骨。三因方。
Anal prolapse of the large intestine. Burn *mu zei* with its nature retained. [Grind this into] powder, apply it [to the prolapsed intestine], and firmly press it into [the anus]. This ends [the ailment]. Another [recipe] adds dragon bones. *San yin fang*.

婦人血崩，血氣痛不可忍，遠年近日不瘥者，雷氏木賊散主之。木賊一兩，香附子一兩，朴硝半兩，爲末。每服三錢，色黑者，酒一盞煎，紅赤者，水一盞煎，和滓服，日二服。臍下痛者，加乳香、没藥、當歸各一錢，同煎。忌生冷、硬物、豬魚油膩、酒麪。醫壘元戎。

Blood collapse[390] of women, and blood and qi [disorder] with unbearable pain, that has not been cured for long years or just some recent days is controlled by "Mr. Lei's powder with *mu zei.*" [Grind] one *liang* of *mu zei*, one *liang* of nutgrass and half a *liang* of mirabilite into powder. Each time [let the patient] ingest three *qian*. If [the blood] is black, boil [the powder] in one cup of wine. If it is red, boil it in one cup of water. [Ingest the liquid] with the dregs. To be ingested twice a day. If [the patient] feels pain below the navel, add one *qian* each of frankincense, myrrh, and Chinese *angelica* [root] and boil all these together [with the powder]. [During this therapy] fresh and cold [food], hard items, pork, fish, and oily and fat [items], as well as wine and noodles are to be avoided. *Yi lei yuan rong.*

月水不斷。木賊炒三錢，水一盞，煎七分，温服，日一服。聖惠方。

Unending menstruation. Boil three *qian* of *mu zei*, fried, in one cup of water down to 70% and ingest this warm. To be ingested once a day. *Sheng hui fang.*

胎動不安。木賊去節、川芎等分，爲末。每服三錢，水一盞，入金銀一錢，煎服。聖濟總録。

A moving fetus that does never come to rest. [Grind] equal amounts of *mu zei*, with the nodes discarded, and *ligusticum* [root] into powder. Each time ingest three *qian*. Boil the [powder], with one *qian* of gold or silver added, in one cup of water, and ingest [the decoction]. *Sheng ji zong lu.*

小腸疝氣。木賊細剉，微炒爲末，沸湯點服二錢，緩服取效。

Elevation-illness qi[391] of the small intestine. File *mu zei* to fine [pieces], slightly fry it and [grind them into] powder. Drip [the powder] into bubbling hot water and ingest two *qian*. To be ingested slowly until an effect is reached.

一方：用熱酒下。寇氏本草衍義。

Another recipe: Send [the powder] down with hot wine. Kou shi, *Ben cao yan yi.*

---

390 *Xue beng* 血崩, blood collapse. Excessive vaginal bleeding, identical to *beng zhong* 崩中, collapsing center. BCGM Dict I, 594; 58.

391 *Shan [qi]* 疝[氣], "elevation-illness [qi]," a pathological condition of (1) an item having entered the scrotum, with pain, sometimes ascending, sometimes descending, (2) a condition affecting the scrotum or a testicle, (3) of violent abdominal pain, in some cases associated with constipation and anuria. BCGM Dict I, 419, 417.

誤吞銅錢。木賊爲末，鷄子白調服一錢。聖惠方。

Mistakenly having swallowed a copper coin. [Grind] *mu zei* into powder and ingest mixed with chicken egg white one *qian*. *Sheng hui fang*.

【附録】
Appendix.

15-50-A01
問荆 ***Wen jing***
Unidentified.

【藏器曰】味苦，平，無毒。主結氣瘤痛，上氣氣急，煮汁服之。生伊、洛洲渚間，苗如木賊，節節相接，一名接續草。

[Chen] Cangqi: Flavor bitter, balanced, nonpoisonous. To control knotted qi with painful tumors, rising qi and hectic [breath] qi, boil it to obtain a juice and ingest it. It grows on islets in Yi and Luo zhou. The seedling is similar to that of *mu zei*, with one node following another. An alternative name is "connected herb."

15-51
石龍芻本經上品
Shi long chu. FE *Ben jing*, upper rank.

***Juncus setchuensis* L. Soft rush.**

【釋名】龍鬚本經、龍修山海經、龍華別録、龍珠本經、懸莞別録、草續斷本經、縉雲草綱目、方賓別録、西王母簪。【時珍曰】刈草包束曰芻。此草生水石之處，可以刈束養馬，故謂之龍芻。述異記周穆王東海島中養八駿處，有草名龍芻，是矣。故古語云：一束龍芻，化爲龍駒。亦孟子芻豢之義。龍鬚、王母簪，因形也。縉雲，縣名，屬今處州，仙都山產此草，因以名之。崔豹古今注云：世言黄帝乘龍上天，群臣攀龍鬚墜地生草，名曰龍鬚者，謬也。江東以草織席，名西王母席，亦豈西王母騎虎而墮其鬚乎？

Explanation of Names. *Long xu* 龍鬚, "dragon whiskers," *Ben jing*. *Long xiu* 龍修, "dragon's finest," *Shan hai jing*. *Long hua* 龍華, "dragon's splendor," *Bie lu*. *Long zhu* 龍珠, "dragon's pearl," *Ben jing*. *Xuan guan* 懸莞, *Bie lu*. *Cao xu duan* 草續斷, "herb that connects breaks," *Ben jing*. *Jin yun cao* 縉雲草, "herb from Jin yun," *Gang mu*. *Fang bin* 方賓, "upright guest," *Bie lu*. *Xi wang mu zan* 西王母簪, "Queen mother of the West's hairpin." [Li] Shizhen: To cut herbs and tie them into bundles [to be used as fodder], this is called *chu* 芻. This herb grows in places of water and rocks. It can be cut and tied [to bundles] to feed horses. Therefore it is called "dragon fodder," *long chu* 龍芻. According to the *Shu yi ji*, "King Mu of Zhou raised eight steeds on a Dong hai island. There was an herb called 'dragon fodder,' *long chu* 龍芻." This is [the herb discussed] here. Hence, an ancient saying is: "One bundle of dragon fodder transforms to a dragon colt." This is the meaning underlying Meng zi's reference to *chu huan* 芻豢, "fodder to raise [lifestock]." *Long xu* 龍鬚, "dragon whiskers," and *wang mu can* 王母簪, "the Queen mother's hairpin," refer to the [herb's] physical appearance. Jin yun 縉雲 is the name of a county; today it belongs to Chu zhou. This herb grows in the Xian du mountains [of today's Chu zhou, former Jin yun]. Hence this name. Cui Bao in his *Gu jin zhu* states: "A widespread saying is: 'When the Yellow Thearch ascended a dragon to rise to heaven, all his ministers grabbed the dragon's whiskers. Where they fell down to the ground an herb grew and was named 'dragon whiskers,' *long xu* 龍鬚'." This is absurd. In Jiang dong this herb is weaved to mats, and they are called "Queen mother of the West's mats," *xi wang mu xi* 西王母席. Do we have to assume that when the Queen mother of the West [as legend has it] rode a tiger, [the tiger's] whiskers fell [to the ground, too, and generated this herb]?

【集解】【别録曰】石龍芻生梁州山谷濕地，五月、七月采莖，暴乾，以九節多朱者良。【弘景曰】莖青細相連，實赤，今出近道水石處，似東陽龍鬚以作席者，但多節爾。【藏器曰】今出汾州、沁州、石州，亦處處有之。【保昇曰】叢生，莖如綖，所在有之，俗名龍鬚草，可爲席，八月、九月采根，暴乾。【時珍曰】龍鬚叢生，狀如粽心草及鳧茈，苗直上，夏月莖端開小穗花，結細實，並無枝葉。今吴人多栽蒔織席，他處自生者不多也。本經明言龍芻一名龍鬚，而陶弘景言龍芻似龍鬚但多節，似以爲二物者，非矣。

Connected Explanations. *Bie lu*: *Shi long chu* grows on moist ground in the mountain valleys of Liang zhou. The stem is collected in the fifth and seventh month. It is dried in the sun. Those with nine nodes and many pearls are good. [Tao] Hongjing: The stems are greenish, fine and interconnected. The fruits are red. Today [this herb] comes from places with rocks in waters of nearby regions. It resembles the "dragon whiskers" of Dong yang that are used to make mats there, but it has many more nodes. [Chen] Cangqi: Today it can be found at many places in Fen zhou, Qin zhou and Shi zhou. [Han] Baosheng: It grows as a cluster. The stems are similar to tassels on a hat. [*Shi long chu*] can be found everywhere. A common name is "dragon whisker herb." They can be made to mats. The root is collected in the eight month and in the ninth month. It is dried in the sun. [Li] Shizhen: *Long xu* grows as a cluster. Its shape is similar to that of *diarrhena* herb, and *eleocharis*. Its seedling is rising straight up. During the summer months at the tip of the stem a small spike flower opens;

the herb has neither branches nor leaves. Today, in Wu many people plant it and weave it to mats. In other regions where they grow wild there are not many. The *Ben jing* clearly says that "*long chu* 龍芻 is also named *long xu* 龍鬚." But Tao Hongjing says that "*long chu* 龍芻 resembles *long xu* 龍鬚, but has more nodes." It seems he assumed these were two different items, and that is wrong.

15-51-01
莖 *Jing*
Stem [of *shi long chu*].

【氣味】苦，微寒，無毒。【別録曰】微溫。

Qi and Flavor. Bitter, slighly cold, nonpoisonous. *Bie lu*: Slightly warm.

【主治】心腹邪氣，小便不利，淋閉，風濕，鬼疰，惡毒。久服補虛羸，輕身，耳目聰明，延年。本經。補内虛不足，痞滿，身無潤澤，出汗，除莖中熱痛，療蚘蟲及不消食。別録。

Control. Evil qi in the central and abdominal region, blocked urination. Urinary dripping and closure. Wind [intrusion] and moisture. Demon attachment-illness.[392] Malign poison. Ingested over a long time, it supplements depletion emaciation, relieves the body of its weight, clears ears and eyes and extends the years [of life]. *Ben jing*. It supplements insufficient [qi] related to an internal depletion, [serves to cure] obstacle-illness[393] with a sensation of fullness, and desiccation of the body. It stimulates sweating and eliminates painful heat from the stalk (i. e., penis). It heals [ailments related to the presence of] roundworms and failure to digest [food]. *Bie lu*.

15-51-02
敗席 *Bai xi*

Decayed mat.

【主治】淋及小便卒不通，彌敗有垢者方尺，煮汁服之。藏器。

Control. Urinary dripping and suddenly blocked urination. Boil a completely decayed and stained [mat] of the size of one square *chi*, and ingest the juice. [Chen] Cangqi.

---

392 *Zhu* 疰, also *zhu* 注, "attachment-illness," "influx-illnesss," reflects a notion of a foreign pathogenic agent, originally of demonic nature, having attached itself to the human organism. BCGM Dict I, 688-695.

393 *Pi* 痞, "obstacle-illness." 1.) An illness sign of a feeling of uncomfortable fullness and distension. 2). A condition of an uncomfortable distension and fullness in the chest and abdominal region. When pressed there is no pain. BCGM Dict I, 371.

15-52
龍常草別録 有名未用

***Long chang cao*. FE *Bie lu*, [Section] "known by name but not in use."**

***Diarrhena manshurica* Maxim.**

【釋名】粽心草。【時珍曰】俚俗五月采，繫角黍之心，呼爲粽心草是也。

Explanation of Names. *Zong xin cao* 粽心草. [Li] Shizhen: It is a common custom to collect it in the fifth month. It is used to fasten the core of [tri]angular millet [dumplings]. Therefore it is called "dumpling (*zong* 粽) core (*xin* 心) herb (*cao* 草)," *zong xin cao* 粽心草.

【集解】【別録曰】生河水旁，狀如龍芻，冬夏生。【時珍曰】按爾雅云：薜，鼠莞也。鄭樵解爲龍芻。郭璞云：纖細似龍鬚，可爲席，蜀中出者好。恐即此龍常也。蓋是龍鬚之小者爾，故其功用亦相近云。

Collected Explanations. *Bie lu*: It grows to the side of rivers and [other] waters. It is shaped like soft rush. It grows in winter and summer. [Li] Shizhen: According to the *Er ya*, "*bi* 薜 is *shu guan* 鼠莞.[394]" Zheng Qiao identified it as soft rush. Guo Pu: "It is as slender as soft rush and can be made to mats. That coming from Shu is good." Maybe, this is *long chang* [*cao*]. The fact is, this is a small variant of soft rush. Hence their [therapeutic] potentials and usages are quite similar.

15-52-01
莖 *Jing*
Stem [of *long chang cao*].

【氣味】鹹，温，無毒。

Qi and Flavor. Salty, warm, nonpoisonous.

【主治】輕身，益陰氣，療痺寒濕。別録。

Control. It relieves the body of its weight, boosts yin qi and heals blockage/numbness related to the presence of cold and moisture. *Bie lu*.

15-53
燈心草宋開寶

***Deng xin cao*. FE Song, *Kai bao*.**

***Juncus effuses* L. Common rush.**

【釋名】虎鬚草綱目、碧玉草綱目。

---

394 *Shu guan* 鼠莞, presumably an alternative name of common rush, *deng xin cao* 燈心草, 15-53.

Explanation of Names. *Hu xu cao* 虎鬚草, “tiger whisker herb,” *Gang mu*. *Bi yu cao* 碧玉草, “bluish jade herb,” *Gang mu*.

【集解】【志曰】燈心草生江南澤地，叢生，莖圓細而長直，人將爲席。【宗奭曰】陝西亦有之。蒸熟待乾，折取中心白穰燃燈者，是謂熟草。又有不蒸者，但生乾剥取爲生草。入藥宜用生草。【時珍曰】此即龍鬚之類，但龍鬚緊小而瓤實，此草稍粗而瓤虚白。吴人栽蒔之，取瓤爲燈炷，以草織席及蓑。他處野生者不多。外丹家以之伏硫、砂。雷公炮炙論序云：硇遇赤鬚，永留金鼎。注云：赤鬚亦呼虎鬚草，煮硇能住火。不知即此虎鬚否也。

Collected Explanations. [Ma] Zhi: *Deng xin cao* grows in the marshlands of Jiang nan. It grows as clusters. The stems are round, fine and long. People use them to make mats. [Kou] Zongshi: It is also found in Shaan xi. It is steamed, dried and broken to remove the white core. The [remaining] stalk serves to light lamps; it is called “heat prepared herb.” It is also possible to dry the raw [herb] without steaming it first, and peel it [to obtain the white core]. This is the “raw/fresh herb.” The raw/fresh herb is added to medication. [Li] Shizhen. This [herb] belongs to the same group as soft rush. However, soft rush is solid, small and filled with pulp. The present herb is a bit coarser and the interior is hollow and white. The people in Wu plant it. They use the interior part as lamp wick and they use the herb to weave mats and raincoats. In other regions wild growing common rush is rare. The experts in [the art of] “external elixirs” used it to check [the effects] of sulphur and cinnabar. The preface to the *Lei gong pao zhi lun* states: “When sal ammoniac meets with red whiskers it will remain in the golden cauldron forever.” A comment states: “’Red whiskers are also named ‘tiger whisker herb,’ *hu xu cao*. To boil it together with sal ammoniac checks its fire.” [I] do not know whether this is *hu xu* [*cao*], or not.”

15-53-01
莖及根 ***Jing ji gen***
Stem and root [of *deng xin cao*].

【修治】【時珍曰】燈心難研，以粳米粉漿染過，晒乾研末，入水澄之，浮者是燈心也，晒乾用。

Pharmaceutical Preparation. [Li] Shizhen: It is difficult to grind *deng xin*. Mix it with the starch of non-glutinous rice, dry it in the sun and then grind it into powder. Give it into water and wait until it has cleared. That floating on the surface is *deng xin*. It is dried in the sun and can then be used.

【氣味】甘，寒，無毒。【元素曰】辛，甘，陽也。【吴綬曰】淡，平。

Qi and Flavor: Sweet, cold, nonpoisonous. [Zhang] Yuansu: Acrid, sweet; a yang [substance]. Wu Shu: Bland, balanced.

【主治】五淋，生煮服之。敗席煮服，更良。開寶。瀉肺，治陰竅濇不利，行水，除水腫癃閉。元素。治急喉痺，燒灰吹之甚捷。燒灰塗乳上，飼小兒，止夜啼。震亨。降心火，止血通氣，散腫止渴。燒灰入輕粉、麝香，治陰疳。時珍。

Control. The five types of [urinary] dripping. The raw [herb] is boiled to be ingested. Decayed mats are boiled to be ingested, and this is even better. *Kai bao*. It drains the lung and serves to cure rough and hampered passage [of urination and defecation] through the yin orifices. It stimulates the passage of water. It removes water swelling and protuberance-illness with closure.[395] [Zhang] Yuansu. To cure acute throat blockage, burn it and blow the ashes [into the patient's throat]. Very quick [effects]. Burned and the ashes applied to the breast feeding mother's breast nipples when feeding the child ends nightly crying. [Zhu] Zhenheng. It brings down hear fire, ends bleeding, opens qi passages, dispels swelling and ends thirst. Burned to ashes and with calomel and musk added, it serves to cure *gan*-illness[396] in the yin [(i.e., genital) region]. [Li] Shizhen.

【附方】舊一，新九。

Added Recipes. One of old. Nine newly [recorded].

破傷出血。燈心草嚼爛傅之，立止。勝金方。

Bleeding wounds. Chew *deng xin cao* to generate a pulpy [mass] and apply it [to the bleeding wound. The bleeding] stops immediately. *Sheng jin fang*.

衄血不止。燈心一兩，爲末，入丹砂一錢。米飲每服二錢。聖濟總録。

Unending nosebleed. [Grind] one *liang* of *deng xin* into powder, add one *qian* of cinnabar and each time ingest with a rice beverage two *qian*. *Sheng ji zong lu*.

喉風痺塞。瑞竹堂方用燈心一握，陰陽瓦燒存性，又炒鹽一匙，每吹一捻，數次立愈。

395 *Long bi* 癃閉, "protuberance-illness with closure," a condition of passing urine in small amounts; in serious cases passage is completely inhibited. BCGM Dict I, 323.

396 *Gan* 疳, "*gan*-illness," also: "sweets-illness," involves several complaints that affect children and adults, with causes and conditions too different to fall into a known disease category. BCGM Dict I, 180-188.

Throat blockage related to wind [intrusion]. The *Rui zhu tang fang* [recommends to] burn a handful of *deng xin* on a yin yang tile[397] with its nature retained, add [to the residue] one spoon of fried salt, and each time blow as much as is twisted with the fingers [into the patient's throat]. After several [such applications], a cure is achieved.

一方：用燈心灰二錢，蓬砂末一錢，吹之。
Another recipe. [Mix] two *qian* of *deng xin* ashes and one *qian* of borax powder and blow this [into the patient's throat].

一方：燈心、箬葉燒灰，等分，吹之。
Another recipe. Burn equal amounts of *deng xin* and *indocalamus* leaves to ashes and blow [them into the patient's throat].

惠濟方用燈心草、紅花燒灰，酒服一錢，即消。
The *Hui ji fang* [recommends to] burn *deng xin cao* and safflower to ashes and ingest with wine one *qian*. This will dissolve [the throat blockage].

痘瘡煩喘，小便不利者。燈心一把，鼈甲二兩，水一升半，煎六合，分二服。龐安常傷寒論。
Small pox sores with vexing panting and impaired urination. Boil one handful of *deng xin* and two *liang* of a turtle shell in one and a half *sheng* of water down to six *ge* and ingest this in two portions. Pang Anchang, *Shang han lun*.

夜不合眼，難睡。燈草煎湯代茶飲，即得睡。集簡方。
Difficulty to fall asleep related to a failure to close the eyes at night. Boil *deng* [*xin*] *cao* and drink the decoction instead of tea. This will enable one to sleep. *Ji jian fang*.

通利水道。白飛霞自制天一丸：用燈心十斤，米粉漿染，晒乾研末，入水澄去粉，取浮者晒乾，二兩五錢，赤白茯苓去皮共五兩，滑石水飛五兩，猪苓二兩，澤瀉三兩，人參一斤切片熬膏，合藥丸如龍眼大，朱砂爲衣。每用一丸，任病換引。大段小兒生理向上，本天一生水之妙，諸病以水道通利爲捷徑也。韓氏醫通。
To open and free the passage through the pathways of water. Bai Feixian's self devised "heaven's primordial pills." Mix ten *jin* of *deng xin* with the starch of non-glutinous rice, dry this in the sun and grind it into powder. Give [the powder] into water, let it become clear and remove the [rice] powder. Take away that which floats on the surface and dry it in the sun. Mix two *liang* and five *qian* with together five

397 Yin yang tiles 陰陽瓦 are curved tiles layed down alternately oberlapping, one concave and one convex.

liang of red and white *poria*, with the skin discarded, five *liang* of talcum, refined by aqueous sublimation, two *liang* of *polyporus* sclerotium, three *liang* of *alisma* [root], and one *jin* of ginseng [root], all cut into pieces, and form pills the size of dragon eyes/longan seeds, coated with cinnabar. Each time ingest one pill, to be guided [in the body to their preferred venue of acitivity] in accordance with the specific disease [to be healed]. In general, the principle of a child's life is a development upward, based on the wondrous generation of water by "heaven's primordial [working]." In the treatment of all types of diseases to free and open the passage of the pathways of water is a quick shortcut [to success]. *Han shi yi tong.*

濕熱黄疸。燈草根四兩，酒、水各半，入瓶内煮半日，露一夜，温服。集玄方。

Yellow *dan*-illness/jaundice related to the presence of moisture and heat. Fill four liang of *deng* [*xin*] *cao* root with one half each of wine and water into a bottle and boil it for half a day. Then let it uncovered in the open for one night and ingest it warm. *Ji xuan fang.*

15-53-02
燈花燼 *Deng hua jin.*

Lampwick cinder

見火部。

See the section "fire." (06-10)

本草綱目
Ben cao gang mu
草部目録
Section Herbs, Contents
第六卷
Chapter 16

草之五
Herbs V
隰草類下七十三種
Marshland Herbs Group, final, 73 kinds

16-01 *Di huang* 地黄, Chinese foxglove. FE *Ben jing* 本經
  16-01-A01 *Hu mian mang* 胡面莽, unidentified.
16-02 *Niu xi* 牛膝, twotooth achyranthes. FE *Ben jing* 本經
16-03 *Zi wan* 紫菀, purple aster. FE *Ben jing* 本經
16-04 *Nü wan* 女菀, *turczaninowia fastigiata*. FE *Ben jing* 本經
16-05 *Mai men dong* 麥門冬, *ophiopogon japonicas*. FE *Ben jing* 本經
16-06 *Xuan cao* 萱草, yellow day lily. FE *Jia you* 嘉祐
16-07 *Chui hu gen* 槌[398]胡根, unidentified. FE *Shi yi* 拾遺
16-08 *Dan zhu ye* 淡竹葉, bland bamboo leaves. FE *Gang mu* 綱目
16-09 *Ya zhi cao* 鴨跖草, day flower. FE *Jia you* 嘉祐, i. e., *zhu ye cai* 竹葉菜
16-10 *Dong kui* 冬[399]葵, Chinese mallow. FE *Ben jing* 本經
16-11 *Shu kui* 蜀葵, common hollyhock. FE *Jia you* 嘉祐
16-12 *Tu kui* 兔[400]葵, least mallow. FE *Tang ben* 唐本
16-13 *Huang shu kui* 黄蜀葵, okra. FE *Jia you* 嘉祐
16-14 *Long kui* 龍葵, common night-shade. FE *Tang ben* 唐本
16-15 *Long zhu* 龍珠, Japanese wild pepper. FE *Shi yi* 拾遺

398 The name of this substance in entry 16-07 is written *chui hu gen* 搥胡根.

399 The name of this substance in entry 16-10 is given simply as *kui* 葵.

400 The name of this substance in entry 16-12 is written *tu kui* 菟葵.

16-16 *Suan jiang* 酸漿, Chinese lantern plant. FE *Ben jing* 本經, i. e., *deng long cao* 燈籠草
16-17 *Shu yang quan* 蜀羊泉, seven-leaf nightshade. FE *Ben jing* 本經
16-18 *Lu ti cao* 鹿蹄草, deer hoof herb. FE *Gang mu* 綱目
16-19 *Bai jiang* 敗醬, dahurian *patrinia.* FE *Ben jing* 本經, i. e., *ku cai* 即苦菜
16-20 *Ying chun hua* 迎春花, winter jasmine. FE *Gang mu* 綱目
16-21 *Kuan dong hua* 款冬花, coltsfoot. FE *Ben jing* 本經
16-22 *Shu qu cao* 鼠麴草, cudweed. FE *Rihua* 日華, i. e., *mi qu* 米麴, *fo er cao* 佛耳草
16-23 *Jue ming* 决明[401], fetid *cassia.* FE *Ben jing* 本經
16-24 *Di fu* 地膚, broom plant. FE *Ben jing* 本經, i. e., *luo zhou* 落帚
16-25 *Qu mai* 瞿麥, fringed pink. FE *Ben jing* 本經
16-26 *Wang bu liu xing* 王不留行, cowherb. FE *Bie lu* 別録
16-27 *Jian chun luo* 剪春羅, mullein pink. FE *Gang mu* 綱目
16-28 *Jin zhan cao* 金盞草, marigold. FE *Gang mu* 綱目[402]
16-29 *Ting li* 葶藶, wood whitlow grass. FE *Ben jing* 本經
16-30 *Che qian* 車前, asiatic plantain. FE *Ben jing* 本經
16-31 *Gou she cao* 狗舌草, dog's tongue herb. FE *Tang ben* 唐本
16-32 *Ma bian cao* 馬鞭草, vervain. FE *Bie lu* 別録, i. e., *long ya* 龍牙
16-33 *She han* 蛇含, kleinian cinquefoil. FE *Ben jing* 本經
16-34 *Nü qing* 女青, *cynanchum thesinides* FE *Bie lu* 別録[403]
16-35 *Shu wei cao* 鼠尾草, Japanese *salvia.* FE *Bie lu* 別録
16-36 *Lang ba cao* 狼把草, threelobe beggarticks. FE *Kai bao* 開寶
16-37 *Gou wei cao* 狗尾草, green bristlegrass. FE *Gang mu* 綱目
16-38 *Li chang* 鱧腸, ink plant. FE *Tang ben* 唐本, i. e., *han lian cao* 旱蓮草
16-39 *Lian qiao* 連翹, *forsythia suspensa* FE *Ben jing* 本經
16-40 *Lu ying* 陸英, Chinese elder. FE *Ben jing* 本經
16-41 *Shuo diao* 蒴藋, Chinese elder. FE *Bie lu* 別録
16-42 *Shui ying* 水英, water bloom. FE *Tu jing* 圖經
16-43 *Lan* 藍, indigo plant. FE *Ben jing* 本經
16-44 *Lan dian* 藍澱, indigo. FE *Gang mu* 綱目
16-45 *Qing dai* 青黛, natural indigo. FE *Kai bao* 開寶
16-45-A01 *Que qiao* 雀翹, unidentified.
16-46 *Gan lan* 甘藍, cabbage varieties. FE *Shi yi* 拾遺

---

401 Entry 16-23, *jue ming* 决明, contains appendices on *jiang mang* 茳芒 and *he ming cao* 合明草.

402 Entry 16-28, *jin zhan cao* 金盞草, names as source *Jiu huang.*

403 Entry 16-34, *nü* qing 女青, names as source *Ben jing.*

16-47 *Liao* 蓼, water pepper. FE *Ben jing* 本經
16-48 *Shui liao* 水蓼, water pepper. FE *Tang ben* 唐本
16-49 *Ma liao* 馬蓼, lady's thumb. FE *Gang mu* 綱目
16-50 *Hong cao* 葒草, red knotweed. FE *Bie lu* 別録
16-51 *Mao liao* 毛蓼, hairy knotgrass. FE *Shi yi* 拾遺
16-52 *Hai gen* 海根, *polygonum virginicum*. FE *Shi yi* 拾遺
16-53 *Huo tan mu cao* 火炭母草, Chinese knotweed. FE *Tu jing* 圖經
16-54 *San bai cao* 三白草, Chinese lizard's tail. FE *Tang ben* 唐本
16-55 *Can wang cao* 蠶𦽂草, Japanese knotweed. FE *Shi yi* 拾遺
16-56 *She wang cao* 蛇㒰草, hill-buckwheat. FE *Shi yi* 拾遺
16-57 *Hu zhang* 虎杖, bushy knotweed. FE *Bie lu* 別録
16-58 *You cao* 蕕草[404], crabgrass. FE *Shi yi* 拾遺
16-59 *Bian xu* 萹蓄, common knotgrass. FE *Ben jing* 本經
16-60 *Jin cao* 藎草, small carpetgrass. FE *Ben jing* 本經
16-61 *Ji li* 蒺藜[405], calthrop. FE *Ben jing* 本經
16-62 *Gu jing cao* 穀精草, pipewort. FE *Kai bao* 開寶
16-63 *Hai jin sha* 海金沙, climbing fern. FE *Jia you* 嘉祐
16-64 *Di yang mei* 地楊梅, woodrush. FE *Shi yi* 拾遺
16-65 *Shui yang mei* 水楊梅, Chinese button bush. FE *Gang mu* 綱目
16-66 *Di wu gong* 地蜈蚣[406], golden hair starviolet. FE *Gang mu* 綱目
16-67 *Ban bian lian* 半邊蓮, lobelia. FE *Gang mu* 綱目
16-68 *Zi hua di ding* 紫花地丁, purpleflower violet. FE *Gang mu* 綱目
16-69 *Gui zhen cao* 鬼針草, beggar tick. FE *Shi yi* 拾遺
16-70 *Du yong jian jun* 獨用將軍, *triosteum sinuatum* FE *Tang ben* 唐本
16-70-A01 *Liu jun dai* 留軍待, unidentified.
16-71 *Jian zhong xiao* 見腫消, *gynura segetum* FE *Tu jing* 圖經
16-72 *Pan dao zeng* 攀倒甑, unidentified. FE *Tu jing* 圖經
16-73 *Shui gan cao* 水甘草, *amsonia sinensis* FE *Tu jing* 圖經

右附方舊一百七十一，新二百九十一。
Recipes added to the entries above:
171 of old. 291 newly [recorded].

404 Entry 16-58 gives as name *you* 蕕, rather than *you cao* 蕕草.

405 Instead of *ji li* 蒺藜, entry 16-61 writes the name *Ji li* 蒺梨.

406 Entry 16-66 gives as name *di wu gong cao* 地蜈蚣草.

本草綱目
Ben cao gang mu
草部
Section herbs
第六卷
Chapter 16
草之五
Herbs V
隰草類下七十三種
Marshland Herbs Group, final, 73 kinds

16-01
地黄本經上品
Di huang, FE *Ben jing*, upper rank.
Rehmannia glutinosa (Gaertn.) Libosch. ex Fisch et Mey. Chinese foxglove.

【釋名】苄音户、芑音起、地髓本經。【大明曰】生者以水浸驗之。浮者名天黄，半浮半沉者名人黄，沉者名地黄。入藥沉者爲佳，半沉者次之，浮者不堪。【時珍曰】爾雅云：苄，地黄。郭璞云，江東呼爲苄。羅願云：苄以沈下珍爲貴，故字從下。

Explanation of Names. *Hu* 苄, read *hu* 户. *Qi* 芑 read *qi* 起. *Di sui* 地髓, "earth marrow," *Ben jing*. Da Ming: It is tested by immersing fresh/raw specimens in water. When they float on the surface, they are called *tian huang* 天黄, "heaven's yellow." If they half float, half sink into the depth, they are called *ren huan* 人黄, "man's yellow." If they sink into the depth, they are called *di huang* 地黄, "earth's yellow." Those that sink into the depth are excellent for adding them to medication. Those that half float, half sink are second. Those that float are not suitable [for medical applications]. [Li] Shizhen: The *Er ya* states: "*Hu* 苄 is *di huang* 地黄." Guo Pu comments: "In Jiang dong it is called *hu* 苄." Luo Yuan states: "*Hu* 苄 that sinks, *xia* 下, into the depth is considered a precious item. Hence the character [*hu* 苄] is derived from [the character] *xia* 下."

【集解】【别録曰】地黄生咸陽川澤黄土者佳，二月、八月采根，陰乾。【弘景曰】咸陽即長安也。生渭城者乃有子實如小麥。今以彭城乾地黄最好，次歷陽，近用江寧板橋者爲勝。作乾者有法，搗汁和蒸，殊用工意。而此云陰乾，恐以蒸作爲失乎？人亦以牛膝、萎蕤作之，人不能别。【頌曰】今處處有之，以同州者爲上。二月生葉，布地便出似車前葉，上有皺文而不光。高者及尺餘，低者三四寸，其花似油麻花而紅紫色，亦有黄花者。其實作房如連翹，中子甚細而沙褐色。根如人手指，通黄色，粗細長短不常。種之甚易，根入土即生。一説古稱種地黄宜黄土。今不然，大宜肥壤虚地，則根大而多汁。其法以葦席圍編如車輪，徑丈餘，以壤土實葦席中爲壇。壇上又以葦席實土爲一級，比下壇徑減一尺。如此數級，如浮屠。乃以地黄根節多者寸斷之，蒔壇上，層層令滿，逐日水灌，令茂盛。至春秋分時，自上層取之，根皆長大而不斷折，不被斸傷故也。得根暴乾。出同州者光潤甘美。【宗奭曰】地黄葉如甘露子，花如脂麻花，但有細斑點。北人謂之牛奶子花，莖有微細短白毛。【時珍曰】今人惟以懷慶地黄爲上，亦各處隨時興廢不同爾。其苗初生塌地，葉如山白菜而毛濇，葉面深青色，又似小芥葉而頗厚，不叉丫。葉中攛莖，上有細毛。莖稍開小筒子花，紅黄色。結實如小麥粒。根長四五寸，細如手指，皮赤黄色，如羊蹄根及胡蘿蔔根，曝乾乃黑，生食作土氣。俗呼其苗爲婆婆奶。古人種子，今惟種根。王旻山居録云：地黄嫩苗，摘其旁葉作菜，甚益人。本草以二月、八月采根，殊未窮物性。八月殘葉猶在，葉中精氣，未盡歸根。二月新苗已生，根中精氣已滋於葉。不如正月、九月采者殊好，又與蒸曝相宜。禮記云：羊苄豕薇，則自古已食之矣。【嘉謨曰】江、浙壤地種者，受南方陽氣，質雖光潤而力微；懷慶山産者，禀北方純陰，皮有疙瘩而力大。

Collected Explanations. Bielu: *Di huang* that grows on yellow soil in the river marshlands of Xian yang is excellent. The root is collected in the second and eighth month; it is dried in the yin (i. e., shade). [Tao] Hongjing: Xian yang is Chang an. [*Di huang*] growing in Wei cheng has seeds/fruit similar to wheat. Today, dried *di huang* from Peng cheng is considered to be the best. That from Li yang is second. In recent times those used from Ban qiao of Jiang ning are superior. To dry [*di huang*] requires a specific method. Pounding it to obtain a juice and steaming it requires quite a lot of effort. When this is [simply] called "drying in the yin (i. e., shade)," could it be that some might consider the steaming to be a negligible procedure? There are people who [pretend to] prepare [*di huang* but] use *achyranthes* [root] and *polygonatum odoratum* [root instead. Ordinary] people are unable to distinguish them. [Su] Song: Today [*di huang*] can be found everywhere. That from Tong zhou is best. It grows leaves in the second month. They cover the ground similar to Asiatic plantain leaves. On their upper side they have a wrinkled line design, and they are not glossy. Tall [*di huang* plants] reach a height of more than one *chi*. Low ones are three to four *cun* high. Their flowers resemble sesame flowers, but they are of a red-purple color. Some have yellow flowers. Their fruits form capsules similar to those of *forsythia* fruit. They contain very small seeds of a sand brown color. The root is similar to a human finger; it is of yellow color throughout. Some are coarse, others are fine, some are long, others are short – there is no regularity. To plant them is very easy. Stick the root into the soil and it will grow. Some say that in acient times it was claimed that to plant *di huang*, "earth's yellow," requires *huang tu* 黄土, "yellow soil." This is not so today. In general, if the ground it fat and fertile, the root will be big and have much juice. The method [to plant *di huang* is as follows.] Spread a round reed mat shaped like a wheel with a diameter of at least one *zhang* on the ground. With fertile soil fill the center of the reed mat to form an altar. On top of this altar place another reed mat, with a diameter of one *chi* less, and fill it with soil, too. This way continue to build something like a Buddha[407] [pagoda]. Then cut *di huang* roots (rhizomes) with many nodes into pieces of one *cun* length and plant them on the altar, filling level after level, and water them every day. This will stimulate a profuse growth. By spring and autum equinox gather [the *di huang*] beginning with the uppermost level. All the roots are long, big and unbroken because there is no need to cut and damage them. Once the root is obtained it is dried in the sun. Those from Tong zhou are shiny, glossy, sweet and delicious. [Kou] Zongshi: The leaves of *di huang* are similar to those of Chinese artichokes. The flowers are similar to those of sesame, but they have fine dots. The people in the North call them "cow breast/milk flowers." The stem has some fine, short, white hair. [Li] Shizhen: Today, people consider only Huai qing's *di huang* as of top quality. This is related to differences in what is accepted and what is discarded in the course of time and at various locations. When the seedling has just begun to grow, it sinks onto the ground. The leaves are similar to those of Chinese celery, but they are hairy and rough. Their upper side is of a deep greenish color. They also resemble the leaves of celery cabbage, but are a little thicker. They have neither forks nor bifurcations to branches. The stem rises from amidst the leaves, and is covered with fine hair. At the tip of the stem a small tube-shaped flower opens. It is of red-yellow color. It forms fruit similar to wheat grains. The root is four to five *cun* long; it is as fine as a human finger. Its skin is of red-yellow color, similar to the root of Japanese dock and to carrot roots. When it is dried in the sun it turns black. Eaten fresh/raw it emits soil qi. The seedling is commonly called "grandmother's breast/milk." The ancients planted seeds; today only the root is planted. Wang Min in his *Shan ju lu* states: "As long as the seedling of *di huang* is tender, pick its leaves and prepare them as a vegetable. This is very positive

407 *Fu tu* 浮屠 is transcription in Chinese of a Sanskrit term for "Buddha."

for humans. According to the *Ben cao*, 'the root is collected in the second and eighth month.' This may reflect an incomplete familiarity with the nature of things. In the eighth month the dilapidated leaves are still in place, and the essence qi inside the leaves have not fully returned to the root. In the second month new seedlings already grow, and the essence qi inside the root has already begun to nourish the leaves. Hence [to collect the root in the second and eighth month] is not as good as to collect it in the first and ninth month. [These two months] are also suitable for steaming [the root] and drying it in the sun. The *Li ji* states: '*Yang hu* 羊苄豕 and *shi wei*[408] 豕薇 have been eaten since ancient times'."

16-01-01
乾地黄 *Gan di huang*
Dried *di huang*.

【修治】【藏器曰】乾地黄，本經不言生乾及蒸乾。方家所用二物各别，蒸乾即温補，生乾即平宣，當依此法用。【時珍曰】本經所謂乾地黄者，即生地黄之乾者也。其法取地黄一百斤，擇肥者六十斤洗净，晒令微皺。以揀下者洗净，木臼中搗絞汁盡，投酒更搗，取汁拌前地黄，日中晒乾，或火焙乾用。

Pharmaceutical Preparation. [Chen] Cangqi: Dried *di huang*, the *Ben jing* does not speak of "fresh" and "dried" and "steamed and dried" [*di huang*]. Recipe experts use these items differently. Those that are steamed and dried serve to warm and to supplement. Those that are dried raw serve to balance and stimulate diffusion. [*Di huang*] must be used in accordance with these [different] methods [of pharmaceutical preparation]. [Li] Shizhen: When the *Ben cao* speaks of "dried *di huang*," this is dried raw *di huang*. The method [to prepare "dried *di huang*" is as follows]. Get 100 *jin* of *di huang*, select 60 *jin* of fat specimens and wash them clean. Expose them to the sun until they are slightly wrinkled. Then wash the remaining [40 *jin*] clean, pound them in a wooden mortar, and squeeze [the resulting pulp] obtain all their juice. Add wine and pound [and squeeze] them again. Then take all the juice and mix it with the first [portion of 60 *jin* of] *di huang*. Dry this in the sun, or bake it over a slow fire for [therapeutic] usage.

【氣味】甘，寒，無毒。【别録曰】苦。【權曰】甘，平。【好古曰】甘、苦，寒，氣薄味厚，沉而降，陰也。入手足少陰、厥陰及手太陽之經。酒浸，上行外行。日乾者平，火乾者温，功用相同。【元素曰】生地黄大寒，胃弱者斟酌用之。恐損胃氣。【之才曰】得清酒、麥門冬良。惡貝母，畏蕪荑。【權曰】忌葱、蒜、蘿蔔、諸血，令人營衛澀，鬚髮白。

---

408 *Shi wei* 豕薇, alternative name of *cynanchum atratum*, *bai wei* 白薇

【斅曰】忌銅鐵器，令人腎消并髮白，男損營，女損衛。【時珍曰】薑汁浸則不泥膈，酒制則不妨胃。鮮用則寒，乾用則涼。

Qi and Flavor. Sweet, cold, nonpoisonous. *Bie lu*: Bitter. [Zhen] Quan: Sweet, balanced. [Wang] Haogu: Sweet, bitter, cold. The qi are weakly pronounced; the flavor is strongly pronounced. [*Di huang*] sinks and [lets the qi of other substances] descend. It is a yin [substance]. It enters the hand and foot minor yin and ceasin yin [conduits], as well as the hand major yang conduits. Soaked in wine it moves upward and it moves to the outer regions. When it is dried in the sun, [qi and flavor are] balanced. When it is dried over a fire, it is warm. The [therapeutic] potentials and usages [of these two kinds] are similar. [Zhang] Yuansu: Fresh/raw *di huang* is very cold. [Patients] with a weak stomach must think twice about using it. It might harm their stomach qi. [Xu] Zhicai: Combined with clear wine and *ophiopogon* [tuber] it yields good results. [Ingested together,] it abhors *fritillaria* [root], and fears *ulmus* [fruit]. [Zhen] Quan: [During a treatment with *di huang*,] avoid onions, garlic, radish and all types of blood. They would roughen the passage of camp and guardian [qi], and let hair and beard turn white. [Lei] Xiao: [For the preparation and storage of *di huang*] avoid copper and iron utensils. They would let one's kidneys melt and one's hair turn white. In males they injure the camp [qi]; in females they injure the guardian [qi]. [Li] Shizhen: Soaked in ginger juice [*di huang*] does not attach itself to the diaphragm; prepared with wine it does not obstruct the stomach. When it is applied fresh, it is cold; applied dried it is cool.

【主治】傷中，逐血痺，填骨髓，長肌肉。作湯除寒熱積聚，除痺，療折跌絶筋。久服輕身不老，生者尤良。本經。主男子五勞七傷，女子傷中胞漏下血，破惡血，溺血，利大小腸，去胃中宿食，飽力斷絶，補五臟内傷不足，通血脉，益氣力，利耳目。别録。助心膽氣，强筋骨，長志安魂定魄，治驚悸勞劣，心肺損，吐血鼻衄，婦人崩中血運。大明。産後腹痛。久服變白延年。甄權。凉血生血，補腎水真陰，除皮膚燥，去諸濕熱。元素。主心病，掌中熱痛，脾氣痿蹶，嗜卧，足下熱而痛。好古。治齒痛唾血。

Control. Harmed center. It eliminates blockage caused by blood, fills the bones with marrow, and stimulates the growth of muscles and flesh. Prepared as a decoction, it removes cold and heat, accumulations and collections. It removes blockage. It heals fractures resulting from a fall and severed sinews. Ingested over a long time it relieves the body of its weight and prevents aging. Fresh/raw [*di huang*] yields especially good results. *Ben jing*. It controls the five types of exhaustion and seven types of harm affecting males, and harmed center, leaking [urinary] bladder and discharge of blood of females. It breaks through [accumulations of] malign blood, [serves to cure] urination with blood, clears the passage through the large and the small intestines and removes abiding food from within the stomach. [It serves to cure] failing strength to [digest after] having eaten to one's fill, supplements [qi in] the five long-term depots in the case of internal damage and insufficient [qi], clears the passage through the blood vessels, boosts the strength of qi, and frees the ears and the eyes. *Bie lu*. It assists the qi of heart and gallbladder, strengthens sinews and bones, extends one's mind, calms the *hun*[-soul] and stabilizes the *po*[-soul]. It serves to cure palpitation and exhaustion following fright, injuries affecting heart and lung, blood spitting and nosebleed, as well as collapsing center[409] and blood [induced brain] movement of women. Da Ming. Abdominal pain following delivery. Ingested over a long time, it changes white [hair to black hair] and extends the years [of life]. Zhen Quan. It cools blood; it generates blood. It supplements the true yin [qi] of the kidneys [i. e., the depot associated with the phase] water. It removes dryness from the skin, and it eliminates all types of moisture and heat. [Zhang] Yuansu. It controls heart diseases, painful heat in the palms, dysfunction of spleen qi with [a tendency to] fall, a preference for lying in bed, and painful heat below the feet. [Wang] Haogu. It serves to cure toothache and blood spitting.

16-01-02

生地黄 *Sheng di huang*

Fresh/raw *di huang*.

【主治】大寒。治婦人崩中血不止，及產後血上薄心悶絶。傷身胎動下血，胎不落，墮墜踠折，瘀血，留血，鼻衄，吐血。皆擣飲之。別録。解諸熱，通月水，利水道。擣貼心腹，能消瘀血。甄權。

Control. Massive heat. It serves to cure collapsing center of women with unending bleeding, as well as, following delivery, rising blood approaching the heart, causing heart-pressure and interruption [of qi] flow. A damaged body letting a fetus move and causing discharge of blood. Failure of a fetus to come down. Fracture resulting from a fall or a struggle. Stagnating blood. Abiding blood. Nosebleed. Blood spitting. For all these [ailments] pound [fresh/raw *di huang*] and drink the [juice]. *Bie lu*. It resolves all types of heat, frees menstruation, and opens the passage through the pathways of water. It can dissolve stagnating blood. Zhen Quan.

【發明】【好古曰】生地黄入手少陰，又爲手太陽之劑，故錢仲陽瀉丙火與木通同用以導赤也。諸經之血熱，與他藥相隨，亦能治之。溺血、便血皆同。【權曰】病人虛而多熱者，宜加用之。【戴原禮曰】陰微陽盛，相火熾强，來乘陰位，日漸煎熬，爲虛火之證者，宜地黄之屬以滋陰退陽。

409 *Beng zhong* 崩中, "collapsing center," excessive vaginal bleeding outside of a menstruation period. BCGM Dict I, 58.

【宗奭曰】本經只言乾、生二種，不言熟者。如血虛勞熱，產後虛熱，老人中虛燥熱者，若與生乾，當慮太寒，故後世改用蒸曝熟者。生熟之功殊別，不可不詳。【時珍曰】本經所謂乾地黃者，乃陰乾、日乾、火乾者，故又云生者尤良。別録復云生地黃者，乃新掘鮮者，故其性大寒。其熟地黃乃後人復蒸晒者。諸家本草皆指乾地黃爲熟地黃，雖主治證同，而涼血補血之功稍異，故今別出熟地黃一條於下。

Explication. [Wang] Haogu: Fresh/raw *di huang* enters the hand minor yin [conduits], and it is a preparation for the hand major yang [conduits]. Therefore, Qian Zhongyang [recommends to] drain yang fire[410] by combining [*di huang*] with *akebia* [herb] in the "[medication] to lead off the red." [Zhen] Quan: Patients with a depletion and much heat should add it to [the medication] applied. Dai Yuanli: When yin [qi] are weak while yang [qi] abound, the latter arrive to occupy the position of yin [qi]. The heat increases day after day, and this is a sign of depletion fire. In such a situation, it is suitable to resort to *di huang* and related [substances] to nourish the yin [qi] and to push back the yang [qi]. [Kou] Zongshi: The *Ben jing* refers to only the two kinds of dried and fresh [*di huang*]. It says nothing about "heat processed" [*di huang*]. When it comes to depletion heat following delivery, or central depletion of old persons with dryness heat, if these were treated with fresh/raw dried [*di huang*], one should keep in mind its extremely cold [nature]. Therefore, in later times this was changed to a use of heat processed [*di huang*] prepared by means of steaming and drying in the sun. The [therapeutic] potentials of fresh/raw and heat processed [*di huang*] are very different. It is impossible to disregard these details. [Li] Shizhen: When the *Ben jing* speaks of dried *di huang*, this is [*di huang*] dried in the yin (i. e., shade), dried in the sun, dried over a fire. Hence it also states that "fresh/raw [*di huang*] yields especially good results." The *Bie lu* speaks of "fresh/raw *di huang*, these are newly undug, fresh specimens." Hence their nature is very cold. Heat processed *di huang* is [*di huang*] steamed and dried in the sun by people in later times. The *Ben cao* works of all authors refer to dried *di huang* as heat processed *di huang*. The illness signs they control are identical, but they slightly differ in their potential of cooling blood and of supplementing blood. Therefore, here heat processed *di huang* is listed in a separate entry below.

410 *Bing huo* 丙火 may be identified based on different historical calculation schemes. It can also refer to the small intestine, and to the heart. The application of medication "to lead off the red" suggests that here a drainage of "yang fire" or of "heart qi", associated with the color red, is meant.

16-01-03
熟地黄 *Shu di huang*
Heat processed *di huang*.

【修治】【頌曰】作熟地黄法：取肥地黄三二十斤净洗，别以揀下瘦短者三二十斤搗絞取汁，投石器中，浸漉令浹，甑上浸三四過。時時浸濾轉蒸，訖，又暴，使汁盡，其地黄當光黑如漆，味甘如飴。須瓷器收之，以其脂柔喜潤也。【斅曰】采生地黄去皮，瓷鍋上柳木甑蒸之，攤令氣歇，拌酒再蒸，又出令乾。勿犯銅鐵器，令人腎消并髮白，男損營，女損衛也。【時珍曰】近時造法：揀取沉水肥大者，以好酒入縮砂仁末在内，拌匀，柳木甑於瓦鍋内蒸令氣透，[日良]乾。再以砂仁酒拌蒸、[日良]。如此九蒸九[日良]乃止。蓋地黄性泥，得砂仁之香而竄，合和五臟冲和之氣，歸宿丹田故也。今市中惟以酒煮熟售者，不可用。

Pharmaceutical Preparation. [Su] Song: The method to prepare heat processed *di huang*. Get 30 or 20 *jin* of fat *di huang* [rhizomes] and wash them clean. In addition, pound 30 or 20 *jin* of meagre and short [*di huang* rhizomes] not picked [as fat specimens], and squeeze [the resulting pulp] to obtain a juice. Give the [cleaned, fat *di huang*] into a stone vessel and soak it [with the juice] until it is thoroughly wetted. [To achieve this,] pour [the juice] from a bottle three to four times to soak [the fat *di huang* rhizomes]. Repeatedly soak and filter and steam [the filtrate] until the end is reached. Again, dry [the fat roots] in the sun and continue until all the juice be used up. Eventually, the *di huang* will have acquired a black shine like lacquer, with a sweet flavor like sugar. It must be stored in a porcelain vessel to keep its fat soft and moist. [Lei] Xiao: Collect a fresh *di huang* [rhizome] and remove the skin. Give it into a porcelain pot and steam it with a willow wood steamer. Spread [the root] to let the [heat] qi disperse, mix it with wine and steam it again. Then remove it again and let it dry. It must not be offended by copper and iron vessels. That would let one's kidneys melt and the hair turn white. In males it would injure the camp [qi], in females it would injure the guardian [qi]. [Li] Shizhen: A processing method of recent times: Pick a large [*di huang* rhizome] that is fat and sinks deep into the water, and mix it evenly with good wine into which *ammomum villosum* powder was given. Steam it in a willow wood steamer placed into a pottery pot and let the [steam] qi pass through [the *di huang* rhizomes]. Dry it in the sun and again mix it with *ammomum villosum* wine, steam this and dry it in the sun. Do this steaming nine times and the drying in the sun nine times, then stop. The fact is, the nature of *di huang* is sticky. Therefore, [ingested] combined with the fragrance and penetrating [nature] of *ammomum villosum*, it links up with the harmonious qi of the five long-term depots and leads them to settle in the Cinnabar Field. Today, on the markets they sell [*di huang* rhizomes] that are steamed with wine only. They must not be used.

【氣味】甘、微苦，微温，無毒。【元素曰】甘、微苦，寒。假酒力洒蒸，則微温而大補。味厚氣薄，陰中之陽，沉也。入手足少陰、厥陰之經。治外治上，須酒制。忌蘿蔔、葱、蒜、諸血。得牡丹皮、當歸，和血生血凉血，滋陰補髓。

Qi and Flavor. Sweet, slightly bitter, slightly warm, nonpoisonous. [Zhang] Yuansu: Sweet, slightly bitter, cold. If it is given the strength of wine by steaming it with wine, it will become slightly warm and acquire a massive [potential of] supplementation. The flavor is strongly pronounced; the qi are weak. [Heat processed *di huang* rhizome] is a yang in yin [substance]. It enters the hand and foot minor yin and ceasing yin conduits. It serves to cure [diseases] in the body's exterior and in the body's upper region; it must be processed with wine. [During a treatment with heat prepared *di huang* rhizome], radish, onions, garlic, and all types of blood are to be avoided. Combined with *paeonia* root bark and Chinese *angelica* [root] it harmonizes blood, generates blood and cools blood. It nourishes yin [qi] and supplements marrow.

【主治】填骨髓，長肌肉，生精血，補五臟内傷不足，通血脉，利耳目，黑鬚髮，男子五勞七傷，女子傷中胞漏，經候不調，胎産百病。時珍。補血氣，滋腎水，益真陰，去臍腹急痛，病後脛股酸痛。元素。坐而欲起，目䀮䀮無所見。好古。

Control. It fills bone marrow, stimulates the growth of muscles and flesh, generates essence/sperm and blood, supplements insufficient [qi] in the case of internal harm affecting the five long-term depots, penetrates the blood vessels, frees ears and eyes, and blackens hair and beard. [It serves to cure] the five types of exhaustion and seven types of harm of males, and internal harm with bladder leakage, as well as irregular menstruation, of women. Also, the hundreds of diseases related to pregnancy and birth. [Li] Shizhen. It supplements blood and qi, nourishes the kidney water, boosts genuine yin [qi] and removes acute pain at the navel and in the abdomen, as well as soreness and pain in the shins and thighs following a disease. [Zhang] Yuansu. When one sits and wishes to rise and the eyes are blinded and see nothing. [Wang] Haogu.

【發明】【元素曰】地黄生則大寒而凉血，血熱者須用之；熟則微温而補腎，血衰者須用之。又臍下痛屬腎經，非熟地黄不能除，乃通腎之藥也。【好古曰】生地黄治心熱、手足心熱，入手足少陰、厥陰，能益腎水，凉心血，其脉洪實者宜之。若脉虚者，則宜熟地黄，假火力蒸九數，故能補腎中元氣。仲景八味丸以之爲諸藥之首，天一所生之源也。湯液四物湯治藏血之臟，以之爲君者，癸乙同歸一治也。【時珍曰】按王碩易簡方云：男子多陰虚，宜用熟地黄；女子多血熱，宜用生地黄。又云：生地黄能生精血，天門冬引入所生之處；熟地黄能補精血，用麥門冬引入所補之處。虞摶醫學正傳云：生地黄生血，而胃氣弱者服之恐妨食；熟地黄補血，而痰飲多者服之恐泥膈。或云：生地黄酒炒則不妨胃，熟地黄薑汁炒則不泥膈。此皆得用地黄之精微者也。【頌曰】崔元亮海上方：治一切心痛，無問新久。以生地黄一味，隨人所食多少，搗絞取汁，搜麪作[飠丕]飥或冷淘食，良久當利出蟲，長一尺許，頭似壁宫，後不復患矣。昔有人患此病二年，深以爲恨。臨終戒其家人，吾死後當剖去病本。從其言果得蟲，置於竹節中，每所食皆飼之。因食地黄[飠丕]飥亦與之，隨即壞爛，由此得方。劉禹錫傳信方亦紀其事云：貞元十年，通事舍人崔抗女，患心痛垂絶，遂作地黄冷淘食，便吐一物，可方寸匕，狀如蝦蟆，無足目，似有口，遂愈。冷淘勿着鹽。

Explication. [Zhang] Yuansu: As long as *di huang* is fresh/raw, it is very cold and cools blood. For blood heat it must be resorted to. Once it is heat processed, it is slightly warm and supplements kidney [qi]. For blood weakness it must be resorted to. Also, pain below the navel is related to the kidney conduits. It is only with heat processed *di huang* that [such pain] can be eliminated. It is a pharmaceutical drug that penetrates the kidneys. [Wang] Haogu: Fresh/raw *di huang* serves to cure heart heat, and heat of the palms and soles. It enters the hand and foot minor yin and ceasing yin [conduits]. It can boost kidney [qi, i. e., qi of the phase] water and cool the heart blood. It is suitable for cases of a vast and replete [movement in the] vessels. For a depleted [movement in the] vessels, heat processed *di huang* is appropriate. As it has been endowed with the strength of fire by steaming it nine times, it is able to supplement the original qi in the kidneys. [Zhang] Zhongjing uses it in his "pills with eight substances"[411] as the chief of all drugs resorted to. It is the source of all generation by the heaven's primodial [qi]. When the *Tang ye* [recommends] the "decoction with four items" to cure the long-term depots responsible for storing the blood, this is meant to cure *gui* 癸 (i. e., the kidneys) and *yi* 乙 (i. e., the liver] at the same time. [Li] Shizhen: According to Wang Shuo's *Yi jian fang*, "males often have a yin [qi] depletion and for them it is advisable to use heat processed *di huang*. Females often experience blood heat. For them it is advisable to use fresh/raw *di huang*." It is also said, "fresh/raw *di huang* can generate essence/sperm and blood. *Asparagus* [root] guides it to the places where blood is generated. Heat processed *di huang* can supplement essence/sperm and blood. *Ophiopogon* [tuber] is used to guide it to the places where a supplementation is required." Yu Tuan in his *Yi xue zheng chuan* states: "Fresh/raw *di huang* generates blood, but when persons with a stomach weakness ingest it, it may hamper their

411 *Ba wei wan* 八味丸, "pills with eight substances," have the following ingredients: Prepared Chinese foxglove rhizome, Asiatic cornelian cherry, Chinese yam, *poria*, *paeonia* root bark, *alisma* root, *cassia* bark, prepared *fu zi*.

desire to eat. Heat processed *di huang* supplements blood. But when persons with much phlegm rheum ingest it, it may stick to their diagphragm." It also says: "Fresh/raw *di huang* fried in wine does not hamper the [functions of the] stomach. Heat processed *di huang* fried in ginger juice will not cling to the diaphragm." All these are subtle essentials related to the application of *di huang*. [Su] Song: Cui Yuanliang in his *Hai shang fang* [recommends the following recipe] "to cure heart pain, regardless of whether this is a new problem or has lasted for a long time. Pound fresh/raw *di huang*, the amount depending on that person's eating habit, and squeeze [the resulting pulp] to obtain a juice. With flour form rice cakes or prepare a cold dish. When he eats this for a long time, eventually worms/bugs will be released. They are a little longer than one *chi*, with a head similar to that of a gecko. After that he will suffer from [such heart pain] never again. In former times someone suffered from this disease for two years. It was truly regrettable. When his end was in sight, he admonished his relatives: 'After my death you must dissect [my body] to remove the base of this disease.' They followed his words and eventually found these worms/bugs. They put them into a bamboo tube and whenever they ate something they also fed it to them. One day they ate rice cakes prepared with *di huang*, and they gave them [to the worms/bugs], whereupon they immediately rotted. The recipes [with *di huang*] originate from this." Liu Yuxi in his *Chuan xin fang*, too, reports such an event: "In the 10th year of the *zhen yuan* reign period (794 CE), a daughter of Mr. Cui Kang suffered from heart pain and was close to death. She was given to eat a cold dish prepared with *di huang* and immediately spat out an item filling a square *cun* spoon. It had a head like a toad, but no feet and no eyes. Apparently it had a mouth. [The daughter] was cured. No salt must be added to the cold dish."

【附方】舊十三，新五十一。

Added Recipes. 13 of old. 51 newly [recorded].

服食法。地黄根净洗，擣絞汁，煎令稠，入白蜜更煎，令可丸，丸如梧子大。每晨温酒送下三十丸，日三服。亦可以青州棗和丸。或别以乾地黄末入膏丸服亦可。百日面如桃花，三年身輕不老。抱朴子云：楚文子服地黄八年，夜視有光。

Method to ingest [*di huang*] as food. Wash *di huang* roots (rhizomes) clean, pound them and squeeze [the resulting pulp] to obtain a juice. Boil it to generate a paste, add white honey and boil it again until eventually it can be formed to pills. The pills are the size of *wu* seeds. Every morning send down with warm wine 30 pills. To be ingested three times a day. It is also possible to resort to Qing zhou dates to form the pills. And it is also possible to prepare the paste with dried *di huang* powder to form pills and ingest them. After one hundred days the face will [have acquired a complexion] similar to peach flowers. Within three years the body is relieved of its weight and does not age. The *Baopu zi* states: "Chu Wenzi ingested *di huang* for eight years. When he saw [items] at night it was as if they were lighted."

地黃煎。補虛除熱，治吐血唾血，取乳石，去癰癤等疾。生地黃不拘多少，三搗三壓，取汁令盡，以瓦器盛之，密蓋勿洩氣。湯上煮減半，絞去滓，再煎如餳，丸彈子大。每温酒服一丸，日二服。千金方。

Di huang decoct. It supplements depleted [qi] and eliminates heat. It serves to cure blood vomiting and blood spitting. Together with stalactite mineral it serves to eliminate illnesses such as obstruction-illness[412] and pimples. Pound any quantity of fresh/raw *di huang* three times and press it three times to obtain all the juice it may contain. Store it in a stoneware vessel, and tightly seal it lest its qi effuse. Then heat it above hot water until one half remains, and squeeze it to remove the dregs. Boil [the liquid] again until it has taken on a consistency similar to that of malt sugar and form pills the size of a bullet. Each time ingest with warm wine one pill. To be ingested twice a day. *Qian jin fang*.

地髓煎。生地黃十斤，洗浄，搗壓取汁，鹿角膠一斤半，生薑半斤，絞取汁，蜜二升，酒四升。文武火煮地黃汁數沸，即以酒研紫蘇子四兩，取汁入煎一二十沸，下膠，膠化，下薑汁、蜜再煎，候稠，瓦器盛之。每空心酒化一匕服，大補益。同上。

Di sui decoct. Wash ten *jin* of fresh/raw *di huang* clean. Pound them and press [the resulting pulp] to obtain a juice. Also, prepare one and a half *jin* of deer horn glue, half a *jin* of fresh ginger, squeezed to obtain the juice, two *sheng* of honey and four *sheng* of wine. Boil the *di huang* juice over a violent fire [first] and a mild fire [later] several times to bubbling. Also grind four *liang* of *perilla* seeds in wine, add this to the [*di huang*] juice and boil this to bubbling ten to 20 times . Then add the [deer horn] glue, and let the glue dissolve. Then add the ginger juice and the honey and boil this again to eventually generate a paste. Store it in an earthenware vessel. Each time ingest, on an empty stomach, a spoonful dissolved in wine. This results in massive supplementation and boosting. [Source of this recipe] identical to the one above.

412 *Yong* 癰, "obstruction-illness," refers to an obstruction of vessels or other ducts inside the body. Qi rushing against the obstruction may cause a local swelling and eventually break through the surface to cause an abscess. BCGM Dict I, 641.

地黄粥。大能利血生精。地黄切二合，與米同入鑵中煮之。候熟，以酥二合，蜜乙合，同炒香入内，再煮熟食。臞仙神隱。

Di huang congee. It is very much able to free the passage of blood and to generate essence/sperm. Cut two *ge* of *di huang* into pieces, give them together with rice into a jar and boil this until done. Fry two *ge* of butter and one *ge* of honey together until they develop a fragrance and give them into [the jar]. Heat it again until done and eat this. *Qu xian shen yin.*

地黄酒。見穀部酒下。

Di huang wine. See under "wine" in the section "cereals."

瓊玉膏。常服開心益智，髮白返黑，齒落更生，辟穀延年。治癰疽勞瘵，欬嗽唾血等病，乃鐵甕城申先生方也。生地黄十六斤取汁，人參末乙斤半，白伏苓末三斤，白沙蜜十斤，濾净拌匀，入瓶内，箬封，安砂鍋中，桑柴火煮三日夜。再換蠟紙重封，浸井底一夜，取起，再煮一伏時。每以白湯或酒點服一匙。丹溪云：好色虚人，欬嗽唾血者，服之甚捷。國朝太醫院進御服食，議加天門冬、麥門冬、枸杞子末各一斤，賜名益壽永真膏。臞仙方加琥珀、沉香半兩。

The "splendid jade paste." Ingested regularly, it opens the heart and boosts wisdom, lets white hair turn black again, lets teeth that have fallen out grow again, and extends the years [of life] while abstaining from cereals. It serves to cure illnesses such as obstruction-illness and impediment-illness,[413] as well as exhaustion consumption, cough and blood spitting. This is a recipe of Mr. Shen from Tie weng cheng. [Press] Give the juice obtained from 16 *jin* of fresh/raw *di huang*, one and a half *jin* of ginseng [root] powder, three *jin* of white *poria* powder and ten *jin* of honey from Bai sha, strained, cleaned and evenly mixed, into a bottle, and seal it with *indocalamus* [leaves]. Place [the bottle] into a pottery pot and with a mulberry fire heat it for three days and three nights. Then change the sealing [of the bottle] to a double wax-paper layer and lower it to the bottom of a well for one night. Lift it up again and heat it once more for one full day and night. Each time ingest one spoonful dripped into clear, boiled water or wine. [Zhu] Danxi: Men with a depletion related to indulging in sex, when they cough and spit blood, ingest this with very quick effects. The Imperial Medical Office of the present dynasty submitted this [medication] to be eaten by the Emperor. They decided to add one *jin* each of *asparagus* [root], *ophiopogon* [root] and *lycium* seed powder. [The Emperor] granted

413 *Yong ju* 癰疽, "obstruction-illness, impediment-illness." refers to two vaguely distinguished obstructions/impediments of vessels or other ducts inside the body. Qi rushing against the obstruction may cause a local swelling and eventually break through the surface to cause an abscess. BCGM Dict I, 642.

it the name "Paste to boost longevity and secure true [qi] forever." The *Qu xian fang* [recommends to] add half a *liang* [each] of amber and aloes wood.

明目補腎。生苄、熟苄各二兩，川椒紅一兩，爲末，蜜丸梧子大，每空心鹽湯下三十丸。普濟方。

To clear the eyes and supplement the kidneys. [Grind] two *liang* each of fresh/raw *hu* and heat processed *hu* together with one *liang* of Chinese pepper into powder and form with honey pills the size of *wu* seeds. Each time send down on an empty stomach with a salt decoction 30 pills. *Pu ji fang.*

固齒烏鬚。一治齒痛，二生津液，三變白鬚，其功極妙。地黄五斤，柳木甑内以土蓋上，蒸熟晒乾。如此三次，擣爲小餅。每噙嚥一枚。御藥院方。

To stabilize the teeth and blacken the beard. First, it serves to cure toothache. Second, it generates body liquids. Third, it changes white beards [to black beards]. Fill five *jin* of *di huang* into a willow wood steamer, cover it with soil, steam it until done and dry it in the sun. Do this three times. Then pound [the *di huang*] and [use the pulp] to prepare small cakes. Each time hold one [such cake] in the mouth and swallow [the resulting liquid]. *Yu yao yuan fang.*

男女虚損，或大病後，或積勞後，四體沉滯，骨肉酸痛，吸吸少氣，或小腹拘急，腰背强痛，咽乾唇燥，或飲食無味，多卧少起，久者積年，輕者百日，漸至瘦削。用生地黄二斤，麪一斤，搗爛，炒乾爲末。每空心酒服方寸匕，日三服。忌如法。肘後方。

Depletion injury of males and females. Or after a serious disease. Or after continued exhaustion, with the four limbs experiencing deep-seated sluggishness, painful soreness affecting bones and flesh, and limited breath qi, or cramps in the lower abdomen, painful stiffness in the lower back and back, dry throat and dryness of lips, or drinking and eating without sensing a flavor, much lying in bed and seldom getting up, which when it lasts long may extend for years and in light cases a hundred days, with a loss of weight to the point of emaciation. Pound two *jin* of fresh/raw *di huang* with one *jin* of wheat flour into a pulpy [mass], fry it until it is dry and [grind it into] powder. Each time ingest on an empty stomach with wine the amount held by a square *cun* spoon. To be ingested three times a day. As for [items] to be avoided, [follow the usual] method. *Zhou hou fang.*

虚勞困乏。地黄一石，取汁，酒三斗，攪勻煎收。日服。必效方。

Depletion exhaustion and fatigue. [Press] one *dan* of *di huang* to obtain a juice, mix it with three *dou* of wine, boil it and store it. To be ingested daily. *Bi xiao fang.*

病後虛汗，口乾心躁。熟地黄五兩，水三盞，煎一盞半，分三服，一日盡。聖惠方。

Depletion sweating following a disease, with a dry mouth and restless heart. Boil five *liang* of heat processed *di huang* in three cups of water down to one and a half cup, and ingest all of this, divided into three portions, within one day. *Sheng hui fang*.

骨蒸勞熱。張文仲方用生地黄一升，擣三度，絞取汁盡，分再服。若利即減之，以凉爲度。外臺秘要。

Bone steaming[414] and exhaustion heat. A recipe by Zhang Wenzhong [recommends to] pound one *sheng* of fresh/raw *di huang* three times, [each time] squeeze [the resulting pulp] to obtain all its juice, and ingest it divided into two portions. If this causes a free-flux [defecation] lower [the dosage. Continue the treatment] until [the bone steaming] is cooled. *Wai tai mi yao*.

婦人發熱，欲成勞病，肌瘦食減，經候不調。地髓煎：用乾地黄一斤爲末，煉蜜丸梧子大。每酒服五十丸。保慶集。

Heat effusion of women, threatening to develop to an exhaustion disease, with muscle emaciation and less intake of food, and irregular menstruation. The "*di huang* decoct." [Grind] one *jin* of dried *di huang* into powder and form with heat refined honey pills the size of *wu* seeds. Each time ingest with wine 50 pills. *Bao qing ji*.

婦人勞熱，心忪。地黄煎：用生乾地黄、熟乾地黄等分，爲末。生薑自然汁，入水相和，打糊丸梧子大。每服三十丸，用地黄湯下，或酒、醋、茶湯下亦可，日三服。覺臟腑虛冷，則晨服八味丸。地黄性冷壞脾，陰虛則發熱，地黄補陰血故也。婦人良方。

Exhaustion heat of women, with heart agitation. *Di huang* decoct. [Grind] equal amounts of dried fresh/raw *di huang* and of dried heat processed *di huang* into powder. Give this together with the natural juice of fresh ginger into water, mix it, and form with a [wheat flour] paste pills the size of *wu* seeds. Each time ingest 30 pills to be sent down with a *di huang* decoction. Or send them down with wine, vinegar or tea decoction. This is possible, too. To be ingested three times a day. If there is a feeling of depletion cold in the long-term depots and short-term repositories, ingest the "pills with the eight substances"[415] in the morning. *Di huang* has a cold nature

414 *Gu zheng* 骨蒸, "bone steaming." 1.) Condition of an infectious consumptive disease with a development of vexing heat in the afternoon. 2.) Illness sign of heat and vexation with a feeling as if this originated in the bones. BCGM Dict I, 197.

415 *Ba wei wan* 八味丸, "pills with eight substances," have the following ingredients: Prepared Chinese foxglove rhizome, Asiatic cornelian cherry, Chinese yam, *poria*, *paeonia* root bark, *alisma* root, *cassia* bark, prepared *fu zi*.

and may damage the spleen. In the case of yin [qi] depletion heat is effused. Hence *di huang* [is used to] supplement yin [qi and] blood. *Fu ren liang fang.*

欬嗽唾血，勞瘦骨蒸，日晚寒熱。生地黄汁三合，煮白粥，臨熟入地黄汁，攪勻，空心食之。食醫心鏡。

Cough and blood spitting. Exhaustion emaciation and bone steaming,[416] with alternating sensations of cold and heat during the [early] day and in the evening. Boil three *ge* of juice obtained from fresh/raw *di huang*. Cook a white congee. When it is close to well done add the *di huang* juice. Mix it evenly and eat this on an empty stomach. *Shi yi xin jing.*

吐血欬嗽。熟地黄末，酒服一錢，日三。聖惠方。

Vomiting of blood and cough. Ingest one *qian* of heat processed *di huang* powder with wine. Three times a day. *Sheng hui fang.*

吐血不止。生地黄汁一升二合，白膠香二兩，以磁器盛，入甑蒸，令膠消，服之。梅師。

Unending vomiting of blood. Fill one *sheng* and two *ge* of the juice of fresh/raw *di huang* and two *liang* of Chinese sweet gum into a porcelain jar and steam it in a steamer until the [Chinese sweet] gum is dissolved. Then ingest this. *Mei shi.*

肺損吐血，或舌上有孔出血。生地黄八兩取汁，童便五合同煎熱，入鹿角膠炒研一兩，分三服。

Spitting of blood related to an injured lung. Or bleeding out of holes on the tongue. [Squeeze] eight *liang* of fresh/raw *di huang* to obtain a juice and heat it together with five *ge* of boys' urine until it is hot. Add one *liang* of deer horn glue, fried and ground, and ingest this divided into three portions.

心熱吐衄，脉洪數者。生节汁半升，熬至一合，入大黄末一兩，待成膏，丸梧子大，每熟水下五丸至十丸。並聖惠方。

Heart heat, vomiting and nosebleed, with a vast and accelerated [movement in the] vessels. Heat half a *sheng* of the juice obtained from fresh/raw *di huang* down to one *ge*, add one *liang* of rhubarb root powder and wait until a paste has developed. Form pills the size of *wu* seeds. Each time send down with boiled water five pills, or up to ten pills. Both [these recipes:] *Sheng hui fang.*

---

416 *Gu zheng* 骨蒸, "bone steaming," 1.) a condition of an infectious consumptive disease with a development of vexing heat in the afternoon. 2.) An illness sign of heat and vexation with a feeling as if this originated in the bones. BCGM Dict I, 197.

鼻出衄血。乾地黄、地龍薄荷等分，爲末。冷水調下。孫兆秘寶方。

Nosebleed. [Grind] equal amounts of dried *di huang* and camphor mint[417] into powder and send it down mixed with cold water. Sun Zhao, *Mi bao fang*.

吐血便血。地黄汁六合，銅器煎沸，入牛皮膠一兩，待化入薑汁半盃，分三服，便止。或微轉一行，不妨。聖惠方。

Vomiting of blood and [urination/defecation] relief with blood. Boil six *ge* of *di huang* juice in a copper vessel to bubbling, add one *liang* of ox hide glue, wait until it has dissolved and add half a cup of ginger juice. Ingest this divided into three portions, and the [bleeding will] end. In some cases a mild changes happens to one [more] passage [of blood], but this is not harmful. *Sheng hui fang*.

腸風下血。生地黄、熟地黄並酒浸，五味子等分，爲末，以煉蜜丸梧子大，每酒下七十丸。百一選方。

Intestinal wind with a discharge of blood. [Grind] equal amounts of fresh/raw *di huang* and heat processed *di huang*, soaked together in wine, and *schisandra* seeds to powder and form with heat refined honey pills the size of *wu* seeds. Each time send down with wine 70 pills. *Bai yi xuan fang*.

初生便血。小兒初生七八日，大小便血出，乃熱傳心肺。不可服凉藥，只以生地黄汁五七匙，酒半匙，蜜半匙，和服之。全幼心鑑。

[Defecation/urination] relief of a newborn with blood. When a newborn child of seven or eight days releases blood with defecation and urination, this is a case of heat transmitted to heart and lung. It cannot ingest a cooling medication. The only possibility is to feed it with a mixture of five to seven spoons of fresh/raw *di huang* juice, half a spoon of wine and half a spoon of honey. *Quan you xin jian*.

小便尿血，吐血，及耳鼻出血。生地黄汁半升，生薑汁半合，蜜一合，和服。聖惠方。

Urination with blood. Vomiting of blood, and blood coming out of ears and nose. Ingest a mixture of half a *sheng* of fresh/raw *di huang* juice, half a *ge* of fresh ginger juice, and one *ge* of honey. *Sheng hui fang*.

小便血淋。生地黄汁、車前葉汁各三合，和煎服。聖惠方。

Urinary dripping with blood. Mix three *ge* each of fresh/raw *di huang* juice and Asiatic plantain leaf juice, boil this and ingest it. *Sheng hui fang*.

---

417 Instead of *di long bo he* 地龍薄荷, *Zheng lei* ch. 6, *gan di huang* 乾地黄, "dried *di huang*," quoting *Sun Zhao fang* writes *long nao bo he* 龍腦薄荷.

小兒蠱痢。生苄汁一升二合，分三四服，立效。子母秘録。

Free-flux illness related to *gu* [poisoning][418] of children. Divide one *sheng* and two *ge* of fresh/raw *hu* juice into three or four portions and [let the child] ingest this. *Zi mu mi lu*.

月水不止。生地黄汁，每服一盞，酒一盞，煎服，日二次。千金方。

Unending menstruation. Each time ingest one cup of fresh *di huang* juice. To be ingested boiled with one cup of wine, twice a day. *Qian jin fang*.

月經不調，久而無子，乃衝任伏熱也。熟地黄半斤，當歸二兩，黄連一兩，並酒浸一夜，焙研爲末，煉蜜丸梧子大。每服七十丸，米飲、温酒任下。禹講師方。

Irregular menstruation with a long lasting failure to have a child results from heat hidden in the throughway and controller [vessels]. Soak half a *liang* of heat processed *di huang*, two *liang* of Chinese *angelica* [root] and one *liang* of *coptis* [rhizome] for one night in wine. Then bake them over a fire in a pan, grind them into powder and form with heat refined honey pills the size of *wu* seeds. Each time ingest 70 pills, to be sent down with a rice beverage or warm wine, whichever is preferred. *Yu jiang shi fang*.

妊娠漏胎，下血不止。百一方用生地黄汁一升，漬酒四合，煮三五沸服之。不止又服。

Leaking fetus[419] during pregnancy, with an unending discharge of blood. The *Bai yi fang* [recommends to] boil a mixture of one *sheng* of fresh/raw *di huang* juice and four *ge* of wine three to five times to bubbling and [let the woman] ingest this. If [the ailment] does not end, ingest this again.

崔氏方用生地黄爲末，酒服方寸匕，日一夜一。

The *Cui shi fang* [recommends to grind] fresh/raw *di huang* into powder and [let the woman] ingest the amount held by a square *cun* spoon. Once during the day, once during the night.

經心録加乾薑爲末。

The *Jing xin lu* [recommends to] add dried ginger and prepare a powder.

418 *Gu du* 蠱毒, "*gu*-poison[ing]." (1) A poison emitted by certain worms/snakes with an ability to cause varying pathological changes in a person who has taken it in by means of wine or food. (2) Abdominal fullness, in some cases with blood spitting, and blood in the stool and urine. BCGM Dict I, 192 - 193. See BCGM 42-22.

419 *Lou tai* 漏胎, "leaking fetus," a condition of vaginal bleeding during pregnancy.

保命集二黄丸：用生地黄、熟地黄等分，爲末。每服半兩，白术、枳殼煎湯，空心調下，日二服。

The *Bao ming ji* [recommends] the "pills with the two [ingredients named] '*huang*'." [Grind] fresh/raw *di huang* and heat processed *di huang* into powder. Each time ingest half a *liang*, to be ingested on an empty stomach mixed with a decoction of *atractylodes macrocephala* [rhizome] and bitter orange fruit. To be ingested twice a day.

妊娠胎痛。妊婦衝任脉虛，惟宜抑陽助陰。内補丸：用熟地黄二兩，當歸一兩，微炒爲末。蜜丸梧子大，每温酒下三十丸。許學士本事方。

Painful womb during pregnancy. In the case of a depletion in the throughway and controller vessels of a pregnant woman, the only measure suitable is to press down yang [qi] and to support yin [qi]. The "pills for an internal supplementation." Slightly fry two *liang* of heat processed *di huang* and one *liang* of Chinese *angelica* [root] and [grind them into] powder. With honey form pills the size of *wu* seeds. Each time [let the woman] send down 30 pills with warm wine. Xu xueshi, *Ben shi fang*.

妊娠胎動。生地黄搗汁，煎沸，入雞子白一枚，攪服。聖惠方。

Fetal movement during pregnancy. Pound fresh/raw *di huang* [and squeeze the resulting pulp] to obtain a juice. Boil it to bubbling, add one chicken egg white, stir this and ingest it. *Sheng hui fang*.

産後血痛有塊，并經脉行後腹痛不調。黑神散：用熟地黄一斤，陳生薑半斤，同炒乾爲末。每服二錢，温酒調下。婦人良方。

Painful blood [disorder] with a lump after delivery, and abnormal abdominal pain following menstruation. The "black spirit powder." Fry together one *jin* of heat processed *di huang* and half a *jin* of long stored fresh ginger until they have dried and [grind them into] powder. Each time [let the patient] ingest two *qian*, to be sent down mixed with warm wine. *Fu ren liang fang*.

産後惡血不止。乾地黄搗末，每食前熱酒服一錢。連進三服。瑞竹堂方。

Unending [discharge of] malign blood[420] following delivery. Pound dried *di huang* into powder and [let the patient] each time prior to a meal ingest with hot wine one *qian*. To be ingested three times consecutively. *Rui zhu tang fang*.

産後中風，脇不得轉。交加散：用生地黄五兩研汁，生薑五兩取汁，交互相浸一夕，次日各炒黄，浸汁乾，乃焙爲末。每酒服一方寸匕。濟生方。

Struck by wind following delivery, with an inability to turn around in the flanks. The "powder to exchange and add." Grind five *liang* of fresh/raw *di huang* to [remove]

420 *E xue* 惡血, "malign blood," identical to *e lu* 惡露, "malign dew," that is blood or turbid liquid leaving from the birth canal after parturition. BCGM Dict I, 144.

the juice. Obtain the juice of five *liang* of fresh ginger. Exchange the two and let [the *di huang* in the ginger juice and the ginger in the *di huang* juice] soak for one night. The next day fry both until they turn yellow. [Again] soak them in the juices until [the juices] are dry. Then bake them over a slow fire and [grind them into] powder. Each time [let the patient] ingest with wine the amount held by one square *cun* spoon. *Ji sheng fang.*

產後煩悶，乃血氣上冲。生地黄汁、清酒各一升，相和煎沸，分二服。集驗方。

Vexing heart-pressure following delivery. This is a rushing upward of blood and qi. Mix one *sheng* each of fresh/raw *di huang* and clear wine and boil this to bubbling. To be ingested divided into two portions. *Ji yan fang.*

產後百病。地黄酒：用地黄汁漬麴貳升，净秫米二斗，令發，如常釀之。至熟，封七日，取清，常服令相接。忌生冷、酢滑、蒜、雞、猪肉，一切毒物。未產先一月釀成。夏月不可造。千金翼方。

The hundreds of diseases following delivery. The "*di huang* wine." Soak two *sheng* of distiller's yeast in *di huang* juice and add two *dou* of clean, glutinous millet. Let it ferment, just like in a normal brewing process. When it is done, seal it for seven days, save the clear [liquid] and regularly ingest it to let [the effects] be linked with each other. [During this treatment] avoid fresh and cold [items], vinegar and smooth [items], garlic, chicken and pork, as well as all poisonous items. Complete the brewing one month prior to a delivery. [This wine] cannot be prepared during summer months. *Qian jin yi fang.*

胞衣不出。生地黄汁一升，苦酒三合，相和煖服。必效方。

Failure of the placenta to come out. Mix one *sheng* of fresh/raw *di huang* juice and three *ge* of bitter wine and ingest this warm. *Bi xiao fang.*

寒疝絞痛來去。用烏雞一隻，治如常法。生地黄七斤，剉細。甑中同蒸，下以銅器承取汁。清旦服至日晡，令盡。其間當下諸寒澼，訖，作白粥食之。久疝者作三劑。肘後方。

A twisting pain, coming and going, related to an elevation-illness[421] caused by cold. Prepare one black [bone] chicken the usual way. Cut seven *jin* of fresh/raw *di huang* into fine pieces and steam them together [with the chicken] in a pot. Place a copper vessel underneath it to obtain the juice. Begin to ingest it in the morning and end

421 *Shan* [*qi*] 疝[氣], "elevation-illness [qi]," a pathological condition of (1) an item having entered the scrotum, with pain, sometimes ascending, sometimes descending, (2) a condition affecting the scrotum or a testicle, (3) of violent abdominal pain, in some cases associated with constipation and anuria. BCGM Dict I, 419, 417.

it at dusk. [Ingest] all of it. In the course [of this treatment] all types of cold wash-out[422] are discharged. When this process has come to an end, prepare a white gruel for consumption [by the patient]. In the case of a long lasting elevation-illness, [let the patient ingest] three preparations. *Zhou hou fang.*

小兒陰腫。以葱椒湯煖處洗之。唾調地黄末傅之。外腎熱者，雞子清調，或加牡蠣少許。危氏方。

Yin (i. e., scrotum) swelling of children. Select a warm place to wash [the affected region] with an onion and Chinese pepper decoction. Then apply a *di huang* powder mixed with human saliva. If the testicles are hot, mix [the powder with] chicken egg white, or add a small amount of oyster shell [powder]. *Wei shi fang.*

小兒熱病，壯熱煩渴，頭痛。生地黄汁三合，蜜半合，和匀，時時與服。普濟方。

Heat disease of children. Strong heat with a vexing thirst and headache. Evenly mix three *ge* of fresh *di huang* juice and half a *ge* of honey and repeatedly give this [to the child] to ingest. *Pu ji fang.*

熱暍昏沉。地黄汁一盞服之。

Heat stroke with clouding and a sunken [movement in the vessels]. [Force the patient] to ingest one cup of *di huang* juice.

熱瘴昏迷，煩悶，飲水不止，至危者，一服見效。生地黄根、生薄荷葉等分，擂爛，取自然汁，入麝香少許，井花水調下，覺心下頓涼，勿再服。普濟方。

Heat miasma[423] with mental confusion, vexing heart-pressure and an unending [desire to] drink water, eventually reaching a critical status. One ingestion will show an effect. Pound equal amounts of fresh/raw *di huang* root (rhizome) and fresh mint leaves into a pulpy [mass, and squeeze it to] obtain their natural juice. Add a little musk and [let the patient] send it down mixed with the first water drawn from a well. When [the patient] has a sudden cold feeling below his heart, he must not ingest it a second time. *Pu ji fang.*

---

422 *Han pi* 寒澼, "cold wash-out," a condition identical to *han pi* 寒癖, "cold aggregation-illness." *Pi* 澼 is an erroneous writing of *pi* 癖 in the *BCGM*. *Han pi* 寒癖, "cold aggregation-illness" refers to a passage of thin white urine following the intake of medication in the course of a treatment of cold aggregation. BCGM Dict I, 208.

423 *Re zhang* 熱瘴, "heat miasma," a condition of *zhang nüe* 瘴瘧, "miasmatic malaria," with heat spells only and no cold. BCGM Dict I, 405.

温毒發斑。黑膏：治温毒發斑嘔逆。生地黄二兩六錢二字半，好豆豉一兩六錢二字半，以豬膏十兩合之，露一夜，煎減三分之一，絞去滓，入雄黄、麝香如豆大，攪匀，分作三服，毒從皮中出則愈。忌蕪荑。千金方。

Warmth poison causing an effusion of macules. The "black ointment." It serves to cure vomiting with a [qi] countermovement and an effusion of macules caused by warmth poison. Mix two *liang*, six *qian* and two and a half *zi* of fresh/raw *di huang*, one *liang*, six *qian* and two and a half *zi* of good [soybean] relish and ten *liang* of lard. Leave this in the open for one night. Boil it down to two thirds. Squeeze this to remove the dregs. Add realgar and musk, [a piece each] as big as a soybean, and mix this evenly. Ingest this divided into three portion. When the poison leaves through the skin, this is the cure. [During the treatment] *ulmus* [fruit] is to be avoided. *Qian jin fang*.

血熱生癬。地黄汁頻服之。千金方。

Blood heat generating a *xuan*-illness.[424] Repeatedly ingest *di huang* juice. *Qian jin fang*.

疔腫乳癰。地黄搗敷之，熱即易。性涼消腫，無不效。梅師方。

Pin-illness swelling[425] and breast obstruction-illness.[426] Pound *di huang* and apply [the pulp to the affected region]. When it gets hot, replace it [with cold pulp]. [*Di huang*] has a cool nature and dissolves swelling. It never has no effect. *Mei shi fang*.

癰癤惡肉：地黄三斤，水一斗，煮取三升，去滓煎稠，塗紙上貼之，日三易。鬼遺方。

Obstruction-illness,[427] pimples, malign flesh [growth]. Boil three *jin* of *di huang* in one *dou* of water down to three *sheng*. Remove the dregs and continue the boiling

424 *Xuan* 癬, "*xuan*-illness," a condition of dermal lesions with initially erythema, papules, and itching gradually extending in all directions to form an irregular ring with clear boundaries. The skin is slightly elevated with small papules, blisters, and/or scales and scraps. The central lesion may appear to heal spontaneously, and it may reappear. Also, local lesions with itching, release of liquid and shedding of scabs. BCGM Dict I, 592.

425 *Ding* 丁, "pin[-illness]," also *ding* 疔, "pin-illness," refers to a deep-reaching and festering hardness in a tissue, eventually rising above the skin like a pinhead. BCGM Dict I, 127-129.

426 *Ru yong* 乳癰, "breast obstruction-illness," a condition of acute putrefication of a woman's breast. Often encountered if a woman, following delivery, experiences *chui nai* 吹奶, "inflated breast," or *du ru* 妒乳, "jealousy breast." BCGM Dict I, 412.

427 *Yong* 癰, "obstruction-illness,"refers to an obstruction of vessels or other ducts inside the body. Qi rushing against the obstruction may cause a local swelling and eventually break through the surface to cause an abscess. BCGM Dict I, 641.

until a paste has formed. Smear it on a sheet of paper and attach it [to the affected region]. Replace it three times a day. *Gui yi fang.*

一切癰疽，及打撲傷損，未破疼痛者。以生地黄杵如泥，攤在上，摻木香末於中，又攤地黄泥一重貼之，不過三五度即内消也。王袞博濟方。

All types of obstruction-illness and impediment-illness,[428] as well as injuries resulting from blows and falls, when [the related swelling] has not broken open yet, but is painful. Pound fresh/raw *di huang* until it has assumed a mud-like consistency and apply it [to the affected region]. Then give *costus* [root] powder into it and spread another layer of *di huang* mud to cover it. After no more than three to five such applications, the [swelling has] dissolved internally. Wang Gun, *Bo ji fang.*

打撲損傷，骨碎及筋傷爛，用生地黄熬膏裹之。以竹簡編夾急縛，勿令轉動。一日一夕，可十易之，則瘥。類説云：許元公過橋墮馬，右臂臼脱，左右急挼入臼中，昏迷不知痛苦。急召田録事視之，曰：尚可救。乃以藥封腫處，中夜方甦，達旦痛止，痛處已白。日日換貼，其瘀腫移至肩背，乃以藥下去黑血三升而愈。即上方也。出肘後方中。

Injuries resulting from a blow or fall, with bone fracture and ruptured sinews. Heat fresh *di huang* to generate a paste and cover [the affected region] with it. Then fix it tightly with bamboo strips so that it cannot move. Within one day and one night this [application] can be replaced ten times, and this results in a cure. The *Lei shuo* states: Xu Yuangong crossed a bridge and fell from his horse, dislocating his right arm from its shoulder capsule. His entourage quickly reset it into the capsule, but [Xu Yuangong] was mentally confused and did not feel any pain. They quickly called on Tian Lushi to examine him, and he said: "A rescue is still possible." Then he sealed the location of the swelling with some medication. By midnight [Xu Yuangong] regained his consciousness and the next morning the pain had stopped. The location of the pain had already turned white. The application was replaced every day. The stagnating [blood] and the swelling moved to the shoulder and the back. He was given medication causing a discharge of three *sheng* of black blood, and then he was cured. This was based on the recipe recorded above. It is taken from the *Zhou hou fang.*

---

428 *Ju* 疽, "impediment-illness," refers to an obstruction of vessels or other ducts inside the body. Qi rushing against the impediment may cause a local swelling and eventually break through the surface to cause an abscess. BCGM Dict I, 277.

損傷打撲瘀血在腹者，用生地黄汁三升，酒一升半，煮二升半，分三服。出千金方。

Stagnating blood in the abdomen, related to an injury resulting from a blow or fall. Boil three *sheng* of fresh/raw *di huang* juice in one and a half *sheng* of wine down to two and a half *sheng*, and ingest it divided into two portions. [Recipe] taken from the *Qian jin fang*.

物傷睛突。輕者瞼胞腫痛，重者目睛突出，但目系未斷者，即納入。急搗生地黄，綿裹傅之。仍以避風膏藥護其四邊。聖濟總録。

The eyball is harmed by a foreign object and protrudes. In light cases the eyelids are swollen and ache. In severe cases this may cause the eyeballs to protrude. When the eyeribbon is not severed yet, it can be inserted back. Quickly pound fresh/raw *di huang*, wrap [the pulp] in a piece of silk and apply this [to the affected eye]. In addition, protect it on all four sides with a medical ointment serving to repel wind. *Sheng ji zong lu*.

睡起目赤腫起，良久如常者，血熱也。卧則血歸於肝，故熱則目赤腫，良久血散，故如常也。用生地黄汁，浸粳米半升，晒乾，三浸三晒。每夜以米煮粥食一盞，數日即愈。有人病此，用之得效。醫餘。

When the eyes are red and swollen when one wakes up, and when it takes quite a long time before they have returned to normal, this is blood heat. While one sleeps, the blood returns to the liver. Hence, in the case of heat the eyes are red and swollen. After a long time the blood disperses and the situation will return to normal. Soak half a *sheng* of glutinous rice in fresh/raw *di huang* juice. Then dry it in the sun. Perform the soaking and the drying three times. Every night use the rice to boil a congee and [let the patient] eat one bowl. After a few days, a cure is achieved. Someone suffered from this. He applied this [recipe] and it was effective. *Yi yu*.

眼暴赤痛。水洗生地黄、黑豆各二兩，搗膏。卧時以鹽湯洗目，閉目以藥厚罨目上，至曉，水潤取下。聖濟總録。

Eyes suddenly turning red and aching. Pound two *liang* each of fresh *di huang*, washed with water, and black soybeans to a paste. At bedtime wash the eyes with a salt decoction. Then let [the patient] close the eyes and apply [the paste] thickly to his eyes. The next morning moisten [the dried paste] with water and remove it. *Sheng ji zong lu*.

蓐内赤目。生地黄薄切，温水浸貼。小品方。

Red eyes during childbirth. Pound fresh/raw *di huang* to small pieces, soak them in warm water and apply this to [the affected region]. *Xiao pin fang*.

牙疳宣露，膿血口氣。生地黄一斤，鹽二合，末，自搗和團，以麪包煨令烟斷，去麪入麝一分，研匀，日夜貼之。聖濟録。

Dental *gan*-illness[429] and tooth exposure, with festering, bleeding and [bad] oral qi. [Grind] one *jin* of fresh/raw *di huang* and two *ge* of salt into powder and form a ball. Wrap it in wheat dough and simmer it until no more smoke is emitted. Remove the dough, add one *fen* of musk and grind it to an even [mixture] to be applied [to the affected region] day and night. *Sheng ji lu.*

牙齒挺長出一分者。常咋生地黄，甚妙。張文仲備急方。

Growth of teeth coming one *fen* long out [of the gums]. Repeatedly bite on a fresh/raw *di huang* [rhizome]. Very wondrous. Zhang Wenzhong, *Bei ji fang*.

牙動欲脱。生地黄綿裹咂之。令汁漬根，并嚥之，日五六次。千金方。

The teeth move and are about to fall out. Wrap fresh/raw *di huang* in silk floss and suck on this. Let the juice soak the roots [of the teeth] and also swallow it. Five to six times a day. *Qian jin fang*.

食蟹齦腫，肉弩出者。生地黄汁一盌，牙皂角數條火炙，蘸盡地黄汁，爲末傅之。永類方。

Swelling of gums related to eating crabs, with a flesh growth. Prepare one boal of fresh/raw *di huang* juice. Then roast with fire several small *gleditsia* [tree] boughs and dip them into the *di huang* juice until it is used up. [Grind them into] powder and apply this [to the affected region]. *Yong lei fang*.

耳中常鳴。生地黄截，塞耳中，日數易之。或煨熟尤妙。肘後方。

Continous sounds in the ears. Cut fresh/raw *di huang* [into pieces] and insert them into the ears. Replace them several times during one day, or [insert them] hot after simmering them. This is particularly wondrous. *Zhou hou fang*.

鬚髮黄赤。生地黄一斤，生薑半斤，各洗，研自然汁，留滓。用不蛀皂角十條，去皮弦，蘸汁，炙至汁盡爲度。同滓入罐内泥固，煅存性，爲末。用鐵器盛末三錢，湯調，停二日，臨卧刷染鬚髮上，即黑。本事方。

Yellow and red hair and beard. Wash one *jin* of fresh/raw *di huang* and half a *jin* of fresh ginger, grind them to obtain their natural juice and keep the dregs. Take ten *gleditsia* pods that are not eaten by moths, with skin and threads removed, and dip them into the juice. Then bake them [and repeat this] until all the juice is used up. Give [the *gleditsia* pods] with the dregs [of *di huang* and ginger] into a pot and seal

429 *Ya gan* 牙疳, "dental *gan*-illness," with teeth and the gums festering and emitting a bad stench, the teeth aching and becoming lose, and the appearance of pus and blood. BCGM Dict I, 605.

it with mud. Calcine them with their nature retained and [grind the residue into] powder. Fill three *qian* of the powder into an iron vessel and mix it with hot water. Let it rest for two days and then apply it, at bedtime, to hair and beard. This will color them black. *Ben shi fang.*

竹木入肉。生地黄嚼爛罨之。救急方。

A splinter of bamboo or wood has entered the flesh. Chew fresh/raw *di huang* to obtain a pulpy [mass] and apply it [to the wound]. *Jiu ji fang.*

毒箭入肉。煎生地黄汁作丸服，至百日，箭出。千金方。

A poisoned arrow has entered the flesh. Boil fresh/raw *di huang* juice to prepare pills and ingest them for up to 100 days and the arrow will come out. *Qian jin fang.*

猘犬咬傷。地黄搗汁飲，并塗之，百度愈。百一方。

Harm caused by a mad dog bite. Pound *di huang* to obtain a juice and drink it, also apply it [to the wound]. Do this 100 times to achieve a cure. *Bai yi fang.*

16-01-04

葉 *Ye*

Leaf [of *di huang*].

【主治】惡瘡似癩，十年者，擣爛日塗，鹽湯先洗。千金方。【時珍曰】按抱朴子云：韓子治用地黄苗喂五十歲老馬，生三駒，又一百三十歲乃死也。張鷟朝野僉載云：雉被鷹傷，銜地黄葉點之；虎中藥箭，食清泥解之。鳥獸猶知解毒，何況人乎？

Control. Malign sores resembling repudiation-illness.[430] If this has lasted for ten years, pound [the leaves] to obtain a pulpy [mass] and apply it [to the affected region] daily. First, though, wash it with a salt decoction. *Qian jin fang.* [Li] Shizhen: According to the *Baopu zi*, Han Zizhi had fed an old horse with *di huang* seedlings for 50 years. Then it gave birth to three colts. Also, it lived on for 130 years before it died. Zhang Zhuo in his *Chao ye jian zai* states: "When a pheasant is harmed by a goshawk, it holds in its mouth a *di huang* leaf to drip [its juice] onto the [wound]. When a tiger is struck by a medicated arrow, it eats clear mud to resolve the [poison]. Fowl and animals seem to know how to resolve poison. Should this not apply all the more to humans?"

430 *Lai* 癩, "*lai*-illness," "repudiation-illness," including cases of leprosy/Aussatz." BCGM Dict I, 293.

16-01-05
實 *Shi*
Fruit [of *di huang*].

【主治】四月采，陰乾擣末，水服方寸匕，日三服，功與地黄等。蘇頌。○【弘景曰】出渭城者有子，淮南七精丸用之。

Control. Collected in the fourth month, dried in the yin (i. e., shade) and ground into powder, and the amount held by a square *cun* spoon ingested with water, has a [therapeutic] potential equal to that of *di huang* [rhizome]. Su Song. [Tao] Hongjing: Those from Wei cheng have seeds. They are used in the "pills of Huai nan with seven essences."

16-01-06
花 *Hua*
Flower [of *di huang*].

【主治】爲末服食，功同地黄。蘇頌。腎虚腰脊痛，爲末，酒服方寸匕，日三。時珍。

Control. The powder ingested as food has a [therapeutic] potential identical to that of *di huang* [rhizomes]. Su Song. For kidney depletion and aching lower back and back, [grind it into] powder and ingest with wine the amount held by a square *cun* spoon. Three times a day. [Li] Shizhen.

【附方】新一。
Added Recipes. One newly [recorded].

内障青盲，風赤生瞖，及墜睛日久，瞳損失明。地黄花晒、黑豆花晒、槐花晒各一兩，爲末。豬肝一具，同以水二斗，煮至上有凝脂，掠盡瓶收。每點少許，日三四次。聖惠方。

Inner screens with green blindness, [eyes] red because of wind [intrusion] and growing a shade, also, eyeballs having descended for an entire day, and injured pupils with a loss of eyesight. [Grind] one *liang* each of *di huang* flowers, dried in the sun, black soybean flowers, dried in the sun, and *sophora japonica* flowers, dried in the sun, into powder. Boil it together with one pig liver in two *dou* of water until a fat congeals on its surface. Scoop it up completely and store it in a jar. Each time drip a small amount [into the affected eyes]. Three to four times a day. *Sheng hui fang*.

【附録】
Appendix.

16-01-A01
胡面莽拾遺。***Hu mian mang***, FE *Shi yi*.

Unidentified.

【藏器曰】味甘，温，無毒。主去痃癖及冷氣，止腹痛，煮服。生嶺南，葉如地黄。

[Chen] Cangqi: Flavor sweet, warm, nonpoisonous. To control the removal of string-illness[431] and aggregation-illness,[432] as well as cold qi, and to end abdominal pain, boil it [in water and] ingest [the decoction]. It grows in Ling nan. The leaves resemble those of *di huang*.

16-02
牛膝本經上品
Niu xi, FE *Ben jing*, upper rank.

***Achyranthes bidentata* Bl. Twotooth achyranthes.**[433]

【釋名】牛莖廣雅、百倍本經、山莧菜救荒、對節菜。【弘景曰】其莖有節，似牛膝，故以爲名。【時珍曰】本經又名百倍，隱語也。言其滋補之功，如牛之多力也。其葉似莧，其節對生，故俗有山莧、對節之稱。

Explanation of Names. *Niu jing* 牛莖, "ox stem," *Guang ya*. *Bai bei* 百倍, "a hundred times more," *Ben jing*. *Shan xian cai* 山莧菜, "mountain amaranth vegetable," *Jiu huang*. *Dui jie cai* 對節菜, "opposite at the nodes vegetable." [Tao] Hongjing: Its stem has nodes resembling the knees of oxen. Hence the name. [Li] Shizhen: The *Ben jing* also names it *bai bei* 百倍, "a hundred times more." This is a secret name. It refers to [the herb's] ability to nourish and supplement, with a strength manifold exceeding that of oxen. The leaves resemble those of *amaranth* [herbs]; they grow facing each other at the nodes. Hence [the plant] is commonly named *shan xian* 山莧, "mountain *amaranth*" and *dui jie* 對節, "opposite at the nodes."

【集解】【别録曰】牛膝生河内川谷及臨朐，二月、八月、十月采根，陰乾。【普曰】葉如夏藍，莖本赤。【弘景曰】今出近道蔡州者，最長大柔潤。其莖有節，莖紫節大者爲雄，青細者爲雌，以雄爲勝。【大明曰】懷

431 *Xuan* 痃, "string-illness," a condition of acute pain located in the abdomen to the left and right of the umbilicus. BCGM Dict I, 591.

432 *Pi* 癖, "aggregation-illness," of painful lumps emerging from time to time in both flanks. BCGM Dict I, 371.

433 *Niu xi* 牛膝, lit.: "ox knee."

州者長白，蘇州者色紫。【頌曰】今江、淮、閩、粵、關中亦有之，然不及懷慶者爲真。春生苗，莖高二三尺，青紫色，有節如鶴膝及牛膝狀。葉尖圓如匙，兩兩相對。於節上生花作穗，秋結實甚細。以根極長大至三尺而柔潤者爲佳。莖葉亦可單用。【時珍曰】牛膝處處有之，謂之土牛膝，不堪服食。惟北土及川中人家栽蒔者爲良。秋間收子，至春種之。其苗方莖暴節，葉皆對生，頗似莧葉而長且尖[角肖]。秋月開花，作穗結子，狀如小鼠負蟲，有澁毛，皆貼莖倒生。九月末取根，水中浸兩宿。挼去皮，[日良]紮暴乾，雖白直可貴，而挼去白汁入藥，不如留皮者力大也。嫩苗可作菜茹。

Collected Explanations. *Bie lu*: *Niu xi* grows in the river valleys of He nei and in Lin qu. The root is collected in the second, eighth and tenth month. It is dried in the yin (i. e., shade). [Wu] Pu: The leaves are similar to those of Chinese indigo plants in summer; the stem is red. [Tao] Hongjing: Specimens recently coming from nearby Cai zhou are very long, big, soft and moist. The stems have nodes. Those with a purple stem and large nodes are males; those that with a greenish and fine [stem] are females. Males are considered to be superior. Da Ming: Specimens from Huai zhou are long and white. Those from Su zhou are of purple color. [Su] Song: Today, [*niu xi*] is also found in Jiang, Huai, Min, Ao and Guan. But [*niu xi* grown in these regions] is not as genuine as that from Huai qing. In spring it grows a seedling. The stem reaches a height of two to three *chi*; it is of greenish-purple color and has nodes similar to the knees of cranes and oxen. The leaves are pointed and round like a spoon, with always two growing facing each other. Flowers grow from the nodes upward and form spikes. In autumn they form very fine fruit. Those with a soft and moist root of a maximum length of up to three *chi* are considered excellent. Stem and leaves can also be used separately. [Li] Shizhen: *Niu xi* can be found everywhere. It is named *tu niu xi* 土牛膝, "soil/local *niu xi*," and is not suitable for ingestion [as medication] or consumption [as vegetable]. Only those [*niu xi*] that are planted in the North and in Chuan zhong are good. The seeds are gathered in autumn to be planted in spring. The seedlings have square stems with extraordinarily pronounced nodes. All the leaves grow facing each other [at these nodes]. They are quite similar to *amaranth* leaves, but they are longer and pointed at their tip. In autumn [*niu xi*] opens flowers. They form spikes with seeds, shaped like small pill bugs. They have rough hair and they cling to the stem with an inverse growth. The root is collected at the end of autumn. It is soaked in water for two days. Then the skin is peeled off and discarded. Dry [the root] and tie it to bundles, and then dry [these bundles] in the sun. Although it is white and truly valuable, and its white juice can be squeezed out to be added to medication, its strength is not equal to that of [the juice of roots] if their skin is left in place. The tender seedlings can be processed into vegetables.

16-02-01
根 *Gen*
Root [of *niu xi*]

【修治】【斅曰】凡使去頭蘆，以黄精自然汁浸一宿，漉出，剉，焙乾用。【時珍曰】今惟以酒浸入藥，欲下行則生用，滋補則焙用，或酒拌蒸過用。

Pharmaceutical Preparation. [Lei] Xiao: For all applications, remove the tip and the reed [rhizomes]. Then soak [the root] in the natural juice of Solomon's seal [root] for one day. Filter this to remove [the root], cut it, bake it over a slow fire until it is dry, and then use it [for therapeutic purposes]. [Li] Shizhen: Today, it is only soaked in wine before it is added to medication. If it is supposed to move downward, it is used fresh. If it is supposed to nourish and supplement, it is used after baking it over a slow fire. It can also be used steamed mixed with wine.

【氣味】苦、酸，平，無毒。【普曰】神農：甘。雷公：酸，無毒。李當之：温。【之才曰】惡螢火、龜甲、陸英，畏白前，忌牛肉。

Qi and Flavor. Bitter, sour, balanced, nonpoisonous. [Wu] Pu: Shen nong: Sweet. Lei gong: Sour, nonpoisonous. Li Dingzhi: Warm. [Xu] Zhicai: [Ingested together,] it abhors fireflies, tortoise carapaces, and Chinese elder. It fears *cynanchum stauntonii* [root]. [During a treatment with *niu xi* roots] avoid beef.

【主治】寒濕痿痺，四肢拘攣，膝痛不可屈伸，逐血氣，傷熱火爛，墮胎。久服輕身耐老。本經。療傷中少氣，男子陰消，老人失溺，補中續絶，益精，利陰氣，填骨髓，止髮白，除腦中痛及腰脊痛，婦人月水不通，血結。别録。治陰痿，補腎，助十二經脉，逐惡血。甄權。治腰膝軟怯冷弱，破癥結，排膿止痛，産後心腹痛并血運，落死胎。大明。强筋，補肝臟風虚。好古。同蓯蓉浸酒服，益腎。竹木刺入肉，嚼爛罨之，即出。宗奭。治久瘧寒熱，五淋尿血，莖中痛，下痢，喉痺，口瘡，齒痛，癰腫惡瘡，傷折。時珍。

Control. Dysfunction and blockage/numbness related to the presence of cold and moisture, with the four limbs cramped and contracted. The knees ache and cannot be bent or stretched. It eliminates blood and qi [disorders], harm caused by heat and fire, and causes abortion. Ingested over a long time, it relieves the body of its weight and helps to endure aging. *Ben jing*. It heals harmed center and lack of [breath] qi, yin melting[434] of males, and uncontrolled urination of older persons. It supplements [qi in] the center and connects interrupted [passages of blood and qi]. It boosts essence/sperm, frees the flow of yin qi, fills bone marrow, ends the greying of hair, removes pain from inside the brain and pain in the lower back and back. [It serves to cure] blocked menstruation of women and blood nodes. *Bie lu.* It serves to cure yin (i. e., erectile) dysfunction, supplements the kidney [qi], supports the [movement in the] 12 conduit vessels and removes malign blood. Zhen Quan. It serves to cure soft and timid lower back and knees, with cold and weakness. It breaks through concretion-illness nodes, dissipates pus and ends pain, [and heals] pain in the central and abdominal region after birth associated with blood [induced brain] movement. It enables the loss of a dead fetus. Da Ming. It strengthens the sinews. It supplements [qi in] the liver long-term depot in a situation of depletion with wind[-intrusion]. [Wang] Haogu. Soaked with desert broomrape and ingested with wine, it boosts the kidney [qi]. When a bamboo or wood splinter has entered the flesh, chew it to a pulpy [mass] and apply this [to the wound. The splinter] will come out. [Kou] Zongshi. It serves to cure long-lasting malaria with alternating sensations of cold and heat, the five types of urinary dripping with blood, and pain in the stalk (i. e., penis), discharge with free-flux illness, throat closure, oral sores, toothache, swelling and malign sores associated with an obstruction-illness,[435] as well as fractures. [Li] Shizhen.

【發明】【權曰】病人虛羸者，加而用之。【震亨曰】牛膝能引諸藥下行，筋骨痛風在下者，宜加用之。凡用土牛膝，春夏用葉，秋冬用根，惟葉汁效尤速。【時珍曰】牛膝乃足厥陰、少陰之藥。所主之病，大抵得酒則能補肝腎，生用則能去惡血，二者而已。其治腰膝骨痛、足痿陰消、失溺久瘧、傷中少氣諸病，非取其補肝腎之功歟？其癥瘕、心腹諸痛、癰腫惡瘡、金瘡折傷、喉齒、淋痛尿血、經候胎産諸病，非取其去惡血之功歟？按陳日華經驗方云：方夷吾所編集要方，予刻之臨汀。後在鄂渚，得九江守王南强書云：老人久苦淋疾，百藥不效。偶見臨汀集要方中用牛膝者，服之而愈。又葉朝議親人患血淋，流下小便在盆内凝如蒟蒻，久而有變如鼠形，但無足爾，百治不效。一村醫用牛膝根煎濃汁，日飲五服，名地髓湯。雖未即愈，而血色漸淡，久乃復舊。後十年病又作，服之又瘥。因檢本草，見肘後方治小便不利，莖中痛欲死，用牛膝并葉，以酒煮服之。今再拈出，表其神功。又按楊士瀛直指方云：小便淋痛，或尿血，或

434 *Yin xiao* 陰消, "yin melting," is *yin wei* 陰痿, "yin dysfunction," a condition of male adults with partial or complete erectile dysfunction, resulting in an inability to have sexual intercourse. BCGM Dict I, 637.

435 *Yong* 癰, "obstruction-illness," refers to an obstruction of vessels or other ducts inside the body. Qi rushing against the obstruction may cause a local swelling and eventually break through the surface to cause an abscess. BCGM Dict I, 641.

沙石服痛。用川牛膝一兩，水二盞，煎一盞，温服。一婦患此十年，服之得效。杜牛膝亦可，或入麝香、乳香尤良。

Explication. [Zhen] Quan: Patients with depletion emaciation use it added [to their medication]. [Zhu] Zhenheng: *Niu xi* can lead all types of medication to move downward. In the case of painful sinews and bones with the presence of wind in the lower [body parts], it is advisable to use it. For all uses of *tu niu xi*, in spring and summer use the leaves, in autumn and winter use the root. The application of only the juice of the leaves yields especially fast effects. [Li] Shizhen: *Niu xi* is a pharmaceutical drug of the foot ceasing yin and minor yin [conduits]. As for the diseases it controls, in general, [ingested] combined with wine it can supplement liver and kidneys. Applied raw, it can eliminate malign blood. [*Niu xi*] has these two [effects], and there is nothing else to it. Now, when it is applied to cure all types of diseases such as aching bones in the lower back and in the knees, dysfunction of the feet and yin melting, uncontrolled loss of urine and long-lasting malaria, harmed center and shortness of [breath] qi, is this not making use of its potential to supplement liver and kidney [qi]? And when [it is applied to cure] all types of diseases such as concretion-illness and conglomeration-illness, all types of pain in the central section and abdomen, swelling and malign sores associated with an obstruction-illness, wounds caused by metal objects/weapons and fracture harm, throat and tooth [disorders], painful urinary dripping with blood, and [ailments associated with] menstruation and birth, is this not making use of its potential to remove malign blood? According to Chen Rihua's *Jing yan fang*, "I printed the *Ji yao fang* compiled by Fang Yiwu in Lin ding. Later in E zhu, Wang Nanqiang, governor of Jiu jiang, sent me a letter stating: 'As an old person [I] often suffered from urinary dripping illness, and none of the hundreds of medications was effective. It so happened that I read of the use of *niu xi* recorded in the *Ji yao fang* [published in] Ling ding. I ingested it and was cured.' Also, a relative of Ye Chaoyi suffered from urinary dripping with blood. When he urinated into a bucket, it congealed to something like devil's tongue. After a long time this assumed the shape of a rat/mouse, but without legs. A hundred therapies remained without effect. A village doctor boiled *niu xi* roots to obtain a thick juice and [let the patient] drink it five times a day; he called it 'earth marrow decoction.' Even before a cure was achieved, the color of the blood became paler and after a long time [the patient's] former condition was restored. Ten years later he acquired the same disease. He ingested [*niu xi*] and was cured again. When [I] checked the *ben cao* [literature, I] realized that the *Zhou hou fang* to cure blocked urination, with a pain in the stalk (i. e., penis) so severe that one wishes to die, uses *niu xi* with its leaves, to be ingested boiled in wine. Here now I point this out again to make widely known its divine potential". Also, according to Yang Shiyin in his

Zhi zhi fang, "for painful urinary dripping, and also urination with blood, and painful distention with a sand and stone [urinary] dripping, [the following recipe] is to be used. Boil one *liang* of *niu xi* from [Si] chuan in two cups of water down to one cup and ingest this warm. A woman suffered from this for ten years. She ingested this [medication] and it was effective. The use of *carpesium* root (*du niu xi* 杜牛膝) is possible, too. With musk and frankincense added [the effects are] especially good."

【附方】舊十三，新八。
Added Recipes. 13 of old. Eight newly [recorded].

勞瘧積久不止者。長牛膝一握，生切，以水六升，煮二升，分三服。清早一服，未發前一服，臨發時一服。外臺秘要。

Exhaustion with malaria that has accumulated for a long time without coming to an end. Boil one handful of long *niu xi*, cut fresh into pieces, in six *sheng* of water down to two *sheng* and ingest this divided into three portions, to be ingested, first, in the early morning, second prior to an outbreak, and third just at the moment of a beginning outbreak. *Wai tai mi yao.*

消渴不止，下元虛損。牛膝五兩爲末，生地黄汁五升浸之，日曝夜浸，汁盡爲度。蜜丸梧子大，每空心溫酒下三十丸。久服壯筋骨，駐顏色，黑髮，津液自生。經驗後方。

Unending melting with thirst,[436] with an injury related to a depletion of original [qi] in the lower [body part]. [Grind] five *liang* of *niu xi* into powder and soak it in five *sheng* of fresh Chinese floxglove [rhizome] juice. Then dry it in the sun, and at night soak it again, and [continue this] until all the juice is used up. With honey form pills the size of *wu* seeds. Each time send down on an empty stomach 30 pills with wine. Ingested over a long time, they strengthen sinews and bones, maintain one's complexion, let the hair remain black and stimulate the generation of body fluids. *Jing yan hou fang.*

卒暴癥疾，腹中有如石刺，晝夜啼呼。牛膝二斤，以酒一斗漬之，密封，于灰火中溫令味出。每服五合至一升，隨量飲。肘後方。

Sudden, violent concretion-illness with in the abdomen forming something like a stone thorn, letting [the patient] shout and wail day and night. Soak two *jin* of *niu xi* in in one *dou* of wine. Firmly seal [the vessel], place it into fiery ashes and warm it until it emits a flavor. Each time ingest five *ge* up to one *sheng*, drinking as much as you please. *Zhou hou fang.*

436 *Xiao ke* 消渴, "melting with thirst," most likely including cases of diabetes. BCGM Dict Vol I, 567.

痢下腸蠱。凡痢下應先白後赤，若先赤後白爲腸蠱。牛膝二兩搗碎，以酒一升漬經一宿。每飲一兩盃，日三服。肘後方。

Free-flux illness discharge, intestinal *gu*.[437] All free-flux illness discharge should be white first and red later on. If it is red first and white afterwards, it is "intestinal *gu*." Pound two *liang* of *niu xi* to small pieces and soak them in one *sheng* of wine for one night. Each time drink one or two cups, to be ingested three times a day. *Zhou hou fang*.

婦人血塊。土牛膝根洗切，焙搗爲末，酒煎温服，極效。福州人單用之。圖經本草。

Blood clots [discharged] by a woman. Wash the root of *tu niu gen* and cut it into pieces. Bake them over a slow fire, and pound them into powder. Boil it in wine and [let the woman] ingest this warm. Extremely effective. In Fu zhou people use it as a single substance. *Tu jing ben cao*.

女人血病。萬病丸：治女人月經淋閉，月信不來，遶臍寒疝痛，及產後血氣不調，腹中結瘕癥不散諸病。牛膝酒浸一宿，焙，乾漆炒令烟盡，各一兩，爲末，生地黄汁一升，入石器內，慢火熬至可丸，丸如梧子大。每服二丸，空心米飲下。拔萃方。

Blood disease of females. The "pills for a myriad diseases." The serve to cure blocked female menstruation, failure of menses to set in, painful elevation-illness[438] related to the presence of cold surrounding the navel, and blood and qi disorders after delivery, as well as conglomeration-illness and concretion-illness that fail to disperse, all such diseases. [Grind] one *liang* each of *niu xi*, soaked in wine for one night and then baked over a slow fire, and dried lacquer, fried until no more fumes are emitted, into powder. Give [the powder together with] one *sheng* of fresh/raw Chinese foxglove [rhizome] juice into an earthenware vessel, and heat this with a slow fire until it [has reached a consistency] that can be formed to pills. [Prepare] pills the size of *wu* seeds. Each time [let the woman] ingest two pills, to be sent down on an empty stomach with a rice beverage. *Ba cui fang*.

437 *Chang gu* 腸蠱, "intestinal *gu*," a condition of a *li ji* 痢疾, "free-flux illness ailment," which is first red and then white and lasts without healing for many years. BCGM Dict I, 79.

438 *Shan* [*qi*] 疝[氣], "elevation-illness [qi]," a pathological condition of (1) an item having entered the scrotum, with pain, sometimes ascending, sometimes descending, (2) a condition affecting the scrotum or a testicle, (3) of violent abdominal pain, in some cases associated with constipation and anuria. BCGM Dict I, 419, 417.

婦人陰痛。牛膝五兩，酒三升，煮取一升半，去滓，分三服。千金方。

Painful yin [(i. e., genital)] region of women. Boil five *liang* of *niu xi* in three *sheng* of wine down to one and a half *sheng*, remove the dregs and [let the woman] ingest [the liquid] divided into three portions. *Qian jin fang*.

生胎欲去。牛膝一握搗，以無灰酒一盞，煎七分，空心服。仍以獨根土牛膝塗麝香，插入牝户中。婦人良方。

An intention to abort a living fetus. Pound one handful of *niu xi* and boil [the pieces] in one cup of ash-free wine down to 70%. Ingest this on an empty stomach. Also, smear musk on a single root *tu niu xi* and insert this into the vagina. *Fu ren liang fang*.

胞衣不出。牛膝八兩，葵子一合，水九升，煎三升，分三服。延年方。

Failure to release the placenta. Boil eight *liang* of *niu xi* and one *ge* of Chinese malva seeds in nine *sheng* of water down to three *sheng* and [let the woman] ingest this divided into three portions. *Yan nian fang*.[439]

產後尿血。川牛膝水煎頻服。熊氏補遺。

Urination with blood following birth. Boil *niu xi* from [Si] chuan in water and ingest this repeatedly. Xiong shi, *Bu yi*.

喉痺乳蛾。新鮮牛膝根一握，艾葉七片，搗，和人乳，取汁灌入鼻內，須臾痰涎從口鼻出，即愈。無艾亦可。

Blocked throat and nipple moths.[440] Pound one handful of newly gathered, fresh *niu xi* root and seven mugwort leaves, mix this with human milk and [squeeze this] to get a juice. Force-feed it into the [patient's] nose. After a short while phlegm leaves from the mouth and the nose, and this is the cure. If no mugwort is available, this works, too.

一方：牛膝搗汁，和陳酢灌之。

Another recipe. Pound *niu xi* to obtain a juice, mix it with long-stored vinegar and force-feed it [to the patient].

口舌瘡爛。牛膝浸酒含漱，亦可煎飲。肘後方。

Sores and erosion affecting mouth and tongue. Soak *niu xi* in wine, hold it in the mouth and rinse it. It is also possible to boil [the *niu xi*] and drink [the liquid]. *Zhou hou fang*.

439 Instead of *Yan nian fang* 延年方, *Zheng lei* ch. 6, *niu xi* 牛膝, names the *Mei shi fang* 梅师方 as source.

440 *Ru e* 乳蛾, "nipple moth," acute tonsillitis. A condition with red swelling and pain on both sides of the throat, in severe cases including the generation of pus forming white dots, as a major sign. BCGM Dict I, 410.

牙齒疼痛。牛膝研末含漱。亦可燒灰。千金方。

Toothache. Grind *niu xi* into powder, hold it in the mouth and rinse [the affected teeth]. It is also possible to burn it to ashes. *Qian jin fang*.

折傷閃肭。杜牛膝搗罨之。衛生易簡方。

Fracture harm and sprain. Pound *du niu xi* (*carpesium* root, sic!) and apply [the pulp to the affected region]. *Wei sheng yi jian fang*.

金瘡作痛。生牛膝搗敷，立止。梅師方。

Painful wounds caused by metal objects/weapons. Pound fresh *niu xi* [to a pulp] and apply this [to the wound. The pain] ends immediately. *Mei shi fang*.

卒得惡瘡人不識者。牛膝根搗傅之。千金方。

Sudden development of malign sores unknown to everybody. Pound *niu xi* root and apply [the resulting pulp to the affected region]. *Qian jin fang*.

癰癤已潰。用牛膝根略刮去皮，插入瘡口中，留半寸在外，以嫩橘葉及地錦草各一握，搗其上。牛膝能去惡血，二草温凉止痛，隨乾隨換，有十全之功也。陳日華經驗方。

Obstruction-illness[441] and pimples that have begun to fester. Remove the skin from a *niu xi* root and insert it into the opening of the sore, with half a *cun* remaining outside. Pound one handful each of tender tangerine leaves and thyme-leaf spurge herb and apply [the resulting pulp] to [the location of the festering]. The *niu xi* is capable of removing malign blood; the two herbs, warming and cooling, end the pain. As soon as [the pulp] has dried, replace it with [moist pulp]. [This therapy] has a potential of 100% success. Chen Rihua, *Jing yan fang*.

風瘙癮疹及痞瘰。牛膝末，酒服方寸匕，日三服。千金方。

Wind itching[442] and dormant papules, and clustered [seeds] illness.[443] Ingest with wine the amount of *niu xi* powder held by a square *cun* spoon. To be ingested three times a day. *Qian jin fang*.

441 *Yong* 癰, "obstruction-illness,"refers to an obstruction of vessels or other ducts inside the body. Qi rushing against the obstruction may cause a local swelling and eventually break through the surface to cause an abscess. BCGM Dict I, 641.

442 *Feng sao* 風瘙, "wind itching," a condition of wind evil or wind cold entering the skin, with the skin itching, or the emergence of skin papules, as major signs. BCGM Dict I, 167.

443 *Pei lei* 痞瘰, "clustered [seeds]-illness," a condition with small pimples or knots on the skin as its major sign. BCGM Dict I, 370.

骨疽癩病。方同上。

Bone impediment-illness,[444] and repudiation-illness.[445] Recipe identical to the one above.

16-02-02

莖葉 *Jing ye*

Stem and leaf [of *niu xi*].

【氣味】缺。

Qi and Flavor. Missing.

【主治】寒濕痿痺，老瘧淋閟，諸瘡。功同根，春夏宜用之。時珍。

Control. Dysfunction and blockage/numbness related to a presence of cold and moisture. Chronic malaria, urinary dripping and heart-pressure. All types of sores. The [therapeutic] potential is identical to that of the root. In spring and summer it is suitable to use [stem and leaf]. [Li] Shizhen.

【附方】舊三，新一。

Added Recipes. Three of old. One newly [recorded].

氣濕痺痛，腰膝痛。用牛膝葉一斤，切，以米三合，於豉汁中煮粥。和鹽、醬，空腹食之。聖惠方。

Painful blockage related to qi [disorder] and the presence of moisture. Painful lower back and knees. Cut one *jin* of *niu xi* leaves, mix them with three *ge* of rice and boil this in [soybean] relish juice to a congee, to be eaten with salt and soysauce on an empty stomach. *Sheng hui fang.*

老瘧不斷。牛膝莖葉一把切，以酒三升漬服，令微有酒氣。不即斷更作，不過三劑止。肘後方。

Long-lasting malaria that does not end. Soak one handful of *niu xi* stems and leaves, cut into pieces, in three *sheng* of wine and [let the patient] ingest this so that he is slightly [intoxicated by] the wine qi. If this is insufficient, [the disease] will be interrupted and then break out again. After no more than three applications it will end. *Zhou hou fang.*

444 *Ju* 疽, "impediment-illness," refers to an obstruction of vessels or other ducts inside the body. Qi rushing against the impediment may cause a local swelling and eventually break through the surface to cause an abscess. BCGM Dict I, 277.

445 *Lai* 癩, "*lai*-illness," "repudiation-illness," including cases of leprosy/Aussatz." BCGM Dict I, 293.

溪毒寒熱。東間有溪毒中人似射工，但無物。初病惡寒發熱煩懊，骨節强痛。不急治，生蟲食臟殺人。用雄牛膝莖紫色節大者一把，以酒、水各一盃同搗，絞汁溫飲，日三服。肘後方。

Rivulet poison[446] with alternating sensations of cold and heat. In the East exists a rivulet poison that may hit one similar to the [poison emitted by the] archer.[447] But it is immaterial. At the beginning of the disease one has an aversion to cold with an effusion of heat and vexing anguish. Bone joints are stiff and ache. If this is not quickly cured, worms/bugs develop and eat the long-term depots, eventually killing that person. Take one handful of *niu xi* stems of purple color with big nodes and pound them together with one cup each of wine and water. Squeeze [the resulting pulp] to obtain a juice and drink it warm. To be ingested three times a day. *Zhou hou fang.*

眼生珠管。牛膝并葉搗汁，日點三四次。聖惠方。

The eyes develop pearls in a tube.[448] Pound *niu xi* [stems] with their leaves to obtain a juice and drip this [into the affected eyes], three to four times a day. *Sheng hui fang.*

16-03
紫菀本經中品

Zi wan. FE *Ben jing*, middle rank.

***Aster tataricus* L. f. Purple aster.**

【釋名】青菀別録、紫蒨別録、返魂草綱目、夜牽牛。【時珍曰】其根色紫而柔宛。故名，許慎説文作茈菀。斗門方謂之返魂草。

Explanation of Names. *Qing wan* 青菀, *Bie lu. Zi qian* 紫蒨, *Bie lu. Fan hun cao* 返魂草, *Gang mu. Ye qian niu* 夜牽牛, "pulling the oxen at night." [Li] Shizhen: The root is purple, *zi* 紫, soft and curved, *wan* 宛. Hence the name. Xu Shen in his *Shuo wen* writes *ci wan* 茈菀. The *Dou men fang* calls it *fan hun cao* 返魂草, "the herb that lets one's *hun*-soul return."

【集解】【別録曰】紫菀生漢中房陵山谷及真定、邯鄲。二月、三月采根，陰乾。【弘景曰】近道處處有之。其生布地，花紫色，本有白毛，根

446 *Xi du* 溪毒, "rivulet poison," 1.) A tiny bug assumed to live in bodies of water and supposedly capable of striking humans when they enter the water, thereby causing disease. 2.) A condition resulting from being struck by rivulet poison. BCGM Dict I, 548.

447 *She gong* 射工, "archer," 1.) a small bug in ancient times believed to live in water and be capable of "shooting" poison from its mouth at people, thereby causing disease; 2.) a condition caused by the archer's poison. BCGM Dict. I, 432. See 42-15.

448 *Zhu guan* 珠管, "pearls in a tube," a condition of *yan xi* 眼瘜, "tumor-illness on the eye," with a crystal clear color reminiscent of pearls in a tube. BCGM Dict I, 691.

甚柔細。有白者名白菀，不復用。【大明曰】形似重臺，根作節，紫色潤軟者佳。【頌曰】今耀、成、泗、壽、台、孟、興國諸州皆有之。三月内布地生苗，其葉二四相連，五月、六月内開黄白紫花，結黑子。餘如陶說。【恭曰】白菀，即女菀也。療體與紫菀相同，無紫菀時亦用之。【穎曰】紫菀連根葉采之，醋浸，入少鹽收藏，作菜辛香，號名仙菜。鹽不宜多，則腐也。【時珍曰】按陳自明云：紫菀以牢山所出根如北細辛者爲良，沂、兗以東皆有之。今人多以車前、旋復根赤土染過僞之。紫菀肺病要藥，肺本自亡津液，又服走津液藥，爲害滋甚，不可不慎。

Collected Explanations. *Bie lu*: *Zi wan* grows in the mountain valleys of Fang ling, in Han zhong, and also in Zhen ding and Han dang. The root is collected in the second and third month. It is dried in the yin (i. e., shade). [Tao] Hongjing: It can be found everywhere nearby. Its growth covers the ground. The flowers are purple; with white hair at their base. The root is very soft and fine. White specimens are called *bai wan* 白菀. They are no longer used. Da Ming: Their physical appearance resembles that of *scrophularia* [root]. [Su] Song: Today it is present in all the *zhou* of Yao, Cheng, Si, Shou, Tai, Meng and Xing guo. In the third month it grows seedlings covering the ground, with two to four leaves interconnected. In the fifth and sixth month it opens yellow-white-purple flowers, and they form black seeds. The rest is as described by Tao [Hongjing]. [Su] Gong: *Bai wan* 白菀 is *nü wan* 女菀. Its therapeutic [potential] is identical to that of *zi wan* 紫菀. If no *zi wan* 紫菀 is at hand, it is used, too. [Wang] Ying: *Zi wan* is collected with the root and the leaves. Soak it in vinegar, add a little salt and store it. Prepared as a vegetable it is acrid and fragrant, and it is called "hermit/immortal's vegetable." Do not add too much salt, lest [the herb] rot. [Li] Shizhen: According to Chen Ziming, "the roots of *zi wan* coming from Lao shan and resembling those of *asarum heteropoides* are good. They can be found everywhere east of Yi and Yan. Today, people fake them by dying the Asiatic plantain and horseheal roots with red soil. *Zi wan* is an important pharmaceutical drug for lung diseases. If [patients] whose lung have already lost body fluids are ingesting medication that causes further loss of body fluids, it is dangerous and increases [the severity of the disease]. One must be careful!"

16-013-01
根 *Gen*
Root [of *zi wan*].

【修治】【斅曰】凡使先去鬚。有白如練色者，號曰羊鬚草，自然不同。去頭及土，用東流水洗净，以蜜浸一宿，至明於火上焙乾用。一兩用蜜二分。

Pharmaceutical Preparation: [Lei] Xiao: For all applications, first remove the "whiskers." There are specimens that are white like refined silk. They are called "sheep whiskers herb." They are of a different nature. Remove the top [of the root] and the soil and wash it clean with water running eastward. Then soak it in honey for one night and the next morning bake it over a slow fire to let it dry so that it can be used [for therapeutic purposes]. For one *liang* [of the root] use two *fen* of honey.

【氣味】苦，温，無毒。【别録曰】辛。【權曰】苦，平。【之才曰】款冬爲之使，惡天雄、瞿麥、藁本、雷丸、遠志，畏茵蔯。

Qi and Flavor. Acrid, warm, nonpoisonous. *Bie lu*: Acrid. [Zhen] Quan: Bitter, acrid. [Xu[Zhicai: Coltsfoot serves as its guiding [substance]. [Ingested together,] it abhors *aconitum* [root], fringed pink, Chinese *ligusticum*, thunderball fungus, and *polygala* [root]. It fears *artemisia scoparia* [herb].

【主治】欬逆上氣，胸中寒熱結氣，去蠱毒痿躄，安五臟。本經。療欬唾膿血，止喘悸，五勞體虚，補不足，小兒驚癇。别録。治尸疰，補虚下氣，勞氣虚熱，百邪鬼魅。甄權。調中，消痰止渴，潤肌膚，添骨髓。大明。益肺氣，主息賁。好古。

Control. Cough with counterflow of rising qi. Bound qi[449] in the chest with [alternating sensations of] cold and heat. It removes *gu* poison[450] causing dysfunction and lameness.[451] It calms the five long-term depots. *Ben jing*. It heals cough associated with spitting pus and blood. It ends panting with agitation, the five types of exhaustion and body depletion. It supplements insufficient [qi]. [It cures] fright epilepsy of children. *Bie lu*. It serves to cure corpse[-qi] attachment-illness,[452] supplements depleted [qi] and discharges qi. [It serves to cure] exhausted qi and depletion heat,[453] as well as the hundred evil [qi] associated with demons and goblins. Zhen Quan. It regulates the center, dissolves phlegm, ends thirst, moistens the muscles and the

449 *Jie qi* 結氣, "bound qi," are pathological qi halting and congealing at any place in the body. BCGM Dict I, 240.

450 *Gu du* 蠱毒, "*gu*-poison[ing]." (1) A poison emitted by certain worms/snakes with an ability to cause varying pathological changes in a person who has taken it in by means of wine or food. (2) Abdominal fullness, in some cases with blood spitting, and blood in the stool and urine. BCGM Dict I, 192 - 193. See BCGM 42-22.

451 Instead of *bi* 躄, "lameness," *Zheng lei* ch. 8, *zi wan* 紫菀, writes *jue* 蹶, "[tendency to] fall."

452 *Shi zhu* 尸疰, "corpse [qi] attachment-illness," a condition of a slowly developing infectious weakness. BCGM Dict I, 202.

453 *Xu re* 虚熱, "depletion heat," a condition of fever brought about by a depletion of yin, *jin* 津 liquid, qi and blood. BCGM Dict I, 588.

skin, and fills the marrow in the bones. Da Ming. It boosts lung qi, and controls running breath.[454]

【附方】舊三，新四。

Added Recipes. Three of old. Four newly [recorded].

肺傷欬嗽。紫菀五錢，水一盞，煎七分，温服。日三次。衛生易簡方。

Cough because of a harmed lung. Boil five *qian* of *zi wan* in one cup of water down to 70% and ingest this warm, three times a day. *Wei sheng yi jian fang*.

久嗽不瘥。紫菀、款冬花各一兩，百部半兩，搗羅爲末。每服三錢，薑三片，烏梅一箇，煎湯調下，日二，甚佳。圖經本草。

Chronic cough that is not cured. Pound one *liang* each of *zi wan* and coltsfoot, with half a *liang* of *stemona* [root] and give them through a sieve to obtain a powder. Each time ingest three *qian*, to be sent down with a decoction of three slices of ginger and one smoked plum. Twice a day. Very excellent. *Tu jing ben cao*.

小兒欬嗽，聲不出者。紫菀末、杏仁等分，入蜜同研，丸芡子大。每服一丸，五味子湯化下。全幼心鑑。

Cough of children, without sound. Add honey to equal amounts of *zi wan* and apricot kernels and grind this together. Form pills the size of *qian* seeds. Each time [let the child] ingest one pill, to be sent down dissolved in a *schisandra* seed decoction. *Quan you xin jian*.

吐血欬嗽，吐血後欬者。紫菀、五味炒，爲末，蜜丸芡子大，每含化一丸。指南方。

Cough with vomiting of blood. When the cough sets in after the vomiting of blood. [Grind] *zi wan* and *schisandra* [seeds] into powder and form with honey pills the size of *qian* seeds. Each time hold in the mouth one pill and let it dissolve. *Zhi nan fang*.

産後下血。紫菀末，水服五撮。聖惠方。

Blood discharge following delivery. [Let the woman] ingest with water five pinches of *zi wan* powder. *Sheng hui fang*.

---

454 *Xi ben* 息賁, "running breath," a condition of a *ji* 積, "accumulation," associated with the lung. It has the shape of a cup turned upside down. It is located below the ribs on the right. It cannot be cured for a long time. It is accompanied by an aversion to cold and fever, as well as by coughing and panting respiration. BCGM Dict I, 548.

纏喉風痺，不通欲死者。用返魂草根一莖，洗净納入喉中，待取惡涎出即瘥，神效。更以馬牙硝津嚥之，即絶根本。一名紫菀，南人呼爲夜牽牛。斗門方。

Throat constricting wind[455] blockage. [The throat] is blocked and [patients] are close to dying. Always wash one *fan hun cao* root clean and insert it into the [patient's] throat. Eventually he will release a malign saliva and this is the cure. Divinely effective. Also, [let him take into his mouth] mirabilite and swallow [the resulting] liquid. This will sever the root [of the problem]. Another name [of *fan hun cao*] is *zi wan* 紫菀. In the South, people call it *ye qian niu* 夜牽牛. *Dou men fang*.

婦人小便卒不得出者。紫菀爲末，井華水服三撮，即通。小便血者，服五撮立止。千金方。

Suddenly blocked urination of women. [Grind] *zi wan* into powder and ingest three pinches with the first water drawn from a well. This clears the passage [of urine]. If the urine is mixed with blood, ingest five pinches, and it will end immediately *Qian jin fang*.

16-04
女菀本經中品
Nü wan, FE *Ben jing*, middle rank.

Turczaninowia fastigiata **(Fisch.) DC.**

【釋名】白菀別録、織女菀別録、女復廣雅、茆音柳。【時珍曰】其根似女體柔婉，故名。

Explanation of Names. *Bai wan* 白菀, *Bie lu*. *Zhi nü wan* 織女菀, *Bie lu*. *Nü fu* 女復, *Guang ya*. *Liu* 茆, read *liu* 柳. [Li] Shizhen: The root is soft and gracious, *wan* 婉, like a female body. Hence the name.

【集解】【別録曰】女菀生漢中山谷或山陽。正月、二月采，陰乾。【弘景曰】比來醫方無復用之。復有白菀似紫菀，恐非此也。【恭曰】白菀即女菀，有名未用重出一條，故陶説疑之。功與紫菀相似。【宗奭曰】女菀即白菀，非二物也。唐修本草删去白菀，甚合宜。【時珍曰】白菀，即紫菀之色白者也。雷斅言，紫菀白如練色者，名羊鬚草，恐即此物也。

Collected Explanations. *Bie lu*: *Nü wan* grows in the mountain valleys and on the southern side of the mountains of Han zhong. It is collected in the first and second month. It is dried in the yin (i. e., shade).[Tao] Hongjing: In recent times it is no lon-

455 *Chan hou feng* 纏喉風, "throat-constricting wind," a condition of throat blockage, with a rapid onset, a swelling of throat and cheeks, and a closure of the throat that makes it impossible to ingest even a liquid. BCGM Dict I, 74.

ger resorted to in medicinal recipes. There is now a *bai wan* resembling purple aster, but it is not the [item discussed] here. [Su] Gong: *Bai wan* 白菀 is *nü wan* 女菀. It has a separate entry in the [section] "known by name but not in use." This is why Tao [Hongjing] voiced his doubts. [The therapeutic] potential is identical to that of purple aster. [Kou] Zongshi: *Nü wan* 女菀 is *bai wan* 白菀. These are not two different items. The *Tang xiu ben cao* quite appropriately omitted [a separate entry of] *bai wan*. [Li] Shizhen: *Bai wan* 白菀 are purple aster, *zi wan* 紫菀, varieties of white color. When Lei Xiao says "there are white specimens of purple aster resembling refined silk and they are named 'sheep whiskers herb'," then these may be the item [discussed] here.

16-04-01
根 *Gen*
Root [of *nü wan*].

【氣味】辛，温，無毒。【之才曰】畏鹵鹹。

Qi and Flavor. Acrid, warm, nonpoisonous. [Xu] Zhicai: [Ingested together,] it fears bittern salt.

【主治】風寒洗洗，霍亂洩痢，腸鳴上下無常處，驚癇，寒熱百疾。本經。療肺傷欬逆出汗，久寒在膀胱支滿，飲酒夜食發病。别録。

Control. Shivering because of wind [intrusion] and the presence of cold. Cholera with outflow and free-flux illness. Intestinal sounds move up and down, not permanently limited to one place. Fright epilepsy. Alternative sensations of cold and heat associated with any of the hundreds of illnesses. *Ben jing*. It cures cough and [qi] counterflow with sweating related to a harmed lung. Long-lasting presence of cold resulting in a propping fullness in the urinary bladder. Diseases breaking out after one has drunk wine and eaten late at night. *Bie lu*.

【發明】【時珍曰】按葛洪肘後方載治人面黑令白方：用真女菀三分，鉛丹一分，爲末，醋漿服一刀圭，日三服。十日大便黑，十八日面如漆，二十一日全白便止，過此太白矣。年三十後不可服。忌五辛。孫思邈千金方用酒服，男十日，女二十日，黑色皆從大便出也。又名醫録云：宋興國時，有女任氏色美，聘進士王公輔，不遂意，鬱久面色漸黑，母家求醫。一道人用女真散，酒下二錢，一日二服。數日面貌微白，一月如故。懇求其方，則用黄丹、女菀二物等分爾。據此，則葛氏之方已試有驗者矣。然則紫菀治手太陰血分，白菀手太陰氣分藥也。肺熱則面紫黑，肺清則面白。三十歲以後則肺氣漸減，不可復泄，故云不可服之也。

[Li] Shizhen: Ge Hong in his *Zhou hou fang* lists a recipe "to cure a black face and let it turn white. [Grind] three *fen* of genuine *nü wan* and one *fen* of minium into powder and ingest with vinegar and fermented water of foxtail millet the amount held by a knife blade. To be ingested three times a day. After ten days, defecation will assume a black color. After 18 days the face will be black like lacquer. After 21 days it will be all white, and [the treatment] ends. If [the treatment] is extended beyond this time, [the face] will be too white. [Persons] 30 years of age and older must not ingest this. [During the treatment] the five acrid [foods] are to be avoided." Sun Simiao in his *Qian jin fang* [recommends to] "ingest [the powder] with wine. Males after ten days and females after 20 days will release the black color through defecation." Also, the *Ming yi lu* states: "During the reign period *xing guo* of the Song [dynasty] (976 – 984), a beautiful girl of the Ren family was married against her will to a *jin shi* Wang Gong-fu. She was depressed and after a long time her complexion gradually assumed a black color. Her mother sought a medical treatment for her and a Daoist [recommended to] use the "powder letting a female find her true self again." She was to send down with wine two *qian* [of the powder], and it was to be ingested twice a day. After several days the face appeared pale white, and within one month it had assumed its original appearance. [The family] begged [the Daoist] to reveal his recipe and was informed that he had used equal amounts of minium and *nü wan*." That is, the recipe listed by Mr. Ge [Hong] had already been tested with a positive result. Now, *zi wan* serves to cure [diseases related to] the blood section of the hand major yin [conduits], while *bai wan* is a pharmaceutical drug for the qi section of the hand major yin conduits. In the case of lung heat the face turns purple-back. When the lung is cool, the complexion is white. After the age of 30, the lung qi greadually decrease and can no longer be drained. Therefore it is said: "[Such persons] must not ingest this [powder]."

16-05

麥門冬本經上品

Mai men dong. FE _Ben jing_, upper rank.

***Ophiopogon japonicus* (L. f.) Ker-Gawl.**

【釋名】虋冬音門，秦名烏韭，齊名愛韭，楚名馬韭，越名羊韭並別録。禹韭吴普、禹餘粮別録、忍冬吴普、忍凌吴普、不死草吴普、階前草。【弘景曰】根似穬麥，故謂之麥門冬。【時珍曰】麥鬚曰虋，此草根似麥而有鬚，其葉如韭，凌冬不凋，故謂之麥虋冬，及有諸韭、忍冬諸名，俗作門冬，便于字也。可以服食斷穀，故又有餘粮、不死之稱，吴普本草一名僕壘，一名隨脂。

Explanation of Names. *Men dong* 虋冬, read *men* 門. In Qin it is named *wu jiu* 烏韭,[456] "crow leek." In Qi it is named *ai jiu* 愛韭, "amiable leek." In Chu it is named

456 Instead of *wu* 烏, "crow/black," *Zheng lei* ch. 6, *mai men dong* 麥門冬, writes *yang* 羊, "sheep/goat."

ma jiu 馬韭, "horse leek." In Yue it is named *yang jiu* 羊韭,[457] "sheep/goat leek." All listed in *Bie lu*. *Yu jiu* 禹韭, "Yu's leek," Wu Pu. *Yu yu liang* 禹餘粮, "Yu's surplus provisions," *Bie lu*. *Ren dong* 忍冬, "survives winter," Wu Pu. *Ren ling* 忍淩, "survives being iced-up," Wu Pu. *Bu si cao* 不死草,[458] "immortal herb," Wu Pu. *Jie qian cao* 階前草, "herb in front of the steps." [Tao] Hongjing: The root resembles that of naked barley, *kuang mai* 穬麥. Therefore it is called *mai men dong* 麥門冬. [Li] Shizhen: The "whiskers" of barley are called *men* 虋. This herb is similar to *mai* 麥, barley, and has "whiskers." Its leaves are similar to those of Chinese leek, *jiu* 韭, and they do not wither when they are "iced-up," *ling* 淩, in winter, *dong* 冬. Hence the [herb] is called *mai men dong* 麥虋冬, and was given various names with *jiu* 韭, Chinese leek, and *ren dong* 忍冬, "survives winter." It is commonly written *men dong* 門冬, which is a simplification of the character [*men* 虋]. It can be consumed as food to reduce grain consumption. Therefore it also has names such as "surplus provisions," *yu liang* 餘粮, and "[herb that does] not let one die," *bu si* 不死. The *Wu Pu ben cao* has two further alternative names, *pu lei* 僕壘 and *sui zhi* 隨脂.

【集解】【别録曰】麥門冬葉如韭，冬夏長生。生函谷川谷及隄坂肥土石間久廢處。二月、八月、十月采根，陰乾。【普曰】生山谷肥地，叢生，葉如韭，實青黄，采無時。【弘景曰】函谷即秦關，處處有之，冬月作實如青珠，以四月采根，肥大者爲好。【藏器曰】出江寧者小潤，出新安者大白。其苗大者如鹿葱，小者如韭葉，大小有三四種，功用相似，其子圓碧。【頌曰】所在有之。葉青似莎草，長及尺餘，四季不凋。根黄白色有鬚，根如連珠形。四月開淡紅花，如紅蓼花。實碧而圓如珠。江南出者葉大，或云吴地者尤勝。【時珍曰】古人惟用野生者。後世所用多是種蒔而成。其法：四月初采根，於黑壤肥沙地栽之。每年六月、九月、十一月三次上糞及芸薹，夏至前一日取根，洗晒收之。其子亦可種，但成遲爾。浙中來者甚良，其葉似韭而多縱文，且堅韌爲異。

Collected Explanations. *Bie lu*: The leaves of *mai men dong* are similar to those of Chinese leek. They grow and are alive in winter and summer. [*Mai men dong*] grows in the river valleys of Han gu and in deserted places on fertile soil and between rocks on dikes and hillsides. The root is collected in the second, eighth and tenth month. It is dried in the yin (i. e., shade). [Wu] Pu: It grows on fertile ground in mountain valleys. It grows as clusters. The leaves are similar to those of Chinese leek. The fruits are greenish-yellow; they are collected anytime. [Tao] Hongjing:

457 Instead of *jiu* 韭, "Chinese leek," *Qian jin yi* ch. 2, *mai men dong* 麥門冬, writes *qi* 耆, "old age," and *Zheng lei* ch. 6, *mai men dong* 麥門冬, writes *shi* 蓍. *Yu lan* ch. 989, *mai men dong* 麥門冬, quoting *Wu shi ben cao*, writes *ji* 薺.

458 Instead of *cao* 草, "herb," *Zheng lei* ch. 6, *mai men dong* 麥門冬, quoting "Mr. Wu [Pu] states," and *Yu lan* ch. 989 *mai men dong* 麥門冬, quoting *Wu shi ben cao*, write *yao* 藥.

Han gu is Qin guan. [*Mai men dong*] can be found everywhere. During the winter months it forms fruit similar to greenish pearls. The root is collected in the fourth month. Fat, big ones are good. [Chen] Cangqi: Those coming from Jiang ning are small and moist. Those from Xin an are big and white. Those with big seedlings are similar to yellow daylilies. Those with small [seedlings] resemble Chinese leek leaves. They may appear in three to four different sizes, but their [therapeutic] potentials are similar. The seeds are round and jade-green. [Su] Song: [*Mai men dong*] can be found everywhere. The leaves are greenish; they resemble those of *cyperus* herbs. They reach a length of more than one *chi*. The root is yellow-white and has "whiskers." The root looks like a string of pearls. In the fourth month, [*mai men dong*] opens pale red flowers, similar to red knotweed flowers. The fruits are jade-green and round like pearls. Those from Jiang nan have big leaves; some say that those from the region of Wu are especially superior. [Li] Shizhen: The ancients used only those grown in the wild. In later times they often used those cultivated by men. The method is as follows. At the beginning of the fourth month collect a root and plant it in fertile, fat, sandy earth. Every year in the sixth, ninth and eleventh month, three times, add manure and celery cabbage seeds, and water this. One day prior to Summer Solstice take the root, wash it, dry it in the sun, and store it. The seeds can be planted, too. But it takes longer until they form a mature [root]. Those from Zhe zhong are very good. Their leaves resemble those of Chinese leek with a profuse vertical line design, and they are firm and pliable for a difference.

16-05-01

根 *Gen*

Root [of *mai men dong*].

【修治】【弘景曰】凡用取肥大者，湯澤，抽去心，不爾令人煩。大抵一斤須減去四五兩也。【時珍曰】凡入湯液，以滚水潤濕，少頃抽去心，或以瓦焙軟，乘熱去心。若入丸散，須瓦焙熱，即於風中吹冷，如此三四次，即易燥，且不損藥力。或以湯浸擣膏和藥，亦可。滋補藥，則以酒浸擂之。

[Pharmaceutical Preparation]. [Tao] Hongjing: For all uses, take fat, big ones. Moisten them with hot water and take out their heart. If this is not done, it will let one suffer from vexation. In general, of one *jin* four to five *liang* will have to be discarded. [Li] Shizhen: Whenever [the root] is added to a decoction, [first] boil it in water to moisten it. After a short while remove the heart. Or bake it on a tile to soften it and remove the heart as long as it is hot. If it is added to pills or powders, it must be baked on a tile to heat it and it is then exposed to the wind to blow it cold. If this is done three to four times, it will easily dry without losing its therapeutic strength. It is also possible to soak [the root] in hot water, pound it to a paste and mix it with [further] medication. For medication supposed to nourish and supplement, it is soaked in wine and then pounded.

【氣味】甘，平，無毒。【別録曰】微寒。【普曰】神農、岐伯：甘，平。黄帝、桐君、雷公：甘，無毒。李當之：甘、小温。【杲曰】甘、微苦，微寒，陽中微陰，降也。入手太陰經氣分。【之才曰】地黄、車前爲之使。惡款冬、苦瓠、苦芙。畏苦參、青蘘、木耳。伏石鍾乳。

Qi and Flavor. Sweet, balanced, nonpoisonous. *Bie lu*: Slightly cold. [Wu] Pu: Shen nong, Qi Bo: Sweet, balanced. Huang Di, Tong jun, Lei gong: Sweet, nonpoisonous. Li Dangzhi: Sweet, a little warm. [Li] Gao: Sweet, slightly bitter, slightly cold. A slight yin in yang [substance]. It descends. It enters the qi section of the hand major yin conduits. [Xu] Zhicai: Chinese foxglove [rhizome] and Asiatic plantain [root] serve as its guiding [substances]. [Ingested together,] it abhors coltsfoot, calabashs, and linear leaf thistle. It fears *sophora* [root], sesame leaves and *auricularia* fungi. It oppresses [the effects of] stalactites.

【主治】心腹結氣，腸中傷飽，胃絡脉絶，羸瘦短氣。久服輕身，不老不飢。本經。療身重目黄，心下支滿，虚勞客熱，口乾燥渴，止嘔吐，愈痿蹶，强陰益精，消穀調中，保神，定肺氣，安五臟，令人肥健，美顔色，有子。别録。去心熱，止煩熱，寒熱體勞，下痰飲。藏器。治五勞七傷，安魂定魄，止嗽，定肺痿吐膿，時疾熱狂頭痛。大明。治熱毒大水，面目肢節浮腫，下水，主泄精。甄權。治肺中伏火，補心氣不足，主血妄行及經水枯，乳汁不下。元素。久服輕身明目。和車前、地黄丸服，去濕痺，變白，夜視有光。藏器。斷穀爲要藥。弘景。

Control. Bound qi[459] in the central and abdominal region. Harm in the intestines caused by overeating, with the [passage in the] stomach enclosing vessels interrupted, resulting in emaciation and shortness of [breath] qi. Ingested for a long time, it relieves the body of its weight, preventing aging and hunger. *Ben jing*. It heals bodily heaviness and yellow eyes, as well as propping fullness below the heart, depletion exhaustion with visiting heat, and dryness in the mouth with thirst. It ends vomiting, heals dysfunction and lameness, strengthens the yin [qi], boosts essence/sperm, dissolves grain and orders the center, guards the spirit, stabilizes lung qi, calms the five long-term depots, lets one become fat and robust, makes the complexion beautiful and lets one have children. *Bie lu*. It dispels heart heat, ends vexing heat and alternating sensations of cold and heat with bodily exhaustion, and serves to discharge phlegm rheum. [Chen] Cangqi: It serves to cure the five types of ex-

459 *Jie qi* 結氣, "bound qi," are pathological qi halting and congealing at any place in the body. BCGM Dict I, 240.

haustion and seven types of harm, calms the *hun*-soul and stabilizes the *po*-soul. It ends cough, and it stabilizes a lung dysfunction associated with vomiting of pus. [It serves to cure] seasonal illnesses associated with heat, madness and headache. Da Ming. It serves to cure heat poison and water bloating, with the face, the eyes, the limbs, and the joints all affected by a surface swelling. It discharges water and controls outflow of essence/sperm. Zhen Quan. It serves to cure fire lying hidden in the lung. It supplements insufficient heart qi. It controls erratic blood movement, dried up menstrual water and [a nursing mother's] failure to let down milk sap. [Zhang] Yuansu. Ingested for a long time, it relieves the body of its weight and clears the eyes. Ingested in pills combined with Asiatic plantain [root] and Chinese foxglove [rhizome] it eliminates blockage associated with the presence of moisture, lets white [hair/beards] turn [black] and enables one to see at night as if there was a light. [Chen] Cangqi. It is an important pharmaceutical drug enabling one to reduce grain consumption. [Tao] Hongjing.

【發明】【宗奭曰】麥門冬治肺熱之功爲多，其味苦，但專泄而不專收，寒多人禁服。治心肺虛熱及虛勞，與地黄、阿膠、麻仁同爲潤經益血、復脉通心之劑，與五味子、枸杞子同爲生脉之劑。【元素曰】麥門冬治肺中伏火、脉氣欲絶者，加五味子、人參，三味爲生脉散，補肺中元氣不足。【杲曰】六七月間濕熱方旺，人病骨乏無力，身重氣短，頭旋眼黑，甚則痿軟。故孫真人以生脉散補其天元真炁。脉者，人之元氣也。人參之甘寒，瀉熱火而益元氣。麥門冬之苦寒，滋燥金而清水源。五味子之酸温，瀉丙火而補庚金，兼益五臟之氣也。【時珍曰】按趙繼宗儒醫精要云：麥門冬以地黄爲使，服之令人頭不白，補髓，通腎氣，定喘促，令人肌體滑澤，除身上一切惡氣不潔之疾，蓋有君而有使也。若有君無使，是獨行無功矣。此方惟火盛氣壯之人服之相宜。若氣弱胃寒者，必不可餌也。

Explication. [Kou] Zongshi: *Mai men dong* has multiple potentials to cure lung heat. Its flavor is bitter. It is especially able to drain, not to gather. Persons with much cold must not ingest it. It serves to cure depletion heat and depletion exhaustion affecting heart and lung. In the same way as Chinese foxglove [rhizome], donkey hide glue and hemp seeds it is a preparation that moistens the conduits and and boosts blood, revives the [movement in the] vessels and opens the passage through the heart. In the same way as *schisandra* seeds and *lycium* seeds it is a preparation to enliven the [movement in the] vessels. [Zhang] Yuansu: *Mai men dong* serves to cure hidden fire in the lung, with the [movement of] qi in the vessels close to being interrupted. Add [to *mai men dong*] *schisandra* [seeds] and ginseng [root], and prepare these three substances to the "powder to enliven [the movement in] the vessels." It supplments insufficient original qi in the lung. [Li] Gao: When in the sixth and seventh month, at a time of extreme moisture and heat, humans suffer from weariness and lack of strength in their bones, with bodily heaviness and shortness of [breath] qi, vertigo and blackened eyes, this is a condition of extreme dysfunction and softness. Hence Sun zhenren with the "powder to enliven the [movement in the] vessels" supplemented the original, true qi [bestowed on man from] heaven. The [movement in the] vessels is the original qi of man. The sweet [flavor] and cold [qi] of ginseng [root] drain heat and fire and boost original qi. The bitter [flavor] and cold [qi] of *mai men dong* nourish the dryness of metal (i. e., the lung) with moisture and clear the source of water. The sour [flavor] and warm [qi] of *schisandra* seeds drain liver fire and supplement lung metal, and they also boost the qi of the five long-term depots. [Li] Shizhen: According to Zhao Jizong in his *Ru yi jing yao*, "if *mai men dong* [is ingested] with Chinese foxglove [rhizome] as its guiding [substance], it prevents one's head from turning white. It supplements marrow, clears the passage of kidney qi, stabilizes panting, lets one's muscles and body be smooth and moist, and eliminates from the body all illnesses related to malign qi and uncleanliness." The fact is, there are ruler [drugs] and guiding [drugs]. If a ruler has no guide, he will move alone without strength. This recipe is suitable to be ingested only for persons with abounding fire and strong qi. Those with weak qi and stomach cold must by no means consume it.

【附方】舊三，新九。

Added Recipes. Three of old. Nine newly [recorded].

麥門冬煎。補中益心，悦顔色，安神益氣，令人肥健，其力甚駃。取新麥門冬根去心，擣熟絞汁，和白蜜。銀器中重湯煮，攪不停手，候如飴乃成。温酒日日化服之。圖經本草。

Mai men dong decoction. It supplements [qi in] the center and boosts heart [qi]. It brightens the complexion, calms the spirit and boosts the qi. It lets one be fat and robust. Its strength shows very fast. Take a new *mai men dong* root and remove its heart. Pound it and squeeze the resulting pulpy [mass] to obtain its juice. Mix it with white honey and boil it in a water bath in a silver vessel. Stir it without ever letting the hand rest until eventually a mass resembling maltose sugar has formed, and this is the final product. Ingest it daily dissolved in warm wine. *Tu jing ben cao.*

消渴飲水。用上元板橋麥門冬鮮肥者二大兩。宣州黄連九節者二大兩，去兩頭尖三五節，小刀子調理去皮毛了，吹去塵，更以生布摩拭，秤之，擣末。以肥大苦瓠汁浸麥門冬經宿，然後去心，即於臼中擣爛，納黄連末和擣，並手丸如梧子大。食後飲下五十丸，日再。但服兩日，其渴必定。

若重者，即初服一百五十丸，二日服一百二十丸，三日一百丸，四日八十丸，五日五十丸。合藥要天炁晴明之夜方浸藥。須净處，禁婦人、雞、犬見之。如覺可時，只服二十五丸。服訖覺虛，即取白羊頭一枚治净，以水三大斗煮爛，取汁一斗以來，細細飲之。勿食肉，勿入鹽。不過三劑平復也。崔元亮海上集驗方。

Melting with thirst[460] and [a desire] to drink water. Use two generous *liang* of fresh and fat specimens of *mai men dong* from Shang yuan ban qiao. Remove from two generous *liang* of *coptis* [rhizome] with nine nodes from Xuan zhou the two pointed ends with three to five nodes and also remove with a small knife the skin and the hair. Blow away the dusk and rub [the rhizomes] with a new piece of cloth, weigh them and pound them into powder. Then soak the *mai men dong* [roots] in the juice of a fat, big calabash for one night, remove their heart and pound them in a mortar to generate a pulpy [mass]. Add the *coptis* [rhizome] powder and pound them together [to obtain a mass] that is formed with the hands to pills the size of *wu* seeds. Send down with a beverage, after a meal, 50 pills. Twice a day. After ingesting them for only two days, the thirst will end. If it is a serious case, ingest at the beginning 150 pills, on the second day 120 pills, on the third day 100 pills, on the fourth day 80 pills and on the fifth day 50 pills. To prepare this medication, the drugs are soaked during a clear night at a clean location. Married women, chicken and dogs must not be allowed to view this. If one has the impression that this is sufficient,[461] an ingestion of only 25 pills is adequate. If after having ingested them a sensation of depletion sets in, clean the head of a white sheep and boil it in three generous *dou* of water down to a pulpy [mass, from which is extracted] about one *dou* of juice. Drink this in small quantities. [During this treatment] do not eat meat, and do not add salt. A normal condition is restored after [an ingestion of] no more than three preparations. Cui Yuanliang, *Hai shang ji yan fang*.

勞氣欲絶。麥門冬一兩，甘草炙二兩，粇米半合，棗二枚，竹葉十五片，水二升，煎一升，分三服。南陽活人書。

Exhaustion with the [movement of] qi close to being interrupted. Boil one *liang* of *mai men dong*, two *liang* of *glycyrrhiza* [root], roasted, half a *ge* of ordinary rice, two Chinese dates and 15 bamboo leaves in two *sheng* of water down to one *sheng* and ingest this divided into three portions. *Nan yang huo ren shu*.

460 *Xiao ke* 消渴, "melting with thirst," most likely including cases of diabetes. BCGM Dict Vol I, 567.

461 Instead of *ru jue ke shi* 如覺可時, *Zheng lei* ch. 6, *mai men dong* 麥門冬, quoting the *Tu jing*, writes *ru si ke mei ri* 如似可每日. "if it seems that this needs [to be ingested] every day."

虛勞客熱。麥門冬煎湯頻飲。本草衍義。

Depletion exhaustion with visiting heat. Boil *mai men dong* in water and repeatedly drink the decoction. *Ben cao yan yi.*

吐血衄血諸方不效者。麥門冬去心一斤，搗取自然汁，入蜜二合，分作二服。即止。活人心統。

Blood vomiting and nosebleed with all types of recipes showing no effect. Pound one *jin* of *mai men dong*, with the heart removed, to obtain its natural juice. Add two *ge* of honey and ingest this divided into two portions. This ends [the ailments]. *Huo ren xin tong.*

衄血不止。麥門冬去心、生地黄各五錢，水煎服。立止。保命集。

Unending nosebleed. Boil five *qian* each of *mai men dong*, with the heart removed, and fresh/raw Chinese foxglove [rhizome] in water and ingest the decoction. [The nosebleed] ends immediately. *Bao ming ji.*

齒縫出血。麥門冬煎湯漱之。蘭室寶鑑。

Bleeding seams of the teeth. Boil *mai men dong* in water and rinse [the affected region]. *Lan shi bao jian.*

咽喉生瘡。脾肺虛熱上攻也。麥門冬一兩，黄連半兩，爲末。煉蜜丸梧子大。每服二十丸，麥門冬湯下。普濟方。

Sores developing in the throat. This is [the result of] an attack of depletion heat from the spleen and the lung having moved upward. [Grind] one *liang* of *mai men dong* and half a *liang* of *coptis* [rhizome] into powder and form with heat refined honey pills the size of *wu* seeds. Each time ingest 20 pills, to be sent down with a *mai men dong* decoction. *Pu ji fang.*

乳汁不下。麥門冬去心焙，爲末。每用三錢，酒磨犀角約一錢許，温熱調下，不過二服便下。熊氏補遺。

Failure [of a nursing mother] to let down milk sap. [Grind] *mai men dong*, with the heart removed and baked over a slow fire, into powder. Each time use three *qian*. To be sent down mixed with warm wine in which approximately one *qian* of rhinoceros horn was rubbed. After no more than two ingestions [the nursing mother] will let down [milk]. Xiong shi, *Bu yi.*

下痢口渴，引飲無度。麥門冬去心三兩，烏梅肉二十箇，細剉，以水一升，煮取七合，細細呷之。必效方。

Discharge with free-flux illness, thirst and drinking without end. Cut three *liang* of *mai men dong*, with the heart removed, with the meat of 20 smoked plums to fine pieces. Boil them in one *sheng* of water down to seven *ge* and sip the liquid in small portions. *Bi xiao fang.*

金石藥發。麥門冬六兩，人參四兩，甘草炙二兩，爲末，蜜丸梧子大。每服五十丸，飲下，日再服。本草圖經。

Effusion [of illness following an ingestion of] metal and mineral pharmaceutical drugs. [Grind] six *liang* of *mai men dong*, four *liang* of ginseng [root] and two *liang* of *glycyrrhiza* [root], roasted, into powder and form with honey pills the size of *wu* seeds. Each time ingest 50 pills, to be sent down with a beverage. To be ingested twice a day. *Ben cao tu jing.*

男女血虛。麥門冬三斤，取汁熬成膏，生地黄三斤，取汁熬成膏，等分，一處濾過，入蜜四之一，再熬成，瓶收。每日白湯點服。忌鐵器。醫方摘要。

Blood depletion of males and females. Obtain the juice of three *jin* of *mai men dong*, and heat it until it turns into a paste. Obtain the juice of three *jin* of fresh/raw Chinese foxglove [rhizome] and heat it until it turns into a paste. Give equal amounts of both [pastes] through a sieve, add one quarter of this of honey and heat it again. Store the resulting paste in a jar. Every day drip it into clear, boiled water and ingest it. Contact with iron utensils is to be avoided. *Yi fang zhai yao.*

16-06
萱草宋嘉祐
Xuan cao, FE Song, *Jia you.*

***Hemerocallis citrina* Baroni. Yellow day lily.**

【釋名】忘憂說文、療愁綱目、丹棘古今注、鹿葱嘉祐、鹿劍土宿、妓女吴普、宜男。【時珍曰】萱本作諼。諼，忘也。詩云：焉得諼草，言樹之背。謂憂思不能自遣，故欲樹此草玩味以忘憂也。吴人謂之療愁。董子云：欲忘人之憂，則贈之丹棘，一名忘憂故也。其苗烹食，氣味如葱，而鹿食九種解毒之草，萱乃其一，故又名鹿葱。周處風土記云：懷妊婦人佩其花，則生男，故名宜男。李九華延壽書云：嫩苗爲蔬，食之動風，令人昏然如醉，因名忘憂。此亦一說也。嵇康養生論：神農經言中藥養性，故“合歡蠲忿，萱草忘憂”，亦謂食之也。鄭樵通志乃言萱草一名合歡者，誤矣。“合歡”見木部。

Explanation of Names. *Wang you* 忘憂, “to forget sorrow,” *Shuo wen. Liao chou* 療愁, “to heal worries,” *Gang mu. Dan ji* 丹棘, “cinnabar-red spines,” *Gu jin zhu. Lu cong* 鹿葱. “deer's onion,” *Jia you. Lu jian* 鹿劍, “deer's sabre,” *Tu su. Ji nü* 妓女, “whore,” Wu Pu. *Yi nan* 宜男, “suitable for males.” [Li] Shizhen: *Xuan* 萱 originally was written *xuan* 諼, "to forget." *Xuan* 諼 is *wang* 忘, "to forget." The *Shi* states: "Get the 'forget it herb.' That is to say, plant it to get rid of it." That is, when sorrow and pondering cannot be deleted, one should plant this herb and play with it to forget one's worries. The people in Wu call it "that which heals worries." Dong [Zhong-shu] zi states: "If you wish to let someone forget his worries, send him *dan ji* 丹棘 as a present, because they are also named *wang you* 忘憂, 'to forget one's worries'." The seedling is boiled to be eaten. It has qi and flavor similar to onions. There are nine types of herbs eaten by deer to resolve poison, and *xuan cao* is one of them. Therefore it is also called *lu cong* 鹿葱, "deer's onion." Zhou Chu in his *Feng tu ji* states: "When a pregnant woman wears this flower at her belt, she will give birth to a boy." Hence it is named *yi nan* 宜男, "suitable for a male." Liu Jiuhua in his *Yan shou shu* states: "When its tender seedlings are eaten prepared as vegetable, they stimulate the movement of wind and this lets one all of a sudden behave like drunk. Therefore it is named *wang you* 忘憂, 'to forget one's worries'." This is yet another explanation. Ji Kang in his *Yang sheng lun* [states]: "In Shen nong's Classic it is said that 'pharmaceutical drugs of middle [rank] nourish one's nature.' Hence it is also said '*mimosa* lets one overcome anger. *Xuan cao* lets one forget worries'." And [the Classic] also says that it can be eaten." When Zheng Qiao in his *Tong zhi* says "*xuan cao* 萱草, alternative name *he huan* 合歡," he is wrong. For *he huan* 合歡, see the section wood (35-20).

【集解】【頌曰】萱草處處田野有之，俗名鹿葱。五月采花，八月采根。今人多采其嫩苗及花跗作葅食。【時珍曰】萱宜下濕地，冬月叢生。葉如蒲、蒜輩而柔弱，新舊相代，四時青翠。五月抽莖開花，六出四垂，朝開暮蔫，至秋深乃盡，其花有紅、黄、紫三色。結實三角，内有子大如梧子，黑而光澤。其根與麥門冬相似，最易繁衍。南方草木狀言，廣中一種水葱，狀如鹿葱，其花或紫或黄，蓋亦此類也。或言鹿葱花有斑文，與萱花不同時者，謬也。肥土所生，則花厚色深，有斑文，起重臺，開有數月；瘠土所生，則花薄而色淡，開亦不久。嵇含宜男花序亦云荆楚之士號爲鹿葱，可以薦葅，尤可憑據。今東人采其花跗乾而貨之，名爲黄花菜。

Collected Explanations. [Su] Song: *Xuan cao* can be found everywhere in the open country. It is commonly named "deer's onion." The flowers are collected in the fifth month. The root is collected in the eighth month. Today many people collect its tender seedlings and the flowers to prepare a pickled vegetable food. [Li] Shizhen: *Xuan cao* [grows] on low-lying, moist ground. In the winter months it grows as clusters. The leaves are similar to those of cattail and garlic, but they are even softer and weaker. New [leaves] replace old [leaves], one after another, and they remain greenish through all four seasons. In the fifth month a stem rises and opens flowers. Of six that appear, four hang down. They open in the morning and wither in the evening. Deep in autumn they are all gone. The flowers may be of three colors, red, yellow and purple. They form fruits with three edges, with seeds the size of *wu* seeds inside. They are black and shiny moist. The root is similar to that of *ophiopogon* [herb]. It is very easy to multiply. The *Nan fang cao mu zhuang* says: "In Guang zhong is a kind of water onion, *shui cong* 水葱, shaped similar to 'deer's onion,' *lu cong* 鹿葱. Its flowers may be purple or yellow." The fact is, they are of the same group. It is also said: "*Lu cong* flowers have a dotted line design and they are alive at another time than *xuan* [*cao*] flowers." This is wrong. When [the plant] grows on fertile soil, its flowers are thick, the color is deep with a dotted line design and there are many layers [of petals]. [The flowers] remain open for several months. Those growing on poor soil have thin flowers with a pale color, and they do not remain open for a long time. Ji Han in his *Yi nan hua xu* states: "In the land of Jing and Chu it is called *lu cong*. It can be prepared as pickled vegetable." This is most trustworthy. Today, in the East people collect the flowers, dry them and market them. They call them "yellow flower vegetable."

16-06-01

苗、花 ***Miao, Hua.***

Seedling, flower [of *xuan cao*].

【氣味】甘，涼，無毒。

Qi and flavor. Sweet, cool, nonpoisonous.

【主治】煮食，治小便赤澀，身體煩熱，除酒疸。大明。消食，利濕熱。時珍。作菹，利胸膈，安五臟，令人好歡樂，無憂，輕身明目。蘇頌。

Control. Boiled in water and eaten, they serve to cure red and rough urination, and vexing heat affecting the entire body. They eliminate *dan*-illness caused by wine.[462] Da Ming. They dissolve food and free the passage of moisture and heat [to leave the body]. [Li] Shizhen. Prepared as pickled vegetable, they free the passage through chest and diaphragm, calm the five long-term depots and let one be joyous without worries. They relieve the body of its weight and clear the eyes. Su Song.

---

462 *Jiu dan* 酒疸, "*dan*-illness [caused by] wine." A condition of *huang dan* 黃疸, "yellow *dan*-illness/jaundice," resulting from an excessive consumption of wine/alcoholic beverages. BCGM Dict I, 271.

16-06-02
根 *Gen*
Root [of *xuan cao*].

【主治】沙淋，下水氣，酒疸黄色遍身者，擣汁服。藏器。大熱衄血，研汁一大盞，和生薑汁半盞，細呷之。宗奭。吹乳、乳癰腫痛，擂酒服，以滓封之。時珍。

Control. Dripping urination with sand. It discharges water qi. In the case of *dan*-illness caused by wine, with the entire body having assumed a yellow color, pound [the root] to obtain its juice and ingest it. [Chen] Cangqi. Strong heat with nosebleed. Grind [the root] to obtain one large cup of juice, mix it with half a cup of fresh ginger juice and sip this in small portions. [Kou] Zongshi. For inflated breast,[463] and breast obstruction-illness[464] with a painful swelling, pound it, [squeeze the pulp to obtain a juice] and ingest it with wine. Seal [the affected region] with the dregs. [Li] Shizhen.

【發明】【震亨曰】萱屬木，性下走陰分，一名宜男，寧無微意存焉？

Explication. [Zhu] Zhenheng: *Xuan* [*cao*] belongs to [the phase] wood. By its nature it moves down and rushes into the qi section. An alternative name is "suitable for males." Doesn't that have a subtle meaning?

【附方】新四。

Added Recipes. Four newly [recorded]

通身水腫。鹿葱根葉，晒乾爲末。每服二錢，入席下塵半錢，食前米飲服。聖惠方。

Water swelling affecting the entire body. Dry root and leaves of *lu cong* in the sun and [grind them] into powder. Each time ingest two *qian*. Add to it half a *qian* of dust from under a mat and ingest this prior to a meal with a rice beverage. *Sheng hui fang*.

小便不通。萱草根煎水頻飲。杏林摘要。

Blocked urination. Boil *xuan cao* root in water and drink it repeatedly. *Xing lin zhai yao*.

463 *Chui ru* 吹乳, "inflated breast." Identical to *chui nai* 吹奶, "inflated breast." A condition with milk blocked after delivery and the breasts turning red and swelling. BCGM Dict I, 101.

464 *Ru yong* 乳癰, "breast obstruction-illness," a condition of acute putrefication of a woman's breast. Often encountered if a woman, following delivery, experiences *chui nai* 吹奶, "inflated breast," or *du ru* 妒乳, "jealousy breast." BCGM Dict I, 412.

大便後血。萱草根和生薑，油炒，酒衝服。聖濟總録。

Bleeding after defecation. Fry *xuan cao* root and fresh ginger in oil and vigorously ingest it with wine. *Sheng ji zong lu*.

食丹藥毒。萱草根研汁服之。事林廣記。

Poisoning caused by consuming an elixir medication. Grind *xuan cao* to obtain a juice and ingest it. *Shi lin guang ji*.

16-07
搥胡根拾遺
Chui hu gen. FE *Shi yi*.

The root to beat the Hu. Unidentified.

【集解】【藏器曰】生江南川谷蔭地，苗如萱草，其根似天門冬。凡用抽去心。

Collected Explanations. [Chen] Cangqi: It grows on yin (i. e., shady) ground in the river valleys of Jiang nan. The seedling is similar to that of yellow day lily. The root resembles that of *asparagus* [herbs]. For all uses remove the heart.

【氣味】甘，寒，無毒。

Qi and Flavor. Sweet, cold, nonpoisonous.

【主治】潤五臟，止消渴，除煩去熱，明目，功如麥門冬。藏器。

Control. It moistens the five long-term depots. It ends melting with thirst.[465] It dispels vexation and eliminates heat. It clears the eyes. Its [therapeutic] potential is similar to that of *ophiopogon* [tuber]. [Chen] Cangqi.

16-08
淡竹葉綱目
Dan zhu ye. FE *Gang mu*.

***Lopatherum gracile* Brongn. Bland bamboo leaves.**

【釋名】根名碎骨子。【時珍曰】竹葉象形，碎骨言其下胎也。

Explanation of Names. The root is named "bone breaker," *sui gu zi* 碎骨子. [Li] Shizhen: [Its leaves] are shaped like bamboo leaves. "Bone breaker" is to say: It causes abortion.

465 *Xiao ke* 消渴, "melting with thirst," most likely including cases of diabetes. BCGM Dict Vol I, 567.

【集解】【時珍曰】處處原野有之。春生苗，高數寸，細莖緑葉，儼如竹米落地所生細竹之莖葉。其根一窠數十鬚，鬚上結子，與麥門冬一樣，但堅硬爾，隨時采之。八九月抽莖，結小長穗。俚人采其根苗，搗汁和米作酒麴，甚芳烈。

Collected Explanations. [Li] Shizhen: It can be found anywhere in the wild. It grows a seedling in spring, reaching a height of several *cun*. Its fine stem and its green leaves very much resemble the stem and leaves of fine bamboo growing where bamboo seeds have fallen to the ground. The root forms a nest with several tens of "whiskers." Seeds form on these "whiskers." [The roots are] similar to *ophiopogon* [tubers], but they are harder. They are collected any time. The stem comes out in the eighth and ninth month; it forms small, lengthy spikes. Uncultured people collect the root with the seedling. They pound them to obtain a juice and mix it with rice to prepare distiller's yeast. It is extremely fragrant.

【氣味】甘，寒，無毒。

Qi and Flavor. Sweet, cold, nonpoisonous.

【主治】葉去煩熱，利小便，清心。根能墮胎催生。時珍。

Control. The leaves dispel vexing heat, free the passage of urine and cool the heart. The root can bring a fetus down and accelerate the birth. [Li] Shizhen.

16-09

鴨跖草跖音隻宋嘉祐補

Ya zhi cao, with 跖 read *zhi*. FE Song, *Jia you*, added.

***Commelina communis* L. Day flower.**

【釋名】鷄舌草拾遺、碧竹子同上、竹雞草綱目、竹葉菜同上、淡竹葉同上、耳環草同上、碧蟬花同上、藍姑草。【藏器曰】鴨跖生江東、淮南平地。葉如竹，高一二尺，花深碧，好爲色，有角如鳥觜。【時珍曰】竹葉菜處處平地有之。三四月生苗，紫莖竹葉，嫩時可食。四五月開花，如蛾形，兩葉如翅，碧色可愛。結角尖曲如鳥喙，實在角中，大如小豆。豆中有細子，灰黑而皺，狀如蠶屎。巧匠采其花，取汁作畫色及彩羊皮燈，青碧如黛也。

Explanation of Names. *Ji she cao* 鷄舌草, "chicken tongue herb," *Shi yi*. *Bi zhu zi* 碧竹子, "jade-greenish bamboo," [source] identical to the previous one. *Zhu ji cao* 竹雞草, "bamboo chicken herb," *Gang mu*. *Zhu ye cai* 竹葉菜, "bamboo leaf vegetable," [source] identical to the previous one. *Dan zhu ye* 淡竹葉, "bland bamboo leaves," [source] identical to the previous one. *Er huan cao* 耳環草, "earring herb," [source] identical to the previous one. *Bi chan hua* 碧蟬花, "jade-greenish cicada flower," [source] identical to the previous one. *Lan gu cao* 藍姑草, "blue aunt herb." [Chen] Cangqi: *Ya zhi* 鴨跖 grows on the plains of Jiang dong and Huai nan. The leaves are similar to those of bamboo. [The plant] is one or two *chi* tall. The flowers are deeply jade-greenish. They are a good colorant. They have an edge similar to a bird's beak. [Li] Shizhen: *Dan zhu cai* can be found anywhere in the plains. They grow a seedling in the third and fourth month. The stem is purple and has bamboo leaves. As long as they are tender they are edible. Flowers open in the fourth and fifth month. They look like moths with two leaves resembling their wings. They are of an amiable jade-greenish color. They form edges that are pointed and curved like a bird's beak. The fruits are inside these edges; they are of the size of mung beans. Inside these beans are fine seeds. They are of an ash-black color and creased. They look like silkworm feces. Artisans collect their flowers. They use their juice to prepare colorants for paintings and to decorate sheepskin lamps. They have a greenish-jade color similar to indigo.

16-09-01
苗 *Miao*
Seedling [of *ya zhi cao*].

【氣味】苦，大寒，無毒。

Qi and Flavor. Bitter, very cold, nonpoisonous.

【主治】寒熱瘴瘧，痰飲丁腫，肉癥澀滯，小兒丹毒，發熱狂癇，大腹痞滿，身面氣腫，熱痢，蛇犬咬、癰疽等毒。藏器。和赤小豆煮食，下水氣濕痺，利小便。大明。消喉痺。時珍。

Control. Alternating sensations of cold and heat related to miasmatic malaria. Phlegm rheum and pin[-illness][466] swelling. Meat concretion-illness[467] with a rough and sluggish [passage of qi]. Cinnabar poison[468] of children. Heat effusion and madness epilepsy. Abdominal obstacle-illness[469] with a sensation of fullness. Qi swelling of the body and the face. Heat free-flux illness. The poison associated with bites by

466 *Ding* 丁, "pin[-illness]," also *ding* 疔, "pin-illness," refers to a deep-reaching and festering hardness in a tissue, eventually rising above the skin like a pinhead. BCGM Dict I, 127-129.

467 *Rou zheng* 肉癥, "meat concretion-illness," a condition of *zheng* 癥, "concretions," which form when someone continuously consumes meat and never seems to be satisfied. BCGM Dict I, 409.

468 *Dan du* 丹毒, "cinnabar poison," a skin ailment with red rashes. BCGM Dict I, 118

469 *Pi* 痞, "obstacle-illness." 1.) An illness sign of a feeling of uncomfortable fullness and distension. 2). A condition of an uncomfortable distension and fullness in the chest and abdominal region. When pressed there is no pain. BCGM Dict I, 371.

snakes and dogs, as well as obstruction-illness and impediment-illness.[470] [Chen] Cangqi. Eaten boiled with mung beans it serves to discharge water, qi and moisture causing a blockage. It clears the passage of urine. Da Ming. It dissolves throat blockage. [Li] Shizhen.

【附方】新四。

Added Recipes. Four newly [recorded].

小便不通。竹雞草一兩，車前草一兩，搗汁入蜜少許，空心服之。集簡方。

Blocked urination. Pound one *liang* of *zhu ji cao* and one *liang* of Asiatic plantain herb to obtain a juice. Add a little honey and ingest this on an empty stomach. *Ji jian fang*.

下痢赤白。藍姑草，即淡竹葉菜，煎湯日服之。活幼全書。

Red and white discharge with free-flux illness. Boil *lan gu cao*, that is, *dan zhu ye cao*, in water and ingest the decoction every day. *Huo you quan shu*.

喉痺腫痛。鴨跖草汁點之。袖珍方。

Throat blockage with painful swelling. Drip *ya zhi cao* juice [into it]. *Xiu zhen fang*.

五痔腫痛。耳環草一名碧蟬兒花。挼軟納患處，即效。危亦林得效方。

The five types of piles with painful swelling. Rub *er huan cao*, also named *bi chan er hua* 碧蟬兒花, to obtain a soft [mass] and insert it into the ailing location. This is effective. Wei Yilin, *De xiao fang*.

16-10

葵本經上品

Kui. FE *Ben jing*, upper rank.

***Malva verticillata* L. Chinese mallow.**

【校正】自菜部移入此。

Editorial Correction. Moved here from the section "vegetables."

【釋名】露葵綱目、滑菜。【時珍曰】按爾雅翼云：葵者，揆也。葵葉傾日，不使照其根，乃智以揆之也。古人采葵必待露解，故曰露葵。今人呼爲滑菜，言其性也。古者葵爲五菜之主，今不復食之，故移入此。

470 *Yong ju* 癰疽, "obstruction-illness, impediment-illness." refers to two vaguely distinguished obstructions/impediments of vessels or other ducts inside the body. Qi rushing against the obstruction may cause a local swelling and eventually break through the surface to cause an abscess. BCGM Dict I, 642.

Explanation of Names. *Lu kui* 露葵, "dew mallow," *Gang mu*. *Hua cai* 滑菜, "smooth vegetable." [Li] Shizhen: According to the *Er ya yi*, "*kui* 葵 is *kui* 揆, 'to guess.' The leaves of *kui* bend toward the sun so that the sunshine cannot reach its root. Hence its knowledge [of sunshing] rests on a 'guess,' *kui* 揆." The ancients collected *kui* 露 only after the dew, *lu* 露, had dissolved. Hence it was called "dew *kui* 露葵." Today, people call it *hua cai* 滑菜, a reference to its nature. The ancients considered *kui* the most outstanding among the five types of vegetables. Today, it is no longer eaten. Hence it is moved here [from the section "vegetables."]

【集解】【別録曰】冬葵子生少室山。【弘景曰】以秋種葵，覆養經冬，至春作子者，謂之冬葵，入藥性至滑利。春葵子亦滑，不堪藥用，故是常葵耳。術家取葵子微炒燁炨，音畢乍，散着濕地，遍踏之。朝種暮生，遠不過宿。【恭曰】此即常食之葵也。有數種，皆不入藥用。【頌曰】葵處處有之。苗葉作菜茹，更甘美，冬葵子古方入藥最多。葵有蜀葵、錦葵、黄葵、終葵、菟葵，皆有功用。【時珍曰】葵菜古人種爲常食，今之種者頗鮮。有紫莖、白莖二種，以白莖爲勝。大葉小花，花紫黄色，其最小者名鴨脚葵。其實大如指頂，皮薄而扁，實内子輕虛如榆莢仁。四五月種者可留子，六七月種者爲秋葵，八九月種者爲冬葵，經年收采。正月復種者爲春葵。然宿根至春亦生。按王禎農書云：葵，陽草也。其菜易生，郊野甚多，不拘肥瘠地皆有之。爲百菜之主，備四時之饌。本豐而耐旱，味甘而無毒。可防荒儉，可以菹腊，其枯枿可爲榜族，根子又能療疾，咸無遺棄。誠蔬茹之要品，民生之資益者也。而今人不復食之，亦無種者。

Collected Explanations. *Bie lu*: *Dong kui zi*. "winter *kui* seeds," grow on Mount Shao shi shan. [Tao] Hongjing: The *kui* planted in autumn, repeatedly fertilized passing through winter and forming seeds in spring is called "winter *kui*," *dong kui* 冬葵. It is added to medication because of its nature that is extremely smoothing and freeing [passages]. "Spring *kui* seeds," *chun kui zi* 春葵子, too, are smoothing, but they are not suitable for a therapeutic application. Hence, they are just ordinary *kui* [seeds]. The experts in the arts [of longevity] slightly fry *kui* seeds until they hear them crack. Then they spread them on a moist ground and tread on them. This way, they are planted in the morning and grow in the evening. Even if such germination takes long, it will never exceed one night. [Su] Gong: This is the *kui* that is often consumed as food. It has several kinds none of which is used added to medication. [Su] Song: *Kui* can be found anywhere. Seedling and leaves are prepared as a vegetable. They are very sweet and delicious. Winter *kui* seeds were very often added to medication in ancient recipes. The varieties of *kui* include *shu kui*, *jin kui*, *huang kui*, *zhong kui* and *tu kui*. They all have a [therapeutic] potential that can be used. [Li] Shizhen: *Kui* vegetables were planted by the ancients for regular consumption as food. Today, they are planted very seldom. There are two kinds, one with a purple stem and one with a white stem. Those with a white stem are superior. They have large leaves and small flowers. The flowers are of a purple-yellow color, and those with the very smallest [flowers] are called *ya jiao kui* 鴨脚葵, "duck foot *kui*." Their fruits are as big as a finger tip. Their skin is thin, and they are flat. The seeds inside the fruits are light and hollow, similar to Siberian elm [seed] kernels. Those planted in the fourth and fifth month can retain their seeds. Those planted in the sixth and seventh month are "autumn *kui*." Those planted in the eighth and ninth month are "winter *kui*." They are collected in the following year. Those planted again in the first month are "spring *kui*." However, they may also grow out of a perennial root. According to Wang Zhen in his *Nong shu*, "*kui* is a yang herb. This vegetable grows easily. It can be found very often in the wild, regardless of whether the ground is fertile or poor. It is the most outstanding among the hundreds of vegetables. It is food available in all four seasons. It is bestowed with strength and survives droughts. Its flavor is sweet and it is nonpoisonous. It helps to withstand famines and periods of poverty. It can be prepared to pickled vegetables and long-stored provisions. The dried stem can be used for whipping. The root and the seeds can serve to heal illness. Nothing of it is discarded as useless. It is truly an important vegetable, contributing to the wellbeing of people." Today, people no longer eat it, and it is no longer planted.

16-10-01
苗 *Miao*
Seedling [of *kui*].

【氣味】甘，寒，滑，無毒。爲百菜主。其心傷人。别録。【弘景曰】葵葉尤冷利，不可多食。【頌曰】作菜茹甚甘美，但性滑利，不益人。【詵曰】其性雖冷，若熱食之，令人熱悶，動風氣。四月食之，發宿疾。天行病後食之，令人失明。霜葵生食，動五種留飲，吐水。凡服百藥，忌食其心，心有毒也。黄背紫莖者勿食之。不可合鯉魚、黍米、鮓食，害人。【時珍曰】凡被狂犬咬者，永不可食，食之即發。食葵須用蒜，無蒜勿食之。又伏硫黄。

Qi and Flavor. Sweet, cold, smooth, nonpoisonous. It is the most outstanding among the hundreds of vegetables. Its heart harms humans. *Bie lu*. [Tao] Hongjing: *Kui* leaves are especially cold and free [passages]. They must not be eaten in large amounts. [Su] Song: Prepared as a vegetable it is sweet and delicious. But its nature is smooth and frees [passages]. It is not good for humans. [Meng] Shen: Its nature may be cold, but if it is eaten hot it lets one turn hot with heart-pressure and stimulates the movement of wind qi. Eaten in the fourth month,[471] it lets an old illness effuse again. Eaten in the aftermath of an epidemic disease, it causes loss of eyesight. When *kui* that was exposed to frost is eaten raw, it excites the five types of abiding rheums, causing vomiting of water. During an ingestion of any of the hundreds of medications, the heart [of *kui*] must not be eaten. It is poisonous. Those with a yellow back and purple stem must not be eaten. It must not be combined with carp or glutinous millet to prepare preserved food. That would be harmful for humans. [Li] Shizhen: Anybody bitten by a rabid dog must not eat [*kui*] for his entire life. If he were to eat it, [the disease] would effuse again. A consumption of *kui* must be combined with garlic. If no garlic is available, it must not be eaten. Also, it oppresses [the effects of] sulphur.

【主治】脾之菜也。宜脾，利胃氣，滑大腸。思邈。宣導積滯，妊婦食之，胎滑易生。蘇頌。煮汁服，利小腸，治時行黄病。乾葉爲末及燒灰服，治金瘡出血。甄權。除客熱，治惡瘡，散膿血，女人帶下，小兒熱毒，下痢丹毒，並宜食之。汪穎。服丹石人宜食。孟詵。潤燥利竅，功與子同。同上。

Control. It is a vegetable for the spleen. It is suitable for the spleen. It clears the passage of stomach qi and smoothes the large intestine. [Sun] Simiao It stimulates the passage of and leads off accumulated and sluggish [qi]. When pregnant women eat it the fetus will have a smooth and easy birth. Su Song. Boiled in water and the juice ingested, it clears the passage through the small intestine. It serves to cure seasonal jaundice. The dried leaves [ground into] powder and burned to ashes are ingested to cure bleeding wounds caused by metal objects/weapons. Zhen Quan. It dispels visiting heat, cures malign sores and disperses pus and blood. It is suitable to be eaten for all [diseases of] women below the belt, and heat poison of children, as well as discharge with free-flux illness and cinnabar poison.[472] Wang Ying. Persons ingesting elixir minerals are well advised to eat it. Meng Shen. It moistens dryness and clears the passage through the orifices. The [therapeutic] potential [of the seedling] is identical to that of the seeds.

【發明】【張從正曰】凡久病大便澀滯者，宜食葵菜，自然通利，乃滑以養竅也。【時珍曰】按唐王燾外臺秘要云：天行斑瘡，須臾遍身皆戴白漿，此惡毒氣也。高宗永徽四年，此瘡自西域東流於海內。但煮葵菜葉以蒜虀啖之，則止。又聖惠方亦云：小兒發斑，用生葵菜葉絞汁，少少與服，散惡毒氣。按此即今痘瘡也。今之治者，惟恐其大小二便頻數，洩其

471 Instead of *si yue* 四月, "fourth month," *Zheng lei* ch. 27, *dong kui zi* 冬葵子 quoting the Shi liao writes *si ji yue* 四季月, "the four last months of a season."

472 *Dan du* 丹毒, "cinnabar poison," a skin ailment with red rashes. BCGM Dict I, 118

元氣，痘不起發。葵菜滑竅，能利二便，似不相宜，而昔人賴之。豈古今運氣不同，故治法亦隨時變易與？

Explication. Zhang Congzheng: All [patients] suffering from rough and sluggish defecation for a long time already should eat *kui* vegetable. This will free [the passage of defecation] because [*kui*] is smoothing and supports the functions of the orifices. [Li] Shizhen: According to the Tang [author] Wang Tao's *Wai tai mi yao*, "when epidemic macula sores within a short time cover the entire body with white liquid pustules, that is a presence of malign and poisonous qi. In the fourth year of the reign period *yong hui* 永徽 (650 – 655) of Emperor Gao zong, such sores spread from the Western territories into the country. [The therapy consisted of] nothing but boiling *kui* vegtetable leaves with minced garlic, and [the transmission] was stopped." Also, as the *Sheng hui fang* states, "when children develop maculas, squeeze fresh *kui* vegetable leaves to obtain a juice and give this, in small quantities, [to the child] to ingest. It disperses the malign and poisonous qi." Now, these [sores] are what is called smallpox today. When this is treated today, it is to be feared that major and minor relief [i. e., defecation and urination] occur too often, draining [the patient's] original qi so that the smallpox cannot rise and effuse. *Kui* vegetable smoothes the orifices and it is capable of freeing [the passage] of both [major and minor] relief. Obviously, it is not suitable [for treating smallpox], but the ancients relied on it. How can it be that the periodic qi in antiquity and today differ, and that, therefore, the therapeutic approaches have also changed over time?

【附方】舊四，新三。

Added Recipes. Four of old. Three newly [recorded].

天行斑瘡。方見上。

Epidemic macula sores. For a recipe, see above.

肉錐怪疾。有人手足甲忽長，倒生肉刺如錐，痛不可忍者，但食葵菜即愈。夏子益奇疾方。

Flesh awl,[473] a strange illness. Someone's fingernails or toenails suddenly grow long and they grow upside down and sting into the flesh like an awl, with an unbearable pain. All that is required is to eat *kui* vegetable, and this is the cure. Xia Ziyi, *Qi ji fang*.

---

473 *Rou zhui* 肉錐, "flesh awl," a condition identical to *qian jia* 嵌甲, "embedded nail." These are *chuang* 瘡, "sore," conditions with a flaming, painful swelling developing when fingernails or toenails grow too long and enter the flesh, or when one cuts one's nails and injures the flesh. Serious cases are associated with putrescence. BCGM Dict I, 389, 409.

諸瘻不合。先以泔清温洗，拭净，取葵菜微火烘暖貼之。不過二三百葉，引膿盡，即肉生也。忌諸魚、蒜、房事。必效方。

All types of fistula that fail to close. First wash [the affected region] with warm water in which rice has been washed and wipe it clean. Then warm *kui* vegetable over a mild fire and apply it [to the affected region]. After [an application of] no more than two to three hundred leaves all the pus will have been drained and the flesh grows again. [During such a therapy] all types of fish, garlic and sex are to be avoided. *Bi xiao fang.*

湯火傷瘡。葵菜爲末傅之。食物本草。

Sores as harm caused by hot water and fire. [Grind] *kui* vegetable into powder and apply this [to the affected region]. *Shi wu ben cao.*

蛇蠍螫傷。葵菜搗汁服之。千金方。

Harm caused by snake and scorpion stings. Pound *kui* vegetable to obtain a juice and ingest it. *Qian jin fang.*

誤呑銅錢。葵菜擣汁冷飲。普濟方。

Mistakenly having swallowed a copper coin. Pound *kui* vegetable to obtain a juice and drink it cold. *Pu ji fang.*

丹石發動，口乾欬嗽者。每食後飲冬月葵虀汁一盞，便卧少時。食療本草。

Effects caused by elixir minerals, when the mouth is dry and [the patient] coughs. After every meal [let the patient] drink one cup of juice obtained from minced winter *kui*, and then he is to lie down to rest for a short while. *Shi liao ben cao.*

16-10-02

根 *Gen*

Root [of *kui*].

【氣味】甘，寒，無毒。

Qi and Flavor. Sweet, cold, nonpoisonous.

【主治】惡瘡，療淋，利小便，解蜀椒毒。别録。小兒呑錢不出，煮汁飲之，神妙。甄權。治疳瘡出黄汁。孟詵。利竅滑胎，止消渴，散惡毒氣。時珍。

Control. Malign sores. It heals [urinary] dripping. It frees urination. It resolves the poison of [Si] chuan pepper. *Bie lu.* When a child has swallowed a copper coin that fails to leave [the body], boil [a *kui* root and let it] ingest the juice. Divinely wondrous. Zhen Quan. It serves to cure *gan*-illness[474] sores emitting a yellow juice. Meng Shen.

【附方】舊五，新七。

Added Recipes. Five of old. Seven newly [recorded].

二便不通脹急者。生冬葵根二斤，擣汁三合，生薑四兩，取汁一合，和匀，分二服。連用即通也。

Blockage of both [the major (i. e., defecation) and minor (i. e., urination)] relief with a critical [abdominal] bloating. Evenly mix three *ge* of juice obtained by pounding two *jin* of winter *kui* roots, with one *ge* of juice obtained from four *liang* of fresh ginger, and ingest this divided into two portions. Use them one after another and [the passage of defecation and urination] is freed.

消渴引飲，小便不利。葵根五兩，水三大，煮汁，平旦服，日一服。並聖惠方。

Melting with thirst[475] and an urge to drink. The urine does not flow freely. Boil five *liang* of *kui* roots in three large cups of water to obtain a juice and ingest it in the early morning. To be ingested once a day. Both [these recipes:] *Sheng hui fang*.

消中尿多，日夜尿七八升。冬葵根五斤，水五斗，煮三斗。每日平旦服二升。外臺秘要。

Melting center[476] with profuse urination. Seven to eight *sheng* of urine are discharged during day and night. Boil five *jin* of winter *kui* roots in five *dou* of water down to three *dou*. Every morning in the early hours ingest two *sheng*. *Wai tai mi yao*.

漏胎下血，血盡子死。葵根莖燒灰，酒服方寸匕，日三。千金方。

Leaking fetus,[477] with a discharge of blood. When the bleeding ends the child has died. Burn *kui* root and stem to ashes and [let the patient] ingest with wine the amount held by a square *cun* spoon. Three times a day. *Qian jin fang*.

---

474 *Gan* 疳, "*gan*-illness," also: "sweets-illness," involves several complaints that affect children and adults, with causes and conditions too different to fall into a known disease category. BCGM Dict I, 180-188.

475 *Xiao ke* 消渴, "melting with thirst," most likely including cases of diabetes. BCGM Dict I, 567.

476 *Xiao zhong* 消中 "melting center," identical to *zhong xiao* 中消, "central melting." A condition of *xiao ke* 消渴, "melting with thirst," associated with a diseased central burner. Major signs: patients are constantly hungry and drink and eat much. BCGM Dict I, 687.

477 *Lou tai* 漏胎, "leaking fetus," a condition of vaginal bleeding during pregnancy. BCGM Dict I, 327.

瘭疽惡毒。肉中忽生一黤子，大如豆粟，或如梅李，或赤或黑，或白或青，其黶有核，核有深根，應心，能爛筋骨，毒入臟腑即殺人。但飲葵根汁，可折其熱毒。姚僧坦集驗方。

Flaming heat impediment-illness[478] with malign poison. Bluish-black seeds suddenly grow out of the flesh. They may have the size of soybeans or millet [grains], or of plums. They may be red or black, or white or greenish. These are skin moles with a kernel, and the kernels has a deep-reaching root around a heart/core. It can cause the decay of sinews and bones. When the poison enters one's long-term depots and short-term repositories, he will die. But if he drinks *kui* root juice, this will turn back the heat and the poison. Yao Sengtan, *Ji yan fang*.

妬乳乳癰。葵莖及子爲末，酒服方寸匕，日二。昝殷産寶。

Jealousy breast,[479] breast obstruction-illness.[480] [Grind] *kui* stems and seeds into powder and ingest with wine the amount held by a square *cun* spoon. Twice a day. Zan Yin, *Chan bao*.

身面疳瘡出黄汁者。葵根燒灰，和豬脂塗之。食療本草。

Gan-illness[481] sores covering body and face and emitting a yellow juice. Burn *kui* roots to ashes, mix them with lard and apply this [to the affected region]. *Shi liao ben cao*.

小兒蓐瘡。葵根燒末傅之。外臺。

Childbed sores of children.[482] Burn *kui* roots and [grind the residue into] powder. Apply this [to the affected region]. *Wai tai*.

---

478 *Biao ju* 瘭疽, "flaming-heat-illness with impediment-illness," a condition initially emerging like a bean kernel from which a root reaches into the depth of the tissue. This is associated with extreme pain. It slowly increases in size and generates several tips filled with pus that look like clusters of rice grains. The surface of the sores is purple-black, and the pus does not come out unimpeded. They often develop on the back of hands and feet. BCGM Dict I, 67.

479 *Du ru* 妒乳, "jealousy breast," a condition with milk blocked after delivery and the breasts turning red and swelling, being hot and painful, accompanied by fever. BCGM Dict I, 135.

480 *Ru yong* 乳癰, "breast obstruction-illness," a condition of acute putrefication of a woman's breast. Often encountered if a woman, following delivery, experiences *chui nai* 吹奶, "inflated breast," or *du ru* 妒乳, "jealousy breast." BCGM Dict I, 412.

481 *Gan* 疳, "*gan*-illness," also: "sweets-illness," involves several complaints that affect children and adults, with causes and conditions too different to fall into a known disease category. BCGM Dict I, 180-188.

482 *Ru chuang* 蓐瘡, "childbed sores," a condition of *chuang* 瘡, "sores," of newborn children developing within their first seven days of life. BCGM Dict I, 409.

小兒緊唇。葵根燒灰，酥調塗之。聖惠方。

Tight lips of children.[483] Burn *kui* roots to ashes, mix them with vinegar and apply this [to the affected region]. *Sheng hui fang*.

口吻生瘡。用經年葵根燒末傅之。外臺秘要。

Sores growing in the mouth and on the lips. Burn *kui* roots that have been stored for a year, [grind the residue into] powder and apply this [to the affected region]. *Wai tai mi yao*.

蛇虺螫傷。葵根搗塗之。古今録驗。

Harm caused by stings of snakes and venomous vipers. Pound *kui* roots [to obtain a pulp] and apply this [to the affected region]. *Gu jin lu yan*.

解防葵毒。葵根擣汁飲之。千金方。

To resolve the poison of *peucedanum* [root]. Pound *kui* roots to obtain a juice and drink it. *Qian jin fang*.

16-10-03
冬葵子 *Dong kui zi*
Seeds of winter *kui*.

【別録曰】十二月采之。【機曰】子乃春生，不應十二月可采也。

Bie lu: Collect them in the 12th month. [Wang] Ji: The seeds grow in spring. It is unlikely that they could be collected in the 12th month.

【氣味】甘，寒，滑，無毒。黄芩爲之使。

Qi and Flavor. Sweet, cold, smooth, nonpoisonous. *Scutellaria* [root] serves as its guiding substance.

【主治】五臟六腑，寒熱羸瘦，五癃，利小便。久服堅骨長肌肉，輕身延年。本經。療婦人乳難內閉，腫痛。別録。出癰疽頭。孟詵。下丹石毒。弘景。通大便，消水氣，滑胎，治痢。時珍。

Control. Cold and heat affecting the five long-term depots and six short-term repositories, with emaciation. The five types of protuberance-illness.[484] They free the passage of urine. Ingested over a long time, they harden the bones and stimulate the growth of muscles and flesh. They relieve the body of its weight and extend the years [of life]. *Ben jing*. They heal breast disorders of women with internal closure, resulting in pain-

483 *Jin chun* 緊唇, "tight lips," a condition with lips growing sores, as well as swelling, distension, festering, fissures and pain. BCGM Dict I, 254.

484 *Long* 癃, "protuberance-illness," passing of urine in small amounts; in serious cases passage is completely inhibited. BCGM Dict I, 323.

ful swelling. *Bie lu.* They let obstruction-illness and impediment-illness[485] develop a tip [opening as an ulcer]. Meng Shen. They discharge the poison of elixir minerals. [Tao] Hongjing. They free the passage of defecation, dissolve water and qi [accumulation], smooth [the birth of a] fetus and serve to cure free-flux illness. [Li] Shizhen.

【發明】【時珍曰】葵氣味俱薄，淡滑爲陽，故能利竅通乳，消腫滑胎也。其根葉與子功用相同。按陳自明婦人良方云：乳婦氣脉壅塞，乳汁不行，及經絡凝滯，奶房脹痛，留蓄作癰毒者。用葵菜子炒香、縮砂仁等分，爲末，熱酒服二錢。此藥滋氣脉，通營衛，行津液，極驗。乃上蔡張不愚方也。

Explication. [Li] Shizhen: Qi and flavor of *kui* are weakly pronounced. It has bland [qualities], is smoothing and is a yang [substance]. Therefore it can open the orifices and free the passage of a nursing mother's milk. It dissolves swelling and smoothes [the birth of a] fetus. The [therapeutic] potentials and usages of the root, the leaves and the seeds are identical. According to Chen Ziming's *Fu ren liang fang*, "when a nursing mother's qi vessels are obstructed and blocked, and the milk sap fails to pass, with congealed and sluggish [qi/blood] in the conduits and network [vessels], painful swelling of the breasts, and abiding accumulations causing obstruction-illness[486] with poison [the following therapy is recommended]. [Grind] equal amounts of *kui* vegetable seeds, fried until they develop a fragrancy, and basterd cardamom kernels into powder and [let the patient] ingest with hot wine two *qian*. This medication nourishes the qi vessels, clears the passage of camp and guardian [qi], stimulates the passage of body fluids, and is extremely effective. It is a recipe of Zhang Buyu of Shang cai."

【附方】舊八，新一十二。

Added Recipes. Eight of old. 12 newly [recorded].

大便不通，十日至一月者。肘後方：冬葵子三升，水四升，煮取一升服。不瘥更作。

Blocked defecation, lasting from ten days to one month. The *Zhou hou fang* [recommends to] boil three *sheng* of winter *kui* seeds in four *sheng* of water down to one *sheng* and ingest this. If this does not result in a cure, repeat it.

485 *Yong ju* 癰疽, "obstruction-illness, impediment-illness." refers to two vaguely distinguished obstructions/impediments of vessels or other ducts inside the body. Qi rushing against the obstruction may cause a local swelling and eventually break through the surface to cause an abscess. BCGM Dict I, 642.

486 *Yong* 癰, "obstruction-illness,"refers to an obstruction of vessels or other ducts inside the body. Qi rushing against the obstruction may cause a local swelling and eventually break through the surface to cause an abscess. BCGM Dict I, 641.

聖惠用葵子末、人乳汁等分，和服，立通。

The *Sheng hui* [recommends to] mix equal parts of *kui* seed powder and a nursing mother's milk and ingest this. [The bowel movement] is released immediately.

關格脹滿，大小便不通，欲死者。肘後方用葵子二升，水四升，煮取一升，納豬脂如一雞子，頓服。

Blockade[487] with distension and a feeling of fullness, with the passage of stools and urine blocked and [patients] nearing death. The *Zhou hou fang* [recommends to] boil two *sheng* of *kui* seeds in four *sheng* of water down to one *sheng*, add lard, the size of a chicken egg, and ingest this all at once.

千金用葵子爲末，豬脂和丸梧子大。每服五十丸，效止。

The *Qian jin* [recommends to grind] *kui* seeds into powder, mix it with lard and form pills the size of *wu* seeds. Each time ingest 50 pills. If an effect is observed, end [the treatment].

小便血淋。葵子一升，水三升，煮汁，日三服。千金方。

Urinary dripping with blood. Boil one *sheng* of *kui* seeds in three *sheng* of water and ingest the juice three times a day. *Qian jin fang*.

妊娠患淋。冬葵子一升，水三升，煮二升，分服。千金方。

Urinary dripping during pregnancy. Boil one *sheng* of winter *kui* seeds in three *sheng* of water down to two *sheng* and ingest this divided into several portions *Qian jin fang*.

妊娠下血。方同上。

Discharge with blood during pregnancy. Recipe identical to the one above.

產後淋瀝不通。用葵子一合，朴硝八分，水二升，煎八合，下硝服之。集驗方。

Urinary dripping and inability of urine to flow freely after delivery. Boil one *ge* of *kui* seeds - and [keep to the side] eight *fen* of mirabilite - in two *sheng* of water down to eight *ge*. Add the mirabilite, and ingest this. *Ji yan fang*.

妊娠水腫，身重，小便不利，洒淅惡寒，起即頭眩。用葵子、伏苓各三兩，爲糁。飲服方寸匕，日三服。小便利則愈。若轉胞者，加髮灰，神效。金匱要略。

487 *Guan ge* 關格, "blockade," a condition of an inability to pass stools and urine resulting from an irregularity of the qi dynamics in the organism. This may be accompanied by vomiting. BCGM Dict I, 198.

Water swelling during pregnancy. The body feels heavy, urine fails to flow freely, [patients] shiver and have an aversion to cold. When they get up, they feel dizzy. [Grind] three *liang* each of *kui* seeds and *poria* into powder and [let the woman] ingest with a beverage the amount held by a square *cun* spoon. To be ingested three times a day. When the urine flows freely, a cure is achieved. If this is a case of contorted urinary bladder, add ashes of burned hair. Divinely effective. *Jin kui yao lüe.*

生產困悶。冬葵子一合，搗破，水二升，煮汁半升，頓服，少時便產。昔有人如此服之，登厠，立撲兒于厠中也。食療。

Difficult birth process with heart-pressure. Pound one *ge* of winter *kui* seeds to break them open and boil them in two *sheng* of water to obtain a juice of half a *sheng*. [Let the woman] ingest this all at once. She will give birth shortly. Formerly a person ingested this and then went to the latrine. The child immediately fell into the latrine. *Shi liao.*

倒生口噤。冬葵子炒黄爲末，酒服二錢匕，效。昝殷產寶。

Footling presentation and clenched jaw. Fry winter *kui* seeds until they turn yellow and [grind them into] powder. [Let the woman] ingest with wine the amount held by two *qian* spoons. Zan Yin, *Chan bao.*

乳汁不通。方見發明。

Failure of a nursing mother to let down milk. For a recipe, see under “Explication.”

胎死腹中。葵子爲末，酒服方寸匕。若口噤不開者，灌之，藥下即甦。千金方。

A dead fetus in the abdomen. [Grind] *kui* seeds into powder and [let the woman] ingest with wine the amount held by a square *cun* spoon. In the case she has clenched jaws, force-feed [the medication] to her. When the medication is sent down, she will regain consciousness. *Qian jin fang.*

胞衣不下。冬葵子一合，牛膝一兩，水二升，煎一升服。千金方。

Failure to discharge the placenta. Boil one *ge* of winter *kui* seeds and one *liang* of *achyranthes* [leaves] in water down to one *sheng* and [let the woman] ingest this. *Qian jin fang.*

血痢產痢。冬葵子爲末，每服二錢，入臘茶一錢，沸湯調服，日三。聖惠方。

Bleeding free-flux illness, free-flux illness during birth. [Grind] winter *kui* seeds into powder and each time [let the woman] ingest two *qian*. Add one *qian* of *la* tea[488] and ingest this mixed with water boiled to bubbling. Three times a day. *Sheng hui fang*.

痎瘧邪熱。冬葵子陰乾爲末，酒服二錢。午日取花挼手，亦去瘧。聖惠方。
Malaria with evil heat. Dry winter *kui* seeds in the yin (i.e., shade) and [grind them into] powder. Ingest with wine two *qian*. At noon take [*kui*] flowers and rub them with the hands. This, too, serves to dispel malaria. *Sheng hui fang*.

癰腫無頭。孟詵曰：三日後，取葵子一百粒，水吞之，當日即開也。
Swelling without tip related to an obstruction-illness.[489] Meng Shen: After three days swallow 100 *kui* seeds with water. That same day they will open.

經驗後方云：只吞一粒即破。如吞兩粒，則有兩頭也。
The *Jing yan hou fang* states: When only one [*kui* seed] kernel is swallowed, [one obstruction-swelling tip] opens. When two kernels are swallowed, two tips open.

便毒初起。冬葵子末，酒服二錢。儒門事親。
Poison [in the region of] relief[490] that has just begun to rise. Ingest with wine two *qian* of winter *kui* seed powder. *Ru men shi qin*.

面上皰瘡。冬葵子、柏子仁、伏苓、瓜瓣各一兩，爲末。食後酒服方寸匕，日三服。陶隱居方。
Blister sores on the face. [Grind] one *liang* each of winter *kui* seeds, arborvitae seed kernels, *poria*, and wax gourd petals into powder. Ingest with wine after a meal the amount held by a square *cun* spoon. To be ingested three times a day. A recipe of Tao Yinju.

解蜀椒毒。冬葵子煮汁飲之。千金方。
To resolve the poison of [Si] chuan pepper. Boil winter *kui* seeds and drink the juice. *Qian jin fang*.

傷寒勞復。葵子二升，粱米一升，煮粥食，取汗立安。聖惠。

---

488 *La* tea, *la cha* 臘茶, lit: "tea of the 12th month," mentioned by Ouyang Xiu and Shen Kua during the Song era. As it is colored like melted wax it is also called *la cha* 蠟茶, "wax tea."

489 *Yong* 癰, "obstruction-illness," refers to an obstruction of vessels or other ducts inside the body. Qi rushing against the obstruction may cause a local swelling and eventually break through the surface to cause an abscess. BCGM Dict I, 641.

490 *Bian du* 便毒, "poison [in the region] of relief," a condition of swelling with poison developing in the body region associated with functions of 'minor relief', i.e. urination, and 'major relief', i.e. defecation. BCGM Dict I, 65.

Relapse into harm caused by cold because of exhaustion. Boil two *sheng* of *kui* seeds and one *sheng* of millet and eat the resulting congee. As soon as [the patient] sweats, healing is achieved. *Sheng hui.*

16-11
蜀葵宋嘉祐
Shu kui, FE Song, *Jia you.*

Althaea rosea **(L.) Cav. Common hollyhock.**

【校正】自菜部移入此。併入有名未用別録吴葵華。

Editorial Correction. Moved here from the section "vegetables." Also inserted here: *Wu kui hua* 吴葵華 from the section "known by name but not in use" of the *Bie lu.*

【釋名】戎葵爾雅、吴葵。【藏器曰】爾雅云：菺，音堅，戎葵也。郭璞註云：今蜀葵也。葉似葵，花如木槿花。戎、蜀其所自來，因以名之。【時珍曰】羅願爾雅翼：吴葵作胡葵，云胡，戎也。夏小正云，四月小滿後五日，吴葵華，別録吴葵，即此也。而唐人不知，退入有名未用。嘉祐本草重於菜部出蜀葵條。蓋未讀爾雅註及千金方"吴葵一名蜀葵"之文故也。今併爲一。

Explanation of Names. *Rong kui* 戎葵, *Er ya*. *Wu kui* 吴葵. [Chen] Cangqi: The *Er ya* states: "*Jian* 菺, read *jian* 堅, is *rong kui* 戎葵." Go Pu in his comment states: "This is today's *shu kui* 蜀葵. The leaves resemble those of Chinese mallows, *kui* 葵; the flowers are similar to *hibiscus* flowers. Rong 戎 and Shu 蜀 refer to where they come from. Therefore their names." [Li] Shizhen: Luo Yuan in his *Er ya yi*: *Wu kui* 吴葵 is written *hu kui* 胡葵, "because the Hu 胡 are the Rong 戎." The *Xia xiao zheng* states: "In the fourth month, five days after the [solar term] Grain Budding (21/22 May), [collect] *wu kui hua* 吴葵華." According to the *Bie lu*, *wu kui* 吴葵 is [the item discussed] here. But this was unknown to Tang people and they pushed it off into the section "known by name but not in use." Then the *Jia you ben cao* in the section "vegetables" released a *shu kui* 蜀葵 entry again. The fact is, they had not read the comments on the *Er ya* and the *Qian jin fang* where it says "*wu kui* 吴葵, alternative name *shu kui* 蜀葵." Here now they are combined [in one entry].

【集解】【頌曰】蜀葵似葵，花如木槿花，有五色。小花者名錦葵，功用更强。【時珍曰】蜀葵處處人家植之。春初種子，冬月宿根亦自生苗，嫩時亦可茹食。葉似葵菜而大，亦似絲瓜葉，有歧叉。過小滿後長莖，高五六尺。花似木槿而大，有深紅、淺紅、紫、黑、白色，單葉、千葉之異。昔人謂其疏莖密葉、翠萼艷花、金粉檀心者，頗善狀之。惟紅、白二色入藥。其實大如指頭，皮薄而扁，内仁如馬兜鈴仁及蕪荑仁，輕虛易種。其稭剥皮，可緝布作繩。一種小者名錦葵，即荆葵也。爾雅謂之荍，音喬。其花大如五銖錢，粉紅色，有紫縷文。掌禹錫補注本草謂此即戎葵，非矣。然功用亦相似。

Collected Explanations. [Su] Song: *Shu kui* 蜀葵 is similar to *kui* 葵, Chinese mallows. The flowers resemble *hibiscus* flowers. They appear with all five colors. Those with small flowers are called "brocade *kui*." Their [therapeutic] potential and usage is even stronger. [Li] Shizhen: *Shu kui* is planted by people everywhere. The seeds are planted in early spring. The perennial roots, surviving the winter months, also develop seedlings by themselves. As long as they are tender they are edible as a vegetable. The leaves resemble those of Chinese mallow vegetables, but are bigger. They also resemble loofah leaves, but have forks/bifurcations. After [the solar term] Grain Budding (21./22. May) a long stem grows, reaching a height of five to six *chi*. The flowers resemble those of *hibiscus*, but are bigger. They may be deep red, pale red, purple, black and white, and they differ in that there may be only one leaf or a thousand leaves. When the ancients said of them "sparse stems, dense leaves. Emerald-green calyxes and gorgeous flowers. A golden powder and a reddish-brown heart," this was an appropriate description. Only those of red and white color are added to medication. Their fruits are as big as a fingertip. Their skin is thin, and they are flat. The kernels inside are similar to *aristolochia* kernels, and also *ulmus* fruit. They are light, hollow and easy to plant. The skin peeled off the stalk can be woven to fabrics and made to ropes. A small kind is called "brocade *kui*." This is *jing kui* 荆葵. The *Er ya* calls it *qiao* 荍, read *qiao* 喬. Its flowers are as big as a five *zhu* coin. They are pink, with a line design of purple threads. Zhang Yuxi in his *Bu zhu ben cao* says that this is *rong kui*. He is wrong, Still, there [therapeutic] potentials and uses are similar.

16-11-01

苗 *Miao*

Seedling [of *shu kui*].

【氣味】甘，微寒，滑，無毒。【思邈曰】不可久食，鈍人志性。若被狗齧者食之，永不瘥也。【李廷飛曰】合豬肉食，人無顏色。

Qi and Flavor. Sweet, slightly cold, smoothing, nonpoisonous. [Sun] Simiao: It must not be eaten for a long time. It lets one turn dull-witted. If one eats eat after a dog chewed on it, he will never be cured [of the resulting disease]. Li Tingfei: Eaten together with lard causes a loss of complextion.

【主治】除客熱，利腸胃。思邈。煮食，治丹石發熱，大人小兒熱毒下痢。藏器。作蔬食，滑竅治淋，潤燥易産。時珍。擣爛塗火瘡，燒研傅金瘡。大明。

Control. It disperses visitor heat[491] and clears the passage through the intestines and the stomach. [Sun] Simiao. Eaten boiled in water, it serves to cure heat effusion caused by elixir minerals. Discharge with free-flux illness of adults and children alike caused by heat poison. [Chen] Cangqi. Prepared as a vegetable, it smoothens the [passage through the] orifices and serves to cure urinary dripping. It moistens dryness and makes birth easier. [Li] Shizhen. Pounded into a pulpy [mass] it is applied to fire sores. Burned and [the residue] ground it is applied to wounds caused by metal objects/weapons. Da Ming.

16-11-02
根莖 *Gen jing*
Root, stem [of *shu kui*].

【主治】客熱，利小便，散膿血惡汁。藏器。

Control. Visitor heat. They free urination. They disperse pus, blood [accumulation] and malign juice. [Chen] Cangqi.

【發明】【宗奭曰】蜀葵，四時取紅色單葉者根，陰乾，治帶下，排膿血惡物，極驗也。

Explication. [Kou] Zongshi: *Shu kui*, during all four seasons take the roots of those of red color and with only one leaf, dry them in the yin (i. e., shade) and use them to cure [diseases of women] below the belt. They expel pus, [stagnating] blood and malign items, in a most effective way.

【附方】新七。

Added Recipes. Seven newly [recorded].

小便淋痛。葵花根洗剉，水煎五七沸，服之如神。衛生寶鑒。

Painful urinary dripping. Wash *kui* flower roots clean, boil them in water to bubbling, five to seven times, and ingest this. Divine-like [effect]. *Wei sheng bao jian.*

小便血淋。葵花根二錢，車前子一錢，水煮，日服之。簡便單方。

Urinary dripping with blood. Boil in water two *qian* of *kui* flower roots and one *qian* of Asiatic plantain seeds and ingest this daily. *Jian bian dan fang.*

491 *Ke re* 客熱, "visitor heat," 1.) an etiological agent identified as heat evil intruding into the human organism from outside. 2.) A condition identical to *re* 熱, "heat." BCGM Dict I, 282.

小便尿血。葵莖灰，酒服方寸匕，日三。千金。

Urination with blood. Ingest with wine an amount of *kui* stem ashes held by a square *cun* spoon. Three times a day. *Qian jin.*

腸胃生癰。懷忠丹：治内癰有敗血，腥穢殊甚，臍腹冷痛，用此排膿下血。單葉紅蜀葵根、白芷各一兩，白枯礬、白芍藥各五錢，爲末，黄蠟溶化，和丸梧子大，每空心米飲下二十丸。待膿血出盡，服十宣散補之。坦仙皆效方。

Obstruction-illness[492] in the intestines and the stomach. The "elixir yearning for loyalty." To cure internal obstruction-illness with decayed blood, generating extremely foul and dirty [items], and painful cold in the navel and abdominal region, the application of this [elixir] serves to eliminate pus and to discharge blood. [Grind] one *liang* each of single leaf, red *shu kui* root and *angelica dahurica* [root], and five *qian* each of processed alum and white *paeonia* [root] into powder and form with melted beeswax pills the size of *wu* seeds. Each time send down on an empty stomach 20 pills with a rice beverage until all the pus and the blood have left. Ingest the "powder with ten [ingredients] to lead off [evil qi]"[493] to supplement the [patient's qi]. Tan xian, *Jie xiao fang.*

諸瘡腫痛不可忍者。葵花根去黑皮，搗爛，入井花水調稠貼之。普濟方。

All types of sores with swelling and an unbearable pain. Pound *kui* flower roots, with the black skin discarded, into a pulpy [mass], add the first water drawn from a well in the morning and attach this [to the affected region]. *Pu ji fang.*

小兒吻瘡，經年欲腐。葵根燒研傅之。聖惠方。

Lip sores of children, having lasted for a year with a threat to let [the lips] rot. Burn *kui* roots, grind [the residue into powder] and apply this [to the affected region]. *Sheng hui fang.*

小兒口瘡。赤葵莖炙乾爲末，蜜和含之。聖惠方。

Oral sores of children. Roast red *kui* stems until they are dry and [grind them into] powder. Mix it with honey and [let the child] hold this in its mouth. *Sheng hui fang.*

---

492 *Yong* 癰, "obstruction-illness," refers to an obstruction of vessels or other ducts inside the body. Qi rushing against the obstruction may cause a local swelling and eventually break through the surface to cause an abscess. BCGM Dict I, 641.

493 The ingredients of *shi xuan fang* 十宣散, "powder with ten[ingredients] to lead off [evil qi]," include: Ginseng root, Chinese *angelica* root, *astragalus* root, *platycodon* root, *cassia* bark, *magnolia* bark, *saposhnikovia* root, *ligusticum* root, *angelica dahurica* root, and *glycyrrhiza* root.

16-11-03

吴葵華別録 ***Wu kui hua*** FE *Bie lu.*

Splendor of *kui* from Wu.

【氣味】鹹，寒，無毒。【禹錫曰】蜀葵華：甘，冷，無毒。

Qi and Flavor. Salty, cold, nonpoisonous. [Zhang] Yuxi: *Shu kui hua*[494]: Sweet, cold, nonpoisonous.

【主治】理心氣不足。別録。小兒風瘮，痎瘧。嘉祐。治帶下，目中溜火，和血潤燥，通竅，利大小腸。時珍。

Control. It corrects insufficient heart qi. *Bie lu.* Wind papules[495] and malaria of children. *Jia you.* It serves to cure [women's illnesses] below the belt, fire abiding in the eyes. It harmonizes blood and moistens dryness. It penetrates the orifices and clears the passage through the large and small intestines. [Li] Shizhen.

【發明】【張元素曰】蜀葵花，陰中之陽也。赤者治赤帶，白者治白帶，赤者治血燥，白者治氣燥，皆取其寒滑潤利之功也。又紫葵花，入染髭髮方中用。

Explication. Zhang Yuansu: *Shu kui* flowers are a yang in yin [substance]. Red ones serve to cure red [outflow from below the] belt. White ones serve to cure white [outflow from below the] belt. Red ones serve to cure blood desiccation. White ones serve to cure qi desiccation. For all these [therapeutic purposes] one makes use of their cooling, smoothing, moistening and passage opening potential. There is also a purple *kui* flower. It is added to recipes used to dye beard and hair.

【附方】舊二，新五。

Added Recipes. Two of old. Five newly [recorded].

二便關格，脹悶欲死，二三日則殺人。蜀葵花一兩搗爛，麝香半錢，水一大盞，煎服。根亦可用。

Both [defecation and urination] relief blocked, with a bloating and heart-pressure bringing one close to death. After two or three days, this kills one. Boil one *liang* of *shu kui* flowers, ground to a pulpy [mass], and half a *qian* of musk in one large cup of water and ingest this. The root can be used, too.

---

494 *Shu kui hua* 蜀葵華, "splendor of *kui* from Shu."

495 *Feng zhen* 風瘮, "wind papules," a condition, brought forth by wind evil, of eruptive skin papules of different sizes, accompanied by unbearable itching. If scratched they rise further. BCGM Dict I, 172.

痎瘧邪熱。蜀葵花白者，陰乾爲末。服之。午日取花挼手，亦能去瘧。蘇頌圖經本草。

Malaria with evil heat. [Grind] white *shu kui* flowers, dried in the yin (i. e., shade), into powder and ingest this. To rub the flowers with the hands at noon can also dispel malaria. Su Song, *Tu jing ben cao.*

婦人帶下，臍腹冷痛，面色痿黃，日漸虛困。用葵花一兩，陰乾爲末，每空心溫酒服二錢匕。赤帶用赤葵，白帶用白葵。聖惠方。

Women's [diseases] below the belt, with a painful cold in the navel and abdominal region, and the face taking on a dysfunctional yellow complexion. Dry one *liang* of *kui* flowers in the yin (i. e., shade) and [grind them into] powder. Each time ingest on an empty stomach with wine the amount held by two *qian* spoons. For red [outflow from below the] belt, use red *kui* [flowers]. For white [outflow from below the] belt, use white *kui* [flowers]. *Sheng hui fang.*

橫生倒産。葵花爲末，酒服方寸匕。千金方。

Transverse birth, footling presentation. [Grind] *kui* flowers into powder and [let the woman] ingest with wine the amount held by a square *cun* spoon. *Qian jin fang.*

酒皶赤鼻。蜀葵花研末，臘豬脂和勻，夜傅旦洗。仁存方。

Red nose with wine sediments.[496] Grind *shu kui* flowers into powder, mix it with lard obtained during the twelfth month, apply this [to the affected region] at night and wash it off in the morning. *Ren cun fang.*

誤吞鍼錢。葵花煮汁服之。普濟方。

Mistakenly having swallowed a needle or coin. Boil *kui* flowers in water and ingest it. *Pu ji fang.*

蜂蠍螫毒。五月五日午時，收蜀葵花、石榴花、艾心等分，陰乾爲末，水調塗之。肘後方。

Poison resulting from a bee/wasp or scorpion sting. On the fifth day of the fifth month at noon gather equal amounts of *shu kui* flowers, pomegranate flowers and mugwort leaves, dry them in the yin (i. e., shade) and [grind them into] powder, to be applied, mixed with water, [to the affected region]. *Zhou hou fang.*

---

496 *Jiu zha* 酒皶, "wine sediments," a condition with major signs of a swollen, red nose with papules that may, when squeezed, release white sediments. The condition flares up again and again until eventually the nose has increased in size and has assumed a red color. BCGM Dict I, 275.

16-11-04
子 *Zi*
Seeds [of *shu kui*].

【氣味】甘，冷，無毒。

Qi and Flavor. Sweet, cold, nonpoisonous.

【主治】淋澀，通小腸，催生落胎，療水腫，治一切瘡疥，并瘢疵赤靨。大明。

Control. Rough urinary dripping. It opens the small intestine, hastens birth in that it facilitates the descend of the fetus. It serves to cure all types of sores and *jie*-illness,[497] also scars, blemishes and red pimples. Da Ming.

【發明】【時珍曰】按楊士瀛直指方云：蜀葵子炒，入宣毒藥中最驗。又催生方：用子二錢，滑石三錢，爲末。順流水服五錢，即下。

Explication. [Li] Shizhen: According to Yang Shiying's *Zhi zhi fang*, "fried *shu kui* seeds are very effective when they are added to medication supposed to lead off poison. Also, a recipe to hasten birth: [Grind] two *qian* of [*shu kui*] seeds and three *qian* of talcum into powder and [let the woman] ingest five *qian* with water flowing along its correct flow. This lets [the child] come down."

【附方】舊一，新二。

Added Recipes. One of old. Two newly [recorded].

大小便閉不通者。用白花胡葵子爲末，煮濃汁服之。千金方。

Blocked major and minor (defecaton and urination) relief. [Grind] white flower *hu kui* seeds into powder, boil them to obtain a thick juice and ingest it. *Qian jin fang*.

石淋破血。五月五日，收葵子炒研，食前温酒下一錢，當下石出。聖惠方。

Urinary stone dripping; to break through blood [accumulation]. On the fifth day of the fifth month gather *kui* seeds, roast them, grind them and send down, prior to a meal, with warm wine one *qian*. This serves to discharge the stones. *Sheng hui fang*.

癰腫無頭。蜀葵子爲末，水調傅之。經驗後方。

Obstruction-illness[498] swelling without tips. [Grind] *shu kui* seeds into powder and apply them mixed with water [to the affected region] *Jing yan hou fang*.

---

497 *Jie*-illness 疥, vaguely identifiable skin ailment. BCGM Dict I, 249.

498 *Yong* 癰, "obstruction-illness,"refers to an obstruction of vessels or other ducts inside the body. Qi rushing against the obstruction may cause a local swelling and eventually break through the surface to cause an abscess. BCGM Dict I, 641.

16-12
菟葵唐本草
Tu kui, FE *Tang ben cao.*

***Malva parviflora* L. Least mallow.**

【釋名】天葵圖經、菥音希、雷丸草外丹本草。

Explanation of Names. *Tian kui* 天葵, *Tu jing*. *Xi* 菥, read *xi* 希. *Lei wan cao* 雷丸草, *Wai dan ben cao.*

【集解】【恭曰】菟葵苗如石龍芮而葉光澤，花白似梅，其莖紫黑，煮噉極滑。所在下澤田間皆有，人多識之。六月、七月采莖葉，曝乾入藥。【禹錫曰】郭璞注爾雅云：菟葵似葵而小，葉狀如藜，有毛，汋之可食而滑。【宗奭曰】菟葵，緑葉如黄蜀葵，其花似拒霜，甚雅，其形至小，如初開單葉蜀葵。有檀心，色如牡丹姚黄其蕊，則蜀葵也。唐劉夢得所謂菟葵、燕麥，動揺春風者是也。【時珍曰】按鄭樵通志云：菟葵，天葵也。狀如葵菜。葉大如錢而厚，面青背微紫，生於崖石。凡丹石之類，得此而後能神。所以雷公炮炙論云：如要形堅，豈忘紫背。謂其能堅鉛也。此説得於天台一僧。又按南宫從峋嶁神書云：紫背天葵出蜀中，靈草也，生於水際。取自然汁煮汞則堅，亦能煮八石拒火也。又按初虞世古今録驗云：五月五前齋戒。看桑下有菟葵者，至五日午時至桑下，呪曰繫黎乎俱當蘇婆訶。呪畢，乃以手摩桑陰一遍，口齧菟葵及五葉草嚼熟，以唾塗手，熟揩令遍。再齋七日，不得洗手。後有蛇蟲蠍蠆咬傷者，以此手摩之即愈也。時珍竊謂古有呪由一科，此亦其類，但不知必用菟葵取何義也。若謂其相制，則治毒蟲之草亦多矣。

Collected Explanations. [Su] Gong: *Tu kui* seedlings are similar to cursed crow foot [seedlings], but the leaves are shiny and moist. The flowers are white and resemble those of plums. The stem is purple-black. Eaten boiled in water, they have a smoothing effect. They can be found everywhere in low-lying marshlands and in the open country. Many people are familiar with them. They collect the stem and the leaves in the sixth and seventh month, dry them in the sun and add them to medication. [Zhang] Yuxi: Guo Pu in his comments on the *Er ya* states: "*Tu kui* resemble Chinese mallows, but are smaller. The leaves are shaped like those of lamb's quarters, and they are covered with hair. When burned, [the hair] is edible and has a smoothing effect." [Kou] Zongshi: *Tu kui* have green leaves, resembling those of okra. The flowers resemble those of cotton rose. They are very elegant. Their physical appearance it extremely small, similar to those of single leaf Shu mallows that have just opened. They have a reddish-brown heart; their color is similar to that of the stamens of *paeonia* trees from Yao huang. Actually, this is Shu mallow. These are the [plants] spoken of by the Tang author Liu Mengde as "*tu kui* and Japanese brome waving back and forth in the spring wind." [Li] Shizhen: According to Zheng Qiao's *Tong zhi*, "*tu kui* is *tian kui* 天葵. It is shaped like Chinese mallow. The leaves are shaped like a thick coin. They are greenish on their front and slightly purple on their back. They grow on cliffs and rocks. All elixir minerals can exert divine [effects when they are ingested] in combination with this [herb]." Therefore, the *Lei gong pao zhi* states: "When it is intended to harden its physical appearance, how could one forget the purple back?" What he refers to here is to harden lead. This is a saying obtained from a monk on [Mount] Tian tai. Also, according to Nan Gongcong's *Gou lu shen shu*, "purple back *tian kui* comes from Shu zhong; it is a magic herb. It grows close to waters. When mercury is boiled with its natural juice it hardens. It can also be boiled together with the eight stones/minerals to make them resistant to fire." Furthermore, according to Chu Yushi's *Gu jin lu yan*, "start a vegetarian diet and fasting prior to the fifth [day] of the fifth month and watch out for *tu kui* growing under mulberry trees. On the fifth day at noon proceed to below a mulberry tree and recite the following incantation: Jilihujudansupoke. Following this incantation, rub your hands on the yin/shady side of the mulberry tree and chew in your mouth *tu kui* and common crowfoot to a paste. Spit it into your hands and rub them to distribute it all over [your hands]. Then, again, continue a vegetarian diet for seven days. Do not wash the hands. Thereafter, you will heal those who have been hurt by snake bites, and worm/bug and scorpion stings by stroking them with your hands." I. [Li] Shizhen say: In ancient times there was a discipline "to exorcise the origin [of a disease]." The action just outlined is part of this. However, I do not know what sense it makes to specifically resort to *tu kui* for it. If one were to say that this is a case of mutual checking, then [one should add that] there are many herbs serving to cure [the poison of] worms/bugs.

16-12-01
苗 ***Miao***
Seedling [of *tu kui*].

【氣味】甘，寒，無毒。
Qi and Flavor. Sweet, cold, nonpoisonous.

【主治】下諸石五淋，止虎蛇毒諸瘡，擣汁飲之。塗瘡能解毒止痛。唐本。
Control. To discharge all types of stones, [to cure] the five types of urinary dripping and to end all sores associated with poison resulting from [the bites of] tigers and snakes, pound it to obtain a juice and drink it. Applied to sores it can resolve poison and end pain. *Tang ben*.

16-13
黄蜀葵宋嘉祐
Huang shu kui, FE Song, *Jia you*.

Abelmoschus manihot **(L.) Medic. Okra.**

【校正】自菜部移入此。

Editorial Correction. It has been moved here from the section "vegetables."

【釋名】【時珍曰】黄蜀葵别是一種，宜入草部，而嘉祐本草定入菜部，爲其與蜀葵同名，而氣味主治亦同故也。今移於此。

Explanation of Names: [Li] Shizhen: Okra, "yellow *shu kui*," is a kind [of plant] that should be added to the section "herbs," but the [authors of the] *Jia you ben cao* decided to include it in the section "vegetables" because it has the same name as *shu kui* 蜀葵, and their qi and flavor, as well as their control and therapeutic [potentials] are identical, too. Now it is moved here.

【集解】【禹錫曰】黄蜀葵花，近道處處有之。春生苗葉，頗似蜀葵而葉尖狹多刻缺，夏末開花淺黄色，六七月采，陰乾之。【宗奭曰】黄蜀葵與蜀葵别種，非是蜀葵中黄者也。葉心下有紫檀色，摘下剔散，日乾之。不爾即浥爛也。【時珍曰】黄葵二月下種，或宿子在土自生，至夏始長，葉大如蓖麻葉，深緑色，開岐丫，有五尖如人爪形，旁有小尖。六月開花，大如椀，鵝黄色，紫心六瓣而側，旦開午收暮落，人亦呼爲側金盞花。隨即結角，大如拇指，長二寸許，本大末尖，六稜有毛，老則黑色。其稜自綻，内有六房，如脂麻房。其子纍纍在房内，狀如茼麻子，色黑。其莖長者六七尺，剥皮可作繩索。

Collected Explanations. [Zhang] Yuxi: *Huang shu kui* can be found everywhere nearby. In spring, it grows a seedling and leaves. They are quite similar to those of Shu mallows, but the leaves are pointed and narrow with many indentations. At the end of summer, [okra] opens flowers of a pale yellow color. They are collected in the sixth and seventh month, to be dried in the yin (i. e., shade). [Kou] Zongshi: *Huang shu kui*, "yellow *shu* mallow," and *shu* mallow are two different kinds. [Yellow *shu* mallow] is not simply a yellow kind of *shu* mallows. Below the heart of the leaves is something of a purple-brown-red color. Cut it out and discard it, and then dry [the leaves] in the sun. If this were not done, they would attract moisture and rot. [Li] Shizhen: *Huang shu kui* is planted in the second month. It is also possible that perennial seeds grow [a seedling] by themselves. By summer it begins to grow, with leaves of the size of castor [leaves]. They are deep green and bifurcate to eventually have five ends similar to the shape of a human hand. Flowers, the size of a bowl, open in the sixth month. They are of goose-yellow color, with a purple heart and six petals to the side. They open in the morning, shrink at noon and fall off in the evening. People also call them "flowers with a gold cup to the side." Then they form a "horn"[-like capsule] as big as a thumb, and about two *cun* long. It is big at its base and pointed at its end, with six hairy edges. When it ages it assumes a black color. The "horn" splits open by itself. Inside of it are six chambers, similar to the [seed] chambers of sesame. The seeds are lined up in the chambers; they are shaped like the seeds of Indian mallows. They are black. The stems may reach a length of six or seven *chi*. The skin/bark is sraped off to be made to ropes and strings.

16-13-01
花 ***Hua***
Flower [of *huang shu kui*].

【氣味】甘，寒，滑，無毒。

Qi and Flavor. Sweet, cold, smoothing, nonpoisonous.

【主治】小便淋及催生。治諸惡瘡膿水久不瘥者，作末傅之即愈，爲瘡家要藥。嘉祐。消癰腫。浸油，塗湯火傷。時珍。

Control. Urinary dripping, and hastening birth. It serves to cure all types of malign sores with pus and water that have not been cured for a long time. Prepare them into powder, apply it [to the affected regions] and a cure is achieved. It is an important pharmaceutical drug resorted to by sore specialists. *Jia you*. It dissolves obstruction-illness[499] swelling. Soaked in oil it is applied to harm caused by hot water and fire. [Li] Shizhen.

【附方】新八。

Added Recipes. Eight newly [recorded].

沙石淋痛。黄蜀葵花一兩，炒爲末。每米飲服一錢，名獨聖散。普濟方。

Painful [urinary] dripping with sand and stones. Fry one *liang* of *huang shu kui* flowers and [grind the residue into] powder. Each time ingest with a rice beverage one *qian*. [This recipe] is called "powder with one single sagely [ingredient]." *Pu ji fang*.

難産催生。如聖散：治胎臟乾澀難産，劇者併進三服，良久腹中氣寬，胎滑即下也。用黄葵花焙研末，熟湯調服二錢。無花，用子半合研末，酒淘去滓，服之。産寶鑑。

499 *Yong* 癰, "obstruction-illness," refers to an obstruction of vessels or other ducts inside the body. Qi rushing against the obstruction may cause a local swelling and eventually break through the surface to cause an abscess. BCGM Dict I, 641.

Difficult birth, and to hasten delivery. The "powder with sage-like [effects]." It serves to cure dryness and roughness of the womb long-term depot causing a difficult birth. In serious cases [let the woman] ingest it three times in a row. After quite a while the qi in the abdomen will relax, the fetus will pass with a smooth discharge. Bake *huang* [*shu*] *kui* flowers over a slow fire and grind them into powder. [Let the woman] ingest mixed with boiled water two *qian*. If no flowers are at hand, grind half a *ge* of the seeds into powder, soak them in wine, discard the dregs, and [let the woman] ingest [the liquid]. *Chan bao jian*.

胎死不下。即上方，用紅花酒下。

A dead fetus fails to come down. Recipe identical to the one above, to be sent down with a safflower wine.

癰疽腫毒。黄蜀葵花，用鹽摻，收瓷器中密封，經年不壞，每用傅之，自平自潰。無花，用根葉亦可。直指方。

Poison swelling associated with obstruction-illness and impediment-illness.[500] Mix *huang shu kui* flowers with salt and store them tightly sealed in a porcelain vessel. This way they will not rot even for an entire year. For each [therapy] apply them [to the affected region. The swelling will flatten and it will release its liquid as a result. If no flowers are at hand, the root and the leaves can be used, too. *Zhi zhi fang*.

小兒口瘡。黄葵花燒末傅之。肘後方。

Oral sores of children. Burn *huang* [*shu*] *kui* flowers [and grind the residue into] powder. Apply it [to the affected region]. *Zhou hou fang*.

小兒木舌。黄蜀葵花爲末一錢，黄丹五分，傅之。直指方。

Wooden tongue[501] of children. [Mix] one *qian* of *huang shu kui* flowers, [ground into] powder, with five *fen* of minium, and apply this [to the affected region]. *Zhi zhi fang*.

湯火灼傷。用瓶盛麻油，以筯就樹夾取黄葵花，收入瓶内，勿犯人手，密封收之。遇有傷者，以油塗之，甚妙。經驗方。

Harm caused by hot water and fire. Fill a jar with sesame oil. With chopsticks pick *huang* [*shu*] *kui* flowers directly from the tree and insert them into the jar. They must

500 *Yong ju* 癰疽, "obstruction-illness, impediment-illness." refers to two vaguely distinguished obstructions/impediments of vessels or other ducts inside the body. Qi rushing against the obstruction may cause a local swelling and eventually break through the surface to cause an abscess. BCGM Dict I, 642.

501 *Mu she* 木舌, "wooden tongue," a condition with the body of the tongue massively swollen to an extent that it fills the oral cavity and at the same time is as hard as wood. BCGM Dict I, 344.

not be touched by a human hand. Store them tightly sealed. When you encounter a harm [caused by scalding or a burn], apply the oil [to the affected region]. Very wondrous. *Jing yan fang.*

小兒禿瘡。黄蜀葵花、大黄、黄芩等分，爲末。米泔净洗，香油調搽。普濟方。

Baldness sores of children [Grind] equal amounts of *huang shu kui* flowers, rhubarb root and *scutellaria* [root] into powder. Wash [the affected region] clean with water in which rice has been washed, and apply [the powder] mixed with sesame oil. *Pu ji fang.*

16-13-02

子及根 *Zi ji gen*

Seed and root [of *huang shu kui*].

【氣味】甘，寒，滑，無毒。

Qi and Flavor. Sweet, cold, smoothing, nonpoisonous.

【主治】癰腫，利小便，五淋水腫，産難，通乳汁。時珍。

Control. Obstruction-illness[502] swelling. They free the passage of urine. The five types of [urinary] dripping and water swelling. Difficult birth. They free [the release of a nursing mother's] milk sap. [Li] Shizhen.

【發明】【頌曰】冬葵、黄葵、蜀葵，形狀雖各不同，而性俱寒滑，故所主療不甚相遠。【時珍曰】黄葵子古方少用，今爲催生及利小便要藥。或用，或入湯散皆宜，蓋其性滑，與冬葵子同功故也。花、子與根性功相同，可以互用。無花用子，無子用根。

Explication. [Su] Song: The physical appearances of *dong kui* 冬葵, winter mallows, *huang* [*shu*] *kui* 黄[蜀]葵 and *shu kui* 蜀葵, Chinese *shu* mallows, all differ, but their nature is cold and smoothing. Therefore, the [conditions] they control and heal are not far apart from each other. [Li] Shizhen: Ancient recipes seldom [recommended to] use the seeds of *huang* [*shu*] *kui*. Today, they are an important pharmaceutical drug to hasten birth and to free the passage of urine. Sometimes they are used to ....,[503] or they are added to a decoction or powder. All this is suitable. The fact is, by

502 *Yong* 癰, "obstruction-illness," refers to an obstruction of vessels or other ducts inside the body. Qi rushing against the obstruction may cause a local swelling and eventually break through the surface to cause an abscess. BCGM Dict I, 641.

503 Apparently, in front of or following the character *yong* 用 a piece of the text is missing. The *Hua xia* 華夏, based on the overall meaning of this passage, has added the character *dan* 單, "as a single [substance]," in front of *yong* 用. However, in view of the recipes added below, one might also add *yan lan shui fu* 研爛水服, "ground into a pulpy mass and ingested with water," behind the character *yong* 用.

nature they are smoothing because their [therapeutic] potential is identical to that of winter mallows. The nature and the [therapeutic] potential of flowers and seeds are identical to those of the root; they can be used interchangeably. If no flowers are at hand, resort to the seeds. If no seeds are at hand, resort to the root.

【附方】舊二。新二。
Added Recipes. Two of old. Two newly [recorded].

臨産催生。宗奭曰：臨産時以四十九粒研爛，温水服之，良久即産。
To hasten birth close to the moment of delivery. [Kou] Zongshi: When the time of delivery approaches, grind 49 [*huang shu kui* seed] kernels into a pulpy [mass] and [let the woman] ingest it with warm water. After quite a while, she will give birth.

經驗後方用子焙研三錢，井花水服。無子用根，煎汁服。
The *Jing yan hou fang* [recommends to] bake the seeds over a slow fire and grind three *qian* [to powder] to be ingested with the first water drawn from a well in the morning. If no seeds are at hand, use the root. Boil it [in water] and [let the woman] ingest the juice.

便癰初起。淮人用黄蜀葵子七粒，皂角半挺，爲末，以石灰同醋調塗之。永類鈐方。
Obstruction-illness[504] in the [region of urination and defecation] relief, when [the swelling] is just beginning to rise. People in Huai use seven grains of *huang shu kui* seeds, and grind them with half a *gleditsia* pod into powder. This is mixed with limestone and vinegar to be applied [to the affected region]. *Yong lei qian fang.*

癰腫不破。黄葵子研，酒服，一粒則一頭，神效。衛生易簡方。
An obstruction-illness swelling that fails to break open. Grind *huang* [*shu*] *kui* seeds [to powder] and ingest them with wine. One seed results in [the opening of] one tip. Divinely effective. *Wei sheng yi jian fang.*

打撲傷損。黄葵子研，酒服二錢。海上方。
Harm and injury resulting from a blow or a fall. Grind *huang* [*shu*] *kui* seeds [to powder] and ingest with wine two *qian*. *Hai shang fang.*

504 *Yong* 癰, "obstruction-illness," refers to an obstruction of vessels or other ducts inside the body. Qi rushing against the obstruction may cause a local swelling and eventually break through the surface to cause an abscess. BCGM Dict I, 641.

16-14
龍葵唐本草
Long kui, FE *Tang bèn cao.*

Solanum nigrum L. Common night-shade.

【校正】併入圖經老鴉眼睛草。

Editorial Correction. Inserted here is *lao ya yan jing cao* 老鴉眼睛草, [listed separately in the] *Tu jing.*

【釋名】苦葵圖經、苦菜唐本、天茄子圖經、水茄綱目、天泡草綱目、老鴉酸漿草綱目、老鴉眼睛草圖經。【時珍曰】龍葵，言其性滑如葵也。苦以菜味名，茄以葉形名，天泡、老鴉眼睛皆以子形名也。與酸漿相類，故加老鴉以別之。五爪龍亦名老鴉眼睛草，敗醬、苦苣並名苦菜，名同物異也。

Explanation of Names. *Ku kui* 苦葵, "bitter mallow," *Tu jing*. *Ku cai* 苦菜, "bitter vegetable," *Tang ben*. *Tian qie zi* 天茄子, "heaven's eggplant," *Tu jing*. *Shui qie* 水茄, "water eggplant," *Gang mu*. *Tian pao cao* 天泡草, "celestial blister herb," *Gang mu*. *Lao ya suan jiang cao* 老鴉酸漿草, *Gang mu*. *Lao ya yan jing cao* 老鴉眼睛草, "old crow's eyes herb," *Tu jing*. [Li] Shizhen: *Long kui* 龍葵, "dragon mallow," is to say: Its nature is as slippery/smoothing as that of Chinese mallows. *Ku* 苦, "bitter," is based on the flavor of the vegetable. *Qie* 茄, "eggplant," refers to the physical appearance of the leaves. *Tian pao* 天泡, "celestial blister," and *lao ya yan jing* 老鴉眼睛, "old crow's eyes," both refer to the shape of the seeds. [*Long kui*] belongs to the same group as Chinese lantern plants, *suan jiang* 酸漿. Therefore [the two characters] *lao ya* 老鴉, "old crow," were added to distinguish them. Japanese *cayratia* creeper is also named "old crow's eyes herb," and dahurian *patrinia*, *bai jiang* 敗醬, as well as *sow thistle* [herb] are both called "bitter vegetable," *ku cai* 苦菜. The names are the same, but the items differ.

【集解】【弘景曰】益州有苦菜，乃是苦蘵。【恭曰】苦蘵，即龍葵也。俗亦名苦菜，非荼也。龍葵所在有之，關、河間謂之苦菜，葉圓花白，子若牛李子，生青熟黑。但堪煮食，不任生噉。【頌曰】龍葵近處亦稀，惟北方有之。人謂之苦葵。葉圓似排風而無毛，花白色，子亦似排風子，生青熟黑，其赤者名赤珠，亦可入藥。又曰：老鴉眼睛草，生江湖間。葉如茄子葉，故名天茄子。或云，即漆姑草也。漆姑即蜀羊泉，已見本經草部。人亦不能决識之。【時珍曰】龍葵、龍珠，一類二種也，皆處處有之。四月生苗，嫩時可食，柔滑。漸高二三尺，莖大如筯，似燈籠草而無毛，葉似茄葉而小。五月以後，開小白花，五出黃蕊。結子正圓，大如五味子，上有小蒂，數顆同綴，其味酸。中有細子，亦如茄子之子。但生青熟黑者爲龍葵，生青熟赤者爲龍珠，功用亦相仿佛，不甚遼遠。蘇頌圖經菜部既註龍葵，復於外類重出老鴉眼睛草，蓋不知其即一物也。又謂老鴉眼睛是蜀羊泉，誤矣。蜀羊泉葉似菊，開紫花，子類枸杞，詳見草部本條。楊慎丹鉛録謂龍葵即吴葵，反指本草爲誤，引素問、千金四月吴葵華爲證，蓋不知千金方言吴葵即蜀葵，已自明白矣。今並正之。

Collected Explanations. [Tao] Hongjing: In Yi zhou is a "bitter vegetable," *ku cai* 苦菜; it is *ku shi* 苦蘵. [Su] Gong: *Ku shi* 苦蘵 is *long kui* 龍葵. It is commonly also called *ku cai* 苦菜; it is not *tu* 荼.[505] *Long kui* can be found everywhere. In the region of Guan and He it is called *ku cai* 苦菜. The leaves are round and the flowers are white. The seeds are similar to *niu li* 牛李, "ox plum," seeds. Fresh/raw they are greenish; heat prepared they are black. But they are still edible when boiled in water. They should not be eaten raw. [Su] Song: *Long kui* is not often encountered in nearby regions. It is present only in the North. The people call it *ku kui* 苦葵, "bitter mallow." The leaves are round; they resemble those of climbing nightshade, but they have no hair. The flowers are white. The seeds, too, resemble those of climbing nightshade. When they are fresh/raw they are greenish; when they are heat prepared they are black. When they are red, they are called "red pearls." They, too, can be added to medication. It is also said: *Lao ya yan jing cao* grows in the region of Jiang hu. The leaves are similar to eggplant leaves. Hence [the plant] is named "heaven's eggplant." It is also stated: This is seven-leaf nightshade, *qi gu cao* 漆姑草. *Qi gu* [*cao*] is *shu yang quan* 蜀羊泉; it was already listed in the section "herbs" of the *Ben jing*. People cannot tell which is which. [Li] Shizhen: *Long kui* 龍葵 and *long zhu* 龍珠, "dragon pearl," are two kinds belonging to one group. Both can be found everywhere. They grow a seedling in the fourth month. As long as it is tender, it is edible. It is soft and smooth. It gradually reaches a height of two or three *chi*. The stem has the size of chopsticks. It resembles that of Chinese lantern plants, but has no hair. The leaves resemble eggplant leaves, but are smaller. Beginning with the fifth month they open small, white flowers with five petals and yellow stamens. They form truly round seeds, the size of *schisandra* seeds. Above they have a small fruit base holding several kernels together. Their flavor is sour. Inside are fine seeds; they, too, resemble eggplant seeds. However, those that are greenish as long as they are fresh, and black when they are heat prepared, they are *long kui* 龍葵 [seeds], while those that are greenish as long as they are fresh and turn red when they are heat prepared, they are *long zhu* 龍珠 [seeds]. Their [therapeutic] potentials are quite similar; they are not very far apart from each other. Su Song in his *Tu jing* discusses *long kui* in the vegetables section. And among the [items categorized as] "outer group" he devotes a separate entry to *lao ya yan jing cao*. The fact is, he was

505 Possibly: *Sonchus oleraceus* L.; *Ixeris chinensis* (Thunb.) Nakai. Sow Thistle

not aware that they are one and the same item. It is also said that *lao ya yan jing* is seven-leaf nightshade. That is wrong. The leaves of seven-leaf nightshade resemble *chrysanthemum* [leaves], and it opens purple flowers. The seeds are similar to *lycium* [seeds]. For details, consult the respective entry in the section "herbs." (16-17) Yang Shen in his *Dan qian lu* says: "*Long kui* is *wu kui* 吳葵," pointing out that the *Ben cao* is wrong. He quotes passages from the *Su wen* and the *Qian jin* on *wu kui* of the fourth month as evidence. The fact is, he did not know that the *Qian jin fang* says that "*wu kui* 吳葵 is *shu kui* 蜀葵." So, that was clear enough already. Here, now, this is corrected.

16-14-01
苗 *Miao*
Seedling [of *long kui*].

【氣味】苦、微甘，滑，寒，無毒。

Qi and Flavor. Bitter, slightly sweet, smooth, cold, nonpoisonous.

【主治】食之解勞少睡，去虛熱腫。唐本。治風，補益男子元氣，婦人敗血。蘇頌。消熱散血，壓丹石毒宜食之。時珍。

Control. To eat it resolves exhaustion and drowsiness. It dispels depletion heat swelling. *Tang ben*. It serves to cure wind [intrusion]. It supplements and boosts a male's original qi, and a woman's decayed blood. Su Song. It dissolves heat and disperses blood [accumulations]. To press down the poison of elixir minerals it is advisable to eat it. [Li] Shizhen.

【附方】舊一。
Added Recipes. One of old.

去熱少睡。龍葵菜同米煮作羹粥食之。食醫心鏡。

To dispel heat and drowsiness. Boil *long kui* vegetables together with rice to prepare a congee and eat it. *Shi yi xin jing*.

16-14-02
莖、葉、根 *Jing, Ye, Gen.*
Stem, leaf, root [of *long kui*].

【氣味】同苗。

Qi and Flavor. Identical to those of the seedling.

【主治】擣爛和土傅丁腫火丹瘡，良。孟詵。瘰癧疽腫毒，跌撲傷損，消腫散血。時珍。根與木通、胡荽煎湯服，通利小便。蘇頌。

Control. Pounded into a pulpy [mass], mixed with soil, and applied to swelling associated with a pin[-illness][506] as well as fire cinnabar[507] sores, it yields good results. Meng Shen. It heals swelling with poison related to obstruction-illness and impediment-illness,[508] and harm and injuries caused by a blow or fall. It dissolves swelling and disperses blood [accumulations]. [Li] Shizhen. The root is boiled with *akebia* [herb] and coriander [seeds] to obtain a decoction. To ingest it frees the passage of urine. Su Song.

【附方】舊四，新八。

Added Recipes. Four of old. Eight newly [recorded].

通利小便。方見上。

To free the passage of urine. For the recipe, see above.

從高墜下欲死者。取老鴉眼睛草莖葉擣汁服，以渣傅患處。唐瑶經驗方。

A fall from a high position, bringing one close to death. Pound the stem and leaves of *lao ya yan jing cao* to obtain a juice and [let the patient] ingest it. Apply the dregs to the area harmed. *Tang Yao jing yan fang.*

火焰丹腫。老鴉眼睛草葉，入醋細研傅之，能消赤腫。蘇頌圖經本草。

Flaming cinnabar swelling.[509] Give *lao ya yan jing cao* leaves into vinegar, grind them to a fine [mass] and apply this [to the affected region]. This can dissolve the red swelling. Su Song, *Tu jing ben cao.*

---

506 *Ding* 丁, "pin[-illness]," also *ding* 疔, "pin-illness," refers to a deep-reaching and festering hardness in a tissue, eventually rising above the skin like a pinhead. BCGM Dict I, 127-129.

507 *Huo dan* 火丹, "fire cinnabar," a condition of *dan du* 丹毒, "cinnabar-red poison," displaying a color like fire that rushes through the skin, spreading with great speed. BCGM Dict I, 232.

508 *Yong ju* 癰疽, "obstruction-illness, impediment-illness." refers to two vaguely distinguished obstructions/impediments of vessels or other ducts inside the body. Qi rushing against the obstruction may cause a local swelling and eventually break through the surface to cause an abscess. BCGM Dict I, 642.

509 *Huo yan dan zhong* 火焰丹腫, "flaming cinnabar swelling," a condition of *dan du* 丹毒, "cinnabar red poison," starting from the head and generating a dark red complexion. BCGM Dict I, 235.

癰腫無頭。龍葵莖葉擣傅。經驗方。

Obstruction-illness[510] swelling without tip. Pound *long kui* stem and leaves [into a pulpy mass] and apply it [to the affected region]. *Jing yan fang*.

發背癰疽成瘡者。蘇頌圖經云：用龍葵一兩爲末，麝香一分，研勻塗之甚善。

Obstruction-illness and impediment-illness[511] effusing on the back and generating sores. Su Song in his *Tu jing* states: "[Grind] one *liang* of *long kui* into powder. Grind it together with one *fen* of musk to an even [mixture] and apply this [to the affected region]. Very good."

袖珍方云：一切發背癰疽惡瘡。用蝦蟆一個，同老鴉眼睛草莖葉搗爛，傅之即散。神效。

The *Xiu zhen fang* states: "For all types of obstruction-illness and impediment-illness effusing on the back and generating malign sores. Pound one small toad with seedlings and leaves of *lao ya yan jing cao* into a pulpy [mass]. Apply this [to the affected region] and [the sores] will disperse." Divinely effective.

諸瘡惡腫。老鴉眼睛草擂酒服，以渣傅之。普濟方。

All types of sores with a malign swelling. Pound *lao ya yan jing cao* in wine and ingest the [liquid]. Apply the dregs [to the affected region]. *Pu ji fang*.

丁腫毒瘡。黑色焮腫者，乃服丹石毒也；赤色者，肉麪毒也。用龍葵根一握洗切，乳香末、黄連各三兩，杏仁六十枚。和搗作餅，厚如三錢，依瘡大小傅之，覺痒即換去。痒不可忍，切勿搔動。候炊久，瘡中似石榴子戢戢然，乃去藥。時時以甘草湯温洗，洗後以蠟貼之。終身不得食羊血。如無龍葵，以蔓菁根代之。聖濟總録。

Pin[-illness][512] swelling sores with poison. If they are black with a boiling hot swelling, it is a result of ingesting elixir mineral poison. If they are red, it is the poison of meat and pasta. Wash a handful of *long kui* root and cut it into pieces. Pound them together with three *liang* each of frankincense powder and *coptis* [rhizome], and

---

510 *Yong* 癰, "obstruction-illness," refers to an obstruction of vessels or other ducts inside the body. Qi rushing against the obstruction may cause a local swelling and eventually break through the surface to cause an abscess. BCGM Dict I, 641.

511 *Yong ju* 癰疽, "obstruction-illness, impediment-illness." refers to two vaguely distinguished obstructions/impediments of vessels or other ducts inside the body. Qi rushing against the obstruction may cause a local swelling and eventually break through the surface to cause an abscess. BCGM Dict I, 642.

512 *Ding* 丁, "pin[-illness]," also *ding* 疔, "pin-illness," refers to a deep-reaching and festering hardness in a tissue, eventually rising above the skin like a pinhead. BCGM Dict I, 127-129.

60 bitter apricot seeds into a pulpy [mass] and form a cake about as thick as three coins. Apply this exactly corresponding to the size of the sores. Once [the patient] feels an itch, replace it. Even if the itch is unbearable, do not scratch! Wait for as long as it takes to cook a meal and something like pomegranate seeds accumulates in the sores. Then remove the medication and again and again wash [the sores] with a warm *glycyrrhiza* [root] decoction. After washing them paste beeswax onto them. [Patients] must not consume sheep blood again for their entire life. If no *long kui* is available, simpleleaf chastetree root may be used instead. *Sheng ji zong lu.*

天泡濕瘡。龍葵苗葉搗傅之。

Celestial blister sores[513] with moisture. Pound *long kui* seedlings and leaves [into a pulpy mass] and apply it [to the affected region].

吐血不止。天茄子苗半兩，人參二錢半，爲末。每服二錢，新汲水下。聖濟總録。

Unending vomiting of blood. [Grind] half a *liang* of *tian qie zi* seedlings and two and a half *qian* of ginseng [root] into powder. Each time ingest two *qian*, to be sent down with newly drawn water. *Sheng ji zong lu.*

辟除蚤虱。天茄葉鋪於席下，次日盡死。

To repel lice and fleas. Spread *tian qie* leaves under the [sleeping] mat. The next day they are all dead.

多年惡瘡。天茄葉貼之，或爲末貼。救急良方。

Malign sores of many years. Paste *tian qie* leaves onto them, or [grind them into] powder and apply it [to the affected region]. *Jiu ji liang fang.*

産後腸出不收。老鴉酸漿草一把，水煎，先熏後洗，收乃止。救急方。

Following delivery the [birth] intestine remains outside and is not drawn in again. Boil a handful of *lao ya suan jiang cao* in water. Use it first to steam [the affected region] and then to wash it. End [the treatment] once the [intestine] is drawn in again. *Jiu ji fang.*

16-14-03

子 *Zi*

Seeds [of *long kui*].

七月采之。

Collect them in the seventh month.

---

513 *Tian pao chuang* 天泡瘡, "celestial blister sores," a condition of sores with the appearance of blisters filled with water or pus, especially in children. BCGM Dict I, 503.

【主治】丁腫。唐本。明目輕身甚良。甄權。治風，益男子元氣，婦人敗血。蘇頌。

Control. Pin[-illness][514] swelling. *Tang ben*. They clear the eyes and relieve the body of its weight. Very good. Zhen Quan. They serve to cure wind [intrusion]. They boost the original qi of males and decayed blood of women. Su Song.

16-15
龍珠拾遺
Long zhu. FE *Shi yi*.

Tubocapsicum anomalum (Franch. et Sav.) Makino. Japanese wild pepper.[515]

【釋名】赤珠。【頌曰】龍葵子赤者名赤珠，象形也。

Explanation of Names. *Chi zhu* 赤珠, "red pearl[s]." [Su] Song: Red *long kui* seeds, too, are named *chi zhu* 赤珠. A reference to their physical appearance.

【集解】【甄權曰】龍葵赤珠者名龍珠，挼去汁可食，能變白令黑。【藏器曰】龍珠生道旁，子圓似龍葵，但熟時正赤耳。【時珍曰】龍珠、龍葵，雖以子之黑赤分別，其實一物二色，强分爲二也。

Collected Explanations. Zhen Quan: The red pearls, *chi zhu* 赤珠, of common nightshade, *long kui* 龍葵, are called *long zhu* 龍珠, "dragon pearls." Rub them to remove their juice, and then they are edible. They can turn white [hair] into black [hair again]. [Chen] Cangqi: *Long zhu* grows at the roadside. The seeds are round, resembling those of common nightshade, *long kui* 龍葵, except for that they are properly red when they are ripe. [Li] Shizhen: *Long zhu* and *long kui* differ in that their seeds are black and red, respectively. But in fact they are one identical item with two colors. They are arbitrarily separated as two items.

16-15-01
苗 *Miao*
Seedling [of *long zhu*].

【氣味】苦，寒，無毒。

Qi and Flavor. Bitter, cold, nonpoisonous.

514 *Ding* 丁, "pin[-illness]," also *ding* 疔, "pin-illness," refers to a deep-reaching and festering hardness in a tissue, eventually rising above the skin like a pinhead. BCGM Dict I, 127-129.

515 *Long zhu* 龍珠, lit.: "dragon pearl[s]."

【主治】能變白髮，令人不睡。主諸熱毒，石氣發動，調中解煩。藏器。

Control. It can turn white [hair] into black [hair]. It keeps one awake. It controls all types of heat poison, and excitement caused by the qi of mineral [drugs]. It regulates the center and resolves vexation. [Chen] Cangqi.

【發明】【權曰】龍珠，服之變白令黑，耐老。若能生食得苦者，不食他菜，十日後即有靈異也。不與葱、薤同噉，根亦入藥用。

Explication. [Zhen] Quan: To ingest *long zhu* turns white [hair] into black [hair] and lets one endure aging. If one is able to eat raw [*long zhu* seedlings] with their bitter [flavor], and does not eat any other vegetable, after ten days this results in a magic difference. Do not consume [the seedlings] with onions or Chinese chives. The root is also added to medication for [therapeutic] applications.

16-15-02

子 ***Zi***

[*Long zhu*] seeds.

【氣味】同菜。

Qi and Flavor. Identical to the herb/vegetable.

【主治】丁腫。藏器。

Control. Pin[-illness][516] swelling. [Chen] Cangqi.

16-16

酸漿本經中品

Suan jiang. FE *Ben jing*, middle rank.

***Physalis alkekengi* L. var. *franchetii* (Mast.) Makino. Chinese lantern plant.**

【校正】菜部苦耽，草部酸漿、燈籠草，俱併爲一。

Editorial Correction. *Ku dan* 苦耽 from the "vegetable" section, *suan jiang* 酸漿 and *deng long cao* 燈籠草, both from the "herb" section, are integrated here.

【釋名】醋漿本經、苦葴音針、苦耽嘉祐、燈籠草唐本、皮弁草食療、天泡草綱目、王母珠嘉祐、洛神珠同上。小者名苦蘵。【藏器曰】爾雅云：葴，寒漿也。郭璞注云：即今酸漿，江東人呼爲苦葴。小者爲苦蘵，亦呼爲小苦耽。崔豹古今注云：蘵，一名蘵子，實形如皮弁，其子圓如珠。【時珍曰】酸漿，以子之味名也。苦葴、苦耽，以苗之味名也。燈籠、皮弁，以角之形名也。王母、洛神珠，以子之形名也。按楊慎卮言云：本草

516 *Ding* 丁, "pin[-illness]," also *ding* 疔, "pin-illness," refers to a deep-reaching and festering hardness in a tissue, eventually rising above the skin like a pinhead. BCGM Dict I, 127-129.

燈籠草、苦耽、酸漿，皆一物也。修本草者非一時一人，故重複耳。燕京野果名紅姑孃，外垂絳囊，中含赤子如珠，酸甘可食，盈盈邊砌，與翠草同芳，亦自可愛。蓋姑孃乃瓜囊之訛，古者瓜、姑同音，孃、囊之音亦相近耳。此説得之，故今以本經酸漿、唐本草燈籠草、宋嘉祐本草苦耽，俱併爲一焉。

Explanation of Names. *Cui jiang* 醋漿, "sour *jiang*," *Ben jing*. *Ku zhen* 苦葴, read *zhen* 針; *ku dan* 苦耽, "indulged in sour flavor," *Jia you*. *Deng long cao* 燈籠草, "lantern herb," *Tang ben*. *Pi bian cao* 皮弁草, "leather cap herb," *Shi liao*. *Tian pao cao* 天泡草, "celestial blister herb," *Gang mu*. *Wang mu zhu* 王母珠,"Queen mother pearl[s]," *Jia you*. *Luo shen zhu* 洛神珠, "fallen divine pearl[s]," [source] identical to the one above. Small ones are called *ku zhi* 苦蘵. [Chen] Cangqi: The *Er ya* states: "*Zhen* 葴 is *han jiang* 寒漿." Guo Pu comments: "This is today's *suan jiang* 酸漿. People in Jiang dong call it *ku zhen* 苦葴. Small ones are *ku zhi* 苦蘵. They are also called 'small *ku dan*,' *xiao ku dan* 小苦耽." Cui Bao in his *Gu jin zhu* states: "*Zhi* 蘵 is also called *zhi zi* 蘵子. The fruit have the physical appearance of a leather cap. The seeds are round like pearls." [Li] Shizhen: The name *suan jiang* 酸漿, "sour *jiang*," refers to the flavor of the seeds. *Ku zhen* 苦葴, "bitter *zhen*," and *ku dan* 苦耽, "bitter *dan*," are names referring to the flavor of the seedling. *Deng long* 燈籠, "lantern," and *pi bian* 皮弁, "leather cap," refer to the shape of the pods. *Wang mu* 王母, "queen mother," and "fallen divine pearls," *luo shen zhu* 洛神珠, are names based on the shape of the seeds. According to Yang Shen's *Zhi yan*, "The *deng long cao* 燈籠草, *ku dan* 苦耽 and *suan jiang* 酸漿, listed in the *Ben cao*, are one and the same item." Revisions of the *Ben cao* were carried out at different times and by numerous persons. Hence such multiple listings. In Yan jing is a wild fruit called *hong gu niang* 紅姑孃, "red aunt." It hangs outside [of the herb] like a deep-red pouch with red seeds inside, similar to pearls. It is sour-sweet and edible. It grows profusely and is as fragrant as *cui cao* 翠草. It is lovely. The fact is, *gu niang* 姑孃 is an erroneous reading of *gua nang* 瓜囊. In ancient times, *gua* 瓜 and *gu* 姑 were read identically. The readings of *niang* 孃 and *nang* 囊 are very close. Based on this understanding, the *suan jiang* 酸漿 of the *Ben jing*, the *deng long cao* 燈籠草 of the *Tang ben cao* and the *ku dan* 苦耽 of the Song era *Jia you ben cao* are listed here together.

【集解】【别録曰】酸漿生荆楚川澤及人家田園中，五月采，陰乾。【弘景曰】酸漿處處多有，苗似水茄而小，葉亦可食。子作房，房中有子如梅、李大，皆黄赤色，小兒食之。【保昇曰】酸漿即苦葴也，根如菹芹，白色絶苦。【禹錫曰】苦耽生故墟垣塹間，高二三尺，子作角，如撮口袋，中有子如珠，熟則赤色。關中人謂之洛神珠，一名王母珠，一名皮弁草。一種小者名苦蘵。爾雅謂之黄蒢。【恭曰】燈籠草所在有之。枝榦高三四尺，有紅花，狀若燈籠，內有紅子可愛，根、莖、花、實並入藥用。【宗奭曰】酸漿即苦耽也，嘉祐重出苦耽條。天下有之，苗如天茄子，開小白花，結青殼，熟則深紅，殼中子大如櫻，亦紅色，櫻中復有細子，如落蘇之子，食之有青草氣也。【時珍曰】龍葵、酸漿，一類二種也。酸漿、苦蘵一種二物也。但大者爲酸漿，小者爲苦蘵，以此爲別。敗醬亦名苦蘵，與此不同。其龍葵、酸漿苗葉一樣，但龍葵莖光無毛，五月入秋開小白花，五出黃蕊，結子無殼，纍纍數顆同枝，子有蒂蓋，生青熟紫黑。其酸漿同時開小花黃白色，紫心白蕊，其花如盃狀，無瓣，但有五尖，結一鈴殼，凡五稜，一枝一顆，下懸如燈籠之狀，殼中一子，狀如龍葵子，生青熟赤。以此分別，便自明白。按庚辛玉册云：燈籠草四方皆有，惟川、陝者最大。葉似龍葵，嫩時可食。四五月開花結實，有四葉盛之如燈籠，河北呼爲酸漿。據此及楊慎之說，則燈籠、酸漿之爲一物，尤可證矣。唐慎微以三葉酸草附於酸漿之後，蓋不知其名同物異也。其草見草之八酢漿下。

Collected Explanations. *Bie lu*: *Suan jiang* grows in the river marshlands of Jing chu and in private gardens. It is collected in the fifth month and dried in the yin (i. e., shade). [Tao] Hongjing: *Suan jiang* can be found everywhere. The seedlings resemble those of common nightshade, but are smaller. The leaves, too, are edible. The leaves form capsules. Within the capsules are seeds as big as dark plums and *prunus* plums, all of them of black-red color. Children eat them. [Han] Baosheng: *Suan jiang* is *ku zhen* 苦葴. The root is similar to *ju qin* 菹芹.[517] It is white and extremely bitter. [Zhang] Yuxi: *Ku dan* grows on the walls and in moats of old ruins. It is two to three *chi* tall. The seeds form "horn"[-like capsules], similar to a handbag. Inside are the seeds; they look like pearls. When they are prepared with heat, they assume a red color. People in Guan zhong call the [plant] "fallen divine pearls." Other names are "Queen Mother pearls" and "leather cap herb." A smaller kind is called *ku zhi* 苦蘵. The *Er ya* calls it *huang chu* 黄蒢. [Su] Gong: *Deng long cao* can be found everywhere. The stem with its twigs reaches a height of three to four *chi*. It has red flowers; they are shaped like a lantern. Inside are amiable red seeds. The root, the stem, the flower and the fruit, they all are added to medication for [therapeutic] applications. [Kou] Zongshi: *Suan jiang* is *ku dan* 苦耽. The *Jia you* has a separate *ku dan* 苦耽 entry. It is present all over the country. The seedling is similar to that of common nightshade. It opens small, white flowers. They form greenish [fruit] shells that assume a deep red color when they are prepared with heat. The seeds inside the shells are as big as cherries, and they, too, are red. Inside these cherries are fine seeds again, resembling the seeds of eggplants. When they are eaten, they [effuse] the qi of greenish herbs/grass. [Li] Shizhen: Common nightshade and *suan jiang*

517 Unidentified herb.

are two kinds of one group. *Suan jiang* and *ku zhi* 苦蘵 are two items of one kind. However, large specimens are *suan jiang*; small ones are *ku zhi* 苦蘵. This is how they are distinguished. *Bai jiang* 敗醬, dahurian *patrinia*, is also called *ku zhi* 苦蘵, but it is something different. The stem and leaves of common nightshade and *suan jiang* are identical, with the only [difference] that the stem of common nightshade is shiny and has no hair. In the fifth month, and into autumn, it opens small, white flowers, with five petals and yellow stamens. They form seeds without a shell. Numerous [such seeds] are lined up on one twig. The seeds have a base and a cover. Fresh ones are greenish; prepared with heat they are purple-black. *Suan jiang* opens small flowers of yellow-white color at the same time, with a purple heart and white stamens. The flowers are shaped like a cup; they have no petals. But [these cups] have five pointed tips forming a bell-shaped shell. Each of them has five edges, with one fruit hanging from one twig like a lantern. Inside the shell is one seed, shaped like common nightshade seeds. They are greenish as long as they are fresh; they turn red when they are prepared with heat. This is how they are distinguished. It should be quite clear now. According to the *Geng xin yu ce*, *deng long cao* can be found in all cardinal directions, with most of them present in Chuan and Shaan. The leaves are similar to those of common nightshade; they are edible as long as they are tender. [*Deng long cao*] opens flowers and forms fruit in the fourth and fifth month. The four leaves holding them look like a lantern. In He bei [*deng long cao*] is called *suan jiang*. Based on this and on the record of Yang Shen, *deng long* and *suan jiang* are one and the same item. The evidence is overwhelming. Tang Shenwei added [an entry of] "three leaf *suan cao*", *san ye suan cao* 三葉酸草, to the *suan jiang* [entry]. The fact is, he did not know that these are different items with the same name. For this herb [*san ye suan cao* 三葉酸草] see under the eighth [entry][518] of herbs, *cu jiang* 酢漿 (20-12).

16-16-01

苗、葉、莖、根 *Miao, Ye, Jing, Gen*

Seedling, leaf, stem, root [of *suan jiang*].

【氣味】苦，寒，無毒。【禹錫曰】有小毒。【恭曰】苦，大寒，無毒。【時珍曰】方士取汁煮丹砂，伏白礬，煮三黃，煉硝、硫。

Qi and Flavor. Bitter, cold, nonpoisonous. [Zhang] Yuxi: Slightly poisonous. [Su] Gong: Bitter, very cold, nonpoisonous. [Li] Shizhen: The [longevity] recipe experts take the juice to boil cinnabar. It oppresses [the effects of] alum. It is boiled with

518 Instead of *ba* 八, "eighth entry," this should be *jiu* 九, "ninth entry." See ch. 20, where *cu jiang cao* 酢漿草 is listed in the ninth entry.

the three [items named "yellow",] *huang* 黃.[519] It is used to process mirabilite and sulphur.

【主治】酸漿：治熱煩滿，定志益氣，利水道。本經。搗汁服，治黃病，多效。弘景。燈籠草：治上氣欬嗽，風熱，明目，根莖花實並宜。唐本。苦耽苗子：治傳尸伏連，鬼氣疰忤邪氣，腹內熱結，目黃不下食，大小便澀，骨熱欬嗽，多睡勞乏，嘔逆痰壅，痃癖痞滿，小兒無辜，癧子，寒熱，大腹，殺蟲，落胎，去蠱毒，並煮汁飲，亦生擣汁服。研膏，傅小兒閃癖。嘉祐。

Control. *Suan jiang*: It serves to cure heat, vexation and a [feeling of] fullness. It stabilizes the mind and boosts the qi. It frees the passage through the water pathways. *Ben jing*. Pounded and the juice ingested, it serves to cure jaundice disease, and is often effective. [Tao] Hongjing. *Deng long cao*: It serves to cure rising qi with cough. Wind [intrusion] with heat. It clears the eyes. The root, the stem, the flower and the fruits are all suitable. *Tang ben*. *Ku dan* seedling and seeds: They serve to cure corpse [evil] transmission,[520] [that is,] hidden link.[521] Demon qi attachment-illness and hostile, evil qi, with heat nodes in the abdomen, yellow eyes and an inability to eat. Major (defecation) and minor (urination) relief is rough. The bones are hot. Cough. Sleepiness and fatigue. Vomiting with [qi] counterflow; phlegm obstruction. String-illness,[522] aggregation-illness,[523] obstacle-illness[524] and a feeling of fullness. Innocence [illness][525] of children. Pervasion [illness] seeds.[526] [Alternating sensations of] cold and heat. Abdominal bloating. They kill worms/bugs. They

519 The three [items named "yellow",] *huang* 黃, are sulphur, *liu huang* 硫黃, realgar, *xiong huang* 雄黃, and orpiment, *ci huang* 雌黃.

520 *Chuan shi* 傳屍, "corpse [evil] transmission," a condition of an infectious consumptive disease. BCGM Dict I, 97.

521 *Fu lian* 伏連, "hidden link," identical to *chuan shi* 傳屍, "corpse [evil] transmission." BCGM Dict I, 175.

522 *Xuan* 痃, "string-illness," a condition of acute pain located in the abdomen to the left and right of the umbilicus. BCGM Dict I, 591.

523 *Pi* 癖, "aggregation-illness," of painful lumps emerging from time to time in both flanks. BCGM Dict I, 371.

524 *Pi* 痞, "obstacle-illness." 1.) An illness sign of a feeling of uncomfortable fullness and distension. 2). A condition of an uncomfortable distension and fullness in the chest and abdominal region. When pressed there is no pain. BCGM Dict I, 371.

525 *Wu gu* 無辜, "innocence," a type of *gan*-illness accompanied by scrofula affecting the head and neck. BCGM Dict I, 537.

526 *Li zi* 癧子, "pervasion-illness seeds," identical to *luo li* 瘰癧, "scrofula pervasion-illness," a condition whereby two or three connected swellings of the size of plum or date kernels appear either on the neck or in the armpits, or somewhere else in the body. BCGM Dict I, 316, 329.

cause abortion. They eliminate *gu* poison.[527] For all these [ailments first] boil and then pound them to obtain a juice and [let the patient] ingest it. It is also possible to pound them fresh/raw to obtain a juice and ingest it. Ground to a paste it is applied to sprain with aggregation-illness of children.[528] *Jia you.*

【發明】【震亨曰】燈籠草，苦能除濕熱，輕能治上焦，故主熱欬咽痛。此草治熱痰欬嗽，佛耳草治寒痰欬嗽也。與片芩、清金丸同用，更效。【時珍曰】酸漿利濕除熱。除熱故清肺治咳，利濕故能化痰治疸。一人病虛乏咳嗽有痰，愚以此加入湯中用之，有效。

Explication. [Zhu] Zhenheng: *Deng long cao* is bitter and this enables it to eliminate moisture and heat. It is light and this enable it to cure [ailments affecting the] Upper Burner. Therefore it controls heat and cough with a painful throat. This herb serves to cure heat and phlegm with cough. Cudweed serves to cure cold and phlegm with cough. If used together with the "pills with *pian qin* to cool the metal (i. e., lung],"[529] it is even more effective. [Li] Shizhen: *Suan jiang* frees the passage of moisture and eliminates heat. As it removes heat, it cools the [lung, associated with the phase] metal and serves to cure cough. As it frees the passage of moisture, it serves to transform phlegm and to cure impediment-illness. Once someone had a depletion exhaustion, with cough and phlegm. I added this [herb] to a decoction and used it [to treat him]. It was effective.

【附方】新三。

Added Recipes. Three newly [recorded].

熱欬咽痛。燈籠草爲末，白湯服，名清心丸。仍以醋調傅喉外。丹溪纂要。

Heat, cough, and a painful throat. [Grind] *deng long cao* into powder and ingest it with clear, boiled water. This [medication] is called "pills to cool the heart." In addition mix [the powder] with vinegar and apply it to the throat from outside. *Danxi suan yao.*

---

527 *Gu du* 蠱毒, "*gu*-poison[ing]." (1) A poison emitted by certain worms/snakes with an ability to cause varying pathological changes in a person who has taken it in by means of wine or food. (2) Abdominal fullness, in some cases with blood spitting, and blood in the stool and urine. BCGM Dict I, 192 - 193. See BCGM 42-22.

528 *Shan pi* 閃癖, "sprain with aggregation-illness," a condition of children with swelling below the flanks, loss of appetite, no digestion, yellow complexion, emaciation and desiccation of the hair. This is often accompanied by bone steaming, scrofula, and pervasion-illness. BCGM Dict I, 419.

529 Details of this recipe are unknown.

喉瘡作痛。燈籠草炒焦研末，酒調呷之。醫學正傳。

Painful throat sore. Fry *deng long cao* until it is scorched and grind it into powder. Mix it with wine and sip this. *Yi xue zheng chuan.*

灸瘡不發。酸漿葉貼之。

Sores resulting from cauterization/moxibustion that fail to release [their contents]. Attach *suan jiang* leaves to them.

16-16-02
子 *Zi*
Seeds [of *suan jiang*].

【氣味】酸，平，無毒。【别録曰】寒。

Qi and Flavor. Sour, balanced, nonpoisonous. *Bie lu*: Cold.

【主治】熱煩，定志益氣，利水道。産難，吞之立産。别録。食之除熱，治黄病，尤益小兒。蘇頌。治骨蒸勞熱，尸疰疳瘦，痰癖熱結，與苗莖同功。嘉祐。

Control. Heat and vexation. They stabilize the mind and boost the qi. They free the passage through the water pathways. In the case of difficult delivery, swallow them and the birth will follow immediately. *Bie lu.* To eat them dispels heat. They serve to cure jaundice diseases. They are especially suitable for children. Su Song. They serve to cure bone steaming[530] and exhaustion heat, corpse [qi] attachment illness,[531] and *gan*-illness with emaciation.[532] Phlegm aggregation-illness[533] and heat nodes. The [therapeutic] potential is identical to that of seedling and stem. *Jia you.*

530 *Gu zheng* 骨蒸, "bone steaming," 1.) a condition of an infectious consumptive disease with a development of vexing heat in the afternoon. 2.) An illness sign of heat and vexation with a feeling as if this originated in the bones. BCGM Dict I, 197.

531 *Shi zhu* 尸疰, "corpse [qi] attachment-illness," a condition of a slowly developing infectious weakness. BCGM Dict I, 202.

532 *Gan* 疳, *gan*-illness; sweets-illness. Also: *gan shou* 疳瘦, "*gan*-illness with emaciation." A condition of a chronic malnutrition disease resulting from various causes that harm the spleen and stomach and disturb their functions. The major sign is physical depletion, weakness, and emaciation. It may assume numerous different manifestations, each of which has a specific designation. Until the Tang, this was generally considered a disease affecting adults and children alike. Beginning with the Song, this gradually developed into a disease diagnosed in children only. BCGM Dict I, 180.

533 *Tan pi* 痰癖, "phlegm aggregation-illness," a condition of *pi* 癖, "aggregation-illness," a disease brought forth by stagnant phlegm rheum. BCGM Dict 495.

【附方】新二。
Added Recipes. Two newly [recorded].

酸漿實丸。治三焦腸胃伏熱，婦人胎熱難産。用酸漿實五兩，莧實三兩，馬藺子炒、大鹽、榆白皮炒各二兩，柴胡、黄芩、栝樓根、蔄茹各一兩，爲末。煉蜜丸梧子大。每服三十丸，木香湯下。聖濟總録。

The "pills with *suan jiang* fruit." They serve to cure hidden heat in the Triple Burner, the intestines and the stomach, as well as fetal heat[534] and difficult delivery of women. Use [the following items]. Five *liang* of *suang jiang* fruit. Three *liang* of *amaranth* fruit. Three *liang* of Chinese iris seeds. Two *liang* each of large salt chunks and Siberian elm bark, fried. One *liang* each of *bupleurum* [root], *scutellaria* [root], *trichosanthes* [root] and spurge. [Grind them into] powder and form with heat prepared honey pills the size of *wu* seeds. Each time ingest 30 pills, to be sent down with costus [root] decoction. *Sheng ji zong lu.*

天泡濕瘡。天泡草鈴兒生搗敷之。亦可爲末，油調敷。鄧才雜興方。

Celestial blister sores[535] with moisture. Pound *tian pao cao* bells [into a pulpy mass] and apply it [to the affected region]. It is also possible to [grind them into] powder and apply them mixed with oil [to the affected region]. Deng Cai, *Za xing fang.*

16-17
蜀羊泉本經中品

Shu yang quan, FE *Ben jing*, middle rank.

***Solanum septenlobum* Bunge. Seven-leaf nightshade.**

【釋名】羊泉别録、羊飴别録、漆姑草。【時珍曰】諸名莫解。能治漆瘡，故曰漆姑。

Explanation of Names. *Yang quan* 羊泉, *Bie lu. Yang yi* 羊飴, *Bie lu. Qi gu cao* 漆姑草. [Li] Shizhen: All these names have no explanation. It can cure sores caused by lacquer, *qi* 漆. Hence it is called *qi gu* 漆姑, "lacquer aunt."

【集解】【别録曰】蜀羊泉生蜀郡川谷。【弘景曰】方不復用，人無識者。【恭曰】此草俗名漆姑，葉似菊，花紫色，子類枸杞子，根如遠志，無心有糝。所在平澤有之，生陰濕地，三月、四月采苗葉，陰乾。【藏器

534 *Tai re* 胎熱, "fetal heat," referring to a) a situation where a pregnant woman has been affected by heat that was able to enter the womb, and b) a disease brought forth in children by wind evil that has entered their mother's womb during her pregnancy, with the heat poison abiding in the child's depots and palaces after delivery. BCGM Dict 487.

535 *Tian pao chuang* 天泡瘡, "celestial blister sores," a condition of sores with the appearance of blisters filled with water or pus, especially in children. BCGM Dict I, 503.

曰】陶註杉材云：漆姑葉細細，多生石邊，能療漆瘡。蘇云漆姑是羊泉。按羊泉乃大草，漆姑草如鼠跡大，生堦墀間陰處，氣辛烈，挼付漆瘡，亦主溪毒，乃同名也。【頌曰】或言老鴉眼睛草即漆姑草，漆姑乃蜀羊泉，人不能决識。【時珍曰】漆姑有二種。蘇恭所說是羊泉，陶、陳所說是小草。蘇頌所說老鴉眼睛草，乃龍葵也。又黄蜂作窠，銜漆姑草汁爲蒂，即此草也。

Collected Explanations. *Bie lu*: *Shu yang quan* grows in river valles of Shu prefecture. [Tao] Hongjing: In recipes it is no longer used. And people do not know of it. [Su] Gong: This herb is colloquially called *qi gu* 漆姑. The leaves resemble those of *chrysanthemum*. The flowers are purple. The seeds resemble *lycium* seeds. The root is similar to *polygala* root. It has no heart/core but a powder. It can be found everywhere in marshlands of the plains. It grows on yin/shady, moist ground. The seedling and the leaves are collected in the third, fourth month. They are dried in the yin (i. e., shade). [Chen] Cangqi: In his comments on Chinese cedar wood, Tao [Hongjing] states: "*Qi gu* leaves are very fine. They often grow among rocks and can heal sores caused by lacquer." Su [Gong] states: "*Qi gu* is *yang quan*." Now, *yang quan* is a big herb, while *qi gu* herb has the size of footprints left by a mouse/rat. It grows on staircases in the courtyard, at yin/shady places. Its qi are violently acrid. Rub it with the hands and attach it to sores caused by lacquer. It also controls rivulet poison.[536] [Both items] have the same name. [Su] Song: Some say common nightshade is *qi gu cao* 漆姑草. *Qi gu* is *shu yang quan*. People do not know how to distinguish them. [Li] Shizhen: There are two kinds of *qi gu*. The one mentioned by Su Gong is *yang quan*. The one mentioned by Tao [Hongjing] and Chen [Cangqi] is a small herb. The *lao ya yan jing cao* 老鴉眼睛草 spoken of by Su Song is common nightshade. Also, when yellow bees form their nests they hold *qi gu cao* juice in their mouth to prepare a base. This is the herb [discussed] here.

【氣味】苦，微寒，無毒。

Qi and Flavor. Bitter, slightly cold, nonpoisonous.

【主治】秃瘡，惡瘡熱氣，疥瘙痂癬蟲。本經。療齲齒，女子陰中内傷，皮間實積。别録。主小兒驚，生毛髮，搗塗漆瘡。蘇恭。蚯蚓氣呵者，擣爛入黄丹盦之。時珍。出摘玄方。

536 *Xi du* 溪毒, "rivulet poison," 1.) A tiny bug assumed to live in bodies of water and supposedly capable of striking humans when they enter the water, thereby causing disease. 2.) A condition resulting from being struck by rivulet poison. BCGM Dict I, 548.

Control. Baldness sores. Malign sores. Heat qi. *Jie*-illness[537] with itch. Crusts with *xuan*-illness[538] and worms/bugs. It heals decayed teeth, harm in the yin [(i. e., genital) region] of females and solid accumulations in the skin. *Bie lu*. It controls fright of children and stimulates the growth of hair. Pound [it and] apply [the pulp] to sores caused by lacquer. Su Gong. In the case of [sores resulting from] an exposure to the breath of earthworms pound it into a pulpy mass, add minium and apply it [to the affected region]. Quoted from the *Zhai xuan fang*.

【附方】新。

Added Recipes. [One] newly [recorded].

黃疸疾。漆草一把，搗汁和酒服。不過三五次，即愈。摘玄方。

Jaundice illness. Pound a handful of *qi gu* to obtain a juice and ingest it mixed with wine. After [ingesting this] no more than three to five times a cure is achieved. *Zhai xuan fang*.

16-18

鹿蹄草綱目

Lu ti cao, FE *Gang mu.*

***Pyrola decorata* H. Andr. Deer hoof herb.**

【釋名】小秦王草綱目、秦王試劍草。【時珍曰】鹿蹄象葉形。能合金瘡，故名試劍草。又山慈姑亦名鹿蹄，與此不同。

Explanation of Names. *Xiao qin wang cao* 小秦王草, "small King of Qin's herb," *Gang mu*. *Qin wang shi jian cao* 秦王試劍草, "King of Qin's herb tried on [the wounds caused by] a sword." [Li] Shizhen: The hoofs of deer are shaped like leaves. They are able to close wounds caused by metal objects/weapons. Hence the name "herb tried on [wounds caused by] a sword," *shi jian cao* 試劍草. Also, edible tulips, too, are called *lu ti* 鹿蹄, but they are a different [item].

【集解】【時珍曰】按軒轅述寶藏論云：鹿蹄多生江廣平陸及寺院荒處，淮北絶少，川、陝亦有。苗似堇菜而葉頗大，背紫色。春生紫花。結青實如天茄子。可制雌黃、丹砂。

537 *Jie*-illness 疥, vaguely identifiable skin ailment. BCGM Dict I, 249.

538 *Xuan* 癬, "*xuan*-illness," a condition a) of dermal lesions with initially erythema, papules, and itching gradually extending in all directions to form an irregular ring with clear boundaries. The skin is slightly elevated with small papules, blisters, and/or scales and scraps. The central lesion may appear to heal spontaneously, and it may reappear. b) Designation of local lesions with itching, release of liquid and shedding of scabs. BCGM Dict I, 591.

Collected Explanations. [Li] Shizhen: According to Xuanyuan Shu's *Bao zang lun*, "*Lu ti* grows in large quantities on the plains of Jiang guang and also in deserted temple courtyards. There are very few in Huai bei. It can be found in Chuan and Shaan, too. The seedling resembles that of Chinese celery, but it has much larger leaves. Their back is purple. [*Lu ti*] grows purple flowers in spring. They form fruits similar to those of common nightshade. It checks [the effects of] orpiment and cinnabar."

【氣味】缺。

Qi and Flavor. Missing.

【主治】金瘡出血，擣塗即止。又塗一切蛇蟲犬咬毒。時珍。

Control. Bleeding wounds caused by metal objects/weapons. Pound it, attach it [to the wounds, and the bleeding] ends. Also, apply it to any poison related to the bites of snakes, worms/bugs and dogs. [Li] Shizhen.

16-19
敗醬本經中品

Bai jiang, FE *Ben jing*, middle rank.

***Patrinia scabiosaefolia* Fisch. exTrev.; *P. villosa*. Dahurian *patrinia*.**

【釋名】苦菜綱目、苦蘵綱目、澤敗別録、鹿腸本經、鹿首別録、馬草別録。【弘景曰】根作陳敗豆醬氣，故以爲名。【時珍曰】南人采嫩者暴蒸作菜食，味微苦而有陳醬氣，故又名苦菜，與苦蕒、龍葵同名。亦名苦蘵，與酸醬[539]同名，苗形則不同也。

Explanation of Names. *Ku cai* 苦菜, "bitter vegetable," *Gang mu*. *Ku zhi* 苦蘵, *Gang mu*. *Ze bai* 澤敗, *Bie lu*. *Lu chang* 鹿腸, "deer's intestine," *Ben jing*. *Lu shou* 鹿首, "deer head," *Bie lu*. *Ma cao* 馬草, "horse herb," *Bie lu*. [Tao] Hongjing: The root has qi [smelling like] long-stored rotten soybean sauce, *chen bai dou jiang* 陳敗豆醬. Hence its name *bai jiang* 敗醬, "rotten sauce." [Li] Shizhen: The southerners collect the tender [herb], steam it and eat it prepared as a vegetable. The flavor is slightly bitter and has the qi of long-stored [soybean] sauce. Hence it is also called "bitter vegetable," a name it shares with *sow thistle* [herb] and common nightshade. It is also named *ku zhi* 苦蘵; a name it shares with Chinese lantern plant. Their seedling and physical appearance differ.

【集解】【別録曰】敗醬生江夏川谷，八月采根，暴乾。【弘景曰】出近道。葉似狶薟，根形如柴胡。【恭曰】此藥不出近道，多生岡嶺間。葉似

539 Given the wording of 酸漿、苦蘵一種二物也 further up, the present character *jiang* 醬 must be an erroneous writing of *jiang* 漿.

水茛及薇蘅，叢生，花黄根紫，作陳醬色，其葉殊不似豨薟也。【頌曰】江東亦有之，狀如蘇恭所説。【時珍曰】處處原野有之，俗名苦菜，野人食之。江東人每采收儲焉。春初生苗，深冬始凋。初時葉布地生，似菘菜葉而狹長，有鋸齒，綠色，面深背淺。夏秋莖高二三尺而柔弱，數寸一節，節間生葉，四散如繖。顛頂開白花成簇，如芹花、蛇牀子花狀。結小實成簇。其根白紫，頗似柴胡。吴普言其根似桔梗，陳自明言其根似蛇莓根者，皆不然。

Collected Explanations. *Bie lu*: *Bai jiang* grows in the river valleys of Jiang xia. The root is collected in the eighth month. It is dried in the sun. [Tao] Hongjing: It comes from nearby. The leaves resemble those of St. Paulswort. The root is shaped like *bupleurum* [roots]. [Su] Gong: This pharmaceutical drug does not come from nearby. It mostly grows on hills and mountains. The leaves resemble those of Japanese buttercup and *mei xian* (unidentified, 15-19). It grows as clusters. The flowers are yellow; the root is purple, the color of long stored [soybean] sauce. The leaves are definitely not similar to those of St. Paulswort. [Su] Song: It is also found in Jiang dong, and it is shaped as described by Su Gong. [Li] Shizhen: It can be found everywhere in the wild of the plains. A common name is "bitter vegetable." The people in the wild eat it. The people in Jiang dong collect and store it for later use. At the beginning of spring it grows a seedling which deep in winter begins to wither. At first, the leaves grow covering the ground. They are similar to pak choi leaves, but they are narrow and lengthy, and they have saw teeth. They are green with a deep color on their front and a pale [green] on the back. In summer and autumn the stem reaches a height of two to three *chi*; it is is soft and weak with one node every few *cun*. Between the nodes the leaves grow. They spread in all four directions like an umbrella. White flowers open at the top [of the stem], forming a cluster, similar to the shape of celery flowers and *cnidium* flowers. They form small fruits in clusters. The root is white-purple, very much resembling *bupleurum* [roots]. When Wu Pu says that "its root is similar to *platycodon* [roots]," and Chen Ziming says that "its root resembles the roots of Indian strawberry," this is not so.

16-19-01

根苗同 *Gen, Miao*

Root [of dahurian *patrinia*], identical to the seedling.

【修治】【斅曰】凡收得便粗杵，入甘草葉相拌對蒸。從巳至未，去甘草葉，焙乾用。

Pharmaceutical Preparation. [Lei] Xiao. Whenever it is gathered, immediately pound it roughly, mix it with *glycyrrhiza* leaves and steam [the two items] from *si*

巳 hours (9 – 11) to *wei* 未 hours (13 – 15). Then remove the *glycyrrhiza* leaves, bake [the root] over a slow fire and it is ready for [therapeutic] applications.

【氣味】苦，平，無毒。【別録曰】鹹，微寒。【權曰】辛，苦，微寒。【大明曰】酸。【時珍曰】微苦帶甘。

Qi and Flavor. Bitter, balanced, nonpoisonous. *Bie lu*: Salty, slightly cold. [Zhen] Quan: Acrid, bitter, slightly cold. Da Ming: Sour. [Li] Shizhen: Slightly bitter with some traces of sweetness.

【主治】暴熱火瘡赤氣，疥瘙疽痔，馬鞍熱氣。本經。除癰腫，浮腫，結熱，風痺不足，産後疾痛。別録。治毒風瘰痺，破多年凝血，能化膿爲水，産後諸病，止腹痛餘疹煩渴。甄權。治血氣心腹痛，破癥結，催生落胞，血運，鼻衄，吐血，赤白帶下。赤眼障膜弩肉，聤耳，瘡瘍，疥癬，丹毒，排膿補瘻。大明。

Control. Fire sores[540] and red qi[541] caused by violent heat. *Jie*-illness[542] with itch. Impediment-illness[543] and piles, with the heat qi related to riding on a horse saddle. *Ben jing*. It eliminates obstruction-illness[544] swelling, surface swelling, bound heat,[545] blockage/numbness related to wind [intrusion] with a [qi] insufficiency, and painful ailments following delivery. *Bie lu*. It serves to cure poison wind [intrusion] with numbness blockage,[546] It breaks open blood that has coagulated over many years. It can transform pus to water. All diseases following delivery. It ends abdominal pain, and eliminates papules, vexation and thirst. Zhen Quan. It serves to cure pain in the central and abdominal region related to blood and qi [disorder]. It breaks through concretion-illness nodes, hastens birth and lets the placenta come down. Blood

540 *Huo chuang* 火瘡, "fire sores," a condition of ulcerating sores brought forth by *tang huo shang* 湯火傷, "harm caused by boiling water and fire." BCGM Dict I, 232.

541 *Chi qi* 赤氣, "red qi," a condition referred to only in the *Ben jing* and *Bie lu*. Its meaning remains unclear. The context suggests an ulcerous condition with red skin, swelling, heat and pain. BCGM Dict I, 87.

542 *Jie*-illness 疥, vaguely identifiable skin ailment. BCGM Dict I, 249.

543 *Ju* 疽, "impediment-illness," refers to an obstruction of vessels or other ducts inside the body. Qi rushing against the impediment may cause a local swelling and eventually break through the surface to cause an abscess. BCGM Dict I, 277.

544 *Yong* 癰, "obstruction-illness,"refers to an obstruction of vessels or other ducts inside the body. Qi rushing against the obstruction may cause a local swelling and eventually break through the surface to cause an abscess. BCGM Dict I, 641.

545 *Jie re* 結熱, "bound heat." A condition of blocked depot qi brought about by repletion heat evil, with blocked urine and stools, panting, fullness, and spitting because of [qi] moving contrary to its normal course. BCGM Dict I, 252.

546 *Qun bi* 瘰痺, "numbness blockage." A condition of *bi* 痺, "blockage," with numbness and slackening of the limbs and body. BCGM Dict I, 395.

[related brain] movement. Nosebleed. Blood vomiting. Red and white [discharge] from below the belt. Red eyes, obstructive membranes and tumorous flesh growths. Festering ears. Sores and pimples. *Jie*-illness[547] and *xuan*-illness,[548]. Cinnabar poison.[549] It drives out pus and closes fistulas. Da Ming.

【發明】【時珍曰】敗醬乃手足陽明、厥陰藥也。善排膿破血，故仲景治癰及古方婦人科皆用之。乃易得之物，而後人不知用，蓋未遇識者耳。

Explication. [Li] Shizhen: *Bai jiang* is a pharmaceutical drug for the hand and foot yang brilliance and ceasing yin [conduits]. It is good at driving out pus and breaking open blood [accumulations]. Therefore it was always resorted to by [Zhang] Zhongjing when he cured obstruction-illness and in ancient recipes of the [medical] discipline of [curing the diseases of] women. It is an item that is easily obtained. But people in later times did not know how to use it. Hence one does not encounter someone familiar with it.

【附方】舊二，新三。

Added Recipes. Two of old. Three newly [recorded].

腹癰有膿。薏苡仁附子敗醬湯：用薏苡仁十分，附子二分，敗醬五分，搗爲末。每以方寸匕，水二升，煎一升，頓服。小便當下，即愈。張仲景金匱玉函。

Abdominal obstruction-illness with pus. The "decoction with Job's tears, *aconitum* [accessor tuber] and *bai jiang*." Pound ten *fen* of Job's tears, two *fen* of *aconitum* [accessory tuber] and five *fen* of *bai jiang* into powder. Each time boil the amount held by a square *cun* spoon in two *sheng* of water down to one *sheng*, and ingest it at once. Once the urine has passed, a cure is achieved. Zhang Zhongjing, *Jin kui yu han*.

產後惡露，七八日不止。敗醬、當歸各六分，續斷、芍藥各八分，芎藭、竹茹各四分，生地黄炒十二分，水二升，煮取八合，空心服。外臺秘要。

547 *Jie*-illness 疥, vaguely identifiable skin ailment. BCGM Dict I, 249.

548 *Xuan* 癬, "*xuan*-illness." Conditions of dermal lesions with initially erythema, papules, and itching gradually extending in all directions to form an irregular ring with clear boundaries. The skin is slightly elevated with small papules, blisters, and/or scales and scraps. The central lesion may appear to heal spontaneously, and it may reappear. Also, a designation of local lesions with itching, release of liquid and shedding of scabs. BCGM Dict I, 591.

549 *Dan du* 丹毒, "cinnabar poison," a skin ailment with red rashes. BCGM Dict I, 118

Malign dew[550] following birth, not ending for seven, eight days. Boil six *fen* each of *bai jing* and Chinese *angelica* [root], eight *fen* each of Himalayan teasel herb [root] and *paeonia* [root], four *fen* each of *ligusticum* [root] and bamboo shavings, as well as 12 *fen* of fresh/raw Chinese foxglove [rhizome] in two *sheng* of water down to eight *ge* and [let the patient] ingest this on an empty stomach. *Wai tai mi yao.*

產後腰痛。乃血氣流入腰腿，痛不可轉者。敗醬、當歸各八分，芎藭、芍藥、桂心各六分，水二升，煮八合，分二服。忌葱。廣濟方。

Lower back pain following delivery. This is a situation where blood and qi have flowed into the lower back and thighs, resulting in pain and an inability to turn [one's body] around. Boil eight *fen* each of *bai jiang* and Chinese *angelica* [root], and six *fen* each of *ligusticum* [root], *paeonia* [root] and shaved cinnamom bark in two *sheng* of water down to eight *ge* and [let the patient] ingest this divided into two portions. [During this therapy] avoid onions. *Guang ji fang.*

產後腹痛如錐刺者。敗醬草五兩，水四升，煮二升，每服二合，日三服，良。衛生易簡方。

Abdominal pain following delivery as if pierced by an awl. Boil five *liang* of *bai jiang* herb in four *sheng* of water down to two *sheng*. Each time [let the patient] ingest two *ge*. To be ingested three times a day. Good. *Wei sheng yi jian fang.*

蠼螋尿瘡遶腰者。敗醬煎汁塗之。良。楊氏產乳。

Sores encircling the lower back caused by earwig urine.[551] Boil *bai jiang* to obtain a juice and apply it [to the affected region]. Good. *Yang shi chan ru.*

550 *E lu* 惡露, "malign dew," Blood or turbid liquid (i.e. lochia) leaving from the birth canal after parturition. BCGM Dict I, 141.

551 *Qu sou niao chuang* 蠼螋尿瘡, "earwig-urine sores." A condition forming clusters of blisters on the chest, flanks and lower back with an excruciatingly piercing pain, accompanied by strong heat and an aversion to cold, as a major sign. This condition is reminiscent of the neurological disease herpes zoster. Formerly it was believed that the urine of earwigs, when touched by the shadow of a human, would cause this person to suffer from this disease. BCGM Dict I, 392.

16-20
迎春花綱目
Ying chun hua*, FE *Gang mu.

***Jasminum nudiflorum* Lindl. Winter jasmine.**[552]

【集解】【時珍曰】處處人家栽插之。叢生，高者二三尺，方莖厚葉。葉如初生小椒葉而無齒，面青背淡。對節生小枝，一枝三葉。正月初開小花，狀如瑞香，花黃色，不結實。

Collected Explanations. [Li] Shizhen: It is planted by households everywhere. It grows as clusters and reaches a height of two to three *chi*. The stem is square and the leaves are thick. The leaves resemble small Chinese pepper leaves that have just begun to grow, but they have no teeth. They are greenish on their front and pale on the back. Small twigs grow facing each other at the nodes. One twig has three leaves. At the beginning of the first month small flowers open. They are shaped like those of winter daphne. The flowers are yellow; they do not form fruit.

16-20-01
葉 *Ye*
Leaf [of *ying chun hua*].

【氣味】苦，濇，平，無毒。

Qi and Flavor. Bitter, astringent, balanced, nonpoisonous.

【主治】腫毒惡瘡，陰乾研末，酒服二三錢，出汗便瘥。衛生易簡方。

Control. For malign sores with swelling and poison, dry [the leaves] in the yin (i. e., shade) and grind them into powder. Ingest with wine two or three *qian*. As soon as sweating begins, a cure is achieved. *Wei sheng yi jian fang*.

16-21
款冬花本經中品
***Kuan dong hua*, FE *Ben jing*, middle rank.**

***Tussilago farfara* L. Coltsfoot.**

【釋名】款凍郭璞、顆凍爾雅、氐冬别録、鑽凍衍義、菟奚爾雅、橐吾本經、虎鬚本經。【時珍曰】按述征記云：洛水至歲末凝厲時，款冬生于草冰之中，則顆凍之名以此而得。後人訛爲款冬，即款凍爾。款者至也，至冬而花也。【宗奭曰】百草中惟此不顧冰雪最先春也，故世謂之鑽凍。雖在冰雪之下，至時亦生芽，春時人采以代蔬。入藥須微見花者良。如已芬芳，則都無氣力。今人多使如筯頭者，恐未有花也。

---

552 *Ying chun hua* 迎春花, lit.: "Flower welcoming spring."

Explanation of Names. *Kuan dong* 款凍, Guo Pu. *Ke dong* 顆凍, *Er ya. Di dong* 氐冬, *Bie lu. Zuan dong* 鑽凍, *Yan yi. Tu xi* 菟奚, *Er ya. Tuo wu* 橐吾, *Ben jing. Hu xu* 虎鬚, "a tiger's whiskers," *Ben jing*. [Li] Shizhen: According to the *Shu zheng ji*, when the river Luo shui toward the end of the year freezes in extreme [cold], *kuan dong* grows among herbs and ice. The name *ke dong* 顆凍, "pellets freezing," is based on this. In later times, people changed this to *kuan dong* 款冬, which is *kuan dong* 款凍. *Kuan* 款 is *zhi* 至, "utmost." In utmost winter [cold], it has flowers. [Kou] Zongshi: Of all the hundreds of herbs only this one predates spring despite ice and snow. Therefore it is widely called "ice borer," *zuan dong* 鑽凍. Even below ice and snow, when its time has come it develops sprouts. They are collected in spring as a substitute for vegetables. When it is added to medication, the flowers should already be slightly visible. As soon as they have turned fragrant, their qi are completely without strength. Today, people often use them when they resemble the tips of chopsticks. It may well be that they have not yet developed a flower.

【集解】【別録曰】款冬生常山山谷及上黨水旁，十一月采花，陰乾。【弘景曰】第一出河北，其形如宿蓴未舒者佳，其腹裏有絲。次出高麗百濟，其花乃似大菊花。次亦出蜀北部宕昌而並不如。其冬月在冰下生，十二月、正月旦取之。【恭曰】今出雍州南山溪水，及華州山谷澗間。葉似葵而大，叢生，花出根下。【頌曰】今關中亦有之。根紫色，葉似萆薢，十二月開黄花，青紫萼，去土一二寸，初出如菊花萼，通直而肥實無子。則陶氏所謂出高麗百濟者，近此類也。又有紅花者，葉如荷而斗直，大者容一升，小者容數合，俗呼爲蜂斗葉，又名水斗葉。則蘇氏所謂大如葵而叢生者是也。傅咸款冬賦序云："予曾逐禽，登於北山，于時仲冬之月，冰凌盈谷，積雪被厓，顧見款冬煒然，始敷華艷"，是也。

Collected Explanations. *Bie lu. Kuan dong* grows in the mountain valleys of Mount Chang shan, and near waters in Shang dang. The flowers are collected in the eleventh month. They are dried in the yin (i. e., shade). [Tao] Hongjing: A first degree [quality *kuan dong*] comes from He bei. It is excellent when it is shaped like *zingiber mioga* that has not yet unfolded. It has fibers in its "abdomen." Second degree [*kuan dong*] comes from Bai ji in Gao li. Its flowers resemble big *chrysanthemum* flowers. A still inferior [degree *kuan dong*] comes from Dang chang in the northern region of Shu, but it does not come close [to the others]. [*Kuan dong*] grows in winter below the ice, and is gathered in the early morning in the 12th and first month. [Su] Gong: Today it comes from small streams and rivers of Nan shan in Yong zhou, and also from ravines and river valleys of Hua zhou. The leaves resemble those of Chinese mallows, but are bigger. They grow as clusters, and the flowers come up from below the roots. [Su] Song: Today [*kuan dong hua*] is also present in Guan zhong. The root is purple. The leaves resemble those of *dioscorea* [plants]. It opens yellow flowers in the 12th month with a greenish-purple calyx one or two *cun* above the ground. When they have just come out they are similar to the calyx of *chrysanthemum* [flowers]. They grow straight up, are fat and solid and have no seeds. That is, those said by Mr. Tao [Hongjing] to "come from Bai ji in Gao li," they are very similar. There are also those with red flowers. Their leaves are like those of lotus. They form a cup situated straight upward. Big ones hold one *sheng*; small ones hold several *ge*. They are commonly called "bee cup leaves," and also "water cup leaves." They are the ones said by Mr. Su [Gong] to "have the size of Chinese mallows and to grow as clusters." When Fu Xian in his *Kuan dong fu* states: "Once I went after animals. I climbed on the northern mountain. It was a mid-winter month. Ice filled the valley; snow covered the shores. When I saw the shine of *kuan dong* just about to spread its beautiful splendor," then this is correct.

【修治】【斅曰】凡采得，須去向裏裹花蕊殼，并向裏實如栗零殼者。并枝葉，以甘草水浸一宿，却取款冬葉相拌裛一夜，晒乾去葉用。

Pharmaceutical Preparation. [Lei] Xiao. Whenever [*kuan dong hua*] is collected, remove, reaching toward inside, the shell covering the flower and its stamens, and also reaching toward inside the fruit similar to the shells of *li ling*.[553] And also [put aside] twigs and leaves. Then soak [the herb] in *glycyrrhiza* water for one night, take the *kuan dong* leaves and use them to tie the [*kuan dong* herbs] together for one night. [The next day] dry them in the sun, remove the leaves and [the *kuan dong* herb] may be used [for therapeutic ends].

【氣味】辛，温，無毒。【别録曰】甘。【好古曰】純陽，入手太陰經。【之才曰】杏仁爲之使，得紫菀良，惡皂莢、消石、玄參，畏貝母、辛夷、麻黄、黄耆、黄芩、連翹[554]、青葙。

Qi and Flavor. Acrid, warm, nonpoisonous. *Bie lu*: Sweet. [Wang] Haogu: A pure yang [substance]. It enters the hand major yin conduits. [Xu] Zhicai: Bitter almond kernels serve as its guiding substance. Combined with purple aster [root] it yields good results. [Ingested together,] it abhors *gleditsia* pods/seeds, salpetre and *scrophularia* [root]. It fears *fritillaria* [root], *magnolia* flower buds, *ephedra* [herb], *astragalus* [root], *scutellaria* [root], *forsythia* [fruit], and Prince's feather.

553 Instead of *li* 栗, "Chinese chestnut," *Zheng lei* ch. 9, *kuan dong hua* 款冬花, quoting Lei gong writes *mi* 粟, "millet."

554 Instead of *lian qiao* 連翹, "*forsythia* [fruit]," *Zheng lei* ch. 9, *kuan dong hua* 款冬花, writes *huang lian* 黄連, "*coptis* [rhizome]."

【主治】欬逆，上氣善喘，喉痺，諸驚癇，寒熱邪氣。本經。消渴，喘息呼吸。别録。療肺氣心促急，熱勞欬，連連不絶，涕唾稠粘，肺痿肺癰，吐膿血。甄權。潤心肺，益五臟，除煩消痰，洗肝明目及中風等疾。大明。

Control. Cough with [qi] counterflow. Rising qi with a likelihood to pant. Throat blockage. All types of fright epilepsy. [Alternating sensations of] cold and heat evil qi. *Ben jing*. Melting with thirst.[555] Pant breathing. *Bie lu*. It heals heart [qi] irritation caused by lung qi [disorder]. Exhaustion with continuing, unending cough related to heat. Thick and glue-like snivel and spittle. Lung dysfunction and lung obstruction-illness.[556] Vomiting of pus and blood. Zhen Quan. It moistens the heart and the lung. It boosts the five long-term depots. It dispels vexation and dissolves phlegm. It serves to rinse the liver, clear the eyes and [cure] being struck by wind, all such illnesses. Da Ming.

【發明】【頌曰】本經主欬逆古方用爲温肺治嗽之最。崔知悌療久欬熏法：每旦取款冬花如雞子許，少蜜拌花使潤，納一升鐵鐺中。又用一瓦盌鑽一孔，孔内安一小筆管，以麪泥縫，勿令漏氣。鐺下着炭火，少時烟從筒出，以口含吸，嚥之。如胸中少悶，須舉頭，即將指頭按住筒口，勿使漏，至煙盡乃止。如是五日一爲之。待至六日，飽食羊肉餺飥一頓，永瘥。【宗奭曰】有人病嗽多日，或教然款冬花三兩，於無風處以筆管吸其烟，滿口則嚥之，數日果效。

Explication. [Su] Song: Ancient recipes recorded in the *Ben jing* as controlling cough with [qi] counterflow resort to [*kuan dong hua*] as the most [important ingredient] to warm the lung and cure cough. Cui Zhiti's method of fumigation to heal long-lasting cough is as follows. "Every morning mix as much of *kuan dong* flowers as the size of a chicken egg with a little honey to moisten the flowers and give them into a one *sheng* flat iron pan. Also, take a pottery bowl [to cover the pan] and bore a hole into it. Insert a small tube of a writing brush into [the hole] and tightly seal [the edge where the pan and the bowl meet] with dough or plaster so that no qi can leak. Below the pan light a charcoal fire. After a short while fumes will leave through the tube. Inhale them with the mouth and swallow them. If a slight heart-pressure is felt in the chest, lift the head and press the tip of a finger on the hole of the tube to let no more fumes leave it [for as long as you pause]. Continue [inhaling] until the fumes have come to an end. Perform this once in five days. Wait until the sixth day and have a meal with mutton and rice cakes, eating to repletion.

555 *Xiao ke* 消渴, "melting with thirst," most likely including cases of diabetes. BCGM Dict Vol I, 567.

556 *Fei yong* 肺癰, "lung obstruction-illness," also: *fei yong* 肺壅, "lung obstruction," a condition of abscesses in the lung, with fever, chest pain, and vomiting of bad-smelling pus and blood. BCGM Dict I, 156.

The cure achieved will last forever. [Kou] Zongshi: There was a person who coughed for many days. Someone taught him to ignite three *liang* of *kuan dong hua* and with a writing brush tube inhale the fumes in a windless place. He was to fill his mouth [with the fumes] and then swallow them. Within several days this proved effective."

【附方】新二。

Added Recipes. Two newly [recorded].

痰嗽帶血。款冬花、百合蒸焙，等分爲末。蜜丸龍眼大，每卧時嚼一丸，薑湯下。濟生方。

Cough with phlegm and traces of blood. [Grind] equal amounts of *kuan dong hua* and Brown's lily [bulbs], steamed and baked over a slow fire, into powder. With honey form pills the size of dragon eyes/longan seeds and each time when going to bed chew one pill and send it down with a ginger decoction. *Ji sheng fang*.

口中疳瘡。款冬花、黄連等分，爲細末，用唾津調成餅子。先以蛇牀子煎湯漱口，乃以餅子傅之，少頃確住，其瘡立消也。楊誠經驗方。

Gan-illness[557] sores in the mouth. [Grind] *kuan dong hua* and *coptis* [rhizome] to fine powder. Mix it with human saliva to form cakes. First prepare a *cnidium* seed decoction and rinse the mouth. Then apply the cakes [to the affected region] and exert some pressure for a while. This will dissolve the sores right away. Yang Cheng, *Jing yan fang*.

16-22

鼠麴草日華

***Shu qu cao*, FE *Rihua*.**

***Gnaphalium affine* D. Don. Cudweed.**

【校正】併入有名未用鼠耳及東垣藥類法象佛耳草。

Editorial Correction. *Shu er* 鼠耳, listed [in the *Bie lu*] in the section "known by name but not in use" and *fo er cao* 佛耳草, recorded in [Li] Dongyuan's *Yao lei fa xiang*, are inserted here.

【釋名】米麴綱目、鼠耳别録、佛耳草法象、無心草别録、香茅拾遺、黄蒿會編、茸母。【時珍曰】麴，言其花黄如麴色，又可和米粉食也。鼠耳，言其葉形如鼠耳，又有白毛蒙茸似之，故北人呼爲茸母。佛耳，則鼠

557 *Gan* 疳, "*gan*-illness," also: "sweets-illness," involves several complaints that affect children and adults, with causes and conditions too different to fall into a known disease category. BCGM Dict I, 180-188.

耳之訛也。今淮人呼爲毛耳朵，則香茅之茅，似當作毛。按段成式雜俎云：蚍蜉酒草，鼠耳也，一名無心草。豈蚍蜉食此，故有是名耶。

Explanation of Names. *Mi qu* 米麴, *Gang mu*. *Fo er cao* 佛耳草, *Fa xiang*. *Wu xin cao* 無心草, *Bie lu*. *Xiang mao* 香茅, *Shi yi*. *Huang hao* 黄蒿, *Hui bian*. *Rong mu* 茸母. [Li] Shizhen. *Qu* 麴 is to say: its flowers are yellow like the color of distiller's yeast, *qu* 麴. Also, it can be eaten together with rice, *mi* 米, powder. *Shu er* 鼠耳 is to say, its leaves are shaped like a "mouse/rat ear," *shu er* 鼠耳. Also, because it is covered with soft, white hair, *meng rong* 蒙茸, people in the North call it *rong mu* 茸母, "soft-haired mother." *Fo er* 佛耳, "Buddha's ear," is a misreading of *shu er* 鼠耳. In Huai, people today call it *mao er duo* 毛耳朵, "hairy ear." That is, the *mao* 茅 of *xiang mao* 香茅, "fragrant flossgrass," should probably be written *mao* 毛, "hair." According to Duan Chengshi's *Za zu*, "*pi fu jiu cao* 蚍蜉酒草, 'ant wine herb,' is *shu er* 鼠耳, alternative name: *wu xin cao* 無心草, 'herb without heart/core'. Maybe it was named so because ants eat it."

【集解】【别録曰】鼠耳，一名無心，生田中下地，厚葉肥莖。【藏器曰】鼠麴草，生平崗熟地，高尺餘，葉有白毛，黄花。荆楚歲時記云：三月三日，取鼠麴汁，蜜和爲粉，謂之龍舌粄，以壓時氣。粄音板，米餅也。山南人呼爲香茅，取花雜櫸皮染褐，至破猶鮮。江西人呼爲鼠耳草也。【汪機曰】佛耳草，徽人謂之黄蒿。二三月苗長尺許，葉似馬齒莧而細，有微白毛，花黄。土人采莖葉和米粉擣作粑果食。【時珍曰】日華本草鼠麴，即别録鼠耳也。唐宋諸家不知，乃退"鼠耳"入"有名未用"中。李杲藥類法象用佛耳草，亦不知其即鼠耳也。原野間甚多。二月生苗，莖葉柔軟，葉長寸許，白茸如鼠耳之毛。開小黄花成穗，結細子。楚人呼爲米麴，北人呼爲茸母。故邵桂子甕天語云：北方寒食，采茸母草和粉食。宋徽宗詩"茸母初生認禁煙"者，是也。

Collected Explanations. *Bie lu*: *Shu er* 鼠耳, also named *wu xin* 無心, grows on low-lying ground in the fields. It has thick leaves and a fat stem. [Chen] Cangqi: *Shu qu cao* grows on cultivated land in the plains and on hillocks. It is more than a *chi* tall; its leaves have white hair. The flowers are yellow. The *Jing Chu sui shi ji* states: "On the third day of the third month gather *shu qu* juice, mix it with honey and prepare a powder. This is called 'dragon tongue rice cake' and it serves to hold down seasonal qi." [The character] 粄 is read *ban* 板; it means "rice cake." People in Shan nan call [*shu qu hua*] *xiang mao* 香茅. They mix the flowers with the bark of Schneider's *zelkova* to prepare a brown dyestuff. It stays fresh until [a garment dyed with it] is worn out. It is [the item] called by people in Jiang xi "mouse/rat ear herb." Wang Ji: *Fo er cao* 佛耳草 is called *huang hao* 黄蒿 by people in Hui. During the second and third month the seedling reaches a height of more than a *chi*. The leaves resemble those of purslane, but are finer. They are covered by pale white hair. The flower is yellow. The locals collect the stem and the leaves, pound them with rice powder and prepare them to fruit cakes that they eat. [Li] Shizhen: The *shu qu* 鼠麴 recorded in the *Rihua ben cao* is the *shu er* 鼠耳 of the *Bie lu*. This was unknown to all the authors of the Tang and Song era. Hence they moved *shu er* 鼠耳 into the section "known by name but not in use." When Li Gao in his *Yao lei fa xiang* [recommended to] use *fo er cao* 佛耳草, he, too, did not know that it is *shu er* 鼠耳. There is very much of it in the wild in the plains. It grows a seedling in the second month. The stem and the leaves are soft. The leaves are more than a *cun* long. They are covered by white, soft hair similar to the hair of mouse/rat ears. It opens small, yellow flowers with spikes and forms fine seeds. People in Chu call it *mi qu* 米麴. People in the North call it *rong mu* 茸母. Hence, Shao Guizi in his *Weng tian yu* states: "On the Cold Food [day][558] in the North they collect *rong mu cao* 茸母草 and eat it with [rice] powder." [Emperor] Hui zong of the Song wrote a poem: "*Rong mu* 茸母 that has just begun to grow is adopted [as food] when smoke [rising from a cooking stove] is forbidden." That is correct.

【氣味】甘，平，無毒。【別録曰】鼠耳：酸，無毒。【杲曰】佛耳草：酸，性熱，款冬花爲之使。宜少食之，過則損目。

Qi and Flavor. Sweet, balanced, nonpoisonous. *Bie lu*: *Shu er* 鼠耳: Sour, nonpoisonous. [Li] Gao: *Fo er cao* 佛耳草: Sour, nature hot. Coltsfoot serves as its guiding substance. It should be eaten in small quantities lest it injure the eyes.

【主治】鼠耳：主痺寒寒熱，止欬。別録。鼠麴：調中益氣，止洩，除痰，壓時氣，去熱嗽。雜米粉作糗食，甜美。日華。佛耳：治寒嗽及痰，除肺中寒，大升肺氣。李杲。

Control. *Shu er* 鼠耳: It controls blockage with cold, and [alternating sensations of] cold and heat. It ends cough. *Bie lu*. *Shu qu* 鼠麴: It regulates the center and boosts the qi. It ends outflow, removes phlegm, holds down seasonal qi and dispels heat related to cough. Mixed with rice powder it is prepared to a sweet and delicious food. Rihua. *Fo er* 佛耳: It serves to cure cough related to cold, and phlegm. It dispels cold from within the lung. It is very much able to lift lung qi.

---

558 The "Cold Food Day:" *Jie* [*Zi*]*tui* 介子推 served King Wen of the State of Jin, 5th c. BCE. Eventually he withdrew with his mother to the forests. King Wen summoned him to his court to show his gratitude. When Jie Zitui refused to appear, the king had the forest set on fire to force him to leave his abode. Jie and his mother died in the fire in 476 BCE. The king ordered that no fires were allowed on that day in future, and food was to be consumed cold. Hence the name of that day, *han shi* 寒食, "cold food." BCGM Dict III, 224-225.

【發明】【震亨曰】治寒痰嗽宜用佛耳草，熱痰嗽宜用燈籠草。【時珍曰】别録云治寒熱止欬，東垣云治寒嗽，言其標也；日華云治熱嗽，言其本也。大抵寒嗽多是火鬱於内而寒覆於外也。按陳氏經驗方云：三奇散治一切欬嗽，不問久近晝夜無時。用佛耳草五十文，款冬花二百文，熟地黄二兩，焙研末。每用二錢，於爐中燒之，以筒吸烟嚥下，有涎吐去。予家一僕久病此，醫治不效。偶在沅州得一婢，用此法，兩服而愈也。

Explication. [Zhu] Zhenheng: To cure phlegm and cough related to the presence of cold, it is advisable to use *fo er cao*. For phlegm and cough related to the presence of heat, it is advisable to use lantern herb. [Li] Shizhen: The *Bie lu* states: "It serves to cure [alternating sensations of] cold and heat and ends cough." [Li] Dongyuan states: "It serves to cure cough related to cold." That is to say, [they focus on the] signs [rather than on the root of the problem]. The *Rihua* states: "It serves to cure cough related to heat." That is, [it focusses on] the root [of the problem]. In general, cold cough is mostly related to pent-up heat in the center with the cold covered in the exterior. According to Mr. Chen's *Jing yan fang*, "the 'powder with the three extraordinary [ingredients]' serves to cure all types of cough, regardless of whether this is a long-lasting or a recent issue, whether [the patient coughs] during the day or the night, or any time. Bake 50 *wen* of *fo er cao*, 200 *wen* of coltsfoot, and two *liang* of heat prepared Chinese foxglove [rhizome] over a slow fire and grind them into powder. Each time burn two *qian* in a stove, inhale the fumes [with the mouth] and swallow them. When saliva is produced, spit it out. In my household a servant suffered from this disease for a long time. Therapies introduced by physicians remained without effect. It so happened that while I was in Yuan zhou, a servant-girl applied this method, and after two ingestions a cure was achieved."

16-23
决明本經上品
Jue ming. FE *Ben jing*, upper rank.

***Cassia tora* L. Fetid *cassia*.**

【釋名】【時珍曰】此馬蹄决明也，以明目之功而名。又有草决明、石决明，皆同功者。草决明即青葙子，陶氏所謂萋蒿是也。

Explanation of Names. [Li] Shizhen: This is *ma ti jue ming* 馬蹄决明, "horse hoof *jue ming*." Its name is based on its potential to clear, *ming* 明, the eyes. There are also [herbs called] *cao jue ming* 草决明, "herbal *jue ming*," and *shi jue ming* 石决明, "stone *jue ming*." Their [therapeutic] potentials are identical. *Cao jue ming* 草决明 is *qing xiang zi* 青葙子, "Prince's feather."

【集解】【别録曰】决明子生龍門川澤，十月十日采，陰乾百日。【弘景曰】龍門在長安北。今處處有之。葉如茳芒，子形似馬蹄，呼爲馬蹄决明，用之當搗碎。又别有草决明，是萋蒿草，在下品中。【頌曰】今處處人家園圃所蒔，夏初生苗，高三四尺許。根帶紫色。葉似苜蓿而大。七月開黄花，結角。其子如青緑豆而鋭，十月采之。按爾雅：薢茩，决光。郭璞釋云：藥草决明也。葉黄鋭，赤華，實如山茱萸。或曰蔆也。關西謂之薢茩，音皆苟。其説與此種頗不類。又有一種馬蹄决明，葉如江豆，子形似馬蹄。【宗奭曰】决明，苗高四五尺，春亦爲蔬。秋深結角，其子生角中如羊腎。今湖南、北人家所種甚多。或在村野成段。蜀本圖經言葉似苜蓿而闊大者，甚爲允當。【時珍曰】决明有二種。一種馬蹄决明，莖高三四尺，葉大於苜蓿而本小末奓，晝開夜合，兩兩相帖。秋開淡黄花五出，結角如初生細豇豆，長五六寸。角中子數十粒，參差相連，狀如馬蹄，青緑色，入眼目藥最良。一種茳芒决明，救荒本草所謂山扁豆是也。苗莖似馬蹄决明，但葉之本小末尖，正似槐葉，夜亦不合。秋開深黄花五出，結角大如小指，長二寸許。角中子成數列，狀如黄葵子而扁，其色褐，味甘滑。二種苗葉皆可作酒麴，俗呼爲獨占缸。但茳芒嫩苗及花與角子，皆可瀹茹及點茶食；而馬蹄决明苗角皆韌苦，不可食也。蘇頌言薢茩即决明，殊不類，恐别一物也。

Explication. *Bie lu*: *Jue ming zi* grows in river marshlands of Long men. It is collected on the tenth day of the tenth month, and is dried in the yin (i. e., shade) for 100 days. [Tao] Hongjing: Long men is situated north of Chang an. Today, [*jue ming zi*] can be found everywhere. The leaves are similar to large-leaved senna. The seeds are shaped like horse hoofs. Hence the name "horse hoof *jue ming*." For [therapeutic] applications they must be crushed to pieces. There is also a *cao jue ming* 草决明; it is the *qi hao cao* 萋蒿草, [an herb] of lower rank. [Su] Song: Today, everywhere households plant it in their gardens. At the beginning of summer it grows a seedling reaching a height of more than three to four *chi*. The root has some purple color. The leaves resemble those of alfalfa, but they are bigger. Yellow flowers open in the seventh month. They form horn[-shaped seed capsules]. The seeds [in these capsules] resemble greenish mung beans, but they are pointed. They are collected in the tenth month. According to the *Er ya*, "*jie gou* 薢茩 is *jue guang* 决光[559]." Guo Pu explains: "This is medicinal *cao jue ming*. The leaves are yellow and pointed; the flower is red. Its fruits are similar to Asiatic cornelian cherry [fruit]. They are also called *ling* 蔆. In Guan xi they are called *jie gou* 薢茩, read *jie gou* 皆苟." Their description is very different from the kinds discussed here. There is also a kind [named] "horse hoof *jue ming*." Its leaves are similar to those of cowpea. The

559 Instead of *jue guang* 决光, the Er ya, section *Shi cao* 釋草, "explanation of herbs," writes *jue guang* 英茪.

seeds are shaped like horse hoofs. [Kou] Zongshi: *Jue ming* seedlings are four to five *chi* tall. In spring, they serve as vegetable. Late in autumn they develop horn[-shaped seed capsules]. The seeds grow in these horns and look like sheep kidneys. Today, people in Hu nan and [Hu] bei plant them very often. Sometimes they cover large areas in villages or in the wild. When the *Shu ben tu jing* says that the leaves are similar to those of alfalfa, but are wider and bigger, then this is very accurate. [Li] Shizhen: There are two kinds of *jue ming*. One kind is "horse hoof *jue ming*." Its stem is three to four *chi* tall. The leaves are bigger than those of alfalfa; they are small at their base and very wide at the end. They open during daytime, and are closed at night. They are systematically positioned as pairs of two and two. In autumn, flowers of a pale yellow color open with five petals. They form horn[-shaped seed capsules] resembling those of fine cowpea that have just begun to grow. They are five to six *cun* long. Inside these horns are several tens of seeds, all closely linked to each other and shaped like horse hoofs. They are of a greenish-green color. Added to eye medication they are very good. Then there is a [second] kind, that is, large-leaved senna *jue ming*, it is the *shan bian dou* 山扁豆 mentioned in the *Jiu huang ben cao*. Its seedling and stem resemble those of *ma ti jue ming* 馬蹄决明, except for that the leaves are small at their base and pointed at the end. They really resemble *sophora* [tree] leaves, and they, too, do not close during the night. In autumn it opens deeply yellow flowers with five petals. They form horn[-shaped seed capsules] of the size of a small finger, and more than two *cun* long. The seeds in the horns form several rows. They are shaped like okra seeds, but they are flat. Their color is brown, their flavor is sweet and they are smooth[ing]. The seedling and the leaves of both kinds [of *jue ming*] can be prepared to distiller's yeast. It is commonly called *du zhan gang* 獨占缸, "vat standing alone." However, the tender leaves of large-leaved senna and also the flowers and the seeds in the horns can all be boiled to be eaten as vegetables or consumed as an infusion as tea. In contrast, *ma ti jue ming*'s seedling and horns are hard and bitter and cannot be eaten. Su Song says of *jie gou* 薢茩 that it is *jue ming* 决明. But they are very different. I assume that it is another item.

16-23-01
子 *Zi*
Seeds [of *jue ming*].

【氣味】鹹，平，無毒。【别録曰】苦、甘，微寒。【之才曰】蓍實爲之使，惡大麻子。

Qi and Flavor. Salty, balanced, nonpoisonous. *Bie lu*: Bitter, sweet, slightly cold. [Xu] Zhicai: Siberian milfoil fruit serve as its guiding substance. [Ingested together,] it abhors sesame seeds.

【主治】青盲，目淫膚，赤白膜，眼赤淚出。久服益精光，輕身。本經。療唇口青。别録。助肝氣，益精。以水調末，塗腫毒。熁太陽穴，治頭痛。又貼腦心，止鼻洪。作枕，治頭風明目，甚於黑豆。日華。治肝熱風眼赤淚，每旦取一匙挼净，空心吞之。百日後夜見物光。甄權。益腎，解蛇毒。震亨。葉作菜食，利五臟明目，甚良。甄權。

Control. Green blindness. Excess skin[560] in the eyes. Red and white membranes. Red eyes with tearflow. Ingested for a long time they boost eyesight and relieve the body of its weight. *Ben jing*. They heal greenish lips and mouth. *Bie lu*. They support liver qi and boost essence/sperm. The powder mixed with water is applied to swelling with poison. Applied to cauterize the major yang [needle insertion holes at the temples, the seeds] serve to cure headache. Also, attached to the core of the brain [on the top of the head] they end profuse nosebleed. Prepared as a pillow they serve to cure head wind[561] and brighten the eyes, much better than soybeans. *Rihua*. To cure liver heat and red eyes with tearflow caused by wind [intrusion], every morning rub a spoonful [of seeds] clean and ingest them on an empty stomach. After 100 days items will appear shining at night. Zhen Quan. They boost the kidneys and resolve snake poison. [Zhu] Zhenheng. The leaves are eaten as vegetables. They free the passage through the five long-term depots and clear the eyes. Very good. Zhen Quan.

【發明】【時珍曰】相感志言：圃中種决明，蛇不敢入。丹溪朱氏言决明解蛇毒，本於此也。王旻山居録言：春月種决明，葉生采食，其花陰乾亦可食。切忌泡茶，多食無不患風。按馬蹄决明苗角皆韌而苦，不宜於食。縱食之，有利五臟明目之功，何遂至于患風耶？又鎦績霏雪録言：人家不可種决明，生子多跛。此迂儒誤聽之説也，不可信。

Explication. [Li] Shizhen: The *Xiang gan zhi* says: "When *jue ming* is planted in the garden, snakes will not dare to enter." When Mr. Zhu Danxi says: "*Jue ming* resolves snake poison," he relies on this [saying in the *Xiang gan zhi*]. Wang Min in his *Shan ju lu* says: "During spring months plant *jue ming*. When its leaves grow collect and eat them. The flowers, when dried in the yin (i. e., shade), are also edible. But it is absolutely forbidden to prepare tea at the same time. Eating too much [of *jue ming*] will inevitably let one suffer of wind [intrusion]." Now, the seedling and the horn[-shaped seed capsules] of *ma ti jue ming* are hard and bitter. They are not suitable for eating. When [the leaves of *jue ming*] are eaten, they have a potential of freeing the passage through the five long-term depots and clearing the eyes. How could this

560 *Yin fu* 淫膚, "excess skin," a condition of *xi rou* 瘜肉, "tumorous flesh-growths," developing between the white of the eyeball and the eyelid. BCGM Dict I, 633.

561 *Tou feng* 頭風, "head wind." Condition of wind evil attacking the head followed by pain, dizziness, itching. BCGM Dict I, 509.

result in a "suffering of wind?" Also, Liu Ji in has *Fei xue lu* says: "Households must not plant *jue ming*. [Otherwise] their children will often be lame." This statement is based on an erroneous saying of some narrowminded scholar. It must not be trusted.

【附方】舊一，新七。
Added Recipes. One of old. Seven newly [recorded].

積年失明。决明子二升爲末。每食後粥飲服方寸匕。外臺秘要。

Loss of eyesight over years. [Grind] two *sheng* of *jue ming* seeds into powder. Each time ingest, following a meal, with a congee or beverage the amount held by a square *cun* spoon. *Wai tai mi yao.*

青盲雀目。决明一升，地膚子五兩，爲末。米飲丸梧子大，每米飲下二三十丸。普濟方。

Green blindness and sparrow eyes. [Grind] one *sheng* of *jue ming* and five *liang* of broom plant seeds into powder and form with a rice beverage pills the size of *wu* seeds. Each time send down with a rice beverage 20 to 30 pills. *Pu ji fang.*

補肝明目。决明子一升，蔓菁子二升，以酒五升煮，暴乾爲末。每飲服二錢，温水下。日二服。聖惠方。

To supplement the liver and clear the eyes. Boil one *sheng* of *jue ming* seeds and two *sheng* of rape turnip seeds in five *sheng* of wine. Dry them in the sun and [grind them into] powder. Each time ingest with a beverage two *qian*, to be sent down with warm water. To be ingested twice a day. *Sheng hui fang.*

目赤腫痛。决明子炒研，茶調傅兩太陽穴，乾則易之，一夜即愈。醫方摘玄。

Red eyes with a painful swelling. Fry *jue ming* seeds and grind [them into powder]. Mix [the powder] with tea and apply it to the two major yang [needle insertion] holes [at the temples]. When [the application] has dried, replace it [with a moist application]. A cure is achieved after one night. *Yi fang zhai xuan.*

頭風熱痛。方同上。

Head wind[562] with painful heat. Recipe identical to the one above.

鼻衄不止。方見主治。

Unending nosebleed. For a recipe, see under "Control."

562 *Tou feng* 頭風, "head wind." Condition of wind evil attacking the head followed by pain, dizziness, itching. BCGM Dict I, 509.

癬瘡延蔓。决明子一兩爲末，入水銀、輕粉少許，研不見星，擦破上藥，立瘥，此東坡家藏方也。奇效良方。

Xuan-illness[563] extending and creeping. [Grind] one *liang* of *jue ming* seeds into powder. Add small amounts of mercury and calomel. Grind this until no more [mercury] "stars" are visible. Rub [the affected region] until it opens and apply the medication. An immediate cure is achieved. This is a recipe kept in [Su] Dongpo's family. *Qi xiao liang fang*.

發背初起。草决明生用一升擣，生甘草一兩，水三升，煮一升，分二服。大抵血滯則生瘡，肝主藏血，决明和肝氣，不損元氣也。許學士本事方。

An effusion on the back[564] that has just begun to rise. Boil one *sheng* of fresh *cao jue ming*, pounded [to powder] and one *liang* of fresh *glycyrrhiza* [root] in three *sheng* of water down to one *sheng* and ingest it divided into two portions. In general, stagnating blood generates sores. The liver controls the storage of blood. *Jue ming* harmonizes liver qi and does not harm the original qi. Xu xueshi *Ben shi fang*.

16-23-A01
茳芒拾遺 *Jiang mang*, FE *Shi yi*
***Cassia sophora* L. Large-leaved senna.**

【藏器曰】陶云：决明葉如茳芒。按茳芒生道旁，葉小於决明，性平無毒。火炙作飲極香，除痰止渴，令人不睡，調中，隋稠禪師采作五色飲以進煬帝者，是也。乃草似莞，生海邊，可爲席者，與决明葉不相類。【時珍曰】茳芒亦决明之一種，故俗猶稱獨占缸。説見前集解下。

[Chen] Cangqi: Tao [Hongjing] states: "*Jue ming* (fetid *cassia*, 16-23) leaves are similar to *jiang mang* [leaves]." Now, *jiang mang* grows at the roadside. The leaves are smaller than those of *jue ming*. Its nature is balanced; it is nonpoisonous. Roasted in fire it can be prepared to a most fragrant beverage. It dispels phlegm and ends thirst. It does not let one sleep. It regulates the center. During the Sui dynasty, a Buddhist master Chou collected [an herb] and prepared a five-color beverage that he submitted to Emperor Yang di. That is [the item discussed here]. There is also a *jiang tu* 茳芏, with the character [芏] derived from 土, read *tu* 吐. It is also called *jiang li zi* 江

563 *Xuan* 癬, "*xuan*-illness," a condition of dermal lesions with initially erythema, papules, and itching gradually extending in all directions to form an irregular ring with clear boundaries. The skin is slightly elevated with small papules, blisters, and/or scales and scraps. The central lesion may appear to heal spontaneously, and it may reappear. BCGM Dict I, 591.

564 *Fa bei* 發背, "effusion on/of the back," a condition of *yong* 癰, "obstruction-illnesses," and *ju* 疽, "impediment-illnesses," developing on one's back. As it was believed that the transporter holes of the five depots and six palaces are located on the back, conditions of obstruction-illnesses and impediment-illnesses there, often apparent as abscesses, were considered threatening. BCGM Dict I, 148.

蘺子. Now, this herb resembles *angelica dahurica*; it grows next to the sea and it can be made to mats. It is not similar to *jue ming* leaves. [Li] Shizhen: *Jiang mang* is a kind of *jue ming*. Hence it, too, is commonly called "vat standing alone." For further details see under "Collected Explanations."

16-23-A02

合明草拾遺 ***He ming cao***, FE *Shi yi*

Aeschynomene indica **L., Indian jointvetch.**

【藏器曰】味甘，寒，無毒。主暴熱淋，小便赤澀，小兒瘈病。明目下水，止血痢，擣絞汁服。生下濕地，葉如四出花，向夜葉即合。

[Chen] Cangqi: Flavor sweet, cold, nonpoisonous. It controls sudden heat and [urinary] dripping, with the urine being red and rough. Spasm disease of children. It clears the eyes and discharges water. It ends bleeding free-flux illness. Pound it, squeeze [the resulting pulp to obtain a] juice and ingest it. It grows on low-lying, moist ground. The leaves resemble flowers with four petals. At night, the leaves close.

16-24

地膚本經上品

Di fu, FE *Ben jing*, upper rank.

Kochia scoparia **(L.) Schrad. Broom plant.**[565]

【釋名】地葵本經、地麥别録、落帚日華、獨帚圖經、王篲爾雅、王帚郭璞、掃帚弘景、益明藥性、涎衣草唐本、白地草綱目、鴨舌草圖經、千心妓女土宿本草。【時珍曰】地膚、地麥，因其子形似也。地葵，因其苗味似也。鴨舌，因其形似也。妓女，因其枝繁而頭多也。益明，因其子功能明目也。子落則老，莖可爲帚，故有帚、篲諸名。

Explanation of Names. *Di kui* 地葵, "ground mallow," *Ben jing*. *Di mai* 地麥, "ground wheat," *Bie lu*. *Luo zhou* 落帚, *Rihua*. *Du zhou* 獨帚[566], *Tu jing*. *Wang hui* 王篲, "the king's herbal broom," *Er ya*. *Wang zhou* 王帚, "the king's besom," Guo Pu. *Sao zhou* 掃帚, "Besom to sweep," [Tao] Hongjing. *Yi ming* 益明, "boosting clear [eyesight]," *Yao xing*. *Xian yi cao* 涎衣草, "saliva coated herb," *Tang ben*. *Bai di cao* 白地草, "whitening the ground herb," *Gang mu*. *Ya she cao* 鴨舌草, "duck tongue herb," *Tu jing*. *Qian xin ji nü* 千心妓女, "whore with a thousand hearts," *Tu su ben cao*. [Li] Shizhen: [It is named] *di fu* 地膚, "skin covering the ground," and *di mai* 地麥 because of the shape of its seeds, and *di kui* 地葵 because of the flavor of its

565 *Di fu* 地膚, lit.: "Ground skin."

566 Instead of *du zhou* 獨帚, *Zheng lei* ch. 7, *di fu zi* 地膚子, quoting the *Tu jing* writes *du sao* 獨掃. The same applies below.

seedlings. [It is named] *ya she* 鴨舌 because of its shape, and *ji nü* 妓女 because of its abundance of twigs and numerous heads. [It is named] *yi ming* 益明 because its seeds have the potential of clearing the eyes. When the seeds fall off, *luo* 落, it is old and its stems can be made to besoms, *zhou* 帚. Hence its names *zhou* 帚 and *hui* 簪[567].

【集解】【別録曰】地膚子生荆州平澤及田野，八月、十月采實，陰乾。【弘景曰】今田野間亦多，皆取莖苗爲掃帚。其子微細，入補藥丸散用，仙經不甚用。【恭曰】田野人名爲地麥草，北人名涎衣草。葉細莖赤，出熟田中。苗極弱，不能勝舉。今云堪爲掃帚，恐未之識也。【大明曰】地膚即落帚子也。子色青，似一眠起蠶沙之狀。【頌曰】今蜀川、關中近地皆有之。初生薄地，五六寸，根形如蒿，莖赤葉青，大似荆芥。三月開黄白花，結子青白色，八月、九月采實。神仙七精散云：地膚子，星之精也。或曰其苗即獨帚也，一名鴨舌草。陶弘景所謂莖苗可爲掃帚者，蘇恭言其苗弱不勝舉，二説不同，而今醫家皆以爲帚。密州圖上者，云根作叢生，每窠有二三十莖，莖有赤有黄，七月開黄花，其實地膚也。至八月而藍幹成，可采。此正與獨帚相合。恐西北出者短弱，故蘇説云耳。【時珍曰】地膚嫩苗可作蔬茹，一科數十枝，攢簇團團直上，性最柔弱，故將老時可爲帚，耐用。蘇恭云不可帚，止言其嫩苗而已。其子最繁。爾雅云：葥，王簪。郭璞注云：王帚也，似藜，可以爲掃帚，江東呼爲落帚。此説得之。

Collected Explanations. *Bie lu*: *Di fu zi* grows in the marshlands and the open country of the plains of Jing zhou. The fruit is collected in the eighth and tenth month. It is dried in the yin (i. e., shade). [Tao] Hongjing: Today much of it can be found in the open country. All [people] gather the stems and seedlings to prepare besoms for sweeping. The seeds are rather small/fine; they are added to pills and powders applied as supplementing medication. The classics of the immortals/hermits do not make much use of it. [Su] Gong: People in the open country call it *di mai cao* 地麥草; the northerners call it *xian yi cao* 涎衣草, "saliva coated herb." Its leaves are fine; its stem is red. It comes from cultivated fields. The seedlings are extremely weak and are easily collected. When it is said today that [this herb] is suitable for making besoms for sweeping, [those who say so] may not be familiar with it. Da Ming: *Di fu* 地膚 is *luo zhou zi* 落帚子. The seeds are of greenish color; they are formed like feces excreted by silkworms when they emerge from their first period of sleep. [Su] Song: Today it can be found everywhere nearby in Shu chuan and Guan zhong. It grows on poor ground, five to six *cun* [tall]. The root is shaped like that of wormwood herbs. The stem is red and the leaves are greenish. It is as

567 The character *hui* 簪 combines *cao* 艸, "herb," and *hui* 彗, "broom."

big as that of *schizonepeta* herbs. It opens yellow-white flowers in the third month and forms seeds of greenish-white color. The fruits are collected in the eighth and ninth month. The [recipe of the] "powder with the seven-fold essence of spirits and hermits/immortals" states: "*Di fu zi* is the spirit of the stars." It is also said: "Its seedlings are *du zhou* 獨帚." Another name is *ya she cao* 鴨舌草. Tao Hongjing says that "the stems and seedlings can be made to besoms for sweeping." Su Gong says that "the seedlings are weak and are easily collected." These two statements differ. Now, today's physicians all consider it to be *du zhou* 獨帚. According to illustrations [of this herb] from Mi zhou "the root grows as clusters, and each nest has 20 to 30 stems. The stems may be red or yellow, and they open yellow flowers in the seventh month. Their fruits are *di fu* 地膚. By the eighth month a trunk has formed that can be collected." This is exactly in agreement with [descriptions of] *du zhou* 獨帚. It may well be that because specimens from the North-West are short and weak Su [Gong] has stated [that the seedlings are weak and can be easily collected]. [Li] Shizhen: The tender seedlings of *di fu* can be prepared as a vegetable. One of them develops several tens of twigs. They form round clusters rising straight up. By their nature they are very soft and weak. Hence they can be made to besoms, withstanding [long-term] use, when they have turned old. Su Gong states: "They cannot serve as besoms." This refers only to the tender seedlings. The seeds are plentiful. The *Er ya* states: "*Qian* 葥 [is] *wang hui* 王蔧." Guo Pu in his comment states: "This is *wang zhou* 王帚. It resembles lamb's quarters and can be made to besoms for sweeping. In Jiang dong it is called *luo zhou* 落帚." This is correct.

16-24-01
子 *Zi*
Seeds [of *di fu*].

【氣味】苦，寒，無毒。【時珍曰】甘，寒。

Qi and Flavor. Bitter, cold, nonpoisonous. [Li] Shizhen: Sweet, cold.

【主治】膀胱熱，利小便。補中益精氣，久服耳目聰明，輕身耐老。本經。去皮膚中熱氣，使人潤澤，散惡瘡疝瘕，强陰。別録。治陰卵㿗疾，去熱風，可作湯沐浴。與陽起石同服，主丈夫陰痿不起，補氣益力。甄權。治客熱丹腫。日華。

Control. Urinary bladder heat. It frees the flow of urine. It supplements [qi in] the center and boosts essence/sperm and qi. Ingested over a long time it sharpens the ears and brightens the eyes; it relieves the body of its weight and helps to endure aging. *Ben jing*. It removes heat from from within the skin, provides one with moisture, disperses malign sores, elevation-illness[568] and conglomeration-illness. It strengthens the yin [qi]. *Bie lu.* It serves to cure ailments related to scrotal breakdown-illness.[569] It removes heat and wind. I can be prepared as a decoction for bathing. Ingested together with "the stone-mineral that lets the yang [qi] rise" (10-01) it controls erectile dysfunction of the yin [member (i. e., penis)] of men/husbands. It supplements qi and boosts one's strength. Zhen Quan. It serves to cure visitor heat[570] with cinnabar-red swelling.[571] *Rihua.*

【發明】【藏器曰】衆病皆起于虛。虛而多熱者，加地膚子、甘草。

Explication. [Chen] Cangqi: All diseases emerge from depletion. In the case of a depletion with much heat, add *di fu* seeds and *glycyrrhiza* [root to a medication].

【附方】舊三，新七。

Added Recipes. Three of old. Seven newly [recorded].

風熱赤目。地膚子焙一升，生地黄半斤，取汁和作餅，晒乾研末。每服三錢，空心酒服。聖惠方。

Heat and red eyes related to wind [intrusion]. Obtain the juice of one *sheng* of *di fu* seeds, baked over a slow fire, and half a *jin* of fresh Chinese foxglove [rhizome], mix [it with the dregs] and prepare a cake. Dry it in the sun and grind it into powder. Each time ingest three *qian*. To be ingested with wine on an empty stomach. *Sheng hui fang.*

目痛眯目。凡目痛及眯目中傷有熱瞑者，取地膚子白汁，頻注目中。王燾外臺秘要。

Painful eyes, dust in the eyes. For all cases of painful eyes and harm caused by dust in the eyes with heat and closure of the eyes, obtain the white juice of *di fu* seeds and repeatedly drip it into the [affected] eyes. Wang Dao, *Wai tai mi yao.*

---

568 *Shan* 疝, "elevation-illness," a group of conditions characterized by violent abdominal pain, in some cases associated with constipation and anuria. BCGM Dict I, 417.

569 *Tui* 㿗, "breakdown-illness," identical to *yin tui* 陰㿉, "yin (i.e. scrotal) prominence-illness", a condition of local swelling and pain affecting a male's private parts. BCGM Dict I, 518, 637.

570 *Ke re* 客熱, "visitor heat," 1.) an etiological agent identified as heat evil intruding into the human organism from outside. 2.) A condition identical to *re* 熱, "heat." BCGM Dict I, 282.

571 *Dan zhong* 丹腫, "cinnabar-red swelling," identical to *dan du* 丹毒, "cinnabar poisoning." A condition of skin ailments brought forth by heat poison, manifesting themselves as red rashes as if from burns, as if cinnabar had been pasted there. BCGM Dict I, 118.

雷頭風腫，不省人事。落帚子同生薑研爛，熱冲酒服，取汗即愈。聖濟總録。

Thundering head wind[572] with a swelling; [patients] fail to recognize persons or anything else. Grind *luo zhou* seeds with fresh ginger to obtain a pulp. Pour boiling hot wine on it, and ingest this. Once [the patient] sweats, a cure is achieved. *Sheng ji zong lu.*

脅下疼痛。地膚子爲末，酒服方寸匕。壽域神方。

Pain underneath the flanks. [Grind] *di fu* seeds into powder and ingest with wine the amount held by a square *cun* spoon. *Shou yu shen fang.*

疝氣危急。地膚子即落帚子，炒香研末。每服一錢，酒下。簡便方。

Critical condition of elevation-illness qi.[573] Fry *di fu* seeds, i. e., *luo zhou* seeds, until a fragrance develops and grind them into powder. Each time ingest one *qian*, to be sent down with wine. *Jian bian fang.*

狐疝陰癩。超越舉重，卒得陰癩，及小兒狐疝，傷損生癩。並用地膚子五錢，白术二錢半，桂心五分，爲末，飲或酒服三錢，忌生葱、桃、李。必效方。

Fox elevation-illness,[574] yin breakdown-illness.[575] When someone has lifted something heavy overexerting himself and is suddenly afflicted with a yin breakdown-illness, and in the case of fox elevation-illness of children with an injury causing a breakdown-illness, [grind] five *qian* of *di fu* seeds, two and a half *qian* of *atractylodes macrocephalla* [rhizome] and five *fen* of shaved cinnamom bark into powder, and ingest with a [rice] beverage or wine three *qian*. [During this treatment] fresh onions, peaches and plums are to be avoided. *Bi xiao fang.*

久疹腰痛積年，有時發動。六月、七月取地膚子，乾末。酒服方寸匕。日五六服。肘後。

---

572 *Lei tou feng* 雷頭風, "thundering head wind," a condition of *tou feng* 頭風, "head wind," characterized by headache together with lumps rising in the face and/or sounds in the head. BCGM Dict I, 303.

573 *Shan qi* 疝氣, "elevation-illness qi," a) a condition of an item having entered the scrotum, with pain, sometimes ascending, sometimes descending, and b) a condition affecting the scrotum or a testicle. BCGM Dict I, 419.

574 *Hu shan* 狐疝, "fox elevation-illness," a condition of *shan* 疝, "elevation-illness," with a sudden swelling and pulling pain affecting the scrotum, and with alternating appearance and disappearance of the swelling. BCGM Dict I, 222 417.

575 *Tui* 癩, "breakdown-illness," identical to *yin tui* 陰㿉, "yin (i.e. scrotal) prominence-illness", a condition of local swelling and pain affecting a male's private parts. BCGM Dict I, 518, 637.

Long-lasting papules and lower back pain for several years, with outbreaks every now and then. Obtain *di fu* seeds in the six or seventh month, dry them and [grind them into] powder. Ingest with wine the amount held by a square *cun* spoon. Ingest this for five to six days. *Zhou hou.*

血痢不止。地膚子五兩，地榆、黄芩各一兩，爲末。每服方寸匕，温水調下。聖惠方。

Unending bleeding free-flux illness. [Grind] five *liang* of *di fu* seeds and one *liang* each of *sanguisorba* [root] and *scutellaria* [root] into powder. Each time ingest the amount held by a square *cun* spoon, to be sent down mixed with warm water. *Sheng hui fang.*

妊娠患淋，熱痛酸楚，手足煩疼。地膚子十二兩，水四升，煎二升半，分服。子母秘録。

Suffering from [urinary] dripping during pregnancy, with heat and severe feelings of pain and soreness. Hands and feet feel a vexing pain. Boil 12 *liang* of *di fu* seeds in four *sheng* of water down to two and a half *sheng*, and ingest this divided into several portions. *Zi mu mi lu.*

肢體疣目。地膚子、白礬等分，煎湯頻洗。壽域神方。

Wart eyes on the limbs and on the body. Boil equal amounts of *di fu* seeds and alum in water and repeatedly wash [the affected region] with the decoction. *Shou yu shen fang.*

16-24-02
苗葉 *Miao ye*
Seedling and leaf [of *di fu*].

【氣味】苦。寒，無毒。【時珍曰】甘、苦。燒灰煎霜，制砒石、粉霜、水銀、硫黄、雄黄、硇砂。

Qi and Flavor. Bitter, cold, nonpoisonous. [Li] Shizhen: Sweet, bitter. Burned to ashes, and boiled in water to obtain a frost, it checks [the effects of] arsenic, sublimed calomel, mercury, sulphur, realgar and sal ammoniac.

【主治】搗汁服，主赤白痢，燒灰亦善。煎水洗目，去熱暗雀盲澁痛。别録。主大腸泄瀉，和氣，澁腸胃，解惡瘡毒。蘇頌。煎水日服，治手足煩疼，利小便諸淋。時珍。

Control. Pound them to obtain a juice and ingest it to control red and white free-flux illness. Burned to ashes they [serve this purpose] well, too. Boiled in water to rinse the eyes they remove dim vision, sparrow blindness, and painful roughness.

Bie lu. They control outflow from the large intestine, harmonize the qi, astringe intestines and stomach, and resolve the poison in malign sores. Su Song. Boiled in water and ingested daily, they serve to cure vexing pain in hands and feet, and free the flow of urine in all cases of [urinary] dripping. [Li] Shizhen.

【發明】【時珍曰】按虞摶醫學正傳云：摶兄年七十，秋間患淋，二十餘日，百方不效。後得一方，取地膚草搗自然汁，服之遂通。至賤之物，有回生之功如此。時珍按：聖惠方治小便不通，用地麥草一大把，水煎服。古方亦常用之。此物能益陰氣，通小腸。無陰則陽無以化，亦東垣治小便不通，用黃蘗、知母滋腎之意。

Explication. [Li] Shizhen: According to Yu Tuan in his *Yi xue zheng chuan*, "my elder brother, aged 70, during autumn suffered from [urinary] dripping. This lasted for more than 20 days and all the hundreds of recipes [applied] remained without effect. Then I obtained a recipe [recommending to] pound *di fu* herbs and ingest their natural juice. It freed [the passage of my brother's urine]. This is a very cheap item and has such a potential of letting one return to [normal] life!" [Li] Shizhen comments: When the *Sheng hui fang* [recommends to] cure blocked urination, it requires one to boil in water one generous handful of *di mai cao* and ingest [the decoction]. Ancient recipes, too, regularly resorted to it. This item can boost yin qi and free the passage through the small instestine. If there are no yin [qi], there is nothing from which yang [qi] can transform. This is also the idea underlying [Li] Dongyuan's treatment of blocked urination when he resorts to *phellodendron* bark and *anemarrhena* [root] to nourish the kidneys.

【附方】新一。

Added Recipes. One newly [recorded].

物傷睛陷，弩肉突出。地膚洗去土二兩，搗絞汁，每點少許，冬月以乾者煮濃汁。聖惠方。

Harm caused by a [foreign] item letting the eyeball cave in. Tumorous flesh growth letting [the eyeball] protrude. Wash two *liang* of *di fu* to remove the soil, pound it and squeeze [the pulp] to obtain its juice. Each time drip a small amount [into the affected eye]. In winter boil dry [*di fu*] to obtain a thick juice. *Sheng hui fang*.

16-25

瞿麥瞿音劬本經中品

Qu mai, 瞿 read *qu*. FE *Ben jing*, middle rank.

***Dianthus superbus* S. Fringed pink.**

【釋名】蘧麥爾雅、巨句麥本經、大菊爾雅、大蘭別録、石竹日華、南天竺草綱目。【弘景曰】子頗似麥，故名瞿麥。【時珍曰】按陸佃解韓詩外傳云：生于兩旁謂之瞿。此麥之穗旁生故也。爾雅作蘧，有渠、衢二音。日華本草云"一名燕麥，一名杜姥草"者，誤矣。燕麥即雀麥，雀、瞿二字相近，傳寫之訛爾。

Explanation of Names. *Qu mai* 蘧麥, *Er ya*. *Ju ju mai* 巨句麥, *Ben jing*. *Da ju* 大菊, *Er ya*. *Da lan* 大蘭, *Bie lu*. *Shi zhu* 石竹, "rock bamboo," *Rihua*. *Nan tian zhu cao* 南天竺草, "southern Tian zhu/India herb," *Gang mu*. [Tao] Hongjing: The seeds very much resemble those of *mai* 麥, "wheat." Hence it is named *qu mai* 瞿麥. [Li] Shizhen: According to Lu Dian in his *Han shi wai zhuan*, "something that grows on two sides is called *qu* 瞿. The spikes of this wheat grow on the sides. Hence [the name]." The *Er ya* writes 蘧. This [character] may be read *ju* 渠 or *qu* 衢. When the *Rihua ben cao* states: "Alternative names *yan mai* 燕麥 and *du lao cao* 杜姥草," this is a mistake. *Yan mai* 燕麥 is *que mai* 雀麥.[576] The two characters *que* 雀 and *qu* 瞿 are quite similar. This is a scribal error.

【集解】【別録曰】瞿麥生太山山谷，立秋采實，陰乾。【弘景曰】今出近道。一莖生細葉，花紅紫赤色可愛，合子葉刈取之。子頗似麥子。有兩種，一種微大，花邊有叉椏，未知何者是也。今市人皆用小者。復一種，葉廣相似而有毛，花晚而甚赤。按經云采實，其中子細，燥熟便脱盡矣。【頌曰】今處處有之。苗高一尺以來，葉尖小青色，根紫黑色，形如細蔓菁。花紅紫. 赤色，亦似映山紅，二月至五月開。七月結實作穗子，頗似麥。河陽、河中府出者，苗可用。淮甸出者根細，村民取作刷帚。爾雅謂之大菊，廣雅謂之茈萎是也。【時珍曰】石竹葉似地膚葉而尖小，又似初生小竹葉而細窄，其莖纖細有節，高尺餘，稍間開花。田野生者，花大如錢，紅紫色。人家栽者，花稍小而嫵媚，有細白、粉紅、紫赤、斑爛數色，俗呼爲洛陽花。結實如燕麥，内有小黑子。其嫩苗煠熟水淘過。可食。

Collected Explanations. *Bie lu*: *Qu mai* grows in the mountain valleys of Mount Tai shan. The fruits are collected at Autum Begins (August 7); they are dried in the yin (i. e., shade). [Tao] Hongjing: Today it comes from nearby. One stem grows fine leaves. The flowers are of amiable deep red, purple and fire red colors. They are collected by cutting them with the seeds and the leaves. The seeds very much resemble wheat seeds. There are two kinds [of *qu mai*]. One kind is a little bigger. The edges

576 *Que mai* 雀麥, *Bromus japonicus* Thunb., Japanese brome.

of the flowers are forked. Nobody knows which kind is the real [*qu mai*]. Today, people on the markets all use the smaller ones. Then there is yet another kind. It has leaves of the same width, but they have hair. Its flowers [open] later and are very red. According to the [*Ben*] *jing*, the fruits are collected. Inside they have fine seeds. When [the plant] is heated they all fall off by themselves. [Su] Song: Today they are found everywhere. The seedlings reach a height of about one *chi*. The leaves are pointed, small and of greenish color. The root is purple-black. It is shaped similar to fine rape turnip [roots]. The flowers are red-purple. When they are of a fire red color, they are similar to those of Chinese *azalea*. They open from the second to the fifth month. In the seventh month they form fruits with spikes and seeds, very much like wheat. The seedlings of specimens from He yang and He zhong can be used [for therapeutic purposes]. Specimens coming from Huai dian have fine roots. The villagers collect them to make brushes and besoms. The *Er ya* calls [*qu mai*] *da ju* 大菊. The *Guang ya* calls it *ci wei* 茈萎. [Li] Shizhen: The leaves of *shi zhu* resemble the leaves of broom plants, but they are pointed and smaller. They also resemble the leaves of small bamboo that have just begun to grow, but are finer and narrower. The stem is very delicate and has nodes; it is more than one *chi* tall. It opens a flower at its end. Those growing in the open country have flowers the size of coins; they are red. Those cultivated by people have small flowers and are quite fascinating. They are of several colors, including fine white, powdery deep red, purple fire red, and multi-colored and bright. They are commonly called *luo yang hua* 洛陽花. They form fruits similar to those of Japanese brome. Inside are small, black seeds. The tender seedlings are washed and then fried in oil, and can be eaten.

16-25-01
穗 *Sui*
Spikes [of *qu mai*].

【修治】【斅曰】凡使只用蕊殼，不用莖葉。若一時同使，即空心令人氣噎，小便不禁也。用時以箽竹瀝浸一伏時，漉晒。

Pharmaceutical Preparation. [Lei] Xiao: For all applications, only the [flower] stamens and their shell are used. Do not use the stem and the leaves. If they happen to be applied simultaneously, an empty stomach will let one have a qi occlusion and an incessant flow of urine. When [the drug] is to be used soak it in bamboo stem juice for one full day, then strain it [to recover the drug] and dry it in the sun.

【氣味】苦，寒，無毒。【别録曰】苦。【權曰】甘。【之才曰】蘘草、牡丹爲之使，惡螵蛸，伏丹砂。

Qi and Flavor. Bitter, cold, nonpoisonous. *Bie lu*: Bitter. [Zhen] Quan: Sweet. [Xu] Zhicai: Japanese ginger and *paeonia* serve as its guiding substances. [Ingested together,] it abhors mantis larvae. It suppresses [the effects of] cinnabar.

【主治】關格，諸癃結，小便不通，出刺，决癰腫，明目去翳，破胎墮子，下閉血。本經。養腎氣，逐膀胱邪逆，止霍亂，長毛髮。别録。主五淋。月經不通，破血塊排膿。大明。

Control. Blockade.[577] Nodes of protuberance-illness.[578] Blocked urination. It lets thorns come out [of the flesh]. It resolves swelling related to an obstruction-illness.[579] It clears the eyes and removes shades. It smashes a fetus and causes abortion of a child. It serves to discharge blocked blood. *Ben jing*. It nourishes kidney qi and repels from the urinary bladder evil [qi] with [qi] counterflow. It ends cholera and stimulates the growth of hair on the body and on the head. *Bie lu*. It controls the five types of dripping and blocked menstruation. It breaks through blood clots and dispels pus. Da Ming.

16-25-02

葉 *Ye*

Leaf [of *qu mai*].

【主治】痔瘻并瀉血，作湯粥食。又治小兒蛔蟲，及丹石藥發，并眼目腫痛及腫毒。搗傅，治浸淫瘡，并婦人陰瘡。大明。

Control. For piles fistula combined with bloody outflow prepare a decoction, or a congee to be eaten. Also, it serves to cure children with roundworms, and effusions related to [an ingestion of] elixirs and mineral drugs. In addition, [it serves to cure] painful eye swelling and swelling with poison. Pound [the leaves] and apply [the pulp to an affected region]. This serves to cure sores soaked [with pus and/or blood] and sores in the yin [(i. e., genital) region] of women. Da Ming.

【發明】【杲曰】瞿麥利小便，爲君主之用。【頌曰】古今方通心經、利小腸爲最要。【宗奭曰】八正散用瞿麥，今人爲至要藥。若心經雖有熱，而小腸虚者服之，則心熱未退，而小腸别作病矣。蓋小腸與心爲傳送，故用此入小腸。本草並不治心熱。若心無大熱，止治其心，或制之不盡，當

---

577 *Guan ge* 關格, "blockade," a condition of an inability to pass stools and urine resulting from an irregularity of the qi dynamics in the organism. This may be accompanied by vomiting. BCGM Dict I, 198.

578 *Long jie* 癃結, "nodes of protuberance-illness." Passing of urine in small amounts; in serious cases passage is completely inhibited. BCGM Dict I, 323.

579 *Yong* 癰, "obstruction-illness," refers to an obstruction of vessels or other ducts inside the body. Qi rushing against the obstruction may cause a local swelling and eventually break through the surface to cause an abscess. BCGM Dict I, 641.

求其屬以衰之可也。【時珍曰】近古方家治産難，有石竹花湯，治九孔出血，有南天竺飲，皆取其破血利竅也。

Explication. [Li] Gao: *Qu mai* frees the flow or urine; [in recipes] it is resorted to as a ruler [drug]. [Su] Song: In ancient and contemporary recipes it is a most important [drug] to open the heart conduits and to free the passage through the small intestine. [Kou] Zongshi: The "powder with the eight rectifying [ingredients]"[580] resorts to *qu mai*. Today, people consider it to be a most important pharmaceutical drug. If it is ingested despite heat in the heart conduits and a depletion in the small intestine, the heat in the heart will not recede and the small intestine will be affected by an additional disease. The fact is, small intestine and heart have a relationship of mutual transmission. Hence, when this [drug, *qu mai*,] is used [for a problem in the heart] it enters the small intestine. The *Ben cao* definitely does not resort to it to cure heart heat. If the heart is not affected by massive heat, [*qu mai*] only serves to cure the heart. If its effects fail to completely end [the problem], it is essential to ask for [assistance by] related [drugs] to weaken [the disease]. [Li] Shizhen: Recently, specialists in the application of ancient recipes in treating difficult delivery resorted to a "rock bamboo flower decoction" to cure bleeding from all the nine orifices. And they also resorted to a "southern Tian zhu/India beverage," always availing themselves of [*qu mai*'s] potential of breaking through blood [accumulation] and opening the orifices.

【附方】舊六，新五。

Added Recipes. Six of old. Five newly [recorded].

小便石淋。宜破血，瞿麥子搗爲末，酒服方寸匕，日三服，三日當下石。外臺秘要。

Urinary stone dripping.[581] It is suitable for breaking through blood [accumulation]. Pound *qu mai* seeds and prepare a powder. Ingest with wine the amount held by a square *cun* spoon. To be ingested three times a day. Within three days the stones will be discharged. *Wai tai mi yao.*

580 Ingredients of the *ba zheng san* 八正散, "powder with eight rectifying[ingredients]," include, in addition to *qu mai*, Asiatic plantain herb seeds, knotgrass, talcum, *gardenia* fruit, prepared *glycyrrhiza* [root], *akebia* herb, and rhubarb root.

581 *Shi lin* 石淋, "stone dripping," a condition of difficult urination, or sudden interruption of urine flow, with an uncomfortable feeling and pain in the urinary tract, an unbearable twisting pain in the lower back and abdomen, and the excreted urine appearing as small stones. BCGM Dict I, 452.

小便不利，有水氣，栝樓瞿麥丸主之。瞿麥二錢半，栝樓根二兩，大附子一箇，伏苓、山芋各三兩，爲末。蜜和丸梧子大。一服三丸，日三。未知，益至七八丸，以小便利、腹中温爲知也。張仲景金匱方。

Blocked urination, with the presence of water qi. This is controlled by the "pills with *trichosanthes* [root] and *qu mai*." [Grind] half a *qian* of *qu mai*, two *liang* of *trichosanthes* root, one large *aconitum* [accessory tuber] and three *liang* each of *poria* and Asiatic cornelian cherry [fruit] into powder and form with honey pills the size of *wu* seeds. One dose consists of three pills, to be ingested three times a day. If this remains without effect, increase [the dose] to seven or eight pills. The effect shows once the urine flow is free and a warm sensation is felt in the abdomen. Zhang Zhongjing, *Jin kui fang*.

下焦結熱。小便淋閟，或有血出，或大小便出血。瞿麥穗一兩，甘草炙七錢五分，山卮子仁炒半兩，爲末。每服七錢，連鬚葱頭七箇，燈心五十莖，生薑五片，水二盌，煎至七分，時時温服，名立效散。千金方。

Bound heat[582] in the lower [section of the Triple] Burner. Urinary dripping with blocked [urination], sometimes with the emission of blood, sometimes with major [defecation] and minor [urination] with the emission of blood. [Grind] one *liang* of *qu mai* spikes, seven *qian* and five *fen* of roasted *glycyrrhiza* [root], and half a *liang* of fried mountain *gardenia* seed kernels into powder. Each time ingest seven *qian*. Boil seven onion tips with the "beard" left, 50 stems of common rush and five slices of fresh ginger in two bowls of water down to 70% and ingest this again and again. *Qian jin fang*.

子死腹中，或産經數日不下。以瞿麥煮濃汁服之。千金方。

A child has died in the abdomen, or it fails to leave [the abdomen] in the course of a delivery lasting several days. Boil *qu mai* to obtain a thick juice and [let the woman] ingest it. *Qian jin fang*.

九竅出血，服藥不住者。南天竺草，即瞿麥，拇指大一把，山卮子仁三十箇，生薑一塊，甘草炙半兩，燈草一小把，大棗五枚，水煎服。聖濟總録。

Bleeding from the nine orifices that has not been stopped by ingesting medication. Boil a thumb-size handful of *nan tian zhu cao*, i. e., *qu mai*, 30 mountain *gardenia* fruit kernels, one piece of fresh ginger, half a *liang* of roasted *glycyrrhiza* [root], one small handful of common rush and five Chinese dates in water and ingest [the decoction]. *Sheng ji zong lu*.

---

582 *Jie re* 結熱, "bound heat." A condition of blocked depot qi brought about by repletion heat evil, with blocked urine and stools, panting, fullness, and spitting because of [qi] moving contrary to its normal course. BCGM Dict I, 252.

目赤腫痛，浸淫等瘡。瞿麥炒黄爲末，以鵝涎調塗眦頭即開。或搗汁塗之。普濟方。

Red eyes with painful swelling. Sores soaked [with pus and/or blood]. Fry *qu mai* until it has assumed a yellow color, and [grind it to [powder]. Mix it with goose saliva and apply it to the canthi [of the affected eyes]. This will open them. Or pound it to obtain a juice and apply it [to the affected region]. *Pu ji fang*.

眯目生翳：其物不出者，生膚翳者。瞿麥、乾薑炮爲末，井花水調服二錢，日二服。聖惠方。

Dust in the eyes with a generation of shades. When the [foreign] object fails to come out and a membrane develops. [Grind] *qu mai* and roasted dried ginger into powder, and ingest, mixed with the first water drawn from a well, two *qian*. To be ingested twice a day. *Sheng hui fang*.

魚臍疔瘡。瞿麥燒灰，和油傅之，甚佳。崔氏方。

Fish belly pin sores.[583] Burn *qu mai* to ashes, mix them with oil and apply this [to the affected region]. Very exquisite. *Cui shi fang*.

咽喉骨哽。瞿麥爲末，水服一寸匕，日二。外臺秘要。

Bone stuck in the throat. [Grind] *qu mai* into powder and ingest with water the amount held by a [square] *cun* spoon. Twice a day. *Wai tai mi yao*.

竹木入肉。瞿麥爲末，水服方寸匕。或煮汁，日飲三次。梅師方。

A bamboo or wooden [splinter] has entered the flesh. [Grind] *qu mai* into powder and ingest with water the amount held by a square *cun* spoon. *Mei shi fang*.

箭刀在肉及咽喉、胸膈諸隱處不出。酒服瞿麥末方寸匕，日三服。千金方。

An arrow or a blade in the flesh, the throat, the chest and diaphragm, all such hidden places, from where they fail to come out. Ingest with wine the amount of *qu mai* powder held by a square *cun* spoon. To be ingested three times a day. *Qian jin fang*.

---

583 *Yu qi ding chuang* 魚臍疔瘡, "fish belly pin sores," identical to *yu qi chuang* 魚臍瘡, "fish belly sores." A condition of *chuang* 瘡, "sores," resembling the long and narrow shape of a fish belly. They have a white or slightly dark spot in their center, and are red on all four sides. Also, the swelling is painful and liquid seeps from it. BCGM Dict I, 650-651.

16-26
王不留行別録上品
Wang bu liu xing, FE *Bie lu*, upper rank.

***Vaccaria segetalis* (Neck.) Garcke. Cowherb.**[584]

【釋名】禁宮花日華、剪金花日華、金盞銀臺。【時珍曰】此物性走而不住，雖有王命不能留其行，故名。吴普本草作一名不流行，蓋誤也。

Explanation of Names. *Jin gong hua* 禁宮花, "forbidden palace flower," *Rihua*. *Jian jin hua* 剪金花, "flower of cut gold," *Rihua*. *Jin zhan yin tai* 金盞銀臺, "silver stand of golden cups." [Li] Shizhen: This item by its nature runs and does not stop. Even if the king has ordered it [to stop] it cannot stop its movement. Hence this name. The *Wu Pu ben cao* writes: "alternative name *bu liu xing* 不流行."[585] The fact is, this is wrong.

【集解】【別録曰】王不留行生太山山谷，二月、八月采。【弘景曰】今處處有之。葉似酸漿，子似菘子，人言是蓼子，不爾。多入癰瘻方用。【保昇曰】所在有之。葉似菘藍。其花紅白色，子殻似酸漿，其中實圓黑似菘子，大如黍粟。三月收苗，五月收子。根、苗、花、子並通用。【頌曰】今江浙及並河近處皆有之。苗莖俱青，高七八寸已來。根黄色如薺根。葉尖如小匙頭，亦有似槐葉者，四月開花，黄紫色，隨莖而生，如菘子狀，又似猪藍花。五月采苗莖，晒乾用。俗謂之剪金草。河北生者，葉圓花紅，與此小別。【時珍曰】多生麥地中。苗高者一二尺，三四月開小花，如鐸鈴狀，紅白色。結實如燈籠草子，殻有五稜，殻内包一實，大如豆。實内細子，大如菘子，生白熟黑，正圓如細珠可愛。陶氏言葉以酸漿，蘇氏言花如菘子狀者，皆欠詳審，以子爲花葉狀也。燈籠草即酸漿也。苗、子皆入藥。

Collected Explanations. *Bie lu*: *Wang bu liu xing* grows in the mountain valleys of Mount Tai shan. It is collected in the second and eighth month. [Tao] Hongjing: Today it can be found everywhere. The leaves resemble those of Chinese lantern plants. The flowers are red-white. The seed shell resembles that of Chinese lantern plants. The fruit inside are round and black, resembling the seeds of celery cabbage. They are as big as glutinous millet. The seedling is gathered in the third month. The seeds are gathered in the fifth month. Root, seedling, flower and seeds are all equally used [for therapeutic purposes]. [Su] Song: Today it is present everywhere, in Jiang, in Zhe and in locations near a river. The seedling and the stem are greenish. They reach a height of about seven or eight *cun*. The root is of yellow color, similar to the

---

584 *Wang bu liu xing* 王不留行, lit.: "The king cannot stop its movement."

585 Instead of *bu liu xing* 不流行, the *Yu lan* ch. 991, *wang bu liu xing* 王不留行, quoting *Wu shi ben cao* writes *wang bu liu xing* 王不流行.

root of sheperd's purse. The leaves are pointed similar to the tip of small spoons. Some are similar to the leaves of *sophora japonica* [trees]. It opens flowers in the fourth month; they are of yellow-purple color. They grow together with the stem and they are shaped like those of celery cabbage, and also like *zhu lan* 猪藍 flowers.[586] Seedling and stem are collected in the fifth month. They are dried in the sun for [therapeutic] use. [The herb] is commony called *jian jin cao* 剪金草. Specimens growing in He bei have round leaves and red flowers. They are a little different from the [item discussed] here. [Li] Shizhen: It often grows in wheat fields. The seedlings are one to two *chi* tall. They open small flowers in the third and fourth month, with a shape resembling bells. They are of red-white color, and they form fruits similar to the seeds of Chinese lantern plants. Their [fruit] shells have five edges; inside the shell is one fruit the size of a soybean. Within this fruits are fine seeds the size of celery cabbage seeds. They are white as long as they are unprepared, and they are black when they are prepared with heat. They are perfectly round like fine pearls; amiable. Mr. Tao [Hongjing] says: "The leaves resemble[587] those of Chinese lantern plants." Mr. Su [Song] says: "The flowers are shaped like those of celery cabbage." Both have failed to examine them carefully. The [shape of the] seeds was confused with the shape of flowers and leaves. *Deng long cao* 燈籠草, Chinese lantern plant, is *suan jiang* 酸漿. Seedling and seeds are used as medication.

16-26-01

苗、子 *Miao, Zi*

Seedling and seeds [of *wang bu liu xing*]

【修治】【斅曰】凡采得拌濕蒸之，從巳至未。以漿水浸一宿，焙乾用。

Pharmaceutical Preparation. [Lei] Xiao: Always after collecting them moisten them and steam them from *si* (9 – 11 hrs.) to *wei* (13 – 15 hrs.). Soak them in fermented water of foxtail millet for one night, bake them over a slow fire and then they may be used [for therapeutic] purposes.

【氣味】苦，平，無毒。【普曰】神農：苦，平。岐伯、雷公：甘。【元素曰】甘、苦，平。陽中之陰。

Qi and Flavor. Bitter, balanced, nonpoisonous. [Wu] Pu: Shen nong: Bitter, balanced. Qi Bo, Lei gong: Sweet. [Zhang] Yuansu: Sweet, bitter, balanced. A yin in yang [substance].

【主治】金瘡止血，逐痛出刺，除風痺内塞，止心煩鼻衄，癰疽惡瘡瘻乳，婦人難産。久服輕身耐老增壽。别録。治風毒，通血脉。甄權。遊風

586 *Zhu lan* 猪藍, unidentified herb.

587 The character *yi* 以 should be an erroneous writing of *si* 似.

風瘮，婦人血經不勻，發背。日華。下乳汁。元素。利小便，出竹木刺。時珍。

Control. It ends bleeding of wounds caused by metal objects/weapons. It expels pain and lets a thorn come out [of the flesh]. It eliminates numbness caused by wind [intrusion] with internal blockage. It ends heart vexation and nosebleed, obstruction-illness and impediment-illness[588] with malign sores and breast fistula. Women with difficult delivery. Ingested for a long time, it relieves the body of its weight, helps to endure aging and extends longevity. *Bie lu*. It serves to cure wind poison and frees the passage through the blood vessels. Zhen Quan. Roaming wind[589] and wind papules.[590] Menstrual irregularity. Effusion on the back. *Rihua*. It serves to let down a nursing mother's milk sap. [Zhang] Yuansu. It frees the passage of urine. It lets bamboo and wooden thorns come out [of the flesh]. [Li] Shizhen.

【發明】【元素曰】王不留行，下乳引導用之，取其利血脉也。【時珍曰】王不留行能走血分，乃陽明衝任之藥。俗有"穿山甲、王不留，婦人服了乳長流"之語，可見其性行而不住也。按王執中資生經云，一婦人患淋卧久，諸藥不效。其夫夜告予。予按既效方治諸淋，用剪金花十餘葉煎湯，遂令服之。明早來云：病減八分矣。再服而愈。剪金花，一名禁宮花，一名金盞銀臺，一名王不留行是也。【頌曰】張仲景治金瘡，有王不留行散。貞元廣利方治諸風痙，有王不留行湯，皆最效。

Explication. [Zhang] Yuansu: *Wang bu liu xing* is used to let down a nursing mother's milk and as a guiding [substance]. This is based on its ability to free the passage through the blood vessels. [Li] Shizhen: *Wang bu liu xing* can run into the blood section. It is a pharmaceutical drug for the yang brilliance, the throughway and the controller [conduits/vessels]. A common saying is: "When a woman has ingested pangolin scales and *wang bu liu* [*xing*], her milk will flow a long way." From this it is obvious that by its nature it moves and does not stop. According to Wang Zhizhong in his *Zi sheng jing*, a woman suffered from [urinary] dripping and lay in bed for a long time. No medication proved effective. One night her husband informed me [of her condition]. I followed the *Ji xiao fang*'s [recommendation on how] to cure all types of [urinary] dripping, and asked him to boil ten or more leaves of *jian jin*

588 *Yong ju* 癰疽, "obstruction-illness, impediment-illness." refers to two vaguely distinguished obstructions/impediments of vessels or other ducts inside the body. Qi rushing against the obstruction may cause a local swelling and eventually break through the surface to cause an abscess. BCGM Dict I, 642.

589 *You feng* 游風," roaming wind," a condition of roaming and sudden pain and itching brought about by *feng xie* 風邪, "wind evil." BCGM Dict I, 645.

590 *Feng zhen* 風疹, "wind papules," a condition, brought forth by wind evil, of eruptive skin papules of different sizes, accompanied by unbearable itching. If scratched they rise further. BCGM Dict I, 172.

hua in water and let [the woman] ingest the decoction. The next day he came early in the morning stating that the disease was diminished by 80%. After a second dose [his wife] was cured. *Jian jin hua* 剪金花, with the alternative names *jin gong hua* 禁宮花 and *jin zhan yin tai* 金盞銀臺, is also known as *wang bu liu xing* 王不留行. [Su] Song: To cure wounds caused by metal objects/weapons, Zhang Zhongjing had the "powder with *wang bu liu xing*." To cure all types of spasms related to wind [intrusion], the *Zhen yuan guang li fang* lists the "decoction with *wang bu liu xing*." Both are very effective.

【附方】舊一，新八。

Added Recipes. One of old. Eight newly [recorded].

鼻衄不止。剪金花連莖葉陰乾，濃煎汁溫服，立效。指南方。

Unending nosebleed. Dry *jian jin hua* with its stem and leaves in the yin (i. e., shade), boil it to obtain a thick juice and ingest it warm. Immediately effective. *Zhi nan fang*.

糞後下血。王不留行末，水服一錢。聖濟總録。

Bleeding after defecation. Ingest with water one *qian* of *wang bu liu xing* powder. *Sheng ji zong lu*.

金瘡亡血。王不留行散：治身被刀斧傷，亡血。用王不留行十分，八月八日采之；蒴藋細葉十分，七月七日采之；桑東南根白皮十分，三月三日采之。川椒三分，甘草十分，黄芩、乾薑、芍藥、厚朴各二分。以前三味燒存性，後六味爲散，合之。每大瘡飲服方寸匕，小瘡但粉之。産後亦可服。張仲景金匱要略。

Blood loss from a wound caused by metal objects/weapons. The "powder with *wang bu liu xing*." It serves to cure bodily harm with blood loss caused by a knife or an axe. Collect on the eighth day of the eighth month ten *fen* of *wang bu liu xing*. Collect on the seventh day of the seventh month ten *fen* of fine leaves of Chinese elder. Collect on the third day of the third month the white skin of a south-eastward stretching root of a mulberry tree. [Also required are] three *fen* of Chinese pepper, ten *fen* of *glycyrrhiza* [root] and two *fen* each of *scutellaria* [root], dried ginger, *paeonia* [root] and *magnolia* bark. Burn the first three substances with their nature retained, [grind] the latter six substances into powder and mix them. Each time ingest for a major wound the amount held by a square *cun* spoon. For small wounds apply the powder [directly to the wound]. It can also be ingested after birth. Zhang Zhongjing, *Jin kui yao lüe*.

婦人乳少，因氣鬱者。涌泉散：王不留行、穿山甲炮、龍骨、瞿麥穗、麥門冬等分，爲末。每服一錢，熱酒調下，後食豬蹄羹。仍以木梳梳乳，一日三次。衛生寶鑑方。

Scant amounts of milk let by a woman because of pent-up qi. The "powder to make a spring gush." [Grind] equal amounts of *wang bu liu xing*, roasted pangolin scales, dragon bones, fringed pink spikes and *ophiopogon* [tuber] into powder. Each time [let the woman] ingest one *qian*, to be sent down mixed with hot wine. Then let her eat a pig trotter gruel and comb her breasts with a wooden comb. Three times a day. *Wei sheng bao jian fang*.

頭風白屑。王不留行、香白芷等分，爲末。乾摻，一夜篦去。聖惠方。

Head wind[591] with white scaling.[592] ['Grind] equal amounts of *wang bu liu xing* and fragrant *angelica dahurica* [root] into powder. Rub it dry into [the hair]. After one night remove it with a comb. *Sheng hui fang*.

癰疽諸瘡。王不留行湯：治癰疽妬乳，月蝕白禿，及面上久瘡，去蟲止痛。用王不留行、東南桃枝、東引茱萸根皮各五兩，蛇牀子、牡荆子、苦竹葉、蒺藜子各三升，大麻子一升。以水二斗半，煮取一斗，頻頻洗之。千金方。

All types of sores associated with obstruction-illness and impediment-illness.[593] The "decoction with *wang bu liu xing*." It serves to cure obstruction-illness and impediment-illness, jealousy breast,[594] lunar eclipse[595], white baldness and long-lasting facial sores. It removes worms/bugs and ends pain. Five *liang* each of *wang bu liu xing*, peach tree twigs reaching toward the South-East and the skin on the eastern side of *zanthoxylum* root, as well as three *sheng* each of *cnidium* seeds, *vitex* seeds, bitter bamboo leaves, calthrop seeds, and one *sheng* of hemp seeds are boiled in two and a half *dou* of water down to one *dou* to repeatedly wash [the affected region].

591 *Lei tou feng* 雷頭風, "thundering head wind," a condition of *tou feng* 頭風, "head wind," characterized by headache together with lumps rising in the face and/or sounds in the head. BCGM Dict I, 303.

592 *Bai xie* 白屑, "white scaling," a condition of fine, small scaling or secretions shed by the skin at locations affected by pathological change. BCGM Dict I, 48.

593 *Yong ju* 癰疽, "obstruction-illness, impediment-illness." refers to two vaguely distinguished obstructions/impediments of vessels or other ducts inside the body. Qi rushing against the obstruction may cause a local swelling and eventually break through the surface to cause an abscess. BCGM Dict I, 642.

594 *Du ru* 妒乳, "jealousy breast," a condition with milk blocked after delivery and the breasts turning red and swelling, being hot and painful, accompanied by fever. BCGM Dict I, 135.

595 *Yue shi* 月蝕, "lunar eclipse," a condition of *chuang* 瘡，"sores" developing on the ears, nose, face, and to the side of the orifices in the anal and genital region. BCGM Dict I, 65.

誤呑鐵石、骨刺不下，危急者。王不留行、黄蘗等分，爲末，湯浸蒸餅，丸彈子大，青黛爲衣，線穿掛風處。用一丸，冷水化灌之。百一選方。

Mistakenly having swallowed an iron item or a stone, or a bone stuck [in the throat] that fails to move down, when this has reached a critical status. [Grind] equal amounts of *wang bu liu xing* and *phellodendron* bark into powder. Soak it in hot water, and prepare a steamed cake. Form pills the size of a bullet, coat them with natural indigo and pierce them with a string to suspend them at a windy location. Dissolve one pill in cold water and force-feed it [to the patient]. *Bai yi xuan fang.*

竹木鍼刺在肉中不出，疼痛。以王不留行爲末，熟水調方寸匕，兼以根傅，即出。梅師方。

A bamboo or wooden [splinter] or a needle is stuck in the flesh and fails to come out. Painful. [Grind] *wang bu liu xing* into powder and [ingest], mixed with hot water, the amount held by a square *cun* spoon. In addition apply the root [directly to the location where the foreign object is situated]. This will let it come out. *Mei shi fang.*

疔腫初起。王不留行子爲末，蟾酥丸黍米大。每服一丸，酒下，汗出即愈。集簡方。

Pin-illness[596] sores that have just begun to rise. [Grind] *wang bu liu xing* seeds into powder and form with toad-cake pills the size of glutinous millet. Each time ingest one pill, to be sent down with wine. Once [the patient] sweats, a cure is achieved. *Ji jian fang.*

16-27
剪春羅綱目
Jian chun luo, FE *Gang mu.*

***Lychnis coronata* Thunb. Mullein pink.**[597]

【釋名】剪紅羅。

Explanation of Names. *Jian hong luo* 剪紅羅, "cut red net."

【集解】【時珍曰】剪春羅二月生苗，高尺餘。柔莖緑葉，葉對生，抱莖。入夏開花，深紅色，花大如錢，凡六出，周回如剪成可愛。結實大如豆，内有細子。人家多種之爲玩。又有剪紅紗花，莖高三尺，葉旋覆，夏秋開花，狀如石竹花而稍大，四圍如剪，鮮紅可愛。結穗亦如石竹，穗中有細子。方書不見用者。計其功，亦應利小便、主癰腫也。

596 *Ding* 丁, "pin[-illness]," also *ding* 疔, "pin-illness," refers to a deep-reaching and festering hardness in a tissue, eventually rising above the skin like a pinhead. BCGM Dict I, 127–129.

597 *Jian chun luo* 剪春羅, lit.: "cut spring net."

Collected Explanations. [Li] Shizhen: *Jian chun luo* grows a seedling in the second month. It is more than a *chi* tall. The stem is soft with green leaves. The leaves grow facing each other, they enclose the stem. By summer flowers of a deep red color open. The flowers are as big as a coin, each with six petals. They form an amiable circle as if cut. They form fruits the size of soybeans with small seeds inside. People often plant them for their joy. Then there is [a plant called] *jian hong sha hua* 剪紅紗花 with a stem three *chi* tall. Its leaves overlap forming a circle. It opens flowers in summer and autumn. They are shaped similar to those of fringed pink, but are a bit larger. On their four sides they look as if cut. They are of a fresh red, amiable color. The spikes they form are also similar to those of fringed pink. Inside the spikes are small seeds. They are not recorded in recipe literature for [therapeutic] use. Presumably their [therapeutic] potential is such that they free the passage of urine and control swelling related to obstruction-illness.[598]

【氣味】甘，寒，無毒。

Qi and Flavor. Sweet, cold, nonpoisonous.

【主治】火帶瘡遶腰生者，采花或葉搗爛，蜜調塗之。爲末亦可。時珍。出證治要訣。

Control. When fire girdle sores grow encircling the waist collect the flowers or the leaves and pound them to a pulp, mix it with honey and apply this [to the affected region]. An application as powder is possible, too. [Li] Shizhen, quoted from the *Zheng zhi yao jue*.

16-28
金盞草救荒
Jin zhan cao, FE *Jiu huang*.

***Calendula arvensis* L. Marigold.**

【校正】併入宋圖經杏葉草。

Editorial Correction. *Xing ye cao* 杏葉草, listed in the Song era *Tu jing*, is integrated here.

【釋名】杏葉草圖經、長春花。【時珍曰】金盞，其花形也。長春，言耐久也。

Explanation of Names. *Xing ye cao* 杏葉草, "apricot leaf herb," *Tu jing*. *Chang chun hua* 長春花, "long-lasting spring flower." [Li] Shizhen: *Jin zhan* 金盞, "golden cup,"

598 *Yong* 癰, "obstruction-illness," refers to an obstruction of vessels or other ducts inside the body. Qi rushing against the obstruction may cause a local swelling and eventually break through the surface to cause an abscess. BCGM Dict I, 641.

refers to the shape of the flowers. *Chang chun* 長春, "long-lasting spring," is to say that it remains alive for a long time.

【集解】【頌曰】杏葉草，一名金盞草，生常州。蔓延籬下，葉葉相對。秋後有子如雞頭實，其中變生一小蟲，脱而能行。中夏采花。【周憲王曰】金盞兒花，苗高四五寸。葉似初生萵苣葉，厚而狹，抱莖而生。莖柔脆。莖頭開花，大如指頭，金黄色，狀如盞子，四時不絶。其葉味酸，煠熟水浸過，油鹽拌食。【時珍曰】夏月結實在萼内，宛如尺蠖蟲數枚蟠屈之狀，故蘇氏言其化蟲，實非蟲也。

Collected Explanations. [Su] Song: *Xing ye cao* 杏葉草, also called *jin zhan cao* 金盞草, grows in Chang zhou. It creeps along below hedges; its leaves face each other. Beginning with autumn it has seeds similar to foxnut fruit. Inside of it small worms develop. [When the fruit] has fallen they can move away. The flowers are collected in mid-summer. Zhou Xian wang: *Jin zhan er hua* 金盞兒花 has a seedling four to five *cun* tall. The leaves resemble the leaves of young garden lettuce. They are thick and narrow; they grow enclosing the stem. The stem is soft and brittle. The flowers open at the top of the stem; they are as big as a finger. They are of golden-yellow color and they are shaped like a cup. Throughout the four seasons they do not wither. The flavor of the leaves is sour. Fried in fat and soaked in water, they are prepared with oil and salt to serve as food. [Li] Shizhen: During summer months it forms fruits in a calyx. They are bent as if these were numerous inchworms. Hence Mr. Su [Song] says: "They transform to worms." These are fruits, not worms.

【氣味】酸，寒，無毒。

Qi and Flavor. Sour, cold, nonpoisonous.

【主治】腸痔下血久不止。蘇頌。

Control. Unending, long-lasting bleeding from intestinal piles. Su Song.

16-29
葶藶本經下品

Ting li, FE *Ben jing*, lower rank.

***Lepidium apetalum* Willd. Wood whitlow grass.**

【釋名】丁歷别録、蕇蒿蕇音典、大室本經、大適本經、狗薺别録。【時珍曰】名義不可强解。

Explanation of Names. *Ding li* 丁歷, *Bie lu*. *Dian hao* 蕇蒿, 蕇 read *dian* 典; *da shi* 大室, *Ben jing*. *Da shi* 大適, *Ben jing*. *Gou ji* 狗薺, *Bie lu*. [Li] Shizhen: The meaning of these names is unexplainable.

【集解】【别録曰】葶藶生藁城平澤及田野，立夏後采實，陰乾。【弘景曰】出彭城者最勝，今近道亦有。母即公薺也，子細黄至苦，用之當熬。【頌曰】今汴東、陜西、河北州郡皆有之。曹州者尤佳。初春生苗葉，高六七寸，似薺。根白色，枝莖俱青。三月開花，微黄。結角，子扁小如黍粒微長，黄色。月令：孟夏之月，靡草死。許慎、鄭玄注皆云，靡草，薺、葶藶之屬是也。一説，葶藶單莖向上，葉端出角，粗且短。又有一種狗芥草，葉近根下作奇，生角細長。取時必須分别此二種也。【斅曰】凡使勿用赤鬚子，真相似，只是味微甘苦耳。葶藶子之苦入頂也。【時珍曰】按爾雅云：蕇，葶藶也。郭璞注云：實葉皆似芥，一名狗薺。然則狗芥即是葶藶矣。蓋葶藶有甜苦二種。狗芥味微甘，即甜葶藶也。或云甜葶藶是菥蓂子，攷其功用亦似不然。

Collected Explanations. *Bie lu*: *Ting li* grows in the marshlands of the plains and in the open country of Gao cheng. The fruits are collected after Summer Begins (May 5); they are dried in the yin (i. e., shade). [Tao] Hongjing: Specimens coming from Peng cheng are the very best. Today, it is also found in regions nearby. The mother [herb] is *gong ji* 公薺. Its seeds are fine, yellow and extremely bitter. Before using them [for therapeutic purposes] they must be simmered. [Su] Song: Today it can be found everywhere in the *zhou* and prefectures of Bian dong, Shaan xi and He bei. That from Cao zhou is especially exquisite. Seedling and leaves grow in early spring, reaching a height of six to seven *cun*. They resemble *adenophora* [herbs]. The root is white; the twigs and the stem are all greenish. Flowers open in the third month; they are a bit yellow. They form horn[-size pods] with flat, small seeds similar to millet, but a little longer and of yellow color. *Yue ling*: "In the first month of summer *mi cao* 靡草 dies." Both Xu Shen and Zheng Xuan in their comments state: "*Mi cao* 靡草 belongs to the group of *adenophora* and *ting li*." It is also said: "*Ting li* has a single stem reaching upward. Horn[-size pods] develop at the end of the leaves. They are coarse and short." Also, there is a kind named *gou jie cao* 狗芥草. Its leaves are close to the root, and they are forked.[599] It grows fine, lengthy horn[-size pods]. When gathering them, these two kinds must be distinguished. [Lei] Xiao: For all [therapeutic] applications, do not use *chi xu zi* 赤鬚子.[600] They are very similar; only the flavor is a bit sweet and bitter. The bitter flavor of *ting li* seeds enters the crown of one's head. [Li] Shizhen: According to the *Er ya*, "*dian* 蕇 is *ting li* 葶藶." Guo Pu in his comment states: "Fruit and leaves all resemble [those of] mustard [herbs]. An alternative name is *gou ji* 狗薺." However, *gou jie* 狗芥 is *ting li*. The fact is,

599 Instead of *qi* 奇, "deviating," "odd," the *Wai tai* ch. 10, *shang qi ke shen mian zhong man fang* 上氣欬身面腫滿方, "recipes of rising qi and cough with bodily and facial swelling and a feeling of fullness," writes *qi* 歧, "forked."

600 *Chi xu zi* 赤鬚子, "red whisker seeds," botanically unidentified.

there are two kinds of *ting li*, one sweet, one bitter. *Gou jie* 狗芥 has a slightly sweet flavor. This is sweet *ting li*. Some say that sweet *ting li* is pennycress. A study of its [therapeutic] potential and usage suggests that this is not the case.

16-29-01
子 *Zi*
Seeds [of *ting li*].

【修治】【斅曰】凡使葶藶，以糯米相合，置於㷉上，微焙，待米熟，去米，搗用。

Pharmaceutical Preparation. [Lei] Xiao: For all [therapeutic] applications, combine *ting li* and glutinous rice and place them above a source of heat[601] to slightly bake them over a slow fire. Then remove the rice and pound [the *ting li* to prepare it for therapeutic] use.

【氣味】辛，寒，無毒。【别録曰】苦，大寒。得酒良。【權曰】酸，有小毒。入藥炒用。【杲曰】沉也。陰中陽也。【張仲景曰】葶藶傅頭瘡，藥氣入腦，殺人。【之才曰】榆皮爲之使，得酒良，惡白僵蠶、石龍芮。【時珍曰】宜大棗。

Qi and Flavor. Acrid, cold, nonpoisonous. *Bie lu*: Bitter, very cold. Combined with wine [its application] yields good results. [Zhen] Quan: Sour, slightly poisonous. For a pharmaceutical application fry it before using it. [Li] Gao: It sinks into the depth. It is a yang in yin [substance]. Zhang Zhongjing: When *ting li* is applied to sores on the head, the qi of this pharmaceutical drug enter the brain and kill that person. [Xu] Zhicao: The bark of Siberian elm trees serves as its guiding substance. Combined with wine it yields good results. [Ingested together,] it abhors white, stiff silkworms and cursed crow foot. [Li] Shizhen: It gets along well with Chinese dates.

【主治】癥瘕積聚結氣，飲食寒熱，破堅逐邪，通利水道。本經。下膀胱水，伏留熱氣，皮間邪水上出，面目浮腫，身暴中風熱痱癢，利小腹。久服令人虛。别録。療肺壅上氣欬嗽，止喘促，除胸中痰飲。甄權。通月經。時珍。

Control. Concretion-illness and conglomeration-illness,[602] accumulations and collections, bound qi, cold and heat resulting from beverages and food. It breaks

601 Instead of *yu* 㷉, "warm," the Qian edition writes *zao* 灶, "cooking stove."

602 *Zheng jia* 癥瘕, "concretion-illness and conglomeration-illness." The two terms are often used interchangeably and do not signify two distinctly different conditions. Concretion-illness and conglomeration-illness result from a disharmony of cold and warmth resulting in a failure to transform beverages and food. Nodes form when the clash with the qi of the long-term depots. BCGM Dict I, 677.

through hardenings and repels evil [qi]. It frees the passage through the pathways of water. *Ben jing*. It discharges water from the urinary bladder, and hidden, abiding heat qi. Evil water ascending from within the skin causing surface swelling of face and eyes. Sudden violent wind and heat stroke affecting the body with seething-rash itching. It benefits/frees the passage through the lower abdomen. Ingested over a long time it causes depletion. *Bie lu*. It heals lung obstruction with rising qi and cough. It ends panting. It eliminates from the chest phlegm rheum. Zhen Quan. It frees the passage of menstruation. [Li] Shizhen.

【發明】【杲曰】葶藶大降氣，與辛酸同用，以導腫氣。本草十劑云：洩可去閉，葶藶、大黄之屬。此二味皆大苦寒，一洩血閉，一洩氣閉。蓋葶藶之苦寒，氣味俱厚，不減大黄，又性過於諸藥，以洩陽分肺中之閉，亦能洩大便，爲體輕象陽故也。【宗奭曰】葶藶有甜、苦二種，其形則一也。經既言味辛苦，即甜者不復更入藥也。大概治體皆以行水走泄爲用，故曰久服令人虛，蓋取苦泄之義，藥性論不當言味酸。【震亨曰】葶藶屬火性急，善逐水。病人稍涉虛者，宜遠之，且殺人甚捷，何必久服而後虛也。【好古曰】苦甜二味主治不同。仲景瀉肺湯用苦，餘方或有用甜者，或有不言甜苦者，大抵苦則下泄，甜則少緩，量病人虛實用之，不可不審。本草雖云治同，而甜苦之味安得不異？【時珍曰】甘苦二種，正如牽牛，黑白二色，急緩不同。又如壺蘆，甘苦二味，良毒亦異。大抵甜者下泄之性緩，雖泄肺而不傷胃。苦者下泄之性急，既泄肺而易傷胃，故以大棗輔之。然肺中水氣膹滿急者，非此不能除。但水去則止，不可過劑爾。既不久服，何至殺人？淮南子云：大戟去水，葶藶愈脹，用之不節，乃反成病。亦在用之有節耳。

Explication. [Li] Gao: *Ting li* massively causes qi to descend. Applied together with acrid and sour [substances] it leads off qi responsible for swelling. The *Ben cao shi ji* states: "Through a release of liquid blockages can be ended. *Ting li* and rhubarb root are of a group [causing such release]." Both these two substances are very bitter and cold. One of them serves to release liquid [to end] a blockage of blood; the other serves to release liquid [to end] a blockage of qi. The fact is, the bitter and cold qi of *ting li* are all strongly pronounced; they are not less pronounced than those of rhubarb root. Also, by its nature it surpasses all other pharmaceutical drugs. By releasing liquid from the yang section it [ends] blockages in the lung; and it can also stimulate defecation. The reason is, its light body reflects the yang. [Kou] Zongshi: *Ting li* has two kinds, one sweet, one bitter. But their physical appearances are identical. The Classic says that its flavor is acrid-bitter, and therefore the sweet kind is no longer used for therapeutic ends. In general, when it is applied to cure the body it serves to stimulate the passage of water and to cause outflow. Hence it is said "used for a long time it causes depletion." The fact is, this is based on the idea of bitter [flavor] causing outflow. The *Yao xing lun* is wrong when it says that "[*ting li*] has a sour flavor." [Zhu] Zhenheng: *Ting li* has a drastic fire nature. It is very good at emitting water. If a patient even slightly nears a condition of depletion, he must stay away from it. It could quickly kill him. How can it be [stated] that one must ingest it for a long time to eventually reach a state of depletion?! [Wang] Haogu: The therapeutic control exerted by the two flavors is not identical. In his "decoction to drain the lung," [Zhang] Zhongjing uses the bitter [kind of *ting li*]. In other recipes he uses the sweet [kind], and sometimes does not specify whether the sweet or the bitter [flavor is meant]. In general, the bitter flavor serves to cause discharge and outflow. The sweet kind is a bit milder. They are to be used taking into regard whether a patient has a condition of depletion or repletion. This must be diagnosed [prior to a treatment]. Although the *Ben cao* states that their curative functions are identical, how could it be that they do not differ given that one is sweet and the other bitter? [Li] Shizhen: The two kinds of sweet [*ting li*] and bitter [*ting li*] are as different as the drastic and mild [effects of] the two differently colored, i. e., black and white, kinds of *pharbitis* [seeds]. Also, the two kinds of flavor of sweet and bitter calabash differ in that one is good and the other is poisonous. In general, the sweet kind has a nature of causing mild discharge and outflow. Even though it serves to drain the lung, it does not harm the stomach. The bitter kind has a nature of causing drastic discharge and outflow. When it is applied to drain the lung, it easily may harm the stomach. Hence it is supported by Chinese dates. Still, in the case of an overwhelming and critical condition of water qi filling the lung, there is no way to emit it without [the bitter kind]. However, once the water is removed, [the application] must end. An overdose is to be avoided. So, when it is not ingested for a long time, how could it kill one? The *Huai nan zi* states: "Peking spurge serves to remove water. *Ting li* cures distension. If their application fails to be moderate, contrary [to one's intention] they generate a disease." Their application should be moderate.

【附方】舊十四，新六。

Added Recipes. 14 of old. Six newly [recorded].

陽水暴腫，面赤煩渴，喘急，小便澀，其效如神。甜葶藶一兩半，炒研末，漢防己末二兩，以緑頭鴨血及頭，合擣萬杵，丸梧子大。甚者空腹白湯下十丸，輕者五丸，日三四服，五日止，小便利爲驗。一加豬苓末二兩。外臺秘要。

Sudden swelling related to yang water.[603] The face is red. A vexing thirst. Hectic panting. Rough urination. The effect [of this recipe] is divine. Fry one and a half

603 *Yang shui* 陽水, "yang water," a condition of a *shui zhong* 水腫, "water swelling," disease with swelling of the entire body, vexation, constipation and difficult urination. BCGM

liang of sweet *ting li* and grind it into powder. Mix it with two *liang* of *stephania tetandra* [root] powder from Han and the blood and the head of a green headed duck. Pound this 10 000 times and [with the pulp] form pills the size of *wu* seeds. For severe cases send down with clear, boiled water on an empty abdomen ten pills. For light cases, five pills. To be ingested three to four times a day. End [the treatment] on the fifth day. When the urine flows freely, this shows the effect. Another [recipe] adds two *liang* of *polyporus sclerotium*. *Wai tai mi yao.*

通身腫滿。苦葶藶炒四兩，爲末，棗肉和丸梧子大。每服十五丸，桑白皮湯下，日三服。此方人不甚信，試之自驗。

Swelling covering the entire body with a sensation of fullness. [Grind] four *liang* of fried, bitter *ting li* into powder and form with the meat of Chinese dates pills the size of *wu* seeds. Each time ingest 15 pills, to be sent down with a white mulberry bark decoction. To be ingested three times a day. This recipe is not very much trusted by people. Test it and it will show its effects.

水腫尿澀。梅師方用甜葶藶二兩，炒爲末，以大棗二十枚，水一大升，煎一小升，去棗入葶藶末，煎至可丸如梧子大。每飲服六十丸。漸加，以微利爲度。

Water swelling and rough urination. The *Mei shi fang* [recommends to] fry two *liang* of sweet *ting li* and [grind them into] powder. Boil 20 Chinese dates in one generous *sheng* of water down to less than one *sheng*. Remove the Chinese dates [from the water], add the *ting li* powder instead and boil this until [a consistency is reached] enabling one to form pills the size of *wu* seeds. Each time ingest with a [rice] beverage 60 pills. Slowly increase the dose until a mild free-flow [of urine/defecation] is reached.

崔氏方用葶藶三兩，絹包飯上蒸熟，搗萬杵，丸梧子大，不須蜜和。每服五丸，漸加至七丸，以微利爲佳，不可多服，令人不堪。若氣發，服之得利，氣下即止。此方治水氣無比，蕭駙馬水腫，服此得瘥。

The *Cui shi fang* [recommends to] wrap three *liang* of *ting li* in thin silk and steam it above rice until done. Then pound it 10 000 times and [with the resulting pulp] form pills the size of *wu* seeds. There is no need to add honey. Each time ingest five pills, and gradually increase this to seven pills. Once a mild free-flow [of uring/defecation] is reached, this is perfect. It must not be ingested in large quantities; that would be detrimental [to one's health]. When a free-flow is reached following an ingestion, with a discharge of qi, end [the treatment]. This recipe has no equal in

Dict I, 619.

curing water qi. Xiao, the Emperor's son in law, had a water swelling. He ingested this [medication] and was cured.

外科精義治男婦大小頭面手足腫，用苦葶藶炒研，棗肉和丸小豆大。每服十丸，煎麻子湯下，日三服。五七日小便多，則消腫也。忌鹹酸生冷。

The *Wai ke jing yi* to cure swelling affecting head, face, hands and feet of males and women, adults and young persons [recommends to] fry and grind bitter *ting li*, mix [the powder] with the meat of Chinese dates and form pills the size of mung beans. Each time ingest ten pills, to be sent down with a hemp seed decoction. To be ingested three times a day. After five to seven days urination will have increased and the swelling will have dissolved. [During the treatment] salty, sour, fresh and cold [food] is to be avoided.

大腹水腫。肘後方用苦葶藶二升炒，爲末。割鵾雄雞血及頭，合擣丸梧子大。每小豆湯下十丸，日三服。

Water swelling of the abdomen. The *Zhou hou fang* [recommends to] fry two *sheng* of bitter *ting li* and [grind them into] powder. Then cut a *kun* 鵾 rooster,[604] mix [the *ting li* powder] with its blood and head, pound this and form [the pulp to] pills the size of *wu* seeds. Each time send down with a mung bean decoction ten pills. To be ingested three times a day.

又方：葶藶二升，春酒五升，漬一夜。稍服一合，小便當利。

Another recipe. Soak for one night two *sheng* of *ting li* in five *sheng* of wine brewed in spring and ingest as little as one *ge*. This will free the flow of urine.

又方：葶藶一兩，杏仁二十枚，並熬黄色，擣。分十服，小便去當瘥。

Another recipe. Simmer one *liang* of *ting li* together with 20 apricot kernels until they have assumed a yellow color, and pound this. Ingest this divided into ten portions. When [the swelling] is removed through urination, this is the cure.

腹脹積聚。葶藶子一升熬。以酒五升浸七日，日服三合。千金方。

Abdominal distention with accumulations and collections. Simmer one *sheng* of *ting li* seeds and soak them in five *sheng* of wine for seven days. Ingest three *ge* daily. *Qian jin fang*.

肺濕痰喘。甜葶藶炒爲末，棗肉丸服。摘玄方。

Lung moisture with phlegm and panting. Fry sweet *ting li* and [grind it into] powder. With Chinese date meat form pills and ingest them. *Zhai xuan fang*.

---

604 *Kun* 鵾, an unidentified fowl.

痰飲欬嗽。含膏丸：用曹州葶藶子一兩，紙襯炒令黑，知母一兩，貝母一兩，爲末。棗肉半兩，砂糖一兩半，和丸彈丸大。每以新綿裹一丸，含之嚥津，甚者不過三丸。篋中方。

Phlegm rheum and cough. The "pills held in the mouth and moistening [the throat]." [Grind] one *liang* of *ting li* seeds from Cao zhou, fried on a piece of paper until they have turned black, one *liang* of *anemarrhena* [root] and one *liang* of *fritillaria* [root] into powder. Add half a *liang* of Chinese date meat and half a *liang* of rock sugar and mix all this to form pills the size of a bullet. Each time wrap in silk one pill and hold it in the mouth. [This will generate] a body fluid [that is to be swallowed]. Even severe cases will require no more than three pills. *Jia zhong fang.*

欬嗽上氣不得卧，或遍體氣腫，或單面腫，或足腫，並主之。葶藶子三升，微火熬研，以絹袋盛，浸清酒五升中，冬七日，夏三日。初服如胡桃許大，日三夜一，冬月日二夜二。量其氣力，取微利一二爲度。如患急者，不待日滿，亦可絞服。崔知悌方。

Cough with rising qi making it impossible to lie down/sleep. Or the entire body has a qi swelling. Or only the face is swollen. Or the feet are swollen. [This recipe] controls all this. Simmer three *sheng* of *ting li* seeds above a weak fire and grind it. Fill [the powder] into a silk pouch and soak it in five *sheng* of clear wine. In winter for seven days, in summer for three days. In the beginning ingest as much as about the size of a walnut. Three times during the day; once at night. During winter months twice during the day and twice during the night. Depending on the strength of the [patient's rising] qi continue this until a minor free-flow occurs, once or twice. If the suffering is critical, do not wait for all the days [required for the soaking] to pass. It is also possible to squeeze [the pouch] and ingest [the resulting juice]. *Cui Zhiti fang.*

肺癰喘急不得卧，葶藶大棗瀉肺湯主之。葶藶炒黄搗末，蜜丸彈丸大。每用大棗二十枚，水三升，煎取二升，乃入葶藶一丸，更煎取一升，頓服。亦主支飲不得息。張仲景金匱玉函方。

Lung obstruction-illness[605] with hectic panting making it impossible to lie down/sleep. This is controlled by the "decoction with *ting li* and Chinese dates to drain the lung." Fry *ting li* until it turns yellow and [grind it into] powder. With honey form pills the size of a bullet. Each time boil 20 Chinese dates in three *sheng* of water down to two *sheng*. Then add one *ting li* pill and boil this again down to one *sheng*.

605 *Fei yong* 肺癰, "lung obstruction-illness," also: *fei yong* 肺壅, "lung obstruction," a condition of abscesses in the lung, with fever, chest pain, and vomiting of bad-smelling pus and blood. BCGM Dict I, 156.

Ingest this at once. It also controls propping rheum[606] making breathing impossible. Zhang Zhongjing, *Ji kui yu han fang*.

月水不通。葶藶一升，爲末，蜜丸彈子大。綿裹納陰中二寸，一宿易之。有汁出，止。千金方。

Blocked menstruation. [Grind] one *sheng* of *ting li* into powder and with honey form pills the size of a bullet. Wrap [one pill] in silk floss and insert it two *cun* deep into the vagina. Replace it after one night. When a sap leaves end [the treatment]. *Qian jin fang*.

卒發顛狂。葶藶一升，搗三千杵，取白犬血和丸麻子大。酒服一丸，三服取瘥。肘後方。

Sudden outbreak of peak[-illness] with madness. Pound one *sheng* of *ting li* 3000 times and form mixed with the blood of a white dog pills the size of hemp seeds. Ingest one pill with wine. A cure is achieved after three [pills] are ingested. *Zhou hou fang*.

頭風疼痛。葶藶子爲末。以湯淋汁沐頭，三四度即愈。肘後方。

Painful head wind.[607] [Grind] *ting li* seeds into powder. Pour hot water over it and use it to wash the head. After three or four applications a cure is achieved. *Zhou hou fang*.

疳蟲蝕齒。葶藶、雄黄等分，爲末。臘月豬脂和成，以綿裹槐枝蘸點。金匱要略。

Gan-illness[608] with bugs/worms gnawing on the teeth. [Grind] equal amounts of *ting li* and realgar into powder. Mix it with lard obtained during the 12th month. Wrap silk floss around a *sophora* tree twig, dip it [into the powder] and then apply it [to the affected teeth]. *Jin kui yao lüe*.

---

606 *Zhi yin* 支飲, "propping rheum," a condition brought forth by rheum flowing into the lung with panting, cough, alternating sensations of cold and heat, vomiting of foam, and a feeling of cold in the back. BCGM Dict I, 681.

607 *Lei tou feng* 雷頭風, "thundering head wind," a condition of *tou feng* 頭風, "head wind," characterized by headache together with lumps rising in the face and/or sounds in the head. BCGM Dict I, 303.

608 *Gan* 疳, "*gan*-illness," also "sweets-illness." A condition of a chronic malnutrition disease resulting from various causes that harm the spleen and stomach and disturb their functions. The major sign is physical depletion, weakness, and emaciation. It may assume numerous different manifestations, each of which has a specific designation. Until the Tang, this was generally considered a disease affecting adults and children alike. Beginning with the Song, this gradually developed into a disease diagnosed in children only. BCGM Dict I, 180.

白禿頭瘡。葶藶末塗之。聖惠方。

White baldness head with sores. Apply *ting li* powder to it. *Sheng hui fang*.

瘰癧已潰。葶藶二合，豉一升，搗作餅子，如錢大，厚二分，安瘡孔上，作艾炷灸之令温熱，不可破肉，數易之而灸。但不可灸初起之瘡，恐葶藶氣入腦傷人也。永類方。

Scrofula pervasion-illness[609] that has begun to fester. Pound two *ge* of *ting li* and one *sheng* of [soybean] relish to prepare a cake, the size of a coin and two *fen* thick. Place it on the opening of the sores and cauterize it with a mugwort wick until it warms up and is hot. The flesh must not be injured. Replace [the cake] several times and cauterize [it anew]. However, sores that have just begun to rise must not be cauterized. The *ting li* qi might enter the brain and harm that person. *Yong lei fang*.

馬汗毒氣入腹。葶藶子一兩炒研，水一升浸湯服，取下惡血。續十全方。

When poisonous qi of horse sweat has entered the abdomen. Fry one *liang* of *ting li* seeds and grind them. Soak [the powder] in one *sheng* of water, boil it and ingest the decoction to stimulate a discharge of malign blood. *Xu shi quan fang*.

16-30
車前本經上品
Che qian, FE *Ben jing*, upper rank

***Plantago asiatica* L. Asiatic plantain.**

【釋名】當道本經、芣苡音浮以、馬舄音昔、牛遺並別録、牛舌詩疏、車輪菜救荒、地衣綱目、蝦蟆衣別録。【時珍曰】按爾雅云：芣苡，馬舄。馬舄，車前。陸機詩疏云：此草好生道邊及牛馬跡中，故有車前、當道、馬舄、牛遺之名。舄，足履也。幽州人謂之牛舌。蝦蟆喜藏伏于下，故江東稱爲蝦蟆衣。又韓詩外傳言：直曰車前，瞿曰芣苡，恐亦强説也。瞿乃生于兩旁者。

Explanation of Names. *Dang dao* 當道, *Ben jing*. *Fu yi* 芣苡, read *fu yi* 浮以; *Ma xi* 馬舄,[610] read *xi* 昔; *niu yi* 牛遺, all: *Bie lu*. *Niu she* 舌, *Shi shu*. *Che lun cai* 車輪菜, "car wheel vegetable," *Jiu huang*. *Di yi* 地衣, "the ground's garment," *Gang mu*. *Ha mo yi* 蝦蟆衣, *Bie lu*. [Li] Shizhen: According to the *Er ya*, *fu yi* 芣苡 [is] *ma xi* 馬舄. *Ma xi* 馬舄 [is] *che qian* 車前." Lu Ji in his *Shi shu* states: "This herb prefers to grow at roadsides and in the hoof prints of oxen and horses. Hence it has names

609 *Luo li* 瘰癧, "scrofula pervasion-illness," when two or more connected swellings of the size of plum or date kernels appear either on the neck or in the armpits, or somewhere else on the body. BCGM Dict I. 329.

610 Instead of *ma xi* 馬舄, *Zheng lei* ch. 6, *che qian zi* 車前子, writes *sheng xi* 勝舄, "equivalent to footsteps."

such as *che qian* 車前, "in front of cars," *dang dao* 當道, "by the road," *ma xi* 馬舄, "a horse's footstep," and *niu yi* 牛遺, "left behind by oxen." *Xi* 舄 is "footstep." People in You zhou call it *niu she* 牛舌, "ox tongue." Small toads, *ha mo* 蝦蟆, love to hide underneath it. Hence in Jiang dong they call it *ha mo yi* 蝦蟆衣, "the small toad's garment." Also, the *Han shi wai zhuan* says: "When they are straight, they are called *che qian* 車前, when they are bent, *ju* 瞿, they are called *fu yi* 芣苡." This may be an arbitrary statement. *Ju* 瞿 is "to grow on two sides."

【集解】【别録曰】車前生真定平澤丘陵阪道中，五月五日采，陰乾。【弘景曰】人家及路邊甚多。韓詩言芣苡是木似李，食其實宜子孫者，謬矣。【恭曰】今出開州者勝。【頌曰】今江湖、淮甸、近汴、北地處處有之。春初生苗，葉布地如匙面，累年者長及尺餘。中抽數莖，作長穗如鼠尾。花甚細密，青色微赤。結實如葶藶，赤黑色。今人五月采苗，七月、八月采實。人家園圃或種之，蜀中尤尚。北人取根日乾，作紫菀賣之，甚誤所用。陸機言嫩苗作茹大滑，今人不復噉之。【時珍曰】王旻山居録有種車前剪苗食法，則昔人常以爲蔬矣。今野人猶采食之。

Collected Explanations. *Bie lu*: *Che qian* grows in the mashlands of the plains, on the slopes of hills and by the road in Zhen ding. It is collected on the fifth day of the fifth month. It is dried in the yin (i. e., shade). [Tao] Hongjing: Very much of it can be found in private gardens and on the roadside. When the *Han shi* says that "*fu yi* is a tree resembling plum trees, and that eating its fruit will have a favorable effect on getting children and grandchildren," it is wrong. [Su] Gong: Today specimens coming from Kai zhou are best. [Su] Song: Today it is present everywhere in the Jiang hu area, in Huai dian, near the capital and in the northern regions. When in spring the seedlings begin to grow, the leaves cover the ground like front sides of spoons. Within a year they grow to reach a length of more than a *chi*. Several stems rise from its center. They form lengthy spikes similar to mouse tails/Japanese *salvia*. The flowers are very fine and dense. They are of greenish color, with some red. They form seeds similar to those of wood whitlow grass; they are red-black. Today people collect the seedlings in the fifth month. They collect the fruit in the seventh and eighth month. Some households plant them in their garden, especially so in Shu zhong. The northerners gather the roots, dry them in the sun and sell them as purple aster root. [This leads to their] very mistaken [therapeutic] use. Lu Ji says that "the tender leaves are prepared to vegetables with a strong smoothing effect." Today people no longer eat it. [Li] Shizhen: Wang Min in his *Shan ju lu* records a method to plant *che qian*, cut its seedlings and eat them. That is, ancient people regularly prepared [*che qian* to be consumed] as a vegetable. Today, people living in the wild still collect and eat it.

16-30-01
子 *Zi*
Seeds [of *che qian*].

【修治】【時珍曰】凡用須以水淘洗去泥沙，晒乾。入湯液，炒過用。入丸散，則以酒浸一夜，蒸熟研爛，作餅晒乾，焙研。

Pharmaceutical Preparation,. [Li] Shizhen: For all applications it must be washed in a pan to remove mud and sand. Then it is dried in the sun. For an application as a decoction it is fried. For an application as pills and powders it is to be soaked in wine for one night. Then it is steamed until done, and ground to a pulp. This is prepared to a cake that is dried in the sun, baked over a slow fire and ground [to powder].

【氣味】甘，寒，無毒。【別録曰】鹹。【權曰】甘，平。【大明曰】常山爲之使。

Qi and Flavor. Sweet, cold, nonpoisonous. *Bie lu*: Salty. [Zhen] Quan: Sweet, balanced. Da Ming: Chinese quinine [root] serves as its guiding substance.

【主治】氣癃止痛，利水道小便，除濕痺。久服輕身耐老。本經。男子傷中，女子淋瀝，不欲食，養肺，强陰益精，令人有子，明目療赤痛。別録。去風毒，肝中風熱，毒風衝眼，赤痛障翳，腦痛淚出，壓丹石毒，去心胸煩熱。甄權。養肝。蕭炳。治婦人難産。陸機。導小腸熱，止暑濕瀉痢。時珍。

Control. It ends the pain of qi protuberance-illness,[611] opens the flow of urination through the water pathways and removes blockage/numbness related to the presence of moisture. Ingested over a long time it relieves the body of its weight and helps to endure aging. *Ben jing*. [It serves to cure] damaged center of males and [urinary] dripping of females with an aversion to eating. It nourishes the lung, strengthens the yin [(i. e., male genital) qi] and boosts the essence/sperm. It lets one have children, clears the eyes and heals painful redness [of the eyes]. *Bie lu*. It eliminates wind poison, wind heat in the liver, poison wind rushing into the eyes, painful redness [of the eyes] with an obstructive shade, and brain pain with tearflow. It suppresses the poison of elixirs and minerals. It removes vexing heat from the heart and the chest. Zhen Quan. It nourishes the liver. Xiao Bing. It serves to cure women with difficult birth. Lu Ji. It leads off heat from the small intestine and ends outflow with free-flux illness caused by summer heat moisture. [Li] Shizhen.

611 *Qi long* 氣癃, "qi protuberance-illness," a condition with an inability to pass urine and a feeling of distension and fullness in the lower abdomen and urinary bladder. BCGM Dict I, 385.

【發明】【弘景曰】車前子性冷利，仙經亦服餌之，云：令人身輕，能跳越岸谷，不老長生也。【頌曰】車前子入藥最多。駐景丸用車前、菟絲二物，蜜丸食下服，古今以爲奇方也。【好古曰】車前子能利小便而不走氣，與伏苓同功。【時珍曰】按神仙服食經：車前一名地衣，雷之精也。服之形化，八月采之。今車前五月子已老，而云七八月者，地氣有不同爾。唐張籍詩云：開州午月車前子，作藥人皆道有神。慚愧文君憐病眼，三千里外寄閑人。觀此亦以五月采開州者爲良，又可見其治目之功。大抵入服食，須佐他藥，如六味地黄丸之用澤瀉可也。若單用則泄太過，恐非久服之物。歐陽公常得暴下病，國醫不能治。夫人買市人藥一帖，進之而愈。力叩其方，則車前子一味爲末，米飲服二錢匕。云此藥利水道而不動氣，水道利則清濁分，而穀藏自止矣。

Explication. [Tao] Hongjing: *Che qian* seeds by their nature are cold and free [the flow of liquids]. The classics of the hermits/immortals, too, [recommend to] consume them, stating "they relieve the human body of its weight, enabling one to jump across banks and gorges, and letting him enjoy a long life without aging." [Su] Song: *Che qian* seeds are very often applied as pharmaceutical drug. The "pills to maintain one's condition" make use of the two items *che qian* [seeds] and *cuscuta* [seeds]. These are pills prepared with honey that are ingested after a meal. They were regarded in the past as an outstanding recipe and are so still today. [Wang] Haogu: *Che qian* seeds can free the flow of urine without stimulating qi to rush. Their [therapeutic] potential is identical to that of *poria*. [Li] Shizhen: According to the *Shen xian fu shi jing*, "*che qian* is also named *di yi* 地衣. It is the essence of thunder. To ingest it lets one's physical appearance transform. It is collected in the eighth month." Today, the seeds of *che qian* are old in the fifth month. When it is said that [they are collected] in the seventh and eight month, the qi of the ground are not the same [as prior to the fifth month]. The Tang author Zhang Ji, in a poem states: "The seeds of *che qian* [collected] in Kai zhou in the fifth month to cure people are gods/spirits positioned on all roads. [I am] grateful to Wenjun, who took pity on my eye disease and sent [this drug] over three thousand Li to a person in need." That shows, in Kai zhou, too, they collect these [seeds] in the fifth month because they are considered to yield good results. Also [from the poem] it is obvious that they have a [therapeutic] potential of curing [the ailments of] the eyes. In general, when they are ingested as food, they should be assisted by other pharmaceutical drugs. The "pills with six substances including Chinese foxglove [rhizome]"[612] are a good example. If used as a single substance they cause too strong an outflow; presumably they are not an item that can be ingested over a long time. Ouyang Gong regularly

612 The ingredients of *liu wei di huang wan* 六味地黄丸, the "pills with six substances, including Chinese foxglove rhizome," are prepared Chinese foxglove rhizome, Asiatic cornelian cherry, Chinese yam, *poria*, *paeonia* root bark, and *alisma* root.

suffered from a sudden/violent discharge disease. The government physicians were unable to cure him. His wife bought on the market a medication. He took it and was cured. Then he tried very hard to [have the merchant disclose] the recipe [and eventually was told "to grind] *che qian* seeds as a single substance into powder and ingest with a rice beverage the amount held by two *qian* spoons." [The merchant] stated: "This drug frees the flow through the water pathways and does not excite the [movement of] qi. Once the flow through the water pathways is free, the clear (i. e., urine) and the turbid (i. e., stool) are separated and the [sudden discharge from the] long-term depot of grain ends."

【附方】舊七，新五。

Added Recipes. Seven of old. Five newly [recorded].

小便血淋作痛。車前子晒乾爲末，每服二錢，車前葉煎湯下。普濟方。

Painful urinary dripping with blood. Dry *che qian* seeds in the sun and [grind them into] powder. Each time ingest two *qian*, to be sent down with a *che qian* leaf decoction. *Pu ji fang*.

石淋作痛。車前子二升，以絹袋盛，水八升，煮取三升，服之，須臾石下。肘後方。

Painful [urinary] dripping with [the presence of] stones. Wrap two *sheng* of *che qian* seeds in a silk pouch and boil it in eight *sheng* of water down to three *sheng*. Ingest [the liquid] and within a short time the stones will be discharged. *Zhou hou fang*.

老人淋病，身體熱甚。車前子五合，綿裹煮汁，入青粱米四合，煮粥食，常服明目。壽親養老書。

[Urinary] dripping disease of old persons, with the entire body feeling very hot. Boil five *ge* of *che qian* seeds wrapped in silk floss to obtain a juice. Add four *ge* of spiked millet, boil this to prepare a congee and eat this. Ingested regularly, it clears the eyes. *Shou qin yang lao shu*.

孕婦熱淋。車前子五兩，葵根切一升，以水五升，煎取一升半，分三服。以利爲度。梅師方。

[Urinary] dripping with heat during pregnancy. Boil five *liang* of *che qian* seeds and one *sheng* of sliced Chinese mallow roots in five *sheng* of water down to one and a half *sheng*, and [let the woman] ingest it divided into three portions for as long as it takes to achieve a free flow [of urine]. *Mei shi fang*.

滑胎易產。車前子爲末。酒服方寸匕。不飲酒者，水調服。詩云采采芣苡，能令婦人樂有子也。陸機注云：治婦人産難故也。婦人良方。

To smoothen [the passage of] a fetus and ease birth. [Grind] *che qian* seeds into powder and [let the woman] ingest with wine the amount held by a square *cun* spoon. If [the woman] does not drink wine, let her ingest it mixed with water. The *Shi* states: "Collect, collect *fu yi*," it can make a woman enjoy having a child. Lu Ji in a comment states: "This is so because it serves to cure women with difficult births." *Fu ren liang fang.*

横産不出。車前子末，酒服二錢。子母秘録。

[A fetus] in a transverse position that fails to come out. [Let the woman] ingest with wine two *qian* of *che qian* seed powder. *Zi mu mi lu.*

陰冷悶疼，漸入囊内，腫滿殺人。車前子末，飲服方寸匕，日二服。千金方。

Cold in the yin [(i. e., genital) section] with heart-pressure and pain, slowly entering the scrotum, eventually causing a swelling and a sensation of fullness that will kill that person. Ingest with a [rice] beverage *che qian* seeds, the amount held by a square *cun* spoon. To be ingested twice a day. *Qian jin fang.*

癮瘮入腹，體腫舌强。車前子末粉之，良。千金方。

Dormant papules[613] that have entered the abdomen. The body is swollen and the tongue is stiff. Apply *che qian* seed powder [to the affected region]. Good. *Qian jin fang.*

陰下痒痛。車前子煮汁頻洗。外臺秘要。

Itch and pain in the yin [(i. e., genital) region] below. Boil *che qian* seeds to obtain a juice and frequently wash [the affected region] with it. *Wai tai mi yao.*

久患内障。車前子、乾地黄、麥門冬等分，爲末。蜜丸如梧子大，服之。累試有效。聖惠方。

Suffering for a long time of an internal shade [in the eyes]. [Grind] equal amounts of *che qian* seeds, dried Chinese foxglove [rhizome] and *ophiopogon* [tuber] into powder, form with honey pills the size of *wu* seeds, and ingest them. Repeated tests have shown that it is effective. *Sheng hui fang.*

613 *Yin zhen* 癮瘮, "dormant papules," identical to *feng zhen* 風瘮, "wind papules," a condition, brought forth by wind evil, of eruptive skin papules of different sizes, accompanied by unbearable itching. If scratched they rise further. BCGM Dict. I, 172.

補虛明目。駐景丸：治肝腎俱虛，眼昏黑花，或生障翳，迎風有淚。久服補肝腎，增目力。車前子、熟地黄酒蒸焙各三兩，兔絲子酒浸五兩，爲末，煉蜜丸梧子大。每温酒下三十丸，日二服。和劑局方。

To supplement a depletion and clear the eyes. The "pills to maintain a condition." They serve to cure a depletion of both liver and kidneys, with a dim vision of black flowers. In some cases this generates an obstructive shade. When exposed to wind, tears are shed. Ingested for a long time, [this medication] supplements liver and kidney [qi] and increases the strength of the eyes. [Grind] three *liang* each of *che qian* seeds and prepared Chinese foxglove [rhizome], steamed in wine and baked over a slow fire, as well as five *liang* of *cuscuta* seeds, soaked in wine, into powder and form with heat refined honey pills the size of *wu* seeds. Each time send down with warm wine 30 pills. To be ingested twice a day. *He ji ju fang.*

風熱目暗，澀痛。車前子、宣州黄連各一兩，爲末。食後温酒服一錢，日二服。聖惠方。

Dim vision with heat caused by wind [intrusion]. The eyes are rough and ache. [Grind] one *liang* each of *che qian* seeds and *coptis* [rhizome] from Xuan zhou into powder. Ingest following a meal one *qian* with warm wine. To be ingested twice a day. *Sheng hui fang.*

16-30-02

草及根 *Cao ji gen*

Herb and root [of *che qian*].

【修治】【斅曰】凡使須一窠有九葉，内有蕊，莖可長一尺二寸者。和蕊葉根，去土了，稱一鎰者，力全。使葉勿使蕊莖，剉細，於新瓦上攤乾用。

Pharmaceutical Preparation. [Lei] Xiao: For all applications it is essential to pick one "nest" [of *che qian*] with nine leaves covering the petals, and a stem of a length of one *chi* and two *cun*. When the petals, the leaves and the root, after removing the soil, weigh one *yi*, their [therapeutic] strength is complete. [Only] the leaves are used for [a therapeutic] application; do not use the petals and the stem. Cut [the leaves] to fine pieces and spread them on a new tile to let them dry. Then they can be used.

【氣味】甘，寒，無毒。【土宿真君曰】可伏硫黄，結草砂，伏五礬、粉霜。

Qi and Flavor: Sweet, cold, nonpoisonous. Tu su zhen jun: They can subdue [the effects of] sulphur. They serve to bind herbs and sand.[614] They subdue the [effects of the] five kinds of alum, and and sublimed calomel.

【主治】金瘡，止血衄鼻，瘀血血瘕，下血，小便赤，止煩下氣，除小蟲。别録。主陰癀。之才。葉主泄精病，治尿血。能補五臟，明目，利小便，通五淋。甄權。

Control. Wounds caused by metal objects/weapons. They end bleeding and nosebleed, stagnant blood and blood accumulation, blood discharge, red urine. They end vexation, discharge qi and repel small worms/bugs. *Bie lu*. They control yin (i. e., scrotal) prominence-illness.[615] [Xu] Zhicai. The leaves control disease of [uncontrolled] outflow of essence/sperm. They serve to cure urination with blood. They can supplement the five long-term depots, clear the eyes, free the flow of urine and open the flow in the case of the five types of [urinary] dripping. Zhen Quan.

【發明】【弘景曰】其葉搗汁服。療泄精甚驗。【宗奭曰】陶説大誤矣。此藥甘滑，利小便，泄精氣，有人作菜頻食，小便不禁，幾爲所誤也。

Explication. [Tao] Hongjing: Pound the leaves and ingest the juice. This is very effective for the treatment of [uncontrolled] outflow of essence/sperm. [Kou] Zongshi: What Tao [Hongjing] says is a great mistake. This pharmaceutical drug is sweet and smooth[ing]. It frees the flow of urine and it drains essence qi. There was someone who prepared it as a vegetable and repeatedly ate it. He experienced an uninhibited flow of urine.

【附方】舊四，新七。

Added Recipes. Four of old. Seven newly [recorded].

小便不通。車前草一斤，水三升，煎取一升半，分三服。一方，入冬瓜汁。一方，入桑葉汁。百一方。

Blocked urination. Boil one *jin* of *che qian* herb in three *sheng* of water down to one and a half *sheng* and ingest this divided into three portions. Another recipe adds wax gourd juice. Still another recipe adds mulberry tree leaf juice. *Bai yi fang*.

614 *Jie cao sha* 結草砂 refers to the chemical method of adding an herbal, *cao* 草, substance to mercury to bind, *jie* 結, it to sulphur and generate cinnabar, *dan sha* 丹砂.

615 *Yin tui* 陰癀, "yin (i.e. scrotal) prominence-illness", a condition of local swelling and pain affecting a male's private parts. BCGM Dict I, 518, 637.

初生尿澀不通。車前搗汁，入蜜少許，灌之。全幼心鑑。

Beginning roughness and blockage of urination. Pound *che qian* [herb] to obtain a juice, add a little honey and force-feed it [to the patient]. *Quan you xin jian.*

小便尿血。車前搗汁五合，空心服。外臺秘要。

Urination with blood. Pound *che qian* [herb] to obtain five *ge* of juice and ingest it on an empty stomach. *Wai tai mi yao.*

鼻衄不止。生車前葉搗汁，飲之甚善。圖經本草。

Unending nosebleed. Pound fresh *che qian* leaves to obtain a juice and drink it. Very good. *Tu jing ben cao.*

金瘡血出。車前葉搗傅之。千金方。

Bleeding wounds caused by metal objects/weapons. Pound *che qian* leaves and apply [the pulp to the affected region]. *Qian jin fang.*

熱痢不止。車前葉搗汁一盞，入蜜一合煎，溫服，聖惠方。

Unending free-flux illness with heat. Pound *che qian* leaves to obtain one small cup of juice, add one *ge* of honey and boil this. To be ingested warm. *Sheng hui fang.*

產後血滲入大小腸。車前草汁一升，入蜜一合，和煎一沸，分二服。崔氏方。

Blood seeping following delivery into the large and the small intestine. Add one *ge* of honey to one *sheng* of the juice obtained from *che qian* herbs, boil this once to bubbling and [let the woman] ingest this divided into two portions. *Cui shi fang.*

濕氣腰痛。蝦蟆草連根七科，葱白連鬚七科，棗七枚，煮酒一瓶，常服，終身不發。簡便方。

Painful lower back related to the presence of moisture. Boil seven *ha mo* herbs with their roots, seven onions with their "whiskers," and seven Chinese dates in one jar of wine and ingest this regularly. [The disease] will not break out in a lifetime. *Jian bian fang.*

喉痺乳蛾。蝦蟆衣、鳳尾草擂爛，入霜梅肉、煮酒各少許，再研絞汁，以鵝翎刷患處，隨手吐痰，即消也。趙溍養疴漫筆。

Throat closure and nipple moths.[616] Add to *ha mo yi* and *dryopteris* [root], pounded to a pulp, the meat of salted plums, boiled in wine, with each [substance] in small amounts, grind them again, and squeeze them to obtain a juice. This is applied with

616 *Ru e* 乳蛾, "nipple moth," acute tonsillitis. A condition with red swelling and pain on both sides of the throat, in severe cases including the generation of pus forming white dots, as a major sign. BCGM Dict I, 410.

a goose feather to the affected location. [The patient] will spit out phlegm right away, and [the problem] is solved. Zhao Jin, *Yang ke man bi*.

目赤作痛。車前草自然汁，調朴硝末，卧時塗眼胞上，次早洗去。小兒目痛，車前草汁，和竹瀝點之。聖濟總録。

Painful, red eyes. Mix the natural juice of *che qian* herbs with mirabilite powder and apply this onto the eyelids at bedtime. Wash it off the next morning. When children have painful eyes, mix the juice of *che qian* herbs with the juice of bamboo stems and drip this [into the affected eyes]. *Sheng ji zong lu*.

目中微翳。車前葉、枸杞葉等分，手中揉汁出，以桑葉兩重裹之。懸陰處一夜，破桑葉取點，不過三五度。十便良方。

A slight shade in the eyes. Knead equal amounts of *che qian* leaves and *lycium* leaves in your hand to let their juice come out. Wrap it with two layers of mulberry tree leaves and suspend this at a shady location for one night. Break the mulberry tree leaves to obtain [the juice] and drop it [into the affected eyes]. No more than three to five [applications required]. *Shi bian liang fang*.

16-31
狗舌草唐本草
Gou she cao, FE *Tang ben cao*.

***Senecio kirilowii* Turcz. Dog's tongue herb.**

【集解】【恭曰】狗舌草生渠塹濕地，叢生。葉似車前而無文理，抽莖開花，黄白色。四月、五月采莖，暴乾。

Collected Explanations. [Su] Gong: *Gou she cao* grows in the marshlands along ditches and moats. It grows as clusters. The leaves resemble those of Asiatic plantain but have no line design. A stem rises and opens flowers of a yellow-white color. The stem is collected in the fourth and fifth month. It is dried in the sun.

【氣味】苦，寒，有小毒。

Qi and Flavor. Bitter, cold, slightly poisonous.

【主治】蟲疥瘙瘡，殺小蟲。爲末和塗之，即瘥。蘇恭。

Control. Gu [poison],[617] *jie*-illness[618] and itching sores. It kills small worms/bugs. [Grind it into] powder and apply it [to the affected region]. This results in a cure. Su Gong.

16-32
馬鞭草别録下品
***Ma bian cao*. FE *Bie lu*, lower rank.**

***Verbena officinalis* L. Vervain.**

【校正】併入圖經龍牙草。

Editorial Correction. *Long ya cao* 龍牙草 from the *Tu jing* is inserted here.

【釋名】龍牙草圖經、鳳頸草。【恭曰】穗類鞭鞘，故名馬鞭。【藏器曰】此説未近，乃其節生紫花如馬鞭節耳。【時珍曰】龍牙、鳳頸，皆因穗取名。蘇頌圖經外類重出"龍牙"，今併爲一。又今方士謬立諸草爲各色龍牙之名，甚爲淆亂，不足憑信。

Explanation of Names. *Long ya cao* 龍牙草, "dragon tooth herb," *Tu jing*. *Feng jing cao* 鳳頸草, "phoenix neck herb." [Su] Gong: The spikes resemble whips, *bian shao* 鞭鞘. Hence the name *ma bian* 馬鞭, "horse whip." [Chen] Cangqi: This statement fails to come close to it. The nodes grow purple flowers resembling the nodes of horsewhips. [Li] Shizhen: *Long ya* 龍牙, "dragon teeth," and *feng jing* 鳳頸, "phoenix neck," are names related to the [shape of the] spikes. In the section *wai lei* 外類, "further [substances]," of the *Tu jing*, Su Song lists *long ya* 龍牙, [thereby listing *ma bian cao*] twice. Here now they are combined in one entry. Also, today recipe experts mistakenly attribute the name *long ya* 龍牙 to several herbs of different color. This causes great confusion. It should not be believed.

【集解】【弘景曰】村墟陌甚多。莖似細辛，花紫色，微似蓬蒿也。【恭曰】葉似狼牙及茺蔚，抽三四穗，紫花，似車前，穗類鞭鞘，都不似蓬蒿也。【保昇曰】花白色，七月、八月采苗葉，日乾用。頌曰】今衡山、廬山、江淮州郡皆有之。苗類益母而莖圓，高二三尺。又曰：龍牙草生施州，高二尺以來。春夏有苗葉，至秋冬而枯。采根，洗净用。【時珍曰】馬鞭下地甚多，春月生苗，方莖，葉似益母，對生，夏秋開細紫花，作穗如車前穗，其子如蓬蒿子而細，根白而小。陶言花似蓬蒿，韓言花色白，蘇言莖圓，皆誤矣。

617 *Gu du* 蠱毒, "*gu*-poison[ing]." (1) A poison emitted by certain worms/snakes with an ability to cause varying pathological changes in a person who has taken it in by means of wine or food. (2) Abdominal fullness, in some cases with blood spitting, and blood in the stool and urine. BCGM Dict I, 192 - 193. See BCGM 42-22.

618 *Jie*-illness 疥, vaguely identifiable skin ailment. BCGM Dict I, 249.

Collected Explanations. [Tao] Hongjing: Very much of it can be found on the paths between village ruins. The stem resembles that of *asarum heterpoides*. The flowers are purple, slightly[619] resembling those of garden daisy herbs. [Su] Gong: The leaves resemble those of *agrimonia* and Siberian motherwort herbs. It develops three to four spikes. The purple flowers resemble those of Asiatic plantain. The spikes are like whips. In no respect [*ma bian cao*] resembles garden daisy herbs. [Han] Baosheng: The flowers are white. Seedling and leaves are collected in the seventh and eighth month. For [therapeutic] application they are dried in the sun. [Su] Song: Today it is found on Mount Heng shan and Mount Lu shan and everywhere in the *zhou* and prefectures of the Jiang Huai region. The seedlings resemble those of Siberian motherwort herbs, but their stem is round. They are two to three *chi* tall. It is also said: *Long ya cao* grows in Shi zhou, reaching a height of about two *chi*. It has seedlings with leaves during spring and summer. By autumn and in winter they wither. The root is collected and washed clean for [therapeutic] use. [Li] Shizhen: Much *ma bian* can be found on low-lying ground. It grows a seedling with a square stem during spring months. The leaves resemble those of Siberian motherwort herbs. They grow facing each other. Fine, purple flowers open during summer and autumn. They form spikes similar to Asiatic plantain spikes. The seeds are similar to those of garden daisy herbs, but are finer. The root is white and small. Tao [Hongjing] says: "The flowers resemble those of garden daisy herbs." Han [Baosheng] says: "The flowers are white." [Su] Song says: "The stem is round." They are all wrong.

16-32-01
苗、葉 *Miao, Ye*
Seedling and leaf [of *ma bian cao*].

【氣味】苦，微寒，無毒。保昇。【大明曰】辛，涼，無毒。【權曰】苦，有毒。伏丹砂、硫黄。

Qi and Flavor. Bitter, slightly cold, nonpoisonous. [Han] Baosheng. Da Ming: Acrid, cool, nonpoisonous. [Zhen] Quan: Bitter, poisonous. They subdue [the effects of] cinnabar and sulphur.

【主治】下部䘌瘡。别録。癥瘕血瘕，久瘧，破血殺蟲。擣爛煎取汁，熬如飴，每空心酒服一匕。藏器。治婦人血氣肚脹，月候不匀，通月經。大明。治金瘡，行血活血。震亨。擣塗癰腫及蠼螋尿瘡，男子陰腫。時珍。

619 In front of *wei* 微, "slightly," *Zheng lei* ch. 11, *ma bian cao* 馬鞭草, writes *ye* 葉, "leaf." However, further down Li Shizhen says: 陶言花似蓬蒿, "Tao [Hongjing] says: 'The flowers resemble those of garden daisy [herbs]'." That is, the edition consulted by Li Shizhen may not have had the character *ye* 葉.

Control. Hidden worms/bugs sores in the lower (i. e., genital) body section. *Bie lu*. . Concretion-illness and conglomeration-illness,[620] Blood conglomeration-illness. Long-lasting malaria. They break through blood [accumulation] and kill worms/bugs. Pound them to a pulp, boil it and take the juice. Simmer it to a consistency similar to sugar. Each time ingest a spoonful with wine on an empty stomach. [Chen] Cangqi. They serve to cure stomach distension of women related to blood and qi [disorder]. Irregular menstruation. Blocked menstruation. Da Ming. They serve to cure wounds caused by metal objects/weapons. They stimulate the flow of blood, and they quicken the flow of blood. [Zhu] Zhenheng. Pound them and apply [the pulp] to swelling related to an obstruction-illness,[621] to earwig urine sores[622] and to swelling in the yin [(i. e., genital) region] of males. [Li] Shizhen.

【附方】舊五，新十。

Added Recipes. Five of old. Ten newly [recorded].

瘧痰寒熱。馬鞭草擣汁五合，酒二合，分二服。千金方。

Malaria with phlegm and alternating sensations of cold and heat. Pound *ma bian cao* to obtain five *ge* of its juice. Mix it with two *ge* of wine and ingest this divided into two portions. *Qian jin fang*.

鼓脹煩渴，身乾黑瘦。馬鞭草細剉，曝乾，勿見火。以酒或水同煮，至味出，去滓溫服。以六月中旬雷鳴時采者有效。衛生易簡方。

Drum-like [abdominal distension] with vexing thirst. The body is dry and black and emaciated. Cut *ma bian cao* to fine pieces. Dry them in the sun; do not expose them to fire. Boil them with wine or water until they emit a flavor. Discard the dregs and ingest the warm [liquid]. [*Ma bian cao*] is effective when it is collected in the middle period of the sixth month at the moment of thunder sounds. *Wei sheng yi jian fang*.

---

620 *Zheng jia* 癥瘕, "concretion-illness and conglomeration-illness." The two terms are often used interchangeably and do not signify two distinctly different conditions. Concretion-illness and conglomeration-illness result from a disharmony of cold and warmth resulting in a failure to transform beverages and food. Nodes form when the clash with the qi of the long-term depots. BCGM Dict I, 677.

621 *Yong* 癰, "obstruction-illness,"refers to an obstruction of vessels or other ducts inside the body. Qi rushing against the obstruction may cause a local swelling and eventually break through the surface to cause an abscess. BCGM Dict I, 641.

622 *Qu sou niao chuang* 蠼螋尿瘡, "earwig-urine sores." A condition forming clusters of blisters on the chest, flanks and lower back with an excruciatingly piercing pain, accompanied by strong heat and an aversion to cold, as a major sign. This condition is reminiscent of the neurological disease herpes zoster. Formerly it was believed that the urine of earwigs, when touched by the shadow of a human, would cause this person to suffer from this disease. BCGM Dict I, 392.

大腹水腫。馬鞭草、鼠尾草各十斤，水一石，煮取五斗，去滓，再煎令稠，以粉和丸大豆大。每服二三丸，加至四五丸，神效。肘後方。

Abdominal water swelling. Boil ten *jin* each of *ma bian cao* and Japanese *salvia* in one *dan* of water down to five *dou*. Remove the dregs and boil [the liquid] again until it is viscous. Mix it with rice powder to form pills the size of soybeans. Each time ingest two or three pills and increase the amount to four or five pills. Divinely effective. *Zhou hou fang*.

男子陰腫大如升，核痛，人所不能治者，馬鞭草搗塗之。集驗方。

A swelling the size of a *sheng* in a male's yin [(i.e., genital) region], with painful testicles, that no one could heal. Pound *ma bian cao* and apply [the pulp to the affected region]. *Ji yan fang*.

婦人疝痛，名小腸氣。馬鞭草一兩，酒煎滚服，以湯浴身取汗，甚妙。纂要奇方。

Painful elevation-illness[623] of women, called "small intestine qi." Boil one *liang* of *ma bian cao* in wine and ingest it hot. Use the decoction to wash the body until it sweats. Very wondrous. *Zuan yao qi fang*.

婦人經閉，結成瘕塊，肋脹大欲死者。馬鞭草根苗五斤，剉細，水五斗，煎至一斗，去滓，熬成膏。每服半匙，食前温酒化下，日二服。聖惠方。

Women with blocked menstruation, forming conglomeration-illness lumps and a distension of the ribs so large that [the patient] wishes to die. Cut five *jin* of *ma bian cao* root and seedling to fine pieces and boil them in five *dou* of water down to one *dou*. Discard the dregs and simmer [the liquid] to generate a paste. Each time [let the woman] ingest a spoonful, to be sent down prior to a meal dissolved in warm wine. *Sheng hui fang*.

酒積下血：馬鞭草灰四錢，白芷灰一錢，蒸餅丸梧子大。每米飲下五十丸。摘玄方。

An accumulation of wine resulting in a discharge with blood. Form with steamed cake four *qian* of *ma bian cao* ashes and *angelica dahurica* [root] ashes to pills the size of *wu* seeds. Each time send down with a rice beverage 50 pills. *Zhai xuan fang*.

623 *Shan* 疝, "elevation-illness," a group of conditions characterized by violent abdominal pain, in some cases associated with constipation and anuria. BCGM Dict I, 417.

魚肉癥瘕。凡食魚鱠及生肉，在胸膈不化，成癥瘕，馬鞭草搗汁，飲一升，即消。千金方。

Concretion-illness and conglomeration-illness[624] caused by fish or meat. Whenever a consumption of minced fish or raw meat, that fail to be transformed in the chest and diaphragm region, results in concretion-illness and conglomeration-illness, pound *ma bian cao* to obtain a juice and drink one *sheng*. This will dissolve [the concretion/conglomeration). *Qian jin fang*.

喉痺風，躁腫連頰，吐氣數者。馬鞭草一握，勿見風，截去兩頭，搗汁飲之，良。千金方。

Throat blockage wind [as fast as a running horse][625] with restlessness, a swelling of the adjoing cheeks and frequent spitting of qi. Take a handful of *ma bian cao*, do not expose it to wind, and cut off the two ends [of the seedlings]. Pound them to obtain a juice and ingest it. Good. *Qian jin fang*.

乳癰腫痛。馬鞭草一握，酒一椀，生薑一塊，擂汁服，渣傅之。衛生易簡方。

Painful swelling related to breast obstruction-illness.[626] Pound a handful of *ma bian cao* in one bowl of wine with one piece of fresh ginger and [let the woman] ingest the juice. Apply the dregs [to the affected region]. *Wei sheng yi jian fang*.

白癩風瘡。馬鞭草爲末。每服一錢，食前荆芥、薄荷湯下，日三服。忌鐵器。太平聖惠方。

White repudiation-illness (i. e., massive) wind[627] sores. [Grind] *ma bian cao* into powder. Each time ingest one *qian*, to be sent down prior to a meal with a *schizonepeta* and mint decoction. To be ingested three times a day. [In the course of this treatment] iron utensils are to be avoided. *Tai ping sheng hui fang*.

---

624 *Zheng jia* 癥瘕, "concretion-illness and conglomeration-illness." The two terms are often used interchangeably and do not signify two distinctly different conditions. Concretion-illness and conglomeration-illness result from a disharmony of cold and warmth resulting in a failure to transform beverages and food. Nodes form when the clash with the qi of the long-term depots. BCGM Dict I, 677.

625 [*Ma*] *hou bi feng* [馬]喉痹風, "throat blockage wind [as fast as a running horse]," identical to *ji hou bi* 急喉痹, "acute throat blockage." BCGM Dict I, 332.

626 *Ru yong* 乳癰, "breast obstruction-illness," a condition of acute putrefication of a woman's breast. Often encountered if a woman, following delivery, experiences *chui nai* 吹奶, "inflated breast," or *du ru* 妒乳, "jealousy breast." BCGM Dict I, 412.

627 *Da feng lai* 大風癩, "massive wind [i. e.,] repudiation-illness," most likely including cases of leprosy/Aussatz. BCGM Dict I, 111, 293

人疥馬疥。馬鞭草不犯鐵器，搗自然汁半盞，飲盡，十日內愈，神效。董炳集驗方。

Jie-illness[628] of humans and of horses. Pound *ma bian cao*, do not allow it to be offended by iron utensils, to obtain half a cup of its natural juice and [let the patient/horse] ingest all of it. A cure is achieved within ten days. Divinely effective. Dong Bing, *Ji yan fang*.

赤白下痢。龍牙草五錢，陳茶一撮，水煎服，神效。醫方摘要。

Red and white discharge with free-flux illness. Boil in water five *qian* of *long ya cao* and a pinch of long-stored tea and ingest this. Divinely effective. *Yi fang zhai yao*.

發背癰毒。痛不可忍，龍牙草搗汁飲之。以滓傅患處。集簡方。

Obstruction-illness[629] poison effusing on the back,[630] with an unbearable pain. Pound *long ya cao* to obtain a juice and drink it. Apply the dregs to the location of the suffering. *Ji jian fang*.

楊梅惡瘡。馬鞭草煎湯，先熏後洗，氣到便爽，痛腫隨減。陳嘉謨本草蒙筌。

Malign red bayberry sores.[631] Boil *ma bian cao* to obtain a decoction. First steam [the affected region with it], then wash [the affected region with it]. Once the qi reach there, [the patient] feels good and the pain and the swelling decrease. Chen Jiamo, *Ben cao meng quan*.

16-32-02

根 *Gen*

Root [of *ma bian cao*].

【氣味】辛、濇，温，無毒。

Qi and Flavor. Acrid, astringent, warm, nonpoisonous.

【主治】赤白下痢初起，焙搗羅末，每米飲服一錢匕，無所忌。蘇頌。

628 *Jie*-illness 疥, vaguely identifiable skin ailment. BCGM Dict I, 249.

629 *Yong* 癰, "obstruction-illness," refers to an obstruction of vessels or other ducts inside the body. Qi rushing against the obstruction may cause a local swelling and eventually break through the surface to cause an abscess. BCGM Dict I, 641.

630 *Fa bei* 發背, "effusion on/of the back," a condition of *yong* 癰, "obstruction-illnesses," and *ju* 疽, "impediment-illnesses," developing on one's back. As it was believed that the transporter holes of the five depots and six palaces are located on the back, conditions of obstruction-illnesses and impediment-illnesses there, often apparent as abscesses, were considered threatening. BCGM Dict I, 148.

631 *Yang mei chuang* 楊梅瘡, "red bayberry sores," A condition of syphilitic sores affecting the entire body resulting from an infectious sores poison. BCGM Dict I, 618.

Control. Red and white discharge with free-flux illness at an early stage. Bake [the root] over a slow fire, pound it, and sieve it through a net to obtain a powder. Each time ingest with a rice beverage the amount held by a one *qian* spoon. [During this treatment] nothing is to be avoided. Su Song.

16-33
蛇含本經下品

She han, FE *Ben jing*, lower rank.

Potentilla kleiniana **Wight et Arn. Kleinian cinquefoil.**

【校正】併入圖經紫背龍牙。

Editorial Correction. *Zi bei long ya* 紫背龍牙, listed [separately] in the *Tu jing*, is included here.

【釋名】蛇銜本經、威蛇大明、小龍牙綱目、紫背龍牙。【恭曰】陶氏本草作蛇合，合乃含字之誤也。含、銜義同。見古本草。【時珍曰】按劉敬叔異苑云：有田父見一蛇被傷，一蛇銜一草着瘡上，經日傷蛇乃去。田父因取草治蛇瘡皆驗，遂名曰蛇銜草也。其葉似龍牙而小，背紫色，故俗名小龍牙，又名紫背龍牙。蘇頌圖經重出"紫背龍牙"，今併爲一。

Explanation of Names. *She xian* 蛇銜, *Ben jing*. *Wei she* 威蛇, "awesome snake," Da Ming. *Xiao long ya* 小龍牙, *Gang mu*. *Zi bei long ya* 紫背龍牙. [Su] Gong: The *Tao shi ben cao* writes *she he* 蛇合. *He* 合 is a mistaken writing of the character *han* 含. The meaning of *han* 含 and *xian* 銜 is identical. See the ancient *Ben cao* works. [Li] Shizhen: According to Liu Jingshu's *Yi yuan*, "a farmer observed a snaked that was harmed. Another snake in its mouth held an herb and attached it to the wound. After one day the harmed snake left. The farmer gathered the herb and used it to cure wounds caused by snakes; it has always been effective and henceforth was named *she xian cao* 蛇銜草, 'herb held by a snake in its mouth'." The leaves resemble small dragon teeth. They are purple on their back. Hence the names *xiao long ya* 小龍牙 "small dragon teeth," and also *zi bei long ya* 紫背龍牙, "teeth of the purple back dragon." Su Song in his *Tu jing* lists *zi bei long ya* 紫背龍牙 [in a separate entry, thereby listing *she han*] twice. They are combined here in one entry.

【集解】【別録曰】蛇含出益州山谷，八月采，陰乾。【弘景曰】蛇銜處處有之。有兩種，並生石上，亦生黄土地。當用細葉有黄花者。【頌曰】出益州，今近處亦有。生土石上或下濕地，蜀中人家亦種之，辟蛇。一莖五葉或七葉，有兩種。八月采根，陰乾。日華子云：莖葉俱用，五月采之。又曰：紫背龍牙，生蜀中，春夏生葉，采無時。【時珍曰】此二種，細葉者名蛇銜，大葉者名龍銜。龍銜亦入瘡膏用。【斅曰】蛇銜只用葉晒乾，勿犯火。根莖不用。勿誤用有蘖尖葉者，號竟命草，其味酸澀。誤服令人吐血不止，速服知時子解之。

Collected Explanations. *Bie lu*: *She han* comes from the mountain valleys of Yi zhou. It is collected in the eighth month; it is dried in the yin (i. e., shade). [Tao] Hongjing: *She xian* can be found everywhere. There are two kinds of it, both growing on rocks, and they also grow on yellow soil ground. For [therapeutic applications] those with fine leaves and yellow flowers are to be used. [Su] Song: It comes from Yi zhou. Today it can also be found nearby. It grows on soil and rocks, and also on low-lying, moist ground. People in Shu zhong also plant it to repel snakes. One stem has five leaves or seven leaves; there are two kinds. The root is collected in the eighth month; it is dried in the yin (i. e., shade). *Rihua zi* states: Stem and leaves are all used [for therapeutic purposes]. They are collected in the fifth month. It is also said: *Zi bei long ya* grows in Shu zhong. It grows leaves in spring and summer; they can be collected anytime. [Li] Shizhen: These two kinds, those with fine leaves are called *she xian* 蛇銜, "snake bit," those with big leaves are called *long xian* 龍銜, "dragon bit." *Long xian* is also used as an ingredient of ointments for sores. [Lei] Xiao: Of *she xian* only the leaves are used [for therapeutic purposes]. They are dried in the sun and must not be exposed to fire. The root and the stem are not used. Do not use those with pointed leaves of their shoots. This [plant] is called *jing ming cao* 竟命草, the "herb that lets one complete the entire lifespan."[632] Its flavor is sour and astringent. If ingested mistakenly it causes unending spitting of blood. To resolve this quickly ingest *zhi shi* seeds.[633]

【氣味】苦，微寒，無毒。【權曰】有毒。【頌曰】紫背龍牙：辛，寒，無毒。

Qi and Flavor. Bitter, slightly cold, nonpoisonous. [Zhen] Quan: Poisonous. [Su] Song: *Zi bei long ya*: Acrid, cold, nonpoisonous.

【主治】驚癎，寒熱邪氣，除熱，金瘡疽痔，鼠瘻惡瘡，頭瘍。本經。療心腹邪氣，腹痛濕痺，養胎，利小兒。别録。治小兒寒熱丹瘮。甄權。止血恊風毒，癰腫赤眼。汁傅蛇虺蜂毒。大明。紫背龍牙：解一切蛇毒。治咽喉中痛，含嚥之便效。蘇頌。

Control. Fright epilepsy. Alternating sensations of cold and heat related to the presence of evil qi. Wounds caused by metal objects/weapons, impediment-illness,[634]

---

632 *Jing ming cao* 竟命草, an unidentified herb.

633 *Zhi shi zi* 知時子, an unidentified substance.

634 *Ju* 疽, "impediment-illness," refers to an obstruction of vessels or other ducts inside the body. Qi rushing against the impediment may cause a local swelling and eventually break through the surface to cause an abscess. BCGM Dict I, 277.

piles, malign mouse fistula sores,[635] head ulcers. *Ben jing*. It heals abdominal evil qi, abdominal pain and blockage/numbness related to moisture. It nourishes a fetus and frees the flow of urine. *Bie lu*. It cures cinnabar-red papules with alternating sensations of cold and heat of children. Zhen Quan. It ends bleeding with wind poison.[636] Swelling related to an obstruction-illness[637] and red eyes. The juice is applied to [regions affected by the] poison of [bites/stings] by snakes, venomous vipers and bees/wasps. Da Ming. *Zi bei long ya*: It resolves all types of snake poison. To cure pain in the throat, hold it in the mouth and swallow [the resulting saliva]. This will be effective. Su Song.

【發明】【藏器曰】蛇含治蛇咬。今以草納蛇口中，縱傷人亦不能有毒也。種之，亦令無蛇。【頌曰】古今治丹毒瘡腫方通用之。古今録驗治赤瘮，用蛇銜草，搗極爛，傅之即瘥。赤瘮由冷濕搏於肌中，甚即爲熱，乃成赤瘮。天熱則劇，冷則減是也。【時珍曰】按葛洪抱朴子云：蛇銜膏連已斷之指。今攷葛洪肘後方載蛇銜膏云：治癰腫瘀血，產後積血，耳目諸病，牛領馬鞍瘡。用蛇銜、大黄、附子、芍藥、大戟、細辛、獨活、黄芩、當歸、莽草、蜀椒各一兩，薤白十四枚。右爲末。以苦酒淹一宿，以豬膏二斤，七星火上煎沸，成膏收之。每温酒服一彈丸，日再服。病在外，摩之傅之。在耳，綿裹塞之。在目，點之。若入龍銜藤一兩，則名龍銜膏也。所謂連斷指者，不知即此膏否。

Explication: [Chen] Cangqi: *She han* serves to cure snake bites. Today the herb is inserted into a snake's mouth and as a result the person harmed will not be affected by its poison. When [this herb] is planted, it repels snakes. [Su] Song: In the past and today all recipes to cure cinnabar-red poison sores and swelling resort to it. To cure red papules, the *Gu jin lu yan* [recommends to] "pound *she xian cao* to obtain a very pulpy pulp and apply it [to the affected region]. This results in a cure." Red papules are caused when cold moisture strikes the inside of the skin. In severe cases, this results in heat and red papules. When the weather is hot, this becomes more severe; when it is cold, it decreases. [Li] Shizhen: According to Ge Hong's *Baopu zi*, "*she xian* ointment rejoins a severed finger." Today, in Ge Hong's *Zhou hou fang* a "*she xian* ointment" is recorded, stating: "It serves to cure swelling related to obstruction

635 *Shu lou* 鼠瘻, "mouse fistula," BCGM Dict I, 466, identical to *luo li* 瘰癧, "scrofula pervasion-illnes." BCGM Dict I. 329

636 Instead of *xie feng du* 恊風毒, *Zheng lei* ch. 10, *she quan* 蛇全, writes [火劦]風瘮.

637 *Yong* 癰, "obstruction-illness,"refers to an obstruction of vessels or other ducts inside the body. Qi rushing against the obstruction may cause a local swelling and eventually break through the surface to cause an abscess. BCGM Dict I, 641.

illness[638] and stagnating blood. Blood accumulation following delivery. All types of diseases of the ears and the eyes. Sores on the neck of oxen and under the saddle of horses. [Ingredients include:] One *liang* each of *she xian*, rhubarb root, *aconitum* [accessory tuber], *paeonia* [root], Peking spurge [root], *asarum heteropoides* [root], *angelica biserrata* [root], *scutellaria* [root], Chinese *angelica* [root], *illiceum* [leaf] and [Si] chuan pepper, as well as 14 stalks of Chinese chives. Grind these into powder. Soak it in bitter wine for one night. Add two *jin* of lard, boil it above a seven stars fire[639] to bubbling until a paste has formed and store it. Each time ingest with warm wine a pill the size of a bullet. To be ingested twice a day. If the disease is situated in the outer region [of the body, i. e., the skin] rub it and then apply [the paste there]. If it is in the ears, wrap [the pill] in silk floss and insert it [into the affected ear]. If it is in the eyes, drop it [into the affected eyes]. If one *liang* of *long xian* vines is added, [the recipe is called] '*long xian* ointment'." When it is said that it rejoins a severed finger, it is not clear whether the present ointment is meant.

【附方】舊三，新一。

Added Recipes. Three of old. One newly [recorded].

產後瀉痢。小龍牙根一握，濃煎服之，甚效，即蛇含是也。斗門方。

Outflow with free-flux illness following delivery. Boil one handful of *xiao long ya* root in water to a thick liquid and [let the woman] ingest it. Very effective. This is *she han*. *Dou men fang*.

金瘡出血。蛇含草搗傅之。肘後方。

Bleeding wounds caused by metal objects/weapons. Pound *she han* and apply [the pulp to the affected region]. *Zhou hou fang*.

---

638 *Yong* 癰, "obstruction-illness," refers to an obstruction of vessels or other ducts inside the body. Qi rushing against the obstruction may cause a local swelling and eventually break through the surface to cause an abscess. BCGM Dict I, 641.

639 The term *qi xing huo* 七星火, "seven stars fire," is attested in Ge Hong's *Zhou hou fang*. It is mentioned in the BCGM only once. All records of a "seven stars fire" in further Chinese medical texts refer to the *Zhou hou fang*. The term *qi xing huo* 七星火 is not uncommon in Daoist literature, as are various other types of fire, but not a single explanation of its meaning has been found. The text in the *Zhou hou fang* suggests that seven separate fires or stoves serve to boil a formula of 11 items to bubbling. The "seven stars" may refer to the Big Dipper, and the stoves may have been arranged similar to the image of the Big Dipper. This would correspond to the so called *qi xing zao* 七星灶, "seven stoves [reflecting the seven] stars," a linear arrangement of seven stoves to boil liquids, transmitted in Chinese folk culture to this day. Based on personal communication with Zheng Jinsheng.

身面惡癬。紫背草入生礬研，傅二三次斷根。直指方。

Malign *xuan*-illness[640] on the body and the face. Add alum to *zi bei cao* and grind [it to a pulp]. Apply this two or three times [to the affected region] to cut the root [of the disease]. *Zhi zhi fang.*

蜈蚣蠍傷。蛇銜挼傅之。古今録驗。

Harm caused by centipedes and scorpions. Rub *she xian* [in the hands to obtain a pulp] and apply it [to the affected region]. *Gu jin lu yan.*

16-34
女青本經下品
Nü qing, FE *Ben jing*, lower rank.

***Cynanchum thesinides* (Freyn) K. Schum.**

【釋名】雀瓢本經。

Explanation of Names. *Que piao* 雀瓢, "sparrow's ladle-gourd," *Ben jing.*

【集解】【別録曰】女青，蛇銜根也。生朱厓，八月采，陰乾。【弘景曰】若是蛇銜根，不應獨生朱厓。俗用者是草葉，别是一物，未詳孰是。術云：帶此屑一兩，則疫癘不犯，彌宜識真者。又云：今市人用一種根，形狀如續斷，莖葉至苦，乃云是女青根，出荆州。【恭曰】此草即雀瓢也。生平澤，葉似蘿摩，兩葉相對，子似瓢形，大如棗許，故名雀瓢。根似白薇。莖葉並臭。其蛇銜都非其類。又別録云：葉嫩時似蘿摩，圓端大莖，實黑，莖葉汁黄白。亦與前說相似。若是蛇銜根，何得苗生益州，根在朱厓，相去萬里餘也。蘿摩葉似女青，故亦名雀瓢。【藏器曰】蘿摩是白環藤，雀瓢是女青，二物相似，不能分别，終非一物也。【機曰】蘿摩以子言，女青以根言，蛇銜以苗言，三者氣味功用大有不同。諸註因其同名雀瓢而疑爲一物。又因其各出州郡，而復疑爲二物。本草明言女青是蛇銜根，豈可以根苗異地而致疑？如靡蕪、芎藭所産不同，亦將分爲二物乎？如赤箭、徐長卿同名鬼督郵，亦將合爲一物耶？【時珍曰】女青有二：一是藤生，乃蘇恭所說似蘿摩者；一種草生，則蛇銜根也。蛇銜有大、小二種：葉細者蛇銜，用苗莖葉；大者爲龍銜，用根。故王燾外臺秘要龍銜膏，用龍銜根煎膏治癰腫金瘡者，即此女青也。陳藏器言女青、蘿摩不能分別，張揖廣雅言女青是葛類，皆指藤生女青，非此女青也。別録明說女青是蛇銜根，一言可據。諸家止因其生朱厓致疑，非矣。方土各有

640 *Xuan* 癬, "*xuan*-illness," a condition of dermal lesions with initially erythema, papules, and itching gradually extending in all directions to form an irregular ring with clear boundaries. The skin is slightly elevated with small papules, blisters, and/or scales and scraps. The central lesion may appear to heal spontaneously, and it may reappear. BCGM Dict I, 591.

相傳不同爾，況又不知有兩女青乎？又羅浮山記云：山有男青似女青。此則不知是草生、藤生者也。

Collected Explanations. *Bie lu*: *Nü qing* is the root of Kleinian cinquefoil. It grows in Zhu ya, is collected in the eighth month and dried in the yin (i. e., shade). [Tao] Hongjing: If this were the root of Kleinen cinquefoil, it should not grow in Zhu ya alone. Commonly used [under this name] are herbs and leaves; but they are something different. It is not clear what they are. [The experts of the longevity] arts state: "Those who wear its scraps on their body, they will not be offended by epidemics. This makes it all the more necessary to know what it really is." It is also stated: "Today, market people resort to a kind of root that is shaped similar to Himalayan teasel herb [root]. Stem and leaves are extremely bitter." And it is stated that this is the root of *nü qing*. It comes from Jing zhou. [Su] Gong: This herb is *que piao* 雀瓢. It grows in the plains and in marshlands. The leaves resemble those of *metaplexis* [herbs]; two leaves grow facing other. The seeds are shaped like a flat ladle-gourd. They are about the size of Chinese dates. Hence the name "sparrow's ladle-gourd," *que piao* 雀瓢. The root resembles that of *cynanchum atratum*. Stem and leaves are malodorous. *She xian*, Kleinian cinquefoil, is definitely not related to it. Also, the *Bie lu* states: "As long as the leaves are tender they resemble *metaplexis* [leaves]. They are round at their tips. The stem is big and the fruits are black. The juice of stem and leaves is yellow-white." This, too, corresponds to what was said above. If this were Kleinian cinquefoil, how could it be that its seedlings grow in Yi zhou, while its root is present in Zhu ya, more than 10 000 *li* away?! The leaves of *metaplexis* [herbs] resemble those of *nü qing*. Hence, they, too, are called *que piao* 雀瓢. [Chen] Cangqi: *Metaplexis* [herb] is *bai huan teng* 白環藤, "vine forming a white ring." *Que piao* 雀瓢 is *nü qing*. These two items resemble each other and cannot be told apart. But they are definitely not the same item. [Wang] Ji: One speaks of the seeds of *metaplexis* [herbs], of the root of *nü qing* and of the seedling of Kleinian cinquefoil. Qi, flavors, [therapeutic] potentials and usages of these three items have nothing in common. Because they all are named *que piao*, commentators considered them to be one identical item. Then, because of the [different] *zhou* and prefectures they come from, they were assumed to be two items. The *Ben cao* clearly states that "*nü qing* is the root of Kleinian cinquefoil." How could this be doubted simply because root and seedling are attributed to different grounds? This is similar to *mi wu* 靡蕪and *xiong qiong* 芎藭 (different names of *ligusticum* root) that are produced at different places. Should they, too, be considered to be two different items? Or, like *gastrodia* [root] and *cynanchum paniculatum* [root], should they, too, be considered to be one identical item because both are also named *gui du you* 鬼督郵? [Li] Shizhen: There are two *nü qing*s. One grows as a vine. This is the one said by Su Gong to resemble *metaplexis*. The other [*nü qing*] grows as an herb. This is the root of Kleinian cinquefoil. Kleinian cinquefoil has two kinds, one large, one small. Those with fine leaves are "snake bit," *she xian* 蛇銜. Of them one uses the seedling, the stem and the leaves. Large specimens are "dragon bit," *long xian* 龍銜. Of them one uses the root. Therefore, when Wang Dao in his *Wai tai mi yao*'s "dragon bit ointment" [recommends to] boil "dragon bit" root to prepare an ointment serving to cure swelling related to an obstruction-illness[641] and wounds caused by metal objects/weapons, this is *nü qing*. Chen Cangqi says that "*nü qing* and *metaplexis* [herbs] cannot be told apart." Zhang Yi in his *Guang ya* says that "*nü qing* is related to *pueraria*." Both refer to the *nü qing* that grows as a vine; it is not the *nü qing* discussed here. The *Bie lu* clearly points out: "*Nü qing* is the root of Kleinian cinquefoil." This is an entirely reliable statement. All authors have doubted it because it grows in Zhu ya. But [such doubts] are wrong. All the recipe masters have their differently transmitted versions. Should this not all the more let one know that there are two [kinds of] *nü qing*? Also, the *Luo fu shan ji* states: "In the mountains is a *nan qing* 男青 resembling *nü qing*." It is not known whether this [*nan qing*] grows as an herb or as a vine.

16-34-01
根 *Gen*
Root [of *nü qing*].

【氣味】辛，平，有毒。【權曰】苦，無毒。蛇銜爲使。

Qi and Flavor. Acrid, balanced, nonpoisonous. [Zhen] Quan: Bitter, nonpoisonous. Kleinian cinquefoil serves as its guiding substance.

【主治】蠱毒，逐邪惡氣，殺鬼温瘧，辟不祥。本經。

Control. *Gu* poison.[642] It repels evil, malign qi, kills demons responsible for warmth malaria, and keeps away the inauspicious. *Ben jing*.

【附方】舊二，新一。

Added Recipes. Two of old. One newly recorded.

人卒暴死。搗女青屑一錢，安咽中，以水或送下，立活也。南岳魏夫人内傳。

641 *Yong* 癰, "obstruction-illness,"refers to an obstruction of vessels or other ducts inside the body. Qi rushing against the obstruction may cause a local swelling and eventually break through the surface to cause an abscess. BCGM Dict I, 641.

642 *Gu du* 蠱毒, "*gu*-poison[ing]." (1) A poison emitted by certain worms/snakes with an ability to cause varying pathological changes in a person who has taken it in by means of wine or food. (2) Abdominal fullness, in some cases with blood spitting, and blood in the stool and urine. BCGM Dict I, 192 - 193. See BCGM 42-22.

Sudden death of a person. Pound *nü qing* to obtain one *qian* of scraps. Place them into [the patient's] throat and send them down with water or [wine]. [The patient] is immediately brought back to life. *Nan yue Wei furen zhuan*.

吐利卒死，及大人小兒，卒腹皮青黑赤，不能喘息。即急用女青末納口中，酒送下。子母秘録。

For spitting/vomiting, free-flux [illness] and sudden death, and when adults or children suddenly have an abdominal skin that assumes a greenish, black or red color, coupled with an inability to breathe, quickly insert *nü qing* powder into [the patient's] mouth and send it down with wine. *Zi mu mi lu*.

辟禳瘟疫。正月上寅日，擣女青末，三角絳囊盛，繫帳中，大吉。肘後方。

To keep away, by means of exorcism, warmth epidemics. On the first *yin* 寅 day of the first month pound *nü qing*, fill it into a triangular, deep red bag and attach it to a curtain. Very auspicious. *Zhou hou fang*.

16-35
鼠尾草別録下品

Shu wei cao, FE *Bie lu*, lower rank.

***Salvia japonica* Th. Japanese *salvia*.**

【釋名】葝音勍、山陵翹吴普、烏草拾遺、水青拾遺。【時珍曰】鼠尾以穗形命名。爾雅云：葝，鼠尾也。可以染皂，故名烏草，又曰水青。蘇頌圖經謂鼠尾一名陵時者，乃陵翹之誤也。

Explanation of Names. *Qing* 葝, read *qing* 勍; *shan ling qiao* 山陵翹, Wu Pu. *Wu cao* 烏草, "black herb," *Shi yi*. *Shui qing* 水青, *Shi yi*. [Li] Shizhen: The name *shu wei* 鼠尾, "mouse tail," refers to the shape of [this herb's] spikes. *Er ya*: "*Qing* 葝 is *shu wei* 鼠尾." It can be used to dye black. Hence the name "black herb," *wu cao* 烏草. It is also called *shui qing* 水青. Su Song in his *Tu jing* says: "*Shu wei* 鼠尾 is also named *Tu jing ling shi* 陵時." That is an erroneous [writing of] *ling qiao* 陵翹.

【集解】【別録曰】鼠尾生平澤中，四月采葉，七月采花，陰乾。【弘景曰】田野甚多，人采作滋染皂。【保昇曰】所在下濕地有之。惟黔中人采爲藥。葉如蒿，莖端夏生四五穗，穗若車前，花有赤、白二種。【藏器曰】紫花，莖葉俱可染皂用。

Collected Explanations. *Bie lu*: *Shu wei* grows in the marshlands of the plains. The leaves are collected in the fourth month. The flowers are collected in the seventh month. They are dried in the yin (i. e., shade). [Tao] Hongjing: Much of it is present in the open country. People collect it to prepare black dyestuff. [Han] Baosheng: It can be found everywhere in low-lying marshlands. Only people in Qian zhong collect it as a pharmaceutical drug. The leaves are similar to those of wormwood herbs. Four or five spikes grow at the end of the stem during summer. The spikes resemble those of Asiatic plantain. [The herb] has two kinds of flowers, red and white. [Chen] Cangqi: The flowers are purple. The stem and the leaves can serve to dye black.

16-35-01
花、葉 *Hua, Ye*
Flower, leaf [of *shu wei cao*].

【氣味】苦，微寒。無毒。【藏器曰】平。

Qi and Flavor. Bitter, slightly cold, nonpoisonous. [Chen] Cangqi: Balanced.

【主治】鼠瘻寒熱，下痢膿血不止。白花者主白下，赤花者主赤下。别録。主瘧疾水蠱。時珍。

Control. Mouse fistula with alternating sensations of cold and heat. Unending discharge of pus and blood with free-flux illness. White flowers control white discharge; red flowers control red discharge. *Bie lu.* They control malaria ailments and water *gu* [poison].[643]

【發明】【弘景曰】古方療痢多用之。當濃煮令可丸服之，或煎如飴服。今人亦用作飲，或末服亦得。日三服。

Explication. [Tao] Hongjing: Ancient recipes often use it to heal free-flux illness. For this purpose it is to be boiled to generate a thick liquid that can be formed to pills for ingestion. Or simmer it until it has acquired the consistency of malt sugar, and ingest this. Today people also use it to prepare beverages. But it can also be ingested as powder. To be ingested three times a day.

【附方】舊一，新三。

Added Recipes. One of old. Three newly [recorded].

大腹水蠱。方見馬鞭草下。

Abdominal water swelling and *gu* [poisoning]. For a recipe, see under vervain (16-32).

643 *Gu du* 蠱毒, "*gu*-poison[ing]." (1) A poison emitted by certain worms/snakes with an ability to cause varying pathological changes in a person who has taken it in by means of wine or food. (2) Abdominal fullness, in some cases with blood spitting, and blood in the stool and urine. BCGM Dict I, 192 - 193. See BCGM 42-22.

久痢休息，時止時作。鼠尾草花擣末，飲服一錢。聖惠方。

Long lasting free-flux illness with intermissions. At times it stops, at time it is active. Pound *shu wei cao* herbs into powder and ingest with a [rice] beverage one *qian*. *Sheng hui fang*.

下血連年。鼠尾草、地榆各二兩，水二升，煮一升，頓服。二十年者，不過再服。亦可爲末，飲服之。千金方。

Discharge with blood lasting years. Boil two *liang* each of *shu wei cao* and *sanguisorba* [root] in two *sheng* of water down to one *sheng*, and ingest this all at once. Even if it has lasted for 20 years, no more than two ingestions are required. It can also be prepared into powder to be ingested with a [rice] beverage. *Qian jin fang*.

反花惡瘡，内生惡肉如飯粒，破之血出，隨生反出于外。鼠尾草根切，同豬脂擣傅。聖濟總録。

Malign reversed blossoms sores,[644] with a malign flesh growth inside similar to rice grains. *Sheng ji zong lu*.

16-36
狼把[645]草宋開寶

***Lang ba cao*. FE Song, *Kai bao*.**

***Bidens tripartite* L. Threelobe beggarticks.**

【校正】併入拾遺郎耶草。

Editorial Correction. *Lang ye cao* 郎耶草, [listed separately in the] *Shi yi*, is included here.

【釋名】郎耶草。【時珍曰】此即陳藏器本草郎耶草也。閩人呼爺爲郎罷，則“狼把”當作“郎罷”乃通。又方士言此草即鼠尾草，功用亦近之，但無的據耳。

Explanation of Names. *Lang ye cao* 郎耶草. [Li] Shizhen: This is the *lang ye cao* 郎耶草 listed in Chen Cangqi's *Ben cao*. People in Min call a grandfather, *ye* 爺, *lang ba* 郎罷. Hence, *lang ba* 狼把 should be written *lang ba* 郎罷. Also, the recipe masters say that "this herb is Japanese *salvia*, *shu wei cao* 鼠尾草." The [therapeutic] potential and use are similar but there is no evidence [that they are identical].

---

644 *Fan hua chuang* 反花瘡, "reversed-blossoms sores," a condition with a festering ulcer generating a flesh growth assuming the shape of a flower. BCGM Dict I, 149.

645 *Zheng lei* ch. 10, *ben yao zheng ming* 本藥正名, "correct naming of this pharmaceutical drug," writes *ba* 杷. Li Shizhen changed this character to its homophone *ba* 把. The same applies to the appearance of this character further below.

【集解】【藏器曰】狼把草生山道旁，與秋穗子並可染皂。【又曰】郎耶草生山澤間，高三四尺，葉作雁齒，如鬼針苗。鬼針，即鬼釵也。其葉有椏，如釵脚狀。【禹錫曰】狼把草出近世，古方未見用者，惟陳藏器言之而不詳。太宗皇帝御書記其主療血痢，甚爲精至。謹用書于本草圖經外類篇首。

Collected Explanations. [Chen] Cangqi: *Lang ba cao* grows at the roadside. With the seeds of its spikes collected in autumn it can serve to dye black. It is also said: *Lang ye cao* grows in mountains and marshlands. It reaches a height of three to four *chi*. The leaves have wild goose teeth [margins], similar to the seedlings of demon needle [herbs]. Demon needle [herb], *gui zhen* 鬼針, is *gui chai* 鬼釵, "demon hairpin [herb]." Its leaves are forked, similar to a forked hairpin. [Zhang] Yuxi: *Lang bao cao* has come into sight only recently. Its usage is not seen in ancient recipes. Only Chen Cangqi refers to it, but not in detail. In the book compiled by Emperor Tai zong [of the Song dynasty] it is recorded as very effectively healing blood free-flux illness. A careful description of its usage is found at the very beginning of the section *wai lei* 外類, "further [substances]," of the *Tu jing*,

【氣味】苦，平，無毒。

Qi and Flavor. Bitter, balanced, nonpoisonous.

【主治】黑人髮，令人不老。又云：郎耶草主赤白久痢，小兒大腹痞滿，丹毒寒熱。取根莖煮汁服。藏器。狼把草主丈夫血痢，不療婦人。根治積年疳痢。取草二斤，搗絞取汁一小升，納白麪半雞子許，和勻，空腹頓服。極重者不過三服。或收苗陰乾，擣末，蜜水半盞，服一方寸匕。圖經。可染鬚髮，治積年癬，天陰即痒，搔出黄水者，擣末摻之。時珍。

Control. It blackens hair and prevents aging. It is also said: *Lang ye cao* controls long-lasting red and white free-flux illness, obstacle-illness[646] and a feeling of abdominal fullness of children, cinnabar poison[647] and an alternating sensation of cold and heat. Boil the root and the stem and ingest the [resulting] juice. [Chen] Cangqi. *Lang ba cao* controls blood free-flux illness of males, it does not serve to heal women. The root serves to cure year-long *gan*-illness[648] and free-flux illness. Pound two *jin* of the herb and squeeze [the pulp] to obtain one small *sheng*. Give as much as the size of a chicken egg of it into white wheat flour and mix this evenly to be ingested

646 *Pi* 痞, "obstacle-illness." 1.) An illness sign of a feeling of uncomfortable fullness and distension. 2). A condition of an uncomfortable distension and fullness in the chest and abdominal region. When pressed there is no pain. BCGM Dict I, 371.

647 *Dan du* 丹毒, "cinnabar poison," a skin ailment with red rashes. BCGM Dict I, 118

648 *Gan* 疳, "*gan*-illness," also: "sweets-illness," involves several complaints that affect children and adults, with causes and conditions too different to fall into a known disease category. BCGM Dict I, 180-188.

on an empty stomach all at once. Even for extremely serious cases no more than three ingestions are required. Or, gather the seedling, dry it in the yin (i. e., shade), pound it into powder and give it into half a cup of honey water. Ingest the amount held by a square *cun* spoon. *Tu jing*. It can serve to dye beard and hair. It serves to cure year-long *xuan*-illness[649] with an itch when the sky is cloudy. If a yellow water leaves [the skin] when it is scratched, pound [the herb] into powder and apply it [to the affected region]. [Li] Shizhen.

16-37
狗尾草綱目
Gou wei cao. FE *Gang mu*.

***Setaria viridis* (L.) Beauv. Green bristlegrass.**

【釋名】莠音酉、光明草綱目、阿羅漢草。【時珍曰】莠草秀而不實，故字從秀。穗形象狗尾，故俗名狗尾。其莖治目痛，故方士稱爲光明草、阿羅漢草。

Explanation of Names. *You* 莠, read *you* 酉; *guang ming cao* 光明草, *Gang mu*. *A luo han cao* 阿羅漢草. [Li] Shizhen: *You cao* 莠草 has elegant flowers, *xiu* 秀, but no fruit. Hence the character [*you* 莠] is derived from [the character] *xiu* 秀. The spikes are shaped like a dog's tail. Therefore it is commonly called "dog's tail," *gou wei* 狗尾. The stem serves to cure painful eyes. Hence recipe masters call it "the herb for brilliant light," *guang ming cao* 光明草, and *a luo han cao* 阿羅漢草, the "Arhat/Lohan's herb."

【集解】【時珍曰】原野垣墻多生之。苗葉似粟而小，其穗亦似粟，黃白色而無實。采莖筒盛，以治目病。惡莠之亂苗，即此也。

Collected Explanations. [Li] Shizhen: It grows profusely in the wild and on walls. The seedling and the leaves resemble those of millet [herbs], but are smaller. The spikes, too, resemble those of millet; they are of yellow-white color and have no fruit. The stem is collected and filled into a bamboo tube; it serves to cure eye diseases. With the "weeds that hate green grass, 莠 *you*," the present [item] is meant.

649 *Xuan* 癬, "*xuan*-illness." Conditions of dermal lesions with initially erythema, papules, and itching gradually extending in all directions to form an irregular ring with clear boundaries. The skin is slightly elevated with small papules, blisters, and/or scales and scraps. The central lesion may appear to heal spontaneously, and it may reappear. Also, a designation of local lesions with itching, release of liquid and shedding of scabs. BCGM Dict I, 591.

16-37-01
莖 *Jing*
Stem [of *gou wei cao*]

【主治】疣目，貫髮穿之，即乾滅也。凡赤眼拳毛倒睫者，翻轉目瞼，以一二莖蘸水戛去惡血，甚良。時珍。

Control. For warts, pass a hair through [the stem] and then pierce the [warts].[650] This will let them dry and vanish. For all red eyes with inverted eyelashes and turned over eyelids, dip one or two [*gou wei cao*] stems into water and tap them [onto the affected region] to remove malign blood. Very good. [Li] Shizhen.

16-38
鱧腸唐本草
Li chang, FE *Tang ben cao*

***Eclipta prostrata*(L.) L. Ink plant.**[651]

【釋名】蓮子草唐本、旱蓮草圖經、金陵草圖經、墨煙草綱目、墨頭草綱目、墨菜綱目、猢孫頭必用、豬牙草。【時珍曰】鱧，烏魚也，其腸亦烏。此草柔莖，斷之有墨汁出，故名，俗呼墨菜是也。細實頗如蓮房狀，故得蓮名。

Explanation of Names. *Lian zi cao* 蓮子草, "lotus seeds herb," *Tang ben*. *Han lian cao* 旱蓮草, "dry ground lotus herb," *Tu jing*. *Jin ling cao* 金陵草, "golden mound herb," *Tu jing*. *Mo yan cao* 墨煙草, "ink/black smoke herb," *Gang mu*. *Mo tou cao* 墨頭草, "ink/black head herb," *Gang mu*. *Mo cai* 墨菜, "ink/black vegetable," *Gang mu*. *Hu sun tou* 猢孫頭, *Bi yong*. *Zhu ya cao* 豬牙草, "pig tooth herb." [Li] Shizhen: *Li* 鱧 is the black (snakehead) fish, *wu yü* 烏魚. Its intestines, *chang* 腸, too, are black. This herb has a soft stem [resembling an intestine]. When it is broken it releases a black juice. Hence the name. This is the commonly called "ink vegetable," *mo cai* 墨菜. The shape of its fine fruit very much resembles that of lotus fruit capsules. Hence the name "lotus," *lian* 蓮.

【集解】【恭曰】鱧腸生下濕地，所在坑渠間多有。苗似旋覆。二月、八月采，陰乾。【頌曰】處處有之，南方尤多。此有二種。一種葉似柳而光澤，莖似馬齒莧，高一二尺，開花細而白，其實若小蓮房，蘇恭謂似旋覆者是也。一種苗梗枯瘦，頗似蓮花而黃色，實亦作房而圓，南人謂之連

650 A long hair is passed through a hollow stem of green bristlegrass, with both ends left out. The stem is hard enough to be pierced through the "wart." Then hold one end of the hair and pull the stem out so that the hair stays in the wart. Then it is possible to tie off the "wart" with the hair. As a result it will dry and vanish.

651 *Li chang* 鱧腸, lit.: "black [snakehead] fish intestine."

翹者。二種折其苗皆有汁出，須臾而黑，俗謂之旱蓮子，亦謂之金陵草。【時珍曰】旱蓮有二種。一種苗似旋覆而花白細者，是鱧腸。一種花黄紫而結房如蓮房者，乃是小連翹也。爐火家亦用之。見連翹條。

Collected Explanations. [Su] Gong: *Li chang* grows in low-lying marshlands. Much of it can be found in pits and ditches. The seedling resembles that of horseheal [herbs]. It is collected in the second and eighth month. It is dried in the yin (i. e., shade). [Su] Song: It can be found everywhere, with especially much of it present in the South. This [herb] has two kinds. The leaves of one kind resemble willow [leaves], but are shiny and moist. The stem resembles that of purslane; it is one or two *chi* tall. It opens fine, white flowers, with fruits resembling small lotus capsules. When Su Gong says that "it resembles horseheal [herbs]," he is right. The stem of the other kind is a skinny stalk. Its [flowers] very much resemble lotus flowers, but are of yellow color. Their fruit, too, develop capsules, but they are round. People in the South call it *lian qiao* 連翹.[652] The seedlings of both kinds when broken release a juice that turns black within short time. [The herb] is commonly called *han lian zi* 旱蓮子; it is also called *jin ling cao* 金陵草. [Li] Shizhen: *Han lian* has two kinds. One kind has a seedling resembling that of horseheal [herbs], with fine, white flowers. This is *li chang* 鱧腸. The other kind has yellow-purple flowers and forms [fruit] capsules like the capsules of lotus [flowers]. This is *xiao lian qiao* 小連翹, "small *forsythia*." It is also used by the experts [preparing elixirs on a] furnace. See the entry "*lian qiao* 連翹," *forsythia*, (16-39).

16-38-01
草 *Cao*
[*Li chang*] herb.

【氣味】甘、酸，平，無毒。

Qi and Flavor. Sweet, sour, balanced, nonpoisonous.

【主治】血痢。鍼灸瘡發，洪血不可止者，傅之立已。汁塗眉髮，生速而繁。唐本。烏髭髮，益腎陰。時珍。止血排膿，通小腸，傅一切瘡并蠶瘑。大明。膏點鼻中，添腦。蕭炳。

Control. Blood free-flux illness. Effusion of sores caused by needle and cauterization [therapies], with profuse bleeding that cannot be stopped. Apply the [herb to the affected region] and the [bleeding] stops immediately. When the juice is applied to eyebrows, they will grow fast and profusely. *Tang ben*. It blackens beard and hair, and boosts the kidney yin [qi]. [Li] Shizhen. It ends bleeding and removes pus. It frees the passage through the small intestine. It is applied to all sores and

652 *Lian qiao* 連翹is also the name of *forsythia.*

to silkworm [caused] lair-illness.[653] Da Ming. Drip the ointment into the nose to strengthen the brain. Xiao Bing.

【附方】舊一，新九。

Added Recipes. One of old. Nine newly recorded.

金陵煎。益髭髮，變白爲黑。金陵草一秤，六月以後收采，揀青嫩無泥土者。不用洗，摘去黄葉，爛擣，新布絞取汁，以紗絹濾過，入通油器鉢盛之，日中煎五日。又取生薑一斤絞汁，白蜜一斤，合和，日中煎。以柳木篦攪勿停手，待如稀餳，藥乃成矣。每旦日及午後各服一匙，以温酒一盞化下。如欲作丸，日中再煎，令可丸，大如梧子，每服三十丸。及時多合爲佳，其效甚速。孫真人千金月令方。

Fried *jin ling*. It boosts beard and hair, changes white to black. One *cheng* of *jin ling* is collected in the sixth month and later. Pick greenish, tender [herbs] without soil. Do not wash them. Discard the yellow leaves and pound [the herb] to a pulp. Squeeze it with a new piece of cloth to obtain the juice. Strain it through a silk fabric and keep it in a container generously prepared with oil. Fry it in the sun for five days. In addition get one *jin* of fresh ginger and squeeze it to obtain the juice. Mix it with white honey and fry it in the sun. Stir it with a willow wood comb, without letting the hand pause, until it has assumed the consistency of thin malt-sugar. The pharmaceutical substance is ready now. Every early morning at sunrise and after noon ingest one spoonful, to be sent down mixed with one cup of warm wine. If one prefers to prepare pills, fry [the substance] in the sun again until [it has assumed a consistency] enabling one to form pills the size of *wu* seeds. Each time ingest 30 pills. To prepare large quantities [of the pills] in time is best. The effects are very fast. Sun zhenren, *Qian jin yue ling fang*.

烏鬚固齒。攝生妙用方：七月取旱蓮草連根一斤，用無灰酒洗净，青鹽四兩，淹三宿，同汁入油鍋中，炒存性，研末。日用擦牙，連津嚥之。

To blacken the beard and stabilize the teeth. The *She sheng miao yong fang* [recommends the following]: In the seventh month get one *jin* of *han lian cao* with its root. Wash it clean with ash-free wine and keep it immersed in four *liang* of greenish salt for three days. Then give it with juice into a pot prepared with oil and fry it with its nature retained. Then grind it into powder. Rub the teeth daily with it and swallow the resulting body liquid.

653 *Guo* 瘑, "lair-illness," a condition of sores affecting both hands and feet, with pain and itching and gradual extension. In some cases crumbs are shed off. BCGM Dict I, 203.

又法：旱蓮取汁，同鹽煉乾，研末擦牙。

Another method. Obtain the juice of *han lian* and heat it together with salt until it has dried. Grind it into powder and rub the teeth [with it].

奉親養老書旱蓮散，烏髭固牙。溫尉云：納合相公用此方，年七十鬚髮不白，懇求始得，後遇張經，始傳分兩也。旱蓮草一兩半，麻枯餅三兩，升麻、青鹽各三兩半，訶子連核二十個，皂角三挺，月蠶沙二兩，爲末，薄醋麪糊丸彈子大。晒乾入泥瓶中，火煨令烟出存性，取出研末，日用揩牙。

The *han lian* powder of the *Feng qin yang lao shu* to blacken the beard and stabilize the teeth. Wen Wei states: Minister Duke Nahe used this recipe and even at the age of 70 his hair had not turned white. He tried very hard to obtain the recipe, and got it, but it was only later through Registrar Zhang[654] that he was informed of the quantities [of its ingredients]. Grind into powder one and a half liang of *han lian cao*, three *liang* of dry sesame seed cakes, three and a half *liang* each of *cimicifuga* [rhizome] and greenish salt, 20 *terminalia* fruit with their kernels, three *gleditsia* seeds/pods, and two *liang* of a one month old silkworm's excrements.[655] Form [the powder] with thin vinegar and wheat flour to pills the size of a bullet, dry them in the sun and fill them into a pottery vase. Simmer it above a fire until smoke is emitted, but with its nature retained. Remove it [from the vase] and grind it into powder. Use it daily to rub the teeth.

偏正頭痛。鱧腸草汁滴鼻中。聖濟總録。

Lateral and common headache. Drip *li chang* herb juice into the nose. *Sheng ji zong lu*.

一切眼疾，瞖膜遮障，凉腦，治頭痛，能生髮。五月五日平旦合之。蓮子草一握，藍葉一握，油一斤，同浸，密封四十九日。每卧時，以鐵匙點藥摩頂上，四十九遍，久久甚佳。聖濟總録。

All eye afflictions. Eye shade blocking vision. It cools the brain and serves to cure headache. It can stimulate hair growth. Prepare [the following recipe] in the early morning hours of the fifth day of the fifth month. Soak a handful of *lian zi cao* 蓮子草 and a handful of *eupatorium* [leaves] in one *jin* of oil. Keep it tightly sealed

654 Following the two characters *Zhang jing* 張經, the *Shou qin yang lao xin shu*, ch. 4, *lao ya wu zi fang* 牢牙烏髭方, "recipes to stabilize the teeth and blacken the beard," has the three characters *li chao qing* 歷朝請. Hence, *jing* is the shortened version of *jing li chao qing* 經歷朝請 is an official title: "Registrar and Audience Attendant."

655 The term *yue can sha* 月蠶沙, or *yue can* 月蠶, is attested in the BCGM only once, and is not found elsewhere in Chinese medical-pharmaceutical literature. The life cycle of silkworms comprises 28 days, that is, in the traditional Chinese calendar, one month. That is, *yue can* 月蠶 may refer to silkworms that have been reared for a full month.

for 49 days. Each time when going to bed, drip [some of it] with an iron spoon on the top of the head and rub it [into the skin]. 49 times. The longer the better. *Sheng ji zong lu*.

繫臂截瘧。旱蓮草搥爛，男左女右，置寸口上，以古文錢壓定，帛繫住，良久起小泡，謂之天灸。其瘧即止，甚效。王執中資生經。

Attaching [medication] to the arm to stop malaria. Pound *han lian cao* 旱蓮草 to a pulp and attach it above the inch opening, for males on the left and for females on the right side. Then press an ancient coin on it and fasten it with a piece of silk. After quite some time small blisters will rise. This is called "heavenly cauterization." The malaria will be stopped. Very effective. Wang Zhizhong, *Zi sheng jing*.

小便溺血。金陵草一名墨頭草、車前草各等分，杵取自然汁。每空心服三盃，愈乃止。醫學正傳。

Urination with blood. Pound equal amounts of *jin ling cao* 金陵草, also named *hei tou cao* 墨頭草, and Asiatic plantain to obtain their natural juice. Ingest three cups on an empty stomach. Stop [the treatment when the disease is] healed. *Yi xue zheng chuan*.

腸風臟毒，下血不止。旱蓮子草瓦上焙，研末。每服二錢，米飲下。家藏經驗方。

Intestinal wind and poison affecting the long-term depots with an unending discharge of blood. Bake *han lian zi cao* 旱蓮子草 on a tile over a slow fire and grind it into powder. Each time ingest two *qian*, to be sent down with a rice beverage. *Jia cang jing yan fang*.

痔漏瘡發。旱蓮草一把，連根鬚洗净，用石臼擂如泥，以極熱酒一盞衝入，取汁飲之，滓傅患處，重者不過三服即安。太僕少卿王鳴鳳患此，策杖方能移步，服之得瘥。累治有驗。劉松石保壽堂方。

An outbreak of leaking piles sores. Wash a handful of *han lian cao* 旱蓮草 with its root and hair clean and pound it in a stone mortar to a pulp. Give it into a small cup with extremely hot wine, drink the juice and apply the dregs to the location of the ailment. Even for serious cases no more than three ingestions will have settled [the problem]. Wang Mingfeng, Vice Minister of the Imperial Stud, suffered from this. He needed a stick to walk a few steps. He ingested this [recipe] and was healed. Repeated therapies [based on this recipe] have shown that it is effective. Liu Songshi, *Bao shou tang fang*.

疔瘡惡腫。五月五日收旱蓮草陰乾，仍露一夜收。遇疾時嚼一葉貼上，外以消毒膏護之，二三日疔脫。聖濟總録。

Pin-illness[656] sores with malign swelling. Gather *han lian cao* 旱蓮草 on the fifth day of the fifth month and dry it in the yin (i. e., shade). Then leave it in the open for one night and store it. Confronted with such an illness, chew it and attach [the pulp to the affected region]. Cover it with a poison dissolving ointment. After two or three days the pin-illness will have vanished. *Sheng ji zong lu.*

風牙疼痛。猢孫頭草，入鹽少許，于掌心揉擦即止。集玄方。

Tootchache because of wind [intrusion]. Add a little salt to *hu sun tou cao* 猢孫頭草, rub this on a palm [to obtain a pulp and use this to] massage [the affected teeth]. This will stop [the pain]. *Ji xuan fang.*

16-39
連翹本經下品
Lian qiao, FE *Ben jing*, lower rank.

***Forsythia suspensa* (Thunb.) Vahl.**

【校正】併入有名未用本經翹根。

Editorial Correction. *Qiao gen* 翹根, listed separately in the *Ben jing*, section "known by name but not in use," is included here.

【釋名】連爾雅、異翹爾雅、旱蓮子藥性、蘭華吴普、三廉别録。根名連軺仲景、折根别録。【恭曰】其實似蓮作房，翹出衆草，故名。【宗奭曰】連翹亦不翹出衆草。太山山谷間甚多。其子折之，片片相比如翹，應以此得名耳。【時珍曰】按爾雅云：連，異翹。則是本名連，又名異翹，人因合稱爲連翹矣。連軺亦作連苕，即本經下品翹根是也。唐蘇恭修本草退入"有名未用"中，今併爲一。旱蓮乃小翹，人以爲鱧腸者，故同名。

Explanation of Names. *Lian* 連, *Er ya*. *Yi qiao* 異翹, *Er ya*. *Han lian zi* 旱蓮子, *Yao xing*. *Lan hua* 蘭華, Wu Pu. *San lian* 三廉, *Bie lu*. The root is named *lian zhao* 連軺, [Zhang] Zhongjing, and *zhe gen* 折根, *Bie lu*. [Su] Gong: Its fruits resemble those of lotus and form capsules. It sticks out, *qiao* 翹, from all the other herbs. Hence its name. [Kou] Zongshi: *Lian qiao* 連翹 does not "stick out," *qiao* 翹, from all the other herbs. Very many [*lian qiao* herbs] can be found in the valleys of Mount Tai shan. When the seeds are broken its pieces resemble a bird's tailfeathers, *qiao* 翹. This should be considered the origin of the name [of *lian qiao*]. [Li] Shizhen: According to the *Er ya*, "*lian* 連 is *yi qiao* 異翹." That is, the original name is *lian* 連 and it is also named *yi qiao* 異翹. Hence, people have combined [the two names] and call it *lian qiao* 連翹. *Lian zhao* 連軺 is also written *lian tiao* 連苕; it is the *qiao gen* 翹根,

656 *Ding* 丁, "pin[-illness]," also *ding* 疔, "pin-illness," refers to a deep-reaching and festering hardness in a tissue, eventually rising above the skin like a pinhead. BCGM Dict I, 127-129.

listed among the lower rank items in the *Ben jing*. When during the Tang, Su Gong revised the *Ben cao*, he moved it into the section "known by name but not in use." Here now they are combined again. *Han lian* 旱蓮 is small [*lian*] *qiao* 翹. People believe it to be ink plant, because they share the same name.

【集解】【別録曰】連翹生太山山谷。八月采。陰乾。【弘景曰】處處有之。今用莖連花實。【恭曰】此物有兩種：大翹，小翹。大翹生下濕地，葉狹長如水蘇。花黄可愛，着子似椿實之未開者，作房翹出衆草。其小翹生岡原之上，葉花實皆似大翹而小細。山南人並用之，今長安惟用大翹子，不用莖花也。【頌曰】今近汴京及河中、江寧、潤、淄、澤、兖、鼎、岳、利諸州，南康軍皆有之。有大小二種。大翹生下濕地或山岡上，青葉狹長，如榆葉、水蘇輩，莖赤色，高三四尺，獨莖。稍間開花黄色，秋結實似蓮，内作房瓣，根黄如蒿根，八月采房。其小翹生岡原之上，花葉實皆似大翹而細。南方生者，葉狹而小，莖短，纔高一二尺，花亦黄，實房黄黑，内含黑子如粟粒，亦名旱蓮，南人用花葉。今南方醫家説，云連翹有兩種。一種似椿實之未開者，殻小堅而外完，無跗蕚，剖之則中解，氣甚芳馥，其實纔乾，振之皆落，不着莖也。一種乃如菡萏，殻柔，外有跗蕚抱之而無解脉，亦無香氣，乾之雖久，着莖不脱，此甚相異，此種江南下澤間極多。如椿實者，乃自蜀中來，入用勝似江南者。據本草則亦以蜀中者爲勝，然未見其莖葉也。

Collected Explanations. *Bie lu*: *Lian qiao* grows in the valleys of Mount Tai shan. It is collected in the eighth month and dried in the yin (i. e., shade). [Tao] Hongjing: It can be found everywhere. Today, the stem together with the flowers and the fruits are used [for therapeutic purposes]. [Su] Gong: This item has two kinds: Big *qiao* 翹 and small *qiao* 翹. Big *qiao* grows in low-lying marshlands. The leaves are narrow and lengthy, similar to those of camphor mint. The flowers are of an amiable yellow. The seeds resemble *ailanthus* fruit before they have opened. The capsules it forms stick out from all other herbs. Small *qiao* grows on the ridges of hills above the open country. Leaves, flowers and fruit, they all resemble those of big *qiao*, but are smaller. People in Shan nan use them all alike. In Chang an, today they use only the seeds of big *qiao*; they do not use the stem and the flowers. [Su] Song: Today it is found near the Capital and also in all the *zhou* of He zhong, Jiang ning, Run, Zi, Ze, Yan, Ding, Yue, and Li, and also in Nan kang jun. It has two kinds, big and small [*qiao*]. Big *qiao* grows on low-lying moist ground or on mountains and hills. Its greenish leaves are narrow and lengthy, similar to those of the Siberian elm and camphor mint. The stem is red; it reaches a height of three to four *chi*. There is one, single stem. At its top flowers of yellow color open. In autumn they form fruits resembling lotus [fruit]. The capsules are formed by petals inside [the flowers]. The root is yellow, similar to the root of wormwood. The capsules are collected in the eighth month. The small *qiao* grows on the slopes of hills above the open land. Flowers, leaves and fruit, they all resemble those of big *qiao*, but are finer. Those that grow in the South have narrow and small leaves and a short stem, only one or two *chi* tall. The leaves are red-yellow; the inside of the fruit capsules is yellow-black. They contain black seeds similar to millet. They, too, are named *han lian* 旱蓮. People in the South use the flowers and the leaves. Today, medical experts in the South say that *lian qiao* has two kinds. One has fruits resembling those of *ailanthus* before they have opened. The shells are small, hard and complete on their outside. When they are cut open, they split in the middle, releasing very fragrant qi. The fruit dry out completely; when [the plant] is shaken, they all fall down and do not remain attached to the stem. The other kind is similar to Indian lotus. Its [fruit] shell is soft. Its outside is enclosed by calyxes and has no veins separating them. Also, the [fruit] do not emit fragrant qi. Even when they have dried for a long time, they remain attached to the stem and do not fall down. This kind is abundant in the low-lying marshlands of Jiang nan. Those with fruits resembling *ailanthus* [fruit] come from Shu zhong. They are much better suited for [medicinal] use than those from Jiang nan. According to the *Ben cao*, that from Shu zhong should also be superior. But I have not seen its stem and leaves.

【氣味】苦，平，無毒。【元素曰】性涼味苦，氣味俱薄，輕清而浮，升也陽也。手搓用之。【好古曰】陰中陽也。入手足少陽、手陽明經，又入手少陰經。【時珍曰】微苦、辛。

Qi and Flavor. Bitter, balanced, nonpoisonous. [Zhang] Yuansu: Its nature is cool; its flavor is bitter. Qi and flavor are weakly pronounced. It is a light and clear [substance] that floats. It rises and is yang. It is rubbed with the hands before it is applied. [Wang] Haogu: It is a yang in yin [substance]. It enters the hand and foot minor yang and hand yang brilliance conduits. It also enters the hand minor yin conduits. [Li] Shizhen: Slightly bitter, acrid.

【主治】寒熱鼠瘻瘰癧，癰腫惡瘡，癭瘤，結熱，蠱毒。本經。去白蟲。別録。通利五淋，小便不通，除心家客熱。甄權。通小腸，排膿，治瘡癤，止痛，通月經。大明。散諸經血結氣聚，消腫。李杲。瀉心火，除脾胃濕熱，治中部血證，以爲使。震亨。治耳聾渾渾焞焞。好古。莖葉：主心肺積熱。時珍。

Control. Mouse fistula,[657] [that is,] scrofula pervasion-illness,[658] with alternating sensations of cold and heat. Swelling and malign sores related to obstruction-illness.[659] Goiter tumor.[660] Bound heat.[661] Gu poison.[662] *Ben jing*. It removes white worms/bugs. *Ben jing*. It frees the flow [of urine in the case of] the five types of urinary drippings and blocked urination. It repels visitor heat in the heart. Zhen Quan. It frees the passage through the small intestine, removes pus, serves to cure sores with pimples, ends pain and frees the flow of menstruation. Da Ming. It disperses all kinds of blood nodes and qi accumulation from the conduits. It dissolves swelling. Li Gao. It drains heart fire, removes moisture and heat from the spleen and the stomach and serves to cure blood [illness] signs in the central region. [For all these issues] it serves as guiding substance. [Zhu] Zhenheng. It serves to cure deafness with unclear [hearing and vision]. [Wang] Haogu. Stem and leaves: They control heat accumulation in heart and lung. [Li] Shizhen.

【發明】【元素曰】連翹之用有三：瀉心經客熱，一也；去上焦諸熱，二也；爲瘡家聖藥，三也。【杲曰】十二經瘡藥中不可無此，乃結者散之之義。【好古曰】手足少陽之藥，治瘡瘍瘤癭結核有神，與柴胡同功，但分氣血之異爾。與鼠粘子同用治瘡瘍，別有神功。【時珍曰】連翹狀似人心，兩片合成，其中有仁甚香，乃少陰心經、厥陰包絡氣分主藥也。諸痛癢瘡瘍皆屬心火，故爲十二經瘡家聖藥，而兼治手足少陽、手陽明三經氣分之熱也。

Explication. [Zhang] Yuansu: *Lian qiao* has three usages. It drains visitor heat from the heart conduits. That is the first. It removes all types of heat from the upper [section of the Triple] Burner. That is the second. It is a pharmaceutical drug with

---

657 *Shu lou* 鼠瘻, "mouse fistula," BCGM Dict I, 466, identical to *luo li* 瘰癧, "scrofula pervasion-illnes." BCGM Dict I. 329

658 *Luo li* 瘰癧, "scrofula pervasion-illness," when two or more connected swellings of the size of plum or date kernels appear either on the neck or in the armpits, or somewhere else on the body. BCGM Dict I. 329.

659 *Yong* 癰, "obstruction-illness,"refers to an obstruction of vessels or other ducts inside the body. Qi rushing against the obstruction may cause a local swelling and eventually break through the surface to cause an abscess. BCGM Dict I, 641.

660 *Ying liu* 癭瘤, "goiter tumor," a swelling at the front side of the neck to the side of the throat. BCGM Dict I, 640.

661 *Jie re* 結熱, "bound heat." A condition of blocked depot qi brought about by repletion heat evil, with blocked urine and stools, panting, fullness, and spitting because of [qi] moving contrary to its normal course. BCGM Dict I, 252.

662 *Gu du* 蠱毒, "*gu*-poison[ing]." (1) A poison emitted by certain worms/snakes with an ability to cause varying pathological changes in a person who has taken it in by means of wine or food. (2) Abdominal fullness, in some cases with blood spitting, and blood in the stool and urine. BCGM Dict I, 192 - 193. See BCGM 42-22.

sage-like effects resorted to by sore [therapy] specialists. That is the third. [Li] Gao: There is no substance that comes close to it among the pharmaceutical drugs for sores developing from the 12 conduits. This is based on its ability to disperse nodes. [Wang] Haogu: It is a pharmaceutical drug for the hand and foot minor yang [conduits]. When used to cure sores, ulcers, tumors, goiter and nodular kernels, [its effects] are divine. It has the same [therapeutic] potential as *bupleurum* [root], but they differ in that one reaches the qi section and the other the blood section. When used together with great burdock to cure sores and ulcers, a particularly divine [therapeutic] potential is realized. [Li] Shizhen: The *lian qiao* [fruit capsule] is shaped like a human heart. It consists of two pieces with a very fragrant kernel in between. It is a major pharmaceutical drug for the qi section of the minor yin heart conduits and the ceasing yin [heart] enclosing network. All types of pain, itch, sores and ulcers are related to heart fire. Therefore it is a pharmaceutical drug with sage-like effects resorted to by specialists in the treatment of sores associated with the 12 conduits. It serves to cure heat in the qi section of the three hand and foot minor yang and hand yang brilliance conduits.

【附方】舊一。新二。

Added Recipes. One of old. Two newly [recorded].

瘰癧結核。連翹、脂麻等分，爲末，時時食之。簡便方。

Scrofula pervasion-illness[663] with nodular kernels. [Grind] equal amounts of *lian qian* and sesame seeds into powder and eat it regularly. *Jian bian fang.*

項邊馬刀。屬少陽經。用連翹二斤，瞿麥一斤，大黄三兩，甘草半兩。每用一兩，以水一盌半，煎七分，食後熱服。十餘日後，灸臨泣穴二七壯，六十日決效。張潔古活法機要。

Saber[664] at the sides of the nape, related to the minor yang conduits. [Mix] two *jin* of *lian qiao*, one *jin* of fringed pink, three *liang* of rhubarb root, and half a *liang* of *glycyrrhiza* [root]. Each time boil one *liang* [of this mixture] in one and a half bowls of water down to 70% and ingest this hot after a meal. More than ten days later, cauterize the *lin qi* 臨泣 [needle insertion] hole (GB-15, or GB-41) with two times

663 *Luo li* 瘰癧, "scrofula pervasion-illness," when two or more connected swellings of the size of plum or date kernels appear either on the neck or in the armpits, or somewhere else on the body. BCGM Dict I. 329.

664 *Ma dao* 馬刀, "saber," a condition of saber-shaped, hard *luo li* 瘰癧, "scrofula with pervasion-illness," developing in the armpits. According to Li Dongyuan 李東垣, the location where this type of scrofula develops is not decisive for its identification. He called 'saber' all types of scrofula that are hard and do not fester. BCGM Dict I, 331.

seven [moxa applications]. An effect will be achieved within 60 days. Zhang Jiegu, *Huo fa ji yao*.

痔瘡腫痛。連翹煎湯熏洗，後以刀上飛過緑礬入麝香貼之。集驗方。
Piles sores with painful swelling. Steam and wash [the affected region] with a *lian qiao* decoction. Then apply melanterite, prepared on a knife blade above a fire, to which is added musk, [to the affected region]. *Ji yan fang*.

16-39-01
翹根 *Qiao gen*
[*Lian*] *qiao* root.

【氣味】甘，寒、平，有小毒。【普曰】神農、雷公：甘，有毒。李當之：苦。【好古曰】苦，寒。
Qi and Flavor. Sweet, cold, balanced, a little poisonous. [Wu] Pu: Shen nong, Lei gong: Sweet, poisonous. Li Dangzhi: Bitter. [Wang] Haogu: Bitter, cold.

【主治】下熱氣，益陰精，令人面悦好，明目。久服輕身耐老。本經。以作蒸飲酒病人。别録。治傷寒瘀熱欲發黄。時珍。
Control. It discharges heat qi, boosts yin [qi] and essence/sperm, lets one's face appear pleasant, and clears the eyes. Ingested for a long time, it relieves the body of its weight and helps to endure aging. *Ben jing*. [The liquid obtained] by steaming it is drunk by persons with a wine disease. *Bie lu*. It serves to cure harm caused by cold with stagnating heat that is about to effuse as jaundice. [Li] Shizhen.

【發明】【本經曰】翹根生嵩高平澤，二月、八月采。【弘景曰】方藥不用，人無識者。【好古曰】此即連翹根也，能下熱氣。故張仲景治傷寒瘀熱在裏，麻黄連軺赤小豆湯用之。注云：即連翹根也。
Explication. *Ben jing*: *Qiao gen* grows in the marshlands of the plains of Song gao. It is collected in the second and eighth month. [Tao] Hongjing: It is not used as a recipe drug. People do not know of it. [Wang] Haogu: This is the root of *lian qiao*. It can discharge heat qi. Hence, when Zhang Zhongjing cured stagnating heat in the interior, related to harm caused by cold, he resorted to it in the "decoction with *ephedra* [herb], *lian zhao* and mung beans." A comment states: "This is the root of *lian qiao*."

【附方】新一。

Added Recipes. One newly [recorded].

癰疽腫毒。連翹草及根各一升，水一斗六升，煮汁三升服取汗。外臺秘要。

Swelling with poison associated with obstruction-illness and impediment-illness.[665] Boil one *sheng* of *lian qiao* herb with the root in one *dou* and six *sheng* of water down to obtain three *sheng* of a juice and ingest it to stimulate sweating. *Wai tai mi yao*.

16-40

陸英本經下品

Lu ying, FE *Ben jing*, lower rank.

***Sambucus chinensis* Lindl. Chinese elder.**

【釋名】解見下文。

Explanation of Names. See the text "[Collected] Explanations" below.

【集解】【别録曰】陸英生熊耳川谷及冤句，立秋采。【恭曰】此即蒴藋也。古方無蒴藋，惟言陸英。後人不識，浪出蒴藋條。此葉似芹及接骨花，三物亦同一類。故芹名水英，此名陸英，接骨名木英樹，此三英也。花葉並相似。【志曰】蘇恭以陸英、蒴藋爲一物。今詳陸英味苦寒無毒，蒴藋味酸温有毒。既此不同，難謂一種，蓋其類爾。【宗奭曰】蒴藋與陸英性味及出産皆不同，治療又别，自是二物，斷無疑矣。【頌曰】本草陸英生熊耳川谷及冤句。蒴藋不載所出州土，但云生田野，所在有之。春抽苗，莖有節，節間生枝，葉大似水芹。春夏采葉，秋冬采根、莖。陶、蘇皆以爲一物，馬志以性味不同，疑非一種，亦不能細别。但爾雅木謂之華，草謂之榮，不榮而實謂之秀，榮而不實謂之英。此物既有英名，當是其花。故本經云，立秋采，正是其花時也。【時珍曰】陶、蘇本草、甄權藥性論，皆言陸英即蒴藋，必有所據。馬志、寇宗奭雖破其説，而無的據。仍當是一物，分根、莖、花、葉用，如蘇頌所云也。

Collected Explanations. *Bie lu*: *Lu ying* grows in the river valleys of Xiong er and in Yuan ju. It is collected at [the solar term] Autumn Begins (August 7). [Su] Gong: This is *shuo diao* 蒴藋. In ancient recipes *shuo diao* is not mentioned. They only speak of *lu ying*. In later times people no longer were familiar with it, and they omitted the *shuo diao* entry. The leaves of this [herb] resemble those of celery and also of Asiatic elder. All these three items are related to each other. This is why celery is called *shui ying* 水英, "water bloom," and the [herb discussed] here is called *lu ying*

665 *Yong ju* 癰疽, "obstruction-illness, impediment-illness." refers to two vaguely distinguished obstructions/impediments of vessels or other ducts inside the body. Qi rushing against the obstruction may cause a local swelling and eventually break through the surface to cause an abscess. BCGM Dict I, 642.

陸英, "land bloom," while Asiatic elder is called *mu ying shu* 木英樹, "wood bloom tree."[666] These are three "blooms," *ying* 英. The flowers and the leaves all resemble each other. [Ma] Zhi: Su Gong considers *lu ying* and *shuo diao* to be one item. A closer look today shows that *lu ying* has a bitter flavor, is cold and nonpoisonous. *Shuo diao* has a sour flavor, is warm and poisonous. Given such differences, it is difficult to say that they are one and the same item. The fact is, they are related. [Kou] Zongshi: *Shuo diao* and *lu ying* differ in terms of nature, flavor and place of origin. Their therapeutic potentials differ, too. Hence there should be no doubt whatsoever that they are two different items. [Su] Song: According to the *Ben cao*, *lu ying* grows in the river valleys of Xiong er and in Yuan ju. [The *Ben cao*] does not specify the *zhou* or soil where *shuo diao* comes from. It only states that it grows in the open country, and that it can be found everywhere. During spring a seedling rises. The seedling has nodes. Twigs grow from between the nodes. The leaves are as big as those of Chinese celery. The leaves are collected in spring and summer; the root and the stem are collected in autumn and winter. Tao [Hongjing] and Su Gong believe that [*lu ying* and *shuo diao*] are one item. Based on their different natures and flavors, Ma Zhi assumes that they may not be one item, but he, too, is unable to clearly distinguish them. However, the *Er ya* calls [the flowers] of trees of *hua* 華, it calls [the flowers] of herbs *rong* 榮, it calls [the flowers of plants] without *rong* 榮 that have fruit *xiu* 秀, and it calls [the flowers of plants] with *rong* 榮 and without fruit *ying* 英. The [plant discussed] here is named *ying* 英. This should refer to its flower. Therefore, when the *Ben jing* states: "it is collected at Autumn Begins," this is the time when it has flowers. [Li] Shizhen: Tao [Hongjing], Su [Gong's] *Ben cao*, Zheng Quan's *Yao xing lun*, they all say that *lu yin* is *shuo diao*. This is definitely based on evidence. Ma Zhi and Kou Zongshi contradict their sayings but they fail to provide evidence. That is, they must be one and the same item, with root, stem, flowers and leaves used differently, just as Su Song states.

【氣味】苦，寒，無毒。【權曰】陸英一名蒴藋，味苦、辛，有小毒。

Qi and Flavor. Bitter, cold, nonpoisonous. [Zhen] Quan: *Lu ying* is also called *shuo diao*. Flavor bitter, acrid. A little poisonous.

【主治】骨間諸痺，四肢拘攣疼酸，膝寒痛，陰痿，短氣不足，脚腫。本經。能捋風毒。脚氣上衝，心煩悶絶，水氣虛腫。風瘙皮肌惡痒，煎湯入少酒浴之，妙。甄權。

Control. All types of blockage in bones. The four limbs affected by cramps, contractions and pain. Painful knee related to the presence of cold. Yin [member (i. e. penis)] dysfunction. Short, insufficient [breath] qi. Swollen legs. *Ben jing*. It can

666 *Zheng lei* ch. 11, *lu ying* 陸英, does not have the character *shu* 樹, "tree."

disperse the poison of wind [intrusion], leg qi[667] rushing upward, heart with vexing heart-pressure threatening to interrupt [the flow of qi]. Hollow swelling with water and qi. Malign itch in the skin and muscles related to wind [intrusion].[668] Boil it to obtain a decoction, add a little wine and use it to bathe [the affected region]. Wondrous. Zhen Quan.

16-41

蒴藋音朔弔別録下品

Shuo diao, read *shuo diao*. FE *Bie lu*, lower rank.

***Sambucus chinensis* Lindl. Chinese elder.**

【釋名】堇草別録、芨別録、接骨草。

Explanation of Names. *Qin cao* 堇草, *Bie lu*. *Ji* 芨, *Bie lu*. *Jie gu cao* 接骨草, "bone setter herb."

【集解】【别録曰】蒴藋生田野。春夏采葉，秋冬采莖、根。【弘景曰】田野墟村甚多。【恭曰】此陸英也，剩出此條。爾雅云：芨，堇草。郭璞注云：烏頭苗也。檢三堇别名亦無此者。别録言此一名堇草，不知所出處。【宗奭曰】蒴藋花白，子初青如緑豆顆，每朶如盞面大，又平生，有一二百子，十月方熟紅。【時珍曰】每枝五葉。説見“陸英”下。

Collected Explanations. *Bie lu*: *Shuo diao* grows in the open country. The leaves are collected in spring and summer. Stem and root are collected in autumn and winter. [Tao] Hongjing: Very much of it can be found in the open country, in deserted villages. [Su] Gong: This is *lu ying* 陸英 (16-40). This entry is redundant. The *Er ya* states: *Ji* 芨 is *qin cao* 堇草. Guo Pu in his comment states: "This is the seedling of aconite." A study of the three [herbs with the name] *qin* 堇 as an alternative name has shown that the present item is not among them. The *Bie lu* speaks of *qin cao* 堇草 as first name [of an herb]. But it remains open where it comes from. [Kou] Zongshi: The flowers of *shuo diao* are white. The seeds are greenish in the beginning, similar to mung beans. Each flower is as big as the surface of a cup; some grow flat. They have 100 to 200 seeds. In the tenth month they ripen and turn red. [Li] Shizhen: Each twig has five leaves. For more details, see under the entry "*lu ying* 陸英33" (16-40).

---

667 *Jiao qi* 脚氣, "leg qi." Painful, weak, swollen legs. BCGM Dict I, 248.

668 *Feng sao yang* 風瘙癢, "wind itching," a condition of wind evil or wind cold entering the skin, with the skin itching, or the emergence of skin papules, as major signs. BCGM Dict I, 167.

【氣味】酸，温，有毒。【大明曰】苦，凉，有毒。

Qi and Flavor. Sour, warm, poisonous. Da Ming. Bitter, cool, poisonous.

【主治】風瘙癮疹，身癢濕痺，可作浴湯。别録。浴瘑癩風痺。大明。

Control. Wind itch and dormant papules.[669] Bodily itch and blockage related to the presence of moisture. It can be prepared to a decoction used for bathing. *Bie lu.* To wash lair-illness,[670] repudiation-illness and blockage related to wind [intrusion].[671] Da Ming.

【附方】舊十二，新七。

Added Recipes. 12 of old. Seven newly [recorded].

手足偏風。蒴藋葉，火燎，厚鋪牀上。趁熱眠於上，冷復易之。冬月取根，舂碎熬熱用。外臺秘要。

Hemilateral wind affecting hands and feet.[672] Burn shuo diao herbs above a fire and spread them in a thick layer on a bed. Then [let the patient] sleep on the hot [leaves], and replace them [with hot leaves again] once they have turned cold. During the winter months take the roots [instead of the leaves]. Pound them into pieces, simmer them and use them hot [for the same purpose as the leaves]. *Wai tai mi yao.*

風濕冷痺。方同上。

Blockage/numbness caused by wind, moisture and cold [intrusion]. Recipe identical to the one above.

寒濕腰痛。方同上。

Painful lower back caused by cold and moisture [intrusion]. Recipe identical to the one above.

---

669 *Yin zhen* 癮疹, "dormant papules," identical to *feng zhen* 風疹, "wind papules," a condition, brought forth by wind evil, of eruptive skin papules of different sizes, accompanied by unbearable itching. If scratched they rise further. BCGM Dict. I, 172.

670 *Guo* 瘑, "lair-illness," a condition of sores affecting both hands and feet, with pain and itching and gradual extension. In some cases crumbs are shed off. BCGM Dict I, 203.

671 *Da feng lai* 大風癩, "massive wind [i. e.,] repudiation-illness," most likely including cases of leprosy/Aussatz. BCGM Dict I, 111, 293

672 *Pian feng* 偏風, "hemilateral wind," a condition of unilateral loss of function and inability to move at one's will. Often an aftereffect of wind stroke. BCGM Dict I, 376.

脚氣脛腫，骨疼。蒴藋根研碎，和酒、醋共三分，根一合蒸熟，封裹腫上，一二日即消。亦治不仁。千金方。

Leg qi[673] with shin swelling and painful bones. Grind *shuo diao* root to pieces, mix three *fen* of wine and vinegar, and use this to steam one *ge* of the roots until done. Attach them to the swelling and bandage it. It will have dissolved within one or two days. It also serves to cure numbness. *Qian jin fang.*

渾身水腫，坐卧不得。取蒴藋根去皮，搗汁一合，和酒一合，煖服，當微吐利。梅師方。

Water swelling covering the entire body, making it impossible to sit or lie down. Take *shuo diao* roots, remove their skin and pound them to obtain one *ge* of juice. Mix it with one *ge* of wine and ingest this warm. This will cause some mild vomiting and free flow. *Mei shi fang.*

頭風作痛。蒴藋根二升，酒二升，煮服，汗出止。千金方。

Painful head wind.[674] Boil two *sheng* of *shuo diao* roots in two *sheng* of wine and ingest this hot. End [the treatment] when [the body] sweats. *Qian jin fang.*

頭風旋運，起倒無定。蒴藋、獨活、白石膏各一兩，枳實炒七錢半，每服三錢，酒一盞，煎六分服。聖惠方。

Head wind with vertigo. The [patient] may fall down when he rises at any time. [Mix] one *liang* each of *shuo diao*, *angelica biserrata* [root] and gypsum with seven and a half *qian* of immature and dried bitter orange fruit, fried. For each dose boil three *qian* [of this mixture] in one small cup of wine down to 60% and ingest this. *Sheng hui fang.*

產後血運，心悶煩熱。用接骨草，即蒴藋，破如算子一握，水一升，煎半升，分二服。或小便出血者，服之亦瘥。衛生易簡方。

Blood [induced brain] movement[675] following delivery, with heart-pressure and vexing heat. Break *jie gu cao* 接骨草, i. e., *shuo diao*, into pieces the size of abacus beads, boil a handful [of these pieces] in one *sheng* of water down to half a *sheng* and [let the woman] ingest this in two portions. Urination with blood can be healed, too, by ingesting this. *Wei sheng yi jian fang.*

673 *Jiao qi* 脚氣, "leg qi." Painful, weak, swollen legs. BCGM Dict I, 248.

674 *Tou feng* 頭風, "head wind," a condition of wind evil attacking the head followed by pain, or dizziness, or itching. BCGM Dict I, 509.

675 *Xue yun* 血運, "blood[-induced brain] movements." A condition of sudden vertigo brought forth by sudden and violent depletion of qi and blood following parturition. [Patients] pant and vomit. In severe cases this includes a clouded mind. BCGM Dict I, 602.

產後惡露不除。續骨木二十兩剉，水一斗，煮三升，分三服，即下。千金方。

Failure to release all malign dew[676] following delivery. File 20 *liang* of *xu gu mu* 續骨木 into pieces and boil them in one *dou* of water down to three *sheng*, to be ingested in three portions. [All lochia] will be discharged. *Qian jin fang*.

瘧疾不止。蒴藋一大握，炙令赤色，以水濃煎一盞，欲發前服。斗門方。

Unending malaria illness. Roast one generous handful of *shuo diao* until it assumes a red color and boil it in water to obtain a small cup of a thick decoction. Ingest it when an outbreak is imminent. *Dou men fang*.

卒暴癥塊，堅如石，作痛欲死。取蒴藋根一小束。洗净細擘，以酒二升，漬三宿，温服五合至一升，日三服。若欲速用，於熱灰中温出藥味服之。此方無毒，已愈十六人矣，神驗。藥盡再作之。古今録驗。

Sudden and violent formation of concretion-illness lumps that are as hard as stones, with pain so strong that one wishes to die. Take a small bunch of *shuo diao* roots, wash them clean, cut them into small pieces and soak them in two *sheng* of wine for three days and nights. Ingest five *ge* up to one *sheng* of the warm [liquid]. To be ingested three times a day. If one wishes to use [this medication] right away, warm [the roots] in hot ashes until they emit a medicinal flavor/smell and ingest them. This recipe is nonpoisonous. It has cured 16 persons and is divinely effective. Once the medication is used up, prepare it again. *Gu jin lu yan*.

鼈瘕堅硬，腫起如盆，眠卧不得。蒴藋根白皮一握，擣汁和水服。千金方。

Turtle[-shaped] conglomeration-illness[677] hardening, with a swelling rising similar to a pot, making it impossible to sleep. Pound a handful of the white skin of *shuo diao* root to obtain a juice and ingest it mixed with water. *Qian jin fang*.

下部閉塞。蒴藋根一把，擣汁水和，絞去滓。强人每服一升。外臺秘要。

The lower [body] part blocked by constipation. Pound a handful of *shuo diao* roots to obtain a juice. Mix it with water and squeeze it to remove the dregs. Strong persons each time ingest one *sheng*. *Wai tai mi yao*.

---

676 *E lu* 惡露, "malign dew," blood or turbid liquid (i.e. lochia) leaving from the birth canal after parturition. BCGM Dict. 141.

677 *Bie jia* 鱉瘕, "turtle[-shaped] conglomeration-illness," a *jia* 瘕, "conglomeration-illness," in the abdomen that is shaped like a turtle and moves if squeezed. It was believed that such a condition could result from eating turtles. BCGM Dict I, 67.

一切風瘮。蒴藋煮湯，和少酒塗之，無不瘥。梅師方。

All types of wind papules.[678] Mix a *shuo diao* decoction with some wine and apply this [to the affected region]. There is not a single case that is not cured. *Mei shi fang*.

小兒赤遊，上下遊行，至心即死。蒴藋煎汁洗之。子母秘録。

Red roaming [cinnabar poison][679] of children. It moves up and down, and is constantly roaming. When it reaches the heart, [the patient] dies. Boil *shuo diao* to obtain a juice and wash the [affected region with it]. *Zi mu mi lu*.

五色丹毒。蒴藋葉搗傅之。千金方。

Cinnabar poison[680] of all five colors. Pound *shuo diao* leaves [to a pulp] and apply it [to the affected region]. *Qian jin fang*.

癰腫惡肉不消者。蒴藋灰、石灰各淋取汁，合煎如膏，傅之。能蝕惡肉，亦去痣疵。此藥過十日即不中用也。千金方。

Swelling related to obstruction-illness[681] with malign flesh [growth] that fails to dissolve. Separately drip water over *shuo diao* ashes and lime, mix the two resulting juices and fry them to obtain a paste. Apply it [to the affected region]. It can eat away malign flesh [growth] and it also serves to remove moles and blemishes. This medication should not be applied for more than ten days. *Qian jin fang*.

手足疣目。蒴藋子揉爛，塗目上。聖惠方。

Warts on hands and feet. Rub *shuo diao* seeds[682] to a pulp and apply it onto the warts. *Sheng hui fang*.

熊羆傷人。蒴藋一大把，以水一升漬，須臾，取汁飲，以滓封之。張文仲備急方。

A human harmed by a bear. Soak one generous handful of *shuo diao* in one *sheng* of water for a short while, get the liquid and [let the patient] drink it. Use the dregs to cover [the wounds]. Zhang Wenzhong, *Bei ji fang*.

678 *Feng zhen* 風疹, "wind papules," a condition, brought forth by wind evil, of eruptive skin papules of different sizes, accompanied by unbearable itching. If scratched they rise further. BCGM Dict I, 172.

679 [*Chi you*] *dan du* [赤游]丹毒, "[red roaming] cinnabar poison," a condition of *dan du* 丹毒, "cinnabar poison," with rashes that seem to be hiding. They move here and there and have no permanent location. BCGM Dict I, 89.

680 *Dan du* 丹毒, "cinnabar poison," a skin ailment with red rashes. BCGM Dict I, 118

681 *Yong* 癰, "obstruction-illness,"refers to an obstruction of vessels or other ducts inside the body. Qi rushing against the obstruction may cause a local swelling and eventually break through the surface to cause an abscess. BCGM Dict I, 641.

682 *Zheng lei* ch. 11, *shuo diao*, quoting Zhang Wenzhong, writes *chi zi* 赤子, "red seeds."

16-42
水英宋圖經
Shui ying, FE Song, *Tu jing*.

Water bloom.

【釋名】魚津草。【頌曰】唐天寶單方圖言：此草原生永陽池澤及河海邊。臨汝人呼爲牛葒草，河北信都人名水節，河内連内黄呼爲水棘，劍南、遂寧等郡名龍移草，淮南諸郡名海荏。嶺南亦有，土地尤宜，莖葉肥大，名海精木，亦名魚津草。【時珍曰】此草不著形狀氣味，無以考證。芹菜亦名水英，不知是此否也。

Explanation of Names. *Yu jin cao* 魚津草, "fish liquid herb." [Su] Song: The Tang era *Tian bao dan fang tu* says: "This herb originally grew at/in the ponds and marshlands of Yong yang and at the shores of rivers and the sea." People in Lin ru call it *niu hong cao* 牛葒草. People in Xin du, in He bei, call it *shui jie* 水節. In both He nei and Nei huang it is called *shui ji* 水棘. In the prefectures of Jian nan and Sui ning it is called *long yi cao* 龍移草. In all the prefectures of Huai nan it is called *hai ren* 海荏. It can also be found in Ling nan. The soil and ground there are particularly advantageous for its [growth]. Stem and leaves are fat and big. It is called *hai jing mu* 海精木, "sea essence wood." Another name is *yu jin cao* 魚津草. [Li] Shizhen: Of this herb, the physical appearance as well as its qi and flavor are not recorded. There is nothing that could be examined. Celery vegetables are also called *shui ying* 水英. It remains open whether this [item] is identical to them or not.

【氣味】缺。

Qi and Flavor. Missing.

【主治】骨風。蘇頌。

Control. Wind [intrusion] in bones. Su Song.

【發明】【頌曰】蜀人采其花合面藥。凡丈夫婦人無故兩脚腫滿，連膝脛中痛，屈申急强者，名骨風。其疾不宜針灸及服藥，惟每日取此草五斤，以水一石，煮三斗，及熱浸脚，并淋膝上，日夜三四度。不經五日即瘥，數用神驗。其藥春取苗，夏采葉及花，秋冬用根。腫甚者，加生椒目三升、水二斗。用畢，即摩粉避風。忌油膩、生菜、豬、魚等物。

Explication. [Su] Song: People in Shu collect its flowers to prepare a medicinal powder. When males or women are affected without apparent reason by swelling and fullness of both legs, with pain encompassing the knees and the shins, and with difficulties to bend and stretch the stiff [legs], this is called "bone wind." For this illness it is not advisable to apply needling and cauterization, or to ingest medication. The only [therapy possible is as follows]. Each day boil five *jin* of this herb in one *dan* of water down to three *dou* and soak the [affected] legs in the hot [liquid]. Also, pour it on the knees. Do this three to four times during day and night. After less then five days a cure is achieved. It is often applied with divine effect. Of this pharmaceutical substance, in spring get its seedlings, in summer collect its leaves and flowers. In autumn and winter resort to its root. In the case of a severe swelling, add three *sheng* of Chinese pepper and two *sheng* of water. When the application is completed, rub powder [on the affected parts] and avoid wind. [During the treatment] oily and fat substances, raw vegetables, pork and fish are forbidden.

16-43
藍本經上品
Lan, FE *Ben jing*, upper rank.

***Polygonum tinctorium* Lour. Indigo plant.**

【釋名】【時珍曰】按陸佃埤雅云：月令仲夏令民無刈藍以染。鄭玄言恐傷長養之氣也。然則刈藍先王有禁，制字從監，以此故也。

Explanation of Names. [Li] Shizhen: According to Lu Dian's *Pi ya*, "the *Yue ling* decrees that 'in mid summer people must not cut *lan* for dying.' Zheng Xuan says 'this was decreed out of fear that the qi of growth and nourishing might be harmed.' Therefore, the kings of former times have forbidden to cut *lan* 藍. This is why the character [*lan* 藍] was devised based on [the character] *jian* 監, 'to supervise'."

【集解】【別録曰】藍實生河内平澤，其莖葉可以染青。【弘景曰】此即今染[糸 禁]碧所用者，以尖葉者爲勝。【恭曰】藍有三種。一種葉圍徑二寸許，厚三四分者，堪染青，出嶺南，太常名爲木藍子。陶氏所説乃是菘藍，其汁抨爲澱，甚青者。本經所用乃是蓼藍實也，其苗似蓼而味不辛，不堪爲澱，惟作碧色爾。【頌曰】藍處處有之，人家蔬圃作畦種。至三月、四月生苗，高三二尺許，葉似水蓼，花紅白色，實亦若蓼子而大，黑色，五月、六月采實。但可染碧，不堪作澱，此名蓼藍，即醫方所用者也。別有木藍，出嶺南，不入藥。有菘藍，可爲澱，亦名馬藍。爾雅所謂葴，馬藍是也。又福州一種馬藍，四時俱有，葉類苦蕒菜，土人連根采服，治敗血。江寧一種吴藍，二月内生，如蒿，葉青花白，亦解熱毒。此二種雖不類，而俱有藍名，且古方多用吴藍，或恐是此，故并附之。【宗奭曰】藍實即大藍實也。謂之蓼藍者，非是。乃爾雅所謂馬藍者，解諸藥毒不可闕也。實與葉兩用，註不解實，只解葉，爲未盡。【時珍曰】藍凡五種，各有主治，惟藍實專取蓼藍者。蓼藍：葉如蓼，五六月開花，成穗細小，淺紅色，子亦如蓼，歲可三刈，故先王禁之。菘藍：葉如白菘。馬藍：葉如苦蕒，即郭璞所謂大葉冬藍，俗中所謂板藍者。二藍花子並如蓼藍。吴藍：長莖如蒿而花白，吴人種之。木藍：長莖如决明，高者三四尺，分枝布葉，葉如槐葉，七月開淡紅花，結角長寸許，纍纍如小豆角，其子亦如馬蹄决明子而微小，迥與諸藍不同，而作澱則一也。別有甘藍，可食，見本條。蘇恭以馬藍爲木藍，蘇頌以菘藍爲馬藍，寇宗奭以藍實爲大葉藍之實，皆非矣。今並開列于下。

Collected Explanations. *Bie lu*: *Lan shi* grows in the marshlands of the plains of He nei. [Tao] Hongjing: It is used to dye something dark red and greenish-blue. [Herbs] with pointed leaves are best. [Su] Gong: There exist three kinds of *lan*. One kind has leaves with a perimeter of more than two *cun*. They are three to four *fen* thick. It is used to dye something greenish, and it comes from Ling nan. It is generally called *mu lan zi* 木藍子. The one Mr. Tao [Hongjing] speaks of is *song lan* 菘藍. Its juice is converted to indigo of a deep greenish color. The one used by the *Ben cao* is *liao lan shi* 蓼藍實. Its seedling resembles that of knotweed, *liao* 蓼, but its flavor is not acrid. It cannot be prepared to indigo dyestuff. It is only made to a bluish-green color. [Su] Song: *Lan* 藍 can be found everywhere. Private households plant it in their vegetable gardens in rectangular patches. By the third and fourth month it grows a seedling reaching a height of more than two or three *chi*. The leaves resemble those of knotweed; the flowers are red-white. The fruit, too, resemble the seeds of knotweed, but are bigger and black. The fruits are collected in the fifth and sixth month. They only serve to dye something bluish-green; they are not suitable for preparing indigo dyestuff. [This kind] is named *liao lan* 蓼藍, it is the one resorted to in medicinal recipes. In addition there is a *mu lan* 木藍; it comes from Ling nan and is not added to medication. Then there is *song lan* 菘藍. It can be prepared to indigo dyestuff. It is also named *ma lan* 馬藍. When the *Er ya* speaks of *xian* 葴, then this is *ma lan* 馬藍. Also, in Fu zhou a kind of *ma lan* 馬藍 is available through all four seasons. Its leaves are similar to those of *sow thistle* [herbs]. The locals collect and ingest them together with the root to cure blood decay. In Jiang ning is a kind [named] *wu lan* 吳藍. It grows in the second month and resembles wormwood. The leaves are greenish, and the flowers are white. It also serves to resolve heat poison. These two kinds are not related, but they both are named *lan* 藍. Also, when ancient recipes often [recommend to] use [*lan* 藍], this may be *wu lan* 吳藍, or it may be [the item discussed] here. Hence [entries of] both [*ma lan* 馬藍 and *wu lan* 吳藍] are added as an appendix. [Kou] Zongshi: *Lan shi* 藍實 refers to *da lan shi* 大藍實. To say that this is *liao lan* 蓼藍, is wrong. The *ma lan* 馬藍 spoken of by the *Er ya* is an indispensable substance for dissolving all types of medicinal poison. Both fruit and leaves are used, but the commentary fails to explain the fruit; it explains only the leaves. It is incomplete. [Li] Shizhen: *Lan* 藍 altogether comprises five kinds. Each exerts its specific therapeutic control. Only for *lan shi* 藍實 specifically *liao lan* 蓼藍 is resorted to. *Liao lan* 蓼藍 has leaves like knotweed.

It opens flowers in the fifth and sixth month. They form fine, small spikes of a pale red color. The seeds, too, are similar to those of knotweed. [*Liao lan* 蓼藍] can be cut three times a year. Hence former kings prohibited it. *Song lan* 菘藍: Its leaves are similar to those of celery cabbage. *Ma lan* 馬藍: Its leaves are similar to those of *ow thistle*. This is the [herb] referred to by Guo Pu as "big leaf winter *lan* 藍." It is commonly called *ban lan* 板藍. The flowers and the seeds of these two *lan* 藍 kinds are similar to those of *liao lan* 蓼藍. *Wu lan* 吴藍: It has a long stem similar to that of wormwood [herbs], and white flowers. Wu people plant it. *Mu lan* 木藍: It has a long stem similar to that of fetid *cassia* [herbs]. Tall specimens reach a height of three to four *chi*. The twigs branch out like leaves, and the leaves are similar to *sophora japonica* tree leaves. [*Mu lan*] opens pale red flowers in the seventh month. It forms horn[-like pods] more than a *cun* long. They form a line similar to mung bean pods. The seeds are red similar to fetid *cassia* seeds, but they are very small. [*Mu lan*] is very different from all the other *lan* kinds, but its usage as an indigo dyestuff is identical. In addition, there is a *gan lan* 甘藍. It is edible. See the respective entry (16-46). Su Gong identifies *ma lan* 馬藍 as *mu lan* 木藍. Su Song identifies *song lan* 菘藍 as *ma lan* 馬藍. Kou Zongshi identifies *lan shi* 藍實 as the fruit of big leaf *lan* 藍. They are all wrong. Today each [of these herbs] is listed below.

16-43-01
藍實 ***Lan shi***
Fruit of *lan*.

【氣味】苦，寒，無毒。【權曰】甘。

Qi and Flavor. Bitter, cold, nonpoisonous. [Zhen] Quan: Sweet.

【主治】解諸毒。殺蠱蚑疰鬼螫毒。久服頭不白，輕身。本經。蚑音其，小兒鬼也。填骨髓，明耳目，利五臟，調六腑，通關節，治經絡中結氣，使人健、少睡，益心力。甄權。療毒腫。蘇恭。

Control. It resolves all types of poison. It kills the poison of *gu*,[683] of qi 蚑 attachment-illness and demonic stings. Ingested over a long time it prevents [the hair from] turning white and relieves the body of its weight. *Ben jing*. Qi 蚑 is read *qi* 其. This is a child demon. [*Lan* fruit] fill bone marrow, clear ears and eyes, free the passage through the five long-term depots, regulate the six short-term repositories, penetrate the joints, serve to cure bound qi in the conduits and network vessels,

683 *Gu du* 蠱毒, "*gu*-poison[ing]." (1) A poison emitted by certain worms/snakes with an ability to cause varying pathological changes in a person who has taken it in by means of wine or food. (2) Abdominal fullness, in some cases with blood spitting, and blood in the stool and urine. BCGM Dict I, 192 - 193. See BCGM 42-22.

let one be robust and sleep only a little, and boost the strength of the heart. Zhen Quan. They heal swelling with poison. Su Gong.

16-43-02
藍葉汁此蓼藍也 *Lan ye zhi*
Juice of *lan* leaves. This is *liao lan*.

【氣味】苦、甘，寒，無毒。

Qi and Flavor. Bitter, sweet, cold, nonpoisonous.

【主治】殺百藥毒。解狼毒、射罔毒。別録。【弘景曰】解毒不得生藍汁，以青[糸 禁]布漬汁亦善。汁塗五心，止煩悶，療蜂螫毒。弘景。斑蝥、芫青、樗雞毒。朱砂、砒石毒。時珍。

Control. It kills the poison of the hundreds of pharmaceutical drugs. It resolves the poison of wolfsbane and *aconitum* [accessory tuber]. *Bie lu*. [Tao] Hongjing: If to resolve poison one is unable to get fresh *lan* juice, the juice obtained by soaking an indigo dyed fabric in water is suitable, too. When the juice is applied to the five "hearts/centers," (the center of the body, the palms and the soles), it ends vexing heart-pressure and cures poisoning by bee/wasp and scorpion [stings]. [Tao] Hongjing. The poison of blister beetles, blister flies and latern flies. The poison of cinnabar and arsenic. [Li] Shizhen.

16-43-03
馬藍 *Ma lan*
***Baphicacanthus cusia* (Nees) Bremek**

【主治】婦人敗血。連根焙，擣下篩，酒服一錢匕。蘇頌。

Control. Blood decay of women. Bake it with its root over a slow fire, pound it and pass [the powder] through a sieve. [Let the woman] ingest with wine the amount held by a one *qian* spoon. Su Song.

16-43-04
吴藍 *Wu lan*

【氣味】苦、甘，冷，無毒。

Qi and Flavor. Bitter, sweet, cold, nonpoisonous.

【主治】寒熱頭痛，赤眼，天行熱狂，丁瘡，遊風熱毒，腫毒風瘮，除煩止渴，殺疳，解毒藥毒箭，金瘡血悶，毒刺蟲蛇傷，鼻衄吐血，排膿，産後血運，小兒壯熱。解金石藥毒、狼毒、射罔毒。大明。

Control. Alternating sensations of cold and heat with headache, red eyes, epidemic heat with madness, pin[-illness][684] sores, roaming wind[685] and heat poison, swelling with poison and wind papules.[686] It eliminates vexation and ends thirst. It kills *gan*-illness[687] [worms/bugs] and dissolves medicinal poison and arrow poison. [It serves to cure] wounds caused by metal objects/weapons and blood [disorder] with heart-pressure, harm caused by poisonous worm/bug and snake bites, nosebleed and blood spitting. It dispels pus and blood induced [brain] movement following delivery. Strong heat of children. It resolves the poison of metal and mineral medication, of wolfsbane and *aconitum* [accessory tuber]. Da Ming.

【發明】【震亨曰】藍屬水，能使敗血分歸經絡。【時珍曰】諸藍形雖不同，而性味不遠，故能解毒除熱。惟木藍葉力似少劣，藍子則專用蓼藍者也。至于用澱與青布，則是刈藍浸水入石灰澄成者，性味不能不少異，不可與藍汁一概論也。有人病嘔吐，服玉壺諸丸不效，用藍汁入口即定，蓋亦取其殺蟲降火爾。如此之類，不可不知。【頌曰】藍汁治蟲豸傷。劉禹錫傳信方著其法云：取大藍汁一盌，入雄黄、麝香二物少許，以點咬處，仍細服其汁，神異之極也。張薦員外住劍南，爲張延賞判官，忽被斑蜘蛛咬頭上，一宿，咬處有二道赤色，細如箸，繞項上，從胸前下至心。經兩宿，頭面腫疼，大如數升盌，肚漸腫，幾至不救。張公出錢五百千，并薦家財又數百千，募能療者。忽一人應召，云可治。張公甚不信之，欲驗其方。其人云：不惜方，但療人性命爾。遂取大藍汁一盌，以蜘蛛投之，至汁而死。又取藍汁加麝香、雄黄，更以一蛛投入，随化爲水。張公因甚異之，遂令點于咬處。兩日悉平，作小瘡而愈。

Explication. [Zhu] Zhenheng. *Lan* 藍 is associated with water. It is able to let decayed blood return to the respective conduits and network [vessels]. [Li] Shizhen: Even though the physical appearance of all the *lan* kinds differs, their nature and flavor are not far apart from each other. Hence all of them are able to resolve poison and dispel heat. Only the strength of *mu lan* 木藍 leaves appears to be rather limited. When *lan* seeds are required, one resorts to only those of *liao lan* 蓼藍. As to

684 *Ding* 丁, "pin[-illness]," also *ding* 疔, "pin-illness," refers to a deep-reaching and festering hardness in a tissue, eventually rising above the skin like a pinhead. BCGM Dict I, 127-129.

685 *You feng* 游風," roaming wind," a condition of roaming and sudden pain and itching brought about by *feng xie* 風邪, "wind evil." BCGM Dict I, 645.

686 *Feng zhen* 風疹, "wind papules," a condition, brought forth by wind evil, of eruptive skin papules of different sizes, accompanied by unbearable itching. If scratched they rise further. BCGM Dict I, 172.

687 *Gan* 疳, "*gan*-illness," also: "sweets-illness," involves several complaints that affect children and adults, with causes and conditions too different to fall into a known disease category. BCGM Dict I, 180-188.

indigo dyestuff and greenish fabric, they are produced by cutting *lan*, soaking it in water, adding lime and using the clear liquid. Nature and flavor [of this liquid] are quite different and cannot be argued about in the same way as *lan* juice. There was a man who suffered from vomiting. He ingested all types of pills from jade bottles, but without effect. When he took *lan zhi*, [the vomiting] ended. The fact is, this, too, is an example of resorting to its ability to kill worms/bugs and to let fire descend. Such things must be known. [Su] Song: *Lan* juice serves to cure harm caused by worms/bugs and insects. Liu Yuxi in his *Chuan xin fang* records the respective method. Take a bowl with big [leaf] *lan* juice, add a little realgar and musk and drip this on the location of the bite. Also, ingest small portions of the juice. This is of divinely, extraordinary [effect]. When Zhang Jian served as a judge under Zhang Yanshang in Jian nan, he was suddenly bitten by a multi-colored spider on his head. During the night two paths of red color developed from the location of the bite. They were as fine as chopsticks and formed a circle on his head. Then they extended from the frontside of his chest to his central region. After the second night his head and face were affected by painful swelling the size of a bowl of several *sheng*, and his belly slowly swelled. He came close to a status where he could not be rescued. Mr. Zhang [Yanshang] took out 500 000 cash and [Zhang] Jian's family added another several hundred thousands to attract someone who could heal him. Then without prior notice a man responded to the call, stating that he could cure [Zhang Jian]. Mr. Zhang did not believe him and wanted to examine his recipe. That man stated: "I do not hesitate [to unveil] this recipe. My only intention is to rescue this person's life." Then he took a bowl of large [leaf] *lan* juice and tossed a spider into it. As soon as it came into contact with the juice it died. Then he took additional *lan* juice, added musk and realgar and once again gave a spider into it. It was immediately transformed to water. As a result, Mr. Zhang [Yanzhang] considered this [recipe] to be something special and had [the liquid] dripped on the location of the bite. Within two days [the swelling] flattened. A small sore formed, and [the patient] was healed.

【附方】舊十一，新六。

Added Recipes. Eleven of old. Six newly [recorded].

小兒赤痢。搗青藍汁二升，分四服。子母秘録。

Red free-flux illness of children. Pound greenish *lan* to obtain two *sheng* of juice and [let the child] ingest it in four portions. *Zi mu mi lu.*

小兒中蠱，下血欲死。搗青藍汁，頻服之。聖惠方。

Children struck by *gu*,[688] with a discharge of blood bringing them close to death. Pound greenish *lan* to obtain a juice and [let the child] repeatedly ingest it. *Sheng hui fang*.

陰陽易病。傷寒初愈，交合陰陽，必病拘急，手足拳，小腹急熱，頭不能舉，名陰陽易，當汗之，滿四日難治。藍一把，雄鼠屎三七枚，水煎服。取汗。聖惠方。

Yin yang exchange[689] disease. To have sexual intercourse when a harm caused by cold was just healed inevitably lets one suffer from contraction and tension. Hands and feet cramp. The lower abdomen is tense and hot. The head cannot be raised. This is called yin yang exchange. It must be treated by sweating. When it has lasted for four full days, it is difficult to cure. Boil a handful of *lan* and three times seven pieces of excrements of a male mouse/rat in water and ingest this to cause a sweating. *Sheng hui fang*.

驚癇發熱。乾藍、凝水石等分，爲末，水調傅頭上。聖惠方。

Fright epilepsy with heat effusion. [Grind] equal amounts of dried *lan* and the "stone that congeals water" (11-05) into powder. Mix it with water and apply it to the [patient's] head. *Sheng hui fang*.

上氣欬嗽，呷呀息氣，喉中作聲，唾粘。以藍葉水浸搗汁一升，空腹頻服。須臾以杏仁研汁，煮粥食之。一兩日將息，依前法更服，吐痰盡方瘥。梅師方。

Rising qi with cough. Breathing qi with creaking. Sounds generated inside the throat. Sticky saliva. Soak *lan* leaves in water and pound them to obtain one *sheng* of juice. Repeatedly ingest it on an empty abdomen. Then boil a congee with the juice obtained by grinding apricot seeds and eat it. Rest for one or two days and then ingest [the medication] the same way as before. When all the phlegm is spit out, this is the cure. *Mei shi fang*.

飛血赤目熱痛。乾藍葉切二升，車前草半兩，淡竹葉切三握，水四升，煎二升，去滓溫洗。冷即再煖，以瘥爲度。聖濟總録。

---

688 *Gu du* 蠱毒, "*gu*-poison[ing]." (1) A poison emitted by certain worms/snakes with an ability to cause varying pathological changes in a person who has taken it in by means of wine or food. (2) Abdominal fullness, in some cases with blood spitting, and blood in the stool and urine. BCGM Dict I, 192 - 193. See BCGM 42-22.

689 *Yin yang yi* 陰陽易, "yin and yang exchange," a condition of a communicable disease acquired through sexual intercourse by persons who had been cured of harm caused by cold only shortly before. BCGM Dict I, 639.

Flying blood[690] with red eyes and painful heat. Cut two *sheng* of dried *lan* leaves and boil them together with half a *liang* of Asiatic plantain [herb] and three handfuls of cut, bland bamboo leaves in four *sheng* of water down to two *sheng*. Discard the dregs and use the warm [liquid] to wash [the affected region]. When it has turned cold, heat it again. Continue until a cure is achieved. *Sheng ji zong lu.*

腹中鼈癥。藍葉一斤，搗，以水三升絞汁，服一升，日二次。千金方。

Turtle[-shaped] concretion-illness[691] Pound one *jin* of *lan* leaves and [soak the resulting pulp] in three *sheng* of water. Squeeze it to obtain a juice. Ingest one *sheng*. Twice a day. *Qian jin fang.*

應聲蟲病。腹中有物作聲，隨人語言，名應聲蟲病。用板藍汁一盞，分五服，效。夏子益奇疾方。

Echo bug disease.[692] When an item in the abdomen creates sounds echoing human voices, this is called "echo bug disease." Divide a small cup of *ban lan* juice into five portions and ingest them. Effective. Xia Ziyi, *Qi ji fang.*

卒中水毒。搗藍青汁，傅頭身令匝。肘後方。

Suddenly being struck by water poison. Pound *lan qing* to obtain a juice. Apply it to cover the entire head and body. *Zhou hou fang.*

服藥過劑，煩悶，及中毒煩悶欲死。搗藍汁服數升。肘後方。

Vexing heart-pressure resulting from a medication overdose. Also, poisoning with vexing heart-pressure bringing one close to death. Pound *lan* to obtain a juice and ingest several *sheng*. *Zhou hou fang.*

卒自縊死。以藍汁灌之。千金方。

Death from suicidal hanging. Force-feed *lan* juice [to the victim]. *Qian jin fang.*

毒箭傷人。藍青搗飲并傅之。如無藍，以青布漬汁飲。肘後方。

A person harmed by a poisoned arrow. Pound *lan qing* [to obtain a juice]. Drink it and apply it [to the affected region]. If no *lan* is at hand, soak a greenish [indigo dyed] cloth [in water] and drink the resulting juice. *Zhou hou fang.*

---

690 *Fei xue* 飛血, "flying blood," an illness sign of red vessels covering the white part of the eyeballs. BCGM Dict I, 156.

691 *Bie zheng* 鼈癥, "turtle[-shaped] concretion-illness," identical to *bie jia* 鱉瘕, "turtle[-shaped] conglomeration-illness," in the abdomen that is shaped like a turtle and moves if squeezed. It was believed that such a condition could result from eating turtles. BCGM Dict I, 67.

692 *Ying sheng chong bing* 應聲蟲病, "echo-bug disease," a disease with something in the abdomen issuing sounds echoing human voices. BCGM Dict I, 641.

唇邊生瘡，連年不瘥。以八月藍葉一斤，搗汁洗之，不過三度瘥。千金方。

Sores developing on the margins of the lips that are not healed for several years. Pound one *jin* of *lan* leaves, [collected] in the eighth month, and wash [the sores] with the resulting juice. A cure is achieved after no more than three [applications]. *Qian jin fang.*

齒䘌腫痛。紫藍燒灰傅之，日五度。聖惠方。

Hidden worms teeth[693] with painful swelling. Burn *zi lan* to ashes and apply them [to the affected region]. Five times a day. *Sheng hui fang.*

頭禿瘡。糞藍煎汁頻洗。聖濟録。

Bald head sores. Boil excrement *lan*[694] to obtain a juice and wash [the affected region]. *Sheng ji lu.*

天泡熱瘡。藍葉搗傅之，良。集簡方。

Celestial blister sores[695] with heat. Pound *lan* leaves [to a pulp] and apply it [to the affected region]. *Ji jian fang.*

瘡疹不快。板藍根一兩，甘草一分，爲末。每服半錢或一錢，取雄雞冠血三二點，同温酒少許調下。錢氏小兒方。

Sores and papules that do not vanish soon. [Grind] one *liang* of *ban lan* root and one *fen* of *glycyrrhiza* [root] into powder. Each time ingest half a *qian* or one *qian*. Add two or three drops of blood from the comb of a cock, and send this down mixed with a little warm wine. Qian shi, *Xiao er fang.*

16-44
澱綱目
Lan dian. FE *Gang mu.*

Indigo. Blue sediment.

【釋名】【時珍曰】澱，石殿也，其滓澄殿在下也。亦作淀，俗作靛。南人掘地作坑，以藍浸水一宿，入石灰攪至千下，澄去水則青黑色。亦可乾收，用染青碧。其攪刘浮沫，掠出陰乾，謂之靛花，即青黛。見下。

693 *Chi ni* 齒䘌, "hidden-worms teeth," a tooth disease with a malodorous liquid excreted. BCGM Dict I, 87.

694 *Fen lan* 糞藍, lit. "excrement *lan*," unidentified substance. A short entry is added to ch. 21: 21-A53.

695 *Tian pao chuang* 天泡瘡, "celestial blister sores," a condition of sores with the appearance of blisters filled with water or pus, especially in children. BCGM Dict I, 503.

Explanation of Names. [Li] Shizhen: *Dian* 澱 is a stone sediment, *dian* 殿. These are dregs that have settled as sediment at the bottom. [The character is] also written *dian* 淀, and it is commonly written *dian* 靛. People in the South dig a pit in the ground. There they soak *lan* in water for one night. Then they add lime and stir this 1000 times. When the sediment has settled, they remove the water and [the sediment] has assumed a greenish-black color. It can be dried and stored and serves to dye greenish and jade-bluish-greenish. The foam generated on the surface during the stirring is removed and dried in the yin (i. e., shade). It is called *dian hua* 靛花; it is natural indigo, *qing dai* 青黛. See the next [entry] (16-45).

【氣味】辛、苦，寒，無毒。

Qi and Flavor. Acrid, bitter, cold, nonpoisonous.

【主治】解諸毒。傅熱瘡，小兒禿瘡熱腫。藏器。止血殺蟲，治噎膈。時珍。

Control. It resolves all types of poison. It is applied to sores with heat, and to baldness sores and swelling with heat of children. [Chen] Cangqi. It ends bleeding and kills worms/bugs. It serves to cure gullet occlusion.[696] [Li] Shizhen.

【發明】【時珍曰】澱乃藍與石灰作成。其氣味與藍稍有不同，而其止血拔毒殺蟲之功，似勝於藍。按廣五行記云：唐永徽中，絳州一僧病噎，不下食數年。臨終命其徒曰：吾死後，可開吾胸喉，視有何物苦我如此。及死，其徒依命，開視胸中，得一物，形似魚而有兩頭，遍體悉似肉鱗，安鉢中，跳躍不已。戲投諸味，雖不見食，悉化爲水。又投諸毒物，亦皆銷化。一僧方作藍澱，因以少澱投之，即怖懼奔走，須臾化成水。世傳澱水能治噎疾，蓋本于此。今方士或以染缸水飲人治噎膈，皆取其殺蟲也。

Explication. [Li] Shizhen: *Dian* 澱 is prepared from indigo plants, *lan* 藍, and lime. Its qi and flavor differ a little from those of indigo plants, and its potential of ending bleeding, pulling out poison and killing worms/bugs seems to be superior to that of indigo plants. According to the *Guang wu xing ji*, during the Tang dynasty, during the *yong hui* reign period (650-655), "a monk in Jiang zhu suffered from gullet occlusion and was unable to eat for several years. When he neared the end of his life, he said to his students: 'When I have died, you may open my chest and throat to find out what kind of an item has let me suffer like this.' When he had died, his students followed his order. They opened him and took a look into his chest. There they obtained an item shaped like a fish with two heads. The entire body seemed to be covered by fleshy scales. They placed it into a cup where it continued to wriggle.

696 *Ye ge* 噎膈, "gullet occlusion," a disease situated in the chest and diaphragm region with a sensation of an obstacle in the chest, heart-pressure, and pain, and a failure of beverages and food to move through a blocked esophagus. BCGM Dict I, 189.

They tossed all types of food into [the cup] and even though it was not seen to eat, all [the food] was transformed to water. Then they threw all types of poisonous items at it and they, too, were all dissolved. A monk happened to prepare indigo dyestuff, *lan dian* 藍澱, and threw a little of it [into the cup]. [The item appeared to be] frightened and to run away, but was dissolved to water right away. The tradition throughout the ages that indigo dyestuff can serve to cure gullet occlusion is, in fact, based on this [anecdote]." Today, recipe experts sometimes cure gullet occlusion with water from a dye vat, availing themselves of its ability to kill worms/bugs.

【附方】新四。

Added Recipes. Four newly [recorded].

時行熱毒，心神煩躁。用藍澱一匙，新汲水一盞服。聖惠方。

Seasonally prevalent heat poison with vexing restlessness affecting heart and spirit. Ingest one spoonful of *lan dian* with a small cup of newly drawn water. *Sheng hui fang*.

小兒熱丹。藍澱傅之。秘録方。

Cinnabar [poison][697] with heat of children. Apply *lan dian* [to the affected region]. *Mi lu fang*.

口鼻急疳，數日欲死。以藍澱傅之令遍，日十度，夜四度。千金翼。

Acute *gan*-illness[698] affecting mouth and nose, and bringing one close to death within a few days. Apply *lan dian* to the entire [affected region], ten times during the day, four times during the night. *Qian jin yi*.

誤吞水蛭。青靛調水飲，即瀉出。普濟方。

Accidentally having swallowed a leech. Drink water mixed with greenish indigo and it will leave with an outflow. *Pu ji fang*.

697 *Dan du* 丹毒, "cinnabar poison," a skin ailment with red rashes. BCGM Dict I, 118

698 *Gan* 疳, "*gan*-illness," also: "sweets-illness," involves several complaints that affect children and adults, with causes and conditions too different to fall into a known disease category. BCGM Dict I, 180–188.

16-45
青黛宋開寶
***Qing dai*. FE Song, *Kai bao*.**

Natural Indigo. Prepared from → Chinese Indigo plants, *lan* 藍.

【釋名】靛花綱目、青蛤粉。【時珍曰】黛，眉色也。劉熙釋名云：滅去眉毛，以此代之，故謂之黛。

Explanation of Names: *Dian hua* 靛花, *Gang mu*. *Qing ge fen* 青蛤粉, "greenish clam powder." [Li] Shizhen: *Dai* 黛 is eyebrow color. Liu Xi in his *Shi ming* states: "When the eyebrows are removed, this is used in their place, *dai* 代. Hence it is called *dai* 黛[699]."

【集解】【志曰】青黛從波斯國來。今以太原并廬陵、南康等處，染澱甕上沫紫碧色者用之，與青黛同功。【時珍曰】波斯青黛，亦是外國藍靛花，既不可得，則中國靛花亦可用。或不得已，用青布浸汁代之。貨者復以乾澱充之，然有石灰，入服餌藥中當詳之。

Collected Explanations. [Ma] Zhi: *Qing dai* comes from Po si guo/Persia. Today, in Tai yuan and also in places such as Lu ling and Nan kang the purple greenish-jade-bluish foam on indigo dye vats is used instead. Its [therapeutic] potential is identical to that of *qing dai*. [Li] Shizhen: Persian *qing dai* is a foreign indigo plant. As it cannot be obtained [easily], *dian hua* from China can be used, too. If it is out of reach, the juice in which a greenish [indigo] fabric was soaked may be used instead. Merchants repeatedly pretend dry indigo sediments to be [*qing dai*]. However, [these sediments] contain lime. Hence one should take a close look [at *qing dai*] before adding it to food or medication.

【氣味】鹹，寒，無毒。【權曰】甘，平。

Qi and Flavor. Salty, cold, nonpoisonous. [Zhen] Quan: Sweet, balanced.

【主治】解諸藥毒，小兒諸熱，驚癇發熱，天行頭痛寒熱，並水研服之。亦磨傅熱瘡惡腫，金瘡下血，蛇犬等毒。開寶。解小兒疳熱，殺蟲。甄權。小兒丹熱，和水服之。同雞子白、大黄末，傅瘡癰、蛇虺螫毒。藏器。瀉肝，散五臟鬱火，解熱，消食積。震亨。去熱煩，吐血咯血，斑瘡陰瘡，殺惡蟲。時珍。

Control. It resolves all types of medicinal poison, all types of heat of children, heat effusion related to fright epilepsy, epidemic headache with alternating sensations of cold and heat. For all these issues, grind it in water and ingest this. It can also be rubbed [to powder] to be applied to heat sores and malign swelling, to bleeding wounds caused by metal objects/weapons, and to the poison of snake and dog

699 *Dai* 黛, a character composed of *dai* 代, "to replace," "to substitute," and *hei* 黑, "black."

[bites]. *Kai bao*. It resolves *gan*-illness[700] heat of children. Zhen Quan. For cinnabar [poison][701] heat of children, mix it with water and [let the child] ingest it. Mixed with egg white and rhubarb powder it is applied to sores related to obstruction-illness[702] and to [regions affected by] the poison of snakes, venomous vipers and scorpions. [Chen] Cangqi: It drains liver [qi] and disperses fire pent-up in the five long-term depots. It resolves heat and dissolves food accumulations. [Zhu] Zhenheng. It eliminates heat with vexation, blood spitting and coughing up of blood, macule sores and sores in the body's yin [(i. e. genital) region]. It kills malign worms/bugs. [Li] Shizhen.

【發明】【宗奭曰】青黛乃藍爲之者。有一婦人患臍下腹上，下連二陰，遍生濕瘡，狀如馬爪瘡，他處並無，痒而痛，大小便澀，出黄汁，食亦減，身面微腫。醫作惡瘡治，用鰻[魚黎]魚、松脂、黄丹之藥塗之，熱痛甚。問其人嗜酒食，喜魚蟹發風等物。急令洗其青藥，以馬齒莧四兩，杵爛，入青黛一兩，再研匀塗之。即時熱減，痛痒皆去。仍以八正散，.日三服之，分敗客熱。藥乾即上。如此二日，減三分之一，五日減三分之二，二十日愈。此蓋中下焦蓄風熱毒氣也。若不出，當作腸癰内痔。仍須禁酒色發風物。然不能禁，後果患内痔。

Explication. [Kou] Zongshi: *Qing dai* is produced from Chinese indigo plants, *lan* 藍. A woman suffered from moisture sores on her abdomen below the navel and extending further down to the two private areas. They were shaped like horse-claw sores, and appeared nowhere else. They itched and were painful. Major (defecation) and minor (urination) relief were rough. The [sores] released a yellow juice. [The woman] ate less; her body and face were slightly swollen. A physician applied a cure for malign sores and applied a medication prepared from Japanese eels, pine resin and minium [to the affected region]. This resulted in a painful heat. [The physician] asked her whether she loved to drink wine and [what she preferred] to eat, and [she told him that she preferred to consume] fish and crabs and items that effuse wind. He quickly asked to wash off the medicinal ointment and had four *liang* of purslane ground to a pulp. To this he added one *liang* of *qing dai* and ground it to obtain an even mixture. This he applied [to the affected region]. Soon afterwards the heat decreased and the pain with the itch were all gone. In addition he let her ingest,

700 *Gan* 疳, "*gan*-illness," also: "sweets-illness," involves several complaints that affect children and adults, with causes and conditions too different to fall into a known disease category. BCGM Dict I, 180-188.

701 *Dan du* 丹毒, "cinnabar poison," a skin ailment with red rashes. BCGM Dict I, 118

702 *Yong* 癰, "obstruction-illness,"refers to an obstruction of vessels or other ducts inside the body. Qi rushing against the obstruction may cause a local swelling and eventually break through the surface to cause an abscess. BCGM Dict I, 641.

three times a day, the "powder with the eight rectifying [ingredients]"[703] to dispel the visitor heat. When the medication had dried, [a moist portion] was applied. When this was continued for two days, [the ailment] weakened by one third. On the fifth day, it had weakened by two thirds. After 20 days, she was cured. This [treatment was based on] the fact that the central and the lower [sections of the Triple] Burner store up wind and heat poison qi. If they fail to be released, they will generate intestinal obstruction-illness[704] and internal piles. [The physician informed her that] she should avoid wine and sex and items effusing wind. But she was unable to avoid all this and later she suffered from internal piles.

【附方】舊六，新七。

Added Recipes. Six of old. Seven newly [recorded].

心口熱痛。薑汁調青黛一錢服之。醫學正傳。

Painful heat at the heart/stomach opening. Mix one *qian* of *qing dai* with ginger juice and ingest this. *Yi xue zheng chuan.*

內熱吐血。青黛二錢，新汲水下。聖惠方。

Internal heat with blood spitting. Send two *qian* of *qing dai* down with newly drawn water. *Sheng hui fang.*

肺熱咯血。青餅子：用青黛一兩，杏仁以牡蠣粉炒過一兩，研勻，黄蠟化和，作三十餅子。每服一餅，以乾柿半個夾定。濕紙裹，煨香嚼食，粥飲送下。日三服。華佗中藏經。

Lung heat associated with coughing up of blood. The "*qing* [*dai*] pancake." Grind one *liang* of *qing dai* and one *liang* of apricot kernels, fried with oyster shell powder, to an even mixture, mix it with yellow beeswax and prepare 30 pancakes. Each time ingest one pancake. It is pressed from both sides with half a dried persimmon fruit to stabilize it and wrapped with moist paper. Simmer it until it releases a fragrance, chew it and eat it. Send it down with a congee beverage. To be ingested three times a day. Hua Tuo, *Zhong cang jing.*

---

703 Ingredients of the *ba zheng san* 八正散, "powder with eight rectifying[ingredients]," include, in addition to fringed pink, Asiatic plantain herb seeds, knotgrass, talcum, *gardenia* fruit, prepared *glycyrrhiza* [root], *akebia* herb, and rhubarb root.

704 *Yong* 癰, "obstruction-illness,"refers to an obstruction of vessels or other ducts inside the body. Qi rushing against the obstruction may cause a local swelling and eventually break through the surface to cause an abscess. BCGM Dict I, 641.

兒驚癎。青黛量大小，水研服之。生生編。

Fright epilepsy of children. Grind an amount of *qing dai* adjusted to the age [of the patient] in water and [let the child] ingest this. *Sheng sheng bian.*

小兒夜啼。方同上。

Crying of children during the night. Recipe identical to the one above.

小兒疳痢。宮氣方歌云：
孩兒雜病變成疳，不問强羸女與男。
煩熱毛焦鼻口燥，皮膚枯槁四肢癱。
腹中時時更下痢，青黄赤白一般般。
眼澀面黄鼻孔赤，穀道開張不可看。
此方便是青黛散，孩兒百病服之安。

Gan-illness[705] and free-flux illness. A song in the *Gong qi fang* states:
"When any child disease develops into a *gan*-illness,
regardless of whether [the patient] is strong or emaciated, a girl or a boy,
whether it has vexing heat, scorched hair and parched nose and mouth,
or withered skin and paralysed four limbs,
with repeated discharge with free-flux illness from the abdomen,
that may be greenish, yellow, red or white,
and rough eyes, a yellow face and red nostrils,
with the anus opened and distended that one does not wish to look at it,
the appropriate recipe is the '*qing dai* powder.'
When children with any of the hundreds of diseases ingest it, they are cured."

耳疳出汁。青黛、黄檗末，乾搽。談埜翁方。

Gan-illness affecting the ears and releasing a juice. Rub [the affected region] with a mixture of *qing dai* and *phellodendron* bark powder. *Tan Yeweng fang.*

爛弦風眼。青黛、黄連泡湯，日洗。明目方。

Wind eyes[706] with festering [eyelid] rims. Macerate *qing dai* and *coptis* [rhizome] in hot water and daily wash [the affection region]. *Ming mu fang.*

---

705 *Gan* 疳, "*gan*-illness," also: "sweets-illness," involves several complaints that affect children and adults, with causes and conditions too different to fall into a known disease category. BCGM Dict I, 180-188.

706 *Feng yan* 風眼, "wind eye," a condition of red and festering canthi and eyelids brought about by harm caused to the eyes by heat. BCGM Dict I, 171.

產後發狂。四物湯加青黛，水煎服。摘玄。

Madness after a delivery. Add *qing dai* to the [ingredients of the] "decoction with four items,"[707] fry this in water and [let the woman] ingest this. *Zhai xuan.*

傷寒赤斑。青黛二錢，水研服。活人書。

Harm caused by cold with red speckles. Grind two *qian* of *qing dai* in water and ingest this. *Huo ren shu.*

豌豆瘡毒未成膿者。波斯青黛一棗許，水研服。梅師方。

Pea sores[708] with poison before they have begun to fester. Grind Persian *qing dai*, about the size of a Chinese date, in water and ingest this. *Mei shi fang.*

瘰癧未穿。靛花、馬齒莧同擣，日日塗傅，取效。簡便方。

Scrofula pervasion-illness[709] before it has opened. Pound equal amounts of *dian hua* and purslane and apply [the resulting pulp to the affected region] day after day until an effect shows. *Jian bian fang.*

諸毒蟲傷。青黛、雄黄等分，研末，新汲水服二錢。古今録驗。

Harm caused by all kinds of poisonous worms/bugs. Grind equal amounts of *qing dai* and realgar into powder and ingest with newly drawn water two *qian*. *Gu jin lu yan.*

【附録】
Appendix

16-45-A01
雀翹 *Que qiao*
Unidentified.

【別録有名未用曰】味鹹。益氣明目。生藍中。葉細黄，莖赤有刺。四月實，鋭黄中黑。五月采，陰乾。一名去母，一名更生。

Bie lu, section "known by name but not in use": Flavor salty. It boosts the qi and clears the eyes. It grows among Chinese indigo plants. The leaves are fine and yellow; the stem is red and has thorns. Fruit develop in the fourth month. They are

707 Ingredients include *paeonia* root skin, Chinese foxglove rhizome, Chinese *angelica* root and *ligusticum* root.

708 *Wan dou chuang* 豌豆瘡, "pea sores," a condition identical to *dou chuang* 痘瘡, "smallpox sores." BCGM Dict I, 523.

709 *Luo li* 瘰癧, "scrofula pervasion-illness," when two or more connected swellings of the size of plum or date kernels appear either on the neck or in the armpits, or somewhere else on the body. BCGM Dict I. 329.

pointed, yellow and black inside. They are collected in the fifth month and dried in the yin (i. e. shade). An alternative name is *qu mu* 去母, "to leave one's mother." Another name is *geng sheng* 更生, "revival."

16-46
甘藍拾遺
Gan lan, FE *Shi yi*.

***Brassica oleracea* L. var. *capitata* L. Cabbage varieties.**

【校正】自菜部移入此。

Editorial Correction. Moved here from the section "vegetables."

【釋名】藍菜千金。

Explanation of Names. *Lan cai* 藍菜, "indigo/blue vegetable," *Qian jin*.

【集解】【藏器曰】此是西土藍也，葉闊可食。【時珍曰】此亦大葉冬藍之類也。案胡洽[710]居士云：河東、隴西羌胡多種食之，漢地少有。其葉長大而厚，煮食甘美。經冬不死，春亦有英。其花黃，生角結子，其功與藍相近也。

Collected Explanations. [Chen] Cangqi: This is *lan* 藍 from Western soil. It has broad, edible leaves. [Li] Shizhen: This, too, is one of the big leaf winter *lan* 藍. According to Hu Qia jushi, "it is often planted and eaten in He dong and Long xi, and in the regions of the Qiang and Hu. It is rarely found on the land of the Han. The leaves are lengthy, big and thick. When they are boiled to be eaten, they are sweet and delicious. [*Gan lan*] remains alive throughout winter, and in spring it blooms. The flowers are yellow and they form horn[-like pods] with seeds. Their [therapeutic] potential is very close to that of *lan* 藍."

【氣味】甘，平，無毒。

Qi and Flavor. Sweet, balanced, nonpoisonous.

【主治】久食，大益腎，填髓腦，利五臟六腑，利關節，通經絡中結氣，心下結伏氣，明耳目，健人，少睡。益心力，壯筋骨。作葅經宿色黃，和鹽食，治黃毒。藏器。

Control. Eaten over a long time it massively boosts kidney [qi], fills marrow and brain, frees the passage through the five long-term depots and six short-term repositories, frees [the movement of/passage through] the joints, penetrates bound qi in the conduits and network[vessels], as well as bound, hidden qi below the heart.

710 Instead of Hu Qia 胡洽, *Zheng lei* ch. 27, *gan lan* 甘藍, writes Hu 壺. *Qian jin fang* ch. 26 writes Hu 胡.

It clears ears and eyes, provides one with strength and lets one require only a little sleep. It boosts the strength of the heart and strengthens sinews and bones. Prepared as a vegetable and left over night until it has assumed a yellow color, and eaten mixed with salt, it serves to cure yellow [*dan*-illness/jaundice] poison. [Chen] Cangqi.

16-46-01
子 *Zi*
Seeds [of *gan lan*].

【主治】人多睡。思邈。

Control. Sleepiness. [Su] Simiao.

16-47
蓼本經中品
Liao, FE *Ben jing*, middle rank.

***Polygonum hydropiper* L. Water pepper.**

【校正】自菜部移入此。

Editorial Correction. Moved here from the section "vegetables."

【釋名】【時珍曰】蓼類皆高揚，故字從翏，音料，高飛貌。

Explanation of Names. [Li] Shizhen: All [herbs] of the group of *liao* 蓼 are tall. Hence the character [*liao* 蓼] is derived from *liao* 翏, read *liao* 料, to reflect the image of "soaring high."

【集解】【别録曰】蓼實生雷澤川澤。【弘景曰】此類多人所食，有三種。一是青蓼，人家常用，其葉有圓有尖，以圓者爲勝，所用即此也。一是紫蓼，相似而紫色。一是香蓼，相似而香。並不甚辛，好食。【保昇曰】蓼類甚多。有青蓼、香蓼、水蓼、馬蓼、紫蓼、赤蓼、木蓼七種。紫、赤二蓼，葉小狹而厚；青、香二蓼，葉亦相似而俱薄；馬、水二蓼，葉俱闊大，上有黑點；木蓼一名天蓼，蔓生，葉似柘葉。六蓼花皆紅白，子皆大如胡麻，赤黑而尖扁。惟木蓼花黄白，子皮青滑。諸蓼並冬死，惟香蓼宿根重生，可爲生菜。【頌曰】木蓼亦有大小二種，皆蔓生。陶氏以青蓼入藥，餘亦無用。三茅君傳有作白蓼醬方，藥譜無白蓼，疑即青蓼也。【宗奭曰】蓼實即草部下品水蓼之子也。彼言水蓼是用莖，此言蓼實是用子也。春初以壺盧盛水浸濕，高挂火上，日夜使暖，遂生紅牙，取爲蔬，以備五辛盤。【時珍曰】韓保昇所説甚明。古人種蓼爲蔬，收子入藥。故禮記烹雞豚魚鼈，皆實蓼于其腹中，而和羹膾亦須切蓼也。後世飲食不用，人亦不復栽，惟造酒麴者用其汁耳。今但以平澤所生香蓼、青蓼、紫蓼爲良。

Collected Explanations. *Bie lu*: *Liao* fruit grow in the river marshlands of Lei ze. [Tao] Hongjing: Many people eat such herbs. There are three kinds. One is greenish *liao*. People often resort to it. Its leaves may be round or pointed, but those with pointed [leaves] are superior. It is [the kind] used [for therapeutic purposes]. Then there is a purple *liao*. It is similar, but of purple color. And there is a fragrant *liao*. It is similar, but fragrant. None of them is very acrid; they taste good. [Han] Baosheng: The group of *liao* comprises very many [kinds]. It includes greenish *liao*, fragrant *liao*, water *liao*, horse *liao*, purple *liao*, red *liao*, and wood *liao*, these seven kinds. The two purple and red [kinds of] *liao* have narrow, thick leaves. The two greenish and fragrant [kinds of] *liao* have similar leaves, but they are thin. Both the two horse and water [kinds of] *liao* have broad, big leaves with black dots on their upper side. Wood *liao* is also called "heaven's *liao*." It grows as a creeper and has leaves similar to silkwormthorn [herbs]. The flowers of six of these [kinds of] *liao* are red-white, and all their seeds have the size of hemp seeds. They are red-black, pointed and flat. Only the flowers of wood *liao* are yellow-white. The skin of their seeds is greenish and smooth. All [kinds of] *liao* die in winter. Only fragrant *liao* has a perennial root that grows again [the next year]. It can serve as fresh vegetable [Su] Song: Wood *liao*, too, has two kinds. Both grow as creepers. Mr. [Tao] Hongjing adds greenish *liao* to medication; all the others are not used [for therapeutic purposes]. The *San mao jun zhuan* has a recipe how to prepare a "white *liao* sauce." There is no "white *liao*" recorded in medical literature; it may be greenish *liao*. [Kou] Zongshi: *Liao* fruits are the seeds of water *liao*, listed as a lower rank item in the section "herbs." There it is said that the stem of water *liao* is used. Here it is said that "*liao* fruit" refers to the use of the seeds. In early spring, they are soaked in a bottle gourd filled with water. This is hung high above a fire to keep it warm day and night. Eventually red germs grow that can be taken as a vegetable for the dish with the five acrid components.[711] [Li] Shizhen: Han Baosheng's statement is very clear. The ancients planted *liao* as a vegetable, and they kept the seeds as a pharmaceutical drug. Hence, according to the *Li ji* when chicken, pigs, fish and turtles were cooked, their abdomen was always filled with *liao*, and for a preparation of meat gruel sliced *liao* was required, too. In later times it was no longer resorted to for beverages and food, and it was no longer planted. Only to produce distiller's yeast, its juice is still used. Today, only the fragrant *liao*, the greenish *liao* and the purple *liao* growing in the marshlands of the plains are good.

711 *Wu xin pan* 五辛盤, "the dish composed of five acrid/hot components," usually including onions, garlic, chives, rape and coriander. A dish traditionally consumed in Chu 楚 on the first day of the year.

16-47-01
實 *Shi*
Fruit [of *liao*].

【氣味】辛，温，無毒。【詵曰】多食吐水，壅氣損陽。

Qi and Flavor. Acrid, warm, nonpoisonous. [Meng] Shen: When it is eaten in large quantities it lets one vomit water. It obstructs qi [flow] and harms the yang [qi].

【主治】明目温中，耐風寒，下水氣面浮腫，癰瘍。本經。歸鼻，除腎氣，去癧瘍，止霍亂，治小兒頭瘡。甄權。

Control. It clears the eyes and warms the center; it helps to endure wind and cold. It serves to discharge water qi causing a surface swelling of the face, and ulcers related to an obstruction-illness.[712] *Ben jing*. It finds its way to the nose. It dispels liver qi. It removes pervasion-illness ulcers,[713] ends cholera and serves to cure sores on the head of children. Zhen Quan.

【附方】舊一，新三。

Added Recipes. One of old. Three newly [recorded].

傷寒勞復。因交後卵腫，或縮入腹痛。蓼子一把，水挼汁，飲一升。肘後方。

Relapse of harm caused by cold because of overexertion. When following sexual intercourse the testicles swell, or are drawn back with pain into the abdomen. Rub a handful of *liao* seeds in water and drink one *sheng* of the resulting juice. *Zhou hou fang*.

霍亂煩渴。蓼子一兩，香薷二兩。每服二錢，水煎服。聖惠。

Cholera with vexing thirst. Each time ingest two *qian* of a mixture of one *liang* of *liao* seeds and two *liang* of *elsholtzia* [herb]. To be ingested boiled in water. *Sheng hui*.

712 *Yong* 癰, "obstruction-illness,"refers to an obstruction of vessels or other ducts inside the body. Qi rushing against the obstruction may cause a local swelling and eventually break through the surface to cause an abscess. BCGM Dict I, 641.

713 *Li yang* 癧瘍, "pervasion-illness with ulcer," identical to *li yang feng* 癧瘍風, "pervasion-illness with ulcer wind," a condition of white macules and dots appearing on the skin in the neck, on the chest, and below the armpits, without itching or pain. BCGM Dict I, 315.

小兒頭瘡。蓼子爲末，蜜和雞子白同塗之，蟲出不作痕。藥性論。

Sores on the head of children. [Grind] *liao* seeds into powder, mix it with honey and egg white and apply this [to the affected region]. A worm/bug will come out, and there will be no scars. *Yao xing lun.*

蝸牛咬毒，毒行徧身者。蓼子煎水浸之，立愈。不可近陰，令弱也。陳藏器本草。

Snail bite with poison, when the poison moves through the entire body. Boil *liao* seeds in water and soak [the affected region] in it. A cure is achieved immediately. [The decoction] must not come close to one's yin [(i. e., genital) region], it would weaken it. *Chen Cangqi ben cao.*

16-47-02
苗、葉 *Miao, Ye*
Seedling and leaf [of *liao*].

【氣味】辛，温，無毒。【思邈曰】黄帝云：食蓼過多，有毒，發心痛。和生魚食，令人脱氣，陰核痛，求死。二月食蓼，傷人胃。扁鵲云：久食令人寒熱，損髓、減氣。少精。婦人月事來時食蓼、蒜，喜爲淋。與大麥麪相宜。

Qi and Flavor. Acrid, warm, nonpoisonous. [Sun] Simiao: Huang Di states: "To eat too much of *liao* is poisonous and causes heart pain. Eaten together with raw fish it causes loss of qi and painful testicles, letting on wish to die. To eat *liao* in the second month harms the stomach.[714]" Bian Que states: "Eaten over a long time it lets one have alternating sensations of cold and heat, decreases qi, and diminishes essence/sperm. When women during menstruation eat *liao* or garlic, they easily experience [urinary] dripping. It is advisable to [eat it] together with barley."

【主治】歸舌，除大小腸邪氣，利中益志。别録。乾之釀酒，主風冷，大良。弘景。作生菜食，能入腰脚。煮湯捋脚，治霍亂轉筋。煮汁日飲，治痃癖。擣爛，傅狐尿瘡。藏器。脚暴軟，赤蓼燒灰淋汁浸之，以桑葉蒸罯，立愈。大明。殺蟲伏砒。時珍。

Control. It finds its way to the tongue and removes evil qi from the large and the small intestine. It frees the passage in the center and boosts the mind. *Bie lu.* Dried and added to wine brewing, it controls wind and cold [intrusion]. Very good. [Tao] Hongjing. Eaten prepared as a vegetable it can enter the lower back and the legs. Boiled and the decoction rubbed on the legs serves to cure twisted sinews related to

714 Instead of *wei* 胃, "stomach," *Zheng lei* ch. 28, *liao shi* 蓼實, quoting *Sun zhenren shi ji* 孫真人食忌, writes *shen* 腎, "kidneys." The origin of this quote attributed to Huang Di is unclear.

cholera. Boiled and the juice daily drunk serves to cure string-illness[715] and aggregation-illness. Pounded to a pulp it is applied to fox urine sores.[716] [Chen] Cangqi. For sudden softness/weakness of legs, burn red *liao* to ashes, let water drip over them and soak [the affected limb] in the resulting juice. Steam mulberry tree leaves and attach them [to the affected limb]. Da Ming. It kills worms/bugs and suppresses [the effects of] arsenic. [Li] Shizhen.

【附方】舊四，新三。

Added Recipes. Four of old. Three newly [recorded].

蓼汁酒。治胃脘冷，不能飲食，耳目不聰明，四肢有氣，冬卧足冷。八月三日取蓼日乾，如五升大，六十把，水六石，煮取一石，去滓，拌米飯，如造酒法，待熟，日飲之。十日後，目明氣壯也。千金方。

Liao juice wine. It serves to cure stomach duct cold making it impossible to drink and eat, with ears and eyes not functioning properly, qi [swelling] affecting the four limbs, and an urge to often lie down with cold feet. On the third day of the eighth month obtain *liao* and dry it in the sun. Then boil 60 handfuls, each amounting to five *sheng*, in six *dan* of water down to one *dan*. Discard the dregs and add cooked rice. Then proceed with the method of wine brewing. Once [the *liao* juice wine] is ready, drink it daily. After ten days, the eyes will be clear and the qi are robust. *Qian jin fang.*

肝虛轉筋，吐瀉。赤蓼莖葉切三合，水一盞，酒三合，煎至四合，分二服。聖惠方

Liver [qi] depletion with contorted sinews, vomiting and outflow. Cut three *ge* of *liao* stems and leaves into pieces and boil them in one small cup of water with three *ge* of wine down to four *ge*. Ingest this divided into two portions. *Sheng hui fang.*

霍亂轉筋。蓼葉一升，水三升，煮取汁二升，入香豉一升，更煮一升半，分三服。藥性論。

Cholera with contorted sinews. Boil one *sheng* of *liao* leaves[717] in three *sheng* of water down to obtain two *sheng* of its juice. Add one *sheng* of [soybean] relish and boil this further down to one and a half *sheng*. To be ingested in three portions. *Yao xing lun.*

715 *Xuan* 痃, "string-illness," a condition of acute pain located in the abdomen to the left and right of the umbilicus. BCGM Dict I, 591.

716 *Hu niao [ci] chuang* 狐尿[刺]瘡, "sores resulting from being pierced by fox urine," conditions resulting from touching poisonous substances left on herbs and trees by all types of poisonous bugs/snakes/insects. BCGM Dict I, 221.

717 Instead of *liao ye yi sheng* 蓼葉一升, *Zheng lei* ch. 28, *liao shi* 蓼實, quoting *Yao xing lun* writes *qu zi yi ba* 取子一把, "take a handful of seeds."

夏月暍死。濃煮蓼汁一盞服。外臺。

Heatstroke death in summer. [Force the patient to] ingest a thick decoction of *liao* juice. *Wai tai.*

小兒冷痢。蓼葉擣汁服。千金。

Free-flux illness of children related to cold [intrusion]. Pound *liao* leaves and let [the child] ingest the resulting juice. *Qian jin.*

血氣攻心，痛不可忍。蓼根洗剉，浸酒飲。斗門。

Blood and qi attacking the heart, with an unbearable pain. Wash a *liao* root clean, cut it [to pieces] and soak them in wine. Drink [the liquid]. *Dou men.*

惡犬咬傷。蓼葉擣泥傅。肘後。

Harm caused by the bite of a malign dog. Pound *liao* leaves and apply the pulp [to the location of the bite]. *Zhou hou.*

16-48
水蓼唐本草
Shui liao. FE *Tang ben cao.*

***Polygonum hydropiper* L. Water pepper.**

【釋名】虞蓼爾雅、澤蓼。【志曰】生于淺水澤中，故名水蓼。【時珍曰】按爾雅云：薔，虞蓼也。山夾水曰虞。

Explanation of Names. *Yu liao* 虞蓼, *Er ya. Ze liao* 澤蓼, "moist *liao.*" [Ma] Zhi: It grows in shallow waters, *shui* 水, and on damp ground/marshlands, *ze* 澤. Hence the name "water *liao* 水蓼." [Li] Shizhen: According to the *Er ya*, *qiang* 薔 is *yu liao* 虞蓼. Water between mountains is called *yu* 虞.

【集解】【恭曰】水蓼生下濕水旁。葉似馬蓼，大于家蓼，莖赤色，水挼食之，勝于蓼子。【宗奭曰】水蓼大概與水葒相似，但枝低耳。今造酒取葉，以水浸汁，和麪作麯，亦取其辛耳。【時珍曰】此乃水際所生之蓼，葉長五六寸，比水葒葉稍狹，比家蓼葉稍大而功用仿佛。故寇氏謂蓼實即水蓼之子者，以此故也。

Collected Explanations. [Su] Gong: Water *liao* grows in low-lying marshlands to the side of waters. The leaves resemble those of horse *liao*; they are larger than those of domestic *liao*. The stem is red. When it is eaten rubbed in water, it is superior to *liao* seeds. [Kou] Zongshi: Water *liao* is more or less similar to red knotweed, but its leaves hang down like ears. When wine is brewed today, they soak the leaves in water and mix the resulting juice with wheat flour to prepare yeast. This is to [let the wine] acquire the acrid flavor [of *liao*]. [Li] Shizhen: This is the *liao* growing at the margins of waters. The leaves are five to six *cun* long; they are a little narrower than those of red knotweed, and a little bigger than those of domestic *liao*. Their [therapeutic] potentials are more or less the same. When Mr. Kou [Zongshi] says that *liao shi* 蓼實, *liao* fruit, refers to the seeds of water *liao*, then this is the reason.

16-48-01
莖、葉 *Jing, Ye*
Stem, leaf [of *shui liao*].

【氣味】辛，無毒。【大明曰】冷。

Qi and Flavor. Acrid, nonpoisonous. Da Ming: Cold.

【主治】蛇傷，擣傅之。絞汁服之，止蛇毒入腹心悶。又治脚氣腫痛成瘡，水煮汁漬捋之。唐本。

Control. For harm caused by snakes, pound it and apply [the pulp to the location of the bite]. Squeeze [the pulp] to obtain a juice and ingest it. This blocks the entrance of the snake poison into the abdomen and the heart where it might cause heart-pressure. Also, to cure leg qi[718] with painful swelling eventually generating sores, boil it in water and soak as well as rub [the affected region with the decoction].

16-49
馬蓼綱目
Ma liao, FE *Gang mu.*

***Polygonum persicaria* L. Lady's thumb.**

【釋名】大蓼綱目、墨記草。【時珍曰】凡物大者，皆以馬名之，俗呼大蓼是也。高四五尺，有大小二種。但每葉中間有黑跡，如墨點記，故方士呼爲墨記草。

Explanation of Names. *Da liao* 大蓼, "big *liao*," *Gang mu*. *Mo ji cao* 墨記草, "ink mark herb." [Li] Shizhen: All big items are called "horse," *ma* 馬. It is the commonly called "big *liao*", *da liao* 大蓼. It is four to five *chi* tall, and has two kinds, one big, one small. However the leaves of both of them have black dots in their middle, similar to marks made with ink drops. Therefore the recipe experts call [this herb] "ink mark herb."

【集解】【弘景曰】馬蓼生下濕地，莖斑，葉大有黑點。亦有兩三種，其最大者名蘢薣，即水葒也。

Collected Explanations. [Tao] Hongjing: *Ma liao* grows on low-lying moist ground. The stem is speckled; the leaves are big and have black dots. There are two or three kinds; the biggest is called *long gu* 蘢薣. This is red knotweed.

---

718 *Jiao qi* 脚氣, "leg qi." Painful, weak, swollen legs. BCGM Dict I, 248.

16-49-01
莖、葉 *Jing, Ye*
Stem, leaf [of *ma liao*].

【氣味】辛，温，無毒。【時珍曰】伏丹砂、雌黄。

Qi and Flavor. Acrid, warm, nonpoisonous. [Li] Shizhen: It suppresses [the effects] of cinnabar and orpiment.

【主治】去腸中蛭蟲，輕身。本經。

Control. It removes leeches and further worms/bugs from inside the intestines. It relieves the body of its weight. *Ben jing*.

16-50
葒草別録中品
Hong cao, FE *Bie lu*, middle rank.

***Polygonum orientale* L. Red knotweed.**

【校正】併入有名未用别録天蓼。

Editorial Correction. *Tian liao* 天蓼, listed in the *Bie lu* section "known by name but not in use," is included here.

【釋名】鴻藹音纈、蘢古一作鼓、遊龍詩經、石龍别録、天蓼别録、大蓼。【時珍曰】此蓼甚大而花亦繁紅，故曰葒，曰鴻。鴻亦大也。别録有名未用草部中有天蓼，云一名石龍，生水中。陳藏器解云：天蓼即水葒，一名遊龍，一名大蓼。據此，則二條乃一指其實，一指莖葉而言也。今併爲一。

Explanation of Names. *Hong xie* 鴻藹, [with 藹] read *xie* 纈; *long gu* 蘢古, also written *gu* 鼓; *you long* 遊龍, "roaming dragon," *Shi jing*. *Shi long* 石龍, "stone dragon," *Bie lu*. *Tian liao* 天蓼, "heaven's *liao*," *Bie lu*. *Da liao* 大蓼, "big *liao*." [Li] Shizhen: This *liao* is very big, and it has many red, *hong* 紅, flowers. Hence it is called *hong* 葒, and also *hong* 鴻, "swan goose." Swan geese, too, are "big." The *Bie lu* in the section "known by name but not in use" among the herbs lists a *tian liao* 天蓼, "heaven's *liao*," stating that "it is also called *shi long* 石龍, 'stone dragon.' It grows in waters." Chen Cangqi explains: "*Tian liao* 天蓼 is red knotweed. It is also called *you long* 遊龍, and also *da liao* 大蓼." Based on this, of the two entries one refers to the fruit, the other refers to stem and leaf. Here now they are combined in one entry.

【集解】【别録曰】葒生水旁，如馬蓼而大，五月采實。【弘景曰】今生下濕地甚多，極似馬蓼而甚長大。詩稱隰有遊龍，郭璞云，即蘢古也。

【頌曰】葒即水葒也，似蓼而葉大。赤白色，高丈餘，爾雅云：葒，蘢古。其大者蘬，音詭。陸機云：遊龍一名馬蓼。然馬蓼自是一種也。【時珍曰】其莖粗如拇指，有毛。其葉大如商陸，色淺紅，成穗，秋深子成，扁如酸棗仁而小，其色赤黑而肉白，不甚辛，炊熇可食。

Collected Explanations. *Bie lu*: *Hong* [*cao*] grows at the side of waters; it is similar to lady's thumb, *ma liao* 馬蓼, but bigger. The fruits are collected in the fifth month. [Tao] Hongjing: Today very much of it grows on low-lying, damp ground. It is very similar to horse *liao*, but very much longer and bigger. The *Shi* says: "In the marshy lands are roaming dragons." Guo Pu states: "This is [the herb] *long gu* 蘢古." [Su] Song: *Hong* [*cao*] is *shui hong* 水葒. It resembles *liao* but its leaves are bigger. It is of red-white[719] color and reaches a height of more than a *zhang*. The *Er ya* states: "Hong 葒 is *long gu* 蘢古. Large specimens of it are *gui* 蘬, read *gui* 詭." Lu Ji states: "*You long* 遊龍, 'roaming dragon,' is also called *ma liao* 馬蓼, 'horse *liao*'." But horse *liao* is a kind of itself. [Li] Shizhen: Its stem is coarse; it is similar to a thumb and has hair. The leaves are as big as those of Indian pokewee [herbs]; the [flowers][720] are pale red and form spikes. The seeds inside form in autumn. They are flat and sour like jujube kernels, but smaller. They are red-black [outside] and their pulp is white. They are not very acrid; cooked or stir-fried they can be eaten.

16-50-01

實 *Shi*

Fruit [of *hong cao*].

【氣味】鹹，微寒，無毒。

Qi and Flavor. Salty, slightly cold, nonpoisonous.

【主治】消渴，去熱，明目，益氣。别録。

Control. Melting with thirst.[721] They dispel heat, clear the eyes and boost the qi. *Bie lu*.

719 *Zheng lei* ch. 9, *hong cao* 葒草, quoting a *Tang ben* comment states: 有毛，花紅白, "it has hair and red-white flowers." Hence the character *chi* 赤 should be preceded by the character *hua* 花, "flower."

720 Based on the same source as the previous note, the character *se* 色 should be preceded by the character *hua* 花, "flower."

721 *Xiao ke* 消渴, "melting with thirst," most likely including cases of diabetes. BCGM Dict Vol I, 567.

【附方】舊一，新一。
Added Recipes. One of old. One newly [recorded].

瘰癧。水葒子不以多少，一半微炒，一半生用，同研末。食後好酒調服二錢，日三服。已破者亦治。久則效，效則止。寇宗奭本草衍義。

Scrofula pervasion-illness.[722] Take any amount of *shui hong* seeds. Slightly fry one half, and use the other fresh. Grind both [halves] into powder and ingest two *qian* mixed with good wine after a meal. To be ingested three times a day. When [the scrofula] has already broken open, this [recipe] serves to cure it, too. After a lengthy period of time it will be effective. Once the effect shows, end [the treatment]. Kou Zongshi, *Ben cao yan yi*.

癖痞腹脹及堅硬如盃盌者。用水葒花子一升，另研獨顆蒜三十箇去皮，新狗腦一箇，皮硝四兩，石臼搗爛，攤在患處上，用油紙以長帛束之。酉時貼之，次日辰時取之。未效，再貼二三次。倘有膿潰，勿怪。仍看虛實，日逐間服錢氏白餅子、紫霜丸、塌氣丸、消積丸，利之磨之。服至半月，甚者一月，無不瘥矣。以喘滿者爲實，不喘者爲虛。藺氏經驗方。

Abdominal distension and hardenings similar to a cup or bowl related to aggregation-illness and obstacle-illness. In a stone mortar pound to a pulp one *sheng* of *shui hong* flower seeds, 30 single clove garlics with the skin removed and ground separately, one brain of a newly [killed] dog, and four *liang* of mirabilite. Apply this to the location of the ailment, cover it with oil paper and fasten it with a lengthy piece of cloth. Apply it during *you* 酉 hours (17 – 19) and remove it the next day during *chen* 辰 hours (7 – 9). If this remains without effect, apply it again another two or three times. If pus is released, do not worry. In the course of this treatment ingest "Mr. Qian's white cake,"[723] the "pills with purple frost,"[724] the "pills to calm down qi,"[725] and the "pills to dissolve accumulations"[726] to free the passage [of blocked qi] and to rub them away. Continue ingesting all this for half a month, or even better for a complete month, and there will always be a cure. When [patients] pant and

722 *Luo li* 瘰癧, "scrofula pervasion-illness," when two or more connected swellings of the size of plum or date kernels appear either on the neck or in the armpits, or somewhere else on the body. BCGM Dict I. 329.

723 *Qian shi bai bing zi* 錢氏白餅子, "Mr. Qian's white cake." Ingredients are talcum, pinellia root, arisaema root, calomel, croton seeds, glutinous rice.

724 *Zi shuang wan* 紫霜丸, "purple frost pills." Ingredients are hematite, red halloysite, croton seeds, apricot seeds.

725 *Ta qi wan* 塌氣丸, "pills to calm down qi." Ingredients are *costus* root, green tangerine peels, croton seeds.

726 *Xiao ji wan* 消積丸, "pills to dissolve accumulations." Ingredients are cloves, bastard cardamom seeds/kernels, smoked plums, croton seeds.

have a sensation of fullness, it is a case of repletion. When they do not pant, it is a depletion. *Lin shi jing yan fang*.

16-50-02
花 *Hua*
Flower [of *hong cao*].

【主治】散血，消積，止痛。時珍。

Control. It disperses blood, dissolves accumulations and ends pain. [Li] Shizhen.

【附方】新三。
Added Recipes. Three newly [recorded].

胃脘血氣作痛。水葒花一大撮，水二鍾，煎一鍾服。百户毛菊莊屢驗方也。董炳避水集驗方。

Painful stomach duct related to blood and qi [disorder]. Boil one generous handful of *shui hong* flowers in two *zhong* of water down to one *zhong* and ingest this. This is a recipe of the *bai hu* official Mao Juzhuang; it has repeatedly proved to be effective. Dong Bing, *Bi shui ji yan fang*.

心氣㽲痛。水葒花爲末，熱酒服二錢。又法：男用酒水各半煎服，女用醋水各半煎服。一婦年三十病此，一服立效。摘玄方。

Painful heart qi disease. [Grind] *shui hong* flowers into powder and ingest with hot wine two *qian*. Another method: Males ingest it boiled with one half each of wine and water. Females ingest it boiled with one half each of vinegar and water. One woman of 30 years had this disease. She ingested [this medication] once, with immediate effect. *Zhai xuan fang*.

腹中痞積。水葒花或子一盌，以水三盌，用桑柴文武火煎成膏，量痞大小攤貼，仍以酒調膏服。忌腥葷油膩之物。劉松石保壽堂方。

Obstacle-illness accumulation in the abdomen. Boil one bowl of *shui hong* flowers or seeds in three bowls of water with first a mild and then a strong fire with mulberry wood to generate a paste. Apply an amount [of this paste] in accordance with the size of the obstacle-illness [to the affected region]. In addition, ingest the paste mixed with wine. [During the treatment] fishy and greasy-oily items are to be avoided. Liu Songshi, *Bao shou tang fang*.

16-50-03

天蓼別録 ***Tian liao***, FE *Bie lu*

【時珍曰】此指莖葉也。

[Li] Shizhen: This [name] refers to the stem and the leaves [of *hong cao*].

【氣味】辛，有毒。

Qi and Flavor. Acrid, poisonous.

【主治】惡瘡，去痺氣。别録。根莖：除惡瘡腫，水氣脚氣，煮濃汁漬之。蘇恭。

Control. Malign sores. It removes blockage qi. *Bie lu*. Root, stem: To eliminate swelling related to malign sores, water qi [swelling] and leg qi,[727] boil them to obtain a thick juice and soak [the affected region]. Su Gong.

【附方】新一。

Added Recipes. One newly [recorded].

生肌肉。水葒花根煎湯淋洗，仍以其葉晒乾研末，撒瘡上，每日一次。談埜翁試驗方。

To stimulate the growth of muscles and flesh. Boil *shui hong* flowers and roots and use the resulting decoction to wash [the respective region]. Then dry its leaves in the sun, grind them into powder and apply it to the sores. Once every day. Tan Yeweng, *Shi yan fang*.

16-51

毛蓼拾遺

Mao liao, FE *Shi yi*.

***Polygonum barbatum* L. Hairy knotgrass.**[728]

【集解】【藏器曰】毛蓼生山足，似馬蓼，葉上有毛，冬根不死。【時珍曰】此即蓼之生于山麓者，非澤隰之蓼也。

Collected Explanations. [Chen] Cangqi: *Mao liao*/hairy *liao* grows at the foot of mountains. It resembles horse *liao*/lady's thumb. The leaves are hairy on their surface. The root does not die in winter. [Li] Shizhen: This is a kind of *liao* growing at the foot of a mountain; it is not a *liao* [growing] on marshlands.

---

727 *Jiao qi* 脚氣, "leg qi." Painful, weak, swollen legs. BCGM Dict I, 248.

728 *Mao liao* 毛蓼, lit.: "hairy *liao*."

16-51-01

莖、葉 *Jing, Ye*

Stem, leaf [of *mao liao*].

【氣味】辛，温，有毒。

Qi and Flavor. Acrid, warm, poisonous.

【主治】癰腫疽瘻瘰癧，杵碎納瘡中，引膿血，生肌，亦作湯洗。兼濯足，治脚氣。藏器。

Control. For swelling related to obstruction-illness,[729] impediment-illness[730] fistula, and scrofula pervasion-illness,[731] pound them to small pieces and insert them into the sores This will draw pus and blood and stimulate [the growth of] muscles. Also, prepare a decoction and wash [the affected region]. Also, washing the feet with it serves to cure leg qi.[732] [Chen] Cangqi.

16-52

海根拾遺

Hai gen, FE *Shi yi*

***Polygonum virginicum* L. var. *filiforme* Nakai.**

【集解】【藏器曰】生會稽海畔山谷，莖赤，葉似馬蓼，根似菝葜而小。胡人蒸而用之也。

Collected Explanations. [Chen] Cangqi: It grows in Kuai ji close to the sea and in mountain valleys. The stem is red. The leaves resemble those of *ma liao* 馬蓼, Lady's thumb. The root resembles that of Chinese *sarsaparilla*, but is smaller. The Hu people steam it before use.

16-52-01

根 *Gen*

Root [of *hai gen*].

【氣味】苦，小温，無毒。

Qi and Flavor. Bitter, slightly warm, nonpoisonous.

729 *Yong* 癰, "obstruction-illness,"refers to an obstruction of vessels or other ducts inside the body. Qi rushing against the obstruction may cause a local swelling and eventually break through the surface to cause an abscess. BCGM Dict I, 641.

730 *Ju* 疽, "impediment-illness," refers to an obstruction of vessels or other ducts inside the body. Qi rushing against the impediment may cause a local swelling and eventually break through the surface to cause an abscess. BCGM Dict I, 277.

731 *Luo li* 瘰癧, "scrofula pervasion-illness," when two or more connected swellings of the size of plum or date kernels appear either on the neck or in the armpits, or somewhere else on the body. BCGM Dict I. 329.

732 *Jiao qi* 脚氣, "leg qi." Painful, weak, swollen legs. BCGM Dict I, 248.

【主治】霍亂中惡心腹痛，鬼氣疰忤飛尸，喉痺蠱毒，癰疽惡腫，赤白遊瘮，蛇咬犬毒。酒及水磨服，并傅之。藏器。

Control. Cholera and being struck by the malign with heartache and abdominal pain. Demon-qi attachment-illness and hostility, flying corpse [qi].[733] Throat closure/numbness and malign swelling. Red and white roaming papules. Poison related to snake and dog bites. Grind [the root] in wine and water and ingest this. Also, apply it [to the affected region]. [Chen] Cangqi.

16-53
火炭母草宋圖經
Huo tan mu cao, FE Song, *Tu jing*.

***Polygonum chinense* L. Chinese knotweed.**[734]

【集解】【頌曰】生南恩州原野中。莖赤而柔，似細蓼。葉端尖，近梗形方。夏有白花。秋實如椒，青黑色，味甘可食。

Collected Explanations. [Su] Song: It grows in the wild of the plains of Nan en zhou. The stem is red and pliable; similar to fine *liao* 蓼, water pepper. The leaves are short and pointed. Close to the stalk they are square. In summer it has white flowers. In autumn it has fruit similar to Chinese pepper. They are greenish-black, sweet and edible.

16-53-01
葉 *Ye*
Leaves [of *huo tan mu cao*]

【氣味】酸，平，有毒。

Qi and Flavor. Sour, balanced, poisonous.

【主治】去皮膚風熱，流注骨節，癰腫疼痛。不拘時采。於坩器中擣爛，以鹽酒炒，傅腫痛處。經宿一易之。蘇頌。

Control. It dispels from the skin wind and heat flowing into the bones and joints, and painful swelling related to an obstruction-illness.[735] Collect it any time and pound it in a crucible to a pulp. Fry it with salt and wine and apply this to the

733 *Fei shi* 飛屍, "flying corpse [qi]," a condition with sudden outbreaks and frequently changing appearances that do not show a regular pattern. BCGM Dict I, 155.

734 *Huo tan mu cao* 火炭母草, lit.: "fire charcoal mother herb."

735 *Yong* 癰, "obstruction-illness,"refers to an obstruction of vessels or other ducts inside the body. Qi rushing against the obstruction may cause a local swelling and eventually break through the surface to cause an abscess. BCGM Dict I, 641.

locations of swelling and pain. Replace it [with a new application] after one night. Su Song.

16-54
三白草唐本草
San bai cao, FE *Tang ben cao.*

***Saururus chinensis* (Lour.) Baill. Chinese lizard's tail.**

【釋名】【弘景曰】葉上有三白點，俗因以名。又見下。

Explanation of Names. [Tao] Hongjing. On the leaves are three white dots. Hence it is commonly named ["three white (dots) herb"]. For more, see further down.

【集解】【恭曰】三白草生池澤畔，高尺許。葉似水葒，亦似蕺，又似菝葜。葉上有三黑點，非白也。古人秘之，隱黑爲白爾。根如芹根，黄白色而粗大。【藏器曰】此草初生無白，入夏葉端半白如粉。農人候之蒔田，三葉白則草便秀。故謂之三白。若云三黑點，蘇未識矣。其葉如薯蕷，亦不似水葒。【保昇曰】今出襄州，二月、八月采根用。【時珍曰】三白草生田澤畔，三月生苗，高二三尺，莖如蓼，葉如章陸及青葙。四月其顛三葉面上三次變作白色，餘葉仍青不變。俗云：一葉白，食小麥；二葉白，食梅杏；三葉白，食黍子。五月開花成穗，如蓼花狀，而色白微香，結細實。根長白虛軟，有節鬚，狀如泥菖蒲根。造化指南云：五月采花及根，可制雄黄。蘇恭言似水葒，有三黑點者，乃馬蓼，非三白也。藏器所説雖是，但葉亦不似薯蕷。

Collected Explanations. [Su] Gong: *San bai cao* grows near ponds and marshland. It is more than a *chi* tall. The leaves resemble those of red knotweed, also those of sheperd's purse and also those of Chinese *sarsaparilla*. The leaves have three black dots on their surface. They are not white. In antiquity people held this [plant] secret, and camouflaged black as white. The root is similar to Chinese celery root. It is yellow-white, rough and big. [Chen] Cangqi: When this plant begins to grow, it has no white color. By summer, half of the tip of the leaves turns white, as if they were covered by a powder. The farmers wait for this and then begin to plant their fields. As soon as three leaves have turned white, the herb looks quite beautiful. Therefore it is called "three whites [herb]." When Su [Gong] says that [its leaves] have three black dots, he is not familiar with it. The leaves are similar to those of Chinese yam. They do not resemble those of red knotweed. [Han] Baosheng: Today, [*san bai cao*] comes from Xiang zhou. The root to be used [for therapeutic purposes] is collected in the second and eighth month. [Li] Shizhen: *San bai cao* grows in the wild near marshland. It grows a seedling in the third month, reaching a height of two or three *chi*. The stem resembles that of water pepper. The leaves are similar to those of Indian pokewee and prince's feather. In the fourth month, three leaves at the top change their surface three times to white. The other leaves remain greenish and do not change [their color]. A common saying is: "When one leaf has turned white, eat wheat. When two leaves have turned white, eat plums and apricots. When three leaves have turned white, eat millet." Flowers forming spikes open in the fifth month; they are shaped like those of water pepper, but their color is white and they are slightly fragrant. They form fine fruit. The root is long, white, hollow and pliable. It has joints and beard hair. It is shaped like the root of mud *acorus*. The *Zao hua zhi nan* states: "Collect the flowers and the root in the fifth month; they are able to check [the effects of] realgar." Su Gong says that it resembles red knotweed and has three black dots. But this is lady's thumb, it is not *san bai* [*cao*]. What [Chen] Cangqi says is correct, except that the leaves do not resemble those of Chinese yam.

【氣味】甘、辛，寒，有小毒。

Qi and Flavor. Sweet, acrid, cold, slightly poisonous.

【主治】水腫脚氣，利大小便，消痰破癖，除積聚，消丁腫，唐本。搗絞汁服，令人吐逆，除瘧及胸膈熱痰，小兒痞滿。藏器。根：療脚氣風毒脛腫，擣酒服，亦甚有驗。又煎湯，洗癬瘡。時珍。

Control. Leg qi[736] with water swelling. It frees the passage of major [defecation] and minor [urination] relief. It dissolves phlegm and breaks through aggregation-illness. It removes accumulations. It dissolves swelling related to pin[-illness].[737] *Tang ben*. Pounded, [the pulp] squeezed and the resulting juice ingested it causes vomiting with [qi] counterflow. It eliminates malaria and heat with phlegm in the chest and diaphragm region, and also obstacle-illness and a feeling of fullness of children. [Chen] Cangqi. The root: To heal shin swelling related to leg qi and wind poison, pound [it to pulp] and ingest it with wine. This, too, is very effective. Also, it is boiled to obtain a decoction that is used to wash *xuan*-illness[738] sores.

---

736 *Jiao qi* 脚氣, "leg qi." Painful, weak, swollen legs. BCGM Dict I, 248.

737 *Ding* 丁, "pin[-illness]," also *ding* 疔, "pin-illness," refers to a deep-reaching and festering hardness in a tissue, eventually rising above the skin like a pinhead. BCGM Dict I, 127-129.

738 *Xuan* 癬, "*xuan*-illness." Conditions of dermal lesions with initially erythema, papules, and itching gradually extending in all directions to form an irregular ring with clear boundaries. The skin is slightly elevated with small papules, blisters, and/or scales and scraps. The central lesion may appear to heal spontaneously, and it may reappear. Also, a designation of local lesions with itching, release of liquid and shedding of scabs. BCGM Dict I, 591.

16-55
蠶蔄草拾遺
Can wang cao, FE *Shi yi.*

Polygonum japonicum **Meissn. Japanese knotweed.**

【集解】【藏器曰】生濕地，如蓼大，莖赤花白，東土亦有之。

Collected Explanations. [Chen] Cangqi: It grows on damp ground, and is as big as water pepper. The stem is red and the flowers are white. It can also be found on eastern soil.

【氣味】辛，平，無毒。

Qi and Flavor. Acrid, balanced, nonpoisonous.

【主治】諸蟲如蠶類咬人，恐毒入腹，煮服之。亦搗傅諸瘡。藏器。

Control. Bites of all worms/bugs such as silkworms. When it is to be feared that the poison enters the abdomen, boil [*can wang cao* in water] and ingest it. Also, pound [it to a pulp] and apply it to sores of any kind. [Chen] Cangqi.

16-56
蛇蔄草拾遺
She wang cao, FE *Shi yi.*

Fagopyrum dibotrys **(D.Don) Hara. Hill-buckwheat.**

【集解】【藏器曰】生平地，葉似苦杖而小，節赤，高一二尺，種之辟蛇。又一種草，莖圓似苧，亦傅蛇毒。【慎微曰】按百一方云：東關有草狀如苧，莖方赤，挼傅蛇毒如摘却然，名蛇繭草。又有鼠蔄草，即後莽草。

Collected Explanations. [Chen] Cangqi: It grows on flat land. The leaves resemble those of bushy knotweed, but are smaller. It has red nodes and is one or two *chi* tall. It is planted to keep snakes away. There is another kind of this herb with a round stem resembling ramie plants. It is also applied to [regions affected by] snake [bite] poison. [Tang] Shenwei: According to the *Bai yi fang*, "in Dong guan is an herb shaped like ramie plants. The stem is square and red. Rubbed between one's hands and applied to [the location of] the poison of a snake [bite its effect] is as if [the poison] were pulled out. It is called *she jian cao* 蛇繭草." There is also a *shu wang cao* 鼠蔄草; this is the *illiceum* herb, discussed further down (17-39).

【氣味】缺。

Qi and Flavor. Missing.

【主治】蛇虺毒蟲等螫。取根葉搗傅咬處，當下黃水。藏器。

Control. Bites of snakes, venomous vipers and poisonous worms/bugs. Pound the root and the leaves and apply [the resulting pulp] to the location of the bite. It will discharge a yellow water. [Chen] Cangqi.

16-57
虎杖別録中品
Hu zhang, FE *Bie lu*, middle rank.
Polygonum cuspidatum Sieb. et Zucc. Bushy knotweed.[739]

【釋名】苦杖拾遺、大蟲杖藥性、斑杖日華、酸杖。【時珍曰】杖言其莖，虎言其斑也。或云一名杜牛膝者，非也。一種斑杖似蒻頭者，與此同名異物。

Explanation of Names. *Ku zhang* 苦杖, "bitter rod," *Shi yi*. *Da chong zhang* 大蟲杖, "big worm/bug rod," *Yao xing*. *Ban zhang* 斑杖, "speckled rod," *Rihua*. *Suan zhang* 酸杖, "sour rod." [Li] Shizhen: *Zhang* 杖, "rod," refers to its stem; *hu* 虎, "tiger," refers to its speckled appearance. It is also stated that its name is *du niu xi* 杜牛膝. This is wrong. There is yet another kind of "speckled rod" resembling *indocalamus*. It has the same name as the one discussed here but is a different item.

【集解】【弘景曰】田野甚多，狀如大馬蓼，莖斑而葉圓。【保昇曰】所在有之。生下濕地，作樹高丈餘，其莖赤根黃。二月、八月采根。日乾。【頌曰】今出汾州、越州、滁州，處處有之。三月生苗，莖如竹笋狀，上有赤斑點，初生便分枝丫。葉似小杏葉，七月開花，九月結實。南中出者，無花。根皮黑色，破開即黃似柳根。亦有高丈餘者。爾雅云：蒤，虎杖。郭璞注云：似葒草而粗大，有細刺，可以染赤是也。【宗奭曰】此草藥也。蜀本言作木高丈餘者，非矣。大率皆似寒菊，然花、葉、莖、蕊差大爲異。仍莖葉有淡黑斑。六七月旋旋開花，至九月中方已。花片四出，其色如桃花，差大而外微深。陝西山麓水次甚多。【斆曰】凡使勿誤用天藍及斑袖根，二味根形味皆相似也。【機曰】諸註或云似葒、似杏、似寒菊，各不相侔，豈所產有不同耶？【時珍曰】其莖似葒蓼，其葉圓似杏，其枝黄似柳，其花狀似菊，色似桃花。合而觀之，未嘗不同也。

Collected Explanations. [Tao] Hongjing: Very many can be found in the open country. It is shaped like big Lady's thumb. The stem is speckled and the leaves are round. [Han] Baosheng: It can be found everywhere. It grows on low-lying, damp ground, as trees taller than one *zhang*. The stem is red; the root is yellow. The root is collected in the second and eighth month. It is dried in the sun. [Su] Song.

739 *Hu zhang* 虎杖, lit.: "tiger rod."

Today it comes from Fen zhou, Yue zhou and Chu zhou. It is present everywhere. In the third month it grows a seedling. The stem is shaped like bamboo shoots, but with red speckles and dots on it. At the very beginning of its growth it develops branches forking to the left and right. The leaves are similar to small apricot leaves. It opens flowers in the seventh month. They form fruits in the ninth month. [*Hu zhang*] coming from Nan zhong has no flowers. The skin of the root is black. When it is opened, a yellow color appears similar to that of willow roots. There are also specimens taller than a *zhang*. The *Er ya* states: "*Tu* 蒤 is *hu zhang*." Guo Pu in his comment states: "It resembles red knotweed, but is rough and bigger. It has fine thorns and can be used to dye [things] red." [Kou] Zongshi: This is an herbal pharmaceutical substance. When the *Shu ben* [*cao*] states that it is a tree taller than a *zhang*, this is wrong. In general, it resembles *han ju* 寒菊[740] in all respects. The only difference is that its flower, leaves, stem and petals are a bit bigger, and the stem and the leaves have bland, black speckles. Beginning with the sixth and seventh month, it opens flowers. This ends by the middle of the ninth month. The flowers have four petals with a color similar to that of peach flowers. They are bigger and the color outside is a little deeper. Very many can be found next to the waters at the foot of the mountains in Shaan xi. [Lei] Xiao: For all applications, do not erroneously use *tian lan* and *ban xiu* root.[741] The root, the shape and the flavor of these two items are all similar [to those of *hu zhang*]. [Wang] Ji: All the comments and some others state that it resembles red knotweed, or apricots, or *han ju*, and that they all differ. Could it be that the locations where they grow differ? [Li] Shizhen: The stem resembles that of red knotweed. The leaves are round like those of apricot [trees]. The branches are yellow like those of willow trees. The flowers are shaped like those of *chrysanthemums*. Their color resembles that of peach flowers. In view of all of this, they certainly do not differ.

16-57-01
根 *Gen*
Root [of *hu zhang*].

【修治】【斅曰】采得細剉，却用葉包一夜，晒乾用。

Pharmaceutical Preparation. [Lei] Xiao: Having collected it, cut it into fine pieces. Then wrap it in leaves for one night, dry it in the sun and use it [for therapeutic purposes].

---

740 *Han ju* 寒菊, lit.: "cold chrysanthemum," an unidentified herb.

741 *Tian lan* 天藍, *ban xiu* 斑袖, unidentified plants.

【氣味】微温。【權曰】甘，平，無毒。【宗奭曰】味微苦。今天下暑月多煎根汁爲飲。不得甘草則不堪飲。本文不言味。藥性論云甘，是甘草之味，非虎杖味也。

Qi and Flavor. Slightly warm. [Wang] Ji: Sweet, balanced, nonpoisonous. [Kou] Zongshi: Flavor, slightly bitter. Today, during the summer months everywhere in the Empire the root is boiled and the resulting juice is drunk. But without *glycyrrhiza* [root it is too bitter and] not good to drink. The original text in the [*Bie lu*] fails to mention the [bitter] favor. The *Yao xing lun* states: "Sweet." This is the flavor of *glycyrrhiza* [root]; it is not the flavor of *hu zhang*.

【主治】通利月水，破留血癥結。别録。漬酒服，主暴瘕。弘景。風在骨節間，及血瘀，煮汁作酒服之。藏器。治大熱煩躁，止渴，利小便，壓一切熱毒。甄權。治産後血運，惡血不下，心腹脹滿，排膿，主瘡癤撲損瘀血，破風毒結氣。大明。燒灰，貼諸惡瘡。焙研，煉蜜爲丸，陳米飲服，治腸痔下血。蘇頌。研末酒服，治産後瘀血血痛，及墜撲昏悶，有效。時珍。

Control. It frees menstruation. It breaks through abiding blood with concretion-illness nodes. *Bie lu*. Ingested soaked in wine it controls sudden conglomeration-illness. [Tao] Hongjing. When wind has intruded into the bones and joints, and in the case of stagnating blood, boil it and use the juice to prepare a wine that is to be ingested. [Chen] Cangqi. It serves to cure massive heat and vexing restlessness. It ends thirst. It frees urination. It suppresses all types of heat poison. Zhen Quan. It serves to cure blood [induced brain] movement following delivery, failure of malign blood to be discharged, and swelling and a feeling of fullness in the central and abdominal region. It disperses pus. It controls sores with pimples and stagnating blood resulting from blows and injuries. It breaks through wind poison and bound qi.[742] Da Ming. Burned to ashes it is applied to all types of malign sores. Bake it over a slow fire and grind it [to powder]. Then form with heat refined honey pills and ingest them with a long-stored rice beverage. This serves to cure intestinal piles with a discharge of blood. Su Song. Ground into powder and ingested with wine it serves to cure stagnating blood after delivery and painful blood [accumulation], also clouding with heart-pressure resulting from a fall or a blow. Effective. [Li] Shizhen.

【發明】【權曰】暑月以根和甘草同煎爲飲，色如琥珀可愛，甚甘美。瓶置井中，令冷澈如冰，時人呼爲冷飲子，啜之且尊於茗，極解暑毒。其汁染米作糜餻益美。搗末浸酒常服，破女子經脉不通。有孕人勿服。【時珍曰】孫真人千金方治女人月經不通，腹内積聚，虚脹雷鳴，四肢沉重，亦

742 *Jie qi* 結氣, "bound qi," are pathological qi halting and congealing at any place in the body. BCGM Dict I, 240.

治丈夫積聚，有虎杖煎。取高地虎杖根，剉二斛，水二石五斗，煮取一斗半，去滓，入醇酒五升，煎如餳。每服一合，以知爲度。又許學士本事方治男婦諸般淋疾。用苦杖根洗净，剉一合，以水五合，煎一盞，去滓，入乳香、麝香少許服之。鄞縣尉耿夢得内人患沙石淋已十三年。每漩痛楚不可忍，溺器中小便下沙石剥剥有聲。百方不效，偶得此方服之，一夕而愈。乃予目擊者。

Explication. [Zhen] Quan: During the summer months its root is boiled together with *glycyrrhiza* [root] to prepare a beverage. The color is that of amber; it is lovely. [The beverage] is sweet and delicious. Keep it in a bottle and store it in a well to make it freezing cold. People tend to call it "ice drink." Sipped it is even better than tea. It is the best [beverage] to resolve summer heat poison. When the juice is used to dye rice for the preparation of cakes, they will be even more delicious. Ground into powder, soaked in wine and drunk on a regular basis, it breaks open blocked female menstruation. Pregnant persons must not ingest it. [Li] Shizhen: When Sun zhenren in his *Qian jin fang* [recommends to] cure blocked female menstruation, abdominal accumulations, depletion swelling with thundering sounds, the four limbs feeling heavy and sinking down, and also how to cure accumulations in males, he [advises to use] a *hu zhang* decoction. Cut two *hu* of *hu zhang* root [collected] at a high elevation and boil them in two *dan* and five *dou* of water down to one and a half *dou*. Discard the dregs and add five *sheng* of pure wine. Simmer this until it has assumed the consistency of malt sugar. Each time ingest one *ge* for as long as it takes to achieve an effect. Also Xu Xueshi in his *Ben shi fang* [recommends to] "cure all types of urinary dripping illness of males and women [as follows]. Wash *ku zhang* roots clean and cut one *ge* into fine pieces. Boil them in five *ge* of water down to one small cup full. Discard the dregs, add small amounts of frankincense and musk, and ingest this. The wife of Geng Mengde, Commandant in Yin jian, suffered from sand and stone [urinary] dripping for 13 years. Each time she [urinated, she] was plagued by an unbearable pain, and when she urinated into a chamber pot, the sound of the sand and stones was heard. None of the hundreds of recipes was effective. It was by chance that she obtained this recipe and ingested it. After one night she was cured. I have witnessed this with my own eyes."

【附方】舊三，新三。

Added Recipes. Three of old. Three newly recorded.

小便五淋。苦杖爲末，每服二錢，用飯飲下。集驗方。

The five types of urinary dripping. [Grind] *ku zhang* into powder. Each time ingest two *qian*, to be sent down with a cooked rice beverage. *Ji jian fang*.

月水不利。虎杖三兩，淩霄花、没藥各一兩，爲末，熱酒每服一錢。又方：治月經不通，腹大如甕，氣短欲死。虎杖一斤，去頭暴乾，切。土瓜根汁、牛膝汁二斗，水一斛，浸虎杖一宿，煎取二斗，入二汁同煎如餳。每酒服一合，日再夜一，宿血當下。聖惠方。

Blocked menstruation. [Grind] three *liang* of *hu zhang* and one *liang* each of trumpet flower and myrrh into powder. Each time ingest with hot wine one *qian*. Another recipe: It serves to cure blocked menstruation with an abdomen bloated to the size of a jar and shortness of [breath] qi so that [the woman] comes close to dying. Take one *jin* of *hu zhang* [root], discard the top section, dry it in the sun and cut it [to pieces]. [Get] two *dou*[743] of Japanese gourd root juice and *achyranthes* [leaf] juice. Soak the *hu zhang* [pieces] in one *hu* of *water* for one night and boil it down to two *dou*. Add the two juices and boil [the liquid] until it has assumed the consistency of malt sugar. Each time [let the woman] ingest one *ge*, to be ingested twice during daytime and once during the night. This will cause a discharge of the abiding blood. *Sheng hui fang*.

時疫流毒攻手足，腫痛欲斷。用虎杖根剉，煮汁漬之。肘後方。

Seasonal epidemic with flowing poison[744] attacking hands and feet with a painful swelling letting one wish they were cut off. Cut *hu zhang* root into pieces, boil them and soak [the affected limbs] in the resulting juice. *Zhou hou fang*.

腹中暴癥，硬如石，痛如刺，不治，百日内死。取虎杖根，勿令影臨水上，可得石餘，洗乾搗末，秫米五升炊飯，納入攪之，好酒五斗漬之，封。候藥消飯浮，可飲一升半。勿食鮭魚及鹽。但取一斗乾者，薄酒浸飲，從少起，日三服，亦佳，癥當下也。此方治癥，大勝諸藥也。外臺秘要。

Sudden concretion-illness in the abdomen, hard like a stone with a pain as if pierced. If this is not cured, [patients] will die within 100 days. Collect more than one *dan* of the roots of *hu zhang*, but see to it that [the herb's] shadow is not reflected on the water [nearby].[745] Wash it clean and pound it into powder. Cook a meal with five *sheng* of glutinous rice, add [the powder] and stir it. Soak [the rice with the powder]

743 Instead of *er dou* 二斗, "two *dou*,", *Sheng hui fang* ch. 72, *Zhi fu ren yue shui bu tong fu nei wdi kuai zhu fang* 據聖惠方卷七十二治婦人月水不通腹内癥塊諸方, "all types of recipes to cure blocked female menstruation with the formation of concretion-illness with lumps in the abdomen," writes *ge er jin* 各二斤, "two *jin* each."

744 *Liu du* 流毒, "flowing poison," etiological agent of *du qi* 毒氣, "poison qi," moving between organs or other regions in the body and causing illness. BCGM Dict 319.

745 This recipe appears first in the *Zhou hou fang*. For reasons unexplained, only those specimens of crabgrass were considered useful for therapeutic purposes that do not grow close to a water, and hence "their shadow is not reflected in a water."

in five *dou* of good wine and seal it. Wait until the pharmaceutical substance has dissolved and the rice floats on the surface. Then one and a half *sheng* [of the liquid] can be drunk. [During this treatment] globefish and salt must not be eaten. [Another recipe.] Take one *dou* of dried [*hu zhang* root], soak it in thin wine and drink this. Begin with a small dose, and ingest it three times a day. This, too, is excellent. The concretion-illness will be discharged. This recipe cures concretion-illness much better than all other medications. *Wai tai mi yao.*

氣奔怪病。人忽遍身皮底混混如波浪聲，痒不可忍，抓之血出不能解，謂之氣奔。以苦杖、人參、青鹽、細辛各一兩，作一服，水煎，細飲盡便愈。夏子益奇疾方。

A strange disease of qi run. People suddenly have something moving in the skin all over their body as if it were a wave, with an unbearable itch. When they scratch [the skin] a bleeding results that cannot be stopped. This is called "qi run."[746] Prepare one dose of one *liang* each of *ku zhang*, ginseng [root], greenish salt/halite and *asarum heteropoides* [root]. Boil it in water and drink the entire [liquid] in small portions. This results in a cure. Xia Ziyi, *Qi ji fang.*

消渴引飲。虎杖燒過、海浮石、烏賊魚骨、丹砂等分，爲末。渴時以麥門冬湯服二錢，日三次。忌酒色、魚、麪、鮓、醬、生冷。衛生家寶方。

Melting with thirst[747] and an urge to drink. [Grind] equal amounts of *hu zhang*, completely burned, pumice, cuttlefish bone and cinnabar into powder. When [the patient] is thirsty let him ingest with an *ophiopogon* [tuber] decoction two *qian*, three times a day. [During this treatment] wine and sex, fish, pasta, preserved fish, soy sauce, fresh and cold [items] are to be avoided. *Wei sheng jia bao fang.*

16-58
蕕拾遺
You, FE *Shi yi.*

***Digitaria sanguinalis* (L.) Scop. Crabgrass.**

【校正】併入有名未用別録馬唐。

Editorial Correction. *Ma tang* 馬唐, listed in the *Bie lu*, section "known by name but not in use," is included here.

【釋名】馬唐別録、馬飯別録、羊麻別録、羊粟別録、蔓于爾雅、軒于。【藏器曰】馬食之如糖如飯，故名馬唐、馬飯。【時珍曰】羊亦食之，故

746 *Qi ben* 氣奔, "qi run." BCGM Dict I, 380.

747 *Xiao ke* 消渴, "melting with thirst," most likely including cases of diabetes. BCGM Dict Vol I, 567.

曰羊麻、羊粟。其氣癅臭，故謂之蕕。蕕者癅也，朽木臭也。此草莖頗似蕙而臭，故左傳云一薰一蕕，十年尚猶有臭是也。孫升談圃以爲香薷者，誤矣。即別録馬唐也，今併爲一。

Explanation of Names. *Ma tang* 馬唐, *Bie lu*. *Ma fan* 馬飯, *Bie lu*. *Yang ma* 羊麻, *Bie lu*. *Yang su* 羊粟, *Bie lu*. *Man yu* 蔓于, *Er ya*. *Xuan yu* 軒于. [Chen] Cangqi: Horses, *ma* 馬, eat it as if it were sugar, *tang* 糖, or cooked rice, *fan* 飯. Hence the names *ma tang* 馬唐 and *ma fan* 馬飯. [Li] Shizhen: Sheep, *yang* 羊, too, eat it. Hence it is called *yang ma* 羊麻, "sheep's sesame," and *yang su* 羊粟, "sheep's millet." Its qi are malodorant like those of sick wood, *you* 癅. Hence it is called *you* 蕕. *You* 蕕 is 癅; it is the bad stench of rotten wood. The stem of this herb is quite similar to that of strong fragrant loosestrife, but it is malodorous. Therefore, when the *Zuo zhuan* states: "one *xun* 薰 (sweet basil) and one *you* 蕕 (strong fragrant loosestrife), their bad stench remains even after ten years," this is correct.. Sun Sheng in his *Tan fu* believes it to be *elsholtzia* herb. He is wrong. It is the *ma tang* 馬唐 mentioned in the *Bie lu*. Here now it is combined [with *you* 蕕] in one entry.

【集解】【別録曰】馬唐生下濕地，莖有節生根，五月采。【藏器曰】生南方廢稻田中，節節有根，着土如結縷草，堪飼馬。又曰：蕕生水田中，狀如結縷草而葉長，馬食之。

Collected Explanations. *Bie lu*: *Ma tang* grows on low-lying damp ground. The stem has nodes from which the roots grow. It is collected in the fifth month. [Chen] Cangqi: It grows in the South on deserted rice fields. Each node has a root. [*Ma tang*] clings to the soil similar to Korean lawngrass. It is suitable for feeding horses. It is also said: *You* grows in water fields. It is shaped like Korean lawngrass, but its leaves are lengthy. Horses eat it.

【氣味】甘，寒，無毒。【藏器曰】大寒。

Qi and Flavor. Sweet, cold, nonpoisonous. [Chen] Cangqi: Very cold.

【主治】馬唐：調中，明耳目。別録。煎取汁，明目潤肺。又曰：蕕，消水氣濕痺，脚氣，，虛腫，小腹急，小便赤澀，並合赤小豆煮食，勿與鹽。絞汁服，止消渴。擣葉，傅毒腫。藏器。

Control. *Ma tang*: It regulates the center and clears ears and eyes. *Bie lu*. Boiled to obtain a juice it clears the eyes and moistens the lung. It is also said: *You* dissolves blockage related to water qi, [i. e.,] dampness, leg qi,[748] stubborn blockage, depletion swelling, tight lower abdomen, as well as red and rough urination. It is eaten boiled with mung beans, but do not add salt. To ingest the juice obtained by squeezing it

748 *Jiao qi* 脚氣, "leg qi." Painful, weak, swollen legs. BCGM Dict I, 248.

ends melting with thirst.[749] Pound the leaves and apply [the pulp] to poison swelling. [Chen] Cangqi.

16-59

萹蓄音楄畜本經下品

Bian xu, read *bian xu*, FE *Ben jing*, lower rank.

***Polygonum aviculare* L. Common knotgrass.**

【釋名】扁竹弘景、扁辨吴普、扁蔓吴普、粉節草綱目、道生草。【時珍曰】許慎説文作扁筑，與竹同音。節間有粉，多生道旁，故方士呼爲粉節草、道生草。

Explanation of Names. *Bian zhu* 扁竹, "flat bamboo," [Tao] Hongjing. *Bian bian* 扁辨, Wu Pu. *Bian man* 扁蔓, "flat creeper," Wu Pu. *Fen jie cao* 粉節草, *Gang mu*. *Dao sheng cao* 道生草. [Li] Shizhen: Xu Shen in his *Shuo wen* writes *bian zhu* 扁筑, "flat structure." [*Zhu* 筑, "structure,"] has the same reading as *zhu* 竹, "bamboo." There is a powder, *fen* 粉, between the nodes, *jie* 節, and it often grows at the roadside. Hence recipe experts call it *fen jie cao* 粉節草, "herb with powdered nodes," and *dao sheng cao* 道生草, "herb growing on roads."

【集解】【别録曰】萹蓄生東萊山谷，五月采，陰乾。【弘景曰】處處有之，布地而生，花節間白，葉細緑，人呼爲扁竹。【頌曰】春中布地生道旁，苗似瞿麥，葉細緑如竹，赤莖如釵股，節間花出甚細，微青黄色，根如蒿根，四五月采苗，陰乾。蜀圖經云：二月、八月採苗，日乾。郭璞注爾雅云：似小藜，赤莖節，好生道旁，可食，殺蟲是也。或云爾雅王芻即此也。【時珍曰】其葉似落帚葉而不尖，弱莖引蔓，促節。三月開細紅花，如蓼藍花，結細子，爐火家燒灰煉霜用。一種水扁筑，名[薄-尃+毒]，音督，出説文。

Collected Explanations. *Bie lu*: *Bian xu* grows in the mountain valleys of Dong lai. It is collected in the fifth month and dried in the yin (i. e., shade). [Tao] Hongjing. It can be found everywhere. It grows spread out on the ground. It is white between the flowers and the nodes. The leaves are fine and green. People call it "flat bamboo." [Su] Song: In spring it grows at the roadside spreading out on the ground. The seedling resembles that of fringed pink. The leaves are fine and green like those of bamboo. The stem is red like a hairpin. Extremely fine flowers appear between the nodes; they are of a slightly greenish-yellow color. The root is similar to the wormwood root. The seedlings are collected in the fourth and fifth month; they are dried in the yin (i. e., shade). The *Shu tu jing* states: "The seedling is collected in the

749 *Xiao ke* 消渴, "melting with thirst," most likely including cases of diabetes. BCGM Dict Vol I, 567.

second and eighth month; it is dried in the sun." Guo Pu in his comment on the *Er ya* states: "It resembles small specimens of lambsquarters. It has a red stem with nodes and prefers to grow at the roadside. It is edible and kills worms/bugs." This is correct. It is also said: This is the *wang chu* 王芻, "royal fodder," mentioned in the *Er ya*. [Li] Shizhen: Its leaves resemble the leaves of broom plants, but they are not pointed. The weak stem is a creeper with nodes. In the third month it opens fine, red flowers, similar to the flowers of indigo plants. They form fine seeds. The experts working with stoves burn it to ashes and use them for a preparation with heat of frost (i. e., sublimed calomel). Another kind of water *bian zhu* 扁筑 is called *du* [薄-専+毒], read *du* 督. A quote from the *Shuo wen*.

【氣味】苦，平，無毒。【權曰】甘、濇。

Qi and Flavor. Bitter, balanced, nonpoisonous. [Zhen] Quan: Sweet, astringent.

【主治】浸淫疥瘙疽痔，殺三蟲。本經。療女子陰蝕。別録。煮汁飲小兒，療蚘蟲有驗。甄權。治霍亂黃疸，利小便，小兒魃病。時珍。

Control. Itching *jie*-illness[750] soaked with moisture, impediment-illness[751] and piles. It kills the three types of worms/bugs. *Ben jing*. It heals erosion in the yin [(i. e., genital) region] of females. *Bie lu*. When children drink the juice obtained by boiling [*bian xu*], this effectively heals a roundworm infestation. Zhen Quan. It serves to cure cholera and yellow *dan*-illness/jaundice. It frees the passage of urine. [It serves to cure] jealousy-demon diseases of children.[752] [Li] Shizhen.

【附方】舊六，新三。

Added Recipes. Six of old. Three newly [recorded].

熱淋濇痛。扁竹煎湯頻飲。生生編。

Urinary dripping with heat and painful roughness. Boil *bian zhu* and repeatedly drink the decoction. *Sheng sheng bian*.

熱黃疸疾。扁竹擣汁，頓服一升。多年者，日再服之。藥性論。

---

750 *Jie*-illness 疥, vaguely identifiable skin ailment. BCGM Dict I, 249.

751 *Ju* 疽, "impediment-illness," refers to an obstruction of vessels or other ducts inside the body. Qi rushing against the impediment may cause a local swelling and eventually break through the surface to cause an abscess. BCGM Dict I, 277.

752 *Xiao er qi bing* 小兒魃病, "children's jealousy-demon disease," a condition of children under two years of age who, following a second pregnancy of their mother, lose weight to emaciation, are tired and have their hair wither. This was believed to result from their being cursed by the jealousy demon. BCGM Dict I, 565.

Yellow *dan*-illness/jaundice with heat. Pound *bian zhu* and ingest one *sheng* of the juice all at once. If [the illness] has lasted for many years, ingest [one *sheng*] twice a day. *Yao xing lun*.

霍亂吐利。扁竹入豉汁中，下五味，煮羹食。食醫心鏡。

Cholera with vomiting and free-flow. Give *bian zhu* into [soybean] relish juice, add the five flavor (spices), boil this and eat the congee. *Shi yi xin jing*.

丹石衝眼。服丹石人毒發，衝眼腫痛。扁竹根一握，洗，搗汁服之。食療本草。

Elixir minerals have rushed into the eyes. When a person who has ingested an elixir mineral develops a poisoning that rushes into his eyes causing a painful swelling. Wash clean a handful of *bian zhu* root, pound it and ingest the resulting juice. *Shi liao ben cao*.

蚘咬心痛。食療治小兒蚘咬心痛，面青，口中沫出臨死者，取扁竹十斤剉，以水一石，煎至一斗，去滓煎如餳。隔宿勿食，空心服一升，蟲即下也。仍常煮汁作飯食。

Heart pain caused by roundworm bites. The *Shi liao* [recommends to] cure children with heart pain caused by roundworm bites when their face is greenish, foam comes out of their mouth, and they are close to dying. Cut ten *jin* of *bian zhu* to fine pieces, boil them in one *dan* of water down to one *dou*, discard the dregs and boil [the liquid] until it has assumed a consistency of malt sugar. [The patient] must not eat in the evening and ingest one *sheng* on an empty stomach [the next day]. The worms will be discharged. Regularly boil [*bian zhu*] to obtain a juice and use it to prepare [the child's] meals.

海上歌云：
心頭急痛不能當，我有仙人海上[753]方。
萹蓄醋煎通口嚥，管教時刻便安康。
The *Hai shang ge* states:
A critical pain at the top of the heart (i. e., stomach). I have an hermit/immortal's very best recipe.
Boil *bian xu* in vinegar and sip it through the mouth. Definitely, this will result in peace and health in a moment.

蟲食下部。蟲狀如蝸牛食下部作痒。取扁竹一把水二升煮熟。五歲兒空腹服三五合。楊氏產乳。

753 *Hai shang* 海上, lit: "from overseas," is to say: the very best.

Worms/bugs eating away one's lower (i. e. genital) region. When worms/bugs shaped like a snail eat away one's lower (i. e., genital) region and cause an itch. Boil one handful of *bian xu* in two *sheng* of water until done. Children five years of age ingest three to five *ge* on an empty stomach. *Yang shi chan ru.*

痔發腫痛。扁竹搗汁，服一升，一二服未瘥，再服。亦取汁和麪作餺飥煮食，日三次。藥性論。

Piles developing a painful swelling. Pound *bian xu* to obtain a juice and ingest one *sheng*. If no cure is achieved after one or two ingestions, ingest it again. Also, prepare with the juice and wheat flour dumplings, boil them and eat them. Three times a day. *Yao xing lun.*

惡瘡痂痒作痛。扁竹搗封，痂落即瘥。肘後方。

Malign sores with painful, itching crust. Pound *bian zhu* and seal [the affected region with the pulp]. Once the crust has come off a cure is achieved. *Zhou hou fang.*

16-60

藎草音燼本經下品

Jin cao, read *jin*, FE *Ben jing*, lower rank.

***Arthraxon hispidus* (Thunb.) Makino. Small carpetgrass.**

【釋名】黄草吴普、菉竹唐本、菉蓐唐本、莀草綱目、盭草音戾、王芻爾雅、鴟脚莎。【時珍曰】此草緑色，可染黄，故曰黄、曰緑也。莀、盭乃北人呼緑字音轉也。古者貢草入染人，故謂之王芻，而進忠者謂之藎臣也。詩云：終朝采緑，不盈一掬。許慎説文云：莀草可以染黄。漢書云：諸侯盭綬。晉灼注云：盭草出瑯琊，似艾可染，因以名綬。皆謂此草也。【禹錫曰】爾雅：菉，王芻。孫炎注云：即緑蓐草也。今呼爲鴟脚莎。詩云"菉竹猗猗"是也。

Explanation of Names. *Huang cao* 黄草, "yellow herb," Wu Pu. *Lü zhu* 菉竹, "green bamboo," *Tang ben. Lü ru* 菉蓐, "greenish carpet," *Tang ben. Li cao* 莀草, *Gang mu. Li cao* 盭草, read *li* 戾; *wang chu* 王芻, "royal fodder," *Er ya. Chi jiao suo* 鴟脚莎, "owl leg grass." [Li] Shizhen: This herb is of green, *lü* 緑, color and can serve to dye yellow. Hence it is called *huang* [*cao*] 黄[草], "yellow [herb]," and also *lü* [*cao*] 緑[草], "green [herb]." *Li* 莀 and *li* 盭 are modified pronunciations of the character *lü* 緑 by people in the North. The ancients submitted this herb [to the Court] as a dyestuff for the persons there. Hence it is called *wang chu* 王芻, "royal fodder." Those who served [the king] loyally were called *jin chen* 藎臣, "loyal subject[754]."

754 *Jin chen* 藎臣, lit. "carpetgrass subject," because these officials were as close, that is: loyal, to the king as carpetgrass is to the ground.

The *Shi* states: "If the green [herb] is collected for an entire morning, one will not have obtained enough to fill both hands." Xu Shen in his *Shuo wen* states: "*Li cao* can serve to dye something yellow." The *Han shu* states: "Dukes with a carpetgrass/loyalty ribbon on a seal." Jin Zhuo comments: *Li cao* 盭草 comes from Lang ye. It resembles common mugwort and can be used for dying. Hence it is named 'ribbons on a seal'." But it is always the herb that is meant. [Zhang] Yuxi: "*Er ya*: *Lü* 菉 is *wang chu* 王芻." Sun Yan in his comment states: "This is *lü ru cao* 綠蓐草. Today it is called *chi jiao suo* 鴟脚莎." The *Shi* states: "*Lü zhu* 菉竹, lush and luxuriant." This is [the item discussed here].

【集解】【别録曰】藎草生青衣川谷，九月、十月采，可以染作金色。【普曰】生太山山谷。【恭曰】青衣縣名，在益州西。今處處平澤溪澗側皆有。葉似竹而細薄，莖亦圓小。荆襄人煮以染黄，色極鮮好。俗名菉蓐草。

Collected Explanations. *Bie lu*: *Jin cao* grows in the river valleys of Qing yi. It is collected in the ninth and tenth month. It can be used to dye something to assume the color of gold. [Wu] Pu: It grows in the valleys of Mount Tai shan. [Su] Gong: Qing yi is the name of a county situated in the West of Yi zhou. Today it is found everywhere in the marshlands of the plains and near rivulets. The leaves resemble those of bamboo, but are finer and thin. The stem, too, is round and small. People in Jiang xiang boil it to dye things yellow. The color obtained is extremely fresh and good. [The herb] is commonly called *lü ru cao* 菉蓐草.

【氣味】苦，平，無毒。【吴氏曰】神農、雷公：苦。【之才曰】畏鼠負。

Qi and Flavor: Bitter,[755] balanced, nonpoisonous. Mr. Wu [Pu]: Shen nong, Lei gong: Bitter. [Xu] Zhicai. [Ingested together,] it fears pill bugs.

【主治】久欬上氣喘逆，久寒驚悸，痂疥白秃瘍氣，殺皮膚小蟲。本經。治身熱邪氣，小兒身熱。吴普。洗一切惡瘡，有效。大明。

Control. Long lasting cough with rising qi; panting with [qi] counterflow. Long lasting cold with fright palpitation. Crusts and *jie*-illness,[756] white baldness ulcer qi. It kills small worms/bugs in the skin. *Ben jing*. It serves to cure body heat with evil qi, and body heat of children. Wu Pu. [A decoction of *jin cao* is used to] wash all types of malign sores. Effective. Da Ming.[757]

---

755 In today's available version of the *Yu lan*, ch. 997, *wang chu* 王芻, quoting the *Wu si ben cao*, the character *ku* 苦 is omitted.

756 *Jie*-illness 疥, vaguely identifiable skin ailment. BCGM Dict I, 249.

757 *Zheng lei* ch. 11, *jin cao* 藎草, does not refer to the *Rihua zi ben cao* of Da Ming as its source. It quotes the statement on "control," *zhu zhi* 主治, from the *Yao xing lun*.

16-61

蒺蔾本經上品

***Ji li*, FE *Ben jing*, upper rank.**

***Tribulus terrestris* R. Calthrop.**

【釋名】茨爾雅、旁通本經、屈人本經、止行本經、犲羽本經、升推。【弘景曰】多生道上及墻上。葉布地，子有刺，狀如菱而小。長安最饒，人行多着木履。今軍家乃鑄鐵作之，以布敵路，名鐵蒺蔾。易云“據于蒺蔾”，言其兇傷。詩云墻有茨，不可掃也，以刺梗穢。方用甚稀。【時珍曰】蒺，疾也；蔾，利也；茨，刺也。其刺傷人，甚疾而利也。屈人、止行，皆因其傷人也。

Explanation of Names. *Ci* 茨, *Er ya*. *Pang tong* 旁通, "[an herb] one walks past on the side," *Ben jing*. *Qu ren* 屈人, "[an herb] that makes one bend down," *Ben jing*. *Zhi xing* 止行, "[an herb] that stops one's movement," *Ben jing*. *Chai yu* 犲羽, "a wolf's feathers," *Ben jing*. *Sheng tui* 升推. [Tao] Hongjing: Much of it grows on roads and on walls. The leaves cover the ground. The seeds have thorns. They are shaped like those of water chestnuts but are smaller. In Chang an it is most abundant. When people walk there, they often wear wooden shoes [to avoid being stung by its thorns]. Today the military uses iron to reproduce the [seeds with thorns] and they spread them on the roads of the enemy. [These devices are] called "iron calthrop," *tie ji li* 鐵蒺蔾. The *Yi* states: "According to *ji li* 蒺蔾." That is: [to foretell] a brutal harm. The *Shi* states: "A wall with *ci* 茨. It cannot be swept away." The thorns are most abominable. In recipes [*ji li*] is seldom resorted to. [Li] Shizhen: *Ji* 蒺 is *ji* 疾. *Li* 蔾 is *li* 利. *Ci* 茨 is *ci* 刺. Its thorns, *ci* 刺, harm people; quickly, *ji* 疾, and with sharp edges, *li* 利. *Qu ren* 屈人, "to make a person bend down," and *zhi xing* 止行, "to stop one's movement," all refer to its potential of harming one.

【集解】【别録曰】蒺蔾子生馮翊平澤或道旁，七月、八月采實，暴乾。頌曰】冬月亦采之，黄白色。郭璞注爾雅云，布地蔓生，細葉，子有三角，刺人是也。又一種白蒺蔾，今生同州沙苑，牧馬草地最多，而近道亦有之。緑葉【細蔓，綿布沙上。七月開花黄紫色，如豌豆花而小，九月結實作莢，子便可采。其實味甘而微腥，褐緑色，與蠶種子相類而差大。又與馬薸子酷相類，但馬薸子微大，不堪入藥，須細辨之。【宗奭曰】蒺蔾有二等。一等杜蒺蔾，即今之道旁布地而生者，開小黄花，結芒刺。一種白蒺蔾，出同州沙苑牧馬處。子如羊内腎，大如黍粒，補腎藥今人多用。風家惟用刺蒺蔾也。【時珍曰】蒺蔾葉如初生皂莢葉，整齊可愛。刺蒺蔾狀如赤根菜子及細菱，三角四刺，實有仁。其白蒺蔾結莢長寸許，内子大如脂麻，狀如羊腎而帶緑色，今人謂之沙苑蒺蔾。以此分别。

Collected Explanations. *Bie lu*: *Ji li* seeds grow in the marshlands of the plains of Feng yi, and also at the roadside. The fruits are collected in the seventh and eighth month. They are dried in the sun. [Su] Song. They are also collected during winter months. They are yellow-white. Guo Pu in his comment on the *Er ya* states: "This is a creeper spreading out on the ground with fine leaves. The seeds have three edges that can pierce humans." There is also a white kind of *ji li*. Today it grows on sandy fields in Tong zhou. Most of it is found on grounds with herbs to raise horses. It is also present near roads. [The herb has] green leaves and fine vines, spreading on the sand like a soft cover. In the seventh month it opens flowers of purple color, similar to garden pea flowers, but smaller. They form fruits in the ninth month. The seeds are easily collected from the pods. The flavor of the fruit is sweet, and a little fishy. They are of a brown-green color. They are similar to silkworm eggs, but quite big. They are also very similar to horse/big duckweed, but horse/big duckweed is a little bigger and is not suitable for use as medication. They have to be carefully distinguished. [Kou] Zongshi: There are two kinds of *ji li*. One is *du ji li* 杜蒺藜. This is the kind that grows spreading out on the ground along roads. It opens small, yellow flowers, and bears awns and thorns. Another kind is white *ji li*. It comes from the sandy fields in Tong zhou where horses are raised. The seeds are similar to sheep kidneys. They have the size of millet. It is often used today as a pharmaceutical drug supplementing the kidneys. Persons affected by wind only resort to thorny *ji li*. [Li] Shizhen: The leaves of *ji li* are similar to *gleditsia* leaves that have just begun to grow. They are regular and lovely. Thorny *ji li* is shaped like Chinese cabbage with a red root and also fine water chestnut. It has three edges with four thorns. The fruit contain kernels. White *ji li* forms pods of a length of more than a *cun*. The seeds inside have the size of sesame seeds. They are shaped like sheep kidneys with a green color. Today people call them "sandy field *ji li*" to distinguish them from the other kind.

16-61-01

子 *Zi*

Seeds [of *ji li*].

【修治】【斅曰】凡使揀净蒸之。從午至酉，日乾，木臼舂令刺盡，用酒拌再蒸，從午至酉，日乾用。【大明曰】入藥不計丸散，並炒去刺用。

Pharmaceutical Preparation. [Lei] Xiao: For all applications, select clean [seeds] and steam them from *wu* 午 hours (11 - 13) to *you* 酉 hours (17 - 19). Dry them in the sun. Pound them in a wooden mortar until no more thorns are discernable. Mix this with wine and steam it again from *wu* hours to *you* hours. Dry it in the sun and then use it [for therapeutic purposes]. Da Ming: Regardless of whether they are prepared as a medication to pills or powders, always fry them and remove the thorns before making use of them.

【氣味】苦，温，無毒。【別録曰】辛，微温。【權曰】甘，有小毒。【志曰】其性宣通，久服不冷而無壅熱，當以性温爲是。【之才曰】烏頭爲之使。

Qi and Flavor. Bitter, warm, nonpoisonous. *Bie lu*: Acrid, slightly warm.[758] [Zhen] Quan: Sweet, slightly poisonous. [Ma] Zhi: By their nature they move and penetrate. Ingesting them over a long time, one does not feel cold and will not be affected by obstruction related to heat. The nature [of the seeds] should be warm, indeed. [Xu] Zhicai: *Aconitum* [main tuber] serves as its guiding substance.

【主治】惡血，破癥積聚，喉痺，乳難。久服長肌肉，明目輕身。本經。身體風癢，頭痛，欬逆傷肺，肺痿，止煩下氣。小兒頭瘡，癰腫陰㿉，可作摩粉。别録。治諸風癧瘍，療吐膿，去燥熱。甄權。治奔豚腎氣，肺氣胸膈滿，催生墮胎，益精，療水藏冷，小便多，止遺瀝泄精，溺血腫痛。大明。痔漏陰汗，婦人發乳帶下。蘇頌。治風秘及蚘蟲心腹痛。時珍。

Control. Malign blood. They break through concretion-illness, accumulation and collection, throat blockage and difficulties of a nursing mother to let milk. Ingested over a long time, they stimulate growth of muscles and flesh. They clear the eyes and relieve the body of its weight. *Ben jing*. Body itch related to wind [intrusion]. Headache. Cough with [qi] counterflow and harmed lung. Lung dysfunction. They end vexation and discharge qi. Sores on the head of children. Swelling related to obstruction-illness[759] and yin prominence-illness.[760] They can be prepared to a powder for a massage. *Bie lu*. They serve to cure all types of pervasion-illness ulcers related to wind [intrusion].[761] They heal spitting/vomiting of pus and remove restlessness with heat. Zhen Quan. They serve to cure running piglet[762] kidney qi, and lung qi causing a feeling of fullness in the chest and diaphragm region. They speed up birth and let a fetus drop out. They boost essence/sperm. They heal cold in the water

758 Instead of *wen* 温, "warm," *Zheng lei* ch. 7, *ji li* 蒺藜, writes *han* 寒, "cold."

759 *Yong* 癰, "obstruction-illness," refers to an obstruction of vessels or other ducts inside the body. Qi rushing against the obstruction may cause a local swelling and eventually break through the surface to cause an abscess. BCGM Dict I, 641.

760 *Yin tui* 陰㿉, "yin (i.e. scrotal) prominence-illness," a condition of local swelling and pain affecting a male's private parts. BCGM Dict I, 637.

761 *Li yang feng* 癧瘍風, "pervasion-illness with ulcer wind," also called *li yang* 癧瘍, "pervasion-illness with ulcer," a condition of white macules and dots appearing on the skin in the neck, on the chest, and below the armpits, without itching or pain. BCGM Dict I, 315.

762 *Ben tun* 賁豚, "running piglet," a condition of an accumulation in the kidneys assuming the shape of a piglet moving up and down at irregular intervals. BCGM Dict I, 57.

long-term depot (i. e., the kidneys) with profuse urination. They end uncontrolled dripping and outflow of essence/sperm, and urination with blood and a painful swelling. Da Ming. Leaking piles and sweat in the yin [(i. e., genital) region]. For women they let down milk and [heal diseases] below the belt. Su Song: They serve to cure wind closure[763] and pain in the central and abdominal region caused by the presence of roundworms and other worms/bugs. [Li] Shizhen.

16-61-02
白蒺藜 *Bai ji li*
White *ji li*.

【氣味】甘，温，無毒。

Qi and Flavor. Sweet, warm, nonpoisonous.

【主治】補腎，治腰痛泄精，虛損勞乏。時珍。

Control. It supplements kidney [qi] and serves to cure lower back pain with outflow of essence/sperm, depletion injury and exhaustion. [Li] Shizhen.

【發明】【頌曰】古方皆用有刺者，治風明目最良。神仙方亦有單服蒺藜法，云不問黑白，但取堅實者，舂去刺用。【時珍曰】古方補腎治風，皆用刺蒺藜。後世補腎多用沙苑蒺藜，或以熬膏和藥，恐其功亦不甚相遠也。刺蒺藜炒黄去刺，磨麪作餅，或蒸食，可以救荒。

Explication. [Su] Song: Ancient recipes [recommend to] use [the seeds] with the thorns as this is best to cure wind eyes.[764] The recipes of the divine immortals also include methods for an ingestion of *ji li* as a single substance. They state that it does not matter whether [the seeds] are black or white; all that is required is to select hard, solid specimens and to remove the thorns in a mortar before making use of them. [Li] Shizhen: Ancient recipes designed to supplement kidney [qi] and to cure wind [intrusion] always resorted to thorny *ji li*. In later times, to supplement kidney [qi] mostly sandy field *ji li* was used. Sometimes the [seeds] are simmered to a paste and mixed with [further] pharmaceutical drugs. Presumably the [therapeutic] potentials [of such preparations] are not far apart from each other. When thorny *ci ji* [seeds] are fried until they turn yellow, their thorns are removed, and they are rubbed with wheat flour to prepare cakes, these [cakes] may be steamed to be eaten to rescue one in times of famine.

---

763 *Feng bi* 風秘, "wind closure, a condition of *bian pi* 便秘, "constipation," brought about by intestinal and stomach dryness and a depletion of body liquids. The notion of wind causing intestinal dryness is associated with the observation that wind in nature disperses moisture. BCGM Dict I, 158.

764 *Feng yan* 風眼, "wind eye," a condition of red and festering canthi and eyelids brought about by harm caused to the eyes by heat. BCGM Dict I, 171.

【附方】舊九，新八。

Added Recipes. Nine of old. Eight newly [recorded].

服食法。蒺藜子一碩，七八月熟時收取，日乾，舂去刺，杵爲末。每服二錢，新汲水調下，日三服，勿令中絶，斷穀長生。服之一年以後，冬不寒，夏不熱。二年，老者復少，髮白復黑，齒落更生。服之三年，身輕長生。神仙秘旨。

The method of ingesting [*ji li*] as food. Collect one *dan* of *ji li* seeds when they are ripe in the seventh and eighth month. Dry them in the sun. [Pound them] in a mortar to remove the thorns and grind them into powder. Each time ingest two *qian*, to be sent down mixed with newly drawn water. To be ingested three times a day. Do not interrupt [this treatment] any time. This way the [intake of] grain is stopped and a long life is achieved. After having ingested this for one year, in winter one will not feel cold and in summer one will not feel the heat. After two years, old persons have turned young again; white hair has turned black again. Teeth that had fallen out have grown again. After having ingested it for three years, the body is relieved of its weight and a long life is reached. *Shen xian mi zhi.*

腰脊引痛。蒺藜子擣末，蜜和丸胡豆大。酒服二丸，日三服。外臺秘要。

Pain pulling on the lower back and the spine. Pound *ji li* seeds into powder and form with honey pills the size of peas. Ingest with wine two pills. To be ingested three times a day. *Wai tai mi yao.*

通身浮腫。杜蒺藜日日煎湯洗之。聖惠方。

Surface swelling covering the entire body. Every day boil *du ji li* and wash [the affected region] with the decoction. *Sheng hui fang.*

卒中五尸。蒺藜子擣末，蜜丸胡豆大。每服二丸，日三服。肘後方。

Suddenly being struck by any of the five types of corpse [qi].[765] Pound *ji li* seeds into powder and form with honey pills the size of peas. Each time ingest two pills. To be ingested three times a day. *Zhou hou fang.*

大便風秘。蒺藜子炒一兩，豬牙皂莢去皮酥炙五錢，爲末。每服一錢，鹽茶湯下。普濟方。

765 *Wu shi* 五屍," the five types of corpse [qi]." BCGM Dict I, 158.

Wind closure[766] of major [defecation] relief. [Grind] one *liang* of fried *ji li* seeds and five *qian* of small *gleditsia* pods/seeds,[767] with their skin discarded and roasted in butter, into powder. Each time ingest one *qian*, to be sent down with a salted tea decoction. *Pu ji fang.*

月經不通。杜蒺藜、當歸等分，爲末，米飲每服三錢。儒門事親。

Blocked menstruation. [Grind] equal amounts of *du ji li* and Chinese *angelica* [root] into powder. Each time ingest with a rice beverage three *qian*. *Ru men shi qin.*

催生下衣。難産，胎在腹中，并包衣不下及胎死者，蒺藜子、貝母各四兩，爲末，米湯服三錢。少頃不下，再服。梅師方。

To speed up birth and discharge the placenta. For difficult births, when the fetus remains in the abdomen and also when the placenta fails to be discharged, and when the fetus has died. [Grind] four *liang* each of *ji li* seeds and *fritillaria* [root] into powder and [let the woman] ingest with a rice decoction three *qian*. If [fetus or placenta] are not discharged right away, let her ingest this a second time. *Mei shi fang.*

蚘蟲心痛，吐清水。七月七日采蒺藜子，陰乾，燒作灰，先食服方寸匕，日三服。外臺秘要。

Heart pain related to the presence of roundworms and other worms/bugs; [patients] spit clear water. On the seventh day in the seventh month collect *ji li* seeds. Dry them in the yin (i. e., shade) and burn them to ashes. Prior to meals ingest the amount held by a square *cun* spoon. To be ingested three times a day. *Wai tai mi yao.*

萬病積聚。七八月收蒺藜子，水煮熟，曝乾，蜜丸梧子大。每酒服七丸，以知爲度。其汁煎如飴，服之。

A myriad of diseases with accumulation and collection. Collect *ji li* seeds in the seventh or eighth month, boil them in water until done, dry them in the sun and with honey form pills the size of *wu* seeds. Each time ingest with wine seven pills for as long as it takes to achieve an effect. Boil the juice until it has assumed a consistency of malt sugar and ingest it.

三十年失明。補肝散：用蒺藜子七月七日收，陰乾搗散。食後水服方寸匕，日二。外臺秘要。

---

766 *Feng bi* 風秘, "wind closure, a condition of *bian pi* 便秘, "constipation," brought about by intestinal and stomach dryness and a depletion of body liquids. The notion of wind causing intestinal dryness is associated with the observation that wind in nature disperses moisture. BCGM Dict I, 158.

767 *Zhu ya zao jia* 豬牙皂莢, lit.: "gleditsia seeds/pots as small as pig teeth."

Loss of eyesight for 30 years. The "powder to supplement liver [qi]." Collect *ji li* seeds on the seventh day of the seventh month, dry them in the yin (i. e., shade) and pound them into powder. Ingest with water following a meal the amount held by a square *cun* spoon. Twice a day. *Wai tai mi yao.*

牙齒動摇，疼痛及打動者。土蒺藜去角生研五錢，淡漿水半盌，蘸水入鹽温漱，甚效。或以根燒灰，貼牙即牢也。御藥院方。

Loose teeth. They ache and they move after being hit. Grind [to powder] five *qian* of unprepared local *ji li* with the [sharp] edges removed, give them into half a bowl with thin fermented water of foxtail millet. Add salt and rinse [the affected teeth with the liquid]. Very effective. Or, burn the root to ashes, and paste them on the teeth to stabilize[768] them. *Yü yao yuan fang.*

牙齒出血不止，動摇。白蒺藜末，旦旦擦之。道藏經。

Unending bleeding of teeth. Loose [teeth]. Rub them with *bai ji li* powder every day. *Dao cang jing.*

打動牙疼。蒺藜子或根爲末，日日揩之。瑞竹堂方。

Loose, painful teeth after being hit. [Grind] *ji li* seeds or roots into powder and rub [the teeth with it] every day. *Rui zhu tang fang.*

鼻塞出水，多年不聞香臭。蒺藜二握，當道車碾過，以水一大盞，煮取半盞。仰卧，先滿口含飯，以汁一合灌鼻中。不過再灌，嚏出一兩箇息肉，似赤蛹蟲，即愈。聖惠方。

Water comes from a stuffy nose, with an inability to smell scent or bad smell. Boil two handfuls of *ji li*, crushed by carts on the road, in one large cup of water down to half a cup. [Let the patient] lie down with his face upward. He is first to fill his mouth with cooked rice and hold it. Then he is force-fed with one *ge* of the juice into his nostrils. If this remains without effect, force-feed [the juice into the nose] again. As a result, he will sneeze out a piece or two of tumorous flesh growth resembling red pupae. This is the cure. *Sheng hui fang.*

面上瘢痕。蒺藜子、山巵子各一合，爲末，醋和，夜塗旦洗。救急方。

Wound scars[769] on the face. [Grind] one *ge* each of *ji li* seeds and *gardenia* fruit into powder, mix it with vinegar and apply it [to the scars] at night. Wash it off the next morning. *Jiu ji fang.*

---

768 The original text does not have the character *lao* 牢 here: 原闕一字。今本御藥院方無此語。今從江西本"牢"補。

769 *Ban hen* 瘢痕, "wound scar," a scar remaining after a wound or sores have healed, leaving the texture of the skin permanently altered. BCGM Dict I, 51.

白癜風疾。白蒺藜子六兩，生擣爲末。每湯服二錢，日二服。一月絶根，服至半月，白處見紅點，神效。孫真人食忌。

White patches wind[770] illness. Pound six *liang* of fresh white *ji li* seeds into powder. Each time ingest with boiled water two *qian*. To be ingested twice a day. Within one month, the root [of the problem] will be severed. If this is ingested for half a month, instead of the white [patches] red spots appear. Divinely effective. *Sun zhenren shi ji.*

一切丁腫。蒺藜子一升，熬擣，以醋和封頭上，拔根。外臺秘要。

All types of pin[-illness][771] swelling. Simmer one sheng of *ji li* seeds and pound them [to a pulp]. Mix it with vinegar and cover [the swelling] on the head. This will pull out the root. *Wai tai mi yao.*

16-61-03
花 *Hua*
Flower [of *ji li*].

【主治】陰乾爲末。每温酒服二三錢，治白癜風。宗奭。

Control. Dry it in the yin (i. e., shade) and [grind it into] powder. Each time ingest with warm wine two or three *qian* to cure white patches wind. [Kou] Zongshi.

16-61-04
苗 *Miao*
Seedling [*of ji li*].

【主治】煮湯，洗疥癬風瘡作癢。時珍。

Control. Boil it to a decoction and use it to wash *jie*-illness,[772] *xuan*-illness,[773] and wind [intrusion] sores with itch. [Li] Shizhen.

---

770 *Bai dian feng* 白癜風, "white patches wind." White skin patches without pain and itching. BCGM Dict I, 46.

771 *Ding* 丁, "pin[-illness]," also *ding* 疔, "pin-illness," refers to a deep-reaching and festering hardness in a tissue, eventually rising above the skin like a pinhead. BCGM Dict I, 127-129.

772 *Jie*-illness 疥, vaguely identifiable skin ailment. BCGM Dict I, 249.

773 *Xuan* 癬, "*xuan*-illness." Conditions of dermal lesions with initially erythema, papules, and itching gradually extending in all directions to form an irregular ring with clear boundaries. The skin is slightly elevated with small papules, blisters, and/or scales and scraps. The central lesion may appear to heal spontaneously, and it may reappear. Also, a designation of local lesions with itching, release of liquid and shedding of scabs. BCGM Dict I, 591.

【附方】舊二，新一。

Added Recipes. Two of old. One newly [recorded].

鼻流清涕。蒺藜苗二握，黄連二兩，水二升，煎一升，少少灌鼻中，取嚏，不過再服。聖惠方。

Clear snivel flowing from the nose. Boil two handfuls of *ji li* seedlings and two *liang* of *coptis* [rhizome] in two *sheng* of water down to one *sheng* and force-feed this in small amounts into the [patient's] nose to stimulate a sneezing. No more than two ingestions required. *Sheng hui fang*.

諸瘡腫毒。蒺藜蔓洗，三寸截之，取得一斗，以水五升，煮取二升，去滓，納銅器中，又煮取一升，納小器中，煮如飴狀，以塗腫處。千金方。

All types of swelling with poison. Wash *ji li* creeper and cut it into pieces of three *cun* length. Boil one *dou* in five *sheng* of water down to two *sheng*. Discard the dregs. Give [the liquid] into a copper vessel. Boil it again, this time down to one *sheng*. Give it into a small vessel and boil it there until it has assumed a consistency of malt sugar. Apply this to the swelling. *Qian jin fang*.

蠼螋尿瘡，遶身匝即死。以蒺藜葉搗傅之。無葉用子。備急方。

Sores caused by earwig urine. When they have formed a perfect circle around [the patient's] body, he will die. Pound *ji li* leaves [to a pulp] and apply it [to the affected region]. If no leaves are at hand, resort to seeds. *Bei ji fang*.

16-62

穀精草宋開寶

Gu jing cao, FE Song, *Kai bao*.

***Eriocaulum buergerianum* Koern. Pipewort.**

【釋名】戴星草開寶、文星草綱目、流星草。【時珍曰】穀田餘氣所生，故曰穀精。【志曰】白花似星，故有戴星諸名。

Explanation of Names. *Dai xing cao* 戴星草, "star bearing herb," Kai bao. *Wen xing cao* 文星草, "star ornate herb," *Gang mu*. *Liu xing cao* 流星草. "star spreading herb." [Li] Shizhen: It grows on grain, *gu* 穀, fields out of a surplus of qi. Hence its name "grain essence [herb]," *gu jing* 穀精. [Ma] Zhi: Its white flowers resemble stars, *xing* 星. Hence all its names including [the character for "star,"] *xing* 星.

【集解】【頌曰】處處有之。春生於穀田中，葉、莖俱青，根、花並白色。二月、三月采花用，花白小圓似星。可餧馬令肥，主蟲顙毛焦病。又有一種，莖梗長有節，根微赤，出秦隴間。【時珍曰】此草收穀後，荒田中生之，江湖南北多有。一科叢生，葉似嫩穀秧。抽細莖，高四五寸。莖頭有小白花，點點如亂星。九月采花，陰乾。云二三月采者，誤也。

Collected Explanations. [Su] Song: It can be found everywhere. In spring it grows in grain fields. The leaves and the stem are greenish. The root and the flowers are white. The flower is collected for [therapeutic] use in the second and third month. The flowers are white, small and round, resembling stars. [The herb] can be used to feed horses and makes them fat. It controls the disease of scorched hair at the forehead caused by worms/bugs. There is another kind with a hard and long stem with nodes, and a slightly red root. It comes from Qin long. [Li] Shizhen: This herb grows in barren fields after the grain was harvested. Much of it can be found in the South and North of Jiang hu. It grows as thickets. The leaves resemble those of tender grain herbs. A fine stem rises upward and reaches a height of four to five *cun*. Small white flowers are situated at the top of the stem. They are dots like disarrayed stars. The flowers are collected in the ninth month; they are dried in the yin (i. e., shade). When it is said that they are collected in the second and third month, this is wrong.

16-62

花。

Flower [of *gu jing cao*].

【氣味】辛，溫，無毒。【藏器曰】甘、平。【大明曰】可結水銀成砂子。

Qi and Flavor. Acrid, warm, nonpoisonous. [Chen] Cangqi: Sweet, balanced. Da Ming: It can serve to crystallize mercury.

【主治】喉痺，齒風痛，諸瘡疥。開寶。頭風痛，目盲翳膜，痘後生翳，止血。時珍。

Control. Throat blockage. Toothache related to wind [intrusion]. All types of sores and *jie*-illness.[774] *Kai bao*. Painful head wind.[775] Eyes blinded by a shade or membrane. Shades forming after smallpox. It ends bleeding. [Li] Shizhen.

【發明】【時珍曰】穀精體輕性浮，能上行陽明分野。凡治目中諸病，加而用之，甚良。明目退翳之功，似在菊花之上也。

Explication. [Li] Shizhen: *Gu jing* [*cao*] has a light weight body and by its nature it floats at the surface. It can rise into the yang brilliance section. Whenever any disease affecting the eyes is cured, [*gu jing cao*] is to be used added [to the medication].

---

774 *Jie*-illness 疥, vaguely identifiable skin ailment. BCGM Dict I, 249.

775 *Tou feng* 頭風, "head wind," a condition of wind evil attacking the head followed by pain, or dizziness, or itching. BCGM Dict I, 509.

It is very good. Its potential of clearing the eyes and pushing back a shade appears to be even better than that of *chrysanthemum* flowers.

【附方】舊一，新七。

Added Recipes. One of old. Seven newly [recorded].

腦痛眉痛。穀精草二錢，地龍三錢，乳香一錢，爲末。每用半錢，燒煙筒中，隨左右熏鼻。聖濟録。

Painful brain; painful eyebrows. [Grind] two *qian* of *gu jing cao*, three *qian* of earthworms and one *qian* of frankincense into powder. Each time use half a *qian*. Burn it to channel the fumes through a tube and lead the steam into the left and right nostrils depending on whether [the pain is on the left or on the right]. *Sheng ji lu.*

偏正頭痛。集驗方用穀精草一兩爲末，以白麪糊調攤紙花上，貼痛處，乾換。

Hemilateral and ordinary headache. The *Ji yan fang* [recommends to grind] one *liang* of *gu jing cao* into powder, mix it with white wheat flour [and water] to make a paste and spread it on a paper flower. Then attach it to the location of the pain. When it has dried, replace it [with a moist paste].

聖濟方用穀精草末、銅緑各一錢，硝石半分，隨左右嗃鼻。

The *Sheng ji fang* [recommends to] mix one *qian* each of *gu jing cao* powder and verdigris and half a *fen* of nitrokalite and, depending on [the location of the pain], blow it into the left or right nostril.

鼻衄不止。穀精草爲末，熟麪湯服二錢。聖惠方。

Unending nosebleed. [Grind] *gu jing cao* into powder and ingest two *qian* with a cooked noodle soup. *Sheng hui fang.*

目中翳膜。穀精草、防風等分，爲末，米飲服之，甚驗。明目方。

Shade membrane in an eye. [Grind] equal amounts of *gu jing cao* and *saposhnikovia* [root] into powder and ingest it with a rice beverage. Very effective. *Ming mu fang.*

痘後目翳，隱澀淚出，久而不退。用穀精草爲末，以柿或猪肝片蘸食。一方，加蛤粉等分，同入豬肝内煮熟，日食之。又方：見“夜明沙”。邵真人濟急方。

A shade in the eyes following smallpox, with roughness and tearflow. It this has lasted for a long time and [the shade] was not pushed back. [Grind] *gu jing cao* into powder. Dip persimmon or pig liver slices into it and eat them. Another recipe:

Add an equal amount of clam shell powder, give this into a pig liver and boil it until done. Eat this every day. Yet another recipe: See the entry on "Asian particolored bat." (48-21). Shao zhenren, *Ji ji fang*.

小兒雀盲。至晚忽不見物。用羯羊肝一具，不用水洗，竹刀剖開，入穀精草一撮，瓦罐煮熟，日食之，屢效。忌鐵器。如不肯食，炙熟，搗作丸綠豆大。每服三十丸，茶下。衛生家寶方。

Sparrow blindness of children.[776] In the evening they suddenly see nothing. Cut one liver of a castrated sheep – do not wash it clean with water - open and insert one handful of *gu jing cao* into it. Boil this in a pottery jar and [let the child] eat it every day. This has often been effective. Avoid the use of iron utensils. If [the child] is unwilling to eat this, roast [the filled liver] until done, pound it and prepare pills the size of mung beans. Each time [let the child] ingest 30 pills, to be sent down with tea. *Wei sheng jia bao fang*.

小兒中暑，吐泄煩渴。穀精草燒存性，用器覆之，放冷爲末。每冷米飲服半錢。保幼大全。

Children struck by summer heat, with vomiting, outflow and a vexing thirst. Burn *gu jing cao* with its nature retained. Cover it with a vessel until it has cooled and [grind it into] powder. Each time [let the child] ingest half a *qian* with a rice beverage. *Bao you da quan*.

16-63
海金沙宋嘉祐
Hai jin sha, FE Song, *Jia you*.

**Lygodium japonicum* (Thunb.) Sw. Climbing fern.*[777]

【釋名】竹園荽。【時珍曰】其色黄如細沙也。謂之海者，神異之也。俗名竹園荽，象葉形也。

Explanation of Names. *Zhu yuan sui* 竹園荽, "bamboo garden coriander." [Li] Shizhen: Its color is as yellow as that of fine sand. To call it ["golden sand of the] sea" is to refer to its divine uniqueness. When it is commonly called *zhu yuan sui*, this is because of the similarity of the shape of its leaves [to that of coriander leaves].

【集解】【禹錫曰】出黔中郡，湖南亦有。生作小株，高一二尺。七月收其全科，於日中暴之，小乾，以紙襯承，以杖擊之，有細沙落紙上，且暴

776 *Que mang* 雀盲, "sparrow blindness," identical to *que mu* 雀目, "sparrow eye." Unimpaired vision during daylight and significantly decreased vision after nightfall. BCGM Dict I, 394.

777 *Hai jin sha* 海金沙, lit.: "golden sand from the sea."

且擊，以盡爲度。【時珍曰】江、浙、湖、湘、川、陜皆有之，生山林下。莖細如線，引于竹木上，高尺許。其葉細如園荽葉而甚薄，背面皆青，上多皺文。皺處有沙子，狀如蒲黄粉，黄赤色。不開花，細根堅强。其沙及草皆可入藥。方士采其草取汁，煮砂、縮賀。

Collected Explanations. [Zhang] Yuxi: It comes from Qian zhong commandery, and can also be found in Hu nan. When it grows it forms a small trunk, one or two *chi* tall. In the seventh month the entire plant is collected and exposed to the bright sun. After it has dried a little, put it on a piece of paper and hit it with a stick. Fine sand will fall on the paper. Alternately dry and hit [the plant] until all [the sand has come out]. [Li] Shizhen: It is present in Jiang, Zhe, Hu, Xiang, Chuan and Shaan. It grows in mountain forests under the trees and stretching upward on bamboo and trees, reaching a height of more than a *chi*. The leaves are fine like the leaves of coriander, and they are very thin. Back side and front are all greenish. On its upper side it has many wrinkled lines. The wrinkled locations include sand, shaped similar to cattail pollen, of a yellow-red color. [*Hai jin sha*] does not open flowers. The fine roots are hard and strong. Both the sand and the herb can be added to medication. The recipe experts collect the herb to get its juice. They use it to boil cinnabar and to shrink tin.

【氣味】甘，寒，無毒。

Qi and Flavor. Sweet, cold, nonpoisonous.

【主治】通利小腸。得巵子、馬牙硝、蓬沙，療傷寒熱狂，或丸，或散。嘉祐。治濕熱腫滿，小便熱淋、膏淋、血淋、石淋莖痛，解熱毒氣。時珍。

Control. It penetrates and frees the passage through the small intestine. Combined with *gardenia* fruit, crystallized sodium sufate and borax, it heals harm caused by cold with [body] heat and madness. It may be prepared to either pills or powders. *Jia you*. It serves to cure swelling and a feeling of fullness related to moisture and heat, hot urinary dripping, creamy urinary dripping, and blood [urinary] dripping with a painful stem (i. e., penis). It resolves heat and poison qi. [Li] Shizhen.

【發明】【時珍曰】海金沙，小腸、膀胱血分藥也。熱在二經血分者宜之。

Explication. [Li] Shizhen: *Hai jin sha* is a pharmaceutical drug for the blood section of the [conduits of the] small intestine and the urinary bladder. It is suitable for heat in the blood section of these two conduits.

【附方】舊一，新五。

Added Recipes. One of old. Five newly [recorded].

熱淋急痛。海金沙草陰乾，爲末，煎生甘草湯調服二錢，此陳總領方也。一加滑水。夷堅志。

Urinary dripping and acute pain. Dry *hai jin sha* in the yin (i.. e., shade) and [grind it into] powder. Boil unprepared *glycyrrhiza* [root] and ingest two *qian* [of the powder] mixed with the decoction. This is a recipe of Overseer-General Chen. In another [recipe] talcum[778] is added. *Yijian zhi.*

小便不通，臍下滿悶。海金沙一兩，臘面茶半兩，擣碎，每服三錢，生薑、甘草煎湯下，日二服。亦可末服。圖經本草。

Blocked urination, with a feeling of fullness below the navel, and heart-pressure. Pound one *liang* of *hai jin sha* and half a *liang* of *la mian* tea[779] to small pieces. Each time ingest two *qian*, to be sent down boiled in a decoction with fresh ginger and *glycyrrhiza* [root]. To be ingested twice a day. It is also possible to ingest the powder. *Tu jing ben cao.*

膏淋如油。海金沙、滑石各一兩，甘草稍二錢半，爲末。每服二錢，麥門冬煎湯服。日二次。仁存方。

Creamy urination, resembling oil. [Grind] one *liang* each of *hai jin sha* and talcum and two and a half *liang* of fine *glycyrrhiza* [roots] into powder. Each time ingest two *qian*, boiled with an *ophiopogon* [tuber] decoction. Ingest this twice a day. *Rencun fang.*

血淋痛澀。但利水道，則清濁自分。海金沙末，新汲水或砂糖水服一錢。普濟方。

Painful, rough urinary dripping with blood. All that is required is to free the passage of the water. As a result the clear and turbid parts will separate. Ingest one *qian* of *hai jin sha* powder with newly drawn water or with a rock sugar water. *Pu ji fang.*

脾濕腫滿，腹脹如鼓，喘不得卧。海金沙散：用海金沙三錢，白术四兩，甘草半兩，黑牽牛頭末一兩半，爲末。每服一錢，煎倒流水調下，得利爲妙。東垣蘭室秘藏。

Swelling and a feeling of fullness related to the presence of moisture in the spleen. The abdomen is bloated like a drum. [Patients] pant and cannot lie down. The "powder with *hai jin sha*." [Grind] three *qian* of *hai jin sha*, four *liang* of *atractylodes*

---

778 In view of the ingredient *hua shi* 滑石, talcum, in the recipe quoted from *Rencun fang* below, the character *shui* 水 may be an erroneous writing here of *shi* 石.

779 *La mian cha* 臘面茶, a tea from Fu jian, famous during the Tang and Song era.

macrocephala [rhizome], half a *liang* of *glycyrrhiza* [root], and one and a half *liang* of *pharbitis* [seeds] into powder. Each time ingest one *qian*, to be sent down boiled with reversely flowing water. A wondrous effect is achieved when a free-flow sets in. *Dongyuan lan shi mi cang*.

痘瘡變黑。歸腎。用竹園荽草煎酒，傅其身，即發起。直指方。

Smallpox sores turning black. [The disease] has found its way to the kidneys. Boil *zhu yuan cai* herbs in wine and apply [the liquid to the patient's] body. As a result, [the smallpox] will effuse [and the papules] emerge. *Zhi zhi fang*.

16-64
地楊梅拾遺
Di yang mei, FE *Shi yi*.

***Luzula capitata* (Miq.) ex Kom. Woodrush.**

【集解】【藏器曰】生江東濕地，苗如莎草，四五月有子，似楊梅也。

Collected Explanations. [Chen] Cangqi: It grows on damp ground in Jiang dong. The seedling is similar to that of *cyperus* herbs. It has seeds in the fourth and fifth month, resembling those of box myrtle.

【氣味】辛，平，無毒。

Qi and Flavor. Acrid, balanced, nonpoisonous.

【主治】赤白痢，取莖、子煎湯服。藏器。

Control. Red and white free-flux illness. Boil the stem and the seeds and ingest the decoction. [Chen] Cangqi.

16-65
水楊梅綱目
Shui yang mei, FE *Gang mu*.

***Adina rubella* Hance. Chinese button bush.**

【釋名】地椒。

Explanation of Names. *Di jiao* 地椒, "ground pepper."

【集解】【時珍曰】生水邊，條葉甚多，生子如楊梅狀。庚辛玉册云：地椒，一名水楊梅，多生近道陰濕處，荒田野中亦有之。叢生，苗葉似菊。莖端開黃花，實類椒而不赤。實可結伏三黃、白礬，制丹砂、粉霜。

Collected Explanations. [Li] Shizhen: It grows at the side of water, with numerous boughs and leaves. It grows seeds resembling the shape of box myrtle [seeds]. The *Geng xin yu ce* states: "*Di jiao* is also named *shui yang mei*. Much of it grows near roads in shady, moist locations. It can also be found in deserted fields in the wild. It grows as thickets; the stem and the leaves resemble chrysanthemums. A yellow flower opens at the top of the stem. The fruits resemble pepper, but they are not red. The fruits can be used to suppress [the effects of] the three [items with the name] *huang* 黄, 'yellow,'[780] and alum. They check [the effects of] cinnabar and calomel."

【氣味】辛，温，無毒。

Qi and Flavor. Acrid, warm, nonpoisonous.

【主治】疔瘡腫毒。時珍。

Control Pin-illness[781] sores with a swelling and poison. [Li] Shizhen

16-66
地蜈蚣草綱目
Di wu gong cao, FE *Gang mu*

***Hedyotis chrysotricha* (Palib) Merr. Golden hair starviolet.**

【集解】【時珍曰】生村落塍野間。左蔓延右，右蔓延左。其葉密而對生，如蜈蚣形，其穗亦長，俗呼過路蜈蚣。其延上樹者，呼飛天蜈蚣。根、苗皆可用。

Collected Explanations. [Li] Shizhen: It grows in villages and on raised paths in the wild. A creeper may spread from the left to the right, or from the right to the left. The leaves are situated close to each other and face each other in pairs. They are shaped like centipedes. They also have long spikes. [The plant is] commony called "centipede crossing the road." Those extending upward into trees are called "centipedes flying into the sky." The root and the stem can be used [for therapeutic purposes].

【氣味】苦，寒，無毒。

Qi and Flavor. Bitter, cold, nonpoisonous.

780 The three [items named "yellow",] *huang* 黄, are sulphur, *liu huang* 硫黄, realgar, *xiong huang* 雄黄, and orpiment, *ci huang* 雌黄.

781 *Ding* 丁, "pin[-illness]," also *ding* 疔, "pin-illness," refers to a deep-reaching and festering hardness in a tissue, eventually rising above the skin like a pinhead. BCGM Dict I, 127-129.

【主治】解諸毒及大便不通，搗汁。瘰癰腫，搗塗，并末服，能消毒排膿。蜈蚣傷者，入鹽少許搗塗，或末傅之。時珍。

Control. It resolves all types of poison and blocked defecation. To heal obstruction-illness[782] swelling, pound it and apply [the resulting powder to the affected region]. In addition, ingest the powder. This can dissolve poison and drive out pus. For harm caused by a centipede, add a little salt, pound it and apply [it to the affected region]. Or rub it with the powder. [Li] Shizhen.

【附方】新一。

Added Recipes. One newly [recorded].

一切癰疽及腸癰奶癰，赤腫未破，或已破而膿血不散，發熱疼痛能食者，並宜排膿托裏散。用地蜈蚣、赤芍藥、當歸、甘草等分，爲末。每服二錢，温酒下。和劑局方。

All types of obstruction-illness and impediment-illness,[783] as well as intestinal obstruction-illness[784] and breast obstruction-illness,[785] with a red swelling that has not broken open yet. Or, when it has broken open already without spreading pus and blood, but with heat effusion and pain, and [patients] are still able to eat. For all these situations it is advisable to apply the "powder to push out pus and support the interior." [Grind] equal amounts of *di wu gong*, red *paeonia* [root], Chinese *angelica* [root] and *glycyrrhiza* [root] into powder. Each time ingest two *qian*, to be sent down with warm wine. *He ji ju fang*.

782 *Yong* 癰, "obstruction-illness,"refers to an obstruction of vessels or other ducts inside the body. Qi rushing against the obstruction may cause a local swelling and eventually break through the surface to cause an abscess. BCGM Dict I, 641.

783 *Ju* 疽, "impediment-illness," refers to an obstruction of vessels or other ducts inside the body. Qi rushing against the impediment may cause a local swelling and eventually break through the surface to cause an abscess. BCGM Dict I, 277.

784 *Chang yong* 腸癰, "intestinal obstruction-illness," a *yong* 癰, "obstruction-illness," developing in the abdominal cavity at the site of the intestines. In general, this is accompanied by fever and spastic pain on the right side of the lower abdomen, where a lump can be felt. BCGM Dict I, 80.

785 *Ru yong* 乳癰, "breast obstruction-illness," a condition of acute putrefication of a woman's breast. Often encountered if a woman, following delivery, experiences *chui nai* 吹奶, "inflated breast," or *du ru* 妒乳, "jealousy breast." BCGM Dict I, 412.

16-67
半邊蓮綱目
Ban bian lian, FE *Gang mu.*

***Lobelia chinensis* Lour. Lobelia.**[786]

【集解】【時珍曰】半邊蓮，小草也。生陰濕塍塹邊。就地細梗引蔓，節節而生細葉。秋開小花，淡紅紫色，止有半邊，如蓮花狀，故名。又呼急解索。

Collected Explanations. [Li] Shizhen: *Ban bian lian* is a small herb. It grows in shady, damp places to the side of raised paths and ditches. Fine, slender stalks creep along the ground, with fine flowers growing from their nodes. Small flowers open in autumn; they are of a pale red-purple color. They have [petals on] one half side only, shaped similar to lotus flowers. Hence the name. It is also called "[the herb that] quickly unties ropes."

【氣味】辛，平，無毒。

Qi and Flavor. Acrid, balanced, nonpoisonous.

【主治】蛇虺傷，搗汁飲，以滓圍塗之。又治寒齁氣喘及瘧疾寒熱，同雄黃各二錢，搗泥，盌内覆之，待色青，以飯丸梧子大。每服九丸，空心鹽湯下。時珍。壽域方。

Control. Harm caused by snakes and roundworms.[787] Pound it and drink the juice. Apply the dregs around [the affected region]. Also, to cure snoring and panting related to cold, as well as alternating sensations of cold and heat related to malaria, pound two *qian* each of [*ban bian lian* and] realgar to a mud and leave it covered in a jar until it has assumed a greenish color. With cooked rice form pills the size of *wu* seeds and each time ingest nine pills, to be sent down on an empty stomach with a salt decoction. [Li] Shizhen [quoted from the] *Shou yu fang*.

16-68
紫花地丁綱目
Zi hua di ding, FE *Gang mu.*

***Viola philipica* Cav. Purpleflower violet.**[788]

【釋名】箭頭草綱目、獨行虎綱目、羊角子秘韞、米布袋。

786 *Ban bian lian* 半邊蓮, lit.: "half-sided lotus flower."

787 *Hui* 虺, "roundworm," may be an erroneous writing of *hui* 虺, "venomous viper."

788 *Zi hua di ding* 紫花地丁, lit.: "purple flower ground pin."

Explanation of Names. *Jian tou cao* 箭頭草, "arrowhead herb," *Gang mu. Du xing hu* 獨行虎, "lonely moving tiger," *Gang mu. Yang jiao zi* 羊角子, "sheep horn," *Mi yun. Mi bu dai* 米布袋, "cloth bag of rice."

【集解】【時珍曰】處處有之。其葉似柳而微細，夏開紫花結角。平地生者起莖，溝壑邊生者起蔓。普濟方云：鄉村籬落生者，夏秋開小白花，如鈴兒倒垂，葉微似木香花之葉。此與紫花者相戾，恐別一種也。

Collected Explanations. [Li] Shizhen: It can be found everywhere. The leaves resemble willow [leaves], but are finer. In summer it opens purple flowers that form horn[-shaped pods]. Those growing on flat ground have a stem rising upward. Those growing on the side of ditches, they extend as creepers. The *Pu ji fang* states: "Those growing in rural regions descending from fences, they open small, white flowers in summer and autumn, hanging upside down similar to bells. The leaves are small and resemble the leaves of costus flowers." It differs from the one with purple flowers discussed here. It may be another kind.

【氣味】苦、辛，寒，無毒。

Qi and Flavor. Bitter, acrid, cold, nonpoisonous.

【主治】一切癰疽發背，疔腫瘰癧，無名腫毒惡瘡。時珍。

Control. All types of obstruction-illness and impediment-illness[789] effusing on the back. Pin-illness[790] swelling. Scrofula pervasion-illness.[791] Nameless swelling with poison. Malign sores. [Li] Shizhen.

【附方】新八。

Added Recipes. Eight newly [recorded].

黃疸內熱。地丁末，酒服三錢。乾坤秘韞。

Yellow *dan*-illness/jaundice. Ingest with wine two *qian* of [*zi hua*] *di ding* powder. *Qian kun mi yun.*

789 *Yong ju* 癰疽, "obstruction-illness, impediment-illness." refers to two vaguely distinguished obstructions/impediments of vessels or other ducts inside the body. Qi rushing against the obstruction may cause a local swelling and eventually break through the surface to cause an abscess. BCGM Dict I, 642.

790 *Ding* 丁, "pin[-illness]," also *ding* 疔, "pin-illness," refers to a deep-reaching and festering hardness in a tissue, eventually rising above the skin like a pinhead. BCGM Dict I, 127-129.

791 *Luo li* 瘰癧, "scrofula pervasion-illness," when two or more connected swellings of the size of plum or date kernels appear either on the neck or in the armpits, or somewhere else on the body. BCGM Dict I. 329.

稻芒粘咽不得出者。箭頭草嚼嚥下。同上方。

A rice awn is stuck in the throat and does not come out. Chew *jian tou cao* and swallow [the resulting liquid]. Source of this recipe identical to the one above.

癰疽惡瘡。紫花地丁連根，同蒼耳葉等分，搗爛，酒一鍾，攪汁服。楊誠經驗方。

Malign sores related to obstruction-illness and impediment-illness.[792] Pound equal amounts of *zi hua di ding* with its root and cocklebur leaves into a pulpy substance, stir it in one *zhong* of wine and ingest the juice. Yang Cheng, *Jing yan fang*.

癰疽發背，無名諸腫，貼之如神。紫花地丁草，三伏時收，以白麪和成，鹽、醋浸一夜，貼之。昔有一尼發背，夢得此方。數日而痊。孫天仁集效方。

Attached to obstruction-illness and impediment-illness effusing on the back, and all types of nameless swelling, the effect is divine. Collect *zi hua di ding* herbs during the three ten day periods of the hottest season in a year, mix them with white wheat flour and soak this in salted vinegar for one night. Then attach it [to the affected region]. Formerly, there was a nun with an effusion on her back. She dreamed of this recipe, and was cured after several days. Sun Tianren, *Ji xiao fang*.

一切惡瘡。紫花地丁根，日乾，以罐盛，燒烟對瘡熏之，出黄水，取盡愈。衛生易簡方。

All types of malign sores. Dry *zi hua di ding* roots in the sun. Fill them into a jar. Heat it and direct the fumes at the sores. They will release a yellow water. A cure is achieved when all [the water] has left. *Wei sheng yi jian fang*.

瘰癧丁瘡，發背諸腫。紫花地丁根去粗皮，同白蒺藜爲末，油和塗神效。乾坤秘韞。

Scrofula pervasion-illness[793] and pin[-illness][794] sores, effusing on the back, and all types of swelling. Discard the rough skin of *zi hua di ding* roots and [grind them]

792 *Yong ju* 癰疽, "obstruction-illness, impediment-illness." refers to two vaguely distinguished obstructions/impediments of vessels or other ducts inside the body. Qi rushing against the obstruction may cause a local swelling and eventually break through the surface to cause an abscess. BCGM Dict I, 642.

793 *Luo li* 瘰癧, "scrofula pervasion-illness," when two or more connected swellings of the size of plum or date kernels appear either on the neck or in the armpits, or somewhere else on the body. BCGM Dict I. 329.

794 *Ding* 丁, "pin[-illness]," also *ding* 疔, "pin-illness," refers to a deep-reaching and festering hardness in a tissue, eventually rising above the skin like a pinhead. BCGM Dict I, 127-129.

together with white calthrop into powder. Mix it with oil and apply it [to the affected region]. Divinely effects. *Qian kun mi yun.*

丁瘡腫毒。永類方用紫花地丁草擣汁服，危極者亦效。
Pin[-illness] sores with swelling and poison. The *Yong lei fang* [recommends to] pound *zi hua di ding* herbs and ingest the juice. This is effective even in extremely critical situations.

楊氏方用紫花地丁草、葱頭、生蜜共擣貼之。若瘤瘡，加新黑牛屎。
The *Yang shi fang* [recommends to] pound *zi hua di ding* herbs and onion stalks with fresh honey and apply this [to the affected region]. In the acase of tumor sores, add fresh dung of black oxen.

喉痺腫痛。箭頭草葉，入醬少許，研膏，點入取吐。普濟方。
Painful swelling related to throat closure. Add a little prepared starch to the leaves of *jian tou* herbs and grind this to a paste. Drop it into [the patient's throat] to stimulate a vomiting. *Pu ji fang.*

16-69
鬼針草拾遺
Gui zhen cao, FE *Shi yi.*

***Bidens pilosa* L. Beggar tick.**[795]

【集解】【藏器曰】生池畔，方莖，葉有椏，子作釵脚，著人衣如針。北人謂之鬼針，南人謂之鬼釵。
Collected Explanations. [Chen] Cangqi: It grows on the brink of ponds. It has a square stem; the leaves are forked. The seeds are formed like the base of a hairpin. They stick to one's garments like needles. People in the North call it "demon's needle." The southerners call it "demon's hairpin."

【氣味】苦，平。無毒。
Qi and Flavor. Bitter, balanced, nonpoisonous.

【主治】蜘蛛、蛇咬，杵汁服，併傅。藏器。塗蠍蠆傷。時珍。
Control. For spider and snake bites, pound it and ingest the juice. In addition apply it [to the affected region]. [Chen] Canqi. Apply it to harm caused by scorpions. [Li] Shizhen.

795 *Gui zhen cao* 鬼針草, lit.: "demon's needle herb."

【附方】新一。

Added Recipes. One newly [recorded].

割甲傷肉不愈。鬼針草苗、鼠粘子根擣汁，和臘猪脂塗。千金。

Damaged nail and harmed flesh that have not been cured. Pound the seedlings of *gui zhen cao* and the root of great burdock to obtain a juice. Mix it with lard from the winter months and apply this [to the affected region]. *Qian jin.*

16-70
獨用將軍唐本草
Du yong jiang jun, FE *Tang ben cao.*

***Triosteum sinuatum* Maxim.**[796]

【集解】【恭曰】生林野中，節節穿葉心生苗，其葉似楠，無時采根、葉用。

Collected Explanations. [Su] Gong: It grows in forests in the wild. All the nodes have leaves and from their center a seedling grows. The leaves resemble those of nanmu trees. The roots and the leaves are collected any time for [therapeutic] use.

【氣味】辛，無毒。

Qi and Flavor. Acrid, nonpoisonous.

【主治】毒腫乳癰，解毒，破惡血。恭。

Control. Breast obstruction-illness[797] with poison swelling. It resolves poison and breaks through malign blood [accumulations]. [Su] Gong.

【附方】新一。

Added Recipes. One newly [recorded].

下痢噤口。獨將軍草根，有珠如豆者，取珠擣汁三匙，以白酒半杯和服。簡便方。

Discharge with free-flux illness and lockjaw. Select *du jiang jun* herb roots with [nodular] "pearls" similar to beans. Pound only these "pearls" to obtain three spoons of juice. Mix it with half a cup of white wine and ingest this. *Jian bian fang.*

---

796 *Du yong jiang yun* 獨用將軍, lit.: "individually employed general."

797 *Ru yong* 乳癰, "breast obstruction-illness," a condition of acute putrefication of a woman's breast. Often encountered if a woman, following delivery, experiences *chui nai* 吹奶, "inflated breast," or *du ru* 妒乳, "jealousy breast." BCGM Dict I, 412.

【附錄】
Appendix

16-70-A01
留軍待 ***Liu jun dai***
Unidentified.

【恭曰】生劍州山谷，葉似楠而細長。采無時。味辛，温，無毒。主肢節風痛，折傷瘀血，五緩攣痛。

[Su] Gong. It grows in mountain valleys of Jian zhou. The leaves resemble those of nanmu trees but are fine and lengthy. It is collected any time. Flavor acrid, warm, nonpoisonous. It serves to cure painful wind [intrusion] into the limbs and their joints, fracture harm and stagnating blood, the five types of slackening, and painful contractions.

16-71
見腫消宋圖經
Jian zhong xiao, FE Song, *Tu jing*.

Gynura segetum **(Lour.) Merr.**

【集解】【頌曰】生筠州。春生苗葉，莖紫色，高一二尺，葉似桑而光，面青紫赤色，采無時。

Collected Explanations. [Su] Song: It grows in Yun zhou. A seedling and leaves grow in spring. The stem is of purple color and one or two *chi* tall. The leaves resemble those of mulberry trees, but are shiny. They are greenish-purple-red on their upper side. [The herb] is collected at all times.

【氣味】酸，澀，有微毒。

Qi and Flavor. Sour, astringent, slightly poisonous.

【主治】消癰疽腫及狗咬，擣葉貼之。頌。

Control. It dissolves obstruction-illness and impediment-illness[798] swelling, and [serves to cure] dog bites. Pound the leaves and apply them [to the affected region]. [Su] Song.

798 *Yong ju* 癰疽, "obstruction-illness, impediment-illness." refers to two vaguely distinguished obstructions/impediments of vessels or other ducts inside the body. Qi rushing against the obstruction may cause a local swelling and eventually break through the surface to cause an abscess. BCGM Dict I, 642.

【附方】新一。

Added Recipes. One newly [recorded].

一切腫毒，及傷寒遺毒，發于耳之前後，及項下腫硬。用見腫消草、生白及、生白斂、土大黄、生大薊根、野苧麻根擣成餅，入芒消一錢，和貼留頭，乾即易之。若加金線重樓及山慈姑尤妙。傷寒蘊要。

All types of swelling with poison, as well as remaining poison from harm caused by cold, effusing in front of or behind the ears, and also a hardened swelling below the nape. Pound *jian zhong xiao* herbs, fresh common *bletilla* [root], fresh *ampelopsis* [root], garden sorrel herb, fresh cat thistle root and ramie plant root and form a cake. Add one *qian* of mirabilite, mix this and apply it to the tip of the remaining [poison swelling]. When it has dried, replace it [with a moist cake]. If *paris polyphylla* and edible tulip are added, [the effects are] especially wondrous. *Shang han yun yao.*

16-72
攀倒甑圖經
Pan dao zeng, FE *Tu jing.*

Unidentified.

【集解】【頌曰】生宜州郊野，莖葉如薄荷。一名班杖，一名接骨。【時珍曰】斑杖名同虎杖，接骨名同蒴藋，不知是一類否。

Collected Explanations. [Su] Song: It grows in the wild of Yi zhou. The stem and the leaves are similar to those of mint. Other names are *ban zhang* 班杖[799] and *jie gu* 接骨.[800]

【氣味】苦，寒，無毒。

Qi and Flavor. Bitter, cold, nonpoisonous.

【主治】解利風熱，煩渴狂躁，擣汁服，甚效。頌。

Control. To resolve and free the flow of wind [intrusion] with heat, vexing thirst, madness and restlessness, pound it and ingest the juice. Very effective. [Su] Song.

799 *Zheng lei* ch. 30 *pan dao zeng* 攀倒甑, writes *ban zhang si* 班杖絲.

800 *Zheng lei* ch. 30 *pan dao zeng* 攀倒甑, writes *ban gu cao* 斑骨草.

16-73
水甘草圖經

Shui gan cao, FE *Tu jing.*

***Amsonia sinensis* Tsiang et P.T.Li.**

【集解】【頌曰】生筠州，多在水旁。春生苗，莖青，葉如柳，無花。土人七月、八月采。單用，不入衆藥。

Collected Explanations. [Su] Song: It grows in Yun zhou, often at the side of waters. In spring it grows a seedling. The stem is greenish. The leaves resemble those of willows. [The plant] has no flower. The locals collect it in the seventh and eighth month. They use it as a single substance and do not add it to other pharmaceutical drugs.

【氣味】甘，寒，無毒。

Qi and Flavor. Sweet, cold, nonpoisonous.

【主治】小兒風熱丹毒，同甘草煎飲。頌。

Control. Cinnabar poisoning[801] of children associated with wind [intrusion] and heat. Boil it together with *glycyrrhiza* [root] and [let the child] drink this. [Su] Song.

---

801 *Dan du* 丹毒, "cinnabar poisoning," a condition of skin ailments brought forth by heat poison, manifesting themselves as red rashes as if from burns, as if cinnabar had been pasted there.BCGM Dict I, 118.

本草綱目
Ben cao gang mu
草部目録
Section Herbs, Contents
第十七卷
Chapter 17

草之六
Herbs VI
毒草類四十七種
Poisonous Herbs Group, 47 kinds

17-01 *Da huang* 大黄, rhubarb. FE *Ben jing* 本經
17-02 *Shang lu* 商陸, Indian pokeweed. FE *Ben jing* 本經
17-03 *Lang du* 狼毒, wolfsbane. FE *Ben jing* 本經
17-04 *Fang kui* 防葵, *peucedanum japonicum*. FE *Ben jing* 本經
17-05 *Lang ya* 狼牙, hairy agrimony. FE *Ben jing* 本經
17-06 *Lü ru* 藺茹, spurge. FE *Ben jing* 本經
17-07 *Da ji* 大戟, Peking purge. FE *Ben jing* 本經
17-08 *Ze qi* 澤漆, wartweed. FE *Ben jing* 本經
17-09 *Gan sui* 甘遂, Kansui. FE *Ben jing* 本經
17-10 *Xu sui zi* 續隨子, caper spurge. FE *Kai bao* 開寶
17-11 *Lang dang* 莨菪, henbane. FE *Ben jing* 本經, i. e., *tian xian zi* 天仙子
17-12 *Yun shi* 雲實, Mysore thorn. FE *Ben jing* 本經
17-13 *Bi ma* 蓖麻, castor oil plant. FE *Tang ben* 唐本
17-13-A01 *Bo luo hui* 博落迴, unidentified.
17-14 *Chang shan* 常山, *shu qi* 蜀漆, Chinese quinine. FE *Ben jing* 本經
17-14-A01 *Du jing shan* 杜莖山, Japanese maesa
17-14-A02 *Tu hong shan* 土紅山, unidentified
17-15 *Li lu* 藜蘆, false hellebore. FE *Ben jing* 本經

17-15-A01 *Shan ci shi* 山慈石, edible tulip
17-15-A02 *Shen guo gen* 參杲[802]根, unidentified
17-15-A03 *Ma chang gen* 馬腸根, unidentified

17-16 *Mu li lu* 木藜蘆, *leucothoe grayana*. FE *Shi yi* 拾遺

17-17 *Fu zi* 附子, *aconitum* [accessory tuber]. FE *Ben jing* 本經

17-18 *Tian xiong* 天雄, Carmichael's monkshood. FE *Ben jing* 本經

17-19 *Ce zi* 側子, *aconitum* [marginal "child" tuber]. FE *Bie lu* 別録

17-20 *Lou lan zi* 漏藍[803]子, *aconitum* [tuber as small as "seeds leaking from a basket."] FE *Gang mu* 綱目

17-21 *Wu tou* 烏頭, *aconitum* [main tuber]. FE *Ben jing* 本經

17-22 *Bai fu zi* 白附子, *aconitum coreanum* Lèvl. FE *Bie lu* 別録

17-23 *Hu zhang, tian nan xing* 虎掌天南星, Indian turnip. FE *Ben jing* 本經

17-24 *You ba* 由跋, small root of Indian turnip. FE *Ben jing* 本經

17-25 *Ju ruo* 蒟蒻, devil's tongue. FE *Kai bao* 開寶
17-25-A01 *Pu sa cao* 菩薩草, Bodhisattva herb

17-26 *Ban xia* 半夏, *pinellia ternata*. FE *Ben jing* 本經

17-27 *Zao xiu* 蚤休, love apple. FE *Ben jing* 本經

17-28 *Gui jiu* 鬼臼, umbrella leaf. FE *Ben jing* 本經

17-29 *She gan* 射干, blackberry lily. FE *Ben jing* 本經

17-30 *Yuan wei* 鳶尾, kite's tail iris. FE *Ben jing* 本經

17-31 *Yu zan* 玉簪, assumption lily. FE *Gang mu* 綱目

17-32 *Feng xian* 鳳仙, touch-me-not. FE *Gang mu* 綱目

17-33 *Zuo na cao* 坐拏草, unidentified. FE *Tu jing* 圖經
17-33-A01 押不蘆, *yabulu*

17-34 *Mantuoluo hua* 曼陀羅花, downy thorn apple. FE *Gang mu* 綱目

17-35 *Yang zhi zhu* 羊躑躅, azalea. FE *Ben jing* 本經
17-35-A01 *Shan zhi zhu* 山躑躅, Chinese azalea
17-35-A02 *Yang bu chi cao* 羊不喫草, unidentified

17-36 *Yuan hua* 芫花, daphne flower. FE *Ben jing* 本經

17-37 *Rao hua* 蕘花, *wikstroemia canescens*. FE *Ben jing* 本經

17-38 *Cui yu cao* 醉魚草, Dr. Lindley's *buddleya*. FE *Gang mu* 綱目

17-39 *Mang cao* 莽草, *illiceum lanceolatum*, FE *Ben jing* 本經

17-40 *Yin yu* 茵蕷[804], *skimmia reevesiana*. FE *Ben jing* 本經

802 Entry 17-15-A02 gives the name *shen guo gen* 參果根.

803 Entry 17-20 gives the name *lou lan zi* 漏籃子.

804 Entry 17-40 gives as name *yin yu* 茵芋, identical to the reference to *yin yu* 茵芋 in *Zheng lei* ch. 10.

17-41 *Shi long rui* 石龍芮, cursed crow foot. FE *Ben jing* 本經, i. e., *hu jiao cai* 胡椒菜

17-42 *Ma gen* 毛茛, Japanese buttercup. FE *Shi yi* 拾遺

17-42-A01 *Hai jiang* 每薑,[805] unidentified

17-43 *Niu bian* 牛扁, *aconitum barbatum* Pers. var. *puberulum*. FE *Ben jing* 本經

17-43-A01 虱建草, unidentified

17-44 *Xun ma* 蕁麻, nettle. FE *Tu jing* 圖經

17-45 *Ge zhu cao* 格注草, unidentified. FE *Tang ben* 唐本

17-46 *Hai yu* 海芋, *alocasia macrorhiza*. FE *Gang mu* 綱目

17-46-A01 *Tou shan gen* 透山根, unidentified

17-47 *Gou wen* 鉤吻, *Gelsemium elegans*. FE *Ben jing* 本經

右附方舊一百三十四，新四百九十五。

Recipes added to the entries above:

134 of old. 495 newly [recorded].

805 Following entry 17-42-A01 *mei jiang* 每薑, the text includes a second appendix: 17-42-A02 *yin ming* 陰命.

本草綱目
Ben cao gang mu
草部第十七卷
Section Herbs, Chaper 17
草之六
Herbs VI
毒草類四十七種
Poisonous Herbs Group, 47 kinds

17-01
大黃本經下品
Da huang, FE *Ben jing*, lower rank.

***Rheum palmatum* L. Rhubarb.**

【釋名】黄良本經、將軍當之、火参吴普、膚如吴普。【弘景曰】大黄，其色也。將軍之號，當取其駿快也。【杲曰】推陳致新，如戡定禍亂，以致太平，所以有將軍之號。

Explanation of Names. *Huang liang* 黄良, "the yellow best," *Ben jing*. *Jiang jun* 將軍, "general," [Li] Dangzhi. *Huo shen* 火参, Wu Pu. *Fu ru* 膚如, Wu Pu. [Tao] Hongjing: [It is named] *da huang* 大黄 because of its [yellow] color. The designation *jiang jun* 將軍, "general," refers to its rapid effects. [Li] Gao: It pushes out what is old and lets arrive what is new. This is like suppressing a revolt and establishing peace. Hence the designation "general," *jiang jun* 將軍.

【集解】【别録曰】大黄生河西山谷及隴西。二月、八月采根，火乾。【普曰】生蜀郡北部或隴西。二月卷生黄赤，其葉四四相當，莖高三尺許。三月花黄，五月實黑，八月采根。根有黄汁，切片陰乾。【弘景曰】今采益州北部汶山及西山者，雖非河西、隴西，好者猶作紫地錦色，味甚苦澀，色至濃黑。西川陰乾者勝。北部日乾，亦有火乾者，皮小焦不如，而耐蛀堪久。此藥至勁利，粗者便不中服。【恭曰】葉、子、莖並似羊蹄，但莖高六七尺而脆，味酸，堪生啖。葉粗長而厚。根細者亦似宿羊蹄，大者乃如盌，長二尺。其性濕潤而易蛀壞，火乾乃佳。作時燒石使熱，横寸截，著石上煿之，一日微燥，以繩穿[日良]乾。今出宕州、凉州、西羌、蜀地者皆佳。幽、并以北者漸細，氣力不及蜀中者。陶言蜀地不及隴西，誤矣。【藏器曰】凡用當分別之。若取和厚深沈能攻病者，可用蜀中似牛舌片緊硬者；苦取瀉洩駿快、推陳去熱者，當取河西錦文者。【頌曰】今蜀川、河東、陝西州郡皆有之。以蜀川錦文者佳。其次秦隴來者，謂之土番大黄。正月内生青葉，似蓖麻，大者如扇。根如芋，大者如盌，長一二尺。其細根如牛蒡，小者亦如芋。四月開黄花，亦有青紅似蕎麥花者。莖青紫色，形如竹。二、八月采根，去黑皮，切作横片，火乾。蜀大黄乃作緊片如牛舌形，謂之牛舌大黄。二者功用相等。江淮出者曰土大黄，二月開花，結細實。【時珍曰】宋祁益州方物圖言蜀大山中多有之，赤莖大葉，根巨若盌，藥市以大者爲枕，紫地錦文也。今人以莊浪出者爲最。莊浪即古涇，原隴西地，與別録相合。

Collected Explanations. *Bie lu*: *Da huang* grows in the mountain valleys of He xi and in Long xi. The root is collected in the second and eighth month; it is dried over fire. [Wu] Pu: It grows in the northern region of Shu jun and in Long xi. It grows curled [leaves of] yellow-red color in the second month. Always four leaves grow facing each other. The stem rises to a height of more than three *chi*. Yellow flowers [open] in the third month. Black fruits [form] in the fifth month. The root is collected in the eighth month. The root has a yellow juice. It is cut to slices and dried in the yin (i. e., shade). [Tao] Hongjing: Those collected these days on Mount Wen shan and Mount Xi shan in the northern section of Yi zhou, even though they are not as good as those from He xi and Long xi, they nevertheless have a brocade surface quality on a purple background. Their flavor is very bitter and astringent and the color reaches a very deep black. Those are superior that come from Xi chuan and are dried in the yin (i. e., shade). In the North, they are dried in the sun, but there are also those that are dried over a fire. When the skin is slightly scorched this is best as it protects them from moth infestation for a long time. This is a most effective and useful pharmaceutical drug. Coarse specimens should not be ingested. [Su] Gong: The leaves, the seeds and the stem all alike resemble those of Japanese dock. However, the stem is six to seven *chi* tall and brittle. It has a sour flavor and can be eaten raw. The leaves are coarse, long and thick. Those with a fine root, they, too, resemble Japanese dock.[806] Big specimens are similar to a bowl, with a length of two *chi*. By their nature they are moist and easily destroyed by moth infestation. If dried over fire, this is excellent. For their preparation, heat a stone to let it turn warm. Cut [*da huang*] into one *cun* long pieces and place them on the stone to bake them. Within one day they are almost dry. Thread them on a rope and hang them up to dry in the shade. Today, those coming from Dang zhou, Liang zhou, Xi qiang and the Shu region are all excellent. Those from You, Bing and the North are

806 Alternative name of *yang ti* 羊蹄, Japanese dock: *dong fang xiu* 東方宿. Hence the reference here to *xiu yang ti* 宿羊蹄.

somewhat finer and the strength of their qi does not reach that of specimens from Shu. When Tao [Hongjing] says that "specimens from the Shu region do not come close to those from Long xi," he is wrong. [Chen] Cangqi: Whenever one intends to resort to [*da huang*], it is essential to distinguish [between different kinds]. If one chooses thick specimens with a deep color that can attack a disease, it is advisable to resort to hard specimens from Shu zhong with slices resembling an ox tongue. If one choses those rapidly causing an outflow, that push out the old and dispel heat, it is advisable to resort to those from He xi with a brocade design. [Su] Song: Today [*da huang*] can be found in all the zhou and prefectures of Shu chuan, He dong and Shaan xi. Those from Shu chuan with a brocade design are excellent. Second in quality are those coming from Qin and Long. They are called *Tu fan da huang* 土番大黃, "Turfan *da huang*." They grow greenish leaves in the first month, resembling those of castor [bean] plants. Big [leaves] are similar to fans. The root is similar to taro roots; it may be as big as a bowl, with a length of one or two *chi*. Their fine roots are similar to those of great burdock; small ones also resemble taro [roots]. [*Da huang*] opens yellow flowers in the fourth month. There are some with greenish-red flowers resembling those of buckwheat. The stem is greenish-purple. It is shaped like bamboo. The root is collected in the second and eighth month. The black skin is discarded; then they are cut into transverse slices that are dried over fire. *Da huang* from Shu is cut into hard slices shaped like an ox tongue. They are called "ox tongue *da huang*." [Therapeutic] potential and usage of both kinds are equal. Those coming from the Jiang Huai region are called *tu da huang* 土大黃, "local *da huang*." In the second month flowers open forming fine fruit. [Li] Shizhen: Song Qi in his *Yi zhou fang wu tu* says that "much [*da huang*] can be found in the big mountains of Shu. It has a red stem and big leaves. The root is huge, like a bowl. On markets of pharmaceutical drugs they offer the big ones as pillows. They have brocade line design on a purple background. Today, people consider those coming from Zhuang lang as best." Zhuang lang is the ancient Jing, a region originally in Long xi. This is in agreement with the report in the *Bie lu*.

【正誤】【頌曰】鼎州出一種羊蹄大黄，治疥瘙甚效。初生苗葉如羊蹄，累年長大，即葉似商陸而狹尖。四月内抽條出穗，五七莖相合，花葉同色。結實如蕎麥而輕小，五月熟即黄色，呼爲金蕎麥。三月采苗，五月采實，陰乾。九月采根，破之亦有錦文。亦呼爲土大黄。【時珍曰】蘇説即老羊蹄根也。因其似大黄，故謂之羊蹄大黄，實非一類。又一種酸模，乃山大黄也。狀似羊蹄而生山上，所謂土大黄或指此，非羊蹄也。倶見本條。

Correction of Errors. [Su] Son: From Ding zhou comes a kind of *yang ti da huang*, "sheep hoof/Japanese dock *da huang*." It serves to very effectively cure *jie*-illness[807] with itch. When it just begins to grow, seedling and leaves are similar to those of Japanes dock (Chinese name: *yang ti* 羊蹄, "sheep hoof"). Over the years it grows longer and bigger and its leaves are similar to those of Indian pokewee [herbs], but they are narrow and pointed. In the fourth month, from its interior a bough rises and releases spikes. Five to seven stems are linked to each other. Flowers and leaves are of the same color. They form fruits like those of buckwheat, but they are light and small. When they are ripe in the fifth month, they assume a yellow color. They are called "golden buckwheat." The seedling is collected in the third month. The fruits are collected in the fifth month; they are dried in the yin (i. e., shade). The root is collected in the ninth month. When it is broken open, [inside] it, too, has a brocade design. It, too, is called *tu di huang* 土大黄, "local *di huang*." [Li] Shizhen: What Su [Song] describes is the root of old *yang ti* 羊蹄, Japanese dock. Because it resembles *da huang*, it is called *yang ti da huang*. But, in fact, they are not related. Then there is a kind of *suan mo* 酸模. This is *shan da huang* 山大黄, "mountain *da huang*." Its shape resembles that of *yang ti* 羊蹄, Japanese dock, but it grows on mountains. Maybe, when *tu da huang* 土大黄 is spoken of, this [mountain *da huang*] is meant. It is not *yang ti* 羊蹄, Japanese dock. For both, see their respective entries.

17-01-01
根 *Gen*

Root [of *da huang*].

【修治】【雷曰】凡使細切。以文如水旋斑緊重者，剉片蒸之，從巳至未，晒乾，又洒臘水蒸之，從未至亥，如此凡七次。晒乾，却洒淡蜜水再蒸一伏時，其大黄必如烏膏樣，乃晒乾用。【藏器曰】凡用有蒸、有生、有熟，不得一概用之。【承曰】大黄采時，皆以火石煿乾貨賣，更無生者，用之亦不須更多炮炙蒸煮。

Pharmaceutical Preparation. [Lei] Xiao: For all applications, cut [the root] into fine pieces. Cut specimens with a line design like whirling water, that are firm and heavy, into slices and steam them from *si* hours (9 – 11) to *wei* hours (13 – 15). Then dry them in the sun. Spray water collected in the 12th months over them and steam them again, from *wei* hours (13 – 15) to *hai* hours (21 – 23). Do this seven times. Dry [the slices] in the sun. Then spray bland honey water over them and steam them for one full day. The *da huang* [roots] must have acquired a consistency of a black paste by now. Dry it in the sun, and then it can be used [for therapeutic purposes]. [Chen]

807 *Jie*-illness 疥, vaguely identifiable skin ailment. BCGM Dict I, 249.

Cangqi: For all usages, the [root] may be steamed, may be left unprepared, or may be prepared with heat. It must not be used in one identical [manner of preparation for different therapeutic ends]. [Chen] Cheng: When *da huang* [root] is collected, it is baked dry on stones heated over a fire and then sold as a commodity. Unprepared ware is no longer offered. When [the roots] are used [for therapeutic purposes] there is no need to roast and steam them again.

【氣味】苦，寒。無毒。【別録曰】大寒。【普曰】神農、雷公：苦，有毒。扁鵲：苦，無毒。李當之：大寒。【元素曰】味苦氣寒，氣味俱厚。沉而降，陰也。用之須酒浸煨熟者，寒因熱用。酒浸入太陽經，酒洗入陽明經，餘經不用酒。【杲曰】大黄苦峻下走，用之于下必生用。若邪氣在上，非酒不至，必用酒浸引上至高之分，驅熱而下。如物在高巔，必射以取之也。若用生者，則遺至高之邪熱，是以愈後或目赤，或喉痺，或頭腫，或膈上熱疾生也。【時珍曰】凡病在氣分，及胃寒血虛，並妊娠産後，並勿輕用。其性苦寒，能傷元氣、耗陰血故也。【之才曰】黄芩爲之使，無所畏。【權曰】忌冷水，惡乾漆。

Qi and Flavor. Bitter, cold, nonpoisonous. *Bie lu*: Very cold. [Wu] Pu: Shen nong, Lei gong: Bitter, poisonous. Bian Que: Bitter, nonpoisonous. Li Dangzhi: Very cold.[808] [Zhang] Yuansu: Flavor bitter, qi cold. Qi and flavor are all strongly pronounced. It sinks and falls. It is a yin [substance]. For [therapeutic] applications it must be soaked in wine and simmered until done. Its cold is used prepared with heat. Soaked in wine it enters the major yang conduits. Washed with wine it enters the yang brilliance conduits. For [use in] all the other conduits, do not prepare it with wine. [Li] Gao: *Da huang* is bitter and endowed with an urgent downward movement. When it is used to act downward it must be used unprepared. In the case of evil qi in the upper [body part], it will not reach there if it is not prepared with wine. It must be soaked in wine to be pulled upward to the highest section and from there to dispel the heat and cause it to descend. This is comparable to something that has occupied a topmost position. It must be shot to get a hold of it. If it were used unprepared, it would leave evil [qi] at the topmost position unrestrained. Hence, after a cure is achieved, [the patient's] eyes may be red, or his throat may be closed, or his head may be bloated, or a heat illness emerges above the diaphragm. [Li] Shizhen. For all diseases in the qi section, for stomach cold and blood depletion, and also during pregnancy and following delivery, [*da huang* root] must not be used carelessly. Its nature is bitter and cold, and it can harm the original qi, because it wastes yin [qi, i. e.,] blood. [Xu] Zhicai: *Scutellaria* [root] serves as its guiding substance. [Ingested together with other pharmaceutical substances,] it fears not

808 Instead of *da han* 大寒, "very cold," *Yu lan* ch. 992, *da huang* 大黄, writes *xiao han* 小寒, "slightly cold."

one of them. [Zhen] Quan: [During a treatment with *da huang*] avoid cold water. [Ingested together,] it abhors dried lacquer.

【主治】下瘀血血閉，寒熱，破癥瘕積聚，留飲宿食，蕩滌腸胃，推陳致新，通利水穀，調中化食，安和五臟。本經。平胃下氣，除痰實，腸間結熱，心腹脹滿，女子寒血閉脹，小腹痛，諸老血留結。别録。通女子經候，利水腫，利大小腸，貼熱腫毒，小兒寒熱時疾，煩熱蝕膿。甄權。通宣一切氣，調血脉，利關節，泄壅滯水氣，温瘴熱瘧。大明。瀉諸實熱不通，除下焦濕熱，消宿食，瀉心下痞滿。元素。下痢赤白，裏急腹痛，小便淋瀝，實熱燥結，潮熱譫語，黄疸諸火瘡。時珍。

Control. It serves to discharge stagnating blood and [to cure menstrual] blood blockage and alternating sensations of cold and heat. It breaks through concretion-illness and conglomeration-illness,[809] accumulations and collections, abiding rheum and food remaining in the body overnight. It cleanses the intestines and the stomach. It pushes out the old and lets arrive the new. It frees the passage of water (i. e., beverages) and grain (i. e., solid food). It regulates the center and serves to transform food. It calms and harmonizes the five long-term depots. *Ben jing*. It balances the stomach [qi] and discharges [evil] qi. It eliminates phlegm repletion, bound heat in the intestines, bloating with a feeling of fullness in the central and abdominal region, and [menstrual] blood blockage related to cold of women with an [abdominal] distension, pain in the lower abdomen, as well as all types of abiding and bound old blood. *Bie lu*. It opens the flow of menstruation, frees the passage [of water from a] water swelling and frees the passage through the large and the small intestines. It can be attached to a heat swelling with poison. [It serves to cure] seasonal illnesses of children with alternating feelings of cold and heat, vexing heat with erosion and festering. Zhen Quan. It frees the passage of all types of qi, regulates the blood vessels, frees the [passage through and the movement of] the joints. It causes an outflow of obstructed, sluggish water qi [and serves to cure] warmth miasma and heat malaria. Da Ming. It causes an outflow of all types of blocked repletion heat. It dispels moisture and heat from the lower [section of the Triple] Burner. It dissolves food remaining in the body overnight. It drains obstacle-illness and fullness from below the heart/stomach. [Zhang] Yuansu. [It serves to cure] discharge with a red and white free-flux illness, internal tension with abdominal pain, urinary dripping, repletion heat with dryness and bound [qi], heat waves and incoherent speech, yellow *dan*-illness and all kinds of sores caused by fire. [Li] Shizhen.

809 *Zheng jia* 癥瘕, "concretion-illness and conglomeration-illness." The two terms are often used interchangeably and do not signify two distinctly different conditions. Concretion-illness and conglomeration-illness result from a disharmony of cold and warmth resulting in a failure to transform beverages and food. Nodes form when the clash with the qi of the long-term depots. BCGM Dict I, 677.

【發明】【之才曰】得芍藥、黄芩、牡蠣、細辛、伏苓，療驚恚怒，心下悸氣。得消石、紫石英、桃仁，療女子血閉。【宗奭曰】張仲景治心氣不足，吐血衄血，瀉心湯，用大黄、黄芩、黄連。或曰心氣既不足，而不用補心湯，更用瀉心何也？答曰：若心氣獨不足，則當不吐衄也。此乃邪熱因不足而客之，故令吐衄。以苦泄其熱，以苦補其心，蓋一舉而兩得之。有是證者，用之無不效。惟在量其虛實而已。【震亨曰】大黄苦寒善泄，仲景用之瀉心湯者，正因少陰經不足，本經之陽亢甚無輔，以致陰血妄行飛越，故用大黄瀉去亢甚之火，使之平和，則血歸經而自安。夫心之陰氣不足，非一日矣，肺與肝俱各受火而病作。故黄芩救肺，黄連救肝。肺者陰之主，肝者心之母、血之合也。肝肺之火既退，則陰血復其舊矣。寇氏不明説而云邪熱客之，何以明仲景之意而開悟後人也？【時珍曰】大黄乃足太陰、手足陽明、手足厥陰五經血分之藥。凡病在五經血分者宜用之。若在氣分用之，是謂誅伐無過矣。瀉心湯治心氣不足吐血衄血者，乃真心之氣不足，而手厥陰心包絡、足厥陰肝、足太陰脾、足陽明胃之邪火有餘也。雖曰瀉心，實瀉四經血中之伏火也。又仲景治心下痞滿按之軟者，用大黄黄連瀉心湯主之。此亦瀉脾胃之濕熱，非瀉心也。病發於陰而反下之，則作痞滿，乃寒傷營血，邪氣乘虛結于上焦。胃之上脘在于心，故曰瀉心，實瀉脾也。素問云太陰所至爲痞滿，又云濁氣在上，則生䐜脹是矣。病發於陽而反下之，則成結胸，乃熱邪陷入血分，亦在上脘分野。仲景大陷胸湯丸皆用大黄，亦瀉脾胃血分之邪而降其濁氣也。若結胸在氣分，則只用小陷胸湯；痞滿在氣分則用半夏瀉心湯矣。成無已註釋傷寒論，亦不知分别此義。【成無已曰】熱淫所勝，以苦泄之。大黄之苦，以蕩滌瘀熱，下燥結而泄胃强。【頌曰】本草稱大黄推陳致新，其效最神，故古方下積滯多用之，張仲景治傷寒用處尤多。古人用毒藥攻病，必隨人之虛實寒熱而處置，非一切輕用也。梁武帝因發熱欲服大黄，姚僧坦曰：大黄乃是快藥，至尊年高，不可輕用。帝弗從，幾至委頓。梁元帝常有心腹疾。諸醫咸謂宜用平藥，可漸宣通。僧坦曰：脉洪而實，此有宿妨，非用大黄無瘥理。帝從之，遂愈。以此言之。今醫用一毒藥而攻衆病，其偶中，便謂此方神奇。其差誤，則不言用藥之失，可不戒哉？

Explication. [Xu] Zhicai: Combined with *paeonia* [root], *scutellaria* [root], oyster shells, *asarum heteropoides* [root] and *poria* it heals fright and rage with palpitating qi below the heart. Combined with nitrokalite, amethyst and peach kernels, it heals blockage of female [menstruation] blood. [Kou] Zongshi: For his treatment of heart qi insufficiency accompanied by blood spitting and nosebleed with the "decoction to drain the heart," Zhang Zhongjing resorts to *da huang*, *scutellaria* [root] and *coptis* [rhizome]. Some say: "For an insufficiency of heart qi, why would he not use the 'decoction to supplement heart [qi]' and uses the '[decoction to] drain the heart' instead?" The answer is: If the heart qi alone are insufficient, this does not result in [blood] spitting and nosebleed. The situation here is one of evil heat visiting [the heart] because of its insufficient [qi] and this results in [blood] spitting and nosebleed. The heat is drained by means of bitter [flavor], and this way [the patient] will no longer spit [blood] and have nosebleed. The fact is, one activity serves to achieve two ends. If this [treatment] is resorted to for such illness signs, it will always be successful. All that is required is to assess [the patient's status of] depletion and repletion. [Zhu] Zhenheng: *Da huang* is bitter and cold and is well suited to cause outflow. When [Zhang] Zhongjing uses it in the "decoction to drain the heart," he does so because in the case of insufficient [qi] in the minor yin conduits, there is nothing to restrain the overly active yang [qi] in these conduits and this eventually results in the yin [qi, i. e., the] blood's uncontrolled movements and flying away. Hence *da huang* is used to drain the overly active fire and let it calm down. As a result, the blood returns to its proper conduits and the [disease] is healed. Now, an insufficiency of the heart's yin qi is not an affair of only one day. The lung and the liver have both received the fire and this leads to the disease. Therefore, *scutellaria* [root is chosen to] save the lung, and *coptis* [rhizome is chosen to] save the liver. The lung is the ruler of the qi; the liver is the mother of the heart and the meeting point of blood. As soon as the fire in the liver and the heart recedes, the yin [qi, i. e., the] blood, have reached their old status again. Mr. Kou [Zongshi's] explanation is not clear when he states that "evil heat visits" the [heart]. How could this serve to explain the meaning underlying [Zhang] Zhongjing's [therapy] and to enlighten people in future? [Li] Shizhen: *Da huang* is a pharmaceutical drug for the blood section of five conduits: the foot major yin, the hand and foot yang brilliance and the hand and foot ceasing yin [conduits]. It is to be used for all diseases in the blood section of these five conduits. If it were used for [disease in] the qi section, this would be called "punishment of those who have done nothing wrong." The "decoction to drain the heart" serves to cure insufficient heart qi associated with blood spitting and nosebleed. In this case the genuine qi of the heart are insufficient and there is surplus evil fire in the hand ceasing yin [conduit of the heart] enclosing network, the foot ceasing yin [conduit of the] liver, the foot major yin [conduit of the] spleen, and the foot yang brilliance [conduit of the] stomach. Even though [this decoction] is said to "drain the heart," it does really drain the fire that lies hidden in the blood of four conduits. Also, when [Zhang] Zhongjing cures obstacle-illness with a feeling of fullness, that is soft when pressed, below the heart, he controls this with the "decoction with *da huang* and *coptis* [rhizome] to drain the heart." This, too, is a drainage of moisture and heat from the spleen and the stomach; it is not a drainage of the heart. When a disease effuses in the yin [section] and contrary to [what is required] a discharging [therapy is given], this will result in an obstacle-illness with a feeling of fullness. This is harm to the camp [qi, i. e., the] blood, committed by cold. The evil qi avail themselves of the depletion and conglomerate in the upper [section of the Triple] Burner. The upper end of the stomach duct is situated at the heart. Hence one speaks of "draining the heart," while in reality this is meant to drain the spleen. The *Su wen* states: "Where the minor yin [qi] arrive there is obstacle-illness and a feeling of fullness."[810] It also correctly states: "When turbid qi are in the upper [regions], then this generates bloating."[811] When a disease effuses in the yang [section] and contrary to [what is required] a discharging [therapy is given], this results in bound [qi] in the chest and the heat evil enters the blood section. In addition it will settle in the upper [stomach] duct. [Zhang] Zhongjing in his "major decoction for [evil qi] stuck in the chest"[812] and in his ["major] pills [for evil qi stuck in the chest"][813] uses *da huang*. Here again it serves to drain evil [qi] in the blood section of spleen and stomach and to let their turbid qi descend. If the bound [qi] in the chest are in the qi section, only the "minor decoction for [evil qi] stuck in the chest"[814] is resorted to. If the obstacle-illness with the feeling of fullness are situated in the qi section, the "decoction with *pinellia* root to drain the heart" [815]is used. When Cheng Wuyi commented to explain the *Shang han lun*, he, too, did not know the underlying meaning of this differentiation. Cheng Wuyi: When heat is excessive and dominates [yin qi], it is to be drained with bitter [flavor]. The bitter [flavor] of *da huang* serves to flush out stagnant heat, to discharge dry, bound [qi (i. e., constipation)] and to drain the stomach to give it back its strength. [Su] Song: The *Ben cao* says of *da huang*: "It pushes back the old and lets the new arrive." Its effects are very divine and therefore ancient recipes often resort to it to discharge accumulated and sluggish [qi]. Zhang Zhongjing used it particularly often to cure harm caused by cold. The ancients resorted to poisonous pharmaceutical drugs to

810 A condensed quote from *Su wen*, ch. 71. Paul U. Unschuld and Hermann Tessenow, *Huang Di Nei Jing Su Wen. An Annotated Translation of Huang Di's Inner Classic*, 2 vols. University of California Press, Berkeley and Los Angeles, 2011. Vol. 1, 516.

811 A literal quote from *Su wen*, ch. 5. Paul U. Unschuld and Hermann Tessenow, *Huang Di Nei Jing Su Wen. An Annotated Translation of Huang Di's Inner Classic*, 2 vols. University of California Press, Berkeley and Los Angeles, 2011. Vol. 1, 97.

812 *Da xian xiong tang* 大陷胸湯, the "major decoction for [evil qi] stuck in the chest," has the following ingredients: *Da huang* root, mirabilite, *kansui* root.

813 *Da xian xiong wan* 大陷胸丸, the "major pills for [evil qi] stuck in the chest," has the following ingredients: *Da huang* root, mirabilite, *kansui* root, wood whitlow-grass, apricot seeds.

814 *Xiao xian xiong tang* 小陷胸湯, the minor decoction for [evil qi] stuck in the chest," has the following ingredients: *Coptis* rhizome, *pinellia* tuber, Japanese snake gourd.

815 *Ban xia xie xin tang* 半夏瀉心湯, the "decoction with *pinellia* root to drain the heart," has the following ingredients: *Pinellia* tuber, *scutellaria* root, dried ginger, ginseng root, prepared *glycyrrhiza* root, *coptis* rhizome and Chinese dates.

attack a disease. This required an approach based on an individual person's status of depletion or repletion, cold or heat. They did not carelessly use [*da huang*] for all [diseases] alike. When the Liang [Emperor] Wu di effused heat, he wished to ingest *da huang*. Yao Sengtan said: "*Da huang* is a rapidly acting pharmaceutical drug. You have reached a high age; it must not be carelessly resorted to." The Emperor did not follow this advice and [having ingested *da huang*] he reached a state of severe exhaustion. Liang [Emperor] Yuan di continuously suffered from an illness in his central and abdominal region. All the physicians advised him to ingest pharmaceutical drugs with a balanced nature so as to gradually free the flow [of the evil qi]. [Yao] Sengtan said: "When the [movement in the] vessels is vast and replete, this shows the presence of food that has remained in the body overnight. Without *da huang*, there is no reason why this could be cured." The Emperor acted accordingly and was cured. These [anecdotes] explain [the proper use of *da huang*. However], today's physicians use one poisonous pharmaceutical drug to attack all types of diseases. If they happen, by chance, to hit the target, they simply claim this recipe to be divinely outstanding. When the [treatment proves to be] wrong, they do not explain it as an erroneous application of a pharmaceutical drug. Shouldn't they be careful?

【附方】舊十四，新三十七。
Added Recipes. 14 of old. 37 newly [recorded].

吐血衄血。治心氣不足，吐血衄血者，瀉心湯主之。大黄二兩，黄連、黄芩各一兩，水三升，煮一升，熱服取利。張仲景金匱玉函。

Blood spitting and nosebleed. To cure insufficient heart qi with blood spitting and nosebleed, the "decoction to drain the heart" will control this. Boil two *liang* of *da huang* and one *liang* each of *coptis* [rhizome] and *scutellaria* [root] in three *sheng* of water down to one *sheng*, and ingest this [liquid] hot to stimulate a free-flow [discharge]. Zhang Zhongjing, *Jin kui yü han*.

吐血刺痛。川大黄一兩，爲散。每服一錢，以生地黄汁一合，水半盞，煎三五沸，無時服。簡要濟衆方。

Blood spitting with a piercing pain. [Grind] one *liang* of [Si] chuan *da huang* into powder. Each time ingest one *qian*. Boil it mixed with one *ge* of fresh Chinese foxglove [rhizome] juice in half a cup of water three to five times to bubbling and ingest it any time. *Jian yao ji zhong fang*.

傷寒痞滿。病發於陰，而反下之，心下滿而不痛，按之濡，此爲痞也，大黄黄連瀉心湯主之。大黄二兩，黄連一兩，以麻沸湯二升漬之，須臾絞汁，分作二次温服。仲景傷寒論。

Obstacle-illness and a feeling of fullness related to harm caused by cold. When this disease effuses in the yin [section] and contrary to [what is required] is treated with a discharging therapy, a feeling of fullness develops below the heart that does not ache and when pressed is flexible. This is an obstacle-illness. The "decoction with *da huang* and *coptis* [rhizome] to drain the heart" controls it. Soak two *liang* of *da huang* and one *liang* of *coptis* [rhizome] in two *sheng* of boiling water. After a short while squeeze it to obtain a juice and ingest it warm divided into to portions. [Zhang] Zhongjing, *Shang han lun*.

熱病譫狂。川大黄五兩，剉炒微赤，爲散。用臘雪水五升，煎如膏。每服半匙，冷水下。聖惠方。

Heat disease with incoherent language and madness. Cut five *liang* of [Si] chuan *da huang* into pieces, fry them until they have a assumed a slightly red color and [grind them into] powder. Boil this in five *sheng* of snow water gathered in the 12th month to a paste and each time [let the patient] ingest half a spoonful, to be sent down with cold water. *Sheng hui fang*.

傷寒發黄。方同上。

Harm caused by cold with an effusion of yellow. Recipe identical to the one above.

氣壯者大黄一兩，水二升，漬一宿，平旦煎汁一升，入芒硝一兩，緩服，須臾當利下。傷寒類要。

For those with robust qi, soak one *liang* of *da huang* in two *sheng* of water for one night. The next morning boil one *sheng* of the juice, add one *liang* of mirabilite, and ingest this warm. After a short while a free-flow discharge will set in. *Shang han lei yao*.

腰脚風氣，作痛。大黄二兩，切如棋子，和少酥炒乾，勿令焦，擣篩。每用二錢，空心以水三大合，入薑三片，煎十餘沸，取湯調服，當下冷膿惡物即痛止。崔元亮海上方。

Painful wind qi [intrusion] in the lower back and legs. Cut two *liang* of *da huang* into pieces the size of chess pieces, mix them with a little butter and fry them until they have dried, but see to it that they are not scorched. Then pound them [to powder and give it] through a sieve. Each time ingest two *qian* on an empty stomach. Mix it with three generous *ge* of water, add three slices of ginger and boil this to bubbling more than ten times. Ingest the decoction. This results in a discharge of cold pus and malign items, whereupon the pain ends. Cui Yuanliang, *Hai shang fang*.

一切壅滯。經驗後方治風熱積壅，化痰涎，治痞悶消食，化氣導血。用大黄四兩，牽牛子半炒半生四兩，爲末，煉蜜丸如梧子大。每服十丸，白湯下，並不損人。如要微利，加一二十丸。

All types of obstruction and sluggishness. The *Jing yan hou fang* [recommends to] cure obstruction related to wind and heat accumulation by transforming phlegm to saliva, and to cure obstacle-illness with a feeling of fullness by transforming qi and leading off blood [with the following recipe]. [Grind] four *liang* of *da huang* and four *liang* of *pharbitis* seeds, one half fried, one half unprepared, into powder and form with heat refined honey pills the size of *wu* seeds. Each time ingest ten pills, to be sent down with clear, boiled water. This will not injure that person. If a slight free-flow is intended, add another ten or 20 pills.

衛生寶鑑用皂莢熬膏和丸，名墜痰丸，又名全真丸。金宣宗服之有驗，賜名保安丸。

The *Wei sheng bao jian* [recommends to] simmer [the *da huang*] with *gleditsia* pods to a paste and form pills. They are called "pills to drop down phlegm," and also "pills to re-establish the genuine [qi]." The Jin [Emperor] Xuan zong ingested them, and they proved to be effective. He conferred upon them the name "pills to safeguard piece."

痰爲百病。滚痰丸：治痰爲百病，惟水瀉、胎前産後不可服用。大黄酒浸蒸熟，切晒八兩，生黄芩八兩，沉香半兩。青礞石二兩，以焰硝二兩，同入砂罐固濟，煅紅研末二兩。右各取末，以水和丸梧子大。常服一二十丸，小病五六十丸，緩病七八十丸，急病一百二十丸，温水吞下，即卧勿動。候藥逐上焦痰滯。次日先下糟粕，次下痰涎，未下再服。王隱君歲合四十餘斤，愈疾數萬也。養生主論。

The hundreds of diseases caused by phlegm. The "pills to chase away phlegm." They serve to cure the hundreds of diseases caused by phlegm. Only in the case of watery outflow and prior to and following delivery they must not be ingested. [Grind] four *liang* of *huang*, soaked in wine, steamed until done, cut into pieces and dried in the sun, eight *liang* of unprepared *scutellaria* [root] and half a *liang* of aloes wood [to powder]. Give two *liang* of micacious schist with two *liang* of nitrokalite into a pottery jar and firmly seal it. Then calcine it until it turns red, grind [the contents to] obtain two *liang* of powder. Take all these powders and form with water pills the size of *wu* seeds. Regularly ingest ten to 20 pills. In the case of a minor disease [the dose is] 50 to 60 pills. In the case of a slow/chronic disease, it is 70 to 80 pills. In the case of a critical disease, it is 120 pills. They are to be swallowed with warm water. Then [the patient] must lie down motionless, waiting for the medication to rise to the upper [section of the Triple] Burner, the location of the phlegm sluggishness.

The next day [the patient] will first discharge ordinary excrements. Next he will discharge phlegm and saliva. If nothing is discharged he is to ingest [the pills] again. Wang Yinjun every year prepared more than 40 *jin* [of these pills] and he cured tens of thousands of patients. *Yang sheng zhu lun.*

男女諸病。無極丸：治婦人經血不通，赤白帶下，崩漏不止，腸風下血，五淋，産後積血，癥瘕腹痛，男子五勞七傷，小兒骨蒸潮熱等證，其效甚速。宜六癸日合之。用錦紋大黄一斤，分作四分。一分用童尿一盌，食鹽二錢，浸一日，切晒。一分用醇酒一盌，浸一日，切晒，再以巴豆仁三十五粒同炒，豆黄，去豆不用。一分用紅花四兩，泡水一盌，浸一日，切晒。一分用當歸四兩，入淡醋一盌，同浸一日，去歸，切晒。爲末，煉蜜丸梧子大。每服五十丸，空心温酒下。取下惡物爲驗，未下再服。此武當高士孫碧雲方也。醫林集要。

All types of diseases of males and females. The "pills that are not topped." They cure a woman's blocked menstruation, red and white [discharge from] below the belt, unending [blood] collapse and leaking, intestinal wind with a discharge of blood, the five types of [urinary] dripping, blood accumulation following delivery, concretion-illness and conglomeration-illness[816] with abdominal pain. In males, the five types of exhaustion and seven types of harm. In children, bone steaming[817] and heat waves, all such conditions. Their effects are very fast. They must be prepared on one of the six *gui* 癸 days [as follows]. Divide one *jin* of *da huang* [roots] with a brocade line design into four portions. Soak one portion in a bowl of boys' urine, with two *qian* of salt, for one day. Cut it into pieces and dry them in the sun. Soak the next portion in a bowl with unmixed wine for one day, cut it into pieces and dry them in the sun. Then fry them together with 35 *croton* kernels until these kernels have turned yellow, and discard the kernels; they are of no further use. A [third] portion is soaked together with four *liang* of safflower in one bowl of water that had been boiled to bubbling for one day. It is then cut into pieces and dried in the sun. A [fourth] portion is given with four *liang* of Chinese *angelica* [root] and light vinegar into a bowl to soak for one day. Then the Chinese *angelica* [root] is discarded and the [*da huang*] is cut into pieces and dried in the sun. [All four portions are ground into] powder and formed with heat refined honey to pills the size of *wu* seeds. Each

816 *Zheng jia* 癥瘕, "concretion-illness and conglomeration-illness." The two terms are often used interchangeably and do not signify two distinctly different conditions. Concretion-illness and conglomeration-illness result from a disharmony of cold and warmth resulting in a failure to transform beverages and food. Nodes form when the clash with the qi of the long-term depots. BCGM Dict I, 677.

817 *Gu zheng* 骨蒸, "bone steaming," 1.) a condition of an infectious consumptive disease with a development of vexing heat in the afternoon. 2.) An illness sign of heat and vexation with a feeling as if this originated in the bones. BCGM Dict I, 197.

time ingest 50 pills, to be sent down on an empty stomach with warm wine until a discharge of malign items signals the effect. In the case of no discharge, ingest [the pills] a second time. This is a recipe of the eminent scholar Sun Biyun of Wu dang. *Yi lin ji yao.*

心腹諸疾。三物備急丸：治心腹諸疾，卒暴百病。用大黄、巴豆、乾薑各一兩，搗篩，蜜和搗一千杵，丸小豆大，每服三丸。凡中惡客忤，心腹脹滿，痛如錐刀，氣急口噤，停尸卒死者，以暖水或酒服之，或灌之。未知更服三丸，腹中鳴轉，當吐下便愈。若口已噤者，折齒灌之，入喉即瘥。此乃仲景方，司空裴秀改爲散用，不及丸也。圖經本草。

All types of illnesses in the central and abdominal region. The "pills with three items to be prepared for urgent situations." They serve to cure all types of illnesses in the central and abdominal region, a sudden and violent affliction with hundreds of diseases. Pound one *liang* each of *da huang*, croton seeds and dried ginger [to powder and] pass it through a sieve. Pound it mixed with honey a thousand times and form pills the size of mung beans. Each time ingest three pills. For all cases of being struck by the malign and visiting hostile agents, distension and a feeling of fullness in the central and abdominal region, pain as if pierced by an awl or a knife, hectic [breath] qi and lockjaw, sudden death resulting from uninterred corpse [qi], ingest them with warm water or wine. Or force-feed them [to the dead patient]. If this fails to show an effect, ingest three pills again. This will result in sounds of a revolving mass in the abdomen, and a vomiting and discharge as signs of a cure. In the case of lockjaw, break [the patient's] teeth and force-feed [the pills] to him. Once they enter his throat, he will be cured. This is a recipe of [Zhang] Zhongjing. Pei Xiu, Minister of Works, modified it to be used as powder. But [ingested as powder] it does not reach [the quality of] the pills. *Tu jing ben cao.*

腹中痞塊。大黄十兩爲散，醋三升，蜜兩匙，和煎，丸梧子大。每服三十丸，生薑湯下，吐利爲度。外臺秘要。

Obstacle-illness with a formation of lumps in the abdomen. [Grind] ten *liang* of *da huang* into powder, mix it with three *sheng* of vinegar and two spoonfulls of honey and boil this [to generate a paste] and to form pills the size of *wu* seeds. Each time ingest 30 pills, to be sent down with a fresh ginger decoction until a vomiting and free-flow [signal the effect]. *Wai tai mi yao.*

腹脇積塊。風化石灰末半斤，瓦器炒極熱，稍冷，入大黄末一兩炒熱，入桂心末半兩略炒，下米醋攪成膏，攤布貼之。

Accumulation and the forming of lumps in the abdomen and the flanks. Half a *jin* of lime transformed by wind is fried in a pottery vessel until it is extremely hot.

When it has cooled a little add one *liang* of *da huang* powder, fried until done, and also add half a *liang* of slightly fried shaved cinnamom bark powder. Add rice vinegar and stir this to generate a paste. Spread it [on the affected region].

又方：大黄二兩，朴硝一兩，爲末，以大蒜同搗膏和貼之。或加阿魏一兩，尤妙。丹溪心法。

Another recipe. [Grind] two *liang* of *da huang* and one *liang* of mirabilite into powder. Pound it together with garlic to generate an ointment and paste it on [the affected region]. Or add one *liang* of asafetida. This is especially wondrous. *Danxi xin fa.*

久患積聚。二便不利，氣上搶心，腹脹滿，害食。大黄、白芍各二兩，爲末。水丸梧子大，每湯下四十丸，日三，以知爲度。千金方。

Suffering from accumulation and collection for a long time, with the free flow of the two [major/defecation and minor/urination] reliefs blocked, qi rising to attack the heart, abdominal bloating and a feeling of fullness, and an aversion to eating. [Grind] two *liang* each of *da huang* and *paeonia* [root] into powder and form with water pills the size of *wu* seeds. Each time send down with hot water 40 pills, three times a day, until an effect shows. *Qian jin fang.*

脾癖疳積。不拘大人小兒，錦紋大黄三兩爲末，醋一盞，沙鍋内文武火熬成膏，傾瓦上，日晒夜露三日，再研。用舶上硫黄一兩形如琥珀者，官粉一兩，同研勻。十歲以下小兒半錢，大人一錢半，米飲下。忌一切生冷、魚肉，只食白粥半月。如一服不愈，半月之後再服。若不忌口，不如勿服。聖濟總録。

Spleen aggregation-illness,[818] *gan*-illness[819] and accumulation, regardless of whether [the patients are] adults or children. [Grind] three *liang* of *da huang* [root] with a brocade line design into powder and simmer it with one cup of vinegar in an earthenware pot with a mild fire first and a violent fire later to a paste. Spread it on a tile and expose it for three days to the sun during the day and to dew during the night. Then grind this again. Now grind it with one *liang* of imported sulphur shaped like amber and one *liang* of lead carbonate to an even mixture. Children ten years old or younger [ingest] half a *qian*, adults one and a half *qian*, to be sent down with a rice beverage. [During this treatment] avoid all types of fresh and cold [items], fish and meat. Only eat white congee for half a month. If one ingestion fails to result in

818 *Pi* 癖, "aggregation-illness," a condition of painful lumps emerging from time to time in both flanks. BCGM Dict I, 371.

819 *Gan* 疳, "*gan*-illness," also: "sweets-illness," involves several complaints that affect children and adults, with causes and conditions too different to fall into a known disease category. BCGM Dict I, 180-188.

a cure, wait for half a month and ingest it again. To not avoid the consumption [of the items mentioned] is worse than not ingesting [the medication] at all.

小兒無辜，閃癖瘰癧，或頭乾黄聳，或乍痢乍瘥，諸狀多者，大黄煎主之。大黄九兩錦紋新實者，若微朽即不中用，削去皮，擣篩爲散。以好米醋三升，和置瓦盌中，於大鐺内浮湯上，炭火慢煮，候至成膏，可丸，乃貯器中。三歲兒一服七丸，梧子大，日再服，以下出青赤膿爲度。若不下，或下少，稍稍加丸。若下多，又須減之。病重者七八劑方盡根。大人亦可用之。此藥惟下宿膿，不令兒利也。須禁食毒物，乳母亦禁之。一加木香一兩半。崔知悌方。

Innocence[820] of children. Sprain with aggregation-illness.[821] Scrofula pervasion-illness.[822] In some cases the head turns dry and yellow. Or a free-flux illness at times occurs and at times recedes. There are many possible illness signs. A *da huang* decoction will control them. Take nine *liang* of *da huang* [roots] with a brocade line design. They must be new/fresh and solid. If they are only slightly decayed, they must not be used. Cut and remove the skin. Pound [the rest] into powder and pass it through a sieve. Mix the powder with rice vinegar and give this into a ceramic bowl. Place [the bowl] into a large, flat pan positioned above hot water, Boil [the water] slowly with a charcoal fire until a paste has formed that can be made to pills, and store it in a vessel. Children three years old ingest a single dose of seven pills, the size of *wu* seeds, twice a day until they discharge greenish-red pus. If this is not discharged, or if only a little is discharged, gradually increase the [amount of] pills. If a lot [of pus] is discharged, the number [of pills ingested] must be decreased. In the case of a severe disease, seven or eight recipe dosages will completely eliminate the root [of the disease]. Adults can resort [to these pills], too. This medication serves only to discharge pus that has remained in the body overnight. It does not let the children have a free flow. They must be kept away from eating poisonous items, and their nursing mother, too, must avoid them. Another [recipe] adds one and a half *liang* of *costus* [root]. *Cui Zhiti fang*.

---

820 *Wu gu* 無辜, "innocence," a type of *gan*-illness accompanied by scrofula affecting the head and neck. BCGM Dict I, 537.

821 *Shan pi* 閃癖, "sprain with aggregation-illness," a condition of children with swelling below the flanks, loss of appetite, no digestion, yellow complexion, emaciation and desiccation of the hair. This is often accompanied by bone steaming, scrofula, and pervasion-illness. BCGM Dict I, 419.

822 *Luo li* 瘰癧, "scrofula pervasion-illness," when two or more connected swellings of the size of plum or date kernels appear either on the neck or in the armpits, or somewhere else on the body. BCGM Dict I. 329.

小兒諸熱。大黄煨熟、黄芩各一兩，爲末，煉蜜丸麻子大。每服五丸至十丸，蜜湯下。加黄連，名三黄丸。錢氏小兒方。

All types of heat of children. [Grind] one *liang* each of *da huang*, simmered until done, and *scutellaria* [root, *huang qin*] into powder and form with heat refined honey pills the size of sesame seeds. Each time [let the child] ingest five up to ten pills, to be sent down with a honey decoction. If *coptis* [rhizome, *huang lian*] is added, they are called the "pills with the three [ingredients having in their name the character for "yellow,"] *huang* 黄.[823] *Qian shi xiao er fang*.

骨蒸積熱，漸漸黄瘦。大黄四分，以童子小便五六合，煎取四合，去滓。空腹分爲二服，如人行五里，再服。廣利方。

Bone steaming[824] with accumulated heat, gradually causing one to appear yellow and emaciated. Boil four *fen* of *da huang* in five or six *ge* of boys' urine down to four *ge*, remove the dregs and ingest [the liquid] on an empty abdomen divided into two portions. After the time it takes one to walk five *li*, ingest it a second time. *Guang li fang*.

赤白濁淋。好大黄爲末。每服六分，以雞子一個，破頂入藥，攪勻蒸熟，空心食之。不過三服愈。簡便方。

Turbid, red and white [urinary] dripping. [Grind] good *da huang* into powder. Each time ingest six *fen*. Break open the top of one chicken egg and insert the pharmaceutical drug. Stir it to generate an even mix [with the egg's contents] and steam it until it is done. Ingest this on an empty stomach. A cure will be achieved after no more than three ingestions. *Jian bian fang*.

相火秘結。大黄末一兩，牽牛頭末半兩，每服三錢。有厥冷者，酒服。無厥冷，五心煩，蜜湯服。劉河間保命集。

Closed in, bound minister fire. [Mix] one *liang* of *da huang* powder and half a *liang* of *pharbitis* seed powder and each time ingest three *qian*. In the case of ceasing [yang qi] with cold [legs] ingest it with wine. If there is no ceasing [yang qi] with cold, but if there is a vexing [heat] in the five centers (i. e., the center of the body, the palms and the soles), ingest it with a honey decoction. Liu Hejian, *Bao ming ji*.

---

823 Usually, the three [items named "yellow",] *huang* 黄, include sulphur, *liu huang* 硫黄, realgar, *xiong huang* 雄黄, and orpiment, *ci huang* 雌黄. Here they are *da huang* 大黄, rhubarb root, *huang qin* 黄芩, scutellaria root, and *huang lian* 黄連, coptis rhizome.

824 *Gu zheng* 骨蒸, "bone steaming," 1.) a condition of an infectious consumptive disease with a development of vexing heat in the afternoon. 2.) An illness sign of heat and vexation with a feeling as if this originated in the bones. BCGM Dict I, 197.

諸痢初起。大黃煨熟、當歸各二三錢，壯人各一兩，水煎服，取利。或加檳榔。集簡方。

All types of free-flux illness that have just emerged. Boil two or three *liang* each – strong persons: one *liang* each – of *da huang*, simmered until done, and Chinese *angelica* [root] and ingest the resulting decoction. This will cause a free flow. Or, add *areca* [nuts]. *Ji jian fang*.

熱痢裹急。大黃一兩，浸酒半日，煎服取利。集簡方。

Free-flux illness related to heat, with internal tension. Soak one *liang* of *da huang* in wine for half a day. Then boil it and ingest [the liquid] to cause a free flow. *Ji jian fang*.

忽喘悶絶，不能語言，涎流吐逆，牙齒動摇，氣出轉大，絶而復蘇，名傷寒併熱霍亂。大黃、人參各半兩，水二盞，煎一盞，熱服，可安。危氏得效方。

Sudden onset of panting with heart-pressure and a [threat of] interrupted [qi flow]. [Patients] are unable to speak. Saliva flows and they vomit with [qi] counterflow. The teeth are loose and move. A massive release of qi turned into the other direction. [The flow of qi] is interrupted and then is activated again. This is called "harm caused by cold together with hot cholera." Boil half a *liang* each of *da huang* and ginseng [root] in two cups of water down to one cup and ingest it warm. This can cure [the patient]. *Wei shi de xiao fang*.

食已即吐。胸中有火也。大黃一兩，甘草二錢半，水一升，煮半升，温服。仲景金匱玉函方。

Vomiting immediately following a meal. A fire is present in the chest. Boil one *liang* of *da huang* and two and a half *qian* of *glycyrrhiza* [root] in one *sheng* of water down to half a *sheng* and ingest this warm. [Zhang] Zhongjing, *Jin kui yu han fang*.

婦人血癖作痛。大黃一兩，酒二升，煮十沸，頓服取利。千金翼。

Painful blood aggregation-illness of woman. Boil one *liang* of *da huang* in two *sheng* of wine ten times to bubbling and ingest [all the liquid] at once to cause a free flow. *Qian jin yi*.

產後血塊。大黃末一兩，頭醋半升，熬膏，丸梧子大。每服五丸，温醋化下，良久當下。千金方。

Blood lumps forming following delivery. Simmer one *liang* of *da huang* powder in half a *sheng* of top-quality vinegar to a paste and form pills the size of *wu* seeds. Each time ingest five pills, to be sent down dissolved in warm vinegar. After an extended period of time [the lumps] are discharged. *Qian jin fang*.

乾血氣痛。錦紋大黃酒浸晒乾四兩，爲末，好醋一升，熬成膏，丸芡子大。卧時酒化一丸服，大便利一二行，紅漏自下，乃調經仙藥也。或加香附。董氏集驗方。

Painful dried blood and qi [disorder]. [Grind] four *liang* of *da huang* with a brocade line design, soaked in wine and dried in the sun, into powder and simmer it in one *sheng* of good vinegar to generate a paste to be formed to pills the size of *qian* seeds. At bedtime ingest one pill dissolved in wine. This results in one or two free-flow bowel movements with a red leakage discharge. This is a divine medication to regulate [the flow in] the conduits. Some add nutgrass [root]. Dong shi, *Ji yan fang*.

婦人嫁痛，小户腫痛也。大黄一兩，酒一升，煮一沸，頓服。千金方。

Marriage pain[825] of women, with a painful swelling of the vagina. Boil one *liang* of *da huang* in one *sheng* of wine to bubbling and [let the woman] ingest this all at once. *Qian jin fang*.

男子偏墜作痛。大黄末和醋塗之，乾則易。梅師方。

Painful unilateral dropping [of the testicles]. Apply a mixture of *da huang* powder and vinegar to [the affected region]. When it has dried, replace it [with a moist mixture]. *Mei shi fang*.

濕熱眩運，不可當者。酒炒大黄爲末，茶清服二錢，急則治其標也。丹溪纂要。

Unbearable dizziness related to the presence of moisture and heat. Fry *da huang* in wine and [grind it into] powder. Ingest two *qian* with clear tea. In the case of a critical [condition] the outer signs [of the underlying disease] are to be cured [first]. *Danxi zuan yao*.

小兒腦熱，常欲閉目。大黄一分，水三合，浸一夜。一歲兒服半合，餘者塗頂上，乾即再上。姚和衆至寶方。

Brain heat of children, with a continuing inclination to close the eyes. Soak one *fen* of *da huang* in three *ge* of water for one night. Children one year of age ingest half a *ge*. The remaining [liquid] is applied on the top of their head. When it has dried, it is applied again. Yao Hezhong, *Zhi bao fang*.

暴赤目痛。四物湯加大黄，酒煎服之。傳信適用方。

825 *Jia tong* 嫁痛, "marriage pain," an injury inflicted on a woman's outer genital parts following crude and violent sexual intercourse. BCGM Dict I, 244.

The eyes suddenly turned red and painful. Add *da huang* to the [recipe of the] "decoction with four items,"[826] boil it in wine and ingest this. *Chuan xin shi yong fang.*

胃火牙痛。口含冰水一口，以紙撚蘸大黄末，隨左右嗃鼻，立止。儒門事親。

Stomach fire and toothache. Hold ice water in the mouth. Twirl paper to a stick and dip it into *da huang* powder. Then [insert it into the left or right] nostril, depending on [the location of the toothache on the left or right] and inhale [the powder]. This ends [the pain] immediately. *Ru men shi qin.*

風熱牙痛。紫金散：治風熱積壅，一切牙痛，去口氣，大有奇效。好大黄瓶内燒存性，爲末，早晚揩牙，漱去。都下一家專貨此藥，兩宫常以數千贖之，其門如市也。千金家藏方。

Toothache related to wind [intrusion] and heat. The "purple gold powder." It serves to cure accumulation and obstruction associated with wind and heat [resulting in] all types of toothache. It removes oral qi, and is very effective. Burn good quality *da huang* in a flask with its nature retained, and [grind it into] powder. Apply this to the teeth early in the morning and in the evening. Then rinse them to remove [the powder again]. A firm in the capital city exclusively markets this medication and the two palaces (i.e. the emperor and the empress dowager) regularly spend thousands to purchase it. The gate [of this firm] resembles a market place. *Qian jin jia cang fang.*

風蟲牙痛，齦常出血，漸至崩落，口臭，極效。大黄米泔浸軟、生地黄各旋切一片，合定貼上，一夜即愈，未愈再貼。忌説話，恐引入風。本事方。

Toothache caused by wind [intrusion] and the presence of worms/bugs, accompanied by continuous bleeding from the gums, gradually increasing to a loss [of teeth], and bad mouth odor. Very effective. Soak *da huang* until it is soft in water that was used to wash rice and cut from it and also from fresh Chinese foxglove [rhizome] one slice each and attach them to the [affected teeth]. A cure is achieved within one night. If this fails to result in a cure, attach them again. [During this treatment, the patient] should not speak to avoid drawing even more wind [into the mouth]. *Ben shi fang.*

口瘡糜爛。大黄、枯礬等分，爲末，擦之吐涎。聖惠方。

Oral sores with festering putrescence. [Grind] equal amounts of *da huang* and processed alum into powder. Apply it [to the affected region] and spit out the saliva. *Sheng hui fang.*

826 Ingredients include *paeonia* root skin, Chinese foxglove rhizome, Chinese *angelica* root and *ligusticum* root.

鼻中生瘡。生大黄、杏仁擣匀，豬脂和塗。

Sores growing in the nose. Pound fresh *da huang* and apricot kernels to an even mixture, add lard and apply [this to the affected region].

又方：生大黄、黄連各一錢，麝香少許，爲末，生油調搽。聖惠方。

Another Recipe. [Grind] one *qian* each of fresh *da huang* and *coptis* [rhizome] with a little musk into powder, mix it with fresh oil and apply this [to the affected region]. *Sheng hui fang*.

仙茅毒發，舌脹出口。方見仙茅下。

Poisoning caused by golden eye grass. The tongue protrudes and comes out of the mouth. For a recipe, see the entry *xian mao* 仙茅 (12-22).

傷損瘀血。三因方雞鳴散：治從高墜下，木石壓傷，及一切傷損，血瘀凝積，痛不可忍，並以此藥推陳致新。大黄酒蒸一兩，杏仁去皮尖三七粒。細研，酒一盌，煎六分，雞鳴時服。至曉取下瘀血，即愈。

Stagnating blood related to harm caused by an injury. The "crowing rooster powder" of the *San yin fang*. It serves to cure all [injuries] related to a fall from a higher elevation and to harm resulting from a contusion by wood or a stone, and all further types of harm caused by injuries, with stagnating blood coagulating and accumulating, and an unbearable pain. For all these conditions, this medication pushes out the old and lets arrive the new. Grind one *liang* of *da huang*, steamed with wine, and three times seven apricot kernels, with their skin and tip discarded, [to powder] and boil it in one bowl of wine down to 60%. This is ingested when the roosters crow. Then, by daybreak, the stagnating blood is discharged. This is the cure.

和劑方治跌壓瘀血在内脹滿。大黄、當歸等分，炒研。每服四錢，温酒服，取下惡物愈。

The *He ji fang* [recommends to] cure stagnating blood resulting from falls or contusion with internal distension and a feeling of fullness [as follows]. Fry equal amounts of *da huang* and Chinese *angelica* [root] and grind [them into powder]. Each time ingest four *qian*, to be ingested with warm wine, to cause a discharge of malign items. This is the cure.

打撲傷痕，瘀血滚注，或作潮熱者。大黄末，薑汁調塗。一夜黑者紫，二夜紫者白也。瀕湖集簡方。

Scars left from harm caused by blows or falls, with stagnating blood pouring [into the skin] or heat weaves. Mix *da huang* powder with ginger juice and apply this [to the affected region]. Within one night black spots will turn purple. After a second night, purple spots will have turned white. *Binhu ji jian fang*.

杖瘡腫痛。大黄末，醋調塗之。童尿亦可調。醫方摘玄。

Painfull sores with swelling from flogging. Mix *da huang* powder with vinegar and apply it [to the affected region]. [The powder] may also be mixed with boys' urine. *Yi fang zhai xuan.*

金瘡煩痛，大便不利。大黄、黄芩等分，爲末，蜜丸。先食水下十丸，日三服。千金方。

Wounds caused by metal objects/weapons with vexing pain and constipation. [Grind] equal amounts of *da huang* and *scutellaria* [root] into powder and form with honey pills. Send down with water prior to a meal ten pills. To be ingested three times a day. *Qian jin fang.*

凍瘡破爛。大黄末，水調塗之。衛生寶鑑。

Open, festering frost sores. Mix *da huang* powder with water and apply this [to the affected region]. *Wei sheng bao jian.*

湯火傷灼。莊浪大黄生研，蜜調塗之。不惟止痛，又且滅瘢。此乃金山寺神人所傳方。洪邁夷堅志。

Harm caused by scalds and burns. Grind fresh *da huang* from Zhuang lang [to powder], mix it with honey and apply this [to the affected region]. This will not only end the pain, it also minimizes the scars. This is a recipe handed over by a divine person from Jin shan monastery. Hong Mai, *Yijian zhi.*

灸瘡飛蝶。因艾灸訖，火痂便退，瘡内鮮肉片飛如蝶形而去，痛不可忍，是火毒也。大黄、朴硝各半兩，爲末，水服取利即愈。張杲醫説。

Butterfly-type sores caused by moxibustion/cauterization. When the cauterization with mugwort is completed and the scabs caused by the fire vanish, fresh flesh in the sores is shaped like a butterfly and leaves [the sore] with an unbearable pain. This is a "fire poisoning." [Grind] half a *liang* each of *da huang* and mirabilite into powder and ingest it with water to stimulate a free flow. This is the cure. Zhang Gao, *Yi shuo.*

蠼螋咬瘡。大黄末塗之。醫説。

Sores caused by earwig bites. Apply *da huang* powder [to the affected region]. *Yi shuo.*

火丹赤腫遍身者。大黄磨水，頻刷之。急救方。

Fire cinnabar[827] with a red swelling covering the entire body. Rub *da huang* in water and repeatedly brush the [body] with [the liquid]. *Ji jiu fang.*

827 火丹, "fire cinnabar," a condition of *dan du* 丹毒, "cinnabar-red poison," displaying a color like fire that rushes through the skin, spreading with great speed. BCGM Dict I,

腫毒初起。大黄、五倍子、黄蘗等分，爲末。新汲水調塗，日四五次。簡便方。

A swelling with poison that has just begun to rise. [Grind] equal amounts of *da huang*, Chinese sumac gallnut, and *phellodendron* bark into powder, mix it with newly drawn water and apply this [to the affected region]. Four to five times a day. *Jian bian fang.*

癰腫焮熱作痛。大黄末，醋調塗之。燥即易，不過數易即退，甚驗，神方也。肘後方。

Painful swelling with a radiating heat related to an obstruction-illness.[828] Mix *da huang* powder with vinegar and apply this [to the affected region]. Replace it [with a moist mixture] when it has dried. [The swelling] will recede after only a few such replacements. Very effective. A divine recipe. *Zhou hou fang.*

乳癰腫毒。金黄散：用川大黄、粉草各一兩爲末，好酒熬成膏收之。以絹攤貼瘡上，仰卧。仍先以温酒服一大匙，明日取下惡物。婦人經驗方。

Breast obstruction-illness[829] with a poison swelling. The "golden yellow powder." [Grind] one *liang* each of [Si] chuan *da huang* and *glycyrrhiza* [root] into powder. Simmer it with good wine to generate a paste and store it. Spread it on a silk fabric and attach it to the sore. Then [let the woman] lie down facing upward. Before this, she is to ingest one generous spoonful of warm wine. The next day she will discharge malign items. *Fu ren jing yan fang.*

大風癩瘡。大黄煨一兩，皂角刺一兩，爲末。每服方寸匕，空心温酒下，取出惡毒物如魚腦狀。未下再服，即取下如亂髮之蟲。取盡，乃服雄黄、花蛇藥，名通天再造散。十便良方。

For massive wind,[830] [i. e.,] repudiation-illness,[831] sores. [Grind] one *liang* of *da huang*, simmered, and one *liang* of *gleditsia* pod spikes into powder. Each time ingest the amount held by a square *cun* spoon, to be sent down on an empty stomach

232.

828 *Yong* 癰, "obstruction-illness,"refers to an obstruction of vessels or other ducts inside the body. Qi rushing against the obstruction may cause a local swelling and eventually break through the surface to cause an abscess. BCGM Dict I, 641.

829 *Ru yong* 乳癰, "breast obstruction-illness," a condition of acute putrefication of a woman's breast. Often encountered if a woman, following delivery, experiences *chui nai* 吹奶, "inflated breast," or *du ru* 妒乳, "jealousy breast." BCGM Dict I, 412.

830 *Da feng* 大風, "massive wind," may refer to sores caused by a massive intrusion of wind evil and also to conditions of leprosy. BCGM Dict I, 111.

831 *Lai* 癩, "*lai*-illness," "repudiation-illness," including cases of leprosy/Aussatz." BCGM Dict I, 293.

with warm wine. [The body] will emit malign, poisonous items similar to the shape of fish brain. If it fails to discharge [such items] ingest [the powder] a second time. This then will lead to a discharge of worms shaped like disheveled human hair. Once this has ended, ingest realgar and embroidered pit-viper as medication. This [recipe] is called the "powder for a second creation in correspondence with heaven." *Shi bian liang fang.*

17-01-02
葉 *Ye*
Leaf [of *da huang*]

【氣味】酸，寒，無毒。

Qi and Flavor. Sour, cold, nonpoisonous.

【主治】置薦下，辟虱蟲。相感志。

Control. Placed underneath a straw mat it keeps away lice and worms/bugs. *Xiang gang zhi.*

17-02
商陸本經下品
Shang lu, FE *Ben jing*, lower rank

***Phytolacca acinosa* Roxb. Indian pokeweed.**

【釋名】蓫募音逐湯、當陸開寶、章柳圖經、白昌開寶、馬尾廣雅、夜呼本經。【時珍曰】此物能逐蕩水氣，故曰蓫募。訛爲商陸，又訛爲當陸，北音訛爲章柳。或云枝枝相值，葉葉相當，故曰當陸。或云多當陸路而生也。

Explanation of Names. *Zhu tang* 蓫募, read *zhu tang* 逐湯, *dang lu* 當陸, *Kai bao. Zhang liu* 章柳, *Tu jing. Bai chang* 白昌, "white and prosperous," *Kai bao. Ma wei* 馬尾, "horse tail," *Guang ya. Ye hu* 夜呼, "night cry," *Ben jing.* [Li] Shizhen: This item can "drive out," *zhu* 逐, and "wash away," *tang* 蕩, water qi. Therefore it is called *zhu tang* 蓫募, which is erroneously modified to *shang lu* 商陸, which in turn is further erroneously modified to *dang lu* 當陸. In the northern pronunciation this is erroneously modified to *zhang liu* 章柳. Some say that because its twigs are interconnected and its leaves grow next to each other, *xiang dang* 相當, it is named *dang lu* 當陸, "next to the road." Still others say that it [is named *dang lu* 當陸 because it] often grows close to roadways, *dang lu lu* 當陸路.

【集解】【别録曰】商陸生咸陽川谷。如人形者有神。【恭曰】此有赤白二種. 白者入藥用，赤者見鬼神, 甚有毒。【保昇曰】所在有之。葉大如牛舌而厚脆，赤花者根赤，白花者根白。二月、八月采根，日乾。【頌曰】俗名章柳根，多生於人家園圃中。春生苗，高三四尺，青葉如牛舌而長。莖青赤，至柔脆。夏秋開紅紫花，作朵。根如蘿蔔而長，八九月采之。爾雅謂之蓫募，廣雅謂之馬尾，易經謂之莧陸。【斅曰】一種赤昌，苗葉絶相類，不可服之，有傷筋骨消腎之毒。惟花白年多者，仙人采之作脯，可下酒也。【時珍曰】商陸昔人亦種之爲蔬，取白根及紫色者擘破，作畦栽之，亦可種子。根、苗、莖並可洗蒸食，或用灰汁煮過亦良。服丹砂、乳石人食之尤利。其赤與黄色者有毒，不可食。按周憲王救荒本草云：章柳幹粗似雞冠花幹，微有線楞，色微紫赤，極易生植。

Collected Explanations. *Bie lu*: *Shang lu* grows in river valleys of Xian yang. Those that are shaped similar to humans include a spirit. [Su] Gong: This [herb] has two kinds, red and white. White specimens are added to medication. Red ones let one see demon spirits; they are very poisonous. [Han] Baosheng: [*Shang lu*] can be found everywhere. The leaves are as big as an ox tongue; they are thick and brittle. Those with red flowers have a red root; those with white flowers have a white root. The root is collected in the second and eighth month; it is dried in the sun. [Su] Song: It is commonly called *zhang liu* 章柳 root and it often grows planted in private gardens. In spring a seedling grows; it is three to four *chi* tall. The greenish leaves are similar to an ox tongue, but longer. The stem is greenish-red; it is extremely soft and brittle. Red-purple flowers open in summer and autumn. They form flower buds. The root is similar to carrots, but longer. It is collected in the eighth and ninth month. The *Er ya* call is *zhu tang* 蓫募. The *Guang ya* calls it *ma wei* 馬尾, "horse tail." The *Yi jing* calls it *xian lu* 莧陸. [Lei] Xiao: There is a *chi chang* 赤昌 with a seedling and leaves very similar [to those of *shang lu*]. But it must not be ingested. It has a poison harming sinews and bones and dissolving the kidneys. Only those that have had white flowers for many years are collected by the hermits/immortals to make prepared food. It can be sent down with wine. [Li] Shizhen: *Shang lu* was also planted by the ancients as a vegetable. They took the white root and also those of purple color, broke them apart and stuck them into a field. The seeds, too, can be planted. The root, the seedling and the stem can be eaten when they are washed and steamed. Some boil them with ash juice; this is good, too. When persons who ingest cinnabar and stalactites eat them, this is especially useful. Red and yellow specimens are poisonous; they are not edible. According to Zhou Xian[832] wang's *Jiu huang ben cao*, the trunk of *zhang liu* is rough and resembles the trunk of cockscomb herbs, but has some slight threads and corners. The color is slightly purple-red. It is very easy to plant.

832 Instead of Zhou xian wang 周憲王, the *Ming shi* 明史 writes Zhou ding wang 周定王.

17-02-01
根 *Gen*
Root [of *shang lu*].

【修治】【斅曰】取花白者根，銅刀刮去皮，薄切，以東流水浸兩宿，漉出，架甑蒸，以黑豆葉一重，商陸一重，如此蒸之，從午至亥，取出去豆葉，暴乾剉用。無豆葉，以豆代之。

Pharmaceutical Preparation. [Lei] Xiao: Take the roots [of *shang lu* herbs] with a white flower. Cut off the bark with a copper knife, and cut [the roots] into thin slices. Soak them for two days and nights in water flowing eastward. Then filter them to remove them [from the water] and give them into a rice steamer where they are placed on one layer each of black soybeans leaves and Indian pokewee [roots]. This way steam it, from *wu* 午 hours (11 – 13) to *hai* 亥 hours (21 – 23). Remove the bean leaves, dry [the *shang lu* pieces] in the sun, and for its use [for therapeutic purposes] cut them even further. If bean leaves are not available, they can be replaced with the beans.

【氣味】辛，平，有毒。【別録曰】酸。【權曰】甘，有大毒。忌犬肉。【大明曰】白者苦冷，得大蒜良。赤者有毒，能伏硇砂、砒石、雌黄，拔錫。【恭曰】赤者但可貼腫，服之傷人，痢血不已殺人，令人見鬼神。【張仲景曰】商陸以水服，殺人。【杲曰】商陸有毒，陽中之陰。其味酸辛，其形類人。其用療水，其效如神。

Qi and Flavor. Acrid, balanced, poisonous. *Bie lu*: Sour. [Zhen] Quan: Sweet, very poisonous. [While it is ingested] avoid dog meat. Da Ming: White ones are bitter and cold. It is good to combine them with garlic. Red ones are poisonous. They are able to subdue [the effects of] sal ammoniac, arsenic and orpiment, and they suck out tin. [Su] Gong: Red ones are suitable only for being attached to a swelling; to ingest them harms one with an unending, fatal free-flow with blood and lets one see demon spirits. Zhang Zhongjing: *Shang lu* ingested with water kills one. [Li] Gao: *Shang lu* is poisonous. It is a yin in yang [substance]. Its flavor is sour and [its qi are] balanced. Its physical appearance is that of humans. It is resorted to to heal water [swelling]. Its effects are divine.

【主治】水腫疝瘕痺，熨除癰腫，殺鬼精物。本經。療胸中邪氣，水腫痿痺，腹滿洪直，疏五臟，散水氣。別録。瀉十種水病。喉痺不通，薄切醋炒，塗喉外，良。甄權。通大小腸，瀉蠱毒，墮胎，熻腫毒，傅惡瘡。大明。

Control. Water swelling, elevation-illness with conglomeration-illness,[833] and blockage. Applied as a hot compression it removes swelling associated with an obstruction-illness.[834] It kills demons and essence/spirit items. *Ben jing*. It heals evil qi in the chest, water swelling, dysfunction and blockage, abdominal fullness with a vast bloating. It clears the five long-term depots and disperses water qi. *Bie lu*. It serves to drain the ten kinds of water diseases. [To cure] throat blockage, fry thin slices in vinegar and attach them to the outside of the throat. Good. Zhen Quan. It frees the passage through the large and the small intestine, drains *gu* poison,[835] causes abortion and [serves to cure] heat swelling with poison. Apply it to malign sores. Da Ming.

【發明】【弘景曰】方家不甚用，惟療水腫，切生根，雜鯉魚煮作湯服。道家乃散用之，及煎釀服，皆能去尸蟲，見鬼神。其實子亦入神藥。花名募花，尤良。【頌曰】古方術家多用之，亦可單服。五月五日采根，竹籮盛，掛屋東北角，陰乾百日，搗篩，井華水調服，云神仙所秘法也。【時珍曰】商陸苦寒，沉也，降也，陰也。其性下行，專於行水。與大戟、甘遂，蓋異性而同功。胃氣虛弱者不可用。方家治腫滿、小便不利者，以赤根搗爛，入麝香三分，貼於臍心，以帛束之，得小便利即腫消。又治濕水以指畫肉上，隨散不成文者。用白商陸、香附子炒乾，出火毒，以酒浸一夜，日乾爲末。每服二錢，米飲下。或以大蒜同商陸煮汁服亦可。其莖葉作蔬食，亦治腫疾。【嘉謨曰】古讚云：

其味酸辛，其形類人。
療水貼腫，其效如神。

斯言盡之矣。

Explication. [Tao] Hongjing: Recipe experts do not use it often. Only to heal water swelling the fresh root is cut into slices, boiled with carps and ingested as a decoction. Daoists use it as a powder, and they ingest it boiled and passed through a brewing process. Both ways, it can eliminate corpse worms/bugs, and it lets one see demons and spirits. The fruit and seeds, too, are added to spirit medication. The flowers are called *tang hua* 募花. They are especially good. [Su] Song: The ancient

833 *Shan jia* 疝瘕, "elevation-illness with conglomeration-illness." A lump-like swelling in the abdomen that alternately collects and then dissolves again. BCGM Dict I, 418.

834 *Yong* 癰, "obstruction-illness,"refers to an obstruction of vessels or other ducts inside the body. Qi rushing against the obstruction may cause a local swelling and eventually break through the surface to cause an abscess. BCGM Dict I, 641.

835 *Gu du* 蠱毒, "*gu*-poison[ing]." (1) A poison emitted by certain worms/snakes with an ability to cause varying pathological changes in a person who has taken it in by means of wine or food. (2) Abdominal fullness, in some cases with blood spitting, and blood in the stool and urine. BCGM Dict I, 192 - 193. See BCGM 42-22.

experts of the recipe art used it often. It can also be ingested as a single substance. The root is collected on the fifth day of the fifth month. Put it in a bamboo basket and hang it at the North-East corner of the house to dry in the yin (i. e., shade) for one hundred days. Then pound it [and give the powder] through a sieve. Mix it with well splendor water[836] and ingest this. This is said to be a secret method of spirits and hermits/immortals. [Li] Shizhen: *Shang lu* is bitter and cold; it sinks into the depth. It is a yin [substance]. By its nature it causes downward movements. In particular, it stimulates the movement of water. The fact is, its nature is different from that of Peking spurge and kansui [root], but the [therapeutic] potential is identical. [Persons] with a depletion and weakness of stomach qi must not use it. Recipe experts who cure swelling with a feeling of fullness, and blocked urination, they pound the red root to a pulp, add three *fen* of musk and attach this to the navel in the center. Then they bandage this with a silk cloth and once the urine flows freely, the swelling dissolves. It is also used to cure [swelling caused by] moisture and water when a finger drawn on [the patient's] flesh does not leave a line design [with the following recipe]. Fry white *shang lu* and nutgrass until they are dry and [wait] until the fire poison has left. Then soak them in wine for one night, dry them in the sun and [grind them into] powder. Each time ingest two *qian*; to be sent down with a rice beverage. Or boil garlic together with *shang lu* and ingest the juice. This is possible, too. The stem and the leaves prepared to and eaten as vegetables, they, too, serve to cure swelling illnesses. [Chen] Jiamo: An ancient eulogy states:

"Its flavor is sour and acrid. Its physical appearance resembles that of humans.
To heal water [illness] attach it to the swelling. Its effects are divine."

That is a comprehensive statement.

【附方】舊九。新六。

Attached Recipes. Nine of old. Six newly [recorded].

濕氣脚軟。章柳根切小豆大，煮熟，更以緑豆同煮爲飯。每日食之，以瘥爲度，最效。斗門方。

Soft legs because of moisture qi presence. Cut *zhang liu* roots into pieces the size of red mung beans and boil them until done. Then boil them further together with mung beans to prepare a meal with cooked rice. Eat this every day until a cure is achieved. Very effective. *Dou men fang.*

水氣腫滿。外臺秘要用白商陸根去皮，切如豆大一大盞，以水二升，煮一升。更以粟米一大盞，同煮成粥。每日空心食之，取微利，不得雜食。

836 *Jing hua shui* 井華水, "well splendor water," i. e., the first water drawn from a well in the morning. BCGM Vol. II, 05-15-01.

Swelling and a feeling of fullness because of water qi presence. The *Wai tai bi yao* [recommends to] remove the skin of white *shang lu* roots and cut one generous *qian* into pieces the size of soybeans. Boil them in two *sheng* of water down to one *sheng*. Then boil them further with one large cup of millet to prepare a congee. Every day eat this on an empty stomach to stimulate a mild free flow. Do not eat [the congee] mixed with further items.

千金髓用白商陸六兩，取汁半合，和酒半升，看人與服。當利下水，取效。

The *Qian jin sui* [recommends to] obtain from six *liang* of white *shang lu* [roots] half a *ge* of juice, mix it with half a *sheng* of wine, and [let the patient] ingest it depending on the appearance of the respective person. This should free a discharge of the water and will be effective.

梅師方用白商陸一升，羊肉六兩，水一斗，煮取六升，去滓，和葱、豉作臛食之。

The *Mei shi fang* [recommends to] boil one *sheng* of white *shang lu* [root] and six *liang* of mutton in one *dou* of water down to six *sheng*, remove the dregs and with onions and fermented soy beans prepare a broth to be eaten [by the patient].

腹中暴癥，有物如石，痛刺啼呼，不治，百日死。多取商陸根擣汁或蒸之，以布藉腹上，安藥，勿覆，冷即易，晝夜勿息。孫真人千金方。

Sudden abdominal concretion-illness, with an item similar to a stone and a piercing pain making one scream out loud. If this is not cured, [the patient] will die within 100 days. Pound a large quantity of *shang lu* roots to obtain a juice, or steam it. Then spread a piece of cloth on the [patient's] abdomen, place the medication on it, and place another layer [of cloth] on top of it.[837] Once [the medication] has cooled, replace it [with a hot application]. Continue day and night without a break. Sun zhenren, *Qian jin fang*.

痃癖如石，在脇下堅硬。生商陸根汁一升，杏仁一兩，浸去皮，擣如泥，以商陸汁絞杏泥，火煎如餳。每服棗許，空腹熱酒服，以利下惡物爲度。聖惠方。

Stone-like string-illness[838] and aggregation-illness with a hardening below the flanks. Prepare one *sheng* of fresh *shang lu* root juice. Also, soak one *liang* of apricot kernels [in water], remove the skin and pound it to a mud-like consistency. Then

837 Instead of *wu* 勿, "do not …", *Qian jin fang* ch. 11, *jian zheng ji ju* 堅癥積聚, "hard concretion-illness, accumulations and collections," writes *yi wu* 衣物, "clothing," "garment." This translation follows the *Qian jin fang* wording.

838 *Xuan* 痃, "string-illness," a condition of acute pain located in the abdomen to the left and right of the umbilicus. BCGM Dict I, 591.

mix the *shang lu* juice with the apricot [kernel] mud and squeeze this [to obtain a liquid]. Boil it until it has assumed a consistency of malt sugar. Each time ingest the amount of a Chinese date. To be ingested on an empty abdomen with hot wine until a free flow discharges malign items. *Sheng hui fang*.

產後腹大，堅滿，喘不能卧。白聖散：用章柳根三兩，大戟一兩半，甘遂炒一兩，爲末。每服二三錢，熱湯調下，大便宜利爲度。此乃主水聖藥也。潔古保命集。

Enlarged abdominen following delivery, with a hardening and a feeling of fullness, panting and an inability to lie down. The "white sage-like powder." [Grind] three *liang* of *zhang liu* root, one and a half *liang* of Peking spurge [root] and one *liang* of fried kansui [root] into powder. Each time ingest two to three *qian*, to be sent down mixed with hot, boiled water until a free flow of defecation is achieved. This is a sage-like medication to control water [disorders]. [Zhang] Jiegu, *Bao ming ji*.

五尸注痛。腹痛脹急，不得喘息，上攻心胸，旁攻兩脅，痛或礫塊涌起。用商陸根熬，以囊盛，更互熨之，取效。肘後方。

Painful influx of the five types of corpse [qi],[839] with an aching, enlarged and tense abdomen, and an inability to breathe. [The corpse qi] rise to attack heart and chest, and they attack the two flanks on the sides. The pain may be accompanied by a violent rise of stone-like lumps. Simmer *shang lu* roots to a paste, fill it into a bag and apply it as a hot compression [to the affected region] until an effect is achieved. *Zhou hou fang*.

小兒痘毒。小兒將痘發熱，失表，忽作腹痛，及膨脹弩氣，乾霍亂，由毒氣與胃氣相搏，欲出不得出也。以商陸根和葱白搗傅臍上，斑止痘出，方免無虞。摘玄方。

Smallpox poison affecting children. When smallpox is about to break out with a heat effusion, and the cure of this illness sign [of heat] is missed, [patients] suddenly develop abdominal pain, swelling, distension and [archer-like] crossbow qi,[840] as well as dry cholera. This is because the poison qi and the stomach qi clash; the [smallpox poison qi] wish to leave [the body] but are unable to leave. Pound *shang lu* root and onion white [to a pulp] and apply this to the [child's] navel. The skin speckles disappear and the pox come out. This is a recipe for a carefree application. *Zhai xuan fang*.

---

839 *Wu shi* 五屍," the five types of corpse [qi]." BCGM Dict I, 158.

840 *She gong* 射工, "archer," (1) a small bug in ancient times believed to live in water and be capable of "shooting" poison from its mouth at people, thereby causing disease; (2) a condition caused by the archer's poison. BCGM Dict. I, 432. See BCGM 42-15.

耳卒熱腫。生商陸，削尖納入，日再易。聖濟録。

Sudden swelling of the ears with heat. Cut a fresh *shang lu* [root] to give it a pointed end and insert it [into the affected ear]. Repeatedly replace it during the day. *Sheng ji lu.*

喉卒攻痛。商陸切根炙熱，隔布熨之，冷即易，立愈。圖經本草。

Sudden, beating pain in the throat. Cut a *shang lu* root, roast it until it is hot and press it, separated by a piece of cloth, [on the affected region]. When it has cooled, replace it [with a hot compress]. A cure is achieved immediately. *Tu jing ben cao.*

瘰癧喉痺，攻痛。生商陸根搗作餅，置癧上，以艾炷于上灸三四壯，良。外臺秘要。

Scrofula pervasion-illness[841] with throat closure and a beating pain. Pound fresh *shang lu* roots to prepare a cake and place it on the [location of the] pervasion-illness. Place a mugwort cone on [the cake] and cauterize this three to four times. Good. *Wai tai mi yao.*

一切毒腫。章陸根和鹽少許，搗傅，日再易之。孫真人千金方。

All kinds of poison swelling. Pound *zhang lu* root with a little salt [to a pulp] and apply this [to the affected region]. Replace it several times a day. Sun zhenren, *Qian jin fang.*

石癰如石，堅硬不作膿者。生章陸根搗擦之，燥即易，取軟爲度。亦治濕漏諸癤。张文仲方。

Stone obstruction-illness similar to a stone. A hardening that does not fester. Pound fresh *zhang lu* root [to a pulp] and apply this [to the affected region]. When it has dried, replace it. Continue this until [the hardening] has softened. This also serves to cure moisture with leakage and all types of pimples. *Zhang Wenzhong fang.*

瘡傷水毒。章陸根搗炙，布裹熨之，冷即易之。千金方。

Sores as harm caused by water poison. Pound *zhang lu* root [to a pulp] and fry it. Wrap it in a piece of cloth and apply it as a hot compress [to the affected region]. When it has cooled, replace it [with a hot compress]. *Qian jin fang.*

---

841 *Luo li* 瘰癧, "scrofula pervasion-illness," when two or more connected swellings of the size of plum or date kernels appear either on the neck or in the armpits, or somewhere else on the body. BCGM Dict I. 329.

17-02-02
募花 ***Tang hua***
Flower [of *shang lu*].

【主治】人心昏塞，多忘喜誤，取花陰乾百日，搗末，日暮水服方寸匕乃卧，思念所欲事，即於眠中醒悟也。蘇頌。

Control. A person's heart affected by clouding and blockage.[842] [Patients] forget a lot and tend to make mistakes. Dry the flowers in the yin (i. e., shade) for 100 days and pound them into powder. In the evening [let the patient] ingest it with the amount of water held by a square *cun* spoon and then go to bed where he is to think about things he longs for. While he sleeps, he will come to his senses. Su Song.

17-03
狼毒本經下品
Lang du, FE *Ben jing*, lower rank.
***Stellaria chamaejasme* L. Wolfsbane.**[843]

【釋名】【時珍曰】觀其名，知其毒矣。

Explanation. [Li] Shizhen: Read the name and you know that it is poisonouns.

【集解】【别録曰】狼毒生秦亭山谷及奉高。二月、八月采根，陰乾。陳而沉水者良。【弘景曰】宕昌亦出之。乃言止有數畝地生，蝮蛇食其根，故爲難得。亦用太山者。今用出漢中及建平。云與防葵同根，但置水中沉者是狼毒，浮者是防葵。俗用亦稀，爲療腹内要藥耳。【恭曰】今出秦州、成州，秦亭原在二州之界。秦隴地寒，元無蝮蛇。此物與防葵都不同類，生處又別，太山、漢中亦不聞有，陶説謬矣。【志曰】狼毒葉似商陸及大黄，莖葉上有毛，根皮黄，肉白。以實重者爲良，輕者爲力劣。秦亭在隴西，奉高是太山下縣。陶云"沉者是狼毒，浮者是防葵"，此不足爲信。假使防葵秋冬采者堅實，得水皆沉；狼毒春夏采者輕虚，得水皆浮。且二物全别，不可比類。此與麻黄、橘皮、半夏、枳實、吴茱萸爲六陳也。【保昇曰】根似玄參，惟浮虚者爲劣也。【頌曰】今陜西州郡及遼、石州亦有之，狀如馬志所説。【時珍曰】狼毒出秦、晉地。今人往往以草蔄茹爲之，誤矣。見蔄茹下也。

Collected Explanations. *Bie lu*: *Lang du* grows in the mountain valleys of Qin ting and in Feng gao. The root is collected in the second and eighth month. It is dried in the yin (i. e., shade). Those are good that have been stored for a long time and sink down in water. [Tao] Hongjing: It also comes from Dang chang. They say that it

842 *Hun sai* 昏塞, "clouding and blockage," an illness sign of slowed down thinking with an obvious decrease of one's faculty of memory. BCGM Dict I, 230.

843 *Lang du* 狼毒, lit.: "its poison is as dangerous as a wolf."

grows only on a few *mu*/acres of land, and because breficaude pit vipers eat its root, it is difficult to obtain [large quantities]. So, [*lang du*] from Mount Tai shan is used, too. Today, specimens coming from Han zhong and Jian ping are used. It is said that the root is equal to *peucedanum* root. However, when the two are placed in a water, *lang du* sinks down, while *fang kui* floats. Common [physicians] seldom resort to it, but it is an important pharmaceutical substance for healing intra-abdominal [disorders]. [Su] Gong: Today it comes from Qin zhou and from the border region of the two *zhou* Cheng zhou and Qing ting. The region of Qin long is cold and basically there are no breficaude pit vipers. This item is not at all related to *peucedanum*. Also, the regions where they grow differ, and it has not been heard of that [it grows] on Mount Tai shan and in Han zhong. What Tao [Hongjing] says is wrong. [Ma] Zhi: The leaves of *lang du* resemble those of Indian pokeweed and rhubarb. Its stem and leaves have hair; the root has a yellow skin; its flesh is white. Those that are solid and heavy are good. Light ones have less strength. Qin ting lies in Long xi; Qin gao is a county at the foot of Mount Tai shan. When Tao [Hongjing] states "those that sink are *lang du*; those that float are *peucedanum* [roots]," this is not reliable. If *peucedanum* [root] is collected for application in autumn and winter, it is hard and solid and it will always sink down in water. *Lang du* collected in spring and summer is light and hollow and will always float in water. Also, these two items are completely different; they cannot be related. [*Lang du*] with *ephedra* [herb], tangerine peels, *pinellia* [root], bitter orange fruit and *zanthoxylum* [fruit] belongs to those six [herbal substances] that are stored for a long time [before they can be used for therapeutic purposes]. [Han] Baosheng: The root resembles that of *scrophularia*. Only when it is hollow and floats, its [strength] is inferior. [Su] Song: Today it is also present in the *zhou* and prefectures of Shaan xi, and in Shi zhou. It is shaped as is told by Ma Zhi. [Li] Shizhen: *Lang du* comes from Qin and Jin. Today many people offer spurge [as *lang du*]. That is wrong. See under [the entry] "*lü ru* 藺茹/spurge" (17-06).

17-03-01
根 *Gen*
Root [of *lang du*].

【氣味】辛，平，有大毒。【大明曰】苦，辛，有毒。【之才曰】大豆爲之使，宜醋炒，惡麥句薑，畏占斯、蜜佗僧也。

Qi and Flavor. Acrid, balanced, very poisonous. Da Ming: Bitter, acrid, poisonous. [Xu] Zhicai: Soybeans serve as its guiding substance. It should be fried in vinegar. [Ingested together,] it abhors common *carpesium*, and fears *taxillus* mistletoe and litharge.

【主治】欬逆上氣，破積聚飲食，寒熱水氣，惡瘡鼠瘻疽蝕，鬼精蠱毒，殺飛鳥走獸。本經。除胸下積僻。别録。治痰飲癥瘕，亦殺鼠。大明。合野葛納耳中，治聾。抱朴子。

Control. Cough with qi rising in counterflow. It breaks through accumulations and collections of beverages and food, alternating sensations of cold and heat with water qi [disorders], malign sores, mouse fistula,[844] and impediment-illness[845] with erosion. [It serves to cure attachment-illnes with] demons and spirit-essence, as well as *gu* poison.[846] It kills flying birds and running animals. *Ben jing*. It removes abnormal accumulations from below the chest. *Bie lu*. It serves to cure phlegm rheum, concretion-illness and conglomeration-illness.[847] Also, it kills mice/rats. Da Ming. Inserted together with *gelsemium* herb into the ears, it serves to cure deafness. *Baopu zi*.

【附方】舊四，新六。

Added Recipes. Four of old. Six newly [recorded].

心腹連痛，作脹。用狼毒二兩，附子半兩，搗篩，蜜丸梧子大。一日服一丸，二日二丸，三日三丸止。又從一丸起，至三丸止，以瘥爲度。肘後方。

Extending pain in the central and abdominal region, with a distension. Pound two *liang* of *lang du* and half a *liang* of *aconitum* [accessory tuber into powder] and pass it through a sieve. Then form with honey pills the size of *wu* seeds. On the first day, ingest one pill. On the second day two pills. On the third day three pills, and stop. Then begin again with one pill and stop [on the third day] with three pills. Continue this until a cure is achieved. *Zhou hou fang*.

九種心痛。一蟲，二蛀，三風，四悸，五食，六飲，七冷，八熱，九氣也。又治連年積冷，流注心胸，及落馬墮車，瘀血中惡等證。九痛丸：用

844 *Shu lou* 鼠瘻, "mouse fistula," BCGM Dict I, 466, identical to *luo li* 瘰癧, "scrofula pervasion-illnes."

845 *Ju* 疽, "impediment-illness," refers to an obstruction of vessels or other ducts inside the body. Qi rushing against the impediment may cause a local swelling and eventually break through the surface to cause an abscess. BCGM Dict I, 277.

846 *Gu du* 蠱毒, "*gu*-poison[ing]." (1) A poison emitted by certain worms/snakes with an ability to cause varying pathological changes in a person who has taken it in by means of wine or food. (2) Abdominal fullness, in some cases with blood spitting, and blood in the stool and urine. BCGM Dict I, 192 - 193. See BCGM 42-22.

847 *Zheng jia* 癥瘕, "concretion-illness and conglomeration-illness." The two terms are often used interchangeably and do not signify two distinctly different conditions. Concretion-illness and conglomeration-illness result from a disharmony of cold and warmth resulting in a failure to transform beverages and food. Nodes form when the clash with the qi of the long-term depots. BCGM Dict I, 677.

狼毒炙香，吴茱萸湯泡，巴豆去心，炒取霜，乾薑炮，人參各一兩，附子炮去皮三兩，爲末，煉蜜丸梧子大，每空腹溫酒下一丸。和劑局方。

The nine kinds of heart pain. First, [caused by] worms/bugs. Second, [caused by] moths. Third, [caused by] wind. Fourth, [related to] palpitation. Fifth, [caused by] food. Sixth, [caused by] a beverage. Seventh, [caused by] cold. Eighth, [caused by] heat. Ninth, [caused by] qi [disorder]. Also, it serves to cure cold accumulation formed over several years that has flowed into the heart and the chest. Furthermore, stagnating blood after a fall from a horse or from a car, and being struck by the malign. The "pills for nine kinds of pain." [Grind the following substances into] powder: One *liang* each of *lang du*, fried until it develops fragrance, *zanthoxylum* [root], macerated in hot water, *croton* seeds with the heart discarded and the rest fried to obtain a frost, dried ginger, roasted in a pan, and ginseng [root], as well as three *liang* of *aconitum* [accessory tuber] with its skin discarded. [Mix the powder] with heat refined honey to form pills the size of *wu* seeds. Each time ingest one pill, to be sent down with warm wine. *He ji ju fang*.

腹中冷痛，水穀陰結，心下停痰，兩脇痞滿，按之鳴轉，逆害飲食。用狼毒三兩，附子一兩，旋復花三兩，搗末，蜜丸梧子大。每服三丸，食前白湯下，日三服。肘後方。

Painful cold in the abdomen. Water and grain have invisibly conglomerated with abiding phlegm below the heart/stomach, and obstacle-illness with a feeling of fullness in the two flanks. When this is pressed, a sound of something revolving is heard. It moves in counterflow and harms [the intake of] beverages and food. Pound three *liang* of *lang du*, one *liang* of *aconitum* [accessory tuber] and three *liang* of horseheal flowers into powder and with honey form pills the size of *wu* seeds. Each time ingest three pills, to be sent down prior to a meal with clear, boiled water. To be ingested three times a day. *Zhou hou fang*.

陰疝欲死。丸縮入腹，急痛欲死。狼毒四兩，防風二兩，附子三兩燒，以蜜丸梧子大。每服三丸，日夜三度，白湯下。肘後方。

Yin elevation-illness[848] letting one wish to die, with the testicles drawn into the abdomen and a painful tension letting one wish to die. Burn four *liang* of *lang du*, two *liang* of *saposhnikovia* [root] and three *liang* of *aconitum* [accessory tuber] and form with honey pills the size of *wu* seeds. Each time ingest three pills; three times during the day and the night, to be sent down with clear, boiled water. *Zhou hou fang*.

848 *Yin shan* 陰疝, "yin elevation-illness," a condition with massive swelling and pain in the scrotum. BCGM Dict I, 635.

兩脅氣結。方同腹中冷痛方。

Bound qi in the two flanks. The recipe is identical to the recipe for painful cold in the abdomen.

一切蟲病。川狼毒杵末，每服一錢，用餳一皂子大，沙糖少許，以水化開，卧時空腹服之，次早即下蟲也。集效方。

All types of diseases related to the presence of worms/bugs. Pound *lang du* from [Si] chuan into powder. Each time ingest one *qian*. Dissolve [the powder] with malt-sugar, the size of a *gleditsia* seed, and a small amount of granulated sugar in water and boil it. Ingest this at bedtime on an empty abdomen. The next morning the worms/bugs are discharged. *Ji xiao fang.*

乾濕蟲疥。狼毒不拘多少，搗爛，以豬油、馬油調搽患處。方睡勿以被蒙頭，恐藥氣傷面。此維揚潘氏所傳方。藺氏經驗方。

Worms/bugs and *jie*-illness[849] with either dryness or moisture. Pound any amount of *lang du* into a pulpy consistency, mix it with lard and horse oil and apply this to the ailing location. If the [patient] happens to sleep, do not cover his head. The qi of the medication might harm his face. This is a recipe handed over by Mr. Pan from Wei yang. *Lan shi jing yan fang.*

積年疥癩。狼毒一兩，一半生研，一半炒研，輕粉三合，水銀三錢，以茶末少許，於瓦器内，以津液擦化爲末，同以清油浸藥，高一寸，三日，待藥沉油清，遇夜不見燈火，蘸油塗瘡上，仍以口鼻於藥盞上吸氣，取效。永類方。

Jie-illness and repudiation-illness[850] that have lasted for several years. Fill one *liang* of *lang du*, one half ground fresh, one half ground fried, two *ge* of calomel and three *qian* of mercury with a little tea powder into a pottery vessel. Rub all this until it has transformed into powder. Let the medicinal [powder] soak in a one *cun* high quantity of clear oil for three days until the medicinal [powder] has sunk to the bottom and the oil is clear again. The next night, where no lamp fire is seen, dip something into the oil and apply it to the sores. In addition, [let the patient] hold his mouth and nose above a cup with the medication and inhale its qi. This will be effective. *Yong lei fang.*

849 *Jie*-illness 疥, vaguely identifiable skin ailment. BCGM Dict I, 249.

850 *Lai* 癩, "*lai*-illness," "repudiation-illness," including cases of leprosy/Aussatz." BCGM Dict I, 293.

積年乾癬生痂，搔之黄水出，每逢陰雨即痒。用狼毒末塗之。聖惠方。

A dry *xuan*-illness[851] that has lasted for years with a formation of crusts that when scratched release a yellow water. When they encounter overcast and rain, they itch. Apply *lang du* powder [to the affected region]. *Sheng hui fang*.

惡疾風瘡。狼毒、秦艽等分，爲末。每服方寸匕，温酒下，日一二服。千金方。

Malign illnesses with wind [intrusion] forming sores. [Grind] equal amounts of *lang du* and large *gentiana* root into powder. Each time ingest the amount held by a square *cun* spoon, to be sent down with warm wine. To be ingested once or twice a day. *Qian jin fang*.

17-04
防葵本經上品
Fang kui, FE *Ben jing*, upper rank.

***Peucedanum japonicum* Thunb.**

【釋名】房苑別録、梨蓋本經、利茹吴普。又名爵離、方蓋、農果。【恭曰】根葉似葵花子根，香味似防風，故名防葵。

Explanation of Names. *Fang yuan* 房苑[852], *Bie lu*. *Li gai* 梨蓋, *Ben jing*. *Li ru* 利茹, Wu Pu. It is also named *jue li* 爵離, *fang gai* 方蓋 and *nong guo* 農果. [Su] Gong: The root and the leaves resemble the flower, seeds and root of Chinese mallow, *kui* 葵. It has a fragrant flavor resembling that of *saposhnikovia*, *fang feng* 防風, Hence its name *fang kui* 防葵.

【集解】【別録曰】防葵生臨淄川谷，及嵩高、太山、少室。三月三日采根，暴乾。【普曰】莖葉如葵，上黑黄。二月生根，根大如桔梗根，中紅白。六月花白，七月、八月實白。三月采根。【恭曰】此物亦稀有，襄陽、望楚、山東及興州西方有之。興州者乃勝南者，爲鄰蜀地也。【頌曰】今惟出襄陽地，他郡不聞也。其葉似葵，每莖三葉，一本十數莖，中發一幹，其端開花，如葱花、景天輩而色白，六月開花即結實。根似防風，香味亦如之，依時采者乃沉水。今乃用枯朽狼毒當之，極爲謬矣。【時珍曰】唐時隴西成州貢之。蘇頌所説詳明可據。

851 *Xuan* 癬, "*xuan*-illness." Conditions of dermal lesions with initially erythema, papules, and itching gradually extending in all directions to form an irregular ring with clear boundaries. The skin is slightly elevated with small papules, blisters, and/or scales and scraps. The central lesion may appear to heal spontaneously, and it may reappear. Also, a designation of local lesions with itching, release of liquid and shedding of scabs. BCGM Dict I, 591.

852 Instead of *fang yuan* 房苑, *Zheng lei* ch. 6, *fang kui* 防葵, quoting the *Bie lu* writes *fang ci* 房慈. *Fang yuan* 房苑 appears in *Yu lan* ch. 993, *fang kui* 房葵, quoting *Wu shi ben cao*.

Collected Explanations. *Bie lu*: *Fang kui* grows in the river valleys of Lin zi, and also in Song gao, on Mount Tai shan, and in Shao shi. The root is collected on the third day of the third month; it is dried in the sun. [Wu] Pu: Steam and leaves [of *fang kui* 防葵] resemble those of *kui* 葵, Chinese mallow. Above [*fang kui*] is black-yellow. The root grows in the second month. The root is as big as the *platycodon* root. It is red-white inside. White flowers [open] in the sixth month; white fruits form in the seventh and eighth month. The root is collected in the third month. [Su] Gong: This item is rare. It can be found in Xiang yang, Wang chu, and Shan dong, and also in the western regions of Xing zhou. Those from Xing zhou are superior to those from the South; it is a region adjacent to Shu. [Su] Song: Today it only comes from Xiang yang; it is not heard of in any other prefecture. Its leaves resemble those of Chinese mallows. Each stem has three leaves; from one base ten or more stems emerge with one trunk in the center. At its end flowers open similar to the flowers of onions and stonecrop, but they are white. When the flowers open in the sixth month, they will form fruits. The root resembles that of *saposhnikovia*; it, too, has a fragrant flavor. Those collected at the right time, they sink down in water. When today withered and decayed *lang du* is used instead, this is extremely mistaken! [Li] Shizhen: During the Tang era, Cheng zhou in Long xi submitted it [to the throne]. Su Song's statement is clear and reliable.

【正誤】【弘景曰】防葵今用建平者。本與狼毒同根，猶如三建，其形亦相似，但置水中不沉爾。而狼毒陳久者亦不能沉矣。【斅曰】凡使防葵，勿誤用狼毒，緣真相似，而驗之有異，效又不同，切須審之，恐誤人疾。其防葵在蔡州沙土中生，采得二十日便生蚛，用之惟輕爲妙。【恭曰】狼毒與防葵都不同類，生處亦別。【藏器曰】二物一是上品，善惡不同，形質又別。陶氏以浮沉爲別，後人因而用之，將以防葵破堅積爲下品之物，與狼毒同功。今古因循，遂無甄別，殊爲謬誤。

Correction of Errors. [Tao] Hongjing: Today the *fang kui* from Jian ping is used. Basically its root is identical to that of wolfsbane, and also similar to that of *san jian*.[853] Their physical appearances are similar. But the latter do not sink down when put into water. Still, *lang du* stored for a long time will not sink down either. [Lei] Xiao: For all applications of *fang kui*, do not use wolfsbane. They are truly very similar, but their [therapeutic] results differ, and their effects differ, too. They need to be carefully examined so that one does not take the wrong medication for the disease. The *fang kui* collected from the sandy soil in Cai zhou will generate moths 20 days later. For a [therapeutic] application, only light specimens are wondrous. [Su] Gong: Wolfsbane and *fang kui* are not related; the locations where they grow,

853 *San jian* 三建, an unidentified plant.

they differ, too. [Chen] Cangqi: Of these two items, only one is recorded as upper rank. They differ in their good and bad qualities and their physical appearance. Their material consistency is different, too. Mr. [Tao] Hongjing distinguished them on the basis of their ability to float or sink down. When people in later times followed him in their application [of these drugs], they used *fang kui* to break open hardened accumulations as if it were an item of lower rank, with the same [therapeutic] potential as wolfsbane. Through the times, [Tao Hongjing's advice] was followed and [the two drugs] were not distinguished. That has led to many errors.

17-04-01
根 *Gen*
Root [of *fang kui*].

【修治】【斅曰】凡使，須揀去蚛末，用甘草湯浸一宿，漉出暴乾，用黃精自然汁一二升拌了，土器中炒至汁盡用。

Pharmaceutical Preparation. [Lei] Xiao: For all [therapeutic] applications, pick those where the dust/powder left by moths is removed. Then soak them in a *glycyrrhiza* [root] decoction for one night. Strain [the liquid] to remove [the root] and dry it in the sun. Mix it with one or two *sheng* of the natural juice of Solomon's seal [root] and fry it in an earthen vessel until all the juice is gone. Then it may be used [for therapeutic ends].

【氣味】辛，寒，無毒。【別録曰】甘、苦。【普曰】神農：辛、寒。桐君、扁鵲：無毒。岐伯、雷公、黃帝：辛、苦，無毒。【權曰】有小毒。

Qi and Flavor. Acrid, cold, nonpoisonous. *Bie lu*: Sweet, bitter. [Wu] Pu: Shen nong: Acrid, cold. Tong jun, Bian Que: Nonpoisonous. Qi Bo, Lei gong, Huang Di: Acrid, bitter, nonpoisonous. [Zhen] Quan: Slightly poisonous.

【主治】疝瘕腸洩，膀胱熱結，溺不下，欬逆温瘧，癲癇驚邪狂走。久服堅骨髓，益氣輕身。本經。療五臟虛氣，小腹支滿臚脹，口乾，除腎邪，强志。中火者不可服，令人恍惚見鬼。別録。久服主邪氣驚狂。蘇恭。主痃癖氣塊，膀胱宿水，血氣瘤大如盌者，悉能消散。治鬼瘧，百邪鬼魅精怪，通氣。甄權。

Control. Elevation-illness with conglomeration-illness[854] and intestinal outflow, bound heat in the urinary bladder, blocked urination. Cough with [qi] counterflow and warmth malaria. Peak-illness,[855] epilepsy, fright evil and mad running. Ingested

854 *Shan jia* 疝瘕, "elevation-illness with conglomeration-illness." A lump-like swelling in the abdomen that alternately collects and then dissolves again. BCGM Dict I, 418.

855 *Dian ji* 癲[疾], "peak ailment," a mental disturbance of depression and unhappiness, with a calm attitude and little incentive to speak. BCGM Dict I, 125.

over a long time, it hardens bones and marrow, boosts the qi and relieves the body of its weight. *Ben jing.* It serves to heal conditions of depletion qi in the five long-term depots, propping fullness in the lower abdomen with a distension of the abdominal wall and a dry mouth. It eliminates evil [qi] from the kidneys, and strengthens the mind. Specimens struck by fire cannot be ingested; they let one be absent-minded and see demons. *Bie lu.* Ingested over a long time, it controls evil qi with fright and madness. Su Gong. It controls string-illness[856] and aggregation-illness[857] with qi lumps, water remaining in the urinary bladder overnight, and blood or qi tumors reaching the size of a bowl. It can dissolve and disperse them all alike. It serves to cure demon malaria, and unusual [ailments] caused by the hundred evil demons, monsters and spirit-essence. It frees the flow of qi. [Zhen] Quan.

【發明】【時珍曰】防葵乃神農上品藥，黄帝、岐伯、桐君、雷公、扁鵲、吴普皆言其無毒。獨别録言中火者服之，令人恍惚見鬼。陳延之小品方云：防葵多服，令人迷惑恍惚如狂。按難經云，重陽者狂，脱陽者見鬼，是豈上品養性所宜乎？是豈寒而無毒者乎？不然，則本經及蘇恭所列者，是防葵功用，而别録所列者，乃似防葵之狼毒功用，非防葵也。狼毒之亂防葵，其來亦遠矣，不可不辨。古方治蛇瘕、鼈瘕大方中，多用防葵，皆是狼毒也。

Explication. [Li] Shizhen: *Fang kui* is listed by Shen nong as an upper rank pharmaceutical drug. Huang Di, Qi Bo, Tong jun, Lei gong, Bian Que and Wu Pu, they all say: "It is nonpoisonous." Only the *Bie lu* states that "when it is ingested after it was struck by fire, it will let one be absent-minded and see demons." Chen Yanzhi in his *Xiao pin fang* states: "*Fang kui* ingested in large amounts lets one experience perplexity[858] and absent-mindedness similar to madness." According to the *Nan jing*, "doubled yang results in madness; loss of yang lets one see demons."[859] Does this agree with the functions of an upper rank [substance serving to] nourish one's nature? Is this [a substance] that is cold and nonpoisonous? This is not so. The *Ben jing* and Su Gong have listed the [therapeutic] potential and use of *fang kui*, while the *Bie lu* lists the [therapeutic] potential and use of wolfsbane that resembles *fang kui* but is not *fang kui*. The confusion of wolfsbane with *fang kui* has a long history. They must be distinguished. When ancient large recipes to cure snake conglom-

856 *Xuan* 痃, "string-illness," a condition of acute pain located in the abdomen to the left and right of the umbilicus. BCGM Dict I, 591.

857 *Pi* 癖, "aggregation-illness," of painful lumps emerging from time to time in both flanks. BCGM Dict I, 371.

858 *Mi huo* 迷惑, "perplexity," an illness sign of slowed thinking and a reduced ability to differentiate. BCGM Dict I, 339.

859 A quote from the 20th difficult issue of the *Nan jing*.

eration-illness[860] or tortoise conglomeration-illness, often resort to *fang kui*, they always [mean to resort to] wolfsbane.

【附方】舊一，新二。
腫滿洪大。防葵研末，温酒服一刀圭，至二三服。身瞤[861]及小不仁爲效。肘後方。
Massive [abdominal] swelling with a feeling of fullness. Ingest with warm wine of *fang kui* ground into powder the amount held by a knife blade. To be ingested twice or three times. When the body twitches and has some minor numbness, this shows the effect [of this therapy]. *Zhou hou fang*.

癲狂邪疾。方同上。
Peak-illness and madness, an evil [qi] illness. Recipe identical to the one above.

傷寒動氣。傷寒汗下後，臍左有動氣。防葵散：用防葵一兩，木香，黄芩、柴胡各半兩。每服半兩，水一盞半，煎八分，温服。雲岐子保命集。
Harm caused by cold and excited qi. When following a treatment of harm caused by cold with a therapy causing sweating and discharge the qi to the left of the navel are excited. The "powder with *fang kui*." Prepare a mixture of one *liang* of *fang kui* and half a *liang* each of *costus* [root], *scutellaria* [root] and *bupleurum* [root]. Each time ingest half a *liang*. Boil it in one and a half small cups of water down to 80% and ingest this warm. Yunqi zi, *Bao ming ji*.

17-05
狼牙本經下品
Lang ya, FE *Ben jing*, lower rank.

Agrimonia pilosa Ledeb. Hairy agrimony.[862]

【釋名】牙子本經、狼齒别録、狼子别録、犬牙吴普、抱牙吴普、支蘭李當之。【弘景曰】其牙似獸之齒牙，故有諸名。
Explanation of Names. *Ya zi* 牙子, *Ben jing*. *Lang chi* 狼齒, "a wolf's teeth," *Bie lu*. *Lang zi* 狼子, *Bie lu*. *Quan ya* 犬牙, "a dog's teeth," Wu Pu. *Bao ya* 抱牙, "hold-

860 *She jia* 蛇瘕, "snake conglomeration-illness," a *jia* 瘕, "conglomeration-illness," in the abdomen that has the shape of a snake and moves when squeezed. It was believed that the formation of such aggregations is associated with the consumption of snakes or an inadvertent ingestion of food contaminated with snake sperm. BCGM Dict I, 433.

861 Instead of *run* 瞤, "to twitch," *Zheng lei* ch. 6, *fang kui* 防葵, and *Zhou hou fang* ch. 3, zhi zu fa dian kuang bing fang 治卒發癲狂病方, "recipes for a sudden outbreak of peak-illness/madness diseases," both write run 潤, "to moisten."

862 *Lang ya* 狼牙, lit.: "a wolf's teeth."

ing teeth," Wu Pu. *Zhi lan* 支蘭, Li Dangzhi. [Tao] Hongjing: These [substances called] *ya* 牙, "teeth," resemble the teeth, *chi ya* 齒牙, of wild animals. Hence all these names.

【集解】【别録曰】狼牙生淮南川谷及冤句。八月采根，暴乾。中濕腐爛生衣者殺人。【普曰】葉青，根黄赤，六月、七月華，八月實黑，正月、八月采根。【保昇曰】所在有之。苗似蛇莓而厚大，深緑色。根黑若獸之牙。三月、八月采根，日乾。【頌曰】今江東、汴東州郡多有之。【時珍曰】范子計然云：建康及三辅，色白者善。

Collected Explanations. *Bie lu*: *Lang ya* grows in the river valleys of Huai nan, and also in Yuan ju. The root is collected in the eighth month; it is dried in the sun. Those with moisture inside, that are rotten and pulpy, and have developed an outer "garment," they kill one. [Wu] Pu: Its leaves are greenish. The root is yellow-red. Flowers blossom in the sixth and seventh month. Black fruits form in the eighth month. The root is collected in the first and eighth month. [Han] Baosheng: It can be found everywhere. The seedling resembles that of Indian strawberry plants, but is thick and big. It has a deep green color. The root is black, similar to the teeth of a wild animal. The root is collected in the third and eighth month. It is dried in the sun. [Su] Song: Today much of it is found in the *zhou* and prefectures of Jiang dong and Bian dong. [Li] Shizhen: The *Fan zi ji ran* states: "[Those from] Jian kang and San fu that are of white color, they are good."

17-05-01
根 *Gen*
Root [of *lang ya*].

【氣味】苦，寒，有毒。【别録曰】酸。【普曰】神農、黄帝：苦，有毒。桐君：辛。岐伯、雷公，扁鵲：苦，無毒。【之才曰】蕪荑爲之使。惡地榆、棗肌。

Qi and Flavor. Bitter, cold, poisonous. *Bie lu*: Sour. [Wu] Pu: Shen nong, Huang Di: Bitter, poisonous. Tong jun: Acrid.[863] Qi Bo, Lei gong, Bian Que: Bitter, nonpoisonous. [Xu] Zhicai: *Ulmus* [fruit] serves as its guiding substance. [Ingested together,] it abhors *sanguisorba* [root] and *cnidium* herb.

【主治】邪氣熱氣，疥瘙，惡瘍，瘡痔，去白蟲。本經。治浮風瘙痒，煎汁洗惡瘡。甄權。殺腹臓一切蟲，止赤白痢，煎服。大明。

863 Instead of *xin* 辛, "acrid," *Yu lan* ch. 993, *lang ya* 狼牙, quoting *Wu shi ben cao jing* writes *xian* 鹹, "salty."

Control. Evil qi, heat qi, itching *jie*-illness,[864], malign ulcers, piles sores. It removes white worms/bugs. *Ben jing*. To cure floating wind[865] with itching, boil it to obtain a juice and use it to wash the malign sores. To kill all types of worms/bugs in the abdomen and in the long-term depots and to end red and white free-flux illness, boil it and ingest [the resulting juice]. Da Ming.

【附方】舊六。新四。

Added Recipes. Six of old. Four newly [recorded].

金瘡出血。狼牙草莖葉，熟擣貼之。肘後方。

Bleeding wounds caused by metal objects/weapons. Boil *lang ya* stem and leaves until done, pound them [to a pulp] and apply this [to the affected region]. *Zhou hou fang*.

小便溺血。金粟狼牙草焙乾，入蚌粉、炒槐花、百藥煎，等分爲末。每服三錢，米泔空心調服。亦治酒病。衛生易簡方。

Urination with blood. Dry *lang ya* herbs with golden color anther bearing filaments in a pan, add equal amounts of fresh water mussel powder, fried *sophora japonica* flowers and ferment prepared from Chinese nutgalls and tea leaves, and [grind this into] powder. Each time ingest three *qian*, to be ingested, on an empty stomach, mixed with water in which rice has been washed. It also serves to cure diseases caused by wine [abuse]. *Wei sheng yi jian fang*.

寸白諸蟲。狼牙五兩擣末，蜜丸麻子大。隔宿不食，明旦以漿水下一合，服盡即瘥。外臺秘要。

All types of tapeworms. Pound five *liang* of *lang ya* into powder and form with honey pills the size of hemp seeds. Do not eat at night the day before. In the early morning send down one *ge* with fermented water of foxtail millet. Once this is completely ingested, healing will be achieved. *Wai tai mi yao*.

蟲瘡瘙癢。六月以前采狼牙葉，以後用根，生㕮咀，以木葉裹之，煻火炮熟，於瘡上熨之，冷即止。楊炎南行方。

Itching sores related to the presence of worms/bugs. Pound fresh *lang ya*, either the leaves collected in the sixth month or before, or the root [collected] after [the sixth month] and wrap [the pulpy mass] with a tree leaf. Warm it over a fire and roast

864 *Jie*-illness 疥, vaguely identifiable skin ailment. BCGM Dict I, 249.

865 *Fu feng* 浮風, "floating wind," a condition a) identical to *feng yang* 風癢, "wind itching," and b) of a feeling of nausea brought forth by wind evil that has settled in the stomach. BCGM Dict I, 173.

it until done. Then press it hot on the sore. End this when it has cooled. Yang Yan, *Nan xing fang*.

小兒陰瘡。狼牙草濃煮汁洗之。千金方。

Sores in the yin [(i. e., genital) region] of children. Boil *lang ya* herb to obtain a thick juice and wash [the affected region] with it. *Qian jin fang*.

婦人陰癢。狼牙二兩，蛇牀子三兩，煎水熱洗。外臺秘要。

Itching yin [(i. e., genital) region] of women. Boil two *liang* of *lang ya* and three *liang* of *cnidium* seeds in water and [use the resulting juice to] wash [the affected region]. *Wai tai mi yao*.

婦人陰蝕瘡爛者。狼牙湯：用狼牙三兩，水四升，煮取半升，以箸纏綿浸湯瀝洗，日四五遍。張仲景金匱玉函。

Festering erosion sores in the yin [(i. e., genital) region] of women. The "*lang ya* decoction." Boil three *liang* of *lang ya* in four *sheng* of water down to half a *sheng*. Wrap a chopstick with silk floss, soak it in the decoction and drip [the liquid on the affected region] to wash it. Four to five times a day. Zhang Zhongjing, *Jin kui yu han*.

聤耳出汁。狼牙研末，綿裹，日塞之。聖惠方。

Festering ears releasing a juice. Grind *lang ya* into powder, wrap it in silk floss and insert this [into the affected ear] during the day. *Sheng hui fang*.

毒蛇傷螫。獨莖狼牙根或葉，搗爛，臘豬脂和塗，立瘥。崔氏方。

Harm caused by the bite of a poisonous snake. Pound the root or the leaves of a single stem *lang ya* plant into a pulpy mass, mix it with lard of a pig obtained in the 12th month and apply [this to the affected region]. A cure is achieved immediately. *Cui shi fang*.

射工中人，有瘡。狼牙，冬取根，夏取葉，搗汁飲四五合，并傅之。千金方。

Sores that result when someone is struck by the archer.[866] Pound *lang ya*, in winter use the root, in summer use the leaves, to obtain a juice and drink four to five *ge* of it. In addition, apply it [to the affected region]. *Qian jin fang*.

866 *She gong* 射工, "archer," 1.) a small bug in ancient times believed to live in water and be capable of "shooting" poison from its mouth at people, thereby causing disease; 2.) a condition caused by the archer's poison. BCGM Dict. I, 432. See 42-15.

17-06
藺茹本經下品
Lü ru, FE *Ben jing*, lower rank.

***Euphorbia ebracteolata* Hayata. Spurge.**

【釋名】離婁别録、掘據音結居。白者名草藺茹。【時珍曰】藺茹本作藘蕠，其根牽引之貌。掘據，當作拮據，詩云："予手拮據。"手口共作之狀也。

Explanation of Names. *Li lou* 離婁, *Bie lu*. *Jie ju* 掘據, read *jie ju* 結居. White specimens are called *cao lü ru* 草藺茹, "herbal *lü ru*." [Li] Shizhen: *Lü ru* 藺茹 originally was written *lü ru* 藘蕠, reflecting the winding appearance of the root. *Jie ju* 掘據 should be written *jie ju* 拮據. The *Shi* states: "With my claws I tore, *jie* 拮, and held, *ju* 據." This is the image of [a bird collecting rushes and building a nest] with its "hands/claws and mouth/beak."[867]

【集解】【别録曰】藺茹生代郡川谷。五月采根，陰乾。黑頭者良。【普曰】草高四五尺，葉圓黄，四四相當。四月華，五月實黑。根黄，有汁亦黄色。三月采葉，四月、五月采根。【弘景曰】今第一出高麗，色黄。初斷時汁出凝黑如漆，故云漆頭。次出近道，名草藺茹，色白，皆燒鐵爍頭令黑，以當漆頭，非真也。【頌曰】今河陽、淄、齊州亦有之。二月生苗，葉似大戟而花黄色。根如蘿蔔，皮赤黄，肉白。初斷時，汁出凝黑如漆。三月開淺紅花，亦淡黄色，不着子。陶隱居謂出高麗者，此近之。又有一種草藺茹，色白。古方兩用之。故姚僧坦治癰疽生惡肉，有白藺茹散，傅之看肉盡便停止，但傅諸膏藥。若不生肉，又傅黄耆散。惡肉仍不盡者，可以漆頭赤皮藺茹爲散半錢，和白藺茹散三錢合傅之。觀此，則赤白皆可用也。【時珍曰】范子計然云：藘茹出武都，黄色者善。草藺茹出建康，白色。今亦處處有之，生山原中。春初生苗，高二三尺。根長大如蘿蔔、蔓菁壯[868]，或有岐出者，皮黄赤，肉白色，破之有黄漿汁。莖葉如大戟，而葉長微闊，不甚尖，折之有白汁。抱莖，有短葉相對，團而出尖。葉中出莖，莖中分二三小枝。二三月開細紫花，結實如豆大，一顆三粒相合，生青熟黑，中有白仁如續隨子之狀。今人往往皆呼其根爲狼毒，誤矣。狼毒葉似商陸、大黄輩，根無漿汁。

Collected Explanations. *Bie lu*: *Lü ru* grows in the river valleys of Dai jun. The root is collected in the fifth month; it is dried in the yin (i. e., shade). Those with a black top are good. [Wu] Pu: The herb is four to five *chi* tall. The leaves are round and yellow. Always four of them grow facing each other. The flower blossoms in the fourth month; black fruits appear in the fifth month. The root is yellow. It has a juice that

867 For the context of this quote, see *Shi jing*, Part I, Bk. XV, Ode 3, Verse 3.

868 The character *zhuang* 壯 is an erroneous writing of *zhuang* 狀, "shape."

is yellow, too. The leaves are collected in the third month. The root is collected in the fourth and fifth month. [Tao] Hongjing: Today, top quality comes from Gao li. It is yellow. When it is cut for the first time a juice is released that coagulates and turns black like lacquer. Hence it is said to be a "lacquer head/top." Secondary quality specimens come from nearby. They are called *cao lü ru*, and are white. [*Cao lü ru*] is always heated/burned in an iron utensil to let its head/top shine black as if it were a "lacquer head/top." But this is not the genuine [black lacquer head/top]. [Su] Song: Today it can also be found in He yang, Zi and Qi zhou. It grows a seedling in the second month. The leaves resemble those of Peking spurge, but the flowers are yellow. The root is similar to that of radish. The skin is red-yellow; the meat is white. When it is cut for the first time, a juice is released that is black like lacquer. In the third month, pale red flowers open; they may also be of a pale yellow color. They have no seeds. Those said by Tao Yinju to come from Gao li are similar to them. Then there is another kind, *cao lü ru*. It is white. Ancient recipes resort to both of them. Hence Yao Sengtan has a "powder with white *lü ru*" to cure the growth of malign flesh related to obstruction-illness and impediment-illness.[869] This is applied [to the affected region]. "When all the [malign] flesh is eliminated, [the application must be] ended, and other medical ointments are to be applied. If [new] flesh fails to grow, in addition apply the 'powder with *astragalus* [root].' If the malign flesh is not eliminated entirely, one can prepare half a *qian* of lacquer head/top *lü ru* with a red skin, mix it with three *qian* of white *lü ru* powder, and apply this [to the affected region]." This shows that both red and white kinds can be used.[Li] Shizhen: The *Fan zi ji ran* states: "*Lü ru* comes from Wu du; that of yellow color is good. *Cao lü ru* comes from Jian kang. It is white." Today it can be found everywhere. It grows on plains in the mountains. In the beginning of spring it grows a seedling reaching a height of two to three *chi*. The root is as long and big as that of radish or turnip. Some [roots] are forked. The skin is yellow-red; the flesh is white. When the [root] is broken open, it releases a yellow sauce-like juice. The stem and the leaves resemble those of Peking spurge, but the leaves are lengthy and slightly broader. They are not very pointed. When they are broken, white juice appears. The short leaves embrace the stem and grow facing each other. They are round and appear with pointed ends. The stem comes out from amidst the leaves; in the middle of the stem two or three small twigs branch out. It opens fine, purple flowers in the second or third month forming fruits the size of soybeans. In one of them three kernels lie together. They are green when they are fresh, and black when they are heat processed. Inside are

869 *Yong ju* 癰疽, "obstruction-illness, impediment-illness." refers to two vaguely distinguished obstructions/impediments of vessels or other ducts inside the body. Qi rushing against the obstruction may cause a local swelling and eventually break through the surface to cause an abscess. BCGM Dict I, 642.

white kernels shaped similar to casper spurge seeds. Today people often call the root *lang du* 狼毒, wolfsbane. That is wrong. The leaves of wolfsbane resemble those of Indian pokewee and rhubarb, and its root does not have a sauce-like juice.

17-06-01
根 *Gen*
Root [of spurge].

【氣味】辛，寒，有小毒。【别録曰】酸。【普曰】神農：辛。岐伯：酸、鹹、有毒。李當之：大寒。【之才曰】甘草爲之使，惡麥門冬。

Qi and Flavor. Acrid, cold, slightly poisonous. *Bie lu*: Sour. [Wu] Pu: Shen nong: Acrid. Qi Bo: Sour, salty, poisonous. Li Dangzhi: Very cold. [Xu] Zhicai: *Glycyrrhiza* [root] serves as its guiding substance. [Ingested together,] it abhors *ophiopogon* [tuber].

【主治】蝕惡肉敗瘡死肌，殺疥蟲，排膿惡血，除大風熱氣，善忘不寐。本經。去熱痺，破癥瘕，除息肉。别録。

Control. It eats away malign flesh, decaying sores and dead muscles. It kills the worms/bugs responsible for *jie*-illness.[870] It dispels pus and malign blood. It removes heat qi associated with massive wind. [It serves to cure] forgetfulness and inability to sleep.[871] *Ben jing*. It removes blockage related to the presence of heat. It breaks through concretion-illness and conglomeration-illness,[872] and removes tumorous flesh growth. *Bie lu*.

【發明】【宗奭曰】治馬疥尤善，服食方用至少。【時珍曰】素問治婦人血枯痛，用烏鰂骨、藘茹二物丸服，方見"烏鰂魚"下。王冰言藘茹取其散惡血。又齊書云：郡王子隆年二十，身體過充。徐嗣伯合藘茹丸服之自消。則藘茹亦可服食，但要斟酌爾。孟詵效方：治甲疽生于脚趾邊腫爛，用藺茹三兩，黄芪二兩，苦酒浸一宿，以豬脂五合合煎，取膏三合。日三塗之，即消。又聖惠方，治頭風旋眩，鴟頭丸中亦用之。

Explication. [Kou] Zongshi: It is especially good for curing *jie*-illness of horses. Recipes for ingesting [elixirs] as food only very seldom resort to it. [Li] Shizhen: The *Su wen* [recommends to] cure painful blood withering of woman by letting

870 *Jie*-illness 疥, vaguely identifiable skin ailment. BCGM Dict I, 249.

871 Instead of *mei* 寐, "to sleep," *Zheng lei* ch. 11, *lü ru* 藺茹, quoting the *Ben jing* writes *le* 樂, "cheerful."

872 *Zheng jia* 癥瘕, "concretion-illness and conglomeration-illness." The two terms are often used interchangeably and do not signify two distinctly different conditions. Concretion-illness and conglomeration-illness result from a disharmony of cold and warmth resulting in a failure to transform beverages and food. Nodes form when the clash with the qi of the long-term depots. BCGM Dict I, 677.

them ingest pills with the two items cuttlefish bones and *lü ru*.[873] For the recipe, see the entry *wu ze yu* 烏鰂魚 (44-50-02). Wang Bing says that this is to make use of *lü ru*'s ability to disperse malign blood. Also, the *Qi shu* states: "Commandery Prince Zi long at the age of 20 was heavily overweight. Xu Sibo prepared pills with *lü ru*. He let him ingest them and [the overweight] dissolved." That is, *lü ru* can also be ingested as food, but this requires careful consideration. Meng Shen in his *Bi xiao fang* states: "To cure nail impediment-illness developing at the side of one's toes with a swelling and festering, soak three *liang* of *lü ru* and two *liang* of *astragalus* [root] in bitter wine for one night, then boil this mixed with five *ge* of lard to obtain a paste of three *ge* and apply this three times a day [to the affected region]. This will dissolve [the swelling]." Also, when the *Sheng hui fang* [recommends to] cure head wind[874] with dizziness, it is resorted to as one of the ingredients of the "pills with the head of a black kite." (49-24-01)

【附方】舊二，新二。

Added Recipes. Two of old. Two newly [recorded].

緩疽腫痛。藺茹一兩爲散，温水服二錢匕。聖惠方。

Painful swelling related to a chronic, progressive impediment-illness.[875] [Grind] one *liang* of *lü ru* into powder and ingest with warm water the amount held by two *qian*-size spoons. *Sheng hui fang*.

傷寒咽痛，毒攻作腫。真藺茹爪甲大，納口中，嚼汁嚥之。當微覺爲佳。張文仲備急方。

Painful throat related to harm caused by cold, with a swelling caused by an attack of poison. Insert genuine *lü ru*, the size of a fingernail, into the [patient's] mouth, let him chew it and swallow the resulting juice. A slight sensation [in the throat] shows a good result. Zhang Wenzhong, *Bei ji fang*.

中焦熱痞，善忘不禁。藺茹三分，甘草炙二兩，消石爲末。每服一錢，雞鳴時温酒下，以知爲度。聖惠方。

---

873 *Su wen* ch. 40. Paul U. Unschuld and Hermann Tessenow, *Huang Di Nei Jing Su Wen. An Annotated Translation of Huang Di's Inner Classic*, 2 vols. University of California Press, Berkeley and Los Angeles, 2011. Vol. 1, 602.

874 *Tou feng* 頭風, "head wind." Condition of wind evil attacking the head followed by pain, dizziness, itching. BCGM Dict I, 509.

875 *Huan ju* 緩疽, "chronic progressive impediment-illness," a *ju* 疽, "impediment-illness," with nodular swelling and deep-reaching pain where the erosion of tissue and festering slowly progress and the prognosis is inauspicious. BCGM Dict I, 224.

An obstacle-illness related to heat in the central [section of the Triple] Burner, with a tendency to be forgetful and neglect prohibitions. [Grind] three *fen* of *lü ru*, two *liang* of roasted *glycyrrhiza* [root] and nitrokalite into powder. Each time ingest one *qian*, to be sent down at cockcrow [in the early morning] with warm wine until an effect shows. *Sheng hui fang.*

疥瘡瘙痒。藺茹末，入輕粉，香油調傅之。多能鄙事。

Itching *jie*-illness[876] sores. Add calomel and sesame oil to *lü ru* powder and apply this mixture [to the affected region]. *Duo neng bi shi.*

17-07
大戟本經下品

***Da ji*, FE *Ben jing*, lower rank.**

***Euphorbia pekinensis* Rupr. Peking spurge.**[877]

【釋名】邛鉅爾雅、下馬仙綱目。【時珍曰】其根辛苦，戟人咽喉，故名。今俚人呼爲下馬仙，言利人甚速也。郭璞注爾雅云：蕎，邛鉅，即大戟也。

Explanation of Names. *Qiong ju* 邛鉅, *Er ya*. *Xia ma xian* 下馬仙, *Gang mu*. [Li] Shizhen: The root is acrid bitter and pierces like a guisarme, *ji* 戟, one's throat. Today, common people call it *xia ma xian* 下馬仙, "an hermit/immortal descending from a horse," to refer to the speed with which it benefits one. Guo Pu comments on the *Er ya*, stating: "*Qiao* 蕎 and *qiong ju* 邛鉅 are *da ji* 大戟."

【集解】【别録曰】大戟生常山。十二月采根，陰乾。【保昇曰】苗似甘遂而高大，葉有白汁，花黄。根似細苦參，皮黄黑，肉黄白。五月采苗，二月、八月采根用。【頌曰】近道多有之。春生紅芽，漸長叢，高一尺以來，葉似初生楊柳小團。三月、四月開黄紫花，團圓似杏花，又似蕪荑。根似細苦參，秋冬采根，陰乾。淮甸出者莖圓，高三四尺，花黄，葉至心亦如百合苗。江南生者葉似芍藥。【時珍曰】大戟生平澤甚多。直莖高二三尺，中空，折之有白漿。葉長狹如柳葉而不團，其稍葉密攢而上。杭州紫大戟爲上，江南土大戟次之。北方綿大戟色白，其根皮柔韌如綿，甚峻利，能傷人。弱者服之，或至吐血，不可不知。

Collected Explanations. *Bie lu*: *Da ji* grows on Mount Chang shan. The root is collected in the 12th month; it is dried in the yin (i. e., shade). [Han] Baosheng: The seedling resembles that of kansui herb, but grows taller and is bigger. The leaves have a white juice; the flowers are yellow. The root resembles fine *sophora* roots, with

876 *Jie*-illness 疥, vaguely identifiable skin ailment. BCGM Dict I, 249.

877 *Da ji* 大戟, lit.: "big guisarme."

a yellow-black skin. The meat is yellow-white. The seedling is collected in the fifth month; the root is collected for [therapeutic] use in the second and eighth month. [Su] Song: It can be found in large quantities nearby. In spring it grows red shoots. They gradually increase in length and form clusters reaching around one *chi* high. The leaves resemble those of willows that have just begun to grow, but are smaller and round. Yellow-purple flowers open in the third and fourth month. They are round and resemble apricot flowers and *ulmus* [flowers]. The root resembles fine *sophora* roots. The root is collected in autumn and winter; it is dried in the yin (i. e., shade). Those coming from Huai dian have a round stem, three to four *chi* tall. The flowers are yellow. The leaves up to the center [of their cluster] are also similar to lily seedlings. The leaves of [*da ji*] growing in Jiang nan resemble those of *paeonia* herbs. [Li] Shizhen: Lots of *da ji* grows in the marshlands of the plains. A straight stem reaches a height of two to three *chi*. It is hollow inside. When it is broken open, a white, thick fluid appears. The leaves are long and narrow like willow leaves; they do not curl up. Small leaves rise in dense clusters. In Hang zhou, purple *da ji* is best; local *da ji* from Jiang nan is second. In the North, brocade *da ji* is white.. The skin of its root is soft and pliable similar to brocade. It causes a dramatic free flow and can harm one. When weak [persons] ingest it they may end up spitting blood. This should be common knowledge.

17-07-01
根 *Gen*
Root [of *da ji*].

【修治】【斅曰】凡使勿用附生者，誤服令人洩氣不禁，即煎薺苨湯解之。采得後，于槐砧上細剉，與海芋葉拌蒸，從巳至申，去芋葉，晒乾用。【時珍曰】凡采得以漿水煮軟，去骨，晒乾用。海芋葉麻而有毒，恐不可用也。

Pharmaceutical Preparation. [Lei] Xiao: For all [therapeutic] applications, do not use those growing attached [to the main root]. Erroneously eaten they let one have unending outflow of qi. This is resolved by a decoction of boiled apricot-leaved *adenophora* [root]. After [the *da ji* root] is collected, cut it on a *sophora japonica* anvil to fine pieces and steam them mixed with *alocasia* leaves from *si* 巳 hours (9 -11) to *shen* 申 hours (15 – 17). Then remove the *alocasia* leaves, dry [the *da ji* roots] in the sun and use them [for therapeutic ends]. [Li] Shizhen: Whenever they are collected, boil them in fermented water of foxtail millet to soften them, discard [those remaining that are as hard as] bones and dry them in the sun for [therapeutic] use. *Alocasia* leaves cause numbness and are poisonous. Presumably this is why they are useless.

【氣味】苦，寒，有小毒。【别録曰】甘，大寒。【權曰】苦、辛，有大毒。【元素曰】苦，甘、辛，陰中微陽。瀉肺，損真氣。【時珍曰】得棗即不損脾。【之才曰】反甘草，用菖蒲解之。【恭曰】畏昌蒲、蘆葦、鼠屎。【大明曰】赤小豆爲之使，惡薯蕷。

Qi and Flavor. Bitter, cold, slightly poisonous. *Bie lu*: Sweet, very cold. [Zhen] Quan: Bitter, acrid, very poisonous. [Zhang] Yuansu: Bitter, sweet, acrid. A slight yang in yin [substance]. It drains the liver and injures the true qi. [Li] Shizhen: Combined with Chinese dates it will not injure the spleen. [Xu] Zhicai: [Ingested together,] it is opposed to *glycyrrhiza* [roots]. This can be resolved with *acorus* [root]. [Su] Gong: [Ingested together,] it fears *acorus* [root], reed and the excrements of mice/rats. Da Ming: Red mung beans serve as its guiding substance. [Ingested together,] it abhors Chinese yam.

【主治】蠱毒，十二水，腹滿急痛，積聚，中風，皮膚疼痛，吐逆。本經。頸腋癰腫，頭痛，發汗，利大小便。别録。瀉毒藥，泄天行黄病温瘧，破癥結。大明。下惡血癖塊，腹内雷鳴，通月水，墮胎孕。甄權。治隱瘮風，及風毒脚腫，並煮水，日日熱淋，取愈。蘇頌。

Control. *Gu* poison.[878] The twelve [diseases related to] water [disorder].[879] A feeling of fullness, tension and pain in the abdomen. Accumulations and collections. Being struck by wind. Painful skin. Vomiting with [qi] counterflow. *Ben jing*. Swelling related to an obstruction-illness[880] in the neck and in the armpits. Headache. It causes sweating and frees the passage of major [defecation] and minor [urination] relief.[881] It drains poisonous medication, causes an outflow of epidemic jaundice and warmth malaria, and breaks through concretion-illness nodes. Da Ming. It discharges aggregation-illness lumps of malign blood, as well as thunderous sounds in the abdomen. It opens the flow of menstruation and causes abortion. Zhen Quan. It serves to cure dormant papules and wind [intrusion], as well as leg swelling related

878 *Gu du* 蠱毒, "*gu*-poison[ing]." (1) A poison emitted by certain worms/snakes with an ability to cause varying pathological changes in a person who has taken it in by means of wine or food. (2) Abdominal fullness, in some cases with blood spitting, and blood in the stool and urine. BCGM Dict I, 192 - 193. See BCGM 42-22.

879 A first reference to *shi er shui* 十二水, "12 [diseases related to] water[disorders]," appears in ch. 36 of the *Zhu bing yuan hou lun* 諸病源候論. An enumeration of these 12 diseases in detail is not given. All the text says is that all of them originate in the "long-term depots and short-term repositories," and that different experts speak of 14, 18, 12 or only five such *shui bing* 水病, "water diseases."

880 *Yong* 癰, "obstruction-illness,"refers to an obstruction of vessels or other ducts inside the body. Qi rushing against the obstruction may cause a local swelling and eventually break through the surface to cause an abscess. BCGM Dict I, 641.

881 Instead of *da xiao bian* 大小便, "major [defecation] and minor [urination] relief," *Zheng lei* ch. 10, *da ji* 大戟, quoting *Bie lu* writes 大小腸, "large and small intestines."

to the presence of wind poison. For all these [ailments], boil it in water and rinse [the affected regions] with the hot decoction day after day until a cure is achieved. Su Song.

【發明】【成無己曰】大戟、甘遂之苦以泄水者，腎所主也。【好古曰】大戟與甘遂同爲泄水之藥，濕勝者苦燥除之也。【時珍曰】痰涎之爲物，隨氣升降，無處不到。入于心，則迷竅而成癲癇，妄言妄見。入于肺，則塞竅而成欬唾稠粘，喘急背冷。入于肝，則留伏蓄聚而成脅痛乾嘔，寒熱往來。入于經絡，則麻痺疼痛。入于筋骨，則頸項、胸背、腰脇、手足牽引隱痛。陳無擇三因方並以控涎丹主之，殊有奇效。此乃治痰之本。痰之本，水也，濕也。得氣與火則凝滯而爲痰，爲飲，爲涎，爲涕，爲癖。大戟能泄臟腑之水濕，甘遂能行經隧之水濕，白芥子能散皮裏膜外之痰氣。惟善用者，能收奇功也。又錢仲陽謂腎爲真水，有補無瀉，而復云痘瘡變黑歸腎一證，用百祥膏下之以瀉腎。非瀉腎也，瀉其腑則臟自不實。愚按：百祥惟用大戟一味。大戟能行水，故曰瀉其腑則臟自不實，腑者膀胱也。竊謂百祥非獨瀉腑，正實則瀉其子也，腎邪實而瀉其肝也。大戟味苦澀，浸水色青緑，肝膽之藥也。故百祥膏又治嗽而吐青緑水。夫青緑者，少陽風木之色也。仲景亦云：心下痞滿，引脅下痛，乾嘔短氣者，十棗湯主之。其中亦有大戟。夫乾嘔脇痛非肝膽之病乎？則百祥之瀉肝膽也，明矣。肝乃東方，宜瀉不宜補。况瀉青、瀉黄皆瀉其子，同一瀉也，何獨腎只瀉腑乎？潔古老人治變黑歸腎證，用宣風散代百祥膏，亦是瀉子之意。蓋毒勝火熾則水益涸，風挾火勢則土受虧。故津血内竭不能化膿，而成青黑乾陷之證。瀉其風火之毒，所以救腎扶脾也。或云脾虛腎旺，故瀉腎扶脾者，非也。腎之真水不可瀉，瀉其陷伏之邪毒爾。

Explication. Cheng Wuji: The [potential of] *da ji* and kansui [root] to drain water is under the control of the kidneys. [Wang] Haogu: Both *da ji* and kansui [root] are pharmaceutical drugs that drain water. Where dampness prevails, bitter [flavor] and dryness will eliminate it. [Li] Shizhen: Phlegm and saliva are two items that follow the rise and descend of qi; there is no place they do not reach. When they enter the heart, they block its openings and this results in peak-illness[882] with epilepsy, absurd speaking and hallucinations. When they enter the lung, they fill its openings and this results in cough with a thick paste of saliva, hectic panting and a cold back. When they enter the liver, they lie there hidden as accumulations and collections causing pain in the flanks and dry retching, with alternating episodes of cold and heat. When they enter the conduits and network [vessels], this results in numbness and pain. When they enter the sinews and bones, then the neck and the nape, the

882 *Dian ji* 癲[疾], "peak ailment," a mental disturbance of depression and unhappiness, with a calm attitude and little incentive to speak. BCGM Dict I, 125.

chest and the back, the lower back and the flanks, as well as hands and feet will feel a hidden, pulling pain. Chen Wuze in his *San yin fang* controls all these [conditions] with the "elixir to let saliva trickle out," which is very effective. It is a cure directed at the root of the phlegm. The root of phlegm is water, which is moisture. When it meets with qi and fire it congeals and coagulates to become phlegm, rheum, saliva, snivel and aggregation-illness. *Da ji* is capable of draining water and moisture from the long-term depots and short-term repositories. Kansui [root] is capable of stimulating the passage of water and moisture through the conduit tunnels. White mustard seeds are capable of dispersing phlegm and qi situated inside the skin, outside the membranes. They just have to be used well and extraordinary [effects of their therapeutic] potential will be obtained. Also, Qian Zhongyang says that "the kidneys are the [long-term depots of] the true water. It needs to be supplemented, not to be drained." He also states that "when smallpox sores turn black, this is a sign of [their poison] having reached the kidneys, and [he advises to] use the 'one hundred times auspicious ointment' to discharge [the poison] and thereby drain it from the kidneys. This is not a drainage of the kidneys. To dredge the short-term repository [associated with the kidneys, i. e., the urinary bladder] will end a repletion [with evil qi] in the long-term depot (i. e., the kidneys)." My own humble comment: The "one hundred times auspicious [ointment]" uses only one ingredient, *da ji*. *Da ji* is capable of stimulating the passage of water. Hence it is said "to dredge the short-term repository will end a repletion in the long-term depot." The short-term repository [alluded to here] is the urinary bladder. I dare to say that the "one hundred times auspicious [ointment]" does not simply drain the short-term repository. In the case of a real repletion the child [depot] is to be drained. That is, in the case of an evil [qi] repletion in the kidneys, the liver is drained. The flavor of *da ji* is bitter and astringent. Soaked in water, its color is greenish-green. It is a pharmaceutical drug for the liver and the gallbladder. Therefore, the "one hundred times auspicious ointment" also serves to cure cough and spitting of greenish-green water. Now, greenish-green is the color of minor yang, wind and wood. [Zhang] Zhongjing, too, says: "In the case of an obstacle-illness with a feeling of fullness below the heart, with pain pulling on the flanks, dry retching and shortness of [breath] qi, this is controlled with the 'ten Chinese dates decoction'."[883] *Da ji* is among its ingredients. Now, is not dry retching with painful flanks a disease in the liver and gallbladder? That is, that the "one hundred times auspicious [ointment]" serves to drain liver and gallbladder, this should be clear now. The liver stands for the East. It may well be drained, but should

883 *Shi zao tang* 十棗湯, "ten Chinese dates decoction," with the following ingredients: Chinese dates, *wikstroemea* flower, kansui root, *da ji*.

not be supplemented. Also, [the "pills] to drain the greenish"[884] and [the "pills] to drain the yellow,"[885] all these are drainages of [the kidneys'] child. The [mother and the child] are drained together. Why in the case of a kidney [repletion] should one drain only the [associated] short-term repository? When Jiegu laoren cures [smallpox sores] turning black as a sign of their [poison] having reached the kidneys, [he recommends to] use the "powder to lead off wind"[886] instead of the "one hundred times auspicious ointment." This, too, is based on the idea of draining the child. The fact is, when a poison dominates with fire and extreme heat, the water will dry up. When wind is joined by the strength of fire, the soil will weaken. Therefore, the body liquids and blood will dry up internally and are unable to transform pus. This in turn causes illness signs such as greenish-black [smallpox sores] that are dry and have sunken in. By draining the poison of wind and fire, the kidneys are assisted and the spleen is supported. Some say that "this is a case of spleen depletion and kidney flourishing, and that the kidneys are to be depleted while the spleen is to be supported," but this is wrong. The true water of the kidneys cannot be drained. The evil poison of [smallpox sores] sunken in and lying hidden in them is to be drained.

【附方】新一十一。

Added Recipes. 11 newly [recorded].

百祥膏。治嗽而吐青綠水，又治痘瘡歸腎，紫黑乾陷，不發寒者，宜下之。不黑者，慎勿下。紅芽大戟不以多少，陰乾，漿水煮極軟，去骨日乾，復納原汁中煮，汁盡，焙爲末，水丸粟米大。每服一二十丸，研赤脂麻湯下。

The "one hundred times auspicious ointment." It serves to cure cough and spitting of greenish-green water. It also serves to cure smallpox sore [poison] having reached the kidneys, [when the sores] have turned purple-black, are dry and sunken in. If this is not associated with an effusion of cold, [the poison] needs to be discharged. If [the sores] have not turned black, be cautious and do not apply a discharging [therapy]. Dry any amount of red shoot *da ji* in the yin (i. e., shade) and boil it with fermented water of foxtail millet until [the root] is soft. Remove [roots that have remained as hard as a] bone and dry [the soft specimens] in the sun. Then give them

884 *Xie qing wan* 瀉青丸, the "pills to drain the greenish," with the following ingredients: Chinese *angelica* root, borneol, *ligusticum* root, *gardenia* fruit, rhubarb root, *notopterygium* root, *saposhnikovia* root.

885 *Xie huang wan* 瀉黄丸, the "pills to drain the yellow," with the following ingredients: *Agastache* herb, *gardenia* fruit, gypsum, *glycyrrhiza* root, *saposhnikovia* root.

886 *Xuan feng san* 宣風散, "the powder to lead off wind," with the following ingredients: *Areca* nuts, tangerine peels, *glycyrrhiza* root, *pharbitis* seeds.

back into the original juice and boil them again until all the juice is gone. Bake them over a slow fire and [grind them into] powder. Form this with water to pills the size of millet. Each time ingest ten to 20 pills, to be sent down with a decoction of ground, red sesame seeds.

潔古活法機要棗變百祥丸：治斑瘡變黑，大便秘結。用大戟一兩，棗三枚，水一盌同煮，暴乾，去大戟，以棗肉焙丸服，從少至多，以利爲度。

[Zhang[Jiegu's *Huo fa ji yao* [recommends] the "one hundred times auspicious pills." They serve to cure [smallpox] macula sores that have turned black, with constipation. Boil one *liang* of *da ji* and three Chinese dates in one bowl of water. Dry them in the sun. Take out the *da ji*, bake the meat of the dates over a slow fire, prepare pills and ingest them. Begin with a small number and increase it until a free flow is achieved.

控涎丹。治痰涎留在胸膈上下，變爲諸病，或頸項、胸背、腰脅、手足、胯髀隱痛不可忍，筋骨牽引釣痛走易，及皮膚麻痺，似乎癱瘓，不可誤作風氣風毒及瘡疽施治。又治頭痛不可舉，或睡中流涎，或欬唾喘息，或痰迷心竅，並宜此藥。數服痰涎自失，諸疾尋愈。紫大戟、白甘遂、白芥子微炒各一兩，爲末，薑汁打麫糊丸梧子大。每服七丸，或二十丸，以津液嚥下。若取利則服五六十丸。三因方。

The "elixir to let saliva trickle off." It serves to cure phlegm and saliva abiding in the chest above and below the diaphragm that undergo changes and then create all types of diseases. This may be an unbearable, hidden pain in the neck or nape, in the chest or back, in the lower back or flanks, in the hands and feet, in the hips or thighs. A wandering pain as if sinews and bones were pulled by a fishing rod. Also numbness of the skin, as if it were paralyzed. In such cases it would be wrong to apply a treatment for wind qi and wind poison, as well as sores related to an impediment-illness.[887] It also serves to cure headache when [the head] can no longer be raised, or the flow of saliva while one is asleep. Or the coughing of saliva and pant breathing. Or the heart openings being blocked by phlegm. For all these [issues] this medication is suitable. Frequently ingested, phlegm and saliva will leave as a result, and all related illnesses will be cured. [Grind] one *liang* each of purple *da ji*, white kansui [root] and white mustard seeds, slighty fried, into powder. Form a paste of ginger juice and wheat flower and form [with the medicinal powder] pills the size of *wu* seeds. Each time ingest seven pills, or 20 pills, and swallow them with your own saliva. If a free flow is intended, ingest 50 to 60 pills. *San yin fang.*

887 *Huan ju* 緩疽, "chronic progressive impediment-illness," a *ju* 疽, "impediment-illness," with nodular swelling and deep-reaching pain where the erosion of tissue and festering slowly progress and the prognosis is inauspicious. BCGM Dict I, 224.

水腫喘急，小便濇及水蠱。大戟炒二兩，乾薑炮半兩，爲散。每服三錢，薑湯下，大小便利爲度。聖濟總録。

Water swelling and hectic panting. Rough urination and water *gu*.[888] [Grind] two *liang* of *da ji*, fried, and half a *liang* of dried ginger, roasted in a pan, into powder. Each time ingest three *qian*, to be sent down with a ginger decoction until major [defecation] and minor [urination] relief flow freely. *Sheng ji zong lu*.

水病腫滿，不問年月淺深。大戟、當歸、橘皮各一兩切，以水二升，煮取七合，頓服。利下水二三升，勿怪。至重者，不過再服便瘥。禁毒食一年，永不復作。此方出張尚客。李絳兵部手集。

Water disease with swelling and a feeling of fullness, regardless of whether this is recent or chronic. Cut one *liang* each of *da ji*, Chinese *angelica* [root] and tangerine peels to pieces and boil them in two *sheng* of water down to seven *ge*, to be eaten all at once. If this results in a free flow of two or three *sheng* of water, this is of no concern. Even with severe conditions, a cure is achieved after a maximum of two ingestions. [Following this therapy,] poisonous food is to be avoided for one year, and [the disease] will never be active again. This recipe comes from Zhang Shangke. Li Jiang, *Bing bu shou ji*.

水氣腫脹。大戟一兩，廣木香半兩，爲末。五更酒服一錢半，取下碧水後，以粥補之。忌鹹物。

Swelling and distension related to the presence of water qi. [Grind] one *liang* of *da ji* and half a *liang* of *costus* [root] from Guang into powder. In the early morning ingest with wine one and a half *qian*. Once a bluish-green water has been discharged, supplement the [patient's qi] with a gruel. [During the treatment, the consumption of] salty items is forbidden.

簡便方用大戟燒存性，研末，每空心酒服一錢匕。

The *Jian bian fang* [recommends to] grind *da ji*, burned with its nature retained, into powder and to ingest each time with wine on an empty stomach the amount held by a one *qian* spoon.

水腫腹大如鼓，或遍身浮腫。用棗一斗，入鍋内以水浸過，用大戟根苗蓋之，瓦盆合定，煮熟，取棗無時食之，棗盡决愈。

If the water swelling of the abdomen has reached the size of a drum, or if the entire body is covered by a surface swelling, give one *dou* of Chinese dates into a pot and soak them with water. Cover them with roots and seedlings of *da ji*, and firmly close

888 *Shui gu* 水蠱, "water *gu*[-distension," identical to *gu zhang* 鼓脹, "drum[-like] distension." A condition of an abdominal distension and big upswell brought forth by stagnant water qi accumulating in the abdomen. BCGM Dict 409, 196.

[the pot] with a pottery bowl. Heat it until done, and remove the Chinese dates to be eaten any time. When the Chinese dates are all used up, a cure is achieved.

又大戟散：用大戟、白牽牛、木香等分，爲末。每服一錢，以猪腰子一對，批開摻末在内，濕紙煨熟，空心食之。左則塌左，右則塌右。張潔古活法機要。

Also, the "powder with *da ji*." [Grind] equal amounts of *da ji*, *pharbitis* [seeds] and *costus* [root] into powder. Each time ingest one *qian*. Cut open a pair of pig kidneys and fill the powder insde. Wrap it in moist paper and simmer it until done. Eat it on an empty stomach. The left [side of the pig's kidneys] will calm down the [illness on the] left. The right [side of the pig's kidneys] will calm down the [illness on the] right. Zhang Jiegu, *Huo ren ji yao*.

牙齒摇痛。大戟咬於痛處，良。生生編。

Painful, lose teeth. Chew *da ji* where the pain is located. Good. *Sheng sheng bian*.

中風發熱。大戟、苦参各四兩，白酢漿一斗，煮熟洗之，寒乃止。千金方。

Heat effusion related to a wind stroke. Boil four *liang* each of *da ji* and *sophora* [root] in one *dou* of white vinegar soy-sauce until done and [use the liquid to] wash the [affected region. When the liquid] has cooled, end [the treatment]. *Qian jin fang*.

17-08
澤漆本經下品
Ze qi, FE *Ben jing*, lower rank.

Euphorbia helioscopia **L. Wartweed.**

【釋名】漆莖本經、貓兒眼睛草綱目、緑葉緑花草綱目、五鳳草。【弘景曰】是大戟苗。生時摘葉有白汁，故名澤漆，亦齧人。餘見下。

Explanation of Names. *Qi jing* 漆莖, "lacquer stem," *Ben jing*. *Mao er yan jing cao* 貓兒眼睛草, "cat eye herb," *Gang mu*. *Lü ye lü hua cao* 緑葉緑花草, "green leaves, green flowers herb," *Gang mu*. *Wu feng cao* 五鳳草, "five phoenixes herb." [Tao] Hongjing: These are *da ji* 大戟 seedlings. When the leaves are picked when they have just grown, they have a white juice. Hence the name "moist lacquer," *ze qi* 澤漆, It may also cause erosions of one's [skin]. For more, see below.

【集解】【别録曰】澤漆，大戟苗也。生太山川澤。三月三日、七月七日，采莖葉，陰乾。【大明曰】此即大戟花也。川澤中有。莖梗小，花黄色，葉似嫩菜，五月采之。【頌曰】今冀州、鼎州、明州及近道皆有之。【時珍曰】别録、陶氏皆言澤漆是大戟苗，日華子又言是大戟花，其苗可食。然大戟苗泄人，不可爲菜。今攷土宿本草及寶藏論諸書，並云澤漆是貓兒眼睛草，一名緑葉緑花草，一名五鳳草。江湖原澤平陸多有之。春生苗，一科分枝成叢，柔莖如馬齒莧，緑葉如苜蓿葉，葉圓而黄緑，頗似猫睛，故名貓兒眼。莖頭凡五葉中分，中抽小莖五枝，每枝開細花青緑色，復有小葉承之，齊整如一，故又名五鳳草、緑葉緑花草。掐莖有白汁粘人，其根白色有硬骨。或以此爲大戟苗者，誤也。五月采汁煮雄黄，伏鍾乳，結草砂。據此，則澤漆是貓兒眼睛草，非大戟苗也。今方家用治水蠱、脚氣有效。尤與神農本文相合。自漢人集別録，誤以爲大戟苗，故諸家襲之爾。用者宜審。

Collected Explanations. *Bie lu*: *Ze qi* is the seedling of Peking spurge, *da ji* 大戟. It grows in the river marshlands of Mount Tai shan. The stem and the leaves are collected on the third day of the third month and on the seventh day of the seventh month; they are dried in the yin (i. e., shade). Da Ming: This is the Peking spurge flower. It is present in river marshlands. The stem/trunk is small; the flowers are yellow. The leaves resemble a tender vegetable. They are collected in the fifth month. [Su] Song: Today it can be found everywhere in Ji zhou, Ding zhou and Ming zhou, and nearby. [Li] Shizhen: Both the *Bie lu* and Mr. Zao [Hongjing] say that "*ze qi* is the seedling of Peking spurge," and *Rihua zi* says that "it is Peking spurge flower, and that its seedling is edible." However, the seedling of Peking spurge causes humans to have outflow; it cannot serve as a vegetable. A study now of the *Tu su ben cao* and the *Bao zang lun* shows, both state that *ze qi* is *mao er yan jing cao* 貓兒眼睛草, also named *lü ye lü hua cao* 緑葉緑花草, also named *wu feng cao* 五鳳草. Much of it is present in the marshlands of the plains of Jiang hu and on the flat land. In spring it grows a seedling, with one stem separating into branches that form a cluster. The stem is soft, similar to purslane; the green leaves are similar to alfalfa [leaves]. The leaves are round and yellow-green, a little reminiscent of cat eyes. Hence the name "cat eye." At the top of the stem are five leaves, grouped around the center. The central, small stem has five branches. Each branch opens a fine flower of greenish-yellow color that in turn is held by small leaves again. They are equal [in size] and arranged in a firm structure. Hence the alternative names: "five phoenixes herb" and "green leaves, green flowers herb." When the stem is pinched, a white juice sticks to [the fingers of] that person. The root is white and has a hard bone. Some consider it to be the seedling of Peking spurge; that is wrong. The juice is collected in the fifth month and boiled with realgar. It subdues [the effects of] stalactites, and serves to bind herbs and sand.[889] With this in mind, *ze qi* is *mao er yan jing cao*; it is not the seedling of Peking spurge. Today's recipe experts resort to

889 *Jie cao sha* 結草砂 refers to the chemical method of adding an herbal, *cao* 草, substance to mercury to bind, *jie* 結, it to sulphur and generate cinnabar, *dan sha* 丹砂.

it to effectively cure water *gu*[890] and leg qi.[891] This is in perfect agreement with Shen nong's writings. Since people during the Han era gathered "additional records," *bie lu* 别録, [*ze qi*] has been mistakenly identified as Peking spurge seedling, and all experts have adopted this [error]. When it is used, it should be carefully examined.

17-08-01
莖葉 *Jing, Ye*
Stem, leaf [of *ze qi*].

【氣味】苦，微寒，無毒。【别録曰】辛。【大明曰】冷，有小毒。【之才曰】小豆爲之使，惡薯蕷。

Qi and Flavor. Bitter, slightly cold, nonpoisonous. *Bie lu*: Acrid. Da Ming: Cold, slightly poisonous. [Xu] Zhicai: Mung beans serves as its guiding substance. [Ingested together,] it abhors Chinese yam.

【主治】皮膚熱，大腹水氣，四肢面目浮腫，丈夫陰氣不足。本經。利大小腸，明目輕身。别録。主蠱毒。蘇恭。止瘧疾，消痰退熱。大明。

Control. Skin heat. Water qi in the abdomen. Surface swelling of the four limbs, the face and the eyes. Insufficient yin qi of husbands. *Ben jing*. It frees [the passage through] the large and small intestines, clears the eyes and relieves the body of its weight. *Bie lu*. It controls *gu* poison.[892] Su Gong. It ends malaria illness, dissolves phlegm and dispels heat. Da Ming.

【發明】【時珍曰】澤漆利水，功類大戟，故人見其莖有白汁，遂誤以爲大戟。然大戟根苗皆有毒洩人，而澤漆根硬不可用，苗亦無毒，可作菜食而利丈夫陰氣，甚不相侔也。

Explication. [Li] Shizhen: *Ze qi* frees the flow of water; its [therapeutic] potential equals that of Peking spurge. Hence, when people see that its stem has a white juice they mistakenly assume it to be Peking spurge. However, the root of Peking spurge always has a poison that lets one have an outflow, while the root of *ze qi* is hard and cannot be used [for therapeutic purposes]. Its seedling, too, has no poison. It can be consumed as vegetable and frees the flow of a husband's yin qi. They are really very different.

---

890 *Shui gu* 水蠱, "water *gu*[-distension," identical to *gu zhang* 鼓脹, "drum[-like] distension." A condition of an abdominal distension and big upswell brought forth by stagnant water qi accumulating in the abdomen. BCGM Dict 409, 196.

891 *Jiao qi* 脚氣, "leg qi." Painful, weak, swollen legs. BCGM Dict I, 248.

892 *Gu du* 蠱毒, "*gu*-poison[ing]." (1) A poison emitted by certain worms/snakes with an ability to cause varying pathological changes in a person who has taken it in by means of wine or food. (2) Abdominal fullness, in some cases with blood spitting, and blood in the stool and urine. BCGM Dict I, 192 - 193. See BCGM 42-22.

【附方】舊二，新六。

Added Recipes. Two of old. Six newly [recorded].

肺欬上氣，脉沉者，澤漆湯主之。澤漆三斤，以東流水五斗，煮取一斗五升，去滓。入半夏半升，紫參、白前、生薑各五兩，甘草、黄芩、人參、桂心各三兩，煎取五升。每服五合，日三服。張仲景金匱要略方。

Lung cough with rising qi and a deep [movement in the] vessels. This is controlled by the "decoction with *ze qi*." Boil three *jin* of *ze qi* in five *dou* of eastward flowing water down to one *dou* and five *sheng*. Discard the dregs, add [to the liquid] half a *sheng* of *pinellia* [root], five *qian* each of common bistort, *cynanchum stauntonii* [root] and fresh ginger, as well as three *liang* each of *glycyrrhiza* [root], *scutellaria* [root], ginseng [root] and shaved cinnamom bark, and boil [the liquid] down to five *sheng*. Each time ingest five *ge*, to be ingested three times a day. Zhang Zhongjing, *Jin kui yao lüe fang*.

心下伏瘕，大如盃，不得食者。澤漆四兩，大黄、葶藶熬各三兩，搗篩，蜜丸梧子大。每服二丸，日三服。葛洪肘後方。

Hidden conglomeration-illness[893] below the heart as big as a bowl and making it impossible to eat. Pound four *liang* of *ze qi* and three *liang* each of rhubarb root and wood whitlow-grass, simmered to a paste, and pass this through a sieve. With honey form pills the size of *wu* seeds. Each time ingest two pills; to be ingested three times a day. Ge Hong, *Zhou hou fang*.

十種水氣。澤漆十斤，夏月取嫩莖葉，入酒一斗，研汁約二斗，於銀鍋内，慢火熬如稀餳，入瓶内收。每日空心温酒調下一匙，以愈爲度。聖惠方。

Ten kinds of water qi [disorders]. Give ten *jin* of *ze qi*, during the summer months take the tender stem and leaves, into one *dou* of wine, grind it to obtain about two dou of juice and pour it into a silver pot. Simmer it above a slow fire until it has assumed a consistency of thick malt sugar and fill this into a jar for storage. Each time send down mixed with warm wine on an empty stomach one spoonful until a cure is achieved. *Sheng hui fang*.

水氣蠱病。生鮮貓眼睛草，晒乾爲末，棗肉丸彈子大。每服二丸，白湯化下，日二服。覺腹中暖，小便利爲度。乾坤秘韞。

A *gu* disease related to the presence of water qi.[894] Dry fresh *mao yan jing cao* in the sun and [grind it into] powder. With Chinese date pulp form pills the size of a bul-

893 *Fu jia* 伏瘕, "hidden conglomeration-illness," a *jia* 瘕, "conglomeration-illness," lying deeply hidden in the abdomen. BCGM Dict I, 175.

894 *Shui qi gu bing* 水氣蠱病, identical to *shui gu* 水蠱, "water *gu*[-distension.]" A condition of an abdominal distension and big upswell brought forth by stagnant water qi accumulating in the abdomen. BCGM Dict 409, 196.

let. Each time ingest two pills, to be sent down dissolved in clear, boiled water. To be ingested twice a day until there is a feeling of warmth in the abdomen associated with a free flow of urine. *Qian kun mi yun.*

脚氣赤腫，行步脚痛。貓兒眼睛草、鷺鷥藤、蜂窠等分。每服一兩，水五盌，煎三盌，薰洗之。衛生易簡方。

Leg qi[895] with a red swelling and painful legs when walking. For each ingestion of one *liang* boil equal amounts of *mao er yan jing cao*, honeysuckle [stem] and ground bee nests in five bowls of water down to three bowls. [Use the liquid to] steam and wash [the affected region]. *Wei sheng yi jian fang.*

牙齒疼痛。貓兒眼睛草一搦，研爛，湯泡取汁，含漱吐涎。衛生易簡方。

Toothache. Grind one handful of *mao er yan jing cao* into a pulpy mass. Macerate it in hot water and take the juice into the mouth to rinse [the affected region]. Spit out the resulting saliva. *Wei sheng yi jian fang.*

男婦瘰癧。貓兒眼睛草一二綑，井水二桶，五月五日午時，鍋内熬至一桶，去滓澄清，再熬至一盌，瓶收。每以椒、葱、槐枝煎湯洗瘡净，乃搽此膏，數次愈。便民圖纂方。

Scrofula pervasion-illness[896] of males and women. On the fifth day of the fifth month at noon simmer one or two bundles of *mao er yan jing cao* with two buckets of well water in a pot down to one bucket. Remove the dregs and wait for the liquid to clear. Then simmer it again, this time down to one bowl, and store [the paste] in a jar. Each time prepare with Chinese pepper, onions and *sophora japonica* tree twigs a decoction to wash [the affected region] clean. Then apply this ointment. A cure is achieved after several applications. *Bian min tu zuan fang.*

癬瘡有蟲。貓兒眼睛草，晒乾爲末，香油調搽之。衛生易簡方。

Xuan-illness[897] sores with the presence of worms/bugs. Dry *mao er yan jing cao* and [grind it into] powder. Mix it with sesame oil and apply this [to the affected region]. *Wei sheng yi jian fang.*

---

895 *Jiao qi* 脚氣, "leg qi." Painful, weak, swollen legs. BCGM Dict I, 248.

896 *Luo li* 瘰癧, "scrofula pervasion-illness," when two or more connected swellings of the size of plum or date kernels appear either on the neck or in the armpits, or somewhere else on the body. BCGM Dict I. 329.

897 *Xuan* 癬, "*xuan*-illness." Conditions of dermal lesions with initially erythema, papules, and itching gradually extending in all directions to form an irregular ring with clear boundaries. The skin is slightly elevated with small papules, blisters, and/or scales and scraps. The central lesion may appear to heal spontaneously, and it may reappear. Also, a designation of local lesions with itching, release of liquid and shedding of scabs. BCGM Dict I, 591.

17-09
甘遂本經下品
Gan sui, FE *Ben jing*, lower rank.
***Euphorbia kansui* T. N. Liou ex T.P. Wang. Kansui.**

【釋名】甘藁別録、陵藁吴普、陵澤別録、甘澤吴普、重澤別録、苦澤吴普、白澤吴普、主田別録、鬼醜吴普。【時珍曰】諸名義多未詳。

Explanation of Names. *Gan gao* 甘藁, *Bie lu*. *Ling gao* 陵藁, Wu Pu. *Ling ze* 陵澤, *Bie lu*. *Gan ze* 甘澤, Wu Pu. *Zhong ze* 重澤, *Bie lu*. *Ku ze* 苦澤, Wu Pu. *Bai ze* 白澤, Wu Pu. *Zhu tian* 主田, *Bie lu*. *Gui chou* 鬼醜, Wu Pu. [Li] Shizhen: The meaning of all these names is not clear.

【集解】【別録曰】甘遂生中山川谷。二月采根，陰乾。【普曰】八月采。【弘景曰】中山在代郡。第一本出太山、江東。比來用京口者，大不相似。赤皮者勝，白皮者都下亦有，名草甘遂，殊惡，蓋贋僞者也。【恭曰】甘遂苗似澤漆，其根皮赤肉白，作連珠實重者良。草甘遂乃是蚤休，療體全別，苗亦不同，俗名重臺，葉似鬼臼、蓖麻，根皮白色。【大明曰】西京者上，汴、滄、吴者次之，形似和皮甘草。【頌曰】今陝西、江東亦有之。苗似澤漆，莖短小而葉有汁，根皮赤肉白，作連珠，大如指頭。

Collected Explanations. *Bie lu*: *Gan sui* grows in the river valleys of Mount Zhong shan. The root is collected in the second month; it is dried in the yin (i. e., shade). [Wu] Pu: It is collected in the eighth month. [Tao] Hongjing: Mount Zhong shan lies in Dai jun. Specimens of top quality come from Mount Tai shan and Jiang dong. Those coming from Jing kou in recent times are very different. Those with a red skin are superior. Specimens with a white skin are also found in the vicinity of the capital. They are called *cao gan sui* and this is very malign because they are faked [and poisonous]. [Su] Gong: The seedling of *gan sui* resembles that of wartweed. The skin of its root is red; the meat [inside] is white. Those are good that are shaped like a string of pearls, and that are solid and heavy. *Cao gan sui* is in fact love apple. Its therapeutic [potential] and physical body are entirely different. Even the seedlings are not alike. It is commonly named *chong tai* 重臺, "multiple platforms." The leaves resemble those of umbrella leaf [herbs] and castor oil plants. The root has a white skin. Da Ming: [*Gan sui*] from Xi jing is top; that from Bian, Cang and Wu is of secondary value. Its physical appearance resembles that of *he pi gan cao*.[898] [Su] Song: Today [*gan sui*] is also present in Shaan xi and Jiang dong. The seedling resembles that of wartweed. The stem is short and small, and the leaves have juice. The skin of the root is red, and its meat is white. It is shaped like a string of pearls the size of a finger tip.

---

898 *He pi gan cao* 和皮甘草, a plant of unclear identity.

17-09-01
根 *Gen*

Root [of *gan sui*].

【修治】【斅曰】凡采得去莖，於槐砧上細剉，用生甘草湯、薺苨自然汁二味，攪浸三日，其水如墨汁，乃漉出，用東流水淘六七次，令水清爲度。漉出，于土器中熬脆用之。【時珍曰】今人多以麪煨熟用，以去其毒。

Pharmaceutical Preparation. [Lei] Xiao: Whenever it is collected, remove the stem and cut [the root] on a *sophora japonica* tree wood anvil to pieces. Then soak them in a mixture of fresh *glycyrrhiza* [root] decoction and the natural juice of apricot leaved *adenophora* root. When the water is similar to a black juice, filter it to remove [the *gan sui* root pieces] and rinse them six or seven times with eastward flowing water until the water is clear. Then filter this again and in an earthenware pot simmer [the *gan sui* root pieces] until they have assumed a brittle consistency. Then they can be used [for therapeutic purposes]. [Li] Shizhen: Today, people often simmer [the root] with wheat flour until they are done and then use them. This serves to eliminate their poison.

【氣味】苦，寒，有毒。【别録曰】甘，大寒。【普曰】神農、桐君：苦，有毒。岐伯、雷公：甘，有毒。【元素曰】純陽也。【之才曰】瓜蒂爲之使，惡遠志，反甘草。

Qi and Flavor. Bitter, cold, poisonous. *Bie lu*: Sweet, very cold. [Wu] Pu: Shen nong, Tong jun: Bitter, poisonous. Qi Bo, Lei gong: Sweet, poisonous. [Zhang] Yuansu: A pure yang [substance]. [Xu] Zhicai: Musk melon fruit base serves as its guiding substance. [Ingested together,] it abhors *polygala* [root] and fears *glycyrrhiza* [root].

【主治】大腹疝瘕，腹滿，面目浮腫，留飲宿食，破癥堅積聚，利水穀道。本經。下五水，散膀胱留熱，皮中痞，熱氣腫滿。别録。能瀉十二種水疾，去痰水。甄權。瀉腎經及隧道水濕，脚氣，陰囊腫墜，痰迷癲癇，噎膈痞塞。時珍。

Control. Abdominal elevation-illness with conglomeration-illness,[899] a feeling of abdominal fullness. Surface swelling of face and eyes. Abiding beverages and food remaining [in the body] overnight. It breaks through concretion-illness hardenings, accumulations and collections; it frees the passage through the pathways of water and grain. *Ben jing*. It serves to discharge five types of water [disorders][900] and dis-

899 *Shan jia* 疝瘕, "elevation-illness with conglomeration-illness." A lump-like swelling in the abdomen that alternately collects and then dissolves again. BCGM Dict I, 418.

900 A first reference to *wu shui* 五水, "five [diseases related to] water[disorders]," appears in ch. 36 of the *Zhu bing yuan hou lun* 諸病源候論. An enumeration of these five diseases in detail is not given. All the text says is that all of them originate in the "long-term depots

perses abiding heat in the urinary bladder, obstacle-illnesses in the skin, and heat qi causing swelling and a feeling of fullness. *Bie lu*. It can drain the 12 kinds of water illnesses, and removes phlegm and water. Zhen Quan. It drains water and moisture in the kidney conduits and the tunnel pathways. [It serves to cure] leg qi, swollen and descended scrotum, phlegm confusion,[901] peak-illness with epilepsy, and gullet occlusion with blockage. [Li] Shizhen.

【發明】【宗奭曰】此藥專于行水攻决爲用。【元素曰】味苦氣寒。苦性泄，寒勝熱，直達水氣所結之處，乃泄水之聖藥。水結胸中，非此不能除，故仲景大陷胸湯用之。但有毒不可輕用。【時珍曰】腎主水，凝則爲痰飲，溢則爲腫脹。甘遂能泄腎經濕氣，治痰之本也。不可過服，但中病則止可也。張仲景治心下留飲，與甘草同用，取其相反而立功也。劉河間保命集云：凡水腫服藥未全消者，以甘遂末塗腹，繞臍令滿，内服甘草水，其腫便去。又王璆百一選方云：脚氣上攻，結成腫核，及一切腫毒。用甘遂末，水調傅腫處，即濃煎甘草汁服，其腫即散。二物相反而感應如此。清流韓詠病脚疾用此，一服病去七八，再服而愈也。

Explication. [Kou] Zongshi: This pharmaceutical drug is particularly used for its potential to stimulate water flow. [Zhang] Yuansu: Bitter flavor; cold qi. The nature of bitter is to drain; cold overcomes heat. It reaches straight to the location of bound water qi. It is a sage-like pharmaceutical drug to drain water. Bound water [qi] in the chest can only be eliminated with this [substance]. Therefore, [Zhang] Zhongjing resorts to it in his "decoction for massive chest defects."[902] Still, it is poisonous and must not be used carelessly. [Li] Shizhen: The kidneys control the water. When it congeals, phlegm rheum forms. When it spills over, swelling and distension result. *Gan sui* is capable of draining moisture qi from the kidney conduits; this serves to cure the origin of the phlegm. It must not be ingested excessively. [The treatment] is to end as soon as the disease is struck. To cure abiding beverages/rheum below the heart, Zhang Zhongjing uses it together with *glycyrrhiza* [root], availing himself of their opposition among each other resulting in an immediate success [against the enemy]. Liu Hejian in his *Bao ming ji* states: "Whenever a water swelling is not entirely dissolved by ingesting medication, externally apply *gan sui* to the abdomen by forming a ring around the navel, while internally ingesting *glycyrrhiza* [root] water. This will remove the swelling." Also, Wang Qiu in his *Bai yi xuan fang* states:

and short-term repositories," and that different experts speak of 14, 18, 12 or only five such *shui bing* 水病, "water diseases."

901 *Tan mi* 痰迷, "phlegm confusion, a condition of mental disturbance with forgetfulness, loss of consciousness, and aphasia brought forth by an abundance of phlegm saliva diminishing the patient's mental capacities. BCGM Dict I, 433.

902 *Da xuan xiong tang* 大陷胸湯, the "decoction for massive chest defects," with the following ingredients: Rhubarb root, mirabilite, gansui root.

"[To cure] rising leg qi[903] attacking above and binding together to form swelling and kernels, and all types of swelling with poison, mix *gan sui* powder with water and apply this to the location of the swelling. Then ingest a thick decoction of *glycyrrhiza* [root] juice, and the swelling will go away. These two items are opposed to each other, but their effects are complementary like this. When Han Ying of Qing liu suffered from a leg illness, he used this [therapy]. He ingested it once, and the disease had disappeared by 70 to 80%. Then he ingested it again, and was cured."

【附方】舊三，新一十九。

Added Recipes. Three of old. 19 newly [recorded].

水腫腹滿。甘遂炒二錢二分，黑牽牛一兩半，爲末，水煎，時時呷之。普濟方。

Water swelling with a sensation of abdominal fullness. [Grind] two *qian* and two *fen* of fried *gan sui* and one and a half *liang* of black *pharbitis* [seeds] into powder, boil it in water and from time to time sip it in small amounts. *Pu ji fang*.

膜外水氣。甘遂末、大麥麪各半兩，水和作餅，燒熟食之，取利。聖濟總録。

Water qi outside of the membranes. Mix half a *liang* each of *gan sui* powder and barley flour with water and form a cake. Heat it until done and eat it to free the flow [of water/urine]. *Sheng ji zong lu*.

身面洪腫。甘遂二錢，生研爲末。以豮豬腎一枚，分爲七臠，入末在內，濕紙包煨令熟，食之，日一服。至四五服，當覺腹鳴，小便利，是其效也。肘後方。

Vast swelling of body and face. Grind two *qian* of fresh *gan sui* into powder. Divide one lobe of the liver of a castrated pig into seven small slices and insert the powder between them. Wrap this with moist paper, simmer it until done and eat this. To be ingested once a day. After four to five ingestions there will be a sensation of noises in the abdomen, and the urine will flow freely. This is the effect of this [therapy]. *Zhou hou fang*.

腎水流注，腿膝攣急，四肢腫痛。即上方加木香四錢。每用二錢，煨熟，温酒嚼下。當利黄水爲驗。御藥院方傳。

Influx of kidney water resulting in contraction and tension of legs and knees, and painful swelling of the four limbs. Add four *qian* of *costus* [root] to the previous recipe. Each time simmer two *qian* until done, chew it and send it down with warm

903 *Jiao qi* 脚氣, "leg qi." Painful, weak, swollen legs. BCGM Dict I, 248.

wine. This will cause a free flow of yellow water, and that is the successful [cure of this disease]. Transmitted by the *Yu yao yuan fang*.

正水脹急，大小便不利欲死。甘遂五錢，半生半炒，胭脂坯子十文，研勻，每以一錢，白麪四兩，水和作棋子大，水煮令浮，淡食之。大小便利後，用平胃散加熟附子，每以二錢煎服。普濟方。

Proper water[904] with bloating and tension, accompanied by blocked minor [urination] and major [defecation] relief letting one wish to die. Grind five *qian* of *gan sui*, one half fresh, one half fried, and ten *wen* of rouge base to an even [powder]. Each time mix one *qian* [of the powder] and four *liang* of white wheat flour with water and form [cakes] the size of chess pieces. Boil them in water until they float, and eat them unseasoned. Once the flow of minor [urination] and major [defecation] relief is freed, add to the "powder to balance the stomach"[905] heat prepared *aconitum* [accessory tuber]. Each time boil two *qian* in water and ingest it. *Pu ji fang*.

小兒疳水。珠子甘遂炒，青橘皮等分，爲末。三歲用一錢，以麥芽湯下，以利爲度。忌酸鹹三五日。名水寶散。總微論。

Gan-illness water[906] of children. [Grind] equal amounts of pearl string *gan sui*, fried, and greenish tangerine peels into powder and [let the child] send it down with a malt decoction until a free flow is achieved. [During this therapy] sour and salty [food] is to be avoided for three to five days. [This recipe] is called the "powder with gems for water." *Zong wei lun*.

水蠱喘脹。甘遂、大戟各一兩，慢火炙研。每服一字，水半盞，煎三五沸服。不過十服。聖濟録。

Water *gu*[907] with panting and distension. Roast one *liang* each of *gan sui* and Peking spurge [root] over a slow fire and grind [this into powder]. Each time ingest one *zi*. Boil it in half a small cup of water three to five times to bubbling and ingest this. No more than ten ingestions [are required to achieve a cure]. *Sheng ji lu*.

---

904 *Zheng shui* 正水, "proper water," a *shui zhong* 水腫, "water swelling," disease brought forth by kidney failure due to depletion, and an absence of water flow. BCGM Dict I, 677.

905 *Ping wei san* 平胃散, "the powder to balance the stomach," with the following ingredients: *magnolia* bark, ginger juice, tangerine peels, *glycyrrhiza* root, *atractylodes lancea* rhizome, fresh ginger, Chinese dates.

906 *Gan shui* 疳水, "*gan*-illness water," a *gan*-illness (BCGM Dict I, 180) where the entire body is swollen and the skin has turned yellow. BCGM Dict I, 186.

907 *Shui gu* 水蠱, "water *gu*[-distension]," identical to *gu zhang* 鼓脹, "drum[-like] distension." A condition of an abdominal distension and big upswell brought forth by stagnant water qi accumulating in the abdomen. BCGM Dict 409, 196.

水腫喘急，大小便不通。十棗丸：用甘遂、大戟、芫花等分，爲末，以棗肉和丸梧子大。每服四十丸，侵晨熱湯下，利去黄水爲度。否則次午再服。三因方。

Water swelling with hectic panting, and blocked minor [urination] and major [defecation] relief. The "pills with ten Chinese dates." [Grind] equal amounts of *gan sui*, Peking spurge [root] and daphne flower into powder. With the meat of Chinese dates form pills the size of *wu* seeds. Each time ingest 40 pills, to be sent down in the early morning with hot water until a free flow of yellow water is achieved. If nothing happens, ingest [the pills] a second time at the following noon. *San yin fang*.

妊娠腫滿，氣急，少腹滿，大小便不利，已服豬苓散不瘥者。用太山赤皮甘遂二兩，搗篩，白蜜和丸梧子大，每服五十丸，得微下，仍服豬苓散，不下再服之。豬苓散見豬苓下。小品方。

Swelling and a feeling of fullness during pregnancy, with hectic [breath] qi, a feeling of fullness in the lower abdomen, and blocked minor [urination] and major [defecation] relief. When [patients] have sent down the "powder with *polyporus* sclerotium"[908] already, but without success. Pound two *liang* of *gan sui* with a red skin from Mount Tai shan and give it through a sieve. With white honey form pills the size of *wu* seeds. Each time ingest 50 pills. They will cause a slight discharge. Then ingest the "powder with *polyporus* sclerotium." If there is no discharge, ingest the [pills] a second time. For the "powder with *polyporus* sclerotium," see the entry on "*zhu ling* 豬苓" (37-04). *Xiao pin fang*.

心下留飲，堅滿脉伏，其人欲自利反快。甘遂半夏湯：用甘遂大者三枚，半夏十二個，以水一升，煮半升，去滓。入芍藥五枚，甘草一節，水二升，煮半升，去滓。以蜜半升，同煎八合，頓服取利。張仲景金匱玉函。

Abiding beverage/rheum below the heart, with a hardening, a feeling of fullness and a hidden [movement in the] vessels. Patients wish to have a free flow to return to wellbeing. The "decoction with *gan sui* and *pinellia* [root]." Boil three large *gan sui* [roots] and 12 *pinellia* [roots] in one *sheng* of water down to half a *sheng*, and discard the dregs. Then add five *paeonia* roots and one *glycyrrhiza* [root] node and boil this in two *sheng* of water down to half a *sheng*. Remove the dregs. Boil [the liquid] with half a *sheng* of honey down to eight *ge* and ingest this all at once to achieve a free flow. Zhang Zhongjing, *Jin kui yu han*.

---

908 *Zhu ling san* 豬苓散, "powder with *polyporus* sclerotium," with the following ingredients: *Polyporus* sclerotium, *poria*, alisma [root], talcum, donkey-hide glue.

脚氣腫痛，腎臟風氣，攻注下部瘡痒。甘遂半兩，木鼈子仁四個，爲末。豬腰子一個，去皮膜，切片，用藥四錢摻在內，濕紙包煨熟，空心食之，米飲下。服後便伸兩足。大便行後，吃白粥二三日爲妙。本事方。

Leg qi[909] with a painful swelling. Wind qi in the kidney long-term depot has flowed down to attack the lower [body] section, causing itching sores. [Grind] half a *liang* of *gan sui* and four *momordica* seeds into powder. Then remove the skin and membranes of a pig kidney, cut it into slices and spread the medicinal [powder] between them. Wrap this with moist paper, and simmer it until done. Eat this on an empty stomach, sent down with a rice beverage. Having ingested this, stretch out the two feet. Following a bowel movement, to eat white gruel for two or three days is wondrous. *Ben shi fang*.

二便不通。甘遂末，以生麪糊調傅臍中及丹田內，仍艾三壯，飲甘草湯，以通爲度。又太山赤皮甘遂末一兩，煉蜜和勻，分作四服，日一服取利。聖惠方。

The two reliefs [of urination and defecation] are blocked. Mix *gan sui* powder with fresh wheat flour paste and apply this to the navel and the cinnabar field. Then apply three moxibustions with mugwort leaves and drink a *glycyrrhiza* [root] decoction to free [the passage of urination and defecation]. Also, evenly mix one *liang* of red skin *gan sui* powder from Mount Tai shan with heat prepared honey and ingest this divided into four portions. To be ingested once a day until a free flow is achieved. *Sheng hui fang*.

小便轉脬。甘遂末一錢，豬苓湯調下，立通。筆峰雜興方。

[Blocked] urination because of a contorted bladder. Send down one *qian* of *gan sui* with a "decoction with *polyporus* sclerotium."[910] [Deng] Bifeng, *Za xing fang*.

疝氣偏腫。甘遂、茴香等分，為末，酒服二錢。儒門事親。

Elevation-illness[911] qi with a unilateral swelling [of the scrotum]. [Grind] equal amounts of *gan sui* and fennel [fruit] into powder and ingest with wine two *qian*. *Ru men shi qin*.

婦人血結。婦人少腹滿如敦狀，小便微難而不渴，此爲水與血俱結在血室。大黄二兩，甘遂、阿膠各一兩，水一升半，煮半升，頓服，其血當下。張仲景方。

909 *Jiao qi* 脚氣, "leg qi." Painful, weak, swollen legs. BCGM Dict I, 248.

910 *Zhu ling san* 豬苓散, "powder with *polyporus* sclerotium," with the following ingredients: *Polyporus* sclerotium, *poria*, alisma [root], talcum, donkey-hide glue.

911 *Shan* 疝, "elevation-illness," a group of conditions characterized by violent abdominal pain, in some cases associated with constipation and anuria. BCGM Dict I, 417.

Blood nodes of women. When women in their lower abdomen have a feeling of fullness as if there were a mass, with slightly difficult urination and no thirst, then this is caused by nodes of water and blood forming in the blood chamber/uterus. Boil two *liang* of rhubarb root and one *liang* each of *gan sui* and donkey-hide glue in one and a half *sheng* of water down to half a *sheng*, and [let the woman] ingest this all at once. This will cause a discharge of the blood. A recipe of Zhang Zhongjing.

膈氣哽噎。甘遂麪煨五錢，南木香一錢，爲末。壯者一錢，弱者五分，水酒調下。怪病奇方。

Occlusion qi[912] and choking from gullet occlusion.[913] [Grind] five *qian* of *gan sui* [root], simmered in wheat flour, and one *qian* of southern *costus* [root] into powder. Robust [persons ingest] one *qian*; weak ones five *fen*. To be sent down mixed with water or wine. *Guai bing qi fang*.

痞證發熱，盜汗，胸背疼痛。甘遂麪包，漿水煮十沸，去麪，以細糠火炒黄爲末。大人三錢，小兒一錢，冷蜜水卧時服。忌油膩魚肉。普濟方。

Signs of an obstacle-illness[914] with heat effusion, robber sweating[915] and aching chest and back. Wrap *gan sui* in wheat flour and boil it in fermented water of foxtail millet ten times to bubbling. Discard the flour, fry [the *gan sui*] over a fire of fine seed-coats of rice until it has turned yellow and [grind] it into powder. Adults ingest three *qian*, children one *qian*, with cold honey water at bedtime. [During this therapy] avoid oily and fat items, fish and meat. *Pu ji fang*.

消渴引飲。甘遂麩炒半兩，黄連一兩，爲末，蒸餅丸緑豆大。每薄荷湯下二丸。忌甘草。楊氏家藏方。

Melting with thirst,[916] longing for beverages. [Grind] half a *liang* of *gan sui*, fried in wheat flour, and one *liang* of *coptis* [rhizome] into powder and form with steamed

912 *Ge qi* 膈氣, "occlusion qi," a *ye ge* 噎膈, "gullet occlusion," a disease situated in the chest and diaphragm region with a sensation of an obstacle in the chest, heart-pressure, and pain, and a failure of beverages and food to move through a blocked esophagus. BCGM Dict I. 189.

913 *Geng ye* 哽噎, "choking from gullet occlusion," a condition of an uncomfortable feeling of distension and pain in the throat and esophagus blocked by some item. BCGM Dict I, 191.

914 *Pi* 痞, "obstacle-illness," a condition of an uncomfortable distension and fullness in the chest and abdominal region. When pressed there is no pain. BCGM Dict I. 371.

915 *Dao han* 盜汗, "robber sweating," (1) an illness sign of a profuse sweating during sleep that ends when one wakes up. (2) A pathological condition with robber sweating as major sign. BCGM Dict I, 122.

916 *Xiao ke* 消渴, "melting with thirst," most likely including cases of diabetes. BCGM Dict Vol I, 567.

cakes pills the size of mung beans. Each time send down with a mint decoction two pills. [During this therapy] *glycyrrhiza* [root] is to be avoided. *Yang shi jia cang fang.*

癲癇心風。遂心丹：治風痰迷心，癲癇，及婦人心風血邪。用甘遂二錢，爲末，以豬心取三管血和藥，入豬心内縛定，紙裹煨熟，取末，入辰砂末一錢，分作四丸。每服一丸，將心煎湯調下。大便下惡物爲效，不下再服。濟生方。

Peak-illness with epilepsy and heart wind.[917] The "elixir to comply with the heart." It serves to cure a heart confused by wind and phlegm, peak-illness with epilepsy, and wind and blood evil affecting the heart of a woman. [Grind] two *qian* of *gan sui* into powder. Then take three tubes of blood from the heart of a pig and mix it with the pharmaceutical drug. Put this into the heart of the pig and tie it firmly. Wrap it in moist paper and simmer it until done. Then remove [the *gan sui*] powder. Add one *qian* of cinnabar and prepare this to four pills. Each time ingest one pill, to be sent down with a decoction obtained by boiling the [pig's] heart. The effect [of this therapy is seen] when malign items are defecated. If no such discharge occurs, ingest [the medication] a second time. *Ji sheng fang.*

馬脾風病。小兒風熱喘促，悶亂不安，謂之馬脾風。甘遂麪包煮一錢半，辰砂水飛二錢半，輕粉一角，爲末。每服一字，漿水少許，滴油一小點，抄藥在上，沉下，去漿灌之。名無價散。全幼心鑑。

Horse liver wind disease.[918] Children pant because of wind [intrusion] and heat. They feel heart-pressure, are disturbed and cannot be calmed. This is called "horse spleen wind." Boil one and a half *qian* of *gan sui*, wrapped in wheat flour, [and grind it] with two and a half *qian* of water sublimated cinnabar and one *jiao* of calomel into powder. Each time ingest one *zi* [as follows]. Drop a little oil into a small amount of fermented water of foxtail millet and spread the medicinal [powder] on it. When it has sunk into the depth, remove the fermented water and forcefeed [the medicinal powder to the child]. This [recipe] is called "priceless powder." *Quan you xin jian.*

麻木疼痛。萬靈膏：用甘遂二兩，蓖麻子仁四兩，樟腦一兩，搗作餅貼之。内飲甘草湯。摘玄方。

---

917 *Xin feng* 心風, "heart wind," a condition of a heart affection by wind evil. BCGM Dict I, 575. See also *Xin xian* 心癇, "heart epilepsy" and *dian xian* 癲癇, "peak-illness with epilepsy," which, at the time of its outbreaks, causes the patient's four limbs to twitch, with a red face, heat below the heart, shortness of qi and a breathing that is weak and fast. BCGM Dict I, 580.

918 *Ma pi feng* 馬脾風, "horse-spleen wind," a condition of qi rising with rapid panting brought about by an overabundance of heat in the lung. BCGM Dict I, 333.

Numbness and pain. The "ointment of a myriad magic results." Pound two *liang* of *gan sui*, four *liang* of castor beans and one *liang* of camphor. Prepare [the pulp to] a cake and attach it [to the affected region]. For internal application, drink a *glycyrrhiza* [root] decoction. *Zhai xuan fang.*

耳卒聾閉。甘遂半寸，綿裹插入兩耳内，口中嚼少甘草，耳卒自然通也。永類方。

Sudden deafness because of a closure of the ears. Wrap half a *cun* long *gan sui* [roots] in silk floss and insert them into both ears. In the mouth chew a small *glycyrrhiza* [root] and the ears will suddenly be open again. *Yong lei fang.*

17-10
續隨子宋開寶
Xu sui zi, FE Song, *Kai bao.*

Euphorbia *lathyris* L. Caper spurge.

【釋名】千金子開寶、千兩金日華、菩薩豆日華、拒冬開寶、聯步。【頌曰】葉中出葉，數數相續而生，故名。冬月始長，故又名拒冬。

Explanation of Names. *Qian jin zi* 千金子, "seeds worth thousands in gold," *Kai bao. Qian liang jin* 千兩金, "[worth] a thousand *liang* of gold," *Rihua. Pu sa dou* 菩薩豆, "Bodhisatva's beans," *Rihua. Ju dong* 拒冬, "resists winter." *Kai bao. Lian bu* 聯步, "step by step." [Su] Song: A leaf comes out of a leaf. Many [leaves] grow one following, *xu* 續, the other.[919] Hence the name ["one following the other," *xu sui zi* 續隨子]. It begins to grow in winter. Hence the other name: *ju dong* 拒冬, "resists winter."

【集解】【志曰】續隨子生蜀郡，處處亦有之。苗如大戟。【頌曰】今南中多有，北土產少。苗如大戟，初生一莖，莖端生葉，葉中復出葉。花亦類大戟，自葉中抽幹而生，實青有殼。人家園亭中多種以爲飾。秋種冬長，春秀夏實。【時珍曰】莖中亦有白汁，可結水銀。

Collected Explanations. [Ma] Zhi: *Xu sui zi* grows in Shu jun; it can also be found everywhere else. The seedling is similar to that of Peking spurge. [Su] Song: Today much of it can be found in the South. Only a little grows in the northern regions. The seedling is similar to that of Peking spurge. In the beginning one stem grows. At the tip of the stem a leaf grows. From within this leaf further leaves appear. The

919 Instead of *ye zhong chu ye shu shu xiang xu* 葉中出葉數數相續, "a leaf comes out of a leaf. Many [leaves] grow one following the other," *Zheng lei* ch. 11, *xu sui zi* 續隨子 quoting the *Tu jing* writes: *jing tuan sheng ye ye zhong fu chu shu jing xiang xu* 莖端生葉葉中復出數莖相續, "At the tip of the stem a leaf grows, and from this leaf in turn numerous stems emerge, with [stems and leaves] succeeding each other."

flowers, too, resemble those of Peking spurge. From the leaves a trunk grows. The fruits are greenish and have a shell. Many households plant them in their gardens for decoration. They plant them in autumn, and they grow in winter. They blossom in spring, and bear fruit in summer. [Li] Shizhen: Inside the stem, too, is white juice. It can bind mercury.

【修治】【時珍曰】凡用去殼，取色白者，以紙包，壓去油，取霜用。

Pharmaceutical Preparation. [Li] Shizhen: For all uses discard the shell. Take those that are white, wrap them in paper and press them to remove their oil. Get the "frost" (i. e., the oil-free pulp) for [therapeutic] use.

【氣味】辛，温，有毒。

Qi and Flavor. Acrid, warm, poisonous.

【主治】婦人血結月閉，瘀血癥瘕痃癖，除蠱毒鬼疰，心腹痛，冷氣脹滿，利大小腸，下惡滯物。開寶。積聚痰飲，不下食，嘔逆，及腹内諸疾。研碎酒服，不過三顆，當下惡物。蜀本。宣一切宿滯，治肺氣水氣，日服十粒。瀉多，以酸水或薄醋粥喫，即止。又塗疥癬瘡。大明。

Control. Blood clots and blocked menstruation of women. Sluggish blood, concretion-illness and conglomeration-illness,[920] string-illness[921] and aggregation-illness. [*Xu sui zi*] removes *gu* poison[922] and demon attachment-illness, pain in the central and abdominal region, as well as cold qi with distension and a feeling of fullness. It frees the passage through the large and the small intestine, and serves to discharge malign, sluggish items. *Kai bao*. Accumulations and collections with phlegm rheum, an inability to pass down food, vomiting with [qi] counterflow, and all types of intra-abdominal illnesses. Break [the fruit] to pieces and ingest them with wine. After [ingesting] no more than three pieces malign items will be discharged. *Shu ben*. To lead off all types of stagnant [food/items remaining in the body] overnight and to cure lung qi and water qi [disorders], ingest ten grains a day. If this causes an excessive outflow, take sour [fermented] water [of foxtail millet] or eat a thin

920 *Zheng jia* 癥瘕, "concretion-illness and conglomeration-illness." The two terms are often used interchangeably and do not signify two distinctly different conditions. Concretion-illness and conglomeration-illness result from a disharmony of cold and warmth resulting in a failure to transform beverages and food. Nodes form when the clash with the qi of the long-term depots. BCGM Dict I, 677.

921 *Xuan* 痃, "string-illness," a condition of acute pain located in the abdomen to the left and right of the umbilicus. BCGM Dict I, 591.

922 *Gu du* 蠱毒, "*gu*-poison[ing]." (1) A poison emitted by certain worms/snakes with an ability to cause varying pathological changes in a person who has taken it in by means of wine or food. (2) Abdominal fullness, in some cases with blood spitting, and blood in the stool and urine. BCGM Dict I, 192 - 193. See BCGM 42-22.

vinegar congee. This will end it. It is also applied to *jie*-illness[923] and *xuan*-illness.[924] Da Ming.

【發明】【頌曰】續隨下水最速，然有毒損人，不可過多。【時珍曰】續隨與大戟、澤漆、甘遂莖葉相似，主療亦相似，其功皆長于利水。惟在用之得法，亦皆要藥也。

Explication. [Su] Song: *Xu shui* discharges water very fast. But it also has poison that is harmful for humans. It must not be used excessively. [Li] Shizhen: The stem and leaves of *xu sui*, Peking spurge, wartweed and gansui herbs resemble each other. Their therapeutic controls are similar, too. They all have an excellent [therapeutic] potential of releasing the flow of water. The only [item to remember] is to use them according to the proper method. They all are important pharmaceutical drugs.

【附方】舊二，新四。

Added Recipes. Two of old. Four newly [recorded].

小便不通，臍腹脹痛不可忍，諸藥不效者，不過再服。用續隨子去皮一兩，鉛丹半兩，同少蜜擣作團，瓶盛埋陰處，臘月至春末取出，研，蜜丸梧子大。每服二三十丸，木通湯下，化破尤妙。病急亦可旋合。聖濟録。

Blocked urination, with an unbearably painful abdominal bloating at the navel. When all medication has remained without effect, [the following recipe] is to be ingested no more than twice [to achieve a cure]. Pound one *liang* of *xu sui zi*, with the skin discarded, and half a *liang* of minium with a little honey to a mixture, store it in a jar and bury it at a yin (i. e., shady) location. Remove it some time between the 12th month and the end of spring, grind it and form with honey pills the size of *wu* seeds. Each time ingest 20 to 30 pills, to be sent down with an *akebia* [herb] decoction. When [the seeds] are broken open and dissolved [in the liquid, the effects will be] particularly wondrous. In the case of an acute disease, the [pills] can be prepared right away. *Sheng ji lu*.

水氣腫脹。聯步一兩，去殼研，壓去油，重研，分作七服。每治一人用一服，丈夫生餅子酒下，婦人荊芥湯。五更服之，當下利，至曉自止，後以

923 *Jie*-illness 疥, vaguely identifiable skin ailment. BCGM Dict I, 249.

924 *Xuan* 癬, "*xuan*-illness." Conditions of dermal lesions with initially erythema, papules, and itching gradually extending in all directions to form an irregular ring with clear boundaries. The skin is slightly elevated with small papules, blisters, and/or scales and scraps. The central lesion may appear to heal spontaneously, and it may reappear. Also, a designation of local lesions with itching, release of liquid and shedding of scabs. BCGM Dict I, 591.

厚朴湯補之。頻喫益善，忌鹽、醋一百日，乃不復作。聯步即續隨子也。斗門方。

Swelling and bloating caused by water qi. Remove the skin of one *liang* of *lian bu* [seeds], grind them and press them to remove the oil. Grind them again and ingest them divided into seven portions. For a treatment of one person, one ingestion is required. Husbands send it down with a "fresh pancake wine,"[925] women with a *schizonepeta* decoction. Ingested in the early morning a free flow discharge follows that ends by itself after daybreak. After this, supplement [the patient's qi] with a *magnolia* bark decoction. The more often it is taken, the better the results. [During this therapy] salt and vinegar are to be avoided for 100 days, and [the disease] will never break out again. *Lian bu* 聯步 is *xu sui zi* 續隨子. *Dou men fang.*

陽水腫脹。續隨子炒去油二兩，大黃一兩，爲末，酒水丸綠豆大。每白湯下五十丸，以去陳莝。摘玄方。

Swelling and bloating caused by yang water.[926] [Grind] two *liang* of *xu sui zi*, fried and the oil removed, and one *liang* of rhubarb root into powder. With wine and water form pills the size of mung beans. Each time send down with clear, boiled water 50 pills to remove the old fodder. *Zhai xuan fang.*

涎積癥塊。續隨子三十枚，膩粉二錢，青黛炒一錢，研勻，糯米飯丸芡子大。每服一丸，打破，以大棗一枚，燒熟去皮核，同嚼，冷茶送下。半夜後，取下積聚惡物爲效。聖濟錄。

Accumulation and concretion-illness lumps caused by saliva. Evenly grind 30 *xu sui* seeds, two *qian* of calomel and one *qian* of fried natural indigo [to powder] and form with cooked glutinous rice pills the size of *qian* seeds. Each time ingest one pill. Break it open, chew it together with one Chinese date, heated until done and the skin discarded, and send it down with cold tea. Half a day later the effect is reached when the malign items that had accumulated are discharged. *Sheng ji lu.*

蛇咬腫悶欲死。用重臺六分，續隨子仁七粒，搗篩爲散。酒服方寸匕。兼唾和少許，塗咬處，立效。崔元亮海上方。

Swelling and heart-pressure following a snake bite that brings one close to death. Pound six *fen* of love apple [root] and seven *xu sui zi* kernels and give them through a sieve to obtain a powder. Ingest with wine the amount held by a square *cun* spoon.

925 *Sheng bing zi jiu* 生餅子酒, "fresh pancake wine," is made from the following ingredients: Lead carbonate, litharge, sulphur, minium, calomel.

926 *Yang shui* 陽水, "yang water," a condition of a *shui zhong* 水腫, "water swelling," disease with swelling of the entire body, vexation, constipation and difficult urination. BCGM Dict I, 619.

In addition, mix it with a little saliva and apply this to the location of the bite. Immediately effective. Cui Yuanliang, *Hai shang fang*.

黑子疣贅。續隨子熟時塗之，自落。普濟方。
Black moles and warts. Apply ripe *xu sui* seeds [to the affected region]. *Pu ji fang*.

17-10-01
葉及莖中白汁 ***Ye ji jing zhong bai zhi***

The white juice within the leaves and the stem.

【主治】剥人面皮，去皯䵳。開寶。傅白癜癧瘍。大明。搗葉，傅蠍螫立止。時珍。

Control. It serves to peel facial skin to remove dermal dark spots. *Kai bao*. It is applied to white patches and pervasion-illness with ulcers.[927] Da Ming. Pound the leaves and apply them to [the location of] scorpion stings. [The pain] ends immediately. [Li] Shizhen.

17-11
莨菪音浪蕩本經下品

Lang dang, read *lang dang*. FE *Ben jing*, lower rank.

***Hyoscyamus niger* F.W.Schmidt. Henbane.**

【釋名】天仙子圖經、横唐本經、行唐別録。【時珍曰】莨菪，一作蘭蕩。其子服之，令人狂狼放宕，故名。

Explanation of Names. *Tian xian zi* 天仙子, "celestial immortal seeds," *Tu jing*. *Heng tang* 横唐, Ben jing. *Xing tang* 行唐, *Bie lu*. [Li] Shizhen: *Lang dang* 莨菪 is also written lang dang 蘭蕩. To ingest the seeds lets one immediately turn mad and wild, *lang* 狼. Hence the name.

【集解】【別録曰】莨菪子生海濱川谷及雍州。五月采子。【弘景曰】今處處有之。子形頗似五味核而極小。【保昇曰】所在皆有之。葉似菘藍，莖葉皆有細毛，花白色，子殻作罌狀，結實扁細，若粟米大，青黄色，六月、七月采子，日乾。【頌曰】處處有之。苗莖高二三尺。葉似地黄、王不留行、紅藍等，而闊如三指。四月開花，紫色，莖莢有白毛。五月結實，有殻作罌子狀，如小石榴。房中子至細，青白色，如粟米粒。【斅曰】凡使勿用蒼蓂子，其形相似，只是微赤，服之無效，時人多以雜之。

927 *Li yang* 癧瘍風, "pervasion-illness with ulcer," identical to *li yang feng* 癧瘍風, "pervasion-illness with ulcer wind," a condition of white macules and dots appearing on the skin in the neck, on the chest, and below the armpits, without itching or pain. BCGM Dict I, 315.

【時珍曰】張仲景金匱要略言：菜中有水莨菪，葉圓而光，有毒，誤食令人狂亂，狀如中風，或吐血，以甘草汁解之。

Collected Explanations. *Bie lu*: *Lang dang* seeds grow in river valleys near the sea and in Yong zhou. The seeds are collected in the fifth month. [Tao] Hongjing: Today, they can be found everywhere. The shape of the seeds is a little reminiscent of *schisandra* fruit, but they are very small. [Han] Baosheng: They can be found everywhere. The leaves resemble those of [the Chinese indigo plant] *isatis indigofera*. Stem and leaves have fine hair. The flowers are white. The seed shell is shaped like a poppy capsule. The fruits formed are flat and fine, similar in size to millet of a greenish-yellow color. The seeds are collected in the sixth and seventh month; they are dried in the sun. [Su] Song: They can be found everywhere. The seedling has a stem reaching a height of two to three *chi*. The leaves resemble those of Chinese foxglove, cowherb and safflower; they are as broad as three fingers. Purple flowers open in the fourth month. Stem and pods have white hair. The fruits are formed in the five month. They have a shell shaped similar to poppy seeds and small pomegranate fruits. The seeds in the "housing" are very fine. They are greenish-white, similar to millet grains. [Lei] Xiao: For all [therapeutic] applications, do not use *cang ming* seeds.[928] Their shape is similar, except for [*cang ming* seeds] being slightly red and when ingested they remain without [therapeutic] effect. Nowadays, people often mix them. [Li] Shizhen: Zhang Zhongjing in his *Jin kui yao lüe* says: "Among vegetables is water *lang dang*. It has round and glossy leaves. They are poisonous. Mistakenly eaten, they let one turn mad and confused, similar to being struck by wind, sometimes with blood spitting. This is resolved with *glycyrrhiza* [root] juice.

17-11-01
子 *Zi*

Seeds [of *lang dang*].

【修治】【斅曰】修事莨菪子十兩，以頭醋一鎰，煮乾爲度。却用黄牛乳汁浸一宿，至明日乳汁黑，即是真者。晒乾搗篩用。

Pharmaceutical Preparation. [Lei] Xiao: To prepare them [for therapeutic use], boil ten *liang* of *lang dang* seeds in one *yi* of top quality vinegar until the liquid has dried. Then soak [the seeds] in the milk of a yellow cow for one night. When the milk has turned black the next morning, this is evidence that the seeds are genuine. Dry them in the sun, pound them, pass [the resulting powder] through a sieve and use them [for therapeutic ends].

928 *Cang ming* 蒼蓂, botanical identification unclear.

【氣味】苦，寒，無毒。【别録曰】甘。【權曰】苦、辛，微熱，有大毒。【藏器曰】性温不寒。【大明曰】温，有毒。服之熱發，以緑豆汁、甘草、升麻、犀角並解之。【斅曰】有大毒。誤服之，衝人心，大煩悶，眼生暹火。【頌曰】本經言性寒，後人多云大熱。而史記淳于意傳云：淄川王美人懷子不乳。飲以浪蕩藥一撮，以酒飲，旋乳。且不乳豈熱藥所治？又古方主卒顛狂亦多單用莨菪，豈果性寒耶？

Qi and Flavor. Bitter, cold, nonpoisonous.[929] *Bie lu*: Sweet- [Zhen] Quan: Bitter, acrid, slightly hot, very poisonous. [Chen] Cangqi: Their nature is warm, not cold. Da Ming: Warm, poisonous. To eat them causes heat effusion. This is resolved with either mung bean juice, *glycyrrhiza* [root], *cimicifuga* [rhizome] or rhinoceros horn. [Lei] Xiao: They are very poisonous. Mistakenly eaten, they rush against the heart causing massive vexation and heart-pressure, [Su] Song: The *Ben jing* says that their nature is cold. Later people often state that they are very hot. The biography of Chunyu Yi in the *Shi ji* states: "Wang, a beauty in Zi chuan, gave birth to a child but did not have milk. She took a beverage with a pinch of *lang dang* [seeds] as pharmaceutical drug and drank it with wine. This enabled her to give milk." How can it be that a pharmaceutical drug of hot [nature] can cure a failure to give milk? Also, ancient recipes often resort to *lang dang* as a single substance to control sudden peak[-illness] with madness. How can this be the effect of [a substance of] cold nature?

【主治】齒痛出蟲，肉痺拘急。久服輕身，使人健行，走及奔馬，强志益力，通神見鬼。多食令人狂走。本經。療癲狂風癇，顛倒拘攣。别録。安心定志，聰明耳目，除邪逐風，變白，主痃癖。取子洗晒，隔日空腹，水下一指捻。亦可小便浸令泣盡，暴乾，如上服。勿令子破，破則令人發狂。藏器。炒焦研末，治下部脱肛，止冷痢。主蛀牙痛，咬之蟲出。甄權。燒熏蟲牙，及洗陰汗。大明。

Control. Toothache with an appearance of worms/bugs. Numbness, contraction and tension of flesh. Ingested for a long time they relieve the body of its weight. They let one walk forcefully, and enable one to run as fast as a horse. They strengthen the mind and boost one's strength. They enable communication with spirits and a vision of demons. Eaten in large amounts makes one run around like crazy. *Ben jing*. They

929 Instead of *wu du* 無毒, "nonpoisonous," *Zheng lei* ch. 10, *lang dang zi* 莨菪子, quoting *Bie lu* writes *you du* 有毒, "poisonous."

heal peak-illness and madness[930] and wind epilepsy.[931] Peak inversion[932] with cramps and contraction. *Bie lu*. They calm the heart and stabilize the mind. They clear the ears and brighten the eyes. They remove evil qi, dispel wind and change white [hair/beards to black again]. They control string-illness[933] and aggregation-illness. Wash the seeds clean and dry them in the sun. Every second day ingest with water the amount picked up with three fingers. It is also possible to soak the [seeds] in urine until all the liquid has gone, dry them in the sun and ingest them as outlined above. The seeds must not be broken open. Broken open they let one turn mad. [Chen] Cangqi. Fried until scorched and ground into powder, they cure anal prolapse in the lower body part and end cold free-flux illness. They control toothache related to the presence of worms/bugs. Chewed up they let the worms/bugs appear. Zhen Quan. Burn them to steam/fumigate teeth infested with worms/bugs. Also, they serve to wash the yin [(i. e., genital) region] when it sweats. Da Ming.

【發明】【弘景曰】入療顛狂方用，然不可過劑。久服自無嫌，通神健行，足爲大益，而仙經不見用。【權曰】以石灰清煮一伏時，掬出，去芽暴乾，以附子、乾薑、陳橘皮、桂心、厚朴爲丸服。去一切冷氣，積年氣痢，甚温暖也。不可生服，傷人見鬼，拾鍼狂亂。【時珍曰】莨菪之功，未見如所説，而其毒有甚焉。煮一二日而芽方生，其爲物可知矣。莨菪、雲實、防葵、赤商陸皆能令人狂惑見鬼者，昔人未有發其義者。蓋此類皆有毒，能使痰迷心竅，蔽其神明，以亂其視聽故耳。唐安禄山誘奚契丹，飲以莨菪酒，醉而坑之。又嘉靖四十三年二月，陝西遊僧武如香，挾妖術至昌黎縣民張柱家，見其妻美。設飯間，呼其全家同坐，將紅散入飯内食之。少頃舉家昏迷，任其奸污。復將魘法吹入柱耳中。柱發狂惑，見舉家皆是妖鬼，盡行殺死，凡一十六人，並無血迹。官司執柱囚之。十餘日，柱吐痰二椀許，聞其故，乃知所殺者皆其父母、兄嫂、妻子、姊姪也。柱與如香皆論死。世宗肅皇帝命榜示天下。觀此妖藥，亦是莨菪之流爾。方其痰迷之時，視人皆鬼矣。解之之法，可不知乎？

Explication. [Tao] Hongjing: They are used in recipes to heal peak[-illness] and madness. However, they must not be administered excessively. Ingested over a long time, they are unproblematic. They let one communicate with spirits and walk

930 *Dian kuang* 癲狂, "peak-illness and madness," a condition of mental disturbance. Based on a patient's condition of silence or restlessness one may distinguish between the two types of *dian* 癲, "peak-illness," and *kuang* 狂, "madness." BCGM Dict I, 125.

931 *Feng xian* 風癇, "wind epilepsy," a kind of *xian* 癇, "epilepsy," resulting from the effects of wind evil. BCGM Dict I, 170.

932 *Dian dao* 顛倒, "peak inversion," a sign of mental or emotional derangement. BCGM Dict I, 124.

933 *Xuan* 痃, "string-illness," a condition of acute pain located in the abdomen to the left and right of the umbilicus. BCGM Dict I, 591.

strongly. They are of sufficiently great benefit but their use is rarely seen in the classics of hermits/immortals. [Zhen] Quan: Boil them in lime for one full day. Pick up a handful, remove the shoots and dry them in the sun. With *aconitum* [accessory tubers], dried ginger, long-stored tangerine peels, shaved cinnamom bark and *magnolia* [bark] prepare pills that are to be ingested. They serve to remove all types of cold qi and qi [disorder] free-flux illness accumulated over years. They are very warm and warming. They must not be ingested raw/unprepared. They harm one and let him see demons. [Patients seem] to stitch [some tissue] with a needle, and are confused. [Li] Shizhen: [I] have not seen any of the [therapeutic] effects *lang dang* is said to have. But [the seeds] are very poisonous. When they are boiled for one or two days they grow shoots. This shows what type of items they are. *Lang dang*, Mysore thorn, *peucedanum* [root] and Indian pokewee [root] are all capable of letting one turn mad and see demons. The ancients had not uncovered the meaning underlying [these effects]. The fact is, all members of this group are poisonous, and they can send phlegm to fill the openings of the heart. This way they hide one's spirit brilliance and this is the reason behind one's confusion in what one sees and hears. During the Tang, An Lushan led a campaign against the Xi and the Qi dan. He let them drink *lang dang* wine to intoxification and entrapped them. Also, in the 43rd year of the *jia qing* reign period (1564), an itinerant monk Wu Ruxiang in Shaan xi practicing black art reached the home of Zhang Zhu in Chang li xian. There he saw the beauty of [Zhang Zhu's] wife. [The monk] arranged a meal and asked the entire family to sit together. He added a red powder to the food and let them eat it. After a short while, everybody was clouded with confusion, and [the monk] carried out his shameful activity [on the woman]. Also, he applied a terrifying method by blowing [the powder] into [Zhang] Zhu's ears whereupon [Zhang] Zhu turned mad. He recognized all his family members to be goblins and demons and went to kill them all, 16 persons. But there were no traces of blood. A judicial official arrested and imprisoned him. Ten days later, [Zhang] Zhu spat out more than two bowls of phlegm. When he learned why [he was in prison], he realized that he had killed his father and mother, his elder brother and his sister-in-law, his wife and his children, his sister and his niece. [Zhang] Zhu and [Wu] Ruxiang were both sentenced to death. Emperor Shi zong Su issued a decree to be publicized in the entire empire. A view on this bewitching medication shows that *dang lang* is part of it. When the phlegm has its confusing effect, other people appear as demons. Is it at all possible not to be familiar with the methods to resolve these [effects]?!

【附方】舊二，新二十。

Added Recipes. Two of old. 20 newly [recorded].

卒發顛狂。莨菪三升爲末，以酒一升漬數日，絞去滓，煎令可丸，如小豆三丸，日三服。當覺面急，頭中如有蟲行，額及手足有赤色處，如此並是瘥候也。未知再服，取盡神良。陳延之小品方。

A sudden outbreak of peak[-illness] and madness. [Grind] three *sheng* of *dang lang* into powder and soak it in wine for several days. Then press it [to obtain a juice] and remove the dregs. Boil [the juice to a consistency] permitting it to form pills. Eat three pills the size of [red] mung beans three times a day. This will cause a facial tightness and a feeling in the head as if there were worms/bugs moving. The forehead, the hands and the feet have red areas. When this is so, it is a sign of the cure. If no such effects are seen, ingest [the pills] a second time. Chen Yanzhi, *Xiao pin fang*.

風痺厥痛。天仙子三錢炒，大草烏頭、甘草半兩，五靈脂一兩，爲末，糊丸梧子大，以螺青爲衣。每服十丸，男子菖蒲酒下，女子芫花湯下。聖濟録。

Blockage related to wind [intrusion] and painful recession [of qi]. [Grind] three *qian* of *tian xian zi*, fried, one large *aconitum* [main tuber], half a *liang* of *glycyrrhiza* [root] and one *liang* of flying squirrel droppings into powder. Form with [wheat flour] paste pills the size of *wu* seeds, and coat them with a dark color.[934] Each time ingest ten pills. Males send them down with *acorus* wine; females send them down with daphne flower decoction. *Sheng ji lu*.

久嗽不止，有膿血。莨菪子五錢，淘去浮者，煮令芽出，炒研，真酥一雞子大，大棗七枚，同煎令酥盡，取棗日食三枚。

Unending, long-lasting cough, with pus and blood. Wash five *qian* of *lang dang* seeds in a basin and discard those floating on the surface. Boil the rest until shoots appear. Fry [the seeds] and grind [them into powder]. Then boil [the powder] with genuine butter, the size of an egg, and seven Chinese dates until all the butter has vanished. Take the Chinese dates out and eat three of them per day.

又方：莨菪子三撮，吞之，日五六度。光祿李丞服之神驗。孟詵必效方。

Another recipe. Swallow three pinches of *lang dang* seeds, five or six times a day. Li Cheng of Guang lu ingested this with divine success. Meng Shen, *Bi xiao fang*.

年久呷嗽，至三十年者。莨菪子、木香、熏黄等分，爲末。以羊脂塗青紙上，撒末於上，卷作筒，燒烟熏吸之。崔行功纂要方。

934 *Luo qing* 螺青, lit.: "spiral shell greenish." Used for a dark, almost black, color.

A wheezing cough for as long as a year, or for as long as 30 years. [Grind] equal amounts of *lang dang* seeds, *costus* [root] and realgar into powder. Smear sheep fat on a greenish piece of paper and distribute the powder on it. Roll [the paper] to form a tube. Burn it and let [the patient] inhale the fumes. Cui Xinggong, *Zuan yao fang*.

水腫蠱脹。方見獸部麢羊下。

Water swelling and *gu* distension.[935] For recipes, see under the entry "antelope," in the section "animals." (51-13)

積冷痃癖，不思飯食，羸困者。莨菪子三分，水淘去浮者，大棗四十九個，水三升，煮乾，只取棗去皮核。每空心食一箇，米飲下，覺熱即止。聖濟録。

String-illness[936] and aggregation-illness related to cold [qi] accumulation, with loss of appetite and emaciation. Wash three *fen* of *lang dang* seeds in a basin and discard those floating on the surface. Boil [the rest] with 49 Chinese dates in three *sheng* of water until the liquid has dried. Pick up the dates without their skin and pits. Each time eat one on an empty stomach, to be sent down with a rice beverage. When a sensation of heat sets in, end [the therapy]. *Sheng ji lu*.

水瀉日久。青州乾棗十個去核，入莨菪子填滿札定，燒存性。每粟米飲服一錢。聖惠方。

Watery outflow lasting for a day or longer. Remove the pits from ten Chinese dates from Qing zhou and fill them with *lang dang* seeds. Fix them on a wooden writing board and burn them with their nature retained. Each time ingest with a millet beverage one *qian*. *Sheng hui fang*.

冷疳痢下。莨菪子爲末，臘豬脂和丸，綿裹棗許，導下部。因痢出，更納新者。不過三度瘥。孟詵必效方。

Gan-illness[937] and free-flux illness discharge related to cold [qi]. [Grind] *lang dang* seeds into powder and form with lard, obtained in the 12th month, pills. Wrap a Chinese date size [pill] in silk floss and insert it into the lower body part. When it is pushed out by the free flow, insert a new one. After no more than three such applications, a cure is achieved. Meng Shen, *Bi xiao fang*.

935 *Shui gu* 水蠱, "water *gu*[-distension," identical to *gu zhang* 鼓脹, "drum[-like] distension." A condition of an abdominal distension and big upswell brought forth by stagnant water qi accumulating in the abdomen. BCGM Dict 409, 196.

936 *Xuan* 痃, "string-illness," a condition of acute pain located in the abdomen to the left and right of the umbilicus. BCGM Dict I, 591.

937 *Gan* 疳, "*gan*-illness," also: "sweets-illness," involves several complaints that affect children and adults, with causes and conditions too different to fall into a known disease category. BCGM Dict I, 180-188.

赤白下痢，腹痛，腸滑後重。大黄煨半兩，莨菪子炒黑一抄，爲末。每服一錢，米飲下。普濟方。

Red and white discharge with free-flux illness, abdominal pain, a smooth passage through the intestines, and a feeling of heaviness in the behind. [Grind] half a *liang* of rhubarb root, simmered, and a pinch of *lang dang* seeds, fried until they have turned black, into powder. Each time ingest one *qian*, to be sent down with a rice beverage. *Pu ji fang*.

久痢不止，變種種痢，兼脱肛。莨菪丸：用莨菪子一升，淘去浮者，煮令芽出，晒乾，炒黄黑色，青州棗一升，去皮核，釅醋二升，同煮，搗膏丸梧子大。每服二十丸，食前米飲下。聖惠方。

Long-lasting, unending free-flux illness, changing into various kinds of free-flux illness, associated with anal prolapse. The "pills with *lang dang*." Wash one *sheng* of *lang dang* seeds in a basin and discard those floating on the surface. Boil [the rest] until sprouts appear and dry them in the sun. Fry them until they have assumed a yellow-black color. Then boil them together with one *sheng* of Chinese dates from Qing zhou, with skin and pits removed, in two *sheng* of strong vinegar. Pound them to a paste and form pills the size of *wu* seeds. Each time ingest 20 pills, to be sent down prior to a meal with a rice beverage. *Sheng hui fang*.

腸風下血。莨菪煎：用莨菪實一升，暴乾搗篩，生薑半斤，取汁，銀鍋中更以無灰酒二升搜之，上火煎如稠餳，即旋投酒。度用酒可及五升即止。慢火煎令可丸，大如梧子，每旦酒飲通下三丸，增至五七丸止。若丸時粘手，則以兔絲粉襯隔之。火候忌緊，藥焦則失力也。初服微熱，勿怪。疾甚者，服過三日，當下利。疾去，利亦止。絶有效。篋中方。

Intestinal wind with discharge of blood. The "decoction with *lang dang*." Dry one *sheng* of *lang dang* fruit in the sun, pound them and [pass the powder] through a sieve. Obtain the juice of half a *jin* of fresh ginger and fill it with [the powder] and two *sheng* of ash-free wine into a silver pot. Boil it above a fire until it has assumed a consistency like malt extract. Add more wine. Gradually use wine up to five *sheng*, then stop. Boil this on a slow fire to reach a consistency permitting it to form pills the size of *wu* seeds. Every morning send down with a wine beverage three pills. This may be increased to five or seven pills. Then stop. If the pills, when they are prepared, stick to the hands coat them with *cuscuta* [seed] powder to keep them separate. See to it that the fire is not too strong. A scorched medication has lost its strength. When it is ingested for the first time, [patients] feel some heat, but this should be of no concern. In the case of a severe illness, after ingesting [the medication] for three days a discharge with free flow occurs. When the illness is eliminated, the free flow ends, too. [This therapy] is definitely effective. *Jia zhong fang*.

脱肛不收。莨菪子炒研傅之。聖惠方。

Prolapsed anus that is not drawn back. Grind fried *lang dang* seeds and apply them [to the affected region]. *Sheng hui fang*.

風牙蟲牙。瑞竹堂方用天仙子一撮，入小口瓶內燒烟，竹筒引煙，入蟲孔內熏之即死，永不發。

Teeth affected by wind; teeth affected by worms/bugs. The *Rui zhu tang fang* [recommends to] insert one pinch of *tian xian zi* into a bottle with a narrow opening and heat it to generate fumes. These [fumes] are guided with a bamboo tube into the hole with the worms/bugs to steam them to death. The [ailment] will never break out again.

普濟方用莨菪子入瓶內，以熱湯淋下，口含瓶口，令氣熏之。冷更作，盡三合乃止。有涎津吐去，甚效。

The *Pu ji fang* [recommends to] fill *lang dang* seeds into a bottle and pour hot, boiled water on them. Then hold the opening of the bottle in the mouth and let the qi steam/fumigate the [affected region]. When [the contents of the bottle have cooled] repeat the process. Stop when three *ge* are used up. Saliva generated [during the treatment] should be spat out. Very effective.

備急方用莨菪子數粒納孔中，以蠟封之，亦效。

The *Bei ji fang* [recommends to] insert several *lang dang* seed grains into the holes and seal them with beeswax. This, too, is effective.

牙齒宣落風痛。莨菪子末，綿裹咬之，有汁勿嚥。必效方。

Painful wind [intrusion] into the teeth. Wrap *lang dang* seed powder in silk floss and chew on it. Do not swallow the juice [generated in the mouth]. *Bi xiao fang*.

風毒咽腫，嚥水不下，及瘰癧咽腫。水服莨菪子末兩錢匕，神良。外臺秘要。

Swollen throat caused by wind poison, with an inability to swallow water, and scrofula pervasion illness[938] with a swollen throat. Ingest with water the amount of *lang dang* seed powder held by a two *qian* spoon. Divinely good. *Wai tai mi yao*.

938 *Luo li* 瘰癧, "scrofula pervasion-illness," when two or more connected swellings of the size of plum or date kernels appear either on the neck or in the armpits, or somewhere else on the body. BCGM Dict I. 329.

乳癰堅硬。新莨菪子半匙，清水一盞，服之。不得嚼破。外臺秘要。

Breast obstruction-illness[939] with a hardening. Ingest half a spoonful of new *lang dang* seeds in one small cup of clear water. Do not chew [the seeds] to break them open. *Wai tai mi yao.*

石癰堅硬，不作膿者。莨菪子爲末，醋和，傅瘡頭，根即拔出。千金方。

Rock hard obstruction-illness[940] without festering. [Grind] *lang dang* seeds into powder, mix it with vinegar and apply it to the tip of the sore. This will pull the root out. *Qian jin fang.*

惡瘡似癩，十年不愈者。莨菪子燒研，傅之。千金方。

Malign sores resembling repudiation-illness[941] that have not been cured for ten years. Burn *lang dang* seeds, grind [the residue into powder] and apply it [to the affected region]. *Qian jin fang.*

打撲折傷。羊脂調莨菪子末，傅之。千金方。

Fracture harm resulting from a blow or fall. Mix sheep fat with *lang dang* seed powder and apply it [to the affected region]. *Qian jin fang.*

惡犬咬傷。莨菪子七枚吞之，日三服。千金方。

Harm caused by the bite of a malign dog. Swallow seven *lang dang* seeds. To be ingested three times a day. *Qian jin fang.*

17-11-02

根 *Gen*

Root [of *lang dang*].

【氣味】苦、辛，有毒。

Qi and Flavor. Bitter, acrid, poisonous.

---

939 *Ru yong* 乳癰, "breast obstruction-illness," a condition of acute putrefication of a woman's breast. Often encountered if a woman, following delivery, experiences *chui nai* 吹奶, "inflated breast," or *du ru* 妒乳, "jealousy breast." BCGM Dict I, 412.

940 *Yong* 癰, "obstruction-illness,"refers to an obstruction of vessels or other ducts inside the body. Qi rushing against the obstruction may cause a local swelling and eventually break through the surface to cause an abscess. BCGM Dict I, 641.

941 *Lai* 癩, "*lai*-illness," "repudiation-illness," including cases of leprosy/Aussatz." BCGM Dict I, 293.

【主治】邪瘧，疥癬，殺蟲。時珍。

Control. Evil malaria, *jie*-illness[942] and *xuan*-illness.[943] It kills worms/bugs. [Li] Shizhen.

【附方】新六。

Added Recipes. Six newly [recorded].

瘧疾不止。莨菪根燒灰，水服一合，量人强弱用。千金方。

Unending malaria ailment. Burn *lang dang* root to ashes and ingest with water one *ge*. The use [of the root] must be consistent with the strong or weak constitution of that person. *Qian jin fang*.

惡癬有蟲。莨菪根搗爛，蜜和傅之。千金翼。

Malign *xuan* illness with the presence of worms/bugs. Pound *lang dang* root into a pulpy mass, mix it with honey and apply this [to the affected region]. *Qian jin yi*.

趾間肉刺。莨菪根搗汁塗之。雷公炮炙論序云：脚生肉刺，裩繫菪根。謂繫于裩帶上也。

Corns between toes. Pound *lang dang* root to obtain a juice and apply this [to the affected region]. The *Lei gong pao zhi lun* in its preface states: "When the legs grow corns, fasten *lang dang* to the underwear." That is to say, they are attached to the belt of the underwear.

狂犬咬人。莨菪根和鹽搗傅，日三上。外臺秘要。

A person bitten by a mad dog. Pound *lang dang* root and salt and apply [this to the affected region]. To be applied three times a day. *Wai tai mi yao*.

惡刺傷人。莨菪根水煮汁浸之，冷即易，神方也。千金方。

A person harmed by a malign thorn. Boil *lang dang* root in water and bathe [the affected region] in the resulting juice. Replace it when [the juice] has turned cold. A divine recipe. *Qian jin fang*.

942 *Jie*-illness 疥, vaguely identifiable skin ailment. BCGM Dict I, 249.

943 *Xuan* 癬, "*xuan*-illness." Conditions of dermal lesions with initially erythema, papules, and itching gradually extending in all directions to form an irregular ring with clear boundaries. The skin is slightly elevated with small papules, blisters, and/or scales and scraps. The central lesion may appear to heal spontaneously, and it may reappear. Also, a designation of local lesions with itching, release of liquid and shedding of scabs. BCGM Dict I, 591.

箭頭不出。萬聖神應丹：端午前一日，不語，尋見莨菪科，根本枝葉花實全好者。道云："先生你却在這裏。"道罷，用柴灰自東南起圍了，以木椑子掘取根下周迴土，次日日未出時，依前不語，用钁頭取出，洗净，勿令雞、犬、婦人見，于净室中，以石臼搗如泥，丸彈子大，黄丹爲衣，以紙袋封，懸高處陰乾。遇有箭頭不出者，先以象牙末貼瘡口，後用緋帛袋盛此藥，放臍中，綿兜肚繫了，當便出也。張子和儒門事親方。

An arrowhead that fails to come out. The "elixir of a myriad of sages with divine responses." One day before the fifth day of the fifth month search, without saying a word, for a *lang dang* specimen that is complete with root, stem, twigs, leaves, flowers and fruit. Then say to it: "Sir, you are here!" Having said this, use firewood ashes to draw a circle [around the plant] beginning in the South-East. Then, with a wooden shovel, dig out the soil around the root. The next morning, prior to sunrise, again without saying a word, remove [the plant] with a billhook and wash it clean. Do not let chicken, dogs or women observe this. Then pound it in a clean room in a stone mortar into a pulp and form pills the size of a bullet, with a coating of minium. Seal them in a paper bag and hang it at a high, shady and dry place. When someone with an arrowhead that fails to come out comes by, first apply ivory powder to the opening of the wound. Then fill a red silk floss pouch with this medication, place it on [that person's] navel and tie it with a silk undergarment [to the abdomen]. [The arrowhead] will come out. A recipe from Zhang Zihe's *Ru men shi qin*.

17-12
雲實本經上品

Yun shi, FE *Ben jing*, upper rank.

***Cesalpinia decapetala* (Roth) Alston. Mysore thorn.**

【釋名】員實別録、雲英別録、天豆吴普、馬豆圖經、羊石子圖經。苗名草雲母唐本、臭草圖經、粘刺綱目。【時珍曰】員亦音雲，其義未詳。豆以子形名。羊石當作羊矢，其子肖之故也。

Explanation of Names. *Yuan shi* 員實, *Bie lu*. *Yun ying* 雲英, *Bie lu*. *Tian dou* 天豆, heavenly beans," Wu Pu. *Ma dou* 馬豆, "horse/big beans," *Tu jing*. *Yang shi zi* 羊石子, "sheep stone seed," *Tu jing*. The seedling is called *cao yun mu* 草雲母, "herbal mica," *Tang ben*. *Chou cao* 臭草, "malodorous herb," *Tu jing*. *Nian ci* 粘刺, "sticky thorns," *Gang mu*. [Li] Shizhen: *Yuan* 員 is also read *yun* 雲; the meaning is unclear. The [designation as] *dou* 豆, "bean," refers to the shape of the seeds. *Yang shi* 羊石, "sheep stone," should be *yang shi* 羊矢, "sheep excrements," as the seeds resemble them.

【集解】【别録曰】雲實生河間川谷。十月采，暴乾。【普曰】莖高四五尺，大莖中空，葉如麻，兩兩相值。六月花，八月、九月實，十月采。【弘景曰】處處有之。子細如葶藶子而小黑，其實亦類莨菪，燒之致鬼，未見其法術。【恭曰】雲實大如黍及大麻子等，黄黑似豆，故名天豆。叢生澤旁，高五六尺。葉如細槐，亦如苜蓿。枝間微刺，俗謂苗爲草雲母。陶云似葶藶者，非也。【保昇曰】所在平澤有之。葉似細槐，花黄白色，其莢如豆，其實青黄色，大若麻子。五月、六月采實。【頌曰】葉如槐而狹長，枝上有刺。苗名臭草，又名羊石子草。實名馬豆。三月、四月采苗，十月采實，過時即枯落也。【時珍曰】此草山原甚多，俗名粘刺。赤莖中空，有刺，高者如蔓。其葉如槐。三月開黄花，纍然滿枝。莢長三寸許，狀如肥皂莢。内有子五六粒，正如鵲豆，兩頭微尖，有黄黑斑紋，厚殻白仁，咬之極堅，重有腥氣。

Collected Explanation. *Bie lu*: *Yun shi* grows in the river valleys of He jian. It is collected in the tenth month and dried in the sun. [Wu] Pu: The stem is four to five *chi* tall. Big stems are hollow. The leaves resemble those of hemp plants, with always two and two growing together. Flowers [open] in the sixth month. Fruit [form] in the eighth and ninth month; they are collected in the tenth month. [Tao] Hongjing: [*Yun shi*] is present everywhere. The fine seeds are similar to wood whitlow-grass seeds, but they are smaller and black. The fruits also resemble henban [fruits]. When they are burned, demons come by, but so far I have not seen this art practiced. [Su] Gong: *Yun shi* [seeds] are as big as glutinous millet and hemp seeds. They are yellow-black, resembling beans. Hence the name "heavenly beans." [The plant] grows in clusters near marshland and reaches a height of five to six *chi*. The leaves are similar to fine *sophora japonica* tree leaves. They are also similar to alfalfa [leaves]. Small thorns are situated between the twigs. The seedling is commonly called "herbal mica." Tao [Hongjing] states that "[the seeds] resemble those of wood whitlow-grass." That is wrong. [Han] Baosheng: [*Yun shi*] can be found everywhere in the marshlands of the plains. The leaves resemble those of fine *sophora japonica* trees. The flowers are of yellow-white color. They have pods similar to beans. The fruits are of a greenish-yellow color, with a size similar to hemp seeds. The fruits are collected in the fifth and sixth month. [Su] Song: The leaves resemble those of *sophora japonica* trees, but are narrow and lengthy. There are thorns on the twigs. The seedling is called "malodorous herb." It is also called "sheep stone seed herb." The fruits are called "horse/big beans." The seedling is collected in the third and fourth month. The fruits are collected in the tenth month. If this time is missed, they wither and fall down. [Li] Shizhen: This herb is found in abundance on the plains in the mountains. It is commonly called "sticky thorns." The red stem is hollow and has thorns. Tall specimens are similar to creepers. The leaves are similar to those of *sophora japonica* trees. Yellow flowers open in the third month; they are closely linked to each other and fill the twigs. A thick shell includes a white kernel. When bitten on it, it proves to be very hard, and it emits strong fishy qi.

17-12-01
實 *Shi*

Fruit [of *yun shi*].

【修治】【斅曰】凡采得，粗搗，相對拌渾顆橡實，蒸一日，揀出暴乾。

Pharmaceutical Preparation. [Lei] Xiao: Whenever [*yun shi* fruits] are collected, pound them roughly and add to them unprepared fruits of sawtooth oak. Steam them for one day, take [the *yun shi* fruits] and dry them in the sun.

【氣味】辛，温，無毒。【别録曰】苦。【普曰】神農：辛，小温。黄帝：鹹。雷公：苦。

Qi and Flavor. Acrid, warm, nonpoisonous. *Bie lu*: Bitter. [Wu] Pu: Shen nong: Acrid, slightly warm. Huang Di: Salty. Lei gong: Bitter.

【主治】泄痢腸澼，殺蟲蠱毒，去邪惡結氣，止痛，除寒熱。本經。消渴。别録。治瘧多用。蘇頌。主下䘌膿血。時珍。

Control. Outflow with free-flux illness and intestinal flush. They kill worms/bugs and *gu* poison,[944] remove evil, malign and bound qi, end pain and dispel cold and heat. *Ben jing*. Melting with thirst.[945] *Bie lu*. They serve to cure malaria, and are often resorted to. Su Song. They control discharge with pus and blood related to hidden worms/bugs. [Li] Shizhen.

【附方】新一。

Added Recipes. One newly [recorded].

䘌下不止。雲實、女萎各一兩，桂半兩，川烏頭二兩，爲末，蜜丸梧子大。每服五丸，水下。日三服。肘後方。

Unending discharge related to hidden worms/bugs. [Grind] one *liang* each of *yun shi* and clematis creeper, half a *liang* of *cassia* bark and two *liang* of [Si] chuan *aconitum* [main tuber] into powder and form with honey pills the size of *wu* seeds.

944 *Gu du* 蠱毒, "*gu*-poison[ing]." (1) A poison emitted by certain worms/snakes with an ability to cause varying pathological changes in a person who has taken it in by means of wine or food. (2) Abdominal fullness, in some cases with blood spitting, and blood in the stool and urine. BCGM Dict I, 192 - 193. See BCGM 42-22.

945 *Xiao ke* 消渴, "melting with thirst," most likely including cases of diabetes. BCGM Dict Vol I, 567.

Each time ingest five pills, to be sent down with water. To be ingested three times a day. *Zhou hou fang*.

17-12-02
花 *Hua*

Flower [of *yun shi*].

【主治】見鬼精。多食令人狂走。久服輕身通神明。本經。殺精物，下水。燒之致鬼。別録。

Control. Visions of demonic spirits. Eaten in large amounts it lets one run around madly. Ingested over a long time it relieves the body of its weight and frees one's spirit brilliance. *Ben jing*. It kills essence-spirit items and serves to discharge water. To burn it lets demons to come by. *Bie lu*.

【發明】【時珍曰】雲實花既能令人見鬼發狂，豈有久服輕身之理？此古書之訛也。

Explication. [Li] Shizhen: *Yun shi* flowers can let one see demons and cause madness. How can it be that ingested over a long time they relieve the body of its weight? That is an error in ancient writings.

17-12-03
根 *Gen*

Root [of *yun shi*].

【主治】骨哽及咽喉痛。研汁嚥之。時珍。

Control. For choking on a bone and painful throat, grind it to obtain a juice and swallow it. [Li] Shizhen.

17-13
蓖麻蓖音卑唐本草
Bi ma, 蓖 read *bi* 卑, FE *Tang ben cao.*

***Ricinus communis* L. Castor oil plant.**

【釋名】【頌曰】葉似大麻，子形宛如牛螕，故名。【時珍曰】蓖亦作螕。螕，牛虱也。其子有麻點，故名蓖麻。

Explanation of Names. The leaves resemble those of hemp, *da ma* 大麻. The seeds are formed like ox ticks, *niu pi* 牛螕. Hence the name. [Li] Shizhen: *Bi* 蓖 is also written *bi* 螕. *Bi* 螕 are ox lice. The leaves are dotted like hemp, *ma* 麻, [leaves]. Hence the name *bi ma* 蓖麻.

【集解】【恭曰】此人間所種者，葉似大麻葉而甚大，結子如牛蜱。今胡中來者，莖赤，高丈餘，子大如皂莢核，用之益良。【保昇曰】今在處有之。夏生苗，葉似葎草而大厚。莖赤有節如甘蔗，高丈餘。秋生細花，隨便結實，殼上有刺，狀類巴豆，青黄斑褐。夏采莖葉，秋采實，冬采根，日乾用。【時珍曰】其莖有赤有白，中空。其葉大如瓠葉，每葉凡五尖。夏秋間椏裏抽出花穗，纍纍黄色。每枝結實數十顆，上有刺，攢族如蝟毛而軟。凡三四子合成一顆，枯時劈開，狀如巴豆，殼内有子大如豆。殼有斑點。狀如牛螕。再去斑殼，中有仁，嬌白如續隨子仁，有油，可作印色及油紙。子無刺者良，子有刺者毒。

Collected Explanations. [Su] Gong: When this [herb] is planted by people, its leaves resemble hemp leaves, but are very big. They form seeds similar to ox ticks. Specimens coming from the [region of the] Hu these days have a red stem and are more than a *zhang* tall. The seeds are as big as *gleditsia* pod kernels. Their application [for therapeutic ends] boosts one's wellbeing. [Han] Baosheng:[946] Today it can be found everywhere. It grows a seedling in summer. The leaves resemble those of wild hop, but are bigger and thick. The stem is red and has nodes like sugar cane. It is more than one *zhang* tall. Fine flowers grow in autumn; immediately afterwards they form fruits with thorns on their shell. Their shape is similar to that of croton seeds, They are greenish-yellow and have brown speckles. The stem and the leaves are collected in summer. The fruits are collected in autumn. The root is collected in winter. It is dried in the sun before being used [for therapeutic purposes]. [Li] Shizhen: The stems may be red or white. They are hollow. The leaves are as big as calabash leaves. Each leaf has five tips. During summer and autumn in the forks of the twigs flower spikes emerge. They are closely situated to each other and of yellow color. Each twig forms tens of fruit [capsules] covered with thorns. They are as close together as hedgehog hair, but soft. Always three to four seeds form one [fruit] capsule. When they wither they are broken open with force; their condition is similar to that of *croton* seeds. The seeds inside the shell have the size of soybeans. Their shell has speckles and dots, resembling ox ticks. When the speckled [seed] shell is removed, too, inside a kernel appears. It is of an amiable white color similar to the seed kernels of casper spurge. They have oil that can be made to printing ink and oil paper. Specimens with seeds without thorns are good. Those with seeds with thorns are poisonous.

946 Instead of to [Han] Baosheng 保昇, *Zheng lei* ch. 11, *bi ma zi* 蓖麻子, "*bi ma* seeds," attributes the following quote to the *Tu jing*.

17-13-01
子 *Zi*

Seeds [of *bi ma*].

【修治】【斅曰】凡使勿用黑天赤利子，緣在地蔞上生，是顆兩頭尖，有毒。其蓖麻子，節節有黄黑斑。凡使以鹽湯煮半日，去皮取子研用。【時珍曰】取蓖麻油法：用蓖麻仁五升搗爛，以水一斗煮之，有沫撇起，待沫盡乃止。去水，以沫煎至點燈不炸、滴水不散爲度。

Pharmaceutical Processing. [Lei] Xiao: For all applications do not resort to *hei tian chi li* seeds;[947] they must grow on *di lou*.[948] [*Hei tian chi li* seed] kernels have two pointed ends; they are poisonous. The *bi ma* seeds are covered with yellow-black speckles all over. For all applications, boil them with a salt decoction for half a day. Remove the skin, take the seeds, grind [them] and use [the pulp for therapeutic uses]. [Li] Shizhen: The method to obtain *bi ma* oil. Pound five *sheng* of *bi ma* kernels into a pulpy mass and boil it in one *dou* of water. Skim off the foam and continue [the boiling] until there is no more foam. Then end [the boiling], discard the water and fry the foam until it no longer crackles when dropped into a candle, and fails to disperse when dropped into water.

【氣味】甘、辛，平，有小毒。【時珍曰】凡服蓖麻者，一生不得食炒豆，犯之必脹死。其油能伏丹砂、粉霜。

Qi and Flavor. Sweet, acrid, balanced, slightly poisonous. [Li] Shizhen: Whenever *bi ma* is ingested, be sure to never eat fried soy beans. If this prohibition is offended, bloating and death are inevitable. The oil is capable of subduing [the effects of] cinnabar and sublimed calomel.

【主治】水癥。以水研二十枚服之，吐惡沫，加至三十枚，三日一服，瘥則止。又主風虛寒熱，身體瘡痒浮腫，尸疰惡氣，榨取油塗之。唐本。研傅瘡痍疥癩。塗手足心，催生。大明。治瘰癧。取子炒熟去皮，每卧時嚼服二三枚，漸加至十數枚，有效。宗奭。主偏風不遂，口眼喎斜，失音口噤，頭風耳聾，舌脹喉痺，齁喘脚氣，毒腫丹瘤，湯火傷，鍼刺入肉，女人胎衣不下，子腸挺出，開通關竅經絡，能止諸痛，消腫追膿拔毒。時珍。

---

947 *Hei tian chi li zi* 黑天赤利子 is a plant of unknown botanical identity. It is referred to in Lei Xiao's *Lei gong pao zhi lun*, a work influenced by Daoist thought using a terminology for quite a few substances that was accessible only to insiders and is not explained elsewhere.

948 *Di lou* 地蔞, a plant of unknown botanical identity. See previous note.

Control. Water concretion-illness.[949] With water grind 12 pieces [of *bi ma* seeds] and ingest them to cause a spitting of malign foam. Add up to 30 pieces and ingest them once every third day. When a cure is reached, end [the treatment]. They also control alternating sensations of cold and heat related to a depletion with wind [intrusion], itching body sores, surface swelling, corpse[-qi] attachment-illness[950] and malign qi. Squeeze [the seeds] to obtain their oil and apply it [to the affected region]. *Tang ben*. Grind them and apply them to cure sores, wounds, *jie*-illness,[951] and repudiation-illness.[952] Apply them to the palms of the hands and the soles of the feet to speed up birth. Da Ming. To cure scrofula pervasion-illness.[953] Take the seeds, fry them until done and remove their skin. Each time you go to bed chew two or three pieces and gradually increase this to ten or more pieces. Effective. [Kou] Zongshi. It controls unilateral wind[-stroke with the body] unable to follow [one's will], slanted mouth and eyes, loss of voice and lockjaw, head wind[954] and deafness, swollen tongue and throat closure, noisy panting and leg qi,[955] poison swelling and vermilion tumor,[956] harm caused by scalds and burns, needles or thorns having entered one's flesh, failure of women to release the placenta, and protrusion of the birth canal. It opens the passage through the orifices, the conduits and the network [vessels] and can end all types of pain, dissolve swelling, dispel pus and pull out poison. [Li] Shizhen.

【發明】【震亨曰】蓖麻屬陰，其性善收，能追膿取毒，亦外科要藥。能出有形之滯物，故取胎產胞衣、剩骨膠血者用之。【時珍曰】蓖麻仁甘辛有毒熱，氣味頗近巴豆，亦能利人，故下水氣。其性善走，能開通諸竅經絡，故能治偏風、失音、口噤、口目喎斜、頭風、七竅諸病，不止于出有

949 *Shui zheng* 水癥, "water concretion-illness," a condition of nodes and hardenings in the abdomen brought forth by accumulations of stagnant water. BCGM Dict I, 474.

950 *Shi zhu* 尸疰, "corpse [qi] attachment-illness," a condition of a slowly developing infectious weakness. BCGM Dict I, 202.

951 *Jie*-illness 疥, vaguely identifiable skin ailment. BCGM Dict I, 249.

952 *Lai* 癩, "*lai*-illness," "repudiation-illness," including cases of leprosy/Aussatz." BCGM Dict I, 293.

953 *Luo li* 瘰癧, "scrofula pervasion-illness," when two or more connected swellings of the size of plum or date kernels appear either on the neck or in the armpits, or somewhere else on the body. BCGM Dict I. 329.

954 *Tou feng* 頭風, "head wind." Condition of wind evil attacking the head followed by pain, dizziness, itching. BCGM Dict I, 509.

955 *Jiao qi* 脚氣, "leg qi." Painful, weak, swollen legs. BCGM Dict I, 248.

956 *Dan liu* 丹瘤, "vermilion tumor," a condition of a red kernel-type swelling without a head developing on the head, in the face, or at the throat. The tumor itself does not ache or itch, but is accompanied by fever with an aversion to cold and pain affecting head and body. BCGM Dict I, 119.

形之物而已。蓋鵜鶘油能引藥氣入內，蓖麻油能拔病氣出外，故諸膏多用之。一人病偏風，手足不舉。時珍用此油同羊脂、麝香、鯪鯉甲等藥，煎作摩膏，日摩數次，一月餘漸復。兼服搜風化痰養血之劑，三月而愈。一人病手臂一塊腫痛，亦用蓖麻搗膏貼之，一夜而愈。一人病氣鬱偏頭痛，用此同乳香、食鹽搗熖太陽穴，一夜痛止。一婦產後子腸不收，搗仁貼其丹田，一夜而上。此藥外用屢奏奇勛，但內服不可輕率爾。或言搗膏以箸點于鵝馬六畜舌根下，即不能食，或點肛內，即下血死，其毒可知矣。

Explication. [Zhu] Zhenheng: *Bi ma* is associated with yin [phenomena]. By its nature it tends to collect. It is capable of dispelling pus and to pick up poison. It is also an important pharmaceutical substance in the field of externally applied [medicine]. It is capable of letting sluggish items with a material shape leave [the body]. Therefore it is resorted to to remove [from the body] the placenta after a birth, remaining bones and thick blood. [Li] Shizhen: *Bi ma* kernels are sweet and acrid, and they have a poisonous heat. Their qi and flavor are quite similar to those of *croton* seeds. They, too, can harm humans. Therefore they serve to discharge water qi. By their nature they tend to run. They can open all orifices, and the conduits and network [vessels]. Hence they are able to cure unilateral wind[-stroke], loss of voice, lockjaw, slanted mouth and eyes, head wind,[957] and all types of diseases of the seven orifices. [Their effects] are not limited to causing material items to leave [one's body]. The fact is, pelican oil can lead the qi of all medication into the [body's] interior. *Bi ma* oil can pull disease qi to leave [the body] toward the outside. Hence it is often resorted to in all types of ointments. There was a man who had a unilateral wind[-stroke]. He was unable to lift hands and feet. [I, Li] Shizhen used this oil and boiled it together with pharmaceutical drugs such as sheep fact, musk, and pangolin scales to prepare a massage ointment. Every day [the patient] was given several massages, and within one month the severity of his disease diminished and [his mobility] was restored. At the same time he ingested preparations to search for [and dispel] wind, transform phlegm and nourish blood. Within three months he was cured. Another person had a painful lump-size swelling on his arm. Here, too, [I recommended to] pound *bi ma* to an ointment and attach it [to the affected region]. Within one night he was cured. Still another person had a unilateral headache related to pent-up qi. [I recommended to] pound [*bi ma*] with frankincense and table salt, heat [the pulp] and apply it to the major yang [needle insertion] holes [at the temples]. Within one night the pain ended. A woman after delivery experienced a prolapsed birth canal that was not drawn in again. [I recommended to] pound [*bi ma*] kernels and paste them on her cinnabar field. Within one night [the birth canal] had risen again. The

957 *Tou feng* 頭風, "head wind." Condition of wind evil attacking the head followed by pain, dizziness, itching. BCGM Dict I, 509.

external use of this pharmaceutical drug has repeatedly offered outstanding service. However, internally it must not be ingested without great care. Some say that when an ointment prepared by pounding [*bi ma* seeds] is inserted with chopsticks underneath the root of the tongue of geese, horses or any of the six domestic animals, they will no longer be able to eat. And if it were inserted into the anus, it caused a discharge of blood resulting in death. From this it can be known how poisonous [*bi ma* seeds] are.

【附方】舊九，新二十九。

Added Recipes. Nine of old. 29 newly [recorded].

半身不遂，失音不語。取蓖麻子油一升，酒一斗，銅鉢盛油，着酒中一日，煮之令熟，細細服之。外臺秘要。

Half of the body does not follow [one's will], with loss of voice and an inability to speak. Place [a vessel with] one *sheng* of *bi ma* seed oil into a copper pot with one *dou* of wine and boil it for one day until done. Then [let the patient] ingest [the oil] in small amounts. *Wai tai bi yao.*

口目喎斜。蓖麻子仁搗膏，左貼右，右貼左，即正。

If mouth and eyes are slanted, pound *bi ma* seed kernels to an ointment. If the slanting is on the left, apply it to the right [side of the face]; if it is on the right, apply it to the left [side of the face]. This will correct [the position of mouth and eyes].

婦人良方用蓖麻子仁七七粒，研作餅。右喎安在左手心，左喎安在右手心，却以銅盂盛熱水坐藥上，冷即換，五六次即正也。

The *Fu ren liang fang* [recommends to] grind seven times seven *bi ma* seed kernels and form cakes. In the case of a slanted right [side, the cake] is to be placed in the palm of the left hand; in the case of a slanted left [side, the cake is to be placed in the palm of right hand. Also, give [the cakes] into a copper pot filled with hot water and [let the patient] sit on the medication. When it has cooled, replace it. After five to six [such applications, the slanting] will be corrected.

一方：用蓖麻子仁七七粒，巴豆十九粒，麝香五分，作餅如上用。

Another recipe. Prepare cakes with 49 *bi ma* seed kernels, 19 *croton* seeds and five *fen* of musk and apply them as outlined above.

風氣頭痛不可忍者。乳香、蓖麻仁等分，搗餅隨左右貼太陽穴，解髮出氣，甚驗。

Unbearable headache related to wind qi [intrusion]. Pound equal amounts of frankincense and *bi ma* kernels to cakes and apply them to the major yang [needle insertion] holes [at the temples] depending on whether [the headache is] on the left or right side. This opens the hair [pores] and lets the qi come out. Very effective.

德生堂方用蓖麻油紙剪花，貼太陽亦效。

The *De sheng tang fang* [recommends to] cut paper soaked in *bi ma* oil and apply it to the major yang [holes at the temples]. This, too, is effective.

又方：蓖麻仁半兩，棗肉十五枚，搗塗紙上，捲筒插入鼻中，下清涕即止。

Another Recipe. Pound half a *liang* of *bi ma* kernels and the meat of 15 Chinese dates [to a pulp] and apply it on paper. Roll [the paper] into a tube and insert it into the nose. When clear snivel is discharged, end [the application].

八種頭風。蓖麻子、剛子各四十九粒去殻，雀腦芎一大塊，搗如泥，糊丸彈子大，線穿掛風處陰乾。用時先將好末茶調成膏子塗盞内，後將炭火燒前藥烟起，以盞覆之。待烟盡，以百沸葱湯點盞内茶藥服之。後以綿被裹頭卧，汗出避風。袖珍方。

Eight kinds of head wind.[958] Remove the shell from 49 grains each of *bi ma* seeds and *croton* seeds and pound them together with one large piece of *ligusticum* root to a pulp. With [wheat flour] paste form pills the size of a bullet, pass a string through them and hang them at a windy place in the shade to let them dry. At the time of their application, first mix good tea powder [with water] to form an ointment and apply it to the inside of a small cup. Then burn the medication mentioned above over a charcoal fire until a smoke rises. Cover it with the cup until no more smoke rises. Then drop an onion decoction, heated to bubbling 100 times, into the bowl and ingest the tea-medication. After this, wrap [the patient's] head with a soft quilt and let him lie down. The sweat released serves to dispel the wind. *Xiu zhen fang*.

鼻窒不通。蓖麻子仁三百粒，大棗去皮一枚，搗勻綿裹塞之。一日一易，三十日聞香臭也。聖濟録。

Stuffed, impenetrable nose. Pound 300 *bi ma* seed kernels and one Chinese date, with its skin removed, to an evenly [mixed pulp], wrap it in silk floss and insert it [into the nose]. Replace it once a day. Within 30 days you will be able to distinguish fragrant and malodorous smells. *Sheng ji lu*.

958 *Tou feng* 頭風, "head wind." Condition of wind evil attacking the head followed by pain, dizziness, itching. BCGM Dict I, 509.

天柱骨倒。小兒疳疾及諸病後，天柱骨倒，乃體虛所致，宜生筋散貼之。木鱉子六箇去殼，蓖麻子六十粒去殼，研勻。先包頭，擦項上令熱，以津調藥貼之。鄭氏小兒方。

Collapse of the heaven's pillar bone (cervical spine). When following a *gan*-illness[959] or any other disease of children the heaven's pillar bone collapses, this is the result of a bodily depletion and requires an application of the "powder to generate the growth of sinews." Grind six *momordica* seeds, with their shells removed, and 60 *bi ma* seeds, with their shells removed, to an evenly [mixed pulp]. First wrap the head [of the patient], rub his neck until it turns hot, mix the pharmaceutical drugs with [body] liquid and apply it [to the neck]. *Zheng shi xiao er fang.*

五種風癇，不問年月遠近。用蓖麻仁二兩，黃連一兩，銀石器內水一盌，文武火煮之。乾即添水，三日兩夜取出，去黃連，只用蓖麻風乾，勿令見日，以竹刀每個切作四段。每服二十段，食後荆芥湯下，日二服。終身忌食豆，犯之必腹脹死。衛生寶鑑。

The five kinds of wind epilepsy,[960] regardless of whether they have lasted for years or months, for a long or for a short time. Give two *liang* of *bi ma* kernels and one *coptis* [rhizom] into a silver or stone pot and place it into one bowl of water. Boil this with a mild fire first and a strong fire later. When [the water has] dried, add more water. Remove [the pot] after two nights on the third day and discard the *coptis* [rhizome]. Dry only the *bi ma* [kernels] at a windy [place] and avoid any exposure to the sun. Then cut with a bamboo knife each [kernel] into four pieces. Each time [let the patient] ingest 12 such pieces, to be sent down with a *schizonepeta* decoction after a meal. To be ingested twice a day. [The patient] is to avoid eating soybeans for the rest of his entire life. If he breaks this [restriction] his abdomen will inflate and he will die. *Wei sheng bao jian.*

舌上出血。蓖麻子油紙撚，燒烟熏鼻中，自止。摘玄方。

Bleeding surface of the tongue. Burn paper soaked with *bi ma* seed oil and expose the interior of the nose to the fumes. This will end [the bleeding]. *Zhai xuan fang.*

舌脹塞口。蓖麻仁四十粒，去殼研油塗紙上，作撚燒烟熏之。未退再熏，以愈爲度。有人舌腫出口外，一村人用此法而愈。經驗良方。

Distended tongue filling the mouth. Remove the shells of 40 *bi ma* kernels, grind them and apply the oil to a piece of paper. Roll [the paper into a stick], burn it

959 *Gan* 疳, "*gan*-illness," also: "sweets-illness," involves several complaints that affect children and adults, with causes and conditions too different to fall into a known disease category. BCGM Dict I, 180-188.

960 *Feng xian* 風癇, "wind epilepsy," a kind of *xian* 癇, "epilepsy," resulting from the effects of wind evil. BCGM Dict I, 170.

and expose [the tongue] to the fumes. If [the distension] fails to recede, fumigate it again. Continue until a cure is achieved. There was someone whose tongue was distended to a degree that it came out of his mouth. A fellow villager applied this method and he was cured. *Jing yan liang fang.*

急喉痺塞，牙關緊急不通，用此即破。以蓖麻子仁研爛，紙卷作筒，燒烟熏吸即通。或只取油作撚，尤妙。名聖烟筒。

Sudden throat blockage with lockjaw. The application of the following [recipe] will break it open. Grind *bi ma* seed kernels to a pulpy mass, [apply it to] paper and form a tube. Burn it and [let the patient] inhale the fumes. This will open [his throat]. Or, simply twist [a paper soaked with] the oil [into a stick and burn it to fumigate the throat]. This is particularly wondrous. It is called "sagely fumes tube."

咽中瘡腫。杜壬方用蓖麻子仁一枚，朴硝一錢，同研，新汲水服之，連進二三服，效。

Sore and swelling in the throat. The *Du Ren fang* [recommends] to grind one *bi ma* seed kernel together with one *qian* of mirabilite and ingest this with newly drawn water. Two or three times to be ingested in a row. Effective.

三因方用蓖麻仁、荆芥穗等分，爲末，蜜丸，綿包噙嚥之。千金。

The *San yin fang* [recommends to grind] equal amounts of *bi ma* kernels and *schizonepeta* spikes into powder, form pills with honey, wrap them in silk floss, hold this in the mouth and swallow the [resulting liquid]. *Qian jin.*[961]

水氣脹滿。蓖麻子仁研，水解得三合。清旦一頓服盡，日中當下青黄水也。或云壯人止可服五粒。外臺秘要。

Bloating and a feeling of fullness related to [the presence of] water qi. Grind *bi ma* seed kernels and dissolve [the pulp] in water to obtain [a liquid of] three *ge*. At a clear morning ingest this all at once. At noon, this will cause a discharge of greenish-yellow water. Some say that even persons of a robust constituency must not ingest more than five kernels. *Wai tai mi yao.*

脚氣作痛。蓖麻子七粒，去殼研爛，同蘇合香丸貼足心，痛即止也。外臺秘要。

961 This recipe is not recorded in *Qian jin fang* versions available today. It can be found in *San yin fang* ch. 16, *yan hou bing zheng zhi* 咽喉病證治, "cures of throat diseases and disease signs."

Painful leg qi.[962] Remove the shells of seven *bi ma* seeds and grind them to a pulpy mass. With storax form pills and apply them to the soles of the feet. The pain will end. *Wai tai mi yao.*

小便不通。蓖麻仁三粒，研細，入紙撚内，插入莖中即通。摘玄方。

Blocked urination. Grind three *bi ma* seeds to a fine [paste] and fill it into a paper roll. Insert it into the penis and the passage [of urine] will be freed. *Zhai xuan fang.*

齁喘咳嗽。蓖麻子去殼炒熟，揀甜者食之，須多服見效，終身不可食炒豆。衛生易簡方。

Wheezing panting and cough. Remove the shells of *bi ma* seeds and fry them until done. Select those that are sweet and eat them. After ingesting many of them the effects will be obvious. [Patients] for the entire rest of their life must not eat fried soybeans. *Wei sheng yi jian fang.*

催生下胞。崔元亮海上集驗方：取蓖麻子七粒，去殼研膏，塗脚心。若胎及衣下，便速洗去，不爾，則子腸出，即以此膏塗頂，則腸自入也。

To speed up birth and discharge of the placenta. Cui Yuanliang's *Hai shang ji yan fang* [recommends the following recipe]. Remove the shells of seven *bi ma* seeds, grind them to a paste and apply it to [the woman's] soles. As soon as the fetus and the placenta are discharged, quickly wash [the soles] to remove [the paste]. If this is not done, the birth intestine/uterus will prolapse. In such a case, apply the paste to the [woman's] neck and the intestine/uterus will be withdrawn into [the abdomen] again.

肘後方云：產難，取蓖麻子十四枚，兩手各把七枚，須臾立下也。

The *Zhou hou fang* states: For difficult births, take 14 *bi ma* seeds and [let the woman] grasp with each hand seven pieces. After a short while [the child] will come down.

子宫脱下。蓖麻子仁、枯礬等分，爲末，安紙上托入。仍以蓖麻子仁十四枚，研膏塗頂心即入。摘玄。

Prolapsed uterus. [Grind] equal amounts of *bi ma* seed kernels and processed alum into powder, spread it on a piece of paper and use it to push [the uterus] back into [the abdomen]. In addition, grind 14 *bi ma* seed kernels to an ointment and apply it to the center of [the woman's] head. This will let [the uterus] enter [the body] again. *Zhai xuan.*

962 *Jiao qi* 脚氣, "leg qi." Painful, weak, swollen legs. BCGM Dict I, 248.

盤腸生產。塗頂方同上。

Birth with a twisted intestine.[963] Recipe [for an ointment] to be applied to the top of the head, identical to the one above.

催生下胎。不拘生胎死胎。蓖麻二個，巴豆一個，麝香一分，研貼臍中并足心。

To speed up birth and discharge of a fetus, regardless of whether the fetus is alive or dead. Grind two *bi ma* [seeds], one *croton* [seed] and one *fen* of musk [to a pulp] and attach it to the center of the [woman's] navel and the soles of her feet.

又下生胎：一月一粒，温酒吞下。集簡方。

Also, to discharge/abort a living fetus. [Let the woman] swallow with warm wine one [*bi ma* seed] kernel per month. *Ji jian fang.*

一切毒腫，痛不可忍。蓖麻子仁搗傅，即止也。肘後方。

All types of swelling with poison, with an unbearable pain. Pound *bi ma* seed kernels [to a paste] and apply it [to the affected region]. This ends [the pain]. *Zhou hou fang.*

癘風鼻塌，手指攣曲，節間痛不可忍，漸至斷落。用蓖麻子一兩去皮，黃連一兩剉豆大，以小瓶子入水一升，同浸。春夏二日，秋冬五日後，取蓖麻子一枚擘破，面東以浸藥水吞之。漸加至四五枚，微利不妨。瓶中水盡更添。兩月後喫大蒜、猪肉試之，如不發是效也。若發動再服，直候不發乃止。杜壬方。

Epidemic wind[964] with a collapse of the bridge of the nose, crooked fingers, and an unbearable pain in the joints. Gradually a state is reached where [the fingers] become severed and fall off. Give one *liang* of *bi ma* seeds, with the skin removed, and one *liang* of *coptis* [rhizome], filed to the size of soybeans, into a bottle filled with one *sheng* of water and let them soak there, in spring and summer for two days; in autumn and winter for five days. Then take out one *bi ma* seed, break it open and swallow it, facing East, with the water used for soaking the pharmaceutical drugs. Gradually increase [the number of *bi ma* seeds swallowd] to four or five. A slight free flow is of no concern. When the water in the bottle is consumed, add new water. After two months eat garlic and pork as a test. If [the epidemic wind and

963 *Pan chang sheng chan* 盤腸生產, "birth with a twisted intestine," a condition at the time of birth with the vaginal wall or rectum appearing first and, after the child was born, being unable to retreat by themselves. BCGM Dict I, 369.

964 *Li feng* 癘風, "epidemic wind," identical to *da feng* 大風, "massive wind." Condition of a chronic, infectious skin disease with insensitive skin, red macules, festering swelling, and, in severe cases, loss of eyebrows, harm to the eyes, and collapse of the patient's nose. Possibly including cases of leprosy. BCGM Dict I, 111, 313.

its illness signs] do not effuse again, [the therapy was] effective. If [the epidemic wind and its illness signs] break out again, ingest [the medication] a second time. Continue until there are no more outbreaks. *Ren Du fang*.

小兒丹瘤。蓖麻子五個，去皮研，入麪一匙，水調塗之，甚效。修真秘旨。

Vermilion tumor of children. Remove the skin of five *bi ma* seeds and grind them. Add one spoonful of wheat flour, mix it with water and apply this [to the affected region]. Very effective. *Xiu zhen mi zhi*.

瘰癧結核。蓖麻子炒去皮，每睡時服二三枚，取效。一生不可喫炒豆。阮氏經驗方。

Scrofula pervasion-illness[965] with nodular kernels. At bedtime ingest two or three *bi ma* seeds, fried and with their skin removed, until an effect is seen. [Patients] must not eat fried soybeans for their entire life. *Ruan shi jing yan fang*.

瘰癧惡瘡及軟癤。用白膠香一兩，瓦器溶化，去滓，以蓖麻子六十四個，去殼研膏，溶膠投之，攪勻，入油半匙頭，柱點水中試軟硬，添減膠油得所，以緋帛量瘡大小攤貼，一膏可治三五癤也。儒門事親。

Scrofula pervasion-illness with malign sores and soft pimples. Dissolve one *liang* of Chinese sweet gum in a pottery vessel and remove the dregs. Remove the shells of 64 *bi ma* seeds, grind them to a paste and give it into the dissolved Chinese sweet gum. Mix [the paste and the Chinese sweet gum] evenly and add half a spoon of oil. Dip a wooden stick into the water to check whether [the mixture] is soft or hard and add more or less Chinese sweet gum and oil to achieve a desired consistency [of the paste]. Take a piece of red silk, measured in accordance with the size of the sore, spread [the paste] on it, and attach it [to the affected region]. One such ointment can serve to cure three to five pimples. *Ru men shi qin*.

肺風面瘡，起白屑，或微有赤瘡。用蓖麻子仁四十九粒，白果、膠棗各三粒，瓦松三錢，肥皂一個，搗爲丸。洗面用之良。吴旻扶壽方。

Lung wind with facial sores that rise as white flakes, or may be accompanied by some red sores. Pound 49 *bi ma* seed kernels, three pieces each of gingko [seeds] and Chinese dates, three *qian* of roof pines, and one Chinese coffee tree [fruit to a pulp] and form pills. [Prepare a decoction with these pills and use it to] wash the face. Good. Wu Min, *Fu shou fang*.

965 *Luo li* 瘰癧, "scrofula pervasion-illness," when two or more connected swellings of the size of plum or date kernels appear either on the neck or in the armpits, or somewhere else on the body. BCGM Dict I. 329.

面上雀斑。蓖麻子仁、密陀僧、硫黄各一錢，爲末。用羊髓和匀，夜夜傅之。摘玄方。

Sparrow speckles on the face.[966] [Grind] one *qian* each of *bi ma* seed kernels, litharge and sulphur into powder and mix it evenly with sheep marrow. Night after night apply [this to the affected region]. *Zhai xuan fang.*

髮黄不黑。蓖麻子仁，香油煎焦，去滓，三日後頻刷之。摘玄方。

When the hair turns yellow and is no longer black. Fry *bi ma* seed kernels in sesame oil until they are scorched and remove the dregs. Three days later repeatedly brush [the hair with the oil]. *Zhai xuan fang.*

耳卒聾閉。蓖麻子一百個去殼，與大棗十五枚擣爛，入乳小兒乳汁，和丸作鋌。每以綿裹一枚塞之，覺耳中熱爲度。一日一易，二十日瘥。千金方。

Sudden closure of the ears with deafness. Remove the shells of 100 *bi ma* seeds and pound them with 15 Chinese dates to a pulpy mass. Add a nursing mother's milk for a child and form pills to prepare small sticks. Each time wrap it with silk floss and insert one [such stick into the affected ear] until you feel heat in this ear. To be replaced once per day. A cure is achieved after 20 days. *Qian jin fang.*

湯火灼傷。蓖麻子仁、蛤粉等分，研膏。湯傷以油調，火灼以水調，塗之。古今録驗。

Harm caused by scalds and burns. Grind equal amounts of *bi ma* seed kernels and clam shell powder to a paste. For harm caused by scalds mix it with oil, for burns mix it with water, and apply this [to the affected region]. *Gu jin lu yan.*

鍼刺入肉。蓖麻子去殼研爛，先以帛襯傷處，傅之。頻看，若見刺出，即拔去，恐藥緊弩出好肉。或加白梅肉同研尤好。衛生易簡方。

A needle has entered the flesh. Remove the shells of *bi ma* seeds and grind them to a pulpy mass. First cover the location of the harm with a piece of cloth. Then apply [the pulpy mass]. Repeatedly [lift the cloth and] take a look whether the needle appears to come out. Then pull it. [The application is shielded from the skin with a piece of cloth because otherwise] the medication could pull out good flesh. Some add the meat of white/salted plums and grind it together with [the pulpy mass]. This is particularly good. *Wei sheng yi jian fang.*

竹木骨哽。蓖麻子仁一兩，凝水石二兩，研匀。每以一捻置舌根噙嚥，自然不見。

966 *Que ban*, "sparrow speckles," identical to *gan zeng* 皯黵, "dermal dark spots," a condition of numerous dark spots appearing on one's face. BCGM Dict I, 118, 394.

Choking on a piece of bamboo or wood. Evenly grind one *liang* of *bi ma* seed kernels and two *liang* of calcite. Each time place a pinch [of the resulting powder] under the root of the tongue, [let the patient] hold it in the mouth and swallow [the resulting liquid]. This will let [the alien items] disappear.

又方：蓖麻油、紅麯等分，研細，沙糖丸皂子大，綿裹含嚥，痰出大良。

Another recipe. Grind equal amounts of *bi ma* oil and medicated red rice to a fine [paste] and form with sugar pills the size of *gleditsia* seeds. Wrap them in silk floss, [let the patient] hold them in the mouth and swallow [the resulting liquid]. Once phlegm is thrown up this is very good.

雞魚骨哽。蓖麻子仁研爛，入百藥煎研，丸彈子大。井花水化下半丸，即下。

Choking on a chicken or fish bone. Grind *bi ma* seed kernels to a pulpy mass. Add ferment prepared from Chinese nutgalls and tea leaves and form pills the size of a bullet. Half a pill is sent down dissolved in well splendor water.[967] This will bring [the bones] down.

惡犬咬傷。蓖麻子五十粒去殼，以井花研膏。先以鹽水洗吹痛處，乃貼此膏。袖珍方。

Harm caused by the bite of a malign dog. Remove the shells of 50 *bi ma* seeds and grind them with well splendor water to an ointment. First wash clean with salt water the painful location and blow at it. Then apply this ointment. *Xiu zhen fang*.

17-13-02

葉 *Ye*

Leaf [of *bi ma*].

【氣味】有毒。

Qi and Flavor. Poisonous.

【主治】脚氣風腫不仁，蒸搗裹之，日二三易，即消。又油塗炙熱，熨顖上，止鼻衄，大驗。蘇恭。治痰喘欬嗽。時珍。

Control. A swelling with numbness related to leg qi[968] and wind [intrusion]. Steam [the leaves], pound them and wrap the [affected region with the pulp]. Replace it twice or three times a day. Also, roast the oil until it is hot and apply it as a hot

967 *Jing hua shui* 井華水, "well splendor water," i. e., the first water drawn from a well in the morning. BCGM Vol. II, 05-15-01.

968 *Jiao qi* 脚氣, "leg qi." Painful, weak, swollen legs. BCGM Dict I, 248.

compress on the fontanel to end nosebleed. Very effective. Su Gong. It serves to cure panting with phlegm and cough. [Li] Shizhen.

【附方】新一。
Added Recipe. One[969] newly [recorded].

齁喘痰嗽。儒門事親方用九尖蓖麻葉三錢，入飛過白礬二錢，以豬肉四兩薄批，摻藥在内，荷葉裹之，文武火煨熟。細嚼，以白湯送下。名九仙散。
Wheezing panting and cough with phlegm. The *Ru men shi qin* [recommends to] cut four *liang* of pork into thin slices and insert three *qian* of *bi ma* leaves with nine pointed ends and two *qian* of white, sublimated alum between them. Then wrap this with lotus leaves and simmer it first with a mild and then with a strong fire until done. Finely chew it and send it down with clear, boiled water. This is called the "nine hermits/immortals powder."

普濟方治欬嗽涎喘，不問年深日近。用經霜蓖麻葉、經霜桑葉、御米殼蜜炒各一兩，爲末，蜜丸彈子大。每服一丸，白湯化下，日一服。名無憂丸。
The *Pu ji fang* [recommends to] cure cough with salivation and panting, regardless of whether this is a [disease] that has lasted for years or just days, [as follows]. [Grind] one *liang* each of *bi ma* leaves that have been exposed to frost, mulberry tree leaves that have been exposed to frost and poppy shells, fried in honey, into powder and form with honey pills the size of a bullet. Each time ingest one pill, to be sent down dissolved in clear, boiled water. To be ingested once a day. [This medication is] called the "pills that make one worry-free."

【附録】
Appendix.

17-13-A01
博落迴拾遺 *Bo luo hui*, FE *Shi yi*
Unidentified.

【藏器曰】有大毒。主惡瘡癭根，，白癜風，蠱毒精魅，溪毒，瘡瘻。和百丈青、雞桑灰等分，爲末傅之。蠱毒精魅當别有法。生江南山谷。莖葉如蓖麻。莖中空，吹之作聲如博落迴。折之有黄汁，藥人立死，不可輕用入口。

969 The text says "one [recipe]" while in fact two recipes are recorded.

[Chen] Cangqi: Very poisonous. It controls malign sores and the root of goiter, tumor redundancy, tumorous flesh growth, white patches wind,[970] *gu* poison[971] and essence goblins, rivulet poison,[972] and sores with fistula. Mix it with equal amounts of *bai zhang qing* 百丈青[973] and *ji sang hui* 雞桑灰,[974] [grind it into] powder and apply this [to the affected region]. For *gu* poison and essence goblins other [therapeutic] methods are available. It grows in mountain valleys of Jiang nan. The stem and the leaves are similar to those of castor plants. The stem is hollow. When one blows into it it emits sounds like *boluohui*. When it is broken, a yellow juice appears. If [the juice] is applied to drug someone, he will die immediately. It must not be used carelessly for oral use.

17-14
常山本經下品
Chang shan, FE *Ben jing*, lower rank.
蜀漆同上
Shu qi, identical to [*chang shan*] above.

***Dichroa febrifuga* Lour. Chinese quinine.**

【釋名】恒山吴普、互草本經、鷄尿草日華、鴨尿草日華。【時珍曰】恒亦常也。恒山乃北岳名，在今定州。常山乃郡名，亦今真定。豈此藥始産于此得名歟？蜀漆乃常山苗，功用相同，今併爲一。

Explanation of Names. *Heng shan* 恒山, Wu Pu. *Hu cao* 互草, Ben jing. *Ji niao cao* 鷄尿草, "chicken urine herb," *Rihua*. *Ya niao cao* 鴨尿草, "duck urine herb," *Rihua*. [Li] Shizhen: *Heng* 恒, "constant," is identical to *chang* 常. Heng shan 恒山 is [one of the five mountain ranges in the North) Bei yue. It is situated in today's Ding zhou. Chang shan 常山 is the name of a prefecture; it, too, is in today's Zhen ding. Could it be that [this herb] was named so because this is where it grew first? *Shu qi* 蜀漆 is the seedling of *chang shan* 常山. Its [therapeutic] potential is identical [to that of *chang shan*]. Here now both are included in one entry.

---

970 *Bai dian feng* 白癜風, "white patches wind," a condition of white skin patches without pain and itching. BCGM Dict I, 46.

971 *Gu du* 蠱毒, "*gu*-poison[ing]." (1) A poison emitted by certain worms/snakes with an ability to cause varying pathological changes in a person who has taken it in by means of wine or food. (2) Abdominal fullness, in some cases with blood spitting, and blood in the stool and urine. BCGM Dict I, 192 - 193. See BCGM 42-22.

972 *Xi du* 溪毒, "rivulet poison," 1.) A tiny bug assumed to live in bodies of water and supposedly capable of striking humans when they enter the water, thereby causing disease. 2.) A condition resulting from being struck by rivulet poison. BCGM Dict I, 548.

973 *Bai zhang qing* 百丈青, a substance of unknown identity.

974 *Ji sang hui* 雞桑灰, a substance of unknown identity.

【集解】【别録曰】常山生益州川谷及漢中。二月、八月采根，陰乾。又曰，蜀漆生江林山川谷及蜀漢中，常山苗也。五月采葉，陰乾。【弘景曰】常山出宜都、建平。細實黄者，呼爲雞骨常山，用之最勝。蜀漆是常山苗而所出又異者，江林山即益州江陽山名，故是同處爾。彼人采得，縈結作丸，得時燥者佳。【恭曰】常山生山谷間。莖圓有節，高者不過三四尺。葉似茗而狹長，兩兩相當。二月生白花，青萼。五月結實青圓，三子爲房。其草暴燥色青白堪用，若陰乾便黑爛鬱壞矣。【保昇曰】今出金州、房州、梁州中江縣。樹高三四尺，根似荆根，黄色而破。五六月采葉，名蜀漆也。【李含光曰】蜀漆是常山莖，八月、九月采之。【頌曰】今汴西、淮、浙、湖南州郡亦有之，並如上説。而海州出者，葉似楸葉。八月有花，紅白色，子碧色，似山楝子而小。今天台山出一種草，名土常山，苗葉極甘。人用爲飲，甘味如蜜，又名蜜香草，性涼益人，非此常山也。

Collected Explanations. *Bie lu*: *Chang shan* grows in river valleys of Yi zhou and in Han zhong. The root is collected in the second and eighth month; it is dried in the yin (i. e., shade). It is also said: *Shu qi* grows in the river valleys of Mount Jiang lin shan and in Shu han. It is the seedling of *chang shan*. The leaves are collected in the fifth month; they are dried in the yin (i. e., shade). [Tao] Hongjing: *Chang shan* comes from Yi du and Jian ping. Specimens with fine, yellow fruits are called *ji gu chang shan* 雞骨常山, "chicken bone *chang shan*." To use them is best. [When it is stated that] *shu qi* is the seedling of *chang shan* but originates from a different region, this is because Mount Jiang lin shan is the name of a mountain in Jiang yang in Yi zhou, and that is the same region. When the people there collect them, they combine [both *chang shan* and *shu qi*] and form pills. They are excellent when they are dry at the time when they are collected. [Su] Gong: *Chang shan* grows in mountain valleys. The stem is round and has nodes. Tall ones do not exceed a height of three to four *chi*. The leaves resemble tea [leaves], but are narrow and lengthy. They grow facing each other in pairs of two. White flowers with a greenish calyx grow in the second month. Greenish, round fruits form in the fifth month. Three seeds are in one "housing." When the herb is quickly dried [in the sun] it assumes a greenish-white color and is then suitable for [therapeutic] use. When it is dried in the yin (i. e., shade), it turns black, rots and is spoiled. [Han] Baosheng: Today it comes from Jin zhou, Fang zhou and Zhong jiang xian in Liang zhou. The tree is three to four *chi* tall. The root resembles the *schizonepeta* root. It is yellow and fragmented. The leaves are collected in the fifth and sixth month. They are named *shu qi* 蜀漆. Li Hanguang: *Shu qi* 蜀漆 is the stem of *chang shan* 常山. It is collected in the eighth and ninth month. [Su] Song: Today it can be found in the *zhou* and prefectures of Bian xi, Huai, Zhe and Hu nan, and also [in regions] described above. Specimens coming from Hai zhou have leaves similar to *catalpa* leaves. [*Chang shan*] has red-white flowers in the eighth month. The seeds are jade-bluish, similar to Persian lilac seeds, but they are smaller. Today one kind of an herb comes from Mount Tian tai shan that is called *tu chang shan* 土常山, *maesa* [plant]. Its seedling and leaves are extremely sweet. People use them to prepare beverages; they are as sweet as honey. [The herb] is also called *mi xiang cao* 蜜香草, "honey fragrance herb." Its nature is cool and it is beneficial for humans. It is not the *chang shan* discussed here.

【修治】【斅曰】采時連根苗收。如用莖葉，臨時去根，以甘草細剉，同水拌溼蒸之。臨時去甘草，取蜀漆細剉，又拌甘草水勻，再蒸，日乾用。其常山，凡用以酒浸一宿，漉出日乾，熬搗用。【時珍曰】近時有酒浸蒸熟或瓦炒熟者，亦不甚吐人。又有醋制者，吐人。

Pharmaceutical Preparation. [Lei] Xiao: When it is collected, [the complete herb] is stored with root and seedling. When the time has come to use [the herb], the root is discarded and [the seedling] is cut together with *glycyrrhiza* [root] to fine pieces. Mix them with water and steam them. Close to the moment [of their application], remove the *glycyrrhiza* [root], cut the *shu qi* into fine pieces, and mix them with *glycyrrhiza* [root] water. Steam them again and dry them in the sun for [therapeutic] use. For all its [therapeutic] uses, soak [the root of] *chang shan* in wine for one night, strain it and dry it in the sun. Then simmer it and pound it to obtain a paste that is ready for [therapeutic] use. [Li] Shizhen: In recent times [*chang shan*] soaked in wine and steamed until done, or fried on a tile until done, does not have a strong effect to let one vomit. That prepared with vinegar lets one vomit.

常山 *Chang shan*

【氣味】苦，寒，有毒。【別録曰】辛，微寒。【普曰】神農、岐伯：苦。桐君：辛，有毒。李當之：大寒。【權曰】苦，有小毒。【炳曰】得甘草，吐瘧。【之才曰】畏玉札。【大明曰】忌葱菜及菘菜。伏砒石。

Qi and Flavor. Bitter, cold, poisonous. *Bie lu*: Acrid, slightly cold. [Wu] Pu: Shen nong, Qi Bo: Bitter. Tong jun: Acrid, poisonous. Li Dangzhi: Very cold. [Zhen] Quan: Bitter, slightly poisonous. [Xiao] Bing: Combined with *glycyrrhiza* [root, it serves to cure] malaria by causing [patients] to vomit. [Xu] Zhicai:: [Ingested together,] it fears jade plates (08-29-02). Da Ming: [During a treatment with *chang shan*] onions and pak choi are to be avoided. It suppresses [the effects of] arsenic.

【主治】傷寒寒熱，熱發温瘧鬼毒，胸中痰結吐逆。本經。療鬼蠱往來，水脹，洒洒惡寒，鼠瘻。別録。治諸瘧，吐痰涎，治項下瘤癭。甄權。

Control. Harm caused by cold with alternating sensations of cold and heat. Heat effusion, warmth malaria and demon poison. Phlegm nodes[975] in the chest with spitting and [qi] counterflow. *Ben jing*. It heals occasional demon [attachment] and *gu* [poison],[976] water bloating, shivering with an aversion to cold, and mouse fistula.[977] *Bie lu*. It serves to cure all types of malaria, and makes you spit out phlegm and saliva. It serves to cure tumorous goiter below the neck. Zhen Quan.

蜀漆。*Shu qi.*

【氣味】辛，平，有毒。【别録曰】微温。【權曰】苦，有小毒。【元素曰】辛，純陽。【炳曰】桔梗爲之使。【之才曰】栝樓爲之使。惡貫衆。

Qi and Flavor. Acrid, balanced, poisonous. *Bie lu*: Slightly warm. [Zhen] Quan: Bitter, slightly poisonous. [Zhang] Yuansu: Acrid, pure yang. [Xiao] Bing: *Platycodon* [root] serves as its guiding substance. [Ingested together,] it abhors *dryopteris* [root].

【主治】瘧及欬逆寒熱，腹中癥堅痞結，積聚邪氣，蠱毒鬼疰。本經。療胸中邪結氣，吐去之。别録。治鬼瘧多時，温瘧寒熱，下肥氣。甄權。破血，洗去腥。與苦酸同用，導膽邪。元素。

Control. Malaria and cough with [qi] counterflow and alternating sensations of cold and heat. Concretion-illness hardening and obstacle-illness[978]nodes in the abdomen, accumulation and collection of evil qi. *Gu* poisoning[979] and demon attachment-illness. *Ben jing*. It heals and removes evil qi nodes in the chest by having them spit out. *Bie lu*. It serves to cure long-time demonic malaria, and warmth malaria with alternating sensations of cold and heat. It discharges fat qi.[980] Zhen Quan. It breaks through blood [accumulation. With water] wash off its fishy smell.

975 *Tan jie* 痰結, "phlegm nodes," a condition brought forth by a non-transformation of phlegm, desiccation of body liquids, and the formation of sticky phlegm nodes. BCGM Dict I, 492.

976 *Gu du* 蠱毒, "*gu*-poison[ing]." (1) A poison emitted by certain worms/snakes with an ability to cause varying pathological changes in a person who has taken it in by means of wine or food. (2) Abdominal fullness, in some cases with blood spitting, and blood in the stool and urine. BCGM Dict I, 192 - 193. See BCGM 42-22.

977 *Shu lou* 鼠瘻, "mouse fistula," BCGM Dict I, 466, identical to *luo li* 瘰癧, "scrofula pervasion-illnes."

978 *Pi* 痞, "obstacle-illness," a condition of an uncomfortable distension and fullness in the chest and abdominal region. When pressed there is no pain. BCGM Dict I. 371.

979 *Gu du* 蠱毒, "*gu*-poison[ing]." (1) A poison emitted by certain worms/snakes with an ability to cause varying pathological changes in a person who has taken it in by means of wine or food. (2) Abdominal fullness, in some cases with blood spitting, and blood in the stool and urine. BCGM Dict I, 192 - 193. See BCGM 42-22.

980 *Fei qi* 肥氣, "fat qi," a condition of pathological *ji ju* 積聚, "accumulation and collection," below the flanks brought forth by liver qi lumps. BCGM Dict I, 155.

Applied together with bitter and sour [items] it leads away evil [qi] from the gallbladder. [Zhang] Yuansu.

【發明】【斅曰】蜀漆春夏用莖葉，秋冬用根。老人久病切忌服之。【頌曰】常山、蜀漆爲治瘧之最要。不可多進，令人吐逆。【震亨曰】常山性暴悍，善驅逐，能傷真氣。病人稍近虛怯，不可用也。外臺乃用三兩作一服，殊昧雷公老人久病切忌之戒。【時珍曰】常山、蜀漆有刼痰截瘧之功，須在發散表邪及提出陽分之後。用之得宜，神妙立見；用失其法，真氣必傷。夫瘧有六經瘧、五臟瘧、痰濕、食積、瘴疫、鬼邪諸瘧，須分陰陽虛實，不可一概論也。常山、蜀漆生用則上行必吐，酒蒸炒熟用則氣稍緩，少用亦不致吐也。得甘草則吐，得大黄則利，得烏梅、鯪鯉甲則入肝，得小麥、竹葉則入心，得秫米、麻黄則入肺，得龍骨、附子則入腎，得草果、檳榔則入脾。蓋無痰不作瘧，二物之功，亦在驅逐痰水而已。楊士瀛直指方云：常山治瘧，人皆薄之。瘧家多蓄痰涎黄水，或停潴心下，或結澼脅間，乃生寒熱。法當吐痰逐水，常山豈容不用？水在上焦，則常山能吐之。水在脇下，則常山能破其澼而下其水。但須行血藥品佐助之，必收十全之功。其有純熱發瘧或蘊熱内實之證，投以常山，大便點滴而下，似泄不泄者，須用北大黄爲佐，泄利數行，然後獲愈也。又待制李燾云：嶺南瘴氣，寒熱所感，邪氣多在營衛皮肉之間。欲去皮膚毛孔中瘴氣根本，非常山不可。但性吐人，惟以七寶散冷服之，即不吐且驗也。

Explication. [Lei] Xiao: Of *shu qi* in spring and summer use the stem and the leaves, in autumn and winter use the root. The elderly and those with a chronic disease must not ingest them. [Su] Song: *Chang shan* and *shu qi* are most important [pharmaceutical drugs] for curing malaria. They must not be taken in large quantities as they cause vomiting with [qi] counterflow. [Zhu] Zhenheng: *Chang shan* has a very violent nature. It is good at driving something out, and is capable of harming one's true qi. Patients with even a slight inclination toward depletion and timidity must not resort to it. The *Wai tai mi yao* [suggests] using three *liang* as one dose of ingestion but this fails to take into account the warnings expressed by Lei gong in regard to what the elderly and those with a chronic disease need to avoid. [Li] Shizhen: *Chang shan* and *shu qi* effectively "rob" phlegm and "cut" malaria. They should be used only after evil [qi] have been dispersed to the outer region [of the body] and the yang section is strengthened. If the application is as required, a divine and wondrous [effect] will be immediately apparent. If the application fails to follow the right approach, [the patient's] true qi will be harmed. Now, malaria may be a malaria in any of the six conduits or a malaria in any of the five long-term depots. [It may be related to] phlegm and moisture, to food accumulation, to epidemic miasma and to demonic evil – there are all such types of malaria. It is essential to distinguish whether it is a condition of yin or yang, of depletion or repletion. It is impossible to make a general statement. When *chang shan* and *shu qi* are used fresh/unprepared, they rise [in the body] and inevitably cause vomiting. Applied steamed with wine and fried until done, their qi are a little slowed down, and used in small quantities they do not cause vomiting. Combined with *glycyrrhiza* [root] they cause vomiting. Combined with rhubarb root, they cause free-flow. Combined with smoked plums and pangolin scales they enter the liver. Combined with wheat and bamboo leaves they enter the heart. Combined with glutinous millet and *ephedra* [herb] they enter the lung. Combined with dragon bones and *aconitum* [accessory tuber] they enter the kidneys. Combined with red cardamom and *areca* [nuts] they enter the spleen. The fact is, without phlegm there can be no malaria. The [therapeutic] potential of the two items [*chang shan* and *shu qi*] is limited to removing phlegm and water. Yang Shiying in his *Zhi zhi fang* states: "All the people belittle the use of *chang shan* to cure malaria. Malaria patients mostly have amassments of phlegm, saliva and yellow water, and these amassments may be located below the heart or collect as a wash-out[981] in the flanks. This then leads to alternating sensations of cold and heat. The appropriate approach [to curing malaria] is to let [patients] spit out the phlegm and dispel the water. Why should *chang shan* not be used for this purpose? When the water is in the upper [section of the Triple] Burner, *chang shan* can have it spit out. When the water is below the flanks, *chang shan* is able to break open the wash-out/aggregation-illness and discharge the water. However, it must be supported by medication stimulating blood movement, and this then guarantees 100% success. If in the case of malaria outbreaks with only a heat effusion, or in the case of signs indicating a repletion of heat collection, *chang shan* is ingested, the stool will appear only as a drop. It seems there is an outflow but there is no outflow. Here northern rhubarb root is to assist [the effects of *chang shan*]. Only when numerous outflows and free flow have occurred, a cure is achieved." Also, Edict Attendent Li Dao[982] states: "In Ling nan where miasmatic qi often cause alternating sensations of cold and heat, the evil qi are often situated in the [region of the] camp and guardian [qi] between skin and flesh. To remove the root of the miasmatic qi through the hair pores in the skin is possible only with *chang shan*. However, by its nature it causes

981 *Han pi* 寒澼, "cold wash-out," a condition identical to *han pi* 寒癖, "cold aggregation-illness." *Pi* 澼 is an erroneous writing of *pi* 癖 in the *BCGM*. *Han pi* 寒癖, "cold aggregation-illness" refers to a passage of thin white urine following the intake of medication in the course of a treatment of cold aggregation. BCGM Dict I, 208.

982 *Ling nan wei sheng fang*, 1st ch., Li dai zhi zhang nüe lun 李待制瘴瘧論, "Edict Attendent Li on miasmatic malaria," writes Li Qiu 李璆 instead of Li Dao 李燾.

vomiting. Hence it is ingested only in combination with the 'powder with seven gems.'[983] This prevents vomiting and is still effective."

【附方】舊三，新二十三。
Added Recipes. Three of old. 23 newly recorded.

截瘧諸湯。外臺秘要用常山三兩，漿水三升，浸一宿，煎取一升，欲發前頓服，取吐。

All decoctions serving to "cut" malaria. The *Wai tai mi yao* [recommends to] soak three *liang* of *chang shan* in three *sheng* of fermented water of foxtail millet for one night. Then boil it down to one *sheng* and ingest this all at once to stimulate vomiting when an outbreak is imminent.

肘後方用常山一兩，秫米一百粒，水六升，煮三升，分三服。先夜未發臨發時服盡。

The *Zhou hou fang* [recommends to] boil one *liang* of *chang shan* and 100 grains of glutinous millet in six *sheng* of water down to three *sheng* and ingest this divided into three portions. They are to be ingested the night before [an outbreak], prior to an outbreak and when the outbreak is immiment.

養生主論王隱者驅瘧湯云：予用此四十年，奇效不能盡述，切勿加減，萬無一吐者。常山酒煮晒乾、知母、貝母、草果各一錢半，水一鍾半，煎半熟，五更熱服。渣以酒浸，發前服。

In the *Yang sheng zhu lun*, Wang, living as an hermit, relates a "decoction to remove malaria" stating: I have used this for 40 years. Its extraordinary effects cannot all be listed. There was not a single vomiting in a myriad cases. Boil one and a half *qian* each of *chang shan*, boiled in wine and dried in the sun, *anamarrhena* [root], *fritillaria* [root] and red cardamom in one and a half *zhong* of water down to one half until done and ingest this hot in the early morning hours. Soak the dregs in wine and ingest it prior to an outbreak.

截瘧諸酒。肘後方用常山一兩，酒一升，漬二三日，分作三服，平旦一服，少頃再服，臨發又服。或加甘草，酒煮服之。

All wines to "cut" malaria. The *Zhou hou fang* [recommends to] soak one *liang* of *chang shan* in one *sheng* of wine for two or three days and ingest [the liquid] divided into three portions. Ingest a first portion in the early morning, and a second portion

983 *Qi bao san* 七寶散, the "powder with seven gems," has the following ingredients: *Chang shan*, *magnolia* bark, tangerine peels, green tangerin peels, *glycyrrhiza* root, *areca* nuts, red cardamom.

a little later. When an outbreak is immiment ingest it again. Some add *glycyrrhiza* [root]. Boil it in wine and ingest this.

宋俠經心録醇醨湯，治間日瘧。支太醫云：乃桂广州方也，甚驗。恒山一錢二分，大黄二錢半，炙甘草一錢二分。水一盞半，煎减半，曰醇，發日五更温服。再以水一盞，煎减半，曰醨，未發時温服。

Song Xia in his *Jing xin lu* [lists a] "decoction of good wine and dregs" that serves to cure malaria with outbreaks every other day. Imperial Physician Zhi states: This is a recipe from Gui and Guang zhou. It is very effective. Boil one *qian* and two *fen* of *heng shan*, two and a half *qian* of rhubarb root and one *qian*, two *fen* of roasted *glycyrrhiza* [root] in one and a half small cups of water down to one half. [Pour the liquid out;] it is the "good wine." It is ingested in the early morning hours of the day of an outbreak. In addition, add [to the dregs] one small cup of water and boil it down to one half. This is the "dregs." Ingest the [liquid] warm prior to an outbreak.

虞摶醫學正傳治久瘧不止。常山一錢半，檳榔一錢，丁香五分，烏梅一個，酒一盞，浸一宿，五更飲之。一服便止，永不再發，如神。

Yu Tuan's *Yi xue zheng chuan* [recommends to] cure unending, chronic malaria [as follows]. Soak in one cup of wine for one night one and a half *qian* of *chang shan*, one *qian* of *areca* [nuts], five *fen* of clove and one smoked plum and drink [the liquid] in the early morning hours. One ingestion will stop [the outbreaks] and there will never be outbreaks again. Divine.

截瘧諸丸。千金方恒山丸：治數年不瘥者，兩劑瘥。一月以來者，一劑瘥。恒山三兩，研末，雞子白和丸梧子大，瓦器煮熟，殺腥氣，則取晒乾收之。每服二十丸，竹葉湯下，五更一服，天明一服，發前一服，或吐或否即止。

All pills to "cut" malaria. The "*heng shan* pills" of the *Qian jin fang*. They serve to cure [malaria] that has continued for several years without being cured. Two preparations will achieve a cure. Those having lasted up to one month will be cured with a single preparation. Grind three *liang* of *heng shan* into powder and with chicken egg white form pills the size of *wu* seeds. Heat them on a tile until done to kill their fishy qi. Then dry them in the sun and store them. Each time ingest 20 pills, to be sent down with a bamboo leaf decoction. Ingest a first portion in the early morning hours. At daybreak ingest another portion. Prior to an outbreak ingest yet another portion. There may or may not be vomiting[984] and [the disease] has ended.

984 *Qian jin fang* ch. 10, *shang han fang* 傷寒方, "recipes for harm caused by cold," section *wen nue* 温瘧, "warmth malaria," instead of *huo tu huo fou* 或吐或否, "there may or may not be vomiting," writes *yu tu dan tu* 欲吐但吐, "if there is an urge to vomit, just vomit."

肘後丹砂丸：恒山搗末三兩，真丹一兩研，白蜜和杵百下，丸梧子大。先發時三丸，少頃再服三丸，臨時服三丸，酒下，無不斷者。

The "pills with cinnabar" of the *Zhou hou*. Mix three *liang* of *heng shan*, pounded into powder, one *liang* of genuine cinnabar, ground, and white honey and pound this one hundred times. Then form pills the size of *wu* seeds. Prior to an outbreak [ingest] three pills. A short time later again ingest three pills. When an outbreak is imminent, once again ingest three pills, all to be sent down with wine. There is not a single case that remains uninterrupted.

曾世榮活幼心書黄丹丸：治大小久瘧。恒山二兩，黄丹半兩，烏梅連核瓦焙一兩，爲末，糯米粉糊丸梧子大。每服三五十丸，凉酒下，隔一夜一服，平旦一服。午後方食。

The "pills with minium" in Zeng Shirong's *Huo you xin shu*. They serve to cure long-lasting malaria of adults and children. [Grind] two *liang* of *heng shan*, half a *liang* of minium and one *liang* of smoked plums with their pits, baked on a tile over a slow fire, into powder. With glutinous rice form pills the size of *wu* seeds. Each time ingest 30 to 50 pills, to be sent down with cool wine. One night before ingest them once; the next morning ingest them again. Have a meal soon after noon.

葛洪肘後方用恒山三兩，知母一兩，甘草半兩，搗末，蜜丸梧子大。先發時服十丸，次服七丸，後服五六丸，以瘥爲度。

Ge Hong in his *Zhou hou fang* [recommends to] pound three *liang* of *heng shan*, one *liang* of *anemarrhena* [root] and half a *liang* of *glycyrrhiza* [root] into powder and form with honey pills the size of *wu* seeds. Prior to an outbreak ingest ten pills, next ingest seven pills, then ingest five or six pills until a cure is achieved.

和劑局方瞻仰丸：治一切瘧。常山四兩，炒存性，草果二兩，炒存性，爲末，薄糊丸梧子大。每卧時冷酒服五十丸，五更再服。忌鵝羊熱物。

The "pills letting one look upward"[985] of the *He ji ju fang*. They serve to cure all types of malaria. [Grind] four *liang* of *chang shan*, fried with their nature retained, and two *liang* of red cardamom [fruits], fried with their nature retained, into powder and form with thin [wheat flour] paste pills the size of *wu* seeds. Each time when going to sleep ingest with cold wine 50 pills. In the early morning hours ingest [50 pills] again. [During this therapy] goose meat, mutton and hot items are to be avoided.

985 *Pu ji fang*, ch. 197, *zhu nue men* 諸瘧門, "section all types of malaria," *dan ying wan* 膽仰丸, "pills to look up with bravery," writes *dan* 膽, "bravery," instead of *zhan* 瞻, "to look upward."

又勝金丸：治一切瘧，胸膈停痰，發不愈者。常山八兩，酒浸蒸焙，檳榔二兩生，研末，糊丸梧子大，如上法服。

Also, the "pills more worth than gold." They serve to cure all types of malaria, with phlegm accumulation in the chest and at the diaphragm, and outbreaks that could not be healed. Soak eight *liang* of *chang shan* in wine, steam it and bake [the *chang shan*] over a slow fire. Grind it with two *liang* of fresh/unprepared *areca* [nuts] into powder and with [wheat flour] form a paste to prepare pills the size of *wu* seeds that are ingested according to the method outlined above.

集簡方二聖丸：治諸瘧不拘遠近大小。雞骨恒山、雞心檳榔各一兩，生研，鯪鯉甲煨焦一兩半，爲末，糯粉糊丸緑豆大，黄丹爲衣。每服三五十丸，如上法服。

The "two sages pills" of the *Ji jian fang*. They serve to cure all types of malaria, regardless of whether these are chronic or recent cases, affecting adults or children. [Grind] into powder one *liang* each of chicken bone [type] *heng shan* and chicken heart [type] *areca* [nuts], ground fresh, and one and a half *liang* of pangolin scales, simmered until scorched. With a glutinous rice paste form pills the size of mung beans and coat them with minium. Each time ingest 30 to 50 pills. To be ingested according to the method outlined above.

厥陰肝瘧。寒多熱少，喘息如死狀，或少腹滿，小便如癃，不問久近，不吐不泄，如神。恒山一兩，醋浸一夜，瓦器煮乾。每用二錢，水一盞，煎半盞，五更冷服。趙真人濟急方。

Malaria affecting the ceasing yin liver [conduits], with much sensation of cold, and little sensation of heat, and pant breathing as if one were to die, occasionally accompanied by a feeling of lower abdominal fullness and a passage of urine similar to protuberance-illness.[986] Regardless of whether this has lasted for long or is only a recent issue, [this recipe] will cause neither vomiting nor outflow; it is divine. Soak one *liang* of *heng shan* in vinegar for one night and heat it on a tile until it has dried. Each time boil two *qian* in one bowl of water down to half a bowl and ingest it cold in the early morning hours. Zhao zhenren, *Ji ji fang*.

太陰肺瘧。痰聚胸中，病至令人心寒，寒甚乃熱，熱間善驚，如有所見。恒山三錢，甘草半錢，秫米三十五粒，水二鍾，煎一鍾，發日早分三次服。千金方。

986 *Qi long* 氣癃, "qi protuberance-illness," a condition with an inability to pass urine and a feeling of distension and fullness in the lower abdomen and urinary bladder. BCGM Dict I, 385.

Malaria affecting the major yin lung [conduits]. With phlegm collection in the chest. When the disease has reached a state where the patient's heart turns cold and when the cold is extreme it changes to heat. During the heat phase [patients] tend to be frightened as if they had seen something [horrifying]. Boil three *qian* of *heng shan*, half a *qian* of *glycyrrhiza* [root] and 35 grains of glutinous millet in two *zhong* of water down to one *zhong* and ingest this, divided into three portions, early in the morning of a day with an [expected] outbreak. *Qian jin fang*.

少陰腎瘧。凄凄然寒，手足寒，腰脊痛，大便難，目眴眴然。恒山二錢半，豉半兩，烏梅一錢，竹葉一錢半，葱白三根，水一升半，煎一升，發前分三服。千金方。

Malaria affecting the minor yin kidney [conduits]. [Patients] feel chills and cold. Hands and feet are cold. Spine and lower back ache. Urination is difficult. The eyes feel as if dazzled. Boil two and a half *qian* of *heng shan*, half a *liang* of [soybean] relish, one *qian* of smoked plums, one and a half *qian* of bamboo leaves and three roots of onion white in one and a half *sheng* of water down to one *sheng* and ingest it divided into three portions prior to an outbreak. *Qian jin fang*.

牝瘧獨寒不熱者。蜀漆散：用蜀漆、雲母煅三日夜、龍骨各二錢，爲末。每服半錢，臨發日旦一服，發前一服，酢漿水調下。温瘧又加蜀漆一錢。張仲景金匱要略。

Female malaria with only sensations of cold, and no heat. The "powder with *shu qi*." [Grind] two *qian* each of *shu qi* and mica, calcined for three days and nights, and dragon bones into powder, Each time ingest half a *qian*. Ingest this once in the early morning of the a day close to an outbreak and ingest it again prior to an outbreak, always to be sent down mixed with vinegar and fermented water of foxtail millet. For warmth malaria add one more *qian* of *shu qi*. Zhang Zhongjing, *Jin kui yao lüe*.

牡瘧獨熱不冷者。蜀漆一錢半，甘草一錢，麻黄二錢，牡蠣粉二錢，水二鍾，先煎麻黄、蜀漆，去沫入藥再煎至一鍾，未發前温服，得吐則止。王燾外臺秘要。

Male malaria with only sensations of heat, and no cold. Prepare one and a half *qian* of *shu qi*, one *qian* of *glycyrrhiza* [root], two *qian* of *ephedra* [herb] and two *qian* of oyster shell powder. First boil the *ephedra* [herb] and the *shu qi* in two *zhong* of water. Remove the foam, add the [remaining] pharmaceutical drugs and boil [the liquid] down to one *zhong*. Ingest this warm prior to an outbreak. Once a vomiting is induced [the outbreak] ends. Wang Dao, *Wai tai mi yao*.

温瘧熱多。恒山一錢，小麥三錢，淡竹葉二錢，水煎，五更服，甚良。藥性論。

Warmth malaria with much heat. Boil one *qian* of *heng shan*, three *qian* of wheat and two *qian* of bland bamboo leaves in water and ingest it in the early morning hours. Very good. *Yao xing lun*.

三十年瘧。肘後方治三十年老瘧及積年久瘧。常山、黄連各一兩，酒三升，漬一宿，以瓦釜煮取一升半。發日早服五合，發時再服。熱當吐，冷當利，無不瘥者。

Malaria that has lasted for 30 years. The *Zhou hou fang* [recommends to] cure chronic malaria that has lasted for 30 years and chronic malaria that has lasted for as long as a year [as follows]. Soak one *liang* each of *chang shan* and *coptis* [rhizome] in three *sheng* of wine for one night and then boil this in an earthenware cauldron down to one and a half *sheng*. Early in the morning of a day of an [expected] outbreak ingest five *ge*. Ingest this again at the time of an outbreak. [Ingested] hot, it will cause vomiting. [Ingested] cold, it will cause free flow. No case will remain without cure.

張文仲備急方用恒山一兩半，龍骨五錢，附子炮二錢半，大黄一兩，爲末，雞子黄和丸梧子大。未發時五丸，將發時五丸，白湯下。支太醫云：此方神驗，無不斷者。

Zhang Wenzhong in his *Bei ji fang* [recommends to grind] one and a half *liang* of *heng shan*, five *qian* of dragon bones, two and a half *qian* of *aconitum* [accessory tuber] and one *liang* of rhubarb root into powder and form with chicken egg yoke pills the size of *wu* seeds. Prior to an outbreak [ingest] five pills. If an outbreak is imminent [take another] five pills, all to be sent down with clear, boiled water. Imperial Physician Zhi states: This recipe is divinely effective. There is not a single [outbreak of malaria] that is not interrupted.

瘴瘧寒熱。劉長春經驗方常山一寸，草果一枚，熱酒一盌，浸一夜，五更望東服之，蓋卧，酒醒即愈。

Miasmatic malaria with alternating sensations of cold and heat. Liu Changchun in his *Jing yan fang* [recommends the following recipe]. Soak a one *cun* long piece of *chang shan* and one red cardamom fruit in one bowl of hot wine for one night and [let the patient] ingest [the liquid] in the early morning hours facing East. Then let him lie down covered [warm] and he will be healed when he wakes up from [the effects of] the wine.

談埜翁試驗方用常山、檳榔、甘草各二錢，黑豆一百粒，水煎服之。乃彭司寇所傳。

Tan Yeweng in his *Shi yan fang* [recommends to] boil two *qian* each of *chang shan*, *areca* [nuts] and *glycyrrhiza* [root] together with one hundred grains of black soybeans in water and ingest it. This [is a recipe] transmitted by the Minister of Justice Peng.

葛稚川肘後方用常山、黄連、香豉各一兩，附子炮七錢，搗末，蜜丸梧子大。空腹飲服四丸，欲發時三丸。至午後乃食。

Ge Zhichuan in his *Zhou hou fang* [recommends to] pound one *liang* each of *chang shan*, *coptis* [rhizome] and [soybean] relish with seven *qian* of *aconitum* [accessory tuber], roasted in a pan, into powder and form with honey pills the size of *wu* seeds. Ingest on an empty stomach with a beverage four pills, and another three pills when an outbreak is imminent. Have a meal after noon.

妊娠瘧疾。酒蒸常山、石膏煅各一錢，烏梅炒五分，甘草四分，水一盞，酒一盞，浸一夜，平旦温服。姚僧坦集驗方。

Malaria illness during pregnancy. Soak one *qian* each of *chang shan*, steamed with wine, and gypsum, calcined, with five *fen* of smoked plums, fried, and four *fen* of *glycyrrhiza* [root] in a mixture of one bowl of water and one bowl of wine, and [let the woman] ingest this warm in the early morning. Yao Sengtan, *Ji yan fang*.

百日兒瘧。水鑑仙人歌曰：

瘧是邪風寒熱攻，直須術治免成空。

常山刻作人形狀，釘在孩兒生氣宮。

如金生人，金生在巳，即釘巳上，木生人釘亥上，火生人釘寅上，水土生人釘申上也。

Malaria of a 100 days young child. The *Shui jian xian ren ge* says:

"Malaria is an attack of evil wind, cold and heat. With the right therapeutic technique applied, it will not be successful.

Carve a *chang shan* [root] in the shape of a human being and insert a nail into the child's palace where its vital qi [are located]."[987]

In the case of a person born during the phase metal, as metal is generated at *si*, insert the nail above the *si*.[988] In the case of a person born during the phase wood, insert

987 *Sheng qi gong* 生氣宮, "the palace of the vital qi," possibly a reference to the "gate of life," i. e., the right kidney. See *Nan jing*, difficult issue 36: "The 'gate of life' is the place where the spirit essence lodges; it is the place to which the original qi are tied." Paul U. Unschuld, *Nan jing. The Classic of Difficult Issues.* University of California Press, Berkeley and Los Angeles, 2016, 320.

988 *Si* 巳 is the earthly branch associated with the phase fire and the South. Fire brings forth soil, and soil brings forth metal. To kill the demon responsible for a malaria of a child

the nail above the *hai*.[989] In the case of a person born during the phase fire, insert the nail above the *yin*.[990] In the case of a person born during the phases water and soil, insert it it above the *shen*.[991]

小兒驚忤。暴驚，卒死，中惡。用蜀漆炒二錢，左顧牡蠣一錢二分，漿水煎服，當吐痰而愈。名千金湯。阮氏。

Children frightened by a demon's hostility.[992] Violent fright, sudden death, being struck by the malign. Boil two *qian* of *shu qi*, fried, and one *qian* and two *fen* of oyster shells with spirals winding toward the left in fermented water of foxtail millet and [let the child] ingest this. It will vomit phlegm and is cured. [This recipe] is called "decoction worth thousands in gold." Ruan shi.

胸中痰飲。恒山、甘草各一兩，水五升，煮取一升，去滓，入蜜二合，温服七合，取吐。不吐更服。千金方。

Phlegm rheum in the chest. Boil one *liang* each of *heng shan* and *glycyrrhiza* [root] in five *sheng* of water down to one *sheng*, discard the dregs, add two *ge* of honey and ingest seven *ge* of this warm to stimulate vomiting. If [the patient] fails to vomit, he is to ingest [the liquid] a second time. *Qian jin fang*.

---

born during the phase metal, the nail is inserted into the "southern" region of the wooden figurine, that is, the heart, where the demon resides.

989 *Hai* 亥 is the earthly branch associated with the phase water and the North. Fire brings forth wood. To kill the demon responsible for a malaria of a child born during the phase wood, the nail is inserted into the "northern" region of the wooden figurine, that is the kidneys, where the demon resides.

990 *Yin* 寅 is the earthly branch associated with the phase wood and the East. Wood brings forth fire. To kill the demon responsible for a malaria of a child born during the phase fire, the nail is inserted into the "eastern" region of the wooden figurine, that is, the gallbladder, where the demon resides.

991 *Shen* 申 is the earthly branch associated with the phase metal and the West. Metal brings forth water. To kill the demon responsible for a malaria of a child born during the phase water, the nail is inserted into the "western" region of the wooden figurine, that is, the large intestine, where the demon resides.

992 *Jing wu* 驚忤, "frightened by [a demon's] hostility," a condition of sudden loss of speech, or a condition of being frightened or experiencing fright epilepsy, believed to be caused by a hostile demon. BCGM Dict I, 268.

【附録】

Appendix.

17-14-A01

杜莖山圖經 *Du jing shan*, FE *Tu jing*

***Maesa japonica* (Thunb.) Moritzi. Japanese Maesa.**

【頌曰】葉味苦性寒，主溫瘴寒熱，作止不定，煩渴，頭痛心躁。杵爛，新酒浸，絞汁服，吐出惡涎，甚效。生宜州。苗高四五尺，葉似苦蕒菜。秋有花，紫色。實如枸杞子，大而白。

[Su] Song: Leaves: flavor bitter, nature cold. It controls warmth malaria with alternating sensations of cold and heat, and irregular phases of activity and pause, vexing thirst, headache and heart restlessness. Pound it to a pulpy mass, soak it in new wine, squeeze it to obtain a juice and ingest it. This lets one vomit malign saliva. Very effective. It grows in Yi zhou. The seedling is four to five *chi* tall. The leaves resemble those of *sow thistle* herbs. Flowers are present in autumn; they are purple. The fruits resemble *lycium* seeds; they are big and white.

17-14-A02

土紅山 *Tu hong shan*

Unidentified.

【頌曰】葉甘，微寒，無毒。主骨節疼痛，勞熱瘴瘧。生南恩州山野中。大者高七八尺，葉似枇杷而小，無毛，秋生白花如粟粒，不實。福州生者作細藤，似芙蓉葉，其葉上青下白，根如葛頭。土人取根，米泔浸一宿，以清水再浸一宿，炒黄爲末。每服一錢，水一盞，生薑一片，同煎服。亦治勞瘴，甚效。【時珍曰】杜莖山即土恒山，土紅山又杜莖山之類，故並附之。

[Su] Song: The leaf is bitter, slightly cold and nonpoisonous. It controls painful bone joints, exhaustion heat and miasmatic malaria. It grows in the wild of the mountains of Nan en zhou. Large specimens are seven to eight *chi* tall. The leaves resemble those of loquat, but are small and have no hair. [*Tu hong shan*] grows white flowers similar to millet kernels in autumn. They bear no fruit. Specimens growing in Fu zhou develop fine vines, resembling Indian lotus leaves. The leaves are greenish on their upper side and white on their lower side. The root is similar to *pueraria* [root]. The locals collect the root, soak it for one night in water that has been used to wash rice and then soak it in clear water for another night, fry it until it has turned yellow and [grind it into] powder. Each time ingest one *qian* to be boiled in one small cup of water together with one slice of fresh ginger, and ingest this. It also serves to cure exhaustion miasma.[993] Very effective. [Li] Shizhen: *Du jing shan* 杜莖山 is *tu heng shan* 土恒山. *Tu hong shan* 土紅山 is related to *du jing shan* 杜莖山. Therefore, both are attached here.

17-15
藜蘆本經下品
Li lu, FE *Ben jing*, lower rank.

***Veratrum nigrum* L. False hellebore.**

【釋名】山葱別録、葱苒同、葱菼音毯。、葱葵普、豐蘆普、憨葱綱目、鹿葱。【時珍曰】黑色曰黎，其蘆有黑皮裹之，故名。根際似葱，俗名葱管藜蘆是矣。北人謂之憨葱，南人謂之鹿葱。

Explanation of Names. *Shan cong* 山葱, "mountain onion," *Bie lu*. *Cong ran* 葱苒, "onion luxuriance," identical [source]. *Cong tan* 葱菼, read *tan* 毯. *Cong kui* 葱葵, [Wu] Pu. *Feng lu* 豐蘆, "abounding reed," [Wu] Pu. *Han cong* 憨葱, *Gang mu*. *Lu cong* 鹿葱, "deer's onion." [Li] Shizhen: Black color is called *li* 黎. This is a reed, *lu* 蘆, with black skin; hence the name [*li lu* 藜蘆, "black reed"]. The roots occasionally resemble onions. This is the meaning underlying the common name "onion tube black reed," *cong guan li lu* 葱管藜蘆. People in the North call it *han cong* 憨葱, "silly onion." The southerners call it "deer's onion," *lu cong* 鹿葱.

【集解】【別録曰】藜蘆生太山山谷。三月采根，陰乾。【普曰】大葉，小根相連。【弘景曰】近道處處有之。根下極似葱而多毛。用之止剔取根，微炙之。【保昇曰】所在山谷皆有。葉似鬱金、秦艽、蘘荷等，根若龍膽，莖下多毛。夏生冬凋，八月采根。【頌曰】今陝西、山南、東、西州郡皆有之，遼州、均州、解州者尤佳。三月生苗葉，似初出椶心，又似車前，莖似葱白，青紫色，高五六寸，上有黑皮裹莖，似椶皮。有花肉紅色，根似馬腸根，長四五寸許，黄白色。二月、三月采根，陰乾。此有二種。一種水藜蘆，莖葉大同，只是生在近水溪澗石上，根鬚百餘莖，不中藥用。今用者名葱白藜蘆，根鬚甚少，只是三二十莖，生高山者爲佳，均州土俗亦呼爲鹿葱。范子計然云：出河東，黄白者善。

Collected Explanations. *Bie lu*: *Li lu* grows in the mountain valleys of Mount Tai shan. The root is collected in the third month; it is dried in the yin (i. e., shade). [Wu] Pu: Its large leaves and small roots are interconnected. [Tao] Hongjing: It can be found everywhere. The lower part of the root is very similar to onions and has much hair. For [therapeutic] applications, cut off the root only and slightly roast it.

993 *Lao zhang* 勞瘴, "exhaustion miasma," identical to *lao nue* 勞瘧, "exhaustion malaria." Condition of a malaria that has not been cured for a long time and leaves people in a state of external and internal depletion, and that breaks out following even a slight exhaustion. BCGM Dict I, 302, 299.

[Han] Baosheng: It is found everywhere in mountain valleys. The leaves resemble those of wild turmeric, large *gentiana* [herb] and zingiber. The root is similar to that of Korean *gentiana* [herb]. The lower part of the stem has much hair. It grows in summer and withers in winter. The root is collected in the eighth month. [Su] Song: Today it can be found in all the *zhou* and prefectures in the East and West in Shaan xi and Shan nan. Specimens from Liao zhou, Jun zhou and Xie zhou are particularly excellent. [*Li lu*] grows a seedling in the third month, resembling *trachycarpus* shoots that have just begun to grow. It also resembles Asiatic plantain [herbs]. The stem resembles that of onion white. It is of greenish-purple color and five to six *cun* tall. Above it has a black bark covering the stem similar to *trachycarpus* palm. The flowers have the red color of meat. The root resembles the *ma chang*[994] root. It is about four to five *cun* long and of yellow-white color. The root is collected in the second and third month; it is dried in the yin (i. e., shade). There exist two kinds. One kind is the water *li lu*. Its stem and leaves are identical [to those of *li lu*]. The only [difference] is that it grows on rocks/stones near waters and mountain streams. The root has more than a hundred hair stems. They are not used as medication. That which is used today is called "onion white *li lu*." The root has only about 20 to 30 whisker stems. Specimens growing in the mountains on a hight altitude are excellent. In Jun zhou locals also call them *lu cong* 鹿葱, "deer's onion." The *Fan zi Ji ran* states: "Yellow-white specimens coming from He dong are good."

17-15-01
根 *Gen*

Root [of *li lu*]

【修治】【雷曰】凡采得去頭，用糯米泔汁煮之。從巳至未，晒乾用。

Pharmaceutical Preparation. [Lei] Xiao: Whenever [the root] is collected, get its upper part and boil it in glutinous rice water from *si* hours (9 – 11) to *wei* hours (13 – 15). Dry it in the sun and use [it for therapeutic ends].

【氣味】辛，寒，有毒。【别録曰】苦，微寒。【普曰】神農、雷公：辛，有毒。岐伯：鹹，有毒。李當之：大寒，大毒。扁鵲：苦，有毒。【之才曰】黄連爲之使。反細辛、芍藥、人參、沙參、紫參、丹參、苦參。惡大黄。【時珍曰】畏葱白。服之吐不止，飲葱湯即止。

Qi and Flavor. Acrid, cold, poisonous. *Bie lu*: Bitter, slightly cold. [Wu] Pu: Shen nong, Lei gong: Acrid, poisonous. Qi Bo: Salty, poisonous. Li Dangzhi: Very cold, very poisonous. Bian Que: Bitter, poisonous. [Xu] Zhicai: *Coptis* [rhizome] serves as its guiding substance. [Ingested together,] it is opposed to *asarum heteropoides*

994 *Ma chang* 馬腸, lit.: "horse/big intestine," remains an unidentified plant.

[root], *paeonia* [root], ginseng [root], *adenophora* [root], common bistort, Chinese sage, and *sophora* [root]. It abhors rhubarb root. [Li] Shizhen: It fears onion white. Incessant vomiting after ingesting it is stopped by drinking an onion decoction.

【主治】蠱毒，欬逆，洩痢腸澼，頭瘍，疥瘙，惡瘡，殺諸蟲毒，去死肌。本經。療噦逆，喉痺不通，鼻中息肉，馬刀爛瘡。不入湯用。别録。主上氣，去積年膿血泄痢。權。吐上膈風涎，暗風癇病，小兒鰕齁痰疾。頌。末，治馬疥癬。宗奭。

Control. *Gu* poison,[995] cough with counterflow, outflow, free flow and intestinal flush, ulcers on the head, *jie*-illness[996] with itch, and malign sores. It kills all types of worms/bugs with poison and removes dead muscles. *Ben jing.* It heals retching with [qi] countermovement, throat blockage, tumorous flesh growth in the nose, and saber-shaped,[997] festering sores. It is not used as decoction. *Bie lu.* It controls rising qi and removes year-long outflow and free flow with pus and blood. [Zhen] Quan. It serves to spit out wind and saliva from the diaphragm, dim-vision wind[998] and epilepsy disease, as well as roaring panting with phlegm illness. [Su] Song. The powder serves to cure horse *jie*-illness[999] and *xuan*-illness.[1000] [Kou] Zongshi.

【發明】【頌曰】藜蘆服錢匕一字則惡吐人，又用通頂令人嚏，而别本云治噦逆，其效未詳。【時珍曰】噦逆用吐藥，亦反胃用吐法去痰積之義。吐藥不一：常山吐瘧痰，瓜丁吐熱痰，烏附尖吐濕痰，萊菔子吐氣痰，藜蘆則吐風痰者也。按張子和儒門事親云：一婦病風癇。自六七歲得驚風

995 *Gu du* 蠱毒, "*gu*-poison[ing]." (1) A poison emitted by certain worms/snakes with an ability to cause varying pathological changes in a person who has taken it in by means of wine or food. (2) Abdominal fullness, in some cases with blood spitting, and blood in the stool and urine. BCGM Dict I, 192 - 193. See BCGM 42-22.

996 *Jie*-illness 疥, vaguely identifiable skin ailment. BCGM Dict I, 249.

997 *Ma dao* 馬刀, "saber," a condition of saber-shaped, hard *luo li* 瘰癧, "scrofula with pervasion-illness," developing in the armpits. According to Li Dongyuan 李東垣, the location where this type of scrofula develops is not decisive for its identification. He called 'saber' all types of scrofula that are hard and do not fester. LSZ adopted this view. BCGM Dict I, 332.

998 *An feng* 暗風, "dim-vision wind," a condition of sudden dizziness or transient unconsciousness. BCGM Dict I, 43.

999 *Ma jie* 馬疥, "horse *jie*-illness," a condition of *jie chuang* 疥瘡, "*jie*-illness sores," whereby the skin forms scales and scraps, while its base is rough and thick. It itches and if scratched one does not feel any pain. BCGM Dict I, 332.

1000 *Xuan* 癬, "*xuan*-illness." Conditions of dermal lesions with initially erythema, papules, and itching gradually extending in all directions to form an irregular ring with clear boundaries. The skin is slightly elevated with small papules, blisters, and/or scales and scraps. The central lesion may appear to heal spontaneously, and it may reappear. Also, a designation of local lesions with itching, release of liquid and shedding of scabs. BCGM Dict I, 591.

後，每一二年一作，至五七年，五七作。三十歲至四十歲則日作，或甚至一日十餘作。【時珍曰】噦逆用吐藥，亦反胃用吐法去痰積之義。吐藥不一：常山吐瘧痰，瓜丁吐熱痰，烏附尖吐濕痰，萊菔子吐氣痰，藜蘆則吐風痰者也。按張子和儒門事親云：一婦病風癇。自六七歲得驚風後，每一二年一作，至五七年，五七作。三十歲至四十歲則日作，或甚至一日十餘作。遂昏癡健忘，求死而已。值歲大飢，采百草食。于野中見草若葱狀，采歸蒸熟飽食。至五更，忽覺心中不安，吐涎如膠，連日不止，約一二斗，汗出如洗，甚昏困。三日後，遂輕健，病去食進，百脉皆和。以所食葱訪人，乃憨葱苗也，即本草藜蘆是矣。圖經言能吐風病，此亦偶得吐法耳。我朝荆和王妃劉氏，年七十，病中風不省人事，牙關緊閉，群醫束手。先考太醫吏目月池翁診視，藥不能入，自午至子，不獲已，打去一齒，濃煎藜蘆湯灌之。少頃，噫氣一聲，遂吐痰而甦，調理而安。藥弗瞑眩，厥疾弗瘳，誠然。

Explication. [Su] Song: To ingest the amount of *li lu* held by a one *qian* spoon, or as much as one *zi*, lets you vomit violently. Also, its application penetrates the crown of one's head and causes sneezing. But when the *Bie lu* states that it causes retching with [qi] counterflow, why it might have this effect is not clear. [Li] Shizhen: For retching with [qi] counterflow medication is used that stimulates vomiting. The approach of causing vomiting is also resorted to in the case of turned over stomach based on the idea that this serves to remove phlegm accumulation. There is not just one pharmaceutical drug stimulating vomiting. Chinese quinine [root] lets one spit out phlegm related to a malaria disease. Musk melon fruit base lets one spit out phlegm related to the presence of heat. The pointed ends of *aconitum* [accessory tuber] let one spit out phlegm related to the presence of moisture. Radish seeds let one spit out phlegm related to qi [disorder], and *li lu* lets one spit out phlegm related to wind [intrusion]. According to Zhang Zihe in his *Ru men shi qin*, "there was a woman who suffered from epilepsy related to wind [intrusion]. When she was six or seven years old, she was affected by fright and wind [intrusion]. After this, [the disease] recurred every year or every second year. From five to seven years later, it recurred five to seven times. From her 30th to her 40th year of age it recurred every day, sometimes in the course of one day more than ten times. Eventually she became lethargic, than succumbed to idiocy and forgetfulness. She just sought to die, and reach an end. That year there was a great famine and she collected hundreds of herbs to eat. In the wild she saw an herb similar in shape to onions. She collected it, took it back, steamed it until done and ate it to her repletion. In the early morning hours of the next day she felt uneasy in her stomach/heart and spat out saliva similar to glue. This did not end for several consecutive days, altogether one or two *dou*. She perspired as if she was washed, eventually she fell into a coma and three days later felt light and healthy. Her disease was gone and she could eat. All the [movements in her] vessels were harmonious. Then she took the onions she had consumed to consult with someone and [was told that] this is the seedling of *han cong*, which is the *li lu* recorded in the *Ben cao*. The *Tu jing* says that it can cure wind [intrusion] disease. This [case of that woman is an example of using this herb] as a method encountered by chance to stimulate vomiting." During our present dynasty, Ms. Liu, a concubine of Prince He of Jing, at the age of 70 suffered from wind stroke and no longer recognized persons or anything else, with severe lockjaw. All physicians were helpless. Eventually [my father] Yuechi weng, an attendant to the Imperial Physicians, examined her. It proved impossible to have her take the medication [he had described]. This continued from *wu* hours (11 – 13) to *zi* hours (23 – 1), but to no avail. Then they struck out one of her teeth and force-fed her with a thick decoction of boiled *li lu*. Within short a sound of belching qi was heard, she spat out phlegm and regained consciousness. She was given harmonizing [medication] and eventually enjoyed health again. [A saying is:] "If a medication fails to cause nausea, illnesses of [qi] recession are not healed." This is true.

【附方】舊六，新十三。

Added Recipes. Six of old. 13 newly [recorded].

諸風痰飲。藜蘆十分，鬱金一分，爲末。每以一字，温漿水一盞和服，探吐。經驗方。

All types of phlegm rheum related to wind [intrusion]. [Grind] ten *fen* of *li lu* and one *fen* of turmeric into powder. Each time ingest one *zi* mixed with a small cup of warm fermented water of foxtail millet and insert [something into the patient's throat to stimulate] vomiting. *Jing yan fang*.

中風不省，牙關緊急者。藜蘆一兩去蘆頭，濃煎防風湯浴過，焙乾切，炒微褐色，爲末。每服半錢，小兒減半，温水調灌，以吐風涎爲效。未吐再服。簡要濟衆。

Wind stroke with a failure to recognize [persons or anything else] and severe lockjaw. Bathe one *liang* of *li lu*, with the top of the root discarded, in a thick decoction of *saposhnikovia* [root], bake it over a slow fire until it is dry and cut it into pieces. Fry them a little until they assume a brown color and [grind them into] powder. Each time [let the patient] ingest half a *qian*, for children this is cut in half, to be force-fed mixed with warm water. When [the patient] spits out wind and saliva, this is the effect. When [the patient] fails to spit/vomit, let him ingest [the medication] a second time. *Jian yao ji zhong*.

中風不語，喉中如曳鋸聲，口中涎沫。取藜蘆一分，天南星一個，去浮皮。于臍上剜一坑，納入陳醋二橡斗，四面火逼黄色，研爲末，生麪丸小豆大。每服三丸，温酒下。經驗。

Wind stroke with loss of ability to speak, hauling sounds from the throat as if sawing and saliva foam in the mouth. Prepare one *fen* of *li lu*. Then remove the superficial skin of one Indian turnip [root] and carve out a cavity in its center. [Insert the *li lu* and] two *dou* of long-stored vinegar, and heat this with a fire on all four sides until it has assumed a yellow color. Then grind it into powder, form with fresh wheat [dough] pills the size of mung beans and each time ingest three pills, to be sent down with warm wine. *Jing yan*.

諸風頭痛。和州藜蘆一莖，日乾研末，入射香少許，吹鼻。

All types of headache related to wind [intrusion] Dry in the sun one stem of *li lu* from He zhou and grind it into powder. Add a little musk and blow this into the [patient's] nose.

又方，通頂散：藜蘆半兩，黄連三分，嗃鼻。聖惠方。

Another recipe. The "powder to penetrate the crown of the head." [Mix] half a *liang* of *li lu* and three *fen* of *coptis* [rhizome] and inhale it through the nose. *Sheng hui fang*.

久瘧痰多，不食，欲吐不吐。藜蘆末半錢，温虀水調下，探吐。保命集。

Long-lasting malaria with much phlegm and an inability to eat. If there is an urge to vomit, [patients] fail to vomit. Send down half a *qian* of *li lu* powder mixed with warm water of minced vegetables. Then insert [something into the throat to stimulate] vomiting. *Bao ming ji*.

痰瘧積瘧。藜蘆、皂莢炙各一兩，巴豆二十五枚，熬黄，研末，蜜丸小豆大。每空心服一丸，未發時一丸，臨發時又服一丸。勿用飲食。肘後。

Phlegm malaria and chronic malaria. Roast one *liang* each of *li lu* and *gleditsia* pods/seeds, roasted, with 25 *croton* [seeds] until they turn yellow and grind them into powder. With honey form pills the size of mung beans. Each time ingest one pill on an empty stomach. One pill prior to an outbreak and another one when an outbreak is imminent. Do not at the same time drink or eat. *Zhou hou*.

黄疸腫疾。藜蘆灰中炮，爲末。水服半錢匕，小吐，不過數服效。百一方。

Swelling illness related to yellow *dan*-illness/jaundice. Roast *li lu* in ashes and [grind them into] powder. Ingest with water the amount held by half a *qian* spoon. This results in a little vomiting. An effect is seen after only a few such ingestions. *Bai yi fang*.

胸中結聚，如駭駭不去者。巴豆半兩，去皮心炒，擣如泥，藜蘆炙研一兩，蜜和擣丸麻子大，每吞一二丸。肘後。

Nodular collections in the chest, like being in shock that will not go away. Remove the skin of half a *liang* of croton [seeds] and fry their hearts/interior. Then pound them to a pulp and pound it further with one *liang* of *li lu*, roasted and ground [to powder], and honey [to a mass] that is formed to pills the size of hemp seeds. Each time swallow one or two pills. *Zhou hou.*

身面黑痣。藜蘆灰五兩，水一大盌淋汁，銅器重湯煮成黑膏，以針微刺破，點之，不過三次效。聖惠。

Black moles on the body and the face. Let one large bowl of water trickle over five *liang* of *li lu* ashes into a copper vessel and boil this in a water bath until a black paste is generated. With a needle slightly pierce [the moles] to open them and drop [the paste into the open moles]. An effect is achieved after no more than three [such applications]. *Sheng hui.*

鼻中息肉。藜蘆三分，雄黄一分，爲末，蜜和點之。每日三上自消，勿點兩畔。聖濟。

Tumorous flesh growth in the nose. [Grind] three *fen* of *li lu* and one *fen* of realgar into powder, mix it with honey and drop it [on the affected region]. Apply this three times every day, and [the flesh growths] will dissolve. Do not drop [the mixture] on the two nasal walls. *Sheng ji.*

牙齒蟲痛。藜蘆末，内入孔中，勿吞汁，神效。千金翼。

Toothache with the presence of worms/bugs. Insert *li lu* powder into the holes. Do not swallow the juice [forming in the mouth]. Divinely effective. *Qian jin yi.*

白秃蟲瘡。藜蘆末，猪脂調塗之。肘後。

White baldness sores with the presence of worms/bugs. Mix *li lu* powder with lard and apply this [to the affected region]. *Zhou hou.*

頭生蟣虱。藜蘆末摻之。直指。

Lice growing on the head. Mix *li lu* powder [into the hair]. *Zhi zhi.*

頭風白屑，痒甚。藜蘆末，沐頭摻之，緊包二日夜，避風，效。本事方。

Head wind[1001] with white scales and an extreme itch. Wash the head and mix *li lu* powder [into the hair]. Tightly wrap [the head] for two days and nights, and shield it against wind. Effective. *Ben shi fang.*

1001 *Tou feng* 頭風, "head wind." Condition of wind evil attacking the head followed by pain, dizziness, itching. BCGM Dict I, 509.

反花惡瘡。惡肉反出如米。藜蘆末，猪脂和傅，日三五上。聖濟録。

Malign reversed blossoms sores.[1002] Malign flesh appears reversed like rice. Mix *li lu* powder with lard and apply this [to the affected region]. To be applied three to five times a day. *Sheng ji lu.*

疥癬蟲瘡。藜蘆末，生油和塗。斗門方

Jie-illness[1003] and *xuan*-illness[1004] sores with the presence of worms/bugs. Mix *li lu* powder with fresh oil and apply this [to the affected region]. *Dou men fang.*

羊疽瘡痒。藜蘆二分，附子八分，爲末傅之，蟲自出也。陶隱居方。

Itching sheep impediment-illness (*sycosis*) sores. [Grind] two *fen* of *li lu* and eight *fen* of *aconitum* [accessory tuber] into powder and apply it [to the affected region]. Tao Yinju's recipe.

誤吞水蛭。藜蘆炒，爲末。水服一錢，必吐出。德生堂方。

Mistakenly having swallowed a leech. Fry *li lu* and [grind it into] powder. Ingest one *qian* with water and it is spat out.

【附録】
Appendix.

17-15-A01
山慈石 *Shan ci shi*
Amana edulis (Miq.) Honda. Edible tulip.[1005]

【別録有名未用曰】苦，平，無毒。主女子帶下。生山之陽。正月生葉如藜蘆，莖有衣。一名爰茈。

Bie lu, section "known by name but not in use." Bitter, balanced, nonpoisonous. It controls [diseases of] women with discharge from below the belt. It grows on the yang (i. e., sunny) side of mountains. In the first month it grows leaves similar to false hellebore/*li lu*.

1002 *Fan hua chuang* 反花瘡, "reversed-blossoms sores, conditions with a festering ulcer generating a fleshgrowth assuming the shape of a flower. BCGM Dict I, 149.

1003 *Jie*-illness 疥, vaguely identifiable skin ailment. BCGM Dict I, 249.

1004 *Xuan* 癬, "*xuan*-illness." Conditions of dermal lesions with initially erythema, papules, and itching gradually extending in all directions to form an irregular ring with clear boundaries. The skin is slightly elevated with small papules, blisters, and/or scales and scraps. The central lesion may appear to heal spontaneously, and it may reappear. Also, a designation of local lesions with itching, release of liquid and shedding of scabs. BCGM Dict I, 591.

1005 *Shan ci shi* 山慈石, lit.: "mountain magnetite."

17-15-A02
參果根 *Shen guo gen*

Unidentified.

【又曰】苦，有毒。主鼠瘻。生百餘根，根有衣裹莖。三月三日采根。一名百連，一名烏蓼，一名鼠莖，一名鹿蒲。

It also says: Bitter, poisonous. It controls mouse fistula.[1006] It grows more than 100 roots. The root has its stem covered by a coating. The root is collected on the third day of the third month. It is also called *bai lian* 百連, *wu liao* 烏蓼, *shu jing* 鼠莖 and *lu pu* 鹿蒲.

17-15-A03
馬腸根宋圖經 ***Ma chang gen***, FE Song, *Tu jing*.
Unidentified.[1007]

【頌曰】苦，辛，寒，有毒。主蠱除風。葉療瘡疥。生秦州。葉似桑。三月采葉，五月、六月采根。

[Su] Song: Bitter, acrid, cold, poisonous. It controls *gu* [poison][1008] and dispels wind. The leaves serve to heal *jie*-illness[1009] sores. It grows in Qin zhou. The leaves resemble those of mulberry trees. The leaves are collected in the third month. The root is collected in the fifth and sixth month.

17-16
木黎蘆拾遺
Mu li lu, FE *Shi yi*.

***Leucothoe grayana* Maxim.**

【釋名】黄黎蘆綱目、鹿驪。

Explanation of Names. *Huang li lu* 黄黎蘆, "yellow false hellebore/*li lu*," *Gang mu*. *Lu li* 鹿驪.

【集解】【藏器曰】陶弘景注漏蘆云：一名鹿驪。山南人用苗，北人用根。按鹿驪乃木黎蘆，非漏蘆也。乃樹生，如茱萸樹，高二尺，有毒。

1006 *Shu lou* 鼠瘻, "mouse fistula," BCGM Dict I, 466, identical to *luo li* 瘰癧, "scrofula pervasion-illness."

1007 *Ma chang gen* 馬腸根, lit.: "horse intestine [shaped] root."

1008 *Gu du* 蠱毒, "*gu*-poison[ing]." (1) A poison emitted by certain worms/snakes with an ability to cause varying pathological changes in a person who has taken it in by means of wine or food. (2) Abdominal fullness, in some cases with blood spitting, and blood in the stool and urine. BCGM Dict I, 192 - 193. See BCGM 42-22.

1009 *Jie*-illness 疥, vaguely identifiable skin ailment. BCGM Dict I, 249.

【時珍曰】鹿驪，俚人呼爲黄黎蘆，小樹也。葉如櫻桃葉，狹而長，多皺文。四月開細黄花。五月結小長子，如小豆大。

Collected Explanations. [Chen] Cangqi: Tao Hongjing commenting on *lou lu* 漏蘆, uniflower swiss centaury, states: "Alternative name: *lu li* 鹿驪. People in Shan nan use the seedling; people in the North use the root." Now, *lu li* 鹿驪 is *mu li lu* 木黎蘆, "wooden false hellebore," it is not *lou lu* 漏蘆. It grows as trees, similar to the Cornelian cherry tree. It is two *chi* tall and poisonous. [Li] Shizhen: Common people refer to *lu li* 鹿驪 as "*huang li lu* 黄黎蘆/yellow false hellebore." It is a small tree. Its leaves are similar to cherry tree leaves; they are narrow and lengthy, with many wrinkled lines. It opens fine, yellow flowers in the fourth month and forms small, lengthy seeds, the size of mung beans, in the fifth month.

【氣味】苦、辛，温，有毒。

Qi and Flavor. Bitter, acrid, warm, poisonous.

【主治】疥癬，殺蟲。藏器。

Control. *Jie*-illness,[1010] *xuan*-illness[1011]. It kills worms/bugs. [Chen] Cangqi.

17-17
附子本經下品
Fu zi, *Ben jing*, lower rank.

***Aconitum carmichaeli* Debx. *Aconitum* [accessory tuber].**

【釋名】其母名烏頭。【時珍曰】初種爲烏頭，象烏之頭也。附烏頭而生者爲附子，如子附母也。烏頭如芋魁，附子如芋子，蓋一物也。别有草烏頭、白附子，故俗呼此爲黑附子、川烏頭以别之。諸家不分烏頭有川、草兩種，皆混雜註解，今悉正之。

Explanation of Names. Its "mother" is called *wu tou* 烏頭, *aconitum* [main tuber]. [Li] Shizhen: What is planted first is *wu tou* 烏頭, "crow head," it looks like the head, *tou* 頭, of a crow, *wu* 烏. Those [tubers] growing attached to the main tuber, they are the "attached children," *fu zi* 附子, just as children, *zi* 子, are attached, *fu* 附, to their mother. The main tuber is similar to taro tuber. The *aconitum* [accessory tuber], *fu zi* 附子, is similar to taro seeds. The fact is, [the main tuber, *wu tou*, and

1010 *Jie*-illness 疥, vaguely identifiable skin ailment. BCGM Dict I, 249.

1011 *Xuan* 癬, "*xuan*-illness." Conditions of dermal lesions with initially erythema, papules, and itching gradually extending in all directions to form an irregular ring with clear boundaries. The skin is slightly elevated with small papules, blisters, and/or scales and scraps. The central lesion may appear to heal spontaneously, and it may reappear. Also, a designation of local lesions with itching, release of liquid and shedding of scabs. BCGM Dict I, 591.

the accessory tuber, *fu zi*] are one item. There are also *cao wu tou* 草烏頭, "herbal *wu tou*," and *bai fu zi* 白附子, "white *fu zi*." Hence [the item discussed here] is commonly called hei *fu zi* 黑附子, "black *fu zi*," and *chuan wu tou* 川烏頭, "[*Si*] *chuan wu tou*," to distinguish them. All authors have have failed to distinguish between the two kinds of [Si] chuan and *cao*/herbal *wu tou* 烏頭. Their comments and explications were all confused. This is corrected here now.

【集解】【别録曰】附子生犍爲山谷及廣漢。冬月采爲附子，春月采爲烏頭。【弘景曰】烏頭與附子同根。附子八月采，八角者良。烏頭四月采。春時莖初生有腦頭，如烏鳥之頭，故謂之烏頭。有兩岐，其蒂狀如牛角者，名烏喙。取汁煎爲射罔。天雄似附子，細而長，乃至三四寸。側子即附子邊角之大者。並是同根，而本經附子出犍爲，天雄出少室，烏頭出朗陵，分生三處，當各有所宜也。今則無别矣。【恭曰】天雄、附子、烏頭，並以蜀道綿州、龍州者佳，俱以八月采造。餘處雖有造得者，力弱，都不相似。江南來者，全不堪用。【大明曰】天雄大而長，少角刺而虛。附子大而短，有角平穩而實。烏喙似天雄，烏頭次于附子，側子小於烏頭，連聚生者名爲虎掌，並是天雄一裔，子母之類，氣力乃有殊等，即宿根與嫩者爾。【斅曰】烏頭少有莖苗，身長而烏黑，少有旁尖。烏喙皮上蒼色，有尖頭，大者孕八九箇，周圍底陷，黑如烏鐵。天雄身全矮，無尖，周匝四面有附子，孕十一箇，皮蒼色。側子只是附子旁，有小顆如棗核者。木鼈子是喙、附、烏、雄、側中毗患者，不入藥用。【保昇曰】正者爲烏頭，兩岐者爲烏喙，細長三四寸者爲天雄，根旁如芋散生者爲附子，旁連生者爲側子，五物同出而異名。苗高二尺許，葉似石龍芮及艾。【宗奭曰】五者皆一物，但依大小長短以象而名之爾。【頌曰】五者今並出蜀土，都是一種所産，其種出于龍州。冬至前，先將陸田耕五七遍，以豬糞糞之，然後布種，逐月耘耔，至次年八月後方成。其苗高三四尺，莖作四稜，葉如艾，其花紫碧色作穗，其實細小如桑椹狀，黑色。本只種附子一物，至成熟後乃有四物。以長二三寸者爲天雄，割削附子旁尖角爲側子，附子之絶小者亦名側子，元種者爲烏頭。其餘大小者皆爲附子，以八角者爲上。綿州彰明縣多種之，惟赤水一鄉者最佳。然收采時月與本草不同。謹按本草冬采爲附子，春采爲烏頭。博物志言：附子、烏頭、天雄一物也。春秋冬夏采之各異。而廣雅云：奚毒，附子也。一歲爲側子，二年爲烏喙，三年爲附子，四年爲烏頭，五年爲天雄。今一年種之，便有此五物。豈今人種蒔之法，用力倍至，故爾繁盛乎？【時珍曰】烏頭有兩種。出彰明者即附子之母，今人謂之川烏頭是也。春末生子，故曰春采爲烏頭。冬則生子已成，故曰冬采爲附子。其天雄、烏喙、側子，皆是生子多者，因象命名；若生子少及獨頭者，即無此數物也。其産江左、山南等處者，乃本經所列烏頭，今人謂之草烏頭者是也，故曰其汁煎爲射罔。陶弘景不知烏頭有二，以附子之烏頭，註射罔之烏頭，遂致諸家疑貳，而雷斅之説尤不近理。宋人楊天惠著附子記甚悉，今撮其要，讀之可不辯而明矣。其説云：綿州乃故廣漢地，領縣八，惟彰明出附子。彰明領鄉二十，惟赤水、廉水、昌明、會昌四鄉産附子，而赤水爲多。每歲以上田熟耕作壟，取種於龍安、龍州、齊歸、木門、青堨、小坪諸處。十一月播種，春月生苗。其莖類野艾而澤，其葉類地麻而厚。其花紫瓣黄蕤，長苞而圓。七月采者，謂之早水，拳縮而小，蓋未長成也。九月采者乃佳。其品凡七，本同而末異。其初種之化者爲烏頭，附烏頭而旁生者爲附子，又左右附而偶生者爲鬲子，附而長者爲天雄，附而尖者爲天錐，附而上出者爲側子，附而散生者爲漏籃子，皆脉絡連貫，如子附母，而附子以貴，故專附名也。凡種一而子六七以上則皆小，種一而子二三則稍大，種一而子特生，則特大。附子之形，以蹲坐正、節角少者爲上，有節多鼠乳者次之，形不正而傷缺風皺者爲下。本草言附子八角者爲良，其角爲側子之説，甚謬矣。附子之色，以花白者爲上，鐵色者次之，青緑者爲下。天雄、烏頭、天錐，皆以豐實盈握者爲勝。漏籃、側子，則園人以乞役夫，不足數也。謹按此記所載漏籃，即雷斅所謂木鼈子，大明所謂虎掌者也。其鬲子即烏喙也。天錐即天雄之類，醫方亦無此名，功用當相同爾。

Collected Explanations. *Bie lu*: *Fu zi* grows in the mountain valleys of Jian wei, and in Guang han. During winter months *fu zi* 附子 is collected. During spring months *wu tou* 烏頭, *aconitum* [main tuber], is collected. [Tao] Hongjing: *Wu tou* and *fu zi* together constitute one root. *Fu zi* is collected in the eighth month; specimens with eight horns/edges are good. *Wu tou* is collected in the fourth month. In spring, when the stem begins to grow, there is something like a head, *tou* 頭, with a brain, shaped like the head of a black/crow, *wu* 烏, bird. Hence it is called *wu tou* 烏頭, "crow head." When it has two diverging branches with a base shaped like the horns of oxen, it is called *wu hui* 烏喙, "crow beak." Its juice is boiled to *she wang* 射罔.[1012] *Tian xiong* 天雄 resembles *fu zi*, but is fine and lengthy, reaching a length of three to four *cun*. *Ce zi* 側子, "lateral children," are the large marginal horns of *fu zi*. Together they all form one root. According to the *Ben jing*, *fu zi* comes from Jian wei, *tian xiong* 天雄 comes from Shao shi, *wu tou* 烏頭 comes from Lang ling. As they grow in three different places, they should have different [therapeutic tasks for which they are] suitable. Today, there is no such differentiation any longer. [Su] Gong: *Tian xiong*, *fu zi* and *wu tou*, no matter whether they come from Mian zhou or Long zhou in Shu dao, they are all excellent. All of them are collected and further processed in the eighth month. Those obtained from and processed in other regions are of weak strength; none of them equals those [from Shu dao]. Specimens from Jiang nan are entirely useless. Da Ming: *Tian xiong* is big and lengthy; it has small piercing horns and is hollow. *Fu zi* is big and short; it has horns that are flat, firm

1012 Instead of *she wang* 射罔, *Zheng lei* ch. 10, *wu tou* 烏頭, writes *she wang* 射罔.

and filled. *Wu hui* 烏喙 resembles *tian xiong*; *wu tou* is of secondary value to *fu zi*, and *ce zi* 側子 is smaller than *wu tou*. The cluster they form when they grow is called *hu zhang* 虎掌, "tiger paw." They are all descendents of *tian xiong* 天雄, similar to a mother and her children. The strength of their qi differs, depending on whether it is a perennial root or a tender [new growth]. [Lei] Xiao: *Wu tou* has few stems and seedlings. Its body is long and black, with only a few pointed ends at the side. *Wu hui* 烏喙 is grey on its skin. It has a pointed head. Large specimens have eight or nine offspring forming a circle around an indented bottom. They are as black as black iron. *Tian xiong* has a short body and no pointed ends. It is surrounded by *fu zi*, bearing 11 of them, with an ash-grey color. *Ce zi* 側子 grow only at the side of *fu zi*. These are small kernels similar to Chinese date pits. *Mu bie zi* are those parts of [*wu*] *hui*, *fu* [*zi*], *wu* [*tou*], [*tian*] *xiong* and *ce* [*zi*] that are damaged. They are not used for medicinal preparations. [Han] Baosheng: The principal [root/tuber] is *wu tou* 烏頭. Those forked into two branches are *wu hui* 烏喙. Those that are fine and three to four *cun* long, they are *tian xiong* 天雄. Those growing spread at the side of the root similar to taro [seeds/tubers], they are *fu zi* 附子. Those growing aligned along the side [of the principal root], they are *ce zi* 側子. These five items [are roots] that come from the same [herb] but have different names. The seedling is about two feet tall. The leaves resemble those of cursed crow foot and common mugwort. [Kou] Zongshi: These five [items] are one and the same item. Still, they are named [differently] related to their size and length. [Su] Song: Today all these five [items] come from Shu soil. They all are products of one planting. This planting has its origin in Long zhou. Prior to Winter Solstice the fields are plowed five to seven times and fertilized with pig dung. Then [the seed] are spread to start the planting. The weeds are removed month after month, and [the planting] will have succeeded in the eighth month of the next year. The seedling is three to four *chi* tall. The stem [is square] with four edges. The leaves resemble those of common mugwort. The flowers are purple-jade-bluish and have spikes. The fruits are fine and small; they are shaped like mulberry fruits. They are black. Originally, the planting aims only at *fu zi*. But after [the *fu zi*] has ripened, there are four items. Those two to three *cun* long are *tian xiong* 天雄. The pointed horns cut from the side of *fu zi* are *ce zi* 側子. Very small specimens of *fu zi* 附子 are also called *ce zi* 側子. The principal [root obtained through the] planting is *wu tou* 烏頭. All the other [segments], regardless of their sizes, are *fu zi* 附子, with those considered best that have eight horns. In Zhang ming xian of Mian zhou they plant lots [of *fu zi*], but only those from the one rural area of Chi shui are the very best. However, the months when they are collected are not identical to [those recorded in] the *ben cao* literature. A [personal] comment: *Fu zi* is collected in winter, while *wu tou* is collected in spring. *Bo wu zhi*: *Fu zi*, *wu tou* and *tian xiong* are one identical item. A difference depends on whether they are collected in spring, autumn, winter or summer. The *Guang ya* states: "*Xi du* 奚毒 is *fu zi* 附子. If it [has grown] for a year, it is *ce zi* 側子. For two years, it is *wu hui* 烏喙. For three years, it is *fu zi* 附子. For four years, it is *wu tou* 烏頭. For five years, it is *tian xiong* 天雄." Nowadays, they plant them and within one year they have all five of these items. Could it be that with today's methods of vegetable farming and much more force applied such abundance is achieved? [Li] Shizhen: There are two kinds of *wu tou*. That coming from Zhang ming is the "mother" of *fu zi*. This is the kind called by people *chuan wu tou* 川烏頭today. At the end of spring it grows "children," *zi* 子. Hence it is said: "In spring collect *wu tou*." In winter the "children" have grown up. Hence it is said: "In winter collect the 'attached children,' *fu zi* 附子. *Tian xiong*, *wu hui* and *ce zi* are the many more "children" that have grown. They are named in accordance with their physical appearance. If [the principal root] gives birth to only a few children, *zi* 子, and has only one "head," *tou* 頭, then there is no such multiplicity of items. Those produced in places such as Jiang zuo and Shan nan, they are the *wu tou* 烏頭 listed in the *Ben jing* and they are what people today call *cao wu tou* 草烏頭, "herbal crow head." Therefore it is said that its juice when boiled is *she wang* 射罔. Tao Hongjing did not know that there are two kinds of *wu tou*. He identified the *wu tou* of *fu zi* as the *wu tou* of *she wang* 射罔 and caused confusion with regard to the two [kinds] among later authors, with the statements of Lei Xiao being particularly far from the truth. When Yang Tianhui, a Song person, wrote his *Fu zi ji*, he was extremely well informed. Here now the essentials [of his book] are concentrated, and readers will have a clear understanding without further argumentation. He says: Mian zhou is the ancient Guang han territory. It has eight counties, but only Zhang ming produces *fu zi*. Zhang ming has 20 rural areas, and only four of them, Chi shui, Lian shui, Chang ming and Hui chang produce *fu zi*, with most of it [produced] in Chi shui. Every year these fields are prepared by plowing them and making ridges. Then the seeds are obtained from numerous locations, such as Long an, Long zhou, Qi gui, Mu men, Qing dui and Xiao ping. The sowing is done in the 11th month; seedlings grow in the months of spring. The seedling is similar to that of wild mugwort, but it is moist. The leaves are similar to those of *di ma*,[1013] but they are thicker. The flowers have purple petals and yellow anther bearing filaments. The "envelopes" are lengthy and round. [When the root] is collected in the seventh month, it is called *zao shui* 早水. It is a small, contracted fist. The fact is, it has not grown to its full length yet. Those collected in the ninth month are excellent. They can be divided into seven ranks. They have an iden-

1013 *Di ma* 地麻, an unidentified herb. The name is mentioned once in the BCGM. It does not appear anywhere else.

tical beginning, but differ in the end. Those having transformed[1014] first after the planting are *wu tou* 烏頭. Those growing attached to *wu tou* from its side are *fu zi* 附子. Those growing attached to the left and right in pairs are *ge zi* 鬲子. Those [growing] attached and being lengthy, they are *tian xiong* 天雄. Those [growing] attached and being pointed, they are *tian zhui* 天錐. Those [growing] attached and ascending, they are *ce zi* 側子. Those growing attached and dispersed, they are *lou lan zi* 漏籃子. All of them are tied to each other through a network of vessels, just like children are tied to their mother. Because "attached children", *fu zi* , are highly valued, *fu* 附, "attached," is the special name given [to all of them]. When from planting one [root] six, seven or more "children" emerge, they are all small. When from planting one [root] two or three "children" emerge, they are somewhat bigger. If from planting one [root] only one "child" is born, it is particularly big. As for the physical appearance of the "attached children," *fu zi* 附子, when they properly sit upright, and when they have few knots and horns, they are best. Those with many knots, similar to mouse/rat teats, they are of secondary value. Those with a physical appearance not [sitting] upright, harmed and wrinkled by wind, they are of low quality. The *Ben cao* says that "*fu zi* with eight horns is good." That is a great mistake. As for the color of *fu zi*, those with white flowers are best. They are followed by those with an iron color. Those that are greenish-green, they are of low quality. *Tian xiong*, *wu tou* and *tian zhui* 天錐 that are very solid and fill one's hand, they are superior. *Lou lan* 漏籃 and *ce zi* 側子 are given by farmers to their workers. They are not worth to be taken into account." A comment: The *lou lan* 漏籃 recorded here is the *mu bie zi* 木鼈子 referred to by Lei Xiao, and the *hu zhang* 虎掌 referred to by Da Ming. The *ge zi* 鬲子 is *wu hui* 烏喙. *Tian zhui* 天錐 is related to *tian xiong* 天雄. These names do not appear in medical recipes. Their [therapeutic] function should be identical.

【修治】【保昇曰】附子、烏頭、天雄、側子、烏喙，采得，以生熟湯浸半日，勿令滅氣，出以白灰裛之，數易使乾。又法：以米粥及糟麴等淹之。並不及前法。【頌曰】五物收時，一處造釀。其法：先於六月内，造大小麪麴。未采前半月，用大麥煮成粥，以麴造醋，候熟去糟。其醋不用太酸，酸則以水解之。將附子去根鬚，於新甕内淹七日，日攪一遍，撈出以疏篩攤之，令生白衣。乃向慢風日中晒之百十日，以透乾爲度。若猛日則皺而皮不附肉。【時珍曰】按附子記云：此物畏恶最多，不能常熟。或種美而苗不茂，或苗秀而根不充，或已釀而腐，或已曝而攣，若有神物陰

1014 Instead of *qi chu zhong zhi hua zhe wei wu tou hua* 其初種之化者爲烏頭, "those having transformed first after the planting are *wu tou* 烏頭," the Song era Yang Tianhui's *Zhang ming fu zi ji* writes: *qi chu zhong zhi xiao zhe wei wu tou hua* 其初種之小者爲烏頭, "small ones resulting from first after the planting are *wu tou* 烏頭."

爲之者。故園人常禱於神，目爲藥妖。其釀法：用醋醅安密室中，淹覆彌月，乃發出晾乾。方出釀時，其大有如拳者，已定輒不盈握，故及一兩者極難得。土人云：但得半兩以上者皆良。蜀人餌者少，惟秦陜、閩、浙人宜之。然秦人纔市其下者，閩、浙纔得其中者，其上品則皆貴人得之矣。【弘景曰】凡用附子、烏頭、天雄，皆熱灰微炮令拆，勿過焦，惟薑附湯生用之。俗方每用附子，須甘草、人參、生薑相配者，正制其毒故也。【斅曰】凡使烏頭，宜文武火中炮令皴拆，擘破用。若用附子，須底平有九角如鐵色，一個重一兩者，即是氣全。勿用雜木火，只以柳木灰火中炮令皴拆，以刀刮去上孕子，并去底尖，擘破，於屋下午地上掘一土坑安之，一宿取出，焙乾用。若陰制者，即生去皮尖底，薄切，以東流水并黑豆浸五日夜，漉出，日中曬乾用。【震亨曰】凡烏、附、天雄，須用童子小便浸透煮過，以殺其毒，并助下行之力，入鹽少許尤好。或以小便浸二七日，揀去壞者，以竹刀每箇切作四片，井水淘净，逐日换水，再浸七日，晒乾用。【時珍曰】附子生用則發散，熟用則峻補。生用者須如陰制之法，去皮臍入藥。熟用者以水浸過，炮令發拆，去皮臍，乘熱切片再炒，令内外俱黄，去火毒入藥。又法：每一箇，用甘草二錢，鹽水、薑汁、童尿各半盞，同煮熟，出火毒一夜用之，則毒去也。

Pharmaceutical Preparation. [Han] Baosheng: *Fu zi*, *wu tou*, *ce zi* and *wu hui*, once collected they are soaked in fresh and processed hot water (05-31) for half a day. Be sure not to lose any of their qi. When they are taken out [of the water again] they are wrapped in lime (07-57). Replace [the lime] several times until [the roots] are dry. Another method: Immerse them in rice gruel or in distillers' yeast. But this method is not equal to the one mentioned before. [Su] Song: When these five items are collected, they are processed together. The method is as follows. Prior to the sixth month prepare a larger or smaller amount of leaven. Half a month prior to collecting [the roots] cook barley to prepare a gruel and with the leaven prepare vinegar. When it is well done remove the dregs. The vinegar should not be overly sour. If it is [too] sour, dilute it with water. Then remove all the hair from *fu zi* roots and soak them in an earthenware jar for seven days. Stir [the liquid] once every day. Then scoop [the roots] up from the water, spread them scattered on a sieve/screen and let them develop a white coating. Next put them in a place with a slow wind and dry them in the sun for 100 days until they are dry inside and outside. If the sun is too strong, their skin folds and no longer adheres to the meat. [Li] Shizhen: According to the *Fu zi ji*, it is to be feared that this item may easily rot; it cannot be kept prepared for a long time. It may well be that the seeds are beautiful, but the seedlings are few. Or the seedling is elegant but the root is incomplete. Or the processing is complete and [the roots] rot. Or [the roots] have been exposed to the sun and contract, as if some spirit item clandestinely was working on them. Hence farmers continuously pray to a spirit and call it "medicine goblin." The method to process [the roots is as follows]. Soak them in vinegar and let them rest in a sealed room for more than a month. Then remove [the root from the vinegar] and dry it. Pieces as big as a fist when they are removed [from the vinegar, when they have dried,] they may have shrunk and no longer fill a hand. Hence it is very difficult to obtain pieces weighing up to one *liang*. The locals states: It is sufficient to obtain those that weigh half a *liang* or more; they all are good. People in Shu only seldom eat [the roots]. Only people in Qin, Shaan, Min and Zhe consider them suitable [for consumption]. While people in Qin market only those of low quality, in Min and Zhe one gets only those of medium quality. Those of top quality are obtained by the nobility. [Tao] Hongjing: Whenever *fu zi*, *wu tou* and *tian xiong* are to be used, slightly wrap them in hot ashes to let them crack. They are used fresh/unprepared only in the "decoction with ginger and *fu* [*zi*]." Whenever *fu zi* is resorted to in commonly used recipes, it must be combined with *glycyrrhiza* [root], ginseng [root] and fresh ginger because this serves to check its poison. [Lei] Xiao: For all applications of *wu tou* 烏頭, it is advisable to roast it on a mild fire first and on a strong fire later in a pan to let them crack and break open. Then break them with your fingers into smaller pieces and this is how they are used [for therapeutic purposes]. When using *fu zi*, those must be chosen that have a flat base with nine horns and a color like iron. When one piece weighs one *liang*, its qi are complete. Do not use [ashes] from a fire of just any wood. Roast them to let them split open only in the ashes left from a fire of willow tree wood. With a knife cut off and remove all the "children," remove the pointed ends from the base and with the fingers break [the roots into small pieces]. In a room, in the afternoon, dig a pit in the soil, place [the pieces] there and remove them again after one night. Bake them over a slow fire, and they can be used [for therapeutic ends]. If they are to be processed according to a yin [method], remove the skin, the pointed ends and the base, and cut [the rest] into thin slices. Then soak them in water flowing eastward with black soybeans for five days and nights, and remove them by straining the water. Dry them in the sun and then they are ready to be used [for therapeutic purposes]. [Zhu] Zhenheng: For all applications of *wu* [*tou*], *fu* [*zi*] and *tian xiong*, soak them in boys' urine to kill their poison and to assist their strength of moving downward. If a small amount of salt is added, this is particularly good. Or, soak them in urine for two times seven days, pick up and remove decayed specimens, and with a bamboo knife cut each [root] into four pieces. Wash them clean with water in a pan, exchanging the water day by day. Then soak them again for seven days. Eventually, dry them in the sun and they are ready to be used [for therapeutic ends]. [Li] Shizhen: When *fu zi* is used fresh/unprepared it has a dispersing effect. When it is used prepared, it has a powerful supplementing effect. For application as a fresh/unprepared item the method of "yin check" must be applied. Remove the skin and the navel[1015] and add the naked interior to medication. For application as a prepared item, after soaking [*fu zi*] in water roast it to let it crack open, remove the skin and the navel, and while it is still hot cut it into slices that are then fried again so that [the root] assumes a yellow color inside and outside. Then remove the fire poison and add it to medication. Another method: Boil each [root] until done with two *qian* of *glycyrrhiza* [root], and half a small cup each of salt water, ginger juice and boys' urine, let the fire poison leave [the *fu zi*] during one night and use [the root for therapeutic ends]. Its poison will have been removed.

【氣味】辛，温，有大毒。【別録曰】甘，大熱。【普曰】神農：辛。岐伯、雷公：甘，有毒。李當之：苦，大温，有大毒。【元素曰】大辛大熱，氣厚味薄，可升可降，陽中之陰，浮中沉，無所不至，爲諸經引用之藥。【好古曰】入手少陽三焦命門之劑，其性走而不守，非若乾薑止而不行。【趙嗣真曰】熟附配麻黄，發中有補，仲景麻黄附子細辛湯、麻黄附子甘草湯是也。生附配乾薑，補中有發，仲景乾薑附子湯、通脉四逆湯是也。【戴原禮曰】附子無乾薑不熱，得甘草則性緩，得桂則補命門。【李燾曰】附子得生薑則能發散，以熱攻熱，又導虚熱下行，以除冷病。【之才曰】地膽爲之使。惡蜈蚣。畏防風、黑豆、甘草、人參、黄耆。【時珍曰】畏緑豆、烏韭、童溲、犀角。忌豉汁。得蜀椒、食鹽，下達命門。

Qi and Flavor. Acrid, warm, very poisonous. *Bie lu*: Sweet, very hot. [Wu] Pu: Shen nong: Acrid, Qi Bo, Lei gong: Sweet, poisonous. Li Dangzhi: Bitter, very warm, very poisonous. [Zhang] Yuansu: Very acrid, very hot, with strongly pronounced qi and weakly pronounced flavor. It can rise and it can descend; it is a yin in yang [substance]. Whether by floating at the surface, being in the middle, or sinking into the depth, there is no place it does not reach. It is a pharmaceutical drug resorted to for guiding [other substances] into all the conduits. [Wang] Haogu: Applications to enter the hand minor yang [conduits], the Triple Burner and the Gate of Life, [make use of] its nature to run rather than hold guard at one place. This is different from dried ginger that is static and fails to move. Zhao Sizhen: Prepared *fu* [*zi*] combined with *ephedra* [herb] has a supplementing effect within its dispersing effect. This is made use of in [Zhang] Zhongjing's "decoction with *ephedra* [herb], *fu zi* and *asarum heteropoides* [root]" and the "decoction with ephedra [herb], *fu zi* and *glycyrrhiza* [root]." Fresh/unprepared *fu* [*zi*] combined with dried ginger has a dispersing effect within its supplementing effect. This is made use of in [Zhang] Zhongjing's "decoction with dried ginger and *fu zi*," and the "decoction to penetrate

1015 *Qi* 臍, "navel," is the indentation at the top of the tuber where it was connected with the stem of the plant. "To remove skin and navel" has the meaning of "to clean thoroughly."

the vessels for [curing] the four countermovements."[1016] Dai Yuanli: Without dried ginger, *fu zi* is not hot. Combined with *glycyrrhiza* [root] its nature is slowed down. Combined with *cassia* it supplements [qi in] the Gate of Life. Li Tao: When *fu zi* is combined with fresh ginger, it is capable of dispersing. As a hot [substance] it serves to attack heat in that it leads depletion heat to move downward, thereby eliminating a cold disease. [Xu] Zhicai: Oil beetles (40-09) serve as its guiding substance. [Ingested together, *fu zi*] abhors centipedes, and fears *saposhnikovia* [root], black soybeans, *glycyrrhiza* [root], ginseng [root] and *astragalus* [root]. [Li] Shizhen: It fears mung beans, Chinese creeping fern, boys's urine, and rhinoceros horn. [During a treatment with *fu zi*] fermented bean juice is to be avoided. Combined with Sichuan pepper and table salt it descends and reaches the Gate of Life.

【主治】風寒欬逆邪氣，寒濕踒躄，拘攣膝痛，不能行步，破癥堅積聚血瘕，金瘡。本經。腰脊風寒，脚氣冷弱，心腹冷痛，霍亂轉筋，下痢赤白，温中强陰，堅肌骨，又墮胎，爲百藥長。别録。温暖脾胃，除脾濕腎寒，補下焦之陽虚。元素。除臟腑沉寒，三陽厥逆，濕淫腹痛，胃寒蚘動，治經閉，補虚散壅。李杲。督脉爲病，脊强而厥。好古。治三陰傷寒，陰毒寒疝，中寒中風，痰厥氣厥，柔痓癲癇，小兒慢驚，風濕麻痺，腫滿脚氣，頭風，腎厥頭痛，暴瀉脱陽，久痢脾泄，寒瘧瘴氣，久病嘔噦，反胃噎膈，癰疽不歛，久漏冷瘡。合葱涕，塞耳治聾。時珍。

Control.. Cough with [qi] counterflow and evil qi, related to wind [intrusion] and the presence of cold. Cold moisture and sprain with loss of mobility, cramps with contraction and aching knees so that one cannot walk. It breaks open concretion-illness hardenings, accumulation and collection, with blood conglomeration-illness, and [cures] wounds inflicted by metal objects/weapons. *Ben jing*. Wind [intrusion] and the presence of cold in the lower back and the spine. Leg qi[1017] with cold and weakness. Painful cold in the central and abdominal region. Cholera with contorted sinews. Red and white discharge with free-flux illness. It warms the center and strengthens the yin [qi]. It hardens muscles and bones. Also, it causes abortion and is the chief among the hundreds of pharmaceutical drugs. *Bie lu*. It warms spleen and stomach, removes moisture from the spleen and cold from the kidneys. It supplements a yang [qi] depletion in the lower [section of the Triple] Burner. [Zhang] Yuansu. It removes cold located deep in the long-term depots and short-term repositories. [It serves to cure] ceasing [qi] and counterflow in the three yang [conduits], painful abdomen because of excessive moisture, stomach cold with

1016 *Tong mai si ni tang* 脉四逆湯, the "decoction to penetrate the vessels for [curing] the four countermovements," has the following ingredients: *Glycyrrhiza* root, dried ginger, *fu zi* and onions white.

1017 *Jiao qi* 脚氣, "leg qi." Painful, weak, swollen legs. BCGM Dict I, 248.

tapeworm movement. It serves to cure blocked menstruation, supplements depleted [qi] and disperses obstructions. Li Gao. [It serves to cure] diseases affecting the supervisor vessel, stiffness of the spine and [yang qi] ceasing [from the extremities]. [Wang] Haogu. It serves to cure the three yin [conduits] harmed by cold, yin poison[1018] and cold elevation-illness,[1019] cold stroke and wind stroke. Phlegm recession[1020] and qi recession.[1021] Soft spasms.[1022] Peak-illness with epilepsy. Slow fright of children.[1023] Numbness and blockage related to wind [intrusion] and the presence of moisture. Swelling with a sensation of fullness and leg qi.[1024] Head wind.[1025] Kidney recession[1026] with headache. Sudden outflow with a loss of yang [qi]. Long-lasting free-flux illness and spleen outflow.[1027] Cold malaria and miasmatic qi. Chronic disease with vomiting and retching. Turned over stomach and gullet occlusion. Obstruction-illness and impediment-illness[1028] that fail to withdraw. Long-lasting,

---

1018 *Yin du* 陰毒, "yin poison," a condition of *shang han* 傷寒, "harm caused by cold," resulting in a flourishing of only yin qi and a diminution of yang qi, with cold extremities and a greenish facial complexion, pain in the abdomen and affecting the entire body, as well as a deep-lying and fine movement in the vessels. BCGM Dict I, 633 (where yang and yin are erroneously exchanged).

1019 *Shan* 疝, "elevation-illness," a group of conditions characterized by violent abdominal pain, in some cases associated with constipation and anuria. BCGM Dict I, 417.

1020 *Tan jue* 痰厥, "phlegm recession," a condition of recession cold affecting the four limbs, brought forth by an abundance of phlegm and closed-in qi. In severe cases this may include the pathological condition of black-out with loss of consciousness, and an inability to recognize things and persons. BCGM Dict I, 493.

1021 *Qi jue* , "qi recession," a condition of *zu jue* 卒厥, sudden fainting, caused by qi weakness or qi blockage. BCGM Dict I, 493.

1022 *Rou jing* 柔痙(= *chi* 痓), "soft spasms," a condition of *jing bing* 痙病, "spasms disease," with the special characteristic of feverish sweating without an aversion to cold. BCGM Dict I, 409.

1023 *Man jing* [*feng*] 慢驚[風], "slow fright [wind]," a condition of a *jing feng* 驚風, "fright wind," characterized by recurrent cramps in the presence or absence of fever. The cramps are slow and not very forceful. Bcgm Dict I, 334.

1024 *Jiao qi* 脚氣, "leg qi." Painful, weak, swollen legs. BCGM Dict I, 248.

1025 *Tou feng* 頭風, "head wind." Condition of wind evil attacking the head followed by pain, dizziness, itching. BCGM Dict I, 509.

1026 *Shen jue* 腎厥, "kidney recession," a condition of headache caused by kidney yang depletion. BCGM Dict I, 441.

1027 *Pi xie* 脾泄, "spleen outflow," a condition of *xie xie* 泄瀉, "outflow," caused by spleen qi depletion and weakness, manifesting itself as abdominal distension and formless stools accompanied by vomiting. BCGM Dict I, 375.

1028 *Yong ju* 癰疽, "obstruction-illness, impediment-illness." refers to two vaguely distinguished obstructions/impediments of vessels or other ducts inside the body. Qi rushing against the obstruction may cause a local swelling and eventually break through the surface to cause an abscess. BCGM Dict I, 642.

leaking, cold sores. Mix it with onion juice and insert it into the ears to cure deafness. [Li] Shizhen.

17-17-01
烏頭即附子母

Wu tou, *aconitum* [main tuber], i. e., the mother of *fu zi*, "attached children," *aconitum* [accessory tuber].

【主治】諸風，風痺，血痺，半身不遂，除寒冷，温養臟腑，去心下堅痞，感寒腹痛。元素。除寒濕，行經，散風邪，破諸積冷毒。李杲。補命門不足，肝風虛。好古。助陽退陰，功同附子而稍緩。時珍。

Control. All types of wind [intrusion]. Blockage related to wind [intrusion]. Blood blockage. Half the body does not follow one's will. It dispels cold. It warms and nourishes the long-term depots and short-term repositories. It removes hardness with obstacle-illness[1029] from below the heart. Abdominal pain related to an affection by cold. [Zhang] Yuansu. It dispels cold and moisture, activates menstruation and disperses wind evil. It breaks through all types of cold poison accumulation. Li Gao. It supplements insufficient [qi] in the Gate of Life and depletion with wind [intrusion] in the liver. [Wang] Haogu. It assists the yang and pushes back the yin. Its [therapeutic] potential is identical to that of *fu zi*, but somewhat slower. [Li] Shizhen.

【發明】【宗奭曰】補虛寒須用附子，風家即多用天雄，大略如此。其烏頭、烏喙、附子，則量其材而用之。【時珍曰】按王氏究原方云：附子性重滯，温脾逐寒。川烏頭性輕疏，温脾去風。若是寒疾即用附子，風疾即用川烏頭。一云：凡人中風，不可先用風藥及烏、附。若先用氣藥，後用烏、附乃宜也。又凡用烏、附藥，並宜冷服者，熱因寒用也。蓋陰寒在下，虛陽上浮。治之以寒，則陰氣益甚而病增；治之以熱，則拒格而不納。熱藥冷飲，下嗌之後，冷體既消，熱性便發，而病氣隨愈。不違其情而致大益，此反治之妙也。昔張仲景治寒疝内結，用蜜煎烏頭。近效方治喉痺，用蜜炙附子，含之嚥汁。朱丹溪治疝氣，用烏頭、巵子。並熱因寒用也。李東垣治馮翰林姪陰盛格陽傷寒，面赤目赤，煩渴引飲，脉來七八至，但按之則散。用薑附湯加人參，投半斤服之，得汗而愈。此則神聖之妙也。【吴綬曰】附子乃陰證要藥。凡傷寒傳變三陰，及中寒夾陰，雖身大熱而脉沉者，必用之。或厥冷腹痛，脉沉細，甚則唇青囊縮者，急須用之，有退陰回陽之力，起死回生之功。近世陰證傷寒，往往疑似，不敢用附子，直待陰極陽竭而用之，已遲矣。且夾陰傷寒，内外皆陰，陽氣頓衰。必須急用人參，健脉以益其原，佐以附子，温經散寒。捨此不用，將

1029 *Pi* 痞, "obstacle-illness," a condition of an uncomfortable distension and fullness in the chest and abdominal region. When pressed there is no pain. BCGM Dict I. 371.

何以救之？【劉完素曰】俗方治麻痺多用烏附，其氣暴能衝開道路，故氣愈麻。及藥氣盡而正氣行，則麻病愈矣。【張元素曰】附子以白朮爲佐，乃除寒濕之聖藥。濕藥宜少加之引經。又益火之原，以消陰翳，則便溺有節，烏、附是也。【虞摶曰】附子稟雄壯之質，有斬關奪將之氣。能引補氣藥行十二經，以追復散失之元陽；引補血藥入血分，以滋養不足之真陰；引發散藥開腠理，以驅逐在表之風寒；引温暖藥達下焦，以祛除在裏之冷濕。【震亨曰】氣虛熱甚者，宜少用附子，以行參、耆。肥人多濕，亦宜少加烏、附行經。仲景八味丸用爲少陰嚮導，後世因以附子爲補藥，誤矣。附子走而不守，取其健悍走下之性，以行地黄之滯，可致遠爾。烏頭、天雄皆氣壯形偉，可爲下部藥之佐。無人表其害人之禍，相習用爲治風之藥及補藥，殺人多矣。【王履曰】仲景八味丸，兼陰火不足者設。錢仲陽六味地黄丸爲陰虛者設。附子乃補陽之藥，非爲行滯也。【好古曰】烏、附非身凉而四肢厥者不可僭用。服附子以補火，必妨涸水。【時珍曰】烏、附毒藥，非危病不用，而補藥中少加引導，其功甚捷。有人纔服錢匕，即發燥不堪，而昔人補劑用爲常藥，豈古今運氣不同耶？荆府都昌王體瘦而冷，無他病。日以附子煎湯飲，兼嚼硫黄，如此數歲。蘄州衛張百户，平生服鹿茸、附子藥，至八十餘，康健倍常。宋張杲醫説載，趙知府耽酒色，每日煎乾薑熟附湯，吞硫黄金液丹百粒，乃能健啖，否則倦弱不支，壽至九十。他人服一粒即爲害。若此數人，皆其臟腑稟賦之偏，服之有益無害，不可以常理概論也。又瑣碎録言：滑臺風土極寒，民啖附子如啖芋、栗。此則地氣使然爾。

Explication. [Kou] Zongshi: To supplement a depletion with cold [qi] it is essential to use *fu zi* 附子, while for patients with wind [intrusion] one often resorts to *tian xiong* 天雄. This is their general [function]. The application of *wu tou* 烏頭, *wu hui* 烏喙 and *fu zi* 附子, though, should be in accordance with their respective specific [therapeutic] abilities. [Li] Shizhen: According to Wang shi's *Jiu yuan fang*, "the nature of *fu zi* is heavy and sluggish; it warms the spleen and dispels cold. The nature of *chuan wu tou* 川烏頭 is light and swift. It warms the spleen and dispels wind. If it is a cold illness, one resorts to *fu zi*; if it is a wind illness, one resorts to *chuan wu tou*. It is also stated: For all persons struck by wind it is not advisable to first use a wind medication and at the same *wu* [*tou*] and *fu* [*zi*]. *Wu* [*tou*] and *fu* [*zi*] are advisable for use only afterwards. Also, when *wu* [*tou*] and *fu* [*zi*] are used, they are to be ingested cold. This is a use of heat because of a condition of cold. The fact is, yin [qi] and cold are below; yang [qi availing themselves of a] depletion rise and float above. When this is cured with [medication of] cold [nature], the yin qi will be extremely boosted and the disease increases in severity. When this is cured with [medication of] hot [nature], there will be resistance [by the yang qi] and [the heat] cannot enter. When a medication of hot [nature] is ingested with a cold beverage, once it is swallowed its cold body dissolves and its hot nature effuses, and this serves to cure the disease. Not to violate the condition and to obtain a great benefit, this is the wondrous [effect] of a cure contrary to [what the nature of the disease might suggest]. Formerly when Zhang Zhongzheng cured cold elevation-illness[1030] with internal nodes, he resorted to *wu tou* boiled in honey. The *Jin xiao fang* [recommends to] cure throat blockage with *fu zi* roasted in honey. It is held in the mouth and the resulting juice is to be swallowed. When Zhu Danxi cures elevation-illness qi, he uses *wu tou* and *gardenia* fruit. They all use [medication of] hot [nature] because of the cold [nature of the disease]. Li Dongyuan cured the niece of Han lin scholar Feng. She suffered from harm caused by cold resulting in yin [qi] exuberance blocking yang [qi]. Her face was red, and her eyes were red, too. She had a vexing thirst and an urge to drink. The [movement in her] vessels arrived seven to eight times [in one breathing period]. It dispersed, when it was pressed. [Li Dongyuan] used the 'decoction with ginger and *fu* [*zi*]' and added ginseng [root]. He let her ingest half a *jin*, whereupon she sweated and was cured. This is one of the wondrous [effects] achieved by spirits and sages!" Wu Shou: *Fu zi* is an important pharmaceutical drug for yin signs [of illness]. Whenever a harm caused by cold has changed into [a harm affecting] the three yin [conduits], and in the case of being struck by cold aggravated by yin [qi], even though the body is very hot and the [movement in the] vessels is in the depth, [*fu zi*] must be used nevertheless. Or, in the case of ceasing [yang qi resulting in] cold with abdominal pain, when the [movement in the] vessels is in the depth and fine, culminating in greenish lips and a contracted scrotum, [*fu zi*] must be resorted to quickly as it has the power of pushing back the yin [qi] and of letting the yang [qi] return, and the potential of raising the dead, bringing them back to life. In recent times, confronted with yin signs of a harm caused by cold [physicians] often are unsure how to proceed. They do not dare to use *fu zi* [from the beginning], and resort to it only when the yin [qi] extremely abound and the yang [qi] are exhausted. But then it is too late. Furthermore, in the case of a harm caused by cold aggravated by yin [qi], when inner and outer [regions of the body] are all [dominated by] yin [qi], only yang [qi] are weak. In such a situation one must quickly resort to ginseng [root] to strengthen the [movement in the] vessels and boost the original [qi]. [The ginseng root] is to be combined with *fu zi* to assist it as it warms the conduits and disperses the cold. If this is neglected, how could it be possible to rescue [a patient]? Liu Wansu: Common recipes to cure numbness and blockage often use *wu* [*tou*] and *fu* [*zi*]. Their qi forcefully opens the pathways [of qi], and their qi will [initially] contribute to fur-

1030 *Shan* 疝, "elevation-illness," a group of conditions characterized by violent abdominal pain, in some cases associated with constipation and anuria. BCGM Dict I, 417.

ther numbness. Eventually, though, wenn the qi of the pharmaceutical drugs is exhausted, and the proper passage of qi is restored, the numbness disease will be healed. Zhang Yuansu: When *fu zi* is assisted by *atractylodes macrocephala* [rhizome] it is a sage-like pharmaceutical drug to dispel cold and moisture. A small amount of pharmaceutical drugs [dispelling] moisture are added as conduit guiding [substances]. Also, when the source of fire is boosted to dissolve yin screens, urination will be controlled again, and this is achieved with *wu* [*tou*] and *fu* [*zi*]. Yu Tuan: *Fu zi* is endowed with a natural disposition of heroic strength. It has the qi of a general who breaks through barriers and seizes the enemy. It is capable of guiding supplementing medication into the 12 conduits to restore dispersed and lost original yang [qi]. It leads blood medication into the blood section to nourish insufficient true qi. It leads effusing and dispersing medication to open the intersticial [skin] structures to dispel wind and cold situated in the body's outer region. It leads warming medication to reach the lower [section of the Triple] Burner to dispel cold moisture situated in the body's inner region. [Zhu] Zhenheng: [Patients] with qi depletion and extreme heat should use *fu zi* in small amounts to promote the movement of ginseng [root] and *astragalus* [root]. Fat persons with much moisture, they, too, should add a little *wu* [*tou*] or *fu* [*zi* to their medications] to lead them into the [appropriate] conduits. [Zhang] Zhongjing designed his "pills with eight substances"[1031] as guides directed toward the minor yin [conduits]. In later times it was believed that they included *fu zi* as a supplementing pharmaceutical drug. That was wrong. *Fu zi* runs and does not hold guard at one place. If one makes use of its nature to forcefully run downward to stimulate the movement of the otherwise sluggish Chinese foxglove [rhizome], this will let its [effect] reach very far. *Wu tou* 烏頭 and *tian xiong* 天雄 are both endowed with robust qi and an imposing physical appearance. They can serve to assist pharmaceutical drugs active in the lower [body] region. No one publicizes their ruinous ability to inflict suffering. In that they are customarily used as pharmaceutical drugs to cure wind [intrusion] and as supplementing medication, they have killed many people. [Wang] Lü: [Zhang] Zhongjing's "pills with eight substances" are designed for conditions of an insufficiency of yin fire. Qian Zhongyang's "pills with six substances including Chinese foxglove [rhizome]"[1032] are designed for conditions of yin [qi] depletion. *Fu zi* is a pharmaceutical drug supplementing yang [qi]; it is not something that stimulates the movement of otherwise

1031 *Ba wei wan* 八味丸, "pills with eight substances," have the following ingredients: Prepared Chinese foxglove rhizome, Asiatic cornelian cherry, Chinese yam, *poria*, *paeonia* root bark, *alisma* root, *cassia* bark, prepared *fu zi*.

1032 *Liu wei di huang wan* 六味地黃丸, "pills with six substances including Chinese foxglove rhizome," have the following ingredients: Prepared Chinese foxglove rhizome, Asiatic cornelian cherry, Chinese yam, *poria*, *paeonia* root bark, *alisma* root.

sluggish [substances]. [Wang] Haogu: *Wu* [*tou*] and *fu* [*zi*] must not be irresponsibly used [to cure patients] who do not have a cold body with ceasing [yang qi] in their four limbs. When *fu zi* is used to supplement fire, one must take care not to dry up the water. [Li] Shizhen: *Wu* [*tou*] and *fu* [*zi*] are poisonous pharmaceutical drugs. If a disease is not dangerous, they must not be used, and they are added in small amounts only as guides to supplementing medication. Their effects are very drastic. Some people after ingesting only as much as is held by a one *qian* spoon develop an unbearable restlessness. Still, the ancients resorted to it in supplementing preparations as an often used pharmaceutical drug. How can it be that the [human] disposition in antiquity differed from that of today? The Prince of Du chang in Jing fu had an emaciated body and was cold, but he had no other disease. Every day, for several years, he drank a decoction with boiled *fu zi* and chew sulphur at the same time. Company Commander Zhang in Qi zhou wei for his entire life ingested a stag's pilose antlers and *fu zi* medication; even when he was 80 years old he was still stronger than average. During the Song era, Zhang Gao in his *Yi shuo* recorded [the following case]. "Prefect Zhao indulged in wine and sex. Every day he [took] the 'decoction with dried ginger and heat processed *fu* [*zi*],' and swallowed one hundred kernels of the 'golden liquid elixir with sulphur.' As a result, his appetite remained strong. Without [these medications] he felt weak and could hardly stand upright. His long life lasted until he reached the 90s." Other people are damaged after eating only one kernel. When the many persons listed here with a one-sided disposition of their long-term depots and short-term repositories that enabled them to ingest [*fu zi*] with a personal benefit and without damage, then this must not be assumed to be normal. Also, the *Suo sui lu* states: "Hua tai is a windy and very cold place. The people eat *fu zi* as if they ate taro [tubers] or Chinese chestnuts." It is the qi of the ground there that allows them [such eating habits].

【附方】舊二十六，新八十七。

Added Recipes. 26 of old. 87 newly [recorded].

少陰傷寒。初得二三日，脉微細，但欲寐，小便色白者，麻黄附子甘草湯微發其汗。麻黄去節二兩，甘草炙二兩，附子炮去皮一枚，水七升，先煮麻黄去沫，納二味，煮取三升，分作三服，取微汗。張仲景傷寒論。

Harm caused by cold affecting the minor yin [conduits]. When during the first two or three days the [movement in the] vessels is weak and fine, and [patients] only wish to sleep and the color of their urine is white, stimulate a mild sweating with the "decoction with *ephedra* [herb], *fu zi* and *glycyrrhiza* [root]." [Prepare] two *liang* of *ephedra* [herb], with the nodes removed. Two *liang* of *glycyrrhiza* [root], roasted.

One *fu zi* [accessory tuber], roasted in a pan and the skin removed. First boil in seven *sheng* of water the *ephedra* [herb] and remove the foam. Then add the remaining two substances, and boil this down to three *sheng*. They are ingested divided into three portions to stimulate a mild sweating. Zhang Zhongjing, *Shang han lun*.

少陰發熱。少陰病始得，反發熱脉沉者，麻黄附子細辛湯發其汗。麻黄去節二兩，附子炮去皮一枚，細辛二兩，水一斗，先煮麻黄去沫，乃納二味，同煮三升，分三服。同上。

Effusion of heat related to [harm caused to] the minor yin [conduits]. When the minor yin [conduits] have just been affected by a disease and contrary to [what might be expected patients] effuse heat with a deep [movement in the] vessels, let them sweat with the "decoction with *ephedra* [herb], *fu zi* and *asarum heteropoides* [root]." [Prepare] two *liang* of *ephedra* [herb] with the nodes removed, one *fu zi* [accessory tuber], roasted in a pan and the skin removed, and two *liang* of *asarum heteropoides* [root]. First boil the *ephedra* [herb] in one *dou* of water and remove the foam. Then add the remaining two substances and boil all this down to three *sheng* to be ingested divided into three portions. [Source of this recipe] identical to the one above.

少陰下利。少陰病，下利清穀，裏寒外熱，手足厥逆，脉微欲絶，身反不惡寒，其人面赤色，或腹痛，或乾嘔，或咽痛，或利止脉不出者，通脉四逆湯。用大附子一個去皮生破八片，甘草炙二兩，乾薑三兩，水三升，煮一升，分温再服，其脉即出者愈。面赤加葱九莖，腹痛加芍藥二兩，嘔加生薑二兩，咽痛加桔梗一兩，利止脉不出，加人參二兩。同上。

Discharge with free-flux illness related to [harm caused to] the minor yin [conduits]. The "decoction to penetrate the vessels for [curing] the four countermovements" [serves to treat the following conditions]. Cold in the interior and heat in the outer [body regions]. Hands and feet with ceasing [yang qi and qi] counterflow. A [movement in the] vessels that is in the depth and threatens to be severed. Contrary to what might be expected the body has no aversion to cold. The face of that person is red. Some [patients] have abdominal pain, some have dry retching, some have throat pain, and in some the free-flow ends and the [movement in the] vessels cannot be determined. Break one large, fresh *fu zi* [accessory tuber], with its skin removed, into eight pieces and boil them together with three *liang* of roasted *glycyrrhiza* [root] and three *liang* of dried ginger in three *sheng* of water down to one *sheng* to be ingested warm divided into two portions. When the [movement in the] vessels appears again, this is the cure. If the [patient's] face is red, add nine onion stems. In the case of abdominal pain, add two *liang* of *paeonia* [root]. If he vomits add two *liang* of fresh ginger. When the free flow has ended and a [movement in the] vessels cannot be determined, add two *liang* of ginseng [root]. [Recipe] identical to the one above.

陰病惡寒。傷寒已發汗不解，反惡寒者，虛也，芍藥甘草附子湯補之。芍藥三兩，甘草炙三兩，附子炮去皮一枚，水五升，煮取一升五合，分服。同上。之。乾薑一兩，生附子一枚。去皮破作八片，水三升，煮取一升，頓服。傷寒論。

A yin disease with an aversion to cold. A harm caused by cold that has resulted in sweating but remains unresolved, with [patients] contrary to [what might be expected having] an aversion to cold, this is a depletion that is supplemented with the "decoction with *paeonia* [root], *glycyrrhiza* [root] and *fu zi*." Boil three *liang* of *paeonia* [root], three *liang* of roasted *glycyrrhiza* [root], and one *fu zi* [accessory tuber] roasted in a pan and with the skin removed, in five *sheng* of water down to one *sheng* and five *ge*, and [let the patient] ingest this divided [into several portions]. Source of the recipe] identical to the one above.

傷寒發躁。傷寒下後，又發其汗，晝日煩躁不得眠，夜而安静，不嘔不渴，無表證，脉沉微，身無大熱者，乾薑附子湯温陰盛格陽。傷寒陰盛格陽，其人必躁熱而不欲飲水，脉沉手足厥逆者，是此證也。霹靂散：用大附子一枚，燒存性，爲末，蜜水調服。逼散寒氣，然後熱氣上行而汗出，乃愈。孫兆口訣。

An effusion of restlessness related to harm caused by cold. When following a harm caused by cold episode [patients] continue to sweat, experience a vexing restlessness the entire day that does not let them sleep, while during the night they are calm and quiet, neither vomit nor have thirst, lack external [disease] signs, have a [movement in the] vessels that is in the depth and weak, and the body does not display great heat, the "decoction with dried ginger and *fu zi*" serves to warm [a condition of] abounding yin [qi] checking yang [qi]. In the case of abounding yin [qi] checking yang [qi] related to harm caused by cold, the signs of the disease are as follows. Patients are restless and hot, but do not wish to drink water. The [movement in their] vessels is in the depth and hands and feet experience ceasing [yang qi and qi] counterflow. The "thunderclap powder." [Grind] one large *fu zi* [accessory tuber], burned with its nature retained, and ingest [the resulting ashes] mixed with honey water. This forcefully disperses cold qi. Then heat qi rise and sweat is released. This is the cure. Sun Zhao, *Kou jue*.

熱病吐下及下利，身冷脉微，發躁不止者。附子炮一枚，去皮臍，分作八片，入鹽一錢，水一升，煎半升，温服，立效。經驗後方。

A heat disease with vomiting and discharge, and discharge with free flow. The body is cold and the [movement in the] vessels is weak, coupled with an endless effusion of restlessness. Roast one *fu zi* [accessory tuber] in a pan, remove the skin and the navel[1033] and divide it into eight pieces. Add one *qian* of salt, heat this in one *sheng* of water down to half a *sheng*, and ingest it warm. Immediately effective. *Jing yan hou fang*.

陰毒傷寒。孫兆口訣云：房後受寒，少腹疼痛，頭疼腰重，手足厥逆，脉息沉細，或作呃逆，並宜退陰散。用川烏頭、乾薑等分，切炒，放冷爲散。每服一錢，水一盞，鹽一撮，煎取半盞，温服，得汗解。

Yin poison related to harm caused by cold. Sun Zhao in his *Kou jue* states: For an affection by cold following sexual intercourse, pain in the lower abdomen, headache and a feeling of heaviness in the lower back, hands and feet with ceasing [yang qi and qi] counterflow, with the [movement in the] vessels in the depth and fine, and in some cases hiccup with [qi] counterflow, for all these conditions the "powder to push back yin [qi]" is suitable. Cut equal amounts of *chuan wu tou* and dried ginger into pieces and fry them. Wait until they have cooled and [grind them into] powder. Each time ingest one *qian*, boiled in one small cup of water with a pinch of salt down to half a cup. This is ingested warm. [The yin poison] is resolved when [the patient] sweats.

本事方玉女散：治陰毒心腹痛，厥逆惡候。川烏頭去皮臍，冷水浸七日，切晒，紙裹收之。遇有患者，取爲末，一錢入鹽八分，水一盞，煎八分服，壓下陰毒如猪血相似，再進一服。

The *Ben shi fang* [recommends] the "jade girl powder." It serves to cure yin poison with painful central region and abdomen, as well as ceasing [yang qi and qi] counterflow, such malign signs.[1034] Remove the skin and the navel[1035] of *chuan wu tou* and soak it in cold water for seven days. Cut it into pieces and dry them in the sun. Then store them wrapped in paper. Confronted with a patient, remove them [from the paper and grind them into] powder. To one *qian* add eight *fen* of salt and boil this in one cup of water down to 80%. This serves to suppress the yin poison and to discharge it resembling pig blood. Then ingest [the medication] a second time.

1033 *Qi* 臍, "navel," is the indentation at the top of the tuber where it was connected with the stem of the plant. "To remove skin and navel" has the meaning of "to clean thoroughly."

1034 *E hou* 惡候, "malign signs," identical to *e bing* 惡病, "malign disease," diseases with diverse illness signs and a bad prognosis. BCGM Dict I, 139, 140.

1035 *Qi* 臍, "navel," is the indentation at the top of the tuber where it was connected with the stem of the plant. "To remove skin and navel" has the meaning of "to clean thoroughly."

濟生回陽散：治陰毒傷寒，面青，四肢厥逆，腹痛身冷，一切冷氣。大附子三枚，炮裂去皮臍，爲末。每服三錢，薑汁半盞，冷酒半盞，調服。良久，臍下如火暖爲度。

The "powder to help life and bring back yang [qi]." It serves to cure yin poison related to harm caused by cold, with a greenish face and the four limbs experiencing ceasing [yang qi and qi] counterflow, abdominal pain and a cold body, as well as all types of cold qi. Roast three big *fu zi* [accessory tubers] in a pan until they crack open, remove their skin and the navel and [grind them into] powder. Each time ingest three *qian* mixed with half a bowl of ginger juice and half a bowl of cold wine until there is a feeling of fiery warmth below the navel.

續傳信方治陰毒傷寒，煩躁迷悶，急者用半兩重附子一個，生破作四片，生薑一大塊作三片，糯米一撮，以水一升，煎六合，温服，暖卧，或汗出，或不出。候心定，則以水解散之類解之，不得與冷水。如渴，更煎滓服。屢用多效。

The *Xu chuan fang* [recommends to] cure serious cases of yin poison related to harm caused by cold with vexing restlessness and perplexity with heart-pressure[1036] [as follows]. Break into four pieces one fresh *fu zi* [accessory tuber] weighing half a *liang* and boil them together with one large piece of fresh ginger, cut into three slices, and one pinch of glutinous rice in one *sheng* of water down to six *ge*. [Let the patient] ingest this warm and then lie down covered with a warm blanket. He may or may not sweat. Wait until his heart has calmed and then resolve [the yin poison] with a [medication] of the same type as the "powder to resolve [poison] to water." [Patients] must not be given cold water. When they are thirsty, boil the dregs again and [let the patient] ingest [the new decoction]. This [recipe] has been used often times and was often effective.

中風痰厥。昏不知人，口眼喎斜，并體虚之人患瘧疾寒多者，三生飲。用生川烏頭、生附子，並去皮臍各半兩，生南星一兩，生木香二錢五分。每服五錢，生薑十片，水二盞，煎一盞，温服。和劑局方。

Wind stroke with phlegm and ceasing [yang qi]. [Patients] are confused and do not know others, their mouth and eyes are slanted, and also for persons with bodily depletion who suffer from malaria with much [sensation] of cold, the "beverage with three fresh [substances]" [is suitable]. [Prepare a mixture of] half a *liang* each

1036 *Mi men* 迷悶, "perplexity with heart-pressure," an illness sign of slowed-down thinking accompanied by an uncomfortable feeling of vexation with heart-pressure. BCGM Dict I, 339.

of fresh *chuan wu tou* and fresh *fu zi*, both with their skin and the navel[1037] removed, one *liang* of fresh Indian turnip [root] and two *qian* and five *fen* of fresh *costus* [root]. Each time ingest five *qian*. Boil them with ten slices of fresh ginger in two bowls of water down to one bowl, and ingest it warm. *He ji ju fang*.

中風氣厥，痰壅，昏不知人，六脉沉伏。生附子去皮、生南星去皮各一兩，生木香半兩。每服四錢，薑九片，水二盞，煎七分，温服之。濟生方。

Wind stroke with qi recession and phlegm obstruction. [Patients] are confused and do not recognize others. The [movement in the] six vessels is in the depth and hidden. Remove the skin of one *liang* each of fresh *fu zi* and fresh *arisaema* [root and mix them] with half a *liang* of fresh *costus* [root]. Each time ingest four *qian*. Boil them with nine slices of ginger in two bowls of water down to 70% and ingest this warm. *Ji sheng fang*.

中風偏廢。羌活湯：用生附子一個，去皮臍，羌活、烏藥各一兩。每服四錢，生薑三片，水一盞，煎七分服。王氏簡易方。

Wind stroke with unilateral disablement. The "decoction with *notopterygium* [root]." Remove the skin and the navel of one fresh *fu zi* [accessory tuber and mix it] with one *liang* each of *notopterygium* [root] and *lindera* [root]. Each time ingest four *qian* boiled with three slices of fresh ginger in one bowl of water down to 70%. Wang shi, *Yi jian fang*.

半身不遂，遂令癖疰。用附子一兩，以無灰酒一升，浸一七日，隔日飲一合。延年秘録。

Half the body does not follow [one's will], eventually resulting in aggregation-illness attachment-illness.[1038] Soak one *liang* of *fu zi* in one *sheng* of ash-free wine for seven days and drink one *ge* every second day. *Yan nian mi lu*.

風病癱緩。手足嚲曳，口眼喎斜，語音蹇澀，步履不正，宜神驗烏龍丹主之。川烏頭去皮臍、五靈脂各五兩，爲末。入龍腦、麝香五分，滴水爲丸，如彈子大。每服一丸，先以生薑汁研化，暖酒調服，一日二服。至五七丸，便覺擡得手，移得步，十丸可以梳頭也。梅師方。

1037 *Qi* 臍, "navel," is the indentation at the top of the tuber where it was connected with the stem of the plant. "To remove skin and navel" has the meaning of "to clean thoroughly."

1038 *Pi zhu* 癖疰, "aggregation-illness attachment-illness," an erroneous writing of *leng pi zhu* 冷痹疰, cold blockage attachment-illness. Identical to *pian feng* 偏風, "unilateral wind." A condition of a unilateral loss of function and inability to move at one's will. Often an aftereffect of wind stroke. BCGM Dict I, 376.

Wind[-stroke] disease with paralysis, drooping hands and feet,[1039] mouth and eyes slanted, an impeded language and [patients] do not walk upright. This is controlled by the "black dragon elixir with divine effects." [Grind] five *liang* each of *chuan wu tou*, with its skin and the navel[1040] removed, and flying squirrel droppings into powder. Add five *fen* of borneol and musk, drip water [into this mixture] and form pills the size of a bullet. Each time [let the patient] ingest one pill. First grind [the pill] in fresh ginger juice until it has dissolved. Then ingest this mixed with warm wine. To be ingested twice on one day. When five to seven pills [are ingested, patients] notice that they can raise their hands and that they are able to walk. When ten pills [are ingested, patients] can comb the hair. *Mei shi fang*.

風寒濕痺。麻木不仁，或手足不遂。生川烏頭末，每以香白米煮粥一碗，入末四錢，慢熬得所，下薑汁一匙，蜜三大匙，空腹啜之。或入薏苡末二錢。左傳云：風淫末疾，謂四末也。脾主四肢，風淫客肝，則侵脾而四肢病也。此湯極有力，予每授人，良驗。許學士本事方。

Blockage related to wind [intrusion] and the presence of cold and moisture. With numbness and in some cases hands and feet not following [one's will]. Each time boil with fragrant, white rice one bowl of a gruel. Add four *qian* of fresh *chuan wu tou* powder to the gruel and simmer it over a slow fire to a paste. Add one spoon of ginger juice and three big spoons of honey and [let the patient] sip this. Or add two *qian* of Job's tears powder. The *Zuo zhuan* states: "When excessive wind causes an illness in the limbs, this is called [an 'illness of] the four limbs'." The spleen controls the four limbs. When excessive wind visits the liver, then it invades the spleen and the four limbs are affected by the disease. This decoction is extremely powerful. For all [such cases] I have given it to others, and it showed good effects. Xu xueshi, *Ben shi fang*.

體虛有風，外受寒濕，身如在空中。生附子、生天南星各二錢，生薑十片，水一盞半，慢火煎服。予曾病此，醫博士張子發授此方，二服愈。本事方。

Bodily depletion with wind [intrusion]. The body has received cold and moisture from outside and seems to exist in the air. Boil in one and a half cup of water over a slow fire two *qian* each of fresh *fu zi* and fresh Indian turnip [root] with ten pieces of fresh ginger and ingest this. I myself have had this disease and was given this

---

1039 *Shou zu duo ye* 手足亸/軃曳, "drooping hands and feet," an illness sign of feeble hands and feet that hang down and cannot be raised. BCGM Dict I, 463.

1040 *Qi* 臍, "navel," is the indentation at the top of the tuber where it was connected with the stem of the plant. "To remove skin and navel" has the meaning of "to clean thoroughly."

recipe by the physician Zhang Zifa. A cure is achieved after two ingestions. *Ben shi fang.*

口眼喎斜。生烏頭、青礬各等分，爲末。每用一字，嗃入鼻内，取涕吐涎，立效無比，名通關散。箧中秘寶方。

Slanted mouth and eyes. [Grind] equal amounts of fresh *wu tou* and greenish alum to powder. Each time ingest one *zi* by inhaling it into the nose. This causes snivel and lets one spit saliva. Immediately effective beyond comparison. [The recipe] is named "powder to open barriers." *Jia zhong mi bao fang.*

口卒噤瘖，卒忤停尸。並用附子末，吹入喉中，瘥。千金翼。

Sudden lockjaw and muteness. Sudden encounter with something hostile that lets one appear like a corpse. For both [these conditions] blow *fu zi* powder into the [patient's] throat and he is cured. *Qian jin yi.*

産後中風。身如角弓反張，口噤不語。川烏頭五兩，剉塊，黑大豆半升，同炒半黑，以酒三升，傾鍋内急攪，以絹濾取酒，微温，服一小盞取汗。若口不開，拗開灌之。未效，加烏雞糞一合炒，納酒中服，以瘥爲度。小品方。

Wind-stroke following delivery. The body is bent backward like a bow, with lock-jaw and an inability to speak. Fry together five *liang* of *chuan wu tou*, cut to pieces, and half a *sheng* of black soybeans until [the *chuan wu tou* is] half black and give them with three *sheng* of wine into a cauldron, stirring vigorously. Then strain this through tough silk to obtain the wine, slightly warm it and [let the woman] ingest a small cup to stimulate sweating. If her mouth fails to open, break it open and force-feed her. If this remains without effect, fry one *ge* of the droppings of black chicken, add it to the wine and [let her, or force her to,] ingest this. [Continue this] until a cure is achieved. *Xiao pin fang.*

諸風血風。烏荆丸：治諸風縱緩，言語蹇澁，遍身麻痛，皮膚瘙痒，及婦人血風，頭痛目眩。腸風臟毒，下血不止者，服之尤效。有痛風攣搐，頤頷不收者，服六七服即瘥也。川烏頭炮去皮臍一兩，荆芥穗二兩，爲末，醋麪糊丸梧子大。温酒或熟水，每服二十丸。和劑方。

All types of wind [intrusion] and blood wind.[1041] The "pills with black *schizonepeta* [spikes]." They serve to cure all types of wind [intrusion] with slackening, impeded language, numbness and/or pain of the entire body, and itching skin. Also, in the case of blood wind of women, headache and dim vision, intestinal wind and poison

1041 *Xue feng* 血風, "blood wind," a condition introduced in *Zhu bing yuan hou lun* ch. 15 as brought about by an intrusion of wind evil qi into an unbalanced state of qi and blood, mostly in women. BCGM Dict I, 594.

in the long-term depots, with unending discharge of blood, to ingest [these pills] is particularly effective. Those with painful wind [intrusion] causing cramps pulling on the cheeks and chin that cannot be contained, they ingest [the pills] six or seven times and are cured. [Grind] one *liang* of *chuan wu tou*, roasted in a pan and the skin and the navel[1042] removed, and two *liang* of *schizonepeta* spikes into powder, mix it with vinegar and wheat flour to a paste and form pills the size of *wu* seeds. Each time ingest with warm wine or with boiled water 20 pills. *He ji fang*.

婦人血風。虛冷，月候不勻，或手脚心煩熱，或頭面浮腫頑麻。用川烏頭一斤，清油四兩，鹽四兩，鐺内同熬，令裂，如桑椹色爲度，去皮臍，五靈脂四兩，爲末，擣勻，蒸餅丸如梧子大。空心温酒、鹽湯下二十丸。亦治丈夫風疾。梅師方。

Blood wind of women. Depletion cold, irregular menstruation. Sometimes with a vexing heat in the palms and soles. Sometimes with a surface swelling of head and face and stubborn hemp[-like] numbness. One *jin* of *chuan wu tou*, four *liang* of clear oil and four *liang* of salt are simmered together in a pot. Let it crack until it has assumed the color of mulberry. Then remove the skin and the navel and grind [the root] with four *liang* of flying squirrel droppings into powder. Stir it evenly and with steamed cakes form pills the size of *wu* seeds. [Let the woman] send down on an empty stomach with warm wine and a salt decoction 20 pills. This also serves to cure wind [intrusion] illnesses of husbands. *Mei shi fang*.

諸風癇疾。生川烏頭去皮二錢半，五靈脂半兩，爲末，猪心血丸梧子大。每薑湯化服一丸。

All types of epilepsy illness related to wind [intrusion]. [Grind] two and a half *qian* of fresh *chuan wu tou* and half a *liang* of flying squirrel droppings into powder, mix it with the blood from a pig's heart and form pills the size of *wu* seeds. Each time ingest one pill dissolved in ginger decoction.

小兒慢驚。搐搦，涎壅，厥逆。川烏頭生去皮臍一兩，全蠍十個去尾，分作三服，水一盞，薑七片，煎服。湯氏嬰孩寶鑑。

Chronic fright of children with convulsions, saliva obstruction[1043] and ceasing [qi] with [qi] counterflow. [Mix] one *liang* of fresh *chuan wu tou*, the skin and the na-

1042 *Qi* 臍, "navel," is the indentation at the top of the tuber where it was connected with the stem of the plant. "To remove skin and navel" has the meaning of "to clean thoroughly."

1043 *Xian yong* 涎壅, saliva obstruction," identical to *xian chao* 涎潮, "saliva upsurge." An illness sign of large quantities of phlegm present in the respiratory tracts evidenced by sounds produced during in- and exhalation. BCGM Dict I, 555.

vel[1044] removed, and ten complete scorpions, the tails removed, and ingest this divided into three portions, boiled with seven ginger slices in one cup of water. Tang shi, *Ying hai bao jian*.

小兒項軟。乃肝腎虛，風邪襲入。用附子去皮臍、天南星各二錢，爲末，薑汁調攤，貼天柱骨。内服瀉青丸。全幼心鑑。

Soft neck of children. This is a liver and kidney depletion invaded by wind evil. [Grind] two *qian* each of *fu zi*, with the skin and the navel removed, and Indian turnip [root] into powder. Mix it with ginger juice and apply it to the [child's] cervical vertebrae. For internal effects let it ingest the "pills to drain the greenish."[1045] *Quan you xin jian*.

小兒顖陷。綿烏頭、附子，並生去皮臍二錢，雄黄八分，爲末，葱根搗和作餅，貼陷處。全幼心鑑。

Sunken fontanel of a child. [Grind] two *qian* of soft *wu tou* and *fu zi*, all fresh with their skin and the navel removed, and eight *fen* of realgar into powder. Pound them with onion roots and with the mixture form cakes to be attached to the location of the sunken [fontanel]. *Quan you xin jian*.

麻痺疼痛。仙桃丸：治手足麻痺，或癱瘓疼痛，腰膝痺痛，或打撲傷損閃肭，痛不可忍。生川烏不去皮、五靈脂各四兩，威靈仙五兩，洗焙，爲末，酒糊丸梧子大。每服七丸至十丸，鹽湯下，忌茶。此藥常服，其效如神。普濟方。

Numbness and pain. The "pills [as effective as] an immortal's peach." They serve to cure numbness of hands and feet, or painful paralysis, with numbness and pain in the lower back and in the knees, or injuries and sprains caused by a blow or fall, with an unbearable pain. First dry over a fire in a pan four *liang* each of fresh *chuan wu* [*tou*], do not remove the skin, and flying squirrel droppings, and five *liang* of Chinese *clematis* [root. Then grind them into] powder. With wine and [wheat flour] make [the powder] to a paste and form pills the size of *wu* seeds. Each time ingest seven pills, up to ten pills, to be sent down with a salt decoction. [During this therapy] tea is to be avoided. When this medication if regularly ingested, its effects are divine. *Pu ji fang*.

1044 *Qi* 臍, "navel," is the indentation at the top of the tuber where it was connected with the stem of the plant. "To remove skin and navel" has the meaning of "to clean thoroughly."

1045 *Xie qing wan* 瀉青丸, "pills to drain the greenish," are made of the following ingredients: Chinese *angelica* root, borneol, *ligusticum* root, *gardenia* fruit, rhubarb root, *notopterygium* root, *saposhnikovia* root.

風痺肢痛，營衛不行。川烏頭炮，去皮，以大豆同炒至汗出爲度，去豆焙乾，全蠍半錢焙，爲末，釅醋熬稠，丸緑豆大。每温酒下七丸，日一服。聖惠方。

Blockage because of wind[-intrusion] and painful limbs, with camp and guardian qi no longer moving. Roast *chuan wu tou*,[1046] remove its skin and fry it together with soybeans until [the soybeans] begin to sweat. Then remove the beans, dry [the *chuan wu tou*] over a fire in a pan and [grind it] together with half a *qian*[1047] of complete scorpions, dried over a fire in a pan, into powder. Simmer it with a dense vinegar until it has reached a thick consistency and form pills the size of mung beans. Each time send down with warm wine seven pills. To be ingested once a day. *Sheng hui fang.*

腰脚冷痺，疼痛，有風。川烏頭三個，生，去皮臍，爲散，醋調塗帛上，貼之。須臾痛止。聖惠方。

Blockage in the lower back and legs with a sensation of cold, associated with pain and the presence of wind. [Grind] three *chuan wu tou* [tubers], fresh, with the skin and the navel[1048] removed, into powder. Mix it with vinegar, spread it on a piece of cloth and attach this to [the affected region]. After a short while the pain will end. *Sheng hui fang.*

大風諸痺，痰澼脹滿。大附子半兩者二枚，炮拆，酒漬之，春冬五日，夏秋三日，每服一合，以瘥爲度。聖惠方。

All types of blockage associated with massive wind.[1049] Phlegm flush[1050] and distension with [a feeling of] fullness. Roast half a *liang* of large *fu zi* [accessory tubers], break them [to pieces] and soak them in wine, in spring and winter for five days, in summer and autumn for three days. Each time ingest one *ge* until a cure is achieved. *Sheng hui fang.*

1046 *Sheng hui fang* ch. 19, *zhi feng bi zhu fang* 治風痺諸方, "all recipes to cure blockage related to wind," writes *chuang wu tou er liang* 川烏頭二兩, "two *liang* of *chuan wu tou.*"

1047 *Sheng hui fang* ch. 19, *zhi feng bi zhu fang* 治風痺諸方, "all recipes to cure blockage related to wind," writes *liang* 兩 instead of *qian* 錢.

1048 *Qi* 臍, "navel," is the indentation at the top of the tuber where it was connected with the stem of the plant. "To remove skin and navel" has the meaning of "to clean thoroughly."

1049 *Da feng* 大風, "massive wind," a chronic, infectious skin disease with insensitive skin, red macules, festering swelling, and, in severe cases, loss of eyebrows, harm to the eyes, and collapse of the patient's nose. Possibly including cases of leprosy. BCGM Dict I, 111.

1050 *Tan pi* 痰澼, "phlegm flush," a condition identical to *tan pi* 痰癖, "phlegm aggregation-illness." BCGM Dict I, 494.

脚氣腿腫，久不瘥者。黑附子一個，生，去皮臍，爲散，生薑汁調如膏，塗之。藥乾再塗，腫消爲度。簡要濟衆。

Leg qi with swollen legs, without cure for a long time. Remove the skin and the navel[1051] of one black *fu zi* [accessory tuber] and [grind it into] powder. Mix [the powder] with fresh ginger juice to obtain a paste and apply it [to the affected region]. When the medication has dried, apply it again and continue this until the swelling is dissolved. *Jian yao ji zhong*.

十指疼痛，麻木不仁。生附子去皮臍、木香各等分，生薑五片，水煎温服。王氏簡易方。

The ten fingers hurt; they are numb and do not feel anything. Boil equal amounts of fresh *fu zi*, with the skin and the navel removed, and *costus* [root] in water and ingest [the liquid] warm. Wang shi, *Jian yi fang*.

搜風順氣。烏附丸：用川烏頭二十個，香附子半斤，薑汁淹一宿，炒焙爲末，酒糊丸梧子大。每温酒下十丸。肌體肥壯有風疾者，宜常服之。瀹寮方。

To sweep away wind and normalize the [movement of] qi. The "pills with *wu* [*tou*] and *fu* [*zi*]." Soak 20 *chuan wu tou* [main tubers] and half a *jin* of fragrant *fu zi* [accessory tubers] in ginger juice for one night. Fry them, bake them over a small fire and [grind them into] powder. Then form [the powder] with wine and [wheat flour] to a paste and prepare pills the size of *wu* seeds. Each time send down with warm wine ten pills. Persons with fat and robust muscles and body suffering from a wind [intrusion] illness are advised to regularly ingest this. *Dan liao fang*.

頭風頭痛。外臺秘要用臘月烏頭一升，炒令黄，末之，以絹袋盛，浸三斗酒中，逐日温服。

Head wind[1052] and headache. The *Wai tai mi yao* [recommends to] fry one *sheng* of *wu tou* collected in the 12th month until it has turned yellow and grind it into powder. Fill [the powder] into a tough silk bag and soak it in three *dou* of wine. Drink [the liquid] warm every day.

孫兆口訣用附子炮、石膏煅等分，爲末，入腦、麝少許。每服半錢，茶、酒任下。

Sun Zhao in his *Kou jue* [recommends to] grind equal amonts of *fu zi*, roasted in a pan, and gypsum, calcined, into powder and add small amounts of camphora and

1051 *Qi* 臍, "navel," is the indentation at the top of the tuber where it was connected with the stem of the plant. "To remove skin and navel" has the meaning of "to clean thoroughly."

1052 *Tou feng* 頭風, "head wind." Condition of wind evil attacking the head followed by pain, dizziness, itching. BCGM Dict I, 509.

musk. Each time ingest half a *qian*, to be sent down with tea or wine, whichever is preferred.

修真秘旨用附子一個，生，去皮臍，綠豆一合，同入銚子内煮，豆熟爲度，去附子，食綠豆，立瘥。每個可煮五次，後爲末服之。

The *Xiu zhen mi zhi* [recommends to] boil in a kettle one fresh *fu zi* [accessory tuber], with the skin and the navel[1053] removed, and one *ge* of mung beans until the beans are done. Then discard the *fu zi* and eat the beans. This results in an immediate cure. Each [*fu zi* accessory tuber] can be boiled five times. Eventually it is [ground into] powder and ingested.

風毒頭痛。聖惠方治風毒攻注頭目，痛不可忍。大附子一枚，炮去皮，爲末。以生薑一兩，大黑豆一合，炒熟，同酒一盞，煎七分，調附末一錢，温服。

Wind poison[1054] with headache. The *Sheng hui fang* [recommends to] cure wind poison that attacked and flowed into the head and the eyes, with an unbearable pain, [as follows]. Roast one large *fu zi* [accessory tuber], remove the skin and [grind it into] powder. Boil one *liang* of fresh ginger with one *ge* of large soybeans, fried until done, in one cup of wine down to 70% and ingest it warm mixed with one *qian* of the *fu* [*zi*] powder.

又方：治二三十年頭風不愈者，用大川烏頭生，去皮四兩，天南星炮一兩，爲末。每服二錢，細茶三錢，薄荷七葉，鹽梅一個，水一盞，煎七分，臨卧温服。

Another recipe. It serves to cure head wind that has lasted for 20 or 30 years without healing. [Grind] four *liang* of fresh, large *chuan wu tou* [main tubers] and one *liang* of Indian turnip [root], roasted, into powder. Each time ingest two *qian*, to be boiled together with three *qian* of fine tea, seven leaves of mint and one salted plum in one cup of water down to 70%. To be ingested warm at bedtime.

朱氏集驗方治頭痛連睛者。生烏頭一錢，白芷四錢，爲末，茶服一字。仍以末嗃鼻。有人用之得效。

The *Zhu shi ji yan fang* [recommends to] cure headache involving the eyeballs [as follows]. [Grind] one *qian* of fresh *wu tou* and four *qian* of *angelica dahurica* [root]

1053 *Qi* 臍, "navel," is the indentation at the top of the tuber where it was connected with the stem of the plant. "To remove skin and navel" has the meaning of "to clean thoroughly."

1054 *Feng du* 風毒, "wind poison," a condition caused by *feng* 風, "wind," and *du* 毒, "poison," resulting in a pathogenic evil qi including the characteristics of both. BCGM Dict I, 160.

into powder and ingest with tea one *zi*. In addition, inhale the powder through the nose. Someone used this [recipe] with success.

風寒頭痛。十便良方治風寒客于頭中，清涕，項筋急硬，胸中寒痰，嘔吐清水。用大附子或大川烏頭二枚，去皮蒸過，川芎藭、生薑各一兩，焙研，以茶湯調服一錢。或剉片，每用五錢，水煎服。隔三四日一服。或加防風一兩。

Headache related to wind [intrusion] and the presence of cold. The *Shi bian liang fang* [recommends to] cure cases of wind and cold visitors present in the head, with clear snivel, tension and hardening of the sinews in the neck, cold phlegm in the chest and vomiting and spitting of clear water [as follows]. Remove the skin of either two large *fu zi* [accessory tubers] or two large *chuan wu tou* [main tubers] and steam them. Then bake them over a slow fire together with one *liang* each of *ligusticum* [root] and fresh ginger, and [grind them into] powder. Ingest one *qian* [of the powder] mixed with a tea decoction. Or, cut [the items] into slices and each time boil five *qian* in water and ingest [the liquid]. To be ingested once every fourth or fifth day. Some add one *liang* of *saphoshnikovia* [root].

三因方必效散：治風寒流注，偏正頭痛，年久不愈，最有神效。用大附子一個，生切四片，以薑汁一盞浸炙，再浸再炙，汁盡乃止，高良薑等分，爲末。每服一錢，臘茶清調下，忌熱物少時。

The *San yin fang*'s "powder with certain effects." It serves to cure with divine effects an influx of wind and cold, with unilateral or proper headache that has remained without healing for years. Soak one large, fresh *fu zi* [accessory tuber], cut into four pieces, in one cup of ginger juice and then fry [the pieces]. Soak them again and fry them again and continue this until all the juice is used up. Then [grind] them with an equal amount of lesser galangal [root] into powder. Each time ingest one *qian*, to be sent down mixed with clear *la* tea.[1055] [During this therapy] hot items are to be avoided for a short time.

頭風摩散。沐頭中風，多汗惡風，當先風一日則痛甚。用大附子一個炮、食鹽等分，爲末。以方寸匕摩顋上，令藥力行。或以油調稀亦可，一日三上。張仲景方。

Massage powder for head wind.[1056] A wind-stroke after one has washed the hair, with much sweating and an aversion to wind. When [the head was] exposed to

1055 *La* tea, *la cha* 臘茶, lit: "tea of the 12th month," mentioned by Ouyang Xiu and Shen Kua during the Song era. As it is colored like melted wax it is also called *la cha* 蠟茶, "wax tea."

1056 *Tou feng* 頭風, "head wind." Condition of wind evil attacking the head followed by pain, dizziness, itching. BCGM Dict I, 509.

wind first and then a day later a strong pain results. [Grind] one large *fu zi* [accessory tuber], roasted, and an equal amount of table salt into powder and massage the fontanel with as much as is held by a square *cun* spoon to stimulate a movement of the medication's strength. Or, mix it with a small amount of oil. To be applied three times a day. A recipe of Zhang Zhongjing.

年久頭痛。川烏頭、天南星等分，爲末。葱汁調塗太陽穴。經驗方。

Headache for years. [Grind] equal amounts of *chuan wu tou* and Indian turnip [root] into powder. Mix it with onion juice and apply it to the major yang [needle insertion] holes [at the temples]. *Jing yan fang.*

頭風斧劈難忍。川烏頭末燒烟熏盌内，温茶泡服之。集簡方。

Head wind with unbearable [pain] as if [the head] was cut in half with an ax. Burn *chuan wu tou* powder and let the smoke steam the inside of an [overturned] bowl. Macerate it in warm tea [in the bowl] and ingest it. *Ji jian fang.*

痰厥頭痛如破，厥氣上衝，痰塞胸膈。炮附子三分，釜墨四錢，冷水調服方寸匕，當吐即愈。忌猪肉、冷水。

Phlegm recession[1057] with a headache as if it had cracked open. Ceasing qi has rushed upward, with phlegm obstructing chest and diaphragm. Mix with cold water three *fen* of roasted *fu zi* and four *qian* of black ashes remaining in or at the bottom of a cauldron after burning herbs and ingest as much as is held by a square *cun* spoon. This will stimulate a vomiting, and this is the cure. [During this therapy] pork and cold water are to be avoided.

腎厥頭痛。指南方用大附子一個，炮熟去皮，生薑半兩，水一升半煎，分三服。

Kidney recession[1058] with headache. The *Zhi nan fang* [recommends to] roast one large *fu zi* [accessory tuber] until done, discard the skin and boil [the tuber] with half a *liang* of fresh ginger in one and a half *sheng* of water. Ingest it divided into three portions.

經驗良方韭根丸：治元陽虚，頭痛如破，眼睛如錐刺。大川烏頭去皮微炮，全蠍以糯米炒過去米，等分爲末，韭根汁丸緑豆大。每薄荷茶下十五丸，一日一服。

1057 *Tan jue* 痰厥, "phlegm recession," a condition of recession cold affecting the four limbs, brought forth by an abundnce of phlegm and closed-in qi. In severe cases this may include the pathological condition of black-out with loss of consciousness, and an inability to recognize things and persons. BCGM Dict I, 493.

1058 *Shen jue* 腎厥, "kidney recession," a condition of headache caused by kidney yang depletion. BCGM Dict I, 441.

The *Jing yan fang*'s "pills with the root of Chinese leek." It serves to cure a depletion of original yang [qi], with the head aching as if it had cracked open, and a feeling as if the eyeballs were pierced with an awl. Remove the skin of a large *chuan wu tou* [main tuber] and slightly roast it. Fry a complete scorpion with glutinous rice and discard the rice. [Grind] equal amounts [of the roasted tuber and the fried scorpion] into powder and form with leek root juice pills the size of mung beans. Each time send down with mint tea 15 pills; to be ingested once a day.

氣虛頭痛。氣虛上壅，偏正頭痛，不可忍者。大附子一枚，去皮臍，研末，葱汁麪糊丸緑豆大。每服十丸，茶清下。

Headache related to qi depletion. A qi depletion associated with an obstruction above causing unbearable unilateral or proper headache. Grind on large *fu zi* [accessory tuber], with the skin and the navel[1059] removed, into powder. Form it with onion juice and wheat flour to a paste and prepare pills the size of mung beans. Each time ingest ten pills, to be sent down with clear tea.

僧繼洪澹寮方蠍附丸：元氣虛頭痛，惟此方最合造化之妙。附子助陽扶虛，鍾乳補陽鎮墜，全蠍取其鑽透，葱涎取其通氣。湯使用椒以達下，鹽以引用，使虛氣下歸。對證用之，無不作效。大附子一枚剜心，入全蠍去毒三枚在内，以餘附末同鍾乳粉二錢半，白麪少許，水和作劑，包附煨熟，去皮研末，葱涎和丸梧子大。每椒鹽湯下五十丸。

The "pills with scorpions and *fu* [*zi*]" in Seng Jihong's *Dan liao fang*. For headache related to an original qi depletion only this recipe is the most wondrous in conformity with Creation. The *fu zi* serves to assist the yang [qi] and support them in a situation of depletion. Stalactites supplement yang [qi] and press down [what has arisen in counterflow. The application of] complete scorpions makes use of their ability to bore through [obstructions. The application of] onion sap makes use of its ability to open passages for the qi. The decoction utilizes Chinese pepper to reach the lower [body region], and salt to guide [the active substances to their preferred place of action]. All this serves to let qi, in a situation of depletion, return to where they belong. Used for the appropriate signs of illness, this is always effective. Take out the "heart" of one large *fu zi* [accessory tuber] and insert three complete scorpions, with their poison removed, into it. Mix the powder of the remains of the *fu* [*zi* "heart"] with two and a half *qian* of stalactite powder and a little white wheat flour and water to prepare [a paste] to wrap the *fu* [*zi* with the scorpions inside] and simmer it until done. Then remove the skin [of the simmered *fu zi*] and grind [the

1059 *Qi* 臍, "navel," is the indentation at the top of the tuber where it was connected with the stem of the plant. "To remove skin and navel" has the meaning of "to clean thoroughly."

rest] into powder to be formed with onion sap to pills the size of *wu* seeds. Each time send down with a Chinese pepper and salt decoction 50 pills.

腎氣上攻，頭項不能轉移，椒附丸。用大熟附子一枚，爲末。每用二錢，以椒二十粒，用白麫填滿椒口，水一盞半，薑七片，煎七分，去椒入鹽，空心點服。椒氣下達，以引逆氣歸經也。本事方。

Kidney qi rise to attack above, resulting in an inability to turn head and neck. The "pills with Chinese pepper and *fu* [*zi*]." [Grind] one large, heat prepared *fu zi* [accessory tuber] into powder. Each time boil two *qian* with 20 Chinese pepper kernels, their openings filled with white wheat flour, in one and a half cups of water together with seven slices of ginger down to 70%. Discard the pepper, add salt and ingest this in small portions on an empty stomach. The pepper qi reach downward leading the counterflow [kidney] qi to return to their appropriate conduits. *Ben shi fang.*

鼻淵腦泄。生附子末，葱涎和如泥，[盦-皿]涌泉穴。普濟方。

Nasal deep-source outflow, [that is,] brain outflow. Mix fresh *fu zi* powder with onion sap to a mud and apply it to the "gushing spring" [needle insertion] hole (KI-1). *Pu ji fang.*

耳鳴不止，無晝夜者。烏頭燒作灰、菖蒲等分，爲末，綿裹塞之，日再用，取效。楊氏産乳。

Unending sounds in the ears, with no difference day and night. Burn *wu tou* to ashes and grind them together with an equal amount of *acorus* [root] into powder. Wrap it in silk floss and insert it [into the ears]. To be applied twice per day until an effect shows. *Yang shi chan ru.*

耳卒聾閉。附子醋浸，削尖插之。或更於上灸二七壯。本草拾遺。

Sudden deafness and closure of the ears. Soak *fu zi* in vinegar, cut off a sharp point and insert it [into the affected ears]. Or in addition practice two times seven times cauterization on/above [the affected ears]. *Ben cao shi yi.*

聤耳膿血。生附子爲末，葱涕和，灌耳中。肘後方。

Festering ears releasing pus and blood. [Grind] fresh *fu zi* into powder, mix it with onion sap and fill it into the [affected ears]. *Zhou hou fang.*

喉痺腫塞。附子去皮，炮令拆，以蜜塗上，炙之令蜜入，含之勿嚥汁。已成者即膿出，未成者即消。本草拾遺。

Blocked throat stuffed with swelling. Remove the skin of *fu zi*, roast it until it breaks, apply honey [to the broken pieces] and fry them to let them absorb the honey. Then [let the patient] hold them in his mouth without swallowing the resulting juice. If pus has formed before, it will be released. If it has not yet formed, it will dissolve. *Ben cao shi yi.*

久患口瘡。生附子爲末，醋麪調貼足心，男左女右，日再換之。經驗後方。
Chronic suffering from mouth sores. [Grind] fresh *fu zi* into powder, mix it with vinegar and wheat flour and apply this to the soles of the feet, for males on the left, for females on the right. Replace it twice a day. *Jing yan hou fang.*

風蟲牙痛。普濟方用附子一兩燒灰、枯礬一分，爲末，揩之。
Toothache related to wind [intrusion] and bugs/worms. The *Pu ji fang* [recommends to] burn one *liang* of *fu zi* to ashes, mix them with one *fen* of dried alum to a powder and apply this to [the affected teeth].

又方：川烏頭、川附子生研，麪糊丸小豆大。每綿包一丸咬之。
Another recipe. Grind fresh *chuan wu tou* and fresh *chuan fu zi* [to powder] and form with a wheat flour paste pills the size of mung beans. Each time wrap one pill in silk floss and bite on it.

删繁方用炮附子末納孔中，乃止。
The *Shan fan fang* [recommends to] insert powder of roasted *fu zi* into the cavities. This ends [the toothache].

眼暴赤腫，磣痛不得開，淚出不止。削附子赤皮，末，如蠶砂大，着眦中，以定爲度。張文仲備急方。
Sudden redness and swelling of the eyes. They are painfully gritty and cannot be opened, with an unending tearflow. Cut the red bark of *fu zi* [into pieces and grind them into] powder, [with grains] similar to the size of silkworm feces. Insert it into the canthi and continue this until [the problem] is settled. Zhang Wenzhong, *Bei ji fang.*

一切冷氣。去風痰，定遍身疼痛，益元氣，强力，固精，益髓，令人少病。川烏頭一斤，用五升大瓷鉢子盛，以童子小便浸七日，逐日添令溢出，揀去壞者不用。餘以竹刀切作四片，新汲水淘七次，乃浸之，日日換水，日足，取焙，爲末，酒煮麪糊丸緑豆大。每服十丸，空心鹽湯下，少粥飯壓之。經驗方。
All types of cold qi. [This recipe serves to] eliminate wind phlegm[1060] and to end pain affecting the entire body. It boosts the original qi, gives strength, stabilizes

1060 *Feng tan* 風痰, "wind phlegm," are pathogenic qi resulting from a combination of *feng* 風, "wind," and *tan* 痰, "phlegm," with the latter being brought about by the former.

essence/sperm, boosts marrow and lets one only seldom fall ill. Fill one *jin* of *chuan wu tou* into a five *sheng* porcelain bowl and soak it in boys' urine for seven days. Day after day add [more urine] until it overflows. Pick out bad [tubers]; they are of no use. Cut the remaining [tubers] with a bamboo knife into four pieces and wash them with newly fetched water in a pan seven times. Then soak them and exchange the water every day. When the time is due remove [the tuber pieces], dry them over a fire in a pan and [grind them into] powder. Boil it in wine and with wheat flour form a paste to prepare pills the size of mung beans. Each time ingest ten pills, to be sent down with a salt decoction, and eat a little rice gruel to press them down. *Jing yan fang*.

升降諸氣。暖則宣流。熟附子一大個，分作二服，水二盞，煎一盞，入沉香汁温服。和劑局方。

To let all types of qi rise and descend. When they are warmed, they flow freely. Divide one large, heat processed *fu zi* [accessory tuber] to be ingested in two portions and boil them in two cups of water down to one cup. Add aloes wood juice and ingest this warm. *He ji ju fang*.

中寒昏困。薑附湯：治體虛中寒，昏不知人，及臍腹冷痛，霍亂轉筋，一切虛寒之病。生附子一兩去皮臍，乾薑炮一兩，每服三錢，水二鍾，煎一鍾，温服。和劑局方。

Being struck by cold, with clouding and dizziness. The "decoction with ginger and *fu* [*zi*]" serves to cure a body depletion struck by cold, with clouding and an inability to recognize other persons, also, cold and pain in the navel and abdominal region, cholera with contorted sinews, all these diseases of being struck by cold. Mix one *liang* of fresh *fu zi*, with the skin and the navel[1061] removed, and one *liang* of dried ginger, roasted, and each time ingest three *qian*. Boil [the mixture] in two *zhong* of water down to one *zhong*, and ingest this warm. *He ji ju fang*.

心腹冷痛。冷熱氣不和。山巵子、川烏頭等分，生研爲末，酒糊丸梧子大。每服十五丸，生薑湯下。小腸氣痛，加炒茴香，葱酒下二十丸。王氏博濟方。

Cold and pain in the central and abdominal region, with an imbalance of cold and hot qi. Grind equal amounts of fresh mountain *gardenia* [fruit] and fresh *chuan wu tou* into powder and form with wine [and wheat flour] a paste to prepare pills the size of *wu* seeds. Each time ingest 15 pills, to be sent down with a fresh ginger

---

BCGM Dict I, 169.

1061 *Qi* 臍, "navel," is the indentation at the top of the tuber where it was connected with the stem of the plant. "To remove skin and navel" has the meaning of "to clean thoroughly."

decoction. In the case of painful qi [disorder] in the lower abdomen, add stir-fried fennel and send down with an onion wine[1062] 20 pills. Wang shi *Bo ji fang*.

心痛疝氣。濕熱因寒鬱而發，用巵子降濕熱，烏頭破寒鬱，烏頭爲巵子所引，其性急速，不留胃中也。川烏頭、山巵子各一錢，爲末。順流水入薑汁一匙，調下。丹溪纂要。

Heart pain and elevation-illness qi.[1063] For an effusion of moisture and heat because of pent-up cold, use *gardenia* [fruit] to let the moisture and the heat descend, and *wu tou* to break open the pent-up cold. The *wu tou* is guided by the *gardenia* [fruit]. By its nature it acts very fast and does not remain in the stomach. [Grind] one *qian* each of *chuan wu tou* and mountain *gardenia* [fruit] into powder. Add one spoonful of ginger juice to properly flowing water and send [the powder] mixed [with the liquid] down. *Danxi zuan yao*.

寒厥心痛，及小腸膀胱痛不可止者。神砂一粒丹：用熟附子去皮、鬱金、橘紅各一兩，爲末，醋麪糊丸如酸棗大，朱砂爲衣。每服一丸，男子酒下，女人醋湯下。宣明方。

Cold with ceasing [yang qi] and heart pain, also an unbearable pain in the urinary bladder in the lower abdomen. The "elixir with one grain of divine sand." [Grind] one *liang* each of heat processed *fu zi*, turmeric and tangerine peels into powder and form with a paste made from vinegar and wheat flour pills the size of jujube kernels, coated with cinnabar. Each time ingest one pill, to be sent down by males with wine and by females with a vinegar decoction. *Xuan ming fang*.

寒疝腹痛繞臍，手足厥冷，白汗出，脉弦而緊，用大烏頭煎主之。大烏頭五枚，去臍，水三升，煮取一升，去滓，納蜜二升，煎令水氣盡。强人服七合，弱人服五合，不瘥，明日更服。張仲景金匱玉函方。

Abdominal pain surrounding the navel related to an elevation-illness with cold. Hands and feet are cold with ceasing [yang qi], white sweating,[1064] [the movement in the] vessels is string-like and firm. This is controlled by an application of boiled, large *wu tou* [main tubers]. Remove the navel[1065] of five large *wu tou* [main tubers] and boil them in three *sheng* of water down to one *sheng*. Discard the dregs. Add

1062 *Cong jiu* 葱酒, an alcoholic beverage made from husked rice, ginger and spring onions.

1063 *Shan* 疝, "elevation-illness," a group of conditions characterized by violent abdominal pain, in some cases associated with constipation and anuria. BCGM Dict I, 417.

1064 *Bai han* 白汗, "white sweat," appears in the BCGM three times. Here possibly a writing error of either *zi han* 自汗, "spontaneous sweating," BCGM Dict I, 46.

1065 *Qi* 臍, "navel," is the indentation at the top of the tuber where it was connected with the stem of the plant. "To remove skin and navel" has the meaning of "to clean thoroughly."

two *sheng* of honey and boil this until all the water has evaporated. Robust persons ingest seven *ge*; weak persons ingest five *ge*. If this does not result in a cure, ingest [the medication] the next day again. Zhang Zhongjing, *Jin kui yu han fang*.

寒疝身痛，腹痛，手足逆冷不仁，或身痛不能眠，用烏頭桂枝湯主之。烏頭一味，以蜜二斤，煎减半，入桂枝湯五合解之，得一升，初服二合，不知再服，又不知加至五合。其知者如醉狀，得吐爲中病也。金匱玉函。

Elevation-illness with cold and body pain and abdominal pain. Hands and feet are cold and without feeling because of [qi] counterflow, or the body aches and one cannot sleep. This is controlled by an application of the "decoction with *wu tou* and *cassia* twigs." Boil one *wu tou* [main tuber] in two *jin* of honey down to one half and dissolve this in five *ge* of *cassia* twig decoction. Take one *sheng* and at first ingest two *ge*. If this remains without effect, ingest [two *ge*] again. If there is still no effect, add the dose up to five *ge*. When eventually the patient appears to be drunk and vomits, this shows the disease is struck. *Jin kui yu han*.

寒疝引脇肋，心、腹皆痛，諸藥不效者。大烏頭五枚，去角四破，以白蜜一斤，煎令透，取焙爲末，别以熟蜜和丸梧子大。每服二十丸，冷鹽湯下，永除。崔氏方。

Elevation-illness with cold [and the pain] pulling on the flanks. The heart/central region and the abdomen all ache, and all types of medication have remained without an effect. Take five big *wu tou* [main tubers], remove their horns and break them into four pieces. Then boil them in one *jin* of honey until they are thoroughly penetrated, dry them over a fire in a pan and [grind them into] powder. Mix it with heat refined honey and form pills the size of *wu* seeds. Each time ingest 20 pills, to be sent down with a cold salt decoction. [The illness] will be eliminated forever. *Cui shi fang*.

寒疝滑泄，腹痛腸鳴，自汗厥逆。熟附子去皮臍、玄胡索炒各一兩，生木香半兩。每服四錢，水二盞，薑七片，煎七分，温服。濟生方。

Cold elevation-illness with a smooth outflow, abdominal pain and sounds in the intestines, spontaneous sweating and ceasing [yang qi with qi] counterflow. Prepare a mixture of one *liang* each of heat processed *fu zi*, with the skin and the navel[1066] removed, and *corydalis* [tuber], fried, and half a *liang* of fresh *costus* [root]. For each ingestion boil four *qian* [of this mixture] with seven slices of ginger in two cups of water down to 70% and ingest the warm [liquid]. *Ji sheng fang*.

1066 *Qi* 臍, "navel," is the indentation at the top of the tuber where it was connected with the stem of the plant. "To remove skin and navel" has the meaning of "to clean thoroughly."

小腸諸疝。倉卒散：治寒疝腹痛，小腸氣、膀胱氣、脾腎諸痛，攣急難忍，汗出厥逆。大附子炒，去皮臍一枚，山巵子炒焦四兩。每用三錢，水一盞，酒半盞，煎七分，入鹽一捻，温服。

All types of elevation-illness involving the small intestine. The "powder for urgent interventions."[1067] It serves to cure cold elevation-illness with abdominal pain, small intestinal qi [disorder], urinary bladder qi [disorder], all types of pain affecting spleen and kidneys, unbearable cramps and spasms, sweating with ceasing [yang qi and qi] counterflow. Prepare a mixture of one big *fu zi* [accessory tuber], fried and the skin and the navel[1068] removed, and four *liang* of mountain *gardenia* [fruit], fried until scorched. For each application boil three *qian* in one cup of water and half a cup of wine down to 70%. Add a pinch of salt and ingest this warm.

宣明方治陰疝小腹腫痛，加蒺藜子等分。虚者加桂枝等分，薑糊爲丸，酒服五十丸。虚寒腰痛。鹿茸去毛酥炙微黄、附子炮去皮臍各二兩，鹽花三分，爲末，棗肉和丸梧子大。每服三十丸，空心温酒下。

The *Xuan ming fang* [recommends to] cure elevation-illness in the yin [(i.e., genital) region] with abdominal swelling and pain by adding an equal amount of calthrop [fruits]. In the case of depletion, it adds an equal amount of *cassia* twigs. With ginger and [wheat flour] paste form pills, and ingest with wine 50 pills. In the case of depletion cold and lower back pain, [grind] two *liang* each of a stag's pilose antlers, with the hair removed and fried in butter until they have assumed a slight yellow color, and *fu zi*, roasted and the skin and the navel removed, and three *fen* of salt into powder. With the meat of Chinese dates form pills the size of *wu* seeds. Each time ingest 30 pills. To be sent down on an empty stomach with warm wine.

夷堅志云：時康祖大夫病心胸一漏，數竅流汁，已二十年。又苦腰痛，行則傴僂，形神憔悴，醫不能治。通判韓子温爲檢聖惠方，得此方令服。旬餘，腰痛減。久服遂瘥，心漏亦瘥。精力倍常，步履輕捷。此方本治腰而效乃如此。

The *Yijian zhi* states: Grand Master Shi Kangzu suffered from [liquids] leaking from his heart and chest. The juice flowed from several of his orifices, and that had already continued for 20 years. In addition he suffered from lower back pain. When he walked he was bent backward, his physical appearance was emaciated and his spirit was exhausted. Physicians were unable to cure him. Controller General Han Ziwen examined the *Sheng hui fang*. He found this recipe and let [the Grand

1067 No source is given here of the *cang cu powder* 倉卒散. It is quoted from *Su Shen liang fang*, ch. 8.

1068 *Qi* 臍, "navel," is the indentation at the top of the tuber where it was connected with the stem of the plant. "To remove skin and navel" has the meaning of "to clean thoroughly."

Master] ingest it. After about ten days, his lower back pain had decreased. After he had ingested it for a long time, he was cured [of the pain] and the heart leakage was cured, too. The strength of his essence/sperm was much better than normal, and his walking was light and easy. Originally this recipe was aimed at curing lower back [pain] but proved to have the effects documented here.

元臟傷冷。經驗方用附子炮，去皮臍，爲末，以水二盞，入藥二錢，鹽、葱、薑、棗同煎，取一盞，空心服。去積冷，暖下元，肥腸益氣，酒食無礙。

The original long-term depot (i. e., the kidneys) harmed by cold. The *Jing yan fang* [recommends to grind] roasted *fu zi*, with the skin and the navel[1069] removed, into powder, give two *qian* into two cups of water and boil it with salt, onions, ginger and Chinese dates down to one cup to be ingested on an empty stomach. This serves to remove the cold [qi] accumulation and warms the original [long-term depot (i. e., the kidneys)] in the lower [body region]. It makes the intestines fat and boosts the qi. Wine and food can be consumed without hesitation.

梅師方二虎丸：補元臟，進飲食，壯筋骨。用烏頭、附子各四兩，釅醋浸三宿，切作片子。掘一小坑，炭火燒赤，以醋三升，同藥傾入坑内，用盆合之。一宿取出，去沙土，入青鹽四兩，同炒赤黄色，爲末，醋打麪糊丸如梧子大。空心冷酒下十五丸。婦人亦宜。

The "pills with two tigers" of the *Mei shi fang*. They serve to supplement [qi in] the original long-term depot and strengthen sinews and bones. Soak four *liang* each of *wu tou* and *fu zi* in thick vinegar for three days and nights, and then cut them into pieces. Dig a small pit and heat it with a charcoal fire until it is hot. Pour the pharmaceutical drugs with three *sheng* of vinegar into the [hot] pit and cover it with a bowl. Take them out again after one night and remove sand and soil. Add four *liang* of halite/greenish salt and roast this together until [the tubers] have assumed a red-yellow color. Then [grind them into] powder. With vinegar and wheat flour make a paste and form pills the size of *wu* seeds. Send down with cold wine 15 pills on an empty stomach. This is also suitable for women.

胃冷有痰，脾弱嘔吐。生附子、半夏各二錢，薑十片，水二盞，煎七分，空心温服。一方：並炮熟，加木香五分。奇效良方。

Stomach cold with phlegm, with spleen weakness and vomiting. Boil two *qian* each of fresh *fu zi* and *pinellia* [root], together with ten ginger slices in two cups of water

1069 *Qi* 臍, "navel," is the indentation at the top of the tuber where it was connected with the stem of the plant. "To remove skin and navel" has the meaning of "to clean thoroughly."

down to 70% and ingest this warm on an empty stomach. Another recipe. Roast both [items] until done and add five *fen* of *costus* [root]. *Qi xiao liang fang.*

久冷反胃。經驗方用大附子一個，生薑一斤，剉細同煮，研如麪糊。每米飲化服一錢。

Long time cold with turned over stomach. The *Jing yan fang* [recommends to] cut one large *fu zi* [accessory tuber] and one *jin* fresh ginger into fine pieces and boil them together. Then grind them into [a paste] similar to wheat flour paste. Each time ingest one *qian* dissolved in a rice beverage.

衛生家寶方用薑汁打糊，和附子末爲丸，大黄爲衣。每温水服十丸。

The *Wei sheng bao fang* [recommends to] prepare ginger juice with [wheat flour] to a paste, add *fu zi* powder and form pills. Coat them with rhubarb root [powder]. Each time ingest with warm wine ten pills.

斗門方用長大附子一個，坐于磚上，四面着火漸逼，以生薑自然汁淬之。依前再逼再淬，約薑汁盡半盌乃止，研末。每服一錢，粟米飲下，不過三服瘥。或以猪腰子切片，炙熟蘸食。

The *Dou men fang* [recommends to] place one long, big *fu zi* [accessory tuber] on a brick and heat it on all four sides with a fire gradually closing in on it. Then extinguish the fire with the natural juice of fresh ginger, enclose [the tuber] with fire as before and extinguish it [with ginger juice] again. Continue this until one half a bowl of ginger juice is used up, and stop. Grind [the tuber] into powder. Each time ingest one *qian*, to be sent down with a millet beverage. A cure is achieved after no more than three ingestions. Or cut a pig's kidneys into pieces, roast them until done, dip them into [the powder] and eat them.

方便集用大附子一個，切下頭子，剜一竅，安丁香四十九個在内，仍合定，線紥，入砂銚内，以薑汁浸過，文火熬乾，爲末。每挑少許，置掌心舐喫，日十數次。忌毒物、生冷。

The *Fang bian ji* [recommends to] cut from one [accessory tuber] the tip, cut out a hole there and insert 49 cloves into it. Close the hole with a string and place [the tuber] into an eartherware kettle where it is soaked in ginger juice. Heat it with a mild fire until the liquid has dried, and [grind the residue] into powder. Each time pick a small amount up with a stick, apply it to the palm and lick it to consume it. Tens of times a day. [During this therapy] poisonous, fresh and cold items are to be avoided.

脾寒瘧疾。濟生方云：五臟氣虛，陰陽相勝，發爲痎瘧，寒多熱少，或但寒不熱，宜七棗湯主之。用附子一枚，炮七次，鹽湯浸七次，去皮臍，分作二服。水一盌，生薑七片，棗七枚，煎七分，露一宿。發日空心温服，未久再進一服。

Malaria illness related to spleen cold. The *Ji sheng fang* states: In the case of a qi depletion in the five long-term depots when yin and yang [qi] strive to mutually overcome each other, and when this effuses as malaria with much cold and little heat, or with cold only and no heat, the "decoction with seven Chinese dates" is appropriate to control this. Roast one *fu zi* [accessory tuber] seven times, soak it in a salt decoction seven times, discard its skin and the navel[1070] and ingest it divided into two portions. Boil them in one bowl of water with seven slices of fresh ginger and seven Chinese dates down to 70% and let this remain in the open for one night. On the day of an outbreak ingest it warm on an empty stomach, and ingest it again shortly afterwards.

王璆百一選方云：寒痰宜附子，風痰宜烏頭。若用烏頭，則寒多者火炮七次，熱多者湯泡七次，去皮焙乾，如上法用。烏頭性熱，炮多則熱散也。

Wang Qiu's *Bai yi xuan fang* states: For cold with phlegm, *fu zi* is suitable; for wind phlegm,[1071] *wu tou* is suitable. If one prefers to use *wu tou*, for [malaria cases with] much cold it is to be roasted on a fire seven times. For [malaria with] much heat steep it in hot water seven times. Then remove the skin, bake it over a fire in a pan until it is dry and use it as described above. *Wu tou* is by nature hot. When it is thoroughly roasted its heat will be dispersed.

又果附湯：用熟附子去皮、草果仁各二錢半，水一盞，薑七片，棗一枚，煎七分，發日早温服。

Also, the "decoction with red cardamom and *fu* [*zi*]." Boil two and a half *qian* each of heat processed *fu zi*, with the skin removed, and red cardamom kernels in one cup of water together with seven slices of ginger and one Chinese date down to 70%. Ingest this in the early morning of the day of an [expected] outbreak.

肘後方：臨發時，以醋和附子塗于背上。

The *Zhou hou fang* [recommends to] mix *fu zi* with vinegar and apply it to the [patient's] back shortly prior to an [expected] outbreak.

1070 *Qi* 臍, "navel," is the indentation at the top of the tuber where it was connected with the stem of the plant. "To remove skin and navel" has the meaning of "to clean thoroughly."

1071 *Feng tan* 風痰, "wind phlegm," are pathogenic qi resulting from a combination of *feng* 風, "wind," and *tan* 痰, "phlegm," with the latter being brought about by the former. BCGM Dict I, 169.

寒熱瘧疾。附子一枚重五錢者，麪煨，人參、丹砂各一錢，爲末，煉蜜丸梧子大。每服二十丸，未發前連進三服。中病則吐，或身體麻木。未中病，來日再服。龐安常傷寒論。

Malaria with alternating sensations of cold and heat. [Grind] one *fu zi* [accessory tuber] weighing five *qian*, coated with wheat flour and roasted, and one *qian* each of ginseng [root] and cinnabar into powder and form with heat refined honey pills the size of *wu* seeds. Each time ingest 20 pills three times in a row prior to an outbreak. When the disease is struck [the patient] vomits, in some cases with bodily numbness, without feeling. When [a first ingestion] failed to strike the disease, ingest [the pills] the next day again. Pang Anchang, *Shang han lun*.

瘴瘧寒熱。冷瘴，寒熱往來，頭痛身疼，嘔痰，或汗多引飲，或自利煩躁，宜薑附湯主之。大附子一枚，四破，每以一片，水一盞，生薑十片，煎七分，温服。李待制云：此方極妙。章傑云：嶺南以啞瘴爲危急，不過一二日而死。醫謂極熱感寒也，用生附子一味治之多愈。得非以熱攻熱而發散寒邪乎？真起死回生之藥也。嶺南衞生方。

Miasmatic malaria with alternating sensations of cold and heat. In the case of cold miasma, cold and heat sensations come and go alternately, with headache, bodily pain, and vomiting of phlegm, in some cases with profuse sweating and an urge to drink; in some cases with spontaneous free flow and vexing restlessness. The "decoction with ginger and *fu* [*zi*]" is suitable to control all this. Break one big *fu zi* [accessory tuber] into four pieces. Boil each piece together with ten slices of fresh ginger in one cup of water down to 70% and ingest this warm. Li Daizhi states: This recipe is extremely wondrous. Zhang Jie states: In Ling nan, miasma with muteness is considered a very serious issue, ending in death within one or two days. Physicians say that this is an extreme heat resulting from an affection with cold, and they resort to only one substance, fresh *fu zi*, to treat it and often achieve a cure. How could [such cures] be achieved if it were not [based on the approach] to attack heat with heat and this way disperse the cold evil? [*Fu zi*] is really a pharmaceutical drug that raises the dead and returns them to life. *Ling nan wei sheng fang*.

小便虚閉，兩尺脉沉微，用利小水藥不效者，乃虚寒也。附子一個炮，去皮臍，鹽水浸良久，澤瀉一兩。每服四錢，水一盞半，燈心七莖，煎服即愈。普濟方。

Blocked urination related to a depletion. When the [movement in the] vessels at the two "foot"/*chi* [locations at the wrists] is in the depth and weak, and when medications to free the flow of urine have had no effect, this is a case of depletion cold. Prepare for one ingestion one *fu zi* [accessory tuber], its skin and the navel[1072] removed and soaked in brine for a long time, and one *liang* of *alisma* [root], and boil four *qian* [of this mixture] in one and a half cups of water, with seven stems of common rush. To ingest this results in a cure. *Pu ji fang*.

腫疾喘滿。大人小兒男女腫因積得，既取積而腫再作，小便不利。若再用利藥性寒，而小便愈不通矣，醫者到此多束手。蓋中焦、下焦氣不升降，爲寒痞隔，故水凝而不通。惟服沉附湯，則小便自通，喘滿自愈。用生附子一個，去皮臍，切片，生薑十片，入沉香一錢，磨水同煎，食前冷飲。附子雖三五十枚亦無害。小兒每服三錢，水煎服。朱氏集驗方。

An illness of swelling with panting and a feeling of fullness. Adults, children, males and females have a swelling resulting from an accumulation. The accumulation may have been eliminated, but the swelling returns, and urination is blocked. If medication is used to free the flow of urine, its passage will be blocked even more. When physicians are confronted with such cases, they are mostly helpless. The fact is, when the qi of the central and the lower [sections of the Triple] Burner fail to rise and descend, this is because of a cold obstacle-illness[1073] barrier. As a result, the water congeals and fails to pass. The only [possible treatment is to let patients] ingest the "decoction with aloes wood and *fu* [*zi*]." It frees the passage of urine, and cures panting and feelings of fullness. Boil one fresh *fu zi* [accessory tuber], with the skin and the navel[1074] removed and cut into pieces, together with ten slices of ginger in water in which one *qian* of aloes wood was rubbed and ingest it cold before a meal. Even if altogether 30 or 50 *fu zi* [accessory tubers are ingested], no harm is to be expected. Children each time ingest three *qian*. Boil them in water and ingest [the liquid]. *Zhu shi ji yan fang*.

脾虛濕腫。大附子五枚，去皮四破，以赤小豆半升，藏附子于中，慢火煮熟，去豆，焙研末，以薏苡仁粉打糊丸梧子大。每服十丸，蘿蔔湯下。朱氏集驗方。

Swelling with moisture related to a spleen depletion. Enclose five big *fu zi* [accessory tubers], with the skin removed and broken into four pieces, with red mung beans and heat them over a slow fire until they are done. Remove the beans, dry [the tubers] over a fire in a pan and grind them into powder. With Job's tears [seed]

1072 *Qi* 臍, "navel," is the indentation at the top of the tuber where it was connected with the stem of the plant. "To remove skin and navel" has the meaning of "to clean thoroughly."

1073 *Pi* 痞, "obstacle-illness," a condition of an uncomfortable distension and fullness in the chest and abdominal region. When pressed there is no pain. BCGM Dict I. 371.

1074 *Qi* 臍, "navel," is the indentation at the top of the tuber where it was connected with the stem of the plant. "To remove skin and navel" has the meaning of "to clean thoroughly."

powder and [wheat flour] prepare a paste and form pills the size of *wu* seeds. Each time ingest 10 pills, to be sent down with a radish decoction. *Zhu shi ji yan fang.*

陰水腫滿。烏頭一升，桑白皮五升，水五升，煮一升，去滓，銅器盛之，重湯煎至可丸，丸小豆大。每服三五丸，取小便利爲佳。忌油膩、酒、麪、魚肉。

Swelling related to water and a feeling of fullness in the yin [region]. Boil one *sheng* of *wu tou* with five *sheng* of white mulberry tree bark in five *sheng* of water down to one *sheng*, remove the dregs and fill [the liquid] into a copper vessel. Then heat it in a water bath until [it has assumed a consistency] permitting it to form pills. The pills are of the size of mung beans. Each time ingest three to five pills until their excellent effect is shown in a free flow of urine. [During this therapy] oil and fat items, wine, wheat flour, fish and meat are to be avoided.

又方：大附子童便浸三日夜，逐日換尿，以布擦去皮，搗如泥，酒糊和丸小豆大。每服三十丸，煎流氣飲送下。普濟方。

Another recipe. Soak one large *fu zi* [accessory tuber] in boys' urine for three days and nights, with the urine exchanged every day. Rub it with a piece of cloth to remove the skin, pound it to a pulp and with wine and [wheat flour] prepare a paste to form pills the size of mung beans. Each time ingest 30 pills, to be sent down with the boiled "beverage to let the qi flow."[1075] *Pu ji fang.*

大腸冷秘。附子一枚炮，去皮，取中心如棗大，爲末二錢，蜜水空心服之。聖濟總録。

Blocked large intestine related to a presence of cold. Roast one *fu zi* [accessory tuber] and remove the skin. Then take out of its center a piece as big as a Chinese date and [grind it to obtain] a powder. Ingest two *qian* [of the powder] with honey water on an empty stomach. *Sheng ji zong lu.*

老人虛泄不禁。熟附子一兩，赤石脂一兩，爲末，醋糊丸梧子大。米飲下五十丸，楊氏家藏方。

Depletion of old persons with an unstoppable outflow. [Grind] one *liang* of heat processed *fu zi* and one *liang* of red halloysite into powder, make a paste with vinegar [and wheat flour] to form pills the size of *wu* seeds, and send down with a rice beverage 50 pills. *Yang shi jia cang fang.*

1075 *Liu qi yin* 流氣飲 is prepared by boiling the following ingredients. Rhubarb root, *ligusticum* root, *chrysanthemum* flowers, great burdock seeds, *asarum heteropoides* root, *saphoshnikovia* root, *gardenia* fruit, white calthrop fruit, *scutellaria* root, *glycyrrhiza* root, *scrophularia* root, simpleleaf chastetree seeds, *schizonepeta* herb, winter horsetail herb, *atractylodes lancea* rhizome, fetid *cassia* seeds.

冷氣洞泄。生川烏頭一兩，木香半兩，爲末，醋糊丸梧子大。每陳皮湯下二十丸。本事方。

Outflow related to cold qi. [Grind] one *liang* of fresh *chuan wu tou* and half a *liang* of *costus* [root] into powder, make a paste with vinegar [and wheat flour] and form pills the size of *wu* seeds. Each time send down with a tangerine peel decoction 20 pills. *Ben shi fang.*

臟寒脾泄，及老人中氣不足，久泄不止。肉豆蔻二兩煨熟，大附子去皮臍一兩五錢，爲末，粥丸梧子大。每服八十丸，蓮肉煎湯下。

Spleen outflow related to a presence of cold in the long-term depots, and also insufficient central qi of old persons related to an unstoppable, long-lasting outflow. [Grind] two *liang* of nutmeg, slowly roasted until done, and one *liang* five *qian* of big *fu zi* [accessory tubers] with their skin and the navel[1076] removed into powder and form with a rice gruel pills the size of *wu* seeds. Each time ingest 80 pills, to be sent down with a decoction of Indian lotus seed germs.

十便良方治脾胃虛冷，大腸滑泄，米穀不化，乏力。用大附子十兩連皮，同大棗二升，於石器內以水煮一日，常令水過兩指。取出，每個切作三片，再同煮半日，削去皮，切焙爲末。别以棗肉和丸梧子大。每空心米飲服三四十丸。

The *Shi bian liang fang* [recommends to] cure depletion of spleen and stomach with the presence of cold, slippery outflow from the large intestine, a failure to digest rice and grain, and a lack of strength [as follows]. Give ten *liang* of big *fu zi* [accessory tubers], with their skin retained, together with two *sheng* of large Chinese dates into a stone vessel and boil them with water for one day. The water level should always exceed [the pharmaceutical drugs] by two fingers. Then take them out and cut each of them into three pieces. Again boil them together, this time for half a day. Cut off their skin, cut them [into small pieces], dry them over a fire in a pan and [grind them into] powder. With the meat of Chinese dates form them to pills the size of *wu* seeds. Each time ingest on an empty stomach with a rice beverage 30 to 40 pills.

小兒吐泄，注下，小便少。白龍丸：用熟附子五錢，白石脂煅、龍骨煅各二錢半，爲末，醋麪糊丸黍米大。每米飲，量兒大小服。全幼心鑑。

Vomiting and outflow of children; an outpour discharge with only a little urination. The "white dragon pills." [Grind] five *qian* of heat processed *fu zi* and two and a half *qian* each of calcined white halloysite and calcined dragon bones into powder and form with a vinegar and wheat flour paste pills the size of glutinous millet. Each

1076 *Qi* 臍, "navel," is the indentation at the top of the tuber where it was connected with the stem of the plant. "To remove skin and navel" has the meaning of "to clean thoroughly."

time let the child ingest with a rice beverage [a quantity of pills] corresponding to its age. *Quan you xin jian.*

霍亂吐泄不止。附子重七錢者，炮去皮臍，爲末。每服四錢，水二盞，鹽半錢，煎一盞，温服，立止。孫兆秘寶方。

Cholera with unending vomiting and outflow. Roast a *fu zi* [accessory tuber] weighing seven *qian*, remove its skin and the navel and [grind it into] powder. Each time ingest four *qian*, boiled in two cups of water with half a *qian* of salt down to one cup. To be ingested warm. [The disease] is stopped immediately. Sun Zhao, *Mi bao fang.*

水泄久痢。川烏頭二枚，一生用，一以黑豆半合同煮熟，研，丸緑豆大。每服五丸，黄連湯下。普濟方。

Watery outflow and long-lasting free-flux illness. Grind two *chuan wu tou* [main tubers], one to be applied fresh, the other one boiled with half a *ge* of soybeans until done, [to powder] and form pills the size of mung beans. Each time ingest five pills, to be sent down with a *coptis* [rhizome] decoction. *Pu ji fang.*

久痢赤白。獨聖丸：用川烏頭一個，灰火燒烟盡，取出地上，盞蓋良久，研末，酒化蠟丸如大麻子大，每服三丸。赤痢，黄連、甘草、黑豆煎湯，放冷吞下。白痢，甘草、黑豆煎湯，冷吞。如瀉及肚痛，以水吞下。並空心服之。忌熱物。經驗方。

Long-lasting free-flux illness with red and white [discharge]. The "single sage pills." Heat one *chuan wu tou* [main tuber] in fiery ashes until no more smoke emerges. Then take it out [of the ashes], place it on the ground and cover it with a cup for an extended period of time. Eventually grind it into powder and with beeswax dissolved in wine form pills the size of hemp seeds. Each time ingest three pills. In the case of a free-flux illness with a red [discharge] swallow them sent down with a decoction, left to cool, of *coptis* [rhizome], *glycyrrhiza* [root] and soybeans. In the case of a free-flux illness with a white [discharge] swallow them with a cold decoction of *glycyrrhiza* [root] and soybeans. If the outflow is accompanied by stomach pain, swallow them with water. In all cases ingest [the pills] on an empty stomach. [During this therapy] hot items are to be avoided. *Jing yan fang.*

久痢休息。熟附子半兩，研末，雞子白二枚，擣和丸梧子大。傾入沸湯，煮數沸，漉出，作兩服，米飲下。聖濟總録。

Long-lasting free-flux illness with periods of remission. Grind half a *liang* of heat processed *fu zi* into powder, pound it with the egg white of two chicken eggs and form pills the size of *wu* seeds. Pour them into bubbling hot water and heat it several times to bubbling. Then pass the liquid through a filter to obtain the pills again and ingest them in two portions, to be sent down with a rice beverage. *Sheng ji zong lu.*

下痢欬逆，脉沈陰寒者，退陰散主之。陳自明云：一人病此不止，服此兩服而愈。方見前陰毒傷寒下。

Discharge with a free-flux illness, and cough with [qi] counterflow. The [movement in the] vessels is in the depth, and there is a presence of cold in the yin [region]. The "powder to push back yin [qi]" controls this. Chen Ziming states: "A person had this disease and it could not be stopped. He ingested two portions of this [powder] and was cured." For the recipe see above under under "yin poison with harm caused by cold."[1077]

下血虛寒：日久腸冷者。熟附子一兩去皮、枯白礬一兩，爲末。每服三錢，米飲下。

Discharge with blood, with a depletion and the presence of cold. When the intestines have been cold for days. [Grind] one *liang* of heat processed *fu zi*, with the skin removed, and one *liang* of processed alum into powder. Each time ingest three *qian*, to be sent down with a rice beverage.

又方：熟附子一枚去皮，生薑三錢半，水煎服。或加黑豆一百粒。並聖惠方。

Another recipe. Boil in water one heat processed *fu zi* [accessory tuber] and three and a half *qian* of fresh ginger, and ingest [the liquid]. Some add one hundred black soybeans. Both [recipes quoted from the] *Sheng hui fang.*

陽虛吐血。生地黄一斤，擣汁，入酒少許，以熟附子一兩半，去皮臍，切片入汁内，石器煮成膏。取附片焙乾，入山藥三兩，研末，以膏和擣丸梧子大。每空心米飲下三十丸。昔葛察判妻苦此疾，百藥皆試，得此而愈，屢發屢效。余居士選奇方。

Yang [qi] depletion with vomiting of blood. Pound one *jin* of fresh Chinese foxglove [rhizome] to obtain a juice, add a little wine. Then remove the skin and the navel[1078] from one and a half *liang* of heat processed *fu zi*, cut them into small pieces and give them into the [Chinese foxglove rhizome] juice. Heat it in a stone vessel to generate a paste. Remove the *fu* [*zi*] pieces, dry them over a fire in a pan, add three *liang* of Chinese yam and grind this into powder. This is pounded mixed with the paste to form pills the size of *wu* seeds. [Patients] send down on an empty stom-

1077 For the *tui yin san* 退陰散, "powder to push back yin [qi]," see above, p. 713.

1078 *Qi* 臍, "navel," is the indentation at the top of the tuber where it was connected with the stem of the plant. "To remove skin and navel" has the meaning of "to clean thoroughly."

ach with a rice beverage 30 pills. Formerly, the wife of Judge Ge suffered from this illness. Hundreds of pharmaceutical drugs were tested, but only after she took this [recipe] she was cured. It was used often and was often effective. Yu Jushi, *Xuan qi fang*.

溲數白濁。熟附子爲末，每服二錢，薑三片，水一盞，煎六分，温服。普濟方。

Frequent white and turbid urination. [Grind] heat processed *fu zi* into powder. Each time ingest two *qian*. Boil them with three slices of ginger in one cup of water down to 60%. To be ingested warm. *Pu ji fang*.

虛火背熱。虛火上行，背内熱如火炙者。附子末，津調，塗涌泉穴。摘玄方。

Depletion fire with a hot back. When a fire resulting from a [yin qi] depletion moves upward and there is heat in the back as if it were roasted by fire. Mix *fu zi* powder with [the patient's saliva] body fluid and apply this to the "gushing spring" [needle insertion] hole (KI-1). *Zhai xuan fang*.

經水不調，血臟冷痛，此方平易捷徑。熟附子去皮、當歸等分。每服三錢，水煎服。普濟方。

Irregular menstruation. Painful presence of cold in the blood long-term depot (i. e., the uterus). This recipe offers an easy shortcut [to a cure. Prepare a mixture of] equal amounts of heat processed *fu zi*, with the skin removed, and Chinese *angelica* [root] and each time ingest three *qian*. Boil it in water and ingest [the decoction]. *Pu ji fang*.

斷産下胎。生附子爲末，淳酒和塗右足心，胎下去之。小品方。

To initiate an abortion. [Grind] fresh *fu zi* into powder, mix it with pure wine[1079] and apply it to the sole of the right foot. Remove it again after the fetus is discharged. *Xiao pin fang*.

折腕損傷。卓氏膏：用大附子四枚，生切，以猪脂一斤，三年苦醋同漬三宿，取脂煎三上三下，日摩傅之。深師方。

Broken wrists, harm caused by an injury. "Mr. Zhuo's ointment." Cut four fresh big *fu zi* [accessory tubers] to pieces and soak them for three days and nights with one *jin* of lard in vinegar stored for three years. Remove the lard and boil the liquid three times until bubbling and let it cool three times. Then apply it by massaging [the affected region] every day. *Shen shi fang*.

1079 The *Wai tai mi yao* ch. 34, *fu ren yu duan chan fang* 婦人欲斷產方, "recipes for women intending to initiate an abortion," writes *ku jiu* 苦酒, "bitter wine."

癰疽腫毒。川烏頭炒、黄蘗炒各一兩，爲末，唾調塗之，留頭，乾則以米泔潤之。同上。

Swelling with poison related to an obstruction-illness or impediment-illness.[1080] [Grind] one *liang* each of fried *chuan wu tou* and fried *phellodendron* bark into powder, mix it with human saliva and apply this [to the affected region]. Leave it on the tip [of the swelling] until it dries. Then moisten it again with water in which rice has been washed. [Source of this recipe] identical to the one above.

癰疽久漏。瘡口冷，膿水不絶，内無惡肉。大附子以水浸透，切作大片，厚三分，安瘡口上，以艾灸之。隔數日一灸，灸至五七次。仍服内托藥，自然肌肉長滿。研末作餅子，亦可。薛己外科心法。

Obstruction-illness and impediment-illness with long-lasting leaking. The opening of the sores is cold, with an uninterrupted [flow of] pus and water, but no malign flesh [growth] inside. Soak one big *fu zi* [accessory tuber] in water until it is entirely penetrated [by the water] and cut it into large slices, three *fen* thick. Place them on the opening of the sores and cauterize them with common mugwort. Perform this once a day, every few days. Perform the cauterization up to five or seven times. In addition, ingest medication to internally drive out [evil matter]. The muscles and the flesh will grow as a result. It is also possible to grind [the substance] into powder and prepare a cake. Xue Ji, *Wai ke xin fa*.

癰疽弩肉，如眼不歛，諸藥不治，此法極妙。附子削如棋子大，以唾粘貼上，用艾火灸之。附子焦，復唾濕再灸，令熱氣徹内，即瘥。千金方。

Obstruction-illness and impediment-illness with tumorous flesh growth protruding similar to an eye. It cannot be retracted and all medication applied fails to cure this. This method is extremely wondrous. Cut a *fu zi* [accessory tuber] in pieces the size of chess pieces and apply them with saliva to [the affected region]. Then cauterize them with a common mugwort [leaf] fire. When the *fu zi* is scorched, apply more saliva to moisten it again and cauterize it again. This way hot qi are led to penetrate the interior, and this results in a cure. *Qian jin fang*.

癰疽肉突。烏頭五枚，濃醋三升，漬三日，洗之，日夜三四度。古今録驗。

Obstruction-illness and impediment-illness with a flesh protrusion. Soak five *wu tou* [main tubers] in three *sheng* of viscous vinegar for three days. Wash [the affected region] with [the liquid] three or four times day and night. *Gu jin lu yan*.

1080 *Yong ju* 癰疽, "obstruction-illness, impediment-illness." refers to two vaguely distinguished obstructions/impediments of vessels or other ducts inside the body. Qi rushing against the obstruction may cause a local swelling and eventually break through the surface to cause an abscess. BCGM Dict I, 642.

丁瘡腫痛。醋和附子末塗之。乾再上。千金翼。

Pin[-illness][1081] sores with painful swelling. Mix *fu zi* powder with vinegar and apply this [to the affected region]. When it has dried, apply it again. *Qian jin yi.*

久生疥癬。川烏頭生切，以水煎洗，甚驗。聖惠方。

Long-lasting *jie*-illness[1082] and *xuan*-illness.[1083] Cut fresh *chuan wu tou* [into pieces], boil them in water and [with the liquid] wash [the affected region]. Very effective. *Sheng hui fang.*

手足凍裂。附子去皮爲末，以水、麪調塗之，良。談埜翁試驗方。

[Skin] cracks of hands and feet because of frost. [Grind] *fu zi*, with the skin removed, into powder, mix it with water and wheat flour and apply this [to the affected region]. Good. Tan Yeweng, *Shi yan fang.*

足釘怪疾。兩足心凸腫，上生黑豆瘡，硬如釘，脛骨生碎孔，髓流出，身發寒顫，惟思飲酒，此是肝腎冷熱相吞。用炮川烏頭末傅之，内服韭子湯，效。夏氏奇疾方。

The strange ailment of foot pin-illness sores: the soles of both feet have a bulging swelling with soybean sores, as hard as a pin, developing on top of them and holes developing in fracturred shin bones from which marrow flows out. The body shivers from cold, and [patients] only long for drinking wine. This is a struggle between cold and heat affecting liver and kidneys. Roast *chuan wu tou*, [grind it into] powder and apply this [to the affected region]. For internal [effects] ingest a Chinese leek decoction. Effective. Xia shi, *Qi ji fang.*

17-17-02
烏頭附子尖 *Wu tou fu zi jian*

Pointed ends of *wu tou* [main tuber] and *fu zi* [accessory tuber].

【主治】爲末，茶服半錢，吐風痰癲癇。時珍。

1081 *Ding* 丁, "pin[-illness]," also *ding* 疔, "pin-illness," refers to a deep-reaching and festering hardness in a tissue, eventually rising above the skin like a pinhead. BCGM Dict I, 127-129.

1082 *Jie*-illness 疥, vaguely identifiable skin ailment. BCGM Dict I, 249.

1083 *Xuan* 癬, "*xuan*-illness." Conditions of dermal lesions with initially erythema, papules, and itching gradually extending in all directions to form an irregular ring with clear boundaries. The skin is slightly elevated with small papules, blisters, and/or scales and scraps. The central lesion may appear to heal spontaneously, and it may reappear. Also, a designation of local lesions with itching, release of liquid and shedding of scabs. BCGM Dict I, 591.

Control. [Ground into] powder and half a *qian* ingested with tea [they serve to cure] vomiting related to wind [intrusion] and the presence of phlegm; peak-illness epilepsy. [Li] Shizhen.

【發明】【時珍曰】烏、附用尖，亦取其鋭氣直達病所爾，無他義也。保幼大全云：小兒慢脾驚風，四肢厥逆。用附子尖一個，硫黄棗大一個，蠍稍七個，爲末，薑汁、麪糊丸黄米大。每服十丸，米飲下。亦治久瀉尫羸。凡用烏、附，不可執謂性熱。審其手足冷者，輕則用湯，甚則用丸，重則用膏，候手足暖，陽氣回，即爲佳也。按此方乃和劑局方碧霞丹變法也，非真慢脾風不可輒用，故初虞世有金虎碧霞之戒。

Explication. [Li] Shizhen: The use of the pointed ends of *wu* [*tou* main tubers] and *fu* [*zi* accessory tubers] serves to use their sharp qi to reach the location of a disease. It has no other meaning. The *Bao you da quan* states: "In the case of slow spleen wind,[1084] with the four limbs affected by ceasing [yang qi and qi] counterflow, [grind] one pointed end of a *fu zi* [accessory tuber], one Chinese date size piece of sulphur and seven scorpions into powder and with a ginger juice and wheat flour paste form pills the size of millet. Each time ingest 10 pills, to be sent down with a rice beverage. This also serves to cure long-lasting outflow with weakness and emaciation. Whenever *wu* [*tou*] and *fu* [*zi*] are to be used, one must not hold back by pointing out their hot nature. Examine whether [a patient's] hands and feet are cold. If it is a light case, use [the tubers] as a decoction. If it is a severe [case of cold], use them as pills. If it is very severe, apply them as an ointment. Wait for the hands and feet to become warm. This is the return of yang qi, a sign of their excellent [effects]." [My] comment: This recipe is a modified approach based on the "bluish-green morning cloud elixir" of the *He ji ju fang*. If it is not a case of true slow spleen wind, it must not be used. This is why Chu Yushi warned against [the application of] golden tiger and bluish-green morning clouds [elixirs].

【附方】舊一，新七。

Added Recipes. One of old. Seven newly [recorded].

風厥癲癇。凡中風痰厥，癲癇驚風，痰涎上壅，牙關緊急，上視搐搦，並宜碧霞丹主之。烏頭尖、附子尖、蠍稍各七十個，石綠研九度飛過十兩，爲末，麪糊丸芡子大。每用一丸，薄荷汁半盞化下，更服温酒半合，須臾吐出痰涎爲妙。小兒驚癇，加白僵蠶等分。和劑局方。

1084 *Man pi feng* 慢脾風, "slow spleen wind," identical to *man jing feng* 慢驚風, "slow fright wind," a condition characterized by recurrent cramps in the presence or absence of fever. The cramps are slow and not very forceful. BCGM Dict I, 334.

Wind and recession,[1085] peak-illness epilepsy. Whenever [patients are affected by] wind stroke with phlegm and ceasing [yang qi], peak-illness epilepsy and fright wind, with phlegm and saliva rising and causing an obstruction, lockjaw, the eyes turned upward with convulsions, for all these cases the bluish-green morning cloud elixir is suitable to control them. [Grind] into powder [the following substances]. Seventy *wu tou* [main tuber] pointed ends, seventy *fu zi* [accessory tuber] pointed ends, 70 scorpions and ten *liang* of malachite, ground nine times and sublimated. With wheat flour paste form pills the size of *qian* seeds. Each time send down one pill dissolved in half a cup of mint juice. In addition, ingest half a *ge* of warm wine. When after a short while phlegm and saliva are spat out, this is the wondrous [effect of this therapy]. For children suffering from fright epilepsy, add an equal amount of white, stiff silkworms. *He ji ju fang.*

臍風撮口。生川烏尖三個，全足蜈蚣半條，酒浸炙，麝香少許，爲末。以少許吹鼻得嚏，乃以薄荷湯灌一字。永類方。

Navel wind[1086] and pursed mouth. Soak the pointed ends of three fresh *chuan wu* [*tou* main tubers] and one half centipede, complete with all its feet,[1087] in wine. Roast them, add a little musk and [grind them] into powder. Blow a little [of this powder] into [the patient's] nose to stimulate a sneeze. Then force-feed [the patient] with one *zi* of a mint decoction. *Yong lei fang.*

木舌腫脹。川烏尖、巴豆研細，醋調塗刷。集簡方。

Wooden tongue, swollen and bloated. Grind *chuan wu* [main tuber] pointed ends and *croton* [seeds] to fine [powder], mix it with vinegar and apply it to [the affected region]. *Ji jian fang.*

牙痛難忍。附子尖、天雄尖、全蠍各七個，生研爲末，點之。永類方。

Toothache hard to bear. Grind fresh seven *fu zi* [accessory tuber] pointed ends, seven *tian xiong* [tuber] pointed ends, and seven complete scorpions into powder and drip it [on the affected teeth]. *Yong lei fang.*

1085 *Feng jue* 風厥, "wind and recession," a condition brought about by liver qi transformed into wind. BCGM Dict I, 163.

1086 *Qi feng* 臍風, "navel wind," a condition of *po shang feng* 破傷風,"wound wind," brought forth by wind evil affecting the navel region of newborn children. BCGM Dict I, 382.

1087 Instead of *quan zu* 全足, "complete with its feet," the *Yong lei qian fang* ch. 20, *xiao er qi feng cui kou jin feng* 小兒臍風撮口噤風, "navel wind, pursed mouth, lockjaw wind," *ding ming san* 定命散, "powder to stabilize life," writes *jin chi* 金赤, "golden red."

奔豚疝氣作痛，或陰囊腫痛。去鈴丸：用生川烏尖七個，巴豆七枚去皮油，爲末，糕糊丸梧子大，朱砂、麝香爲衣。每服二丸，空心冷酒或冷鹽湯下。三兩日一服，不可多。澹寮方。

Painful running piglet[1088] and elevation-illness[1089] qi, also: painful swelling of the scrotum in the yin [(i. e., genital) region]. The "pills to eliminate bells." [Grind] the pointed ends of seven fresh *chuan wu* [*tou* main tubers] and seven *croton* [seeds], with their skin and oil removed, into powder and form with a steamed cake paste pills the size of *wu* seeds. Coat them with cinnabar and musk. Each time ingest two pills, to be sent down with cold wine or cold salt decoction. To be ingested every second or third day. One must not [ingest too] many. *Dan liao fang*.

割甲成瘡，連年不愈。川烏頭尖、黄蘗等分，爲末。洗了貼之，以愈爲度。古今録驗。

Sores from cutting finger/toenails that have not been cured for several years. [Grind] the pointed ends of *chuan wu tou* [main tubers] and *phellodendron* bark into powder. Wash [the sores] and then continue to apply [the powder] to them for as long as it takes to achieve a cure. *Gu jin lu yan*.

老幼口瘡。烏頭尖一個，天南星一個，研末，薑汁和，塗足心，男左女右，不過二三次即愈。

Sores in the mouth of the elderly and the young. Grind one pointed end of a *wu tou* [main tuber] and one Indian turnip [root] into powder, mix it with ginger juice and apply it to the sole of [one of the patient's] feet. For males, [to the sole] of the left [foot]; for females of the right [foot]. A cure will be achieved after no more than two or three applications.

17-18
天雄本經下品
Tian xiong, FE *Ben jing*, lower rank.
Aconitum carmichaeli Debx. Carmichael's monkshood.

【釋名】白幕本經。【時珍曰】天雄乃種附子而生出或變出，其形長而不生子，故曰天雄。其長而尖者，謂之天錐，象形也。

Explanation of Names. *Bai mu* 白幕, "white screen," *Ben jing*. [Li] Shizhen: *Tian xiong* is a byproduct, occasionally with a modified outcome, of the planting of *aco-*

1088 *Ben tun* 賁豚, "running piglet," a condition of an accumulation in the kidneys assuming the shape of a piglet moving up and down at irregular intervals. BCGM Dict I, 57.

1089 *Shan* 疝, "elevation-illness," a group of conditions characterized by violent abdominal pain, in some cases associated with constipation and anuria. BCGM Dict I, 417.

nitum [accessory tuber]. Its shape is lengthy and it does not grow "children." Hence it is called *tian xiong* 天雄, "heaven's hero." Specimens that are lengthy and pointed are called *tian zhui* 天錐, "heaven's awl," reflecting their shape.

【集解】【别録曰】天雄生少室山谷。二月采根，陰乾。【弘景曰】今采用八月中旬。天雄似附子細而長，乃至三四寸許。此與烏頭、附子三種，本出建平，故謂之三建。今宜都佷山者最好，謂爲西建。錢塘間者謂爲東建，氣力小弱，不相似，故曰西冰猶勝東白也。其用灰殺之時有冰强者，不佳。【恭曰】天雄、附子、烏頭，並以蜀道綿州、龍州出者佳。餘處縱有，力弱不相似。陶以三物俱出建平故名之者，非也。烏頭苗名堇，音靳。爾雅云，芨，堇草是也。今訛堇爲建，遂以建平譯之矣。【承曰】天雄諸説悉備。但始種而不生附子、側子，經年獨長大者是也。蜀人種之，尤忌生此，以爲不利，如養蠶而成白殭之意。【時珍曰】天雄有二種。一種是蜀人種附子而生出長者，或種附子而盡變成長者，即如種芋形狀不一之類。一種是他處草烏頭之類，自生成者，故别録註烏喙云，長三寸已上者爲天雄是也。入藥須用蜀産曾經釀制者。或云須重一兩半有象眼者乃佳。餘見附子下。

Collected Explanations. *Bie lu*: *Tian xiong* grows in the mountain valleys of Shao shi. The root is collected in the second month; it is dried in the yin (i. e., shade). [Tao] Hongjing: Today it is collected in the middle ten days period of the eighth month. *Tian xiong* resembles *fu zi*, *aconitum* [accessory tubers], but is finer and longer, reaching a length of more than three or four *cun*. With *wu tou*, *aconitum* [main tuber], and *fu zi*, *aconitum* [accessory tuber], it constitutes a group of three kinds. Orginally they came from Jian ping. Hence they are called the "three from Jian." Today specimens from Gen shan in Yi du are best. They are called "western Jian." Those from Qian tang are called "eastern Jian." The strength of their qi is minimal and weak. They are not comparable. Hence it is said: "Ice in the West is superior to what is white in the East." When killing its effects by [enclosing it with] ashes causes it to become as stiff as ice, it is no longer excellent. [Su] Gong: *Tian xiong*, *wu tou*, *aconitum* [main tuber], and *fu zi*, *aconitum* [accessory tuber], regardless of whether they come from Mian zhou and Long zhou in Shu dao, they are all excellent. Those from other places have a weak strength and are not comparable. Tao [Hongjing] assumes that their name is traced back to the origin of all three in Jian ping, but this is wrong. The seedling of *aconitum* [accessory tuber] is called *jin* 堇, read *jin* 靳. The *Er ya* states: "*Ji* 芨 is *jin cao* 堇草, 'the herb *jin*'." Today, *jin* 堇 is mispronounced *jian* 建, and this is explained[1090] with [their origin in] Jian ping. [Chen] Cheng: The statements on *tian xiong* are all rather complete. However, it is such that if when

1090 Instead of *yi* 譯, *Zheng lei* ch. 10, *tian xiong* 天雄, writes *shi* 釋, "to explain."

they are first planted no *fu zi, aconitum* [accessory tuber], or *ce zi* 側子, marginal [tuber], grows, and in the course of that year only long and big [specimens develop], then these are the [*tian xiong*]. When people in Shu plant them, they do not like at all to see them grow; they consider them not profitable. The underlying idea is similar to [the dislike of] white, stiff silkworms generated instead of the silkworms supposed to be cultivated. [Li] Shizhen: There are two kinds of *tian xiong*. One kind are lengthy specimens that grow when people in Shu plant *fu zi, aconitum* [accessory tubers]. Or those that when planted as *fu zi, aconitum* [accessory tubers], completely change to lengthy specimens. This is comparable to the planting of taro [tubers that may yield tubers] of different shapes. The other kind is related to the *cao wu tou* of other regions. They grow and develop as such. Hence the *Bie lu* in its comments on *wu zhui* 烏喙 states: "Those longer than three *cun* are *tian xiong*." For medication those must be used that come from Shu and have undergone a processing. Some say that [*tian xiong*] is excellent when it weighs one and a half *liang* and resembles a root. For more, see under *fu zi* 附子, *aconitum* [accessory tuber], (17-17).

【修治】【斅曰】宜炮皴去皮、尖、底用，或陰制如附子法亦得。【大明曰】凡丸散炮去皮用，飲藥即和皮生使甚佳。【時珍曰】熟用一法：每十兩以酒浸七日。掘土坑，用炭半秤煅赤，去火，以醋二升沃之，候乾，乘熱入天雄在内，小盆合一夜，取出，去臍用之。

Pharmaceutical Processing. [Lei] Xiao: *Tian xiong* should be roasted to let it crack. Then remove the skin and the pointed ends. [Only] the heart is used. It is also possible to process it with the yin method applied to *fu zi, aconitum* [accessory tuber]. Da Ming: For an application as pills or powders, roast it and remove the skin. For an application as a liquid to be drunk it is quite excellent when used fresh with its skin retained. [Li] Shizhen: A method for heat processing. Every ten *liang* are soaked in wine for seven days. Then dig a pit in the earth and with half a *cheng* of charcoal calcine it until it is red. Remove the fire and pour two *sheng* of vinegar [into the pit]. Wait until it has dried, give the *tian xiong* into the hot [pit] and leave it there covered with a small bowl for one night. Then take it out, remove the navel[1091] and use it.

【氣味】辛，温，有大毒。【别録曰】甘，大温。【權曰】大熱。宜乾薑制之。【之才曰】遠志爲之使。惡腐婢。忌豉汁。

Qi and Flavor. Acrid, warm, very poisonous. *Bie lu*: Sweet, very warm. [Zhen] Quan: Very hot; dried ginger is required to check its [effects]. [Xu] Zhicai: *Polygala* [root] serves as its guiding substance. [Ingested together,] it abhors Japanese musk maple. [During a treatment with it] the juice of [soybean] relish is to be avoided.

1091 *Qi* 臍, "navel," is the indentation at the top of the tuber where it was connected with the stem of the plant. "To remove skin and navel" has the meaning of "to clean thoroughly."

【主治】大風，寒濕痺，歷節痛，拘攣緩急，破積聚邪氣，金瘡。强筋骨，輕身健行。本經。療頭面風去來疼痛，心腹結聚，關節重，不能行步，除骨間痛。長陰氣，强志，令人武勇，力作不倦。別録。【禹錫曰】按淮南子云：天雄、雄雞志氣益。注云：取天雄一枚，納雄雞腸中，搗食之，令人勇。治風痰冷痺，軟脚毒風，能止氣喘促急，殺禽蟲毒。甄權。治一切風，一切氣，助陽道，暖水臟，補腰膝，益精明目，通九竅，利皮膚，調血脉，四肢不遂，下胸膈水，破痃癖癰結，排膿止痛，續骨，消瘀血，背脊傴僂，霍亂轉筋，發汗，止陰汗。炮含，治喉痺。大明。

Control. Massive wind,[1092] blockage related to the presence of cold and moisture, pervading joints pain, cramps, contractions, tensions. It breaks through accumulations and collections of evil qi. Wounds caused by metal objects/weapons. It strengthens sinews and bones. It relieves the body of its weight and facilitates walking. *Ben jing*. It heals painful intermittend wind [intrusion] in head and face, nodular collections in the central and abdominal region, a feeling of heaviness in the joints, inability to walk. It removes pain in the bones. It stimulates the growth of yin qi, strengthens the mind, and lets one be brave in battles, with an inexhaustible strength. *Bie lu*. [Zhang] Yuxi: According to the *Huai nan zi*, "*Tian xiong* and roosters boost mind and qi." A comment states: "One *tian xiong* [root] inserted into the intestine of a rooster, pounded and eaten, lets one be brave." It serves to cure blockage related to wind [intrusion] and the presence of phlegm and cold, soft legs related to the presence of poison and wind [intrusion]. It can stop panting and hectic [breath] qi. It kills the poison of fowl and worms/bugs. Zhen Quan: It serves to cure all types of wind [intrusion] and all types of qi [disorder]. It supports the yang path (i. e., male sexual potency), warms the water long-term depot (i. e., the kidneys), supplements [the qi in] the lower back and the knees, boosts essence/sperm, clears the eyes, opens the nine orifices, frees the passage through the skin, and regulates the movement in the blood vessels. [It serves to cure cases of] the four limbs not following [one's will], discharges water from the chest and diaphragm region, breaks through string-illness,[1093] aggregation-illness, and obstruction-illness nodes. It dispels pus and ends pain, reconnects bones and dissolves stagnating blood. [It serves to cure] hunchback and cholera with contorted sinews. It stimulates sweating, and ends sweating in the yin [(i. e., genital) region]. Roasted and held in the mouth, it serves to cure throat blockage. Da Ming.

1092 *Da feng* 大風, "massive wind," may refer to sores caused by a massive intrusion of wind evil and also to conditions of leprosy. BCGM Dict I, 111.

1093 *Xuan* 痃, "string-illness," a condition of acute pain located in the abdomen to the left and right of the umbilicus. BCGM Dict I, 591.

【發明】【宗奭曰】補虛寒須用附子。風家多用天雄，亦取其大者，以其尖角多，熱性不肯就下，故取其敷散也。【元素曰】非天雄不能補上焦之陽虛。【震亨曰】天雄、烏頭，氣壯形偉，可爲下部之佐。【時珍曰】烏、附、天雄，皆是補下焦命門陽虛之藥，補下所以益上也。若是上焦陽虛，即屬心肺之分，當用參、芪，不當用天雄也。且烏、附、天雄之尖，皆是向下生者，其氣下行。其臍乃向上生苗之處。寇宗奭言其不肯就下，張元素言其補上焦陽虛，皆是誤認尖爲上爾。惟朱震亨以爲下部之佐者得之，而未發出此義。雷斅炮炙論序云：咳逆數數，酒服熟雄。謂以天雄炮研，酒服一錢也。

Explication. [Kou] Zongshi: To supplement a depletion with the presence of cold *fu zi*, *aconitum* [accessory tubers] are required. Patients with wind [intrusion] often use *tian xiong*. They, too, choose big specimens. Since they have many pointed horns, their hot nature does not tend to descend [in the body]. Hence, there application makes use of their spreading and dispersing [effects]. [Zhang] Yuansu: Without *tian xiong* it is impossible to supplement a yang [qi] depletion in the upper [region of the Triple] Burner. [Zhu] Zhengheng: *Tian xiong* and *wu tou*, *aconitum* [main tuber], have robust qi and a big physical appearance. They can be used to assist [medication aimed at] the lower [body] region. [Li] Shizhen: *Wu* [*tou*], *aconitum* [main] tuber, *fu zi*, *aconitum* [accessory tuber], and *tian xiong* are all pharmaceutical drugs to supplement yang [qi] depletion in the lower [section of the Triple] Burner and the Gate of Life. As they supplement [qi in] the lower [body section] they boost [the qi in] the upper [body section]. A yang [qi] depletion in the upper [section of the Triple] Burner is associated with the heart and lung section. It requires an application of ginseng [root] and *astragalus* [root]. *Tian xiong* must not be used [for such issues]. Also, the pointed ends of *wu tou*, *aconitum* [main tuber], *fu zi*, *aconitum* [accessory tuber], and *tian xiong* grow directed downward and their qi move downward, while their navel[1094] is directed upward to where the seedling grows. Kou Zongshi says that "they do not tend to descend." Zhang Yuansu says: "They supplement a yang [qi] depletion in the upper [section of the Triple] Burner." They both are wrong in their assumption that the pointed ends [and their effects] are directed upward. Only Zhu Zhenheng its right when he assumes that "they assist [medication aimed at] the lower [body] section;" but he failed to disclose the underlying idea. Lei Xiao in the preface to his *Pao zhi lun* states: " For frequent cough with [qi] counterflow ingest with wine heat processed [*tian*] *xiong*." That is to say, roast *tian xiong*, grind [it into powder] and ingest with wine one *qian*.

1094 *Qi* 臍, "navel," is the indentation at the top of the tuber where it was connected with the stem of the plant.

【附方】新三。

Added Recipes. Three newly [recorded].

三建湯。治元陽素虛，寒邪外攻，手足厥冷，大小便滑數，小便白渾，六脉沉微，除固冷，扶元氣，及傷寒陰毒。用烏頭、附子、天雄並炮裂，去皮臍，等分，㕮咀，每服四錢。水二盞，薑十五片，煎八分，温服。肘後方。

The "triple reinforcement decoction." It serves to cure a depletion of original yang [qi] endowment, with an attack by cold evil from the outside, hands and feet affected by ceasing [yang] qi and turning cold, frequent smooth passage of major [defecation] and minor [urination] relief, and white, turbid urine, with the [movement in the] six vessels being in the depth and weak. It removes solid cold, supports the original qi, and [dispels] harm caused by cold with yin poison. Roast equal amounts of *aconitum* [main tuber], *aconitum* [accessory tuber] and *tian xiong* together until they crack, remove their skin and the navel, pound them, and this way for each ingestion prepare four *qian*. Boil this in two cups of water, with 15 slices of ginger, down to 80% and ingest this warm. *Zhou hou fang*.

男子失精。天雄三兩炮，白术八兩，桂枝六兩，龍骨三兩，爲散。每酒服半錢。張仲景金匱要略。

Loss of essence/sperm of males. [Grind] three *liang* of *tian xiong*, roasted, eight *liang* of *atractylodes macrocephala* [rhizome], six *liang* of *cassia* twigs and three *liang* of dragon bones into powder. Each time ingest with wine half a *qian*. Zhang Zhongjing, *Jin kui yao lue*.

大風惡癩。三月、四月采天雄、烏頭苗及根，去土勿洗，搗汁，漬細粒黑豆，摩去皮不落者，一夜取出，晒乾又浸，如此七次。初吞三枚，漸加至六七枚。禁房室、猪、魚、雞、蒜，犯之即死。

Massive wind,[1095] [i. e.,] malign repudiation-illness.[1096] During the third and fourth month collect seedlings and roots of *tian xiong* and *aconitum* [main tuber]. Remove the soil but do not wash them. Pound them to obtain a juice. Soak fine grain soybeans in it. Rub the [soybeans] and discard those whose skin does not fall off. Take them out [of the juice] after one night, dry them in the sun and soak them again. Continue this seven times. In the beginning, [let patients] swallow three pieces. Gradually increase this to six or seven pieces. [During this therapy] sexual inter-

1095 *Da feng* 大風, "massive wind," may refer to sores caused by a massive intrusion of wind evil and also to conditions of leprosy. BCGM Dict I, 111.

1096 *Lai* 癩, "*lai*-illness," "repudiation-illness," including cases of leprosy/Aussatz." BCGM Dict I, 293.

course, pork, fish, chicken and garlic are to be avoided. [Patients] acting against this [prohibition] will die.

17-19
側子別録下品
Ce zi, FE *Bie lu*, lower rank.

***Aconitum carmichaeli* Debx. *Aconitum* [marginal "child" tuber]**

【釋名】荝子。【時珍曰】生于附子之側，故名。許慎説文作荝子。

Explanation of Names. *Ce zi* 荝子. [Li] Shizhen: It grows at the "side," *ce* 側, of *fu zi* 附子, *aconitum* [accessory tuber/attached child]. Hence the name. Xu Shen in his *Shuo wen* writes *ce zi* 荝子.

【集解】【弘景曰】此附子邊角之大者，削取之。昔時不用，比來醫家以療脚氣多驗。【恭曰】側子、附子，皆是烏頭下旁出者。以小者爲側子，大者爲附子。今以附子角爲側子，理必不然。若當陽以下，江左、山南、嵩高、齊魯間，附子時復有角如大豆許。夔州以上，劍南所出者，附子之角但如黍粟，豈可充用？比來都下皆用細附子有效，未嘗取角也。【保昇曰】今附子邊果有角如大棗核及檳榔以來者，形狀自是一顆，且不小。乃烏頭旁出附子，附子旁出側子，甚明。【時珍曰】側子乃附子旁粘連小者爾，故吴普、陶弘景皆指爲附子角之大者。其又小于側子者，即漏籃子矣。故楊氏附子記言：側子、漏籃，園人皆不重之，以乞役夫。

Collected Explanations. [Tao] Hongjing: These are large horns growing at the side of *fu zi* 附子, *aconitum* [accessory tuber]. They are cut off to be obtained. In ancient times, they were not used [for therapeutic purposes]. More recently, physicians have applied them to cure leg qi[1097] with much success. [Su] Gong: *Ce zi* and *fu zi*, *aconitum* [accessor tuber], are both outgrowths from the side of the lower ends of *wu tou*, *aconitum* [main tuber]. Small ones are considered *ce zi*; large ones are identified as *fu zi*. Today, the horns [growing out of] *fu zi* are identified as *ce zi*. But this is definitely not so. For example, from Dan yang on further down/south, in Jiang zuo, Shan nan, Song gao and Qi lu, *fu zi* grows horns about the size of soybeans. From Kui zhou on further up/north, the horns of *fu zi* of specimens coming from Jian nan are only of the size of millet. How could they be good enough for [therapeutic] use? In recent times, in the capital they all use fine *fu zi* with success; they never resort to its horns. [Han] Baosheng: Today there are horns at the side of *fu zi* the size of Chinese date pits or areca nuts. From their physical appearance and shape, they seem to be fruits of themselves, and they are not small. Now, from the side of *wu tou*, *aconitum* [main] tuber]. *fu zi*, *aconitum* [accessory tubers], emerge. From the

1097 *Jiao qi* 脚氣, "leg qi." Painful, weak, swollen legs. BCGM Dict I, 248.

side of *fu zi*, *ce zi* emerge. That is very obvious. [Li] Shizhen: *Ce zi* are small [tubers] linked to each other and attached to the side of *fu zi*. Therefore, both Wu Pu and Tao Hongjing identify them as the big horns of *fu zi*. Those still smaller than *ce zi* are the "seeds leaking from a basket," *lou lan zi* 漏籃子 (17-20). Hence, Yang shi in his *Fu zi ji* says: "*Ce zi* and *lou lan zi* are not planted by gardeners. They give them to laborers begging for them.

【修治】同附子。

Pharmaceutical Preparation. Identical to that of *aconitum* [accessory tuber].

【氣味】辛，大熱，有大毒。【普曰】神農、岐伯：有大毒。八月采。畏惡與附子同。

Qi and Flavor. Acrid, very hot, very poisonous. [Wu] Pu: Shen nong, Qi Bo: Very poisonous. It is collected in the eighth month. [Ingested] together, it both fears and abhors *fu zi*, *aconitum* [accessory tuber].

【主治】癰腫，風痺歴節，腰脚疼冷，寒熱鼠瘻。又墮胎。别録。療脚氣，冷風濕痺，大風筋骨攣急。甄權。冷酒調服，治遍身風瘮神妙。雷斆。

Control. Obstruction-illness[1098] swelling. Pervading joints wind[1099] blockage. Pain and cold in the lower back and legs. Alternating sensations of cold and heat and mouse fistula.[1100] Also, it stimulates abortion. *Bie lu*. It heals leg qi,[1101] blockage related to cold, wind [intrusion] and moisture. Massive wind with spasm and tension of sinews and bones. Zhen Quan. Ingested mixed with cold wine it serves to cure wind papules[1102] covering the entire body. Divinely wondrous. Lei Xiao.

【發明】【機曰】烏頭乃原生之腦，得母之氣，守而不移，居乎中者也。側子散生旁側，體無定在，其氣輕揚，宜其發散四肢，充達皮毛，爲治風之藥。天雄長而尖，其氣親上，宜其補上焦之陽虚。木鼈子則餘氣所結，

1098 *Yong* 癰, "obstruction-illness,"refers to an obstruction of vessels or other ducts inside the body. Qi rushing against the obstruction may cause a local swelling and eventually break through the surface to cause an abscess. BCGM Dict I, 641.

1099 *Li jie [feng]* 歴節[風], pervading joints [wind], a condition of *tong feng* 痛風, "pain wind," characterized by spontaneous sweating, shortness of qi/breath, aching joints, and difficulties in bending and stretching. BCGM Dict I, 314.

1100 *Shu lou* 鼠瘻, "mouse fistula," BCGM Dict I, 466, identical to *luo li* 瘰癧, "scrofula pervasion-illnes."

1101 *Jiao qi* 脚氣, "leg qi." Painful, weak, swollen legs. BCGM Dict I, 248.

1102 *Feng zhen* 風疹, "wind papules," a condition, brought forth by wind evil, of eruptive skin papules of different sizes, accompanied by unbearable itching. If scratched they rise further. BCGM Dict I, 172.

其形摧殘，宜其不入湯服，令人喪目也。【時珍曰】唐元希聲侍郎治癱瘓風，有側子湯，見外臺秘要，藥多不録。

Explication. [Wang] Ji: *Wu tou, aconitum* [main tuber], is the "brain" of the original plant. It has received the qi of its mother; it guards one place and does not move. It resides in the center. *Ce zi*, its "children at the side," grow dispersed at its side; their body has no fixed place and their qi are light and spreading. They are a pharmaceutical drug suitable for dispersing into the four limbs, and reaching into skin and hair, where they serve to cure wind [intrusion]. *Tian xiong* is long and pointed. Its qi tend to rise. It is suitable for supplementing yang [qi] depletion in the upper [section of the Triple] Burner. *Mu bie zi* (i. e., *lou lan zi*, 17-20) is a conglomeration of remnant qi. Its physical appearance is debilitated and incomplete; it must not be ingested as a decoction as it causes loss of vision. [Li] Shizhen: During the Tang, Attendant Gentleman Yuan Xisheng cured paralysis with wind [intrusion] with the "decoction with *ce zi*." [For details] see the *Wai tai mi yao*. As it has a large number of pharmaceutical drugs [as ingredients], it is not recorded here.

17-20
漏籃子綱目
Lou lan zi, FE *Gang mu.*

***Aconitum carmichaeli* Debx. *Aconitum* [tuber as small as "seeds leaking from a basket."]**

【釋名】木鼈子炮炙論、虎掌日華。【時珍曰】此乃附子之瑣細未成者，小而漏籃，故名。南星之最小者名虎掌，此物類之，故亦同名。大明會典載：四川成都府，歲貢天雄二十對，附子五十對，烏頭五十對，漏籃二十斤。不知何用。

Explanation of Names. *Mu bie zi* 木鼈子, "seeds/children of the wooden turtle," *Pao zhi lun*. *Hu zhang* 虎掌, "tiger palm," *Rihua*. [Li] Shizhen: These are very small, incomplete *fu zi, aconitum* [accessory tubers]. They are small enough to "leak from a basket," *lou lan* 漏籃. Hence the name. The smallest specimens of *arisaema* roots are called *hu zhang* 虎掌, "tiger palm." The present item resembles them, hence it has the same name. The *Da Ming hui dian* has the following record: "Cheng du fu in Si chuan in one year sends as tribute 20 pairs of *tian xiong* 天雄, 50 pairs of *fu zi* 附子, 50 pairs of *wu tou* 烏頭, 20 *jin* of *lou lan* 漏籃." It is not known what [the latter] may have been used for.

【氣味】苦、辛，有毒。【斅曰】服之令人喪目。

Qi and Flavor. Bitter, acrid, poisonous. [Lei] Xiao: To ingest them causes loss of vision.

【主治】惡痢，冷漏瘡，惡瘡癘風。時珍。

Control. Malign free-flux illness. Cold, leaking sores, malign sores related to epidemic wind.[1103] [Li] Shizhen.

【發明】【時珍曰】按楊士瀛直指方云：凡漏瘡年久者，復其元陽，當用漏籃子輩，加減用之。如不當用而輕用之，又恐熱氣乘虛變移結核，而爲害尤甚也。又按類編云：一人兩足生瘡，臭潰難近。夜宿五夫人祠下，夢神授方：用漏籃子一枚，生研爲末，入膩粉少許，井水調唾。依法治之，果愈。蓋此物不堪服餌，止宜入瘡科也。

Explication. [Li] Shizhen: According to Yang Shiying in his *Zhi zhi fang*, whenever sores leak for several years, the [patient's] original yang [qi] need to be restored. For this *lou lan zi* is used in varying quantities, in joint [applications with other substances]. That is, if it should not be used but is used in even a small amount only, it may still happen that its hot qi avail themselves of a depletion and transform to nodular kernels, which would be extremely disastrous. Also, as the *Lei bian* states: "Someone developed sores on his two feet. They released a malodorous stench making it difficult to approach [that person]. One night he rested in the Ancestral Temple of the Five Ladies,' and dreamed of a spirit offering him the following recipe. 'Grind one fresh *lou lan zi* [tuber] into powder, add a little calomel, mix it with well water and spit it [on the affected region].[1104]' He started a cure following this advice and eventually was healed." The fact is, this item is not suitable for an ingestion. It is only used [externally] on sores.

【附方】新一。

Added Recipes. One newly [recorded].

一切惡痢雜下及休息痢。百歲丸：用漏籃子一個大者，阿膠、木香、黄連、罌粟殻各半兩，俱炒焦存性，入乳香少許爲末，糊丸梧子大。每一歲一丸，米飲下。羅天益衛生寶鑑。

All types of malign free-flux illness discharge and intermittent free-flux illness. The "pills for 100 years of life." Fry one large *lou lan zi* [tuber], and half a *liang* each of donkey hide glue, *costus* [root], *coptis* [rhizome], and poppy capsule shells until scorched, with their nature retained. Add a little frankincense and [grind this into] powder to be formed with a [wheat flour] paste to pills the size of *wu* seeds. For

1103 *Li feng* 癘風, "epidemic wind," a condition identical to *da feng* 大風, "massive wind," possibly including cases of leprosy. BCGM Dict I, 313, 111.

1104 Instead of *tuo* 唾, "spittle," "to spit," *Yi shuo* ch. 10 quoting *Lei bian* writes *tu* 塗, "to apply," "to smear."

each year of his life [the patient is to ingest] one pill, to be sent down with a rice beverage. Luo Tianyi, *Wei sheng bao jian*.

17-21
烏頭本經下品

Wu tou, FE *Ben jing*, lower rank.

Aconitum carmichaeli **Debx.** ***Aconitum*** **[main tuber].**

【校正】併入拾遺獨白草。

Editorial Correction. *Du bai cao* 獨白草[1105], listed [separately] in the *Shi yi*, is included here.

【釋名】烏喙本經即兩頭尖、草烏頭綱目、土附子日華、奚毒本經、耿子吳普、毒公吳普又名帝秋、金鴉綱目。苗名莨音艮、芨音及、堇音近、獨白草拾遺、鴛鴦菊綱目。汁煎名射罔。【普曰】烏頭，形如烏之頭也。有兩岐相合如烏之喙者，名曰烏喙。喙即烏之口也。【恭曰】烏喙，即烏頭異名也。此有三歧者，然兩歧者少。若烏頭兩歧者名烏喙，則天雄、附子之兩歧者，復何以名之？【時珍曰】此即烏頭之野生于他處者，俗謂之草烏頭，亦曰竹節烏頭，出江北者曰淮烏頭，日華子所謂土附子者是也。烏喙即偶生兩歧者，今俗呼爲兩頭尖，因形而名，其實乃一物也。附子、天雄之偶生兩歧者，亦謂之烏喙，功亦同于天雄，非此烏頭也。蘇恭不知此義，故反疑之。草烏頭取汁，晒爲毒藥，射禽獸，故有射罔之稱。後魏書言遼東塞外秋收烏頭爲毒藥射禽獸，陳藏器所引續漢五行志，言西國生獨白草，煎爲藥，敷箭射人即死者，皆此烏頭，非川烏頭也。菊譜云鴛鴦菊，即烏喙苗也。

Explanation of Names. *Wu hui* 烏喙, "crow beak," *Ben jing*, i. e., *liang tou jian* 兩頭尖, "two pointed ends," and *cao wu tou* 草烏頭, "herbal crow's head," *Gang mu*. *Tu fu zi* 土附子, "local *fu zi*," *Rihua*. *Xi du* 奚毒, "rivulet poison," *Ben jing*. *Geng zi* 耿子, "upright children/seeds," Wu Pu. *Du gong* 毒公, "poisonous duke," Wu Pu. Alternative names: *di qiu* 帝秋[1106] and *jin ya* 金鴉, "golden crow," *Gang mu*. The seedling is called *gen* 莨[1107], read *gen* 艮, *ji* 芨, read *ji* 及, and *jin* 堇, read *jin* 近. *Du bai cao* 獨白草, "single white herb," *Shi yi*. *Yuan yang ju* 鴛鴦菊, "mandarin duck chrysanthemum," *Gang mu*. The juice obtained by boiling it is called *she wang* 射罔, "to cast a net." [Wu] Pu: *Wu tou* 烏頭 has the physical appearance of a crow's, *wu*

1105 Instead of *du bai cao* 獨白草, "single white herb," *Zheng lei* ch. 8 quoting *Shi yi* writes *du zi cao* 獨自草, "isolated herb." 後同不注。

1106 Instead of *di qiu* 帝秋, *Yu lan* ch. 990, *wu tou* 烏頭, quoting *Wu shi ben cao* writes *qian qiu* 千秋, "a thousand autumns."

1107 Instead of *gen* 莨, *Zheng lei* ch. 8 quoting *Shi yi* writes *lang* 莨.

烏, head, *tou* 頭. It has two fork branches united [at their origin] resembling the beak, *hui* 喙, of a crow, *wu* 烏. Therefore the name *wu hui* 烏喙, a "crow's beak." *Hui* 喙 is the mouth of a crow, *wu* 烏. [Su] Gong: *Wu hui* 烏喙 is an alternative name of *wu tou* 烏頭 which has three fork branches. Those with two fork branches are rare. When *wu tou* 烏頭 with two fork branches is called *wu hui* 烏喙, how should *tian xiong* 天雄 and *fu zi* 附子 with their two fork branches be named? [Li] Shizhen: This is *wu tou* 烏頭 growing in the wild at other places. It is commonly called *cao wu tou* 草烏頭, "herbal crow's head." It is also called *zhu jie wu tou* 竹節烏頭, "bamboo node crow's head." Those from Jiang bei are called *huai wu tou* 淮烏頭; they are the ones called *tu fi zi* 土附子 in the *Rihua*. *Wu hui* 烏喙 has two fork branches; today, it is commonly called *liang tou jian* 兩頭尖, "two pointed tips." This name reflects its physical appearance. But in fact, they are all one and the same item. *Fu zi* 附子 and *tian xiong* 天雄 with two fork branches are also called *wu hui* 烏喙, "crow's beak." Their [therapeutic] potential is identical to that of *tian xiong* 天雄, but this is not the *wu tou* 烏頭 discussed here. Su Gong was not familiar with the underlying meaning. Hence he had his doubts. When the juice of *cao wu tou* is extracted and dried in the sun, it becomes a poisonous pharmaceutical drug that is shot/cast at fowl and animals. Hence it is called *she wang* 射罔, "to cast a net." The *Hou Wei shu* says that "in Liao dong, outside the border, in late autumn they collect *wu tou* 烏頭 to prepare a poisonous pharmaceutical drug to be shot at fowl and animals." Chen Cangqi quotes the Treatise on the Five Phases from the *Xu Han* [*shu*] saying that "in western countries a 'single white herb,' *du bai cao* 獨白草, grows that when boiled is made to a pharmaceutical drug. It is applied to arrows and a person shot with it dies. All these are the *wu tou* 烏頭 discussed here; they are not *chuan wu tou* 川烏頭. The *Ju pu* states: *Yuan yang ju* 鴛鴦菊, "mandarin duck *chrysanthemum*." This is the seedling of *wu hui* 烏喙.

【集解】【别録曰】烏頭、烏喙生朗陵山谷。正月、二月采，陰乾。長三寸以上者爲天雄。【普曰】正月始生，葉厚，莖方中空，葉四四相當，與蒿相似。【弘景曰】今采用四月，亦以八月采。搗笮莖汁，日煎爲射罔。獵人以傅箭，射禽獸十步即倒，中人亦死，宜速解之。朗陵屬汝南郡。【大明曰】土附子生去皮搗，濾汁澄清，旋添晒乾取膏，名爲射罔，以作毒箭。【時珍曰】處處有之，根苗花實並與川烏頭相同。但此係野生，又無釀造之法，其根外黑内白，皺而枯燥爲異爾，然毒則甚焉。段成式酉陽雜俎言：雀芋狀如雀頭，置乾地反濕，濕地反乾，飛鳥觸之墮，走獸遇之僵。似亦草烏之類，而毒更甚也。又言：建寧郡烏勾山有牧靡草，烏鵲誤食烏喙中毒，必急食此草以解之。牧靡不知何藥也。

Collected Explanations. *Bie lu*: *Wu tou* 烏頭 and *wu hui* 烏喙 grow in the mountain valleys of Lang ling. They are collected in the first and the second month; they are dried in the yin (i. e., shade). Those longer than three *cun* are *tian xiong*. [Wu] Pu: They begin to grow in the first month. Their leaves are thick; their stem is square and hollow. The leaves grow four and four facing each other, similar to wormwood. Tao Hongjing: Today they are collected in the fourth month, and also in the eighth month. They are pounded to obtain the juice in the stem. It is dried in the sun and then boiled to prepare aconite paste, *she wang* 射罔. Hunters apply it to their arrows to shoot fowl and animals. Those struck move ten more steps and fall to the ground. A person struck will die, too, unless quick measures are taken to resolve [the poison]. Lang ling belongs to Ru nan fu. Da Ming: Remove the skin of *tu fu zi*, pound it, pass the juice through a sieve and wait for the liquid to become clear. Then dry it again in the sun to obtain a paste. This is called *she wang* 射罔 and it serves to prepare poisonous arrows. [Li] Shizhen: It is found everywhere. Its root, seedling, flowers and fruits are all identical to those of *chuan wu tou*. However the item discussed here grows in the wild, and there is no method of processing it. The root is black outside and white inside. Its root is wrinkled, withered and dry, and this is the difference. However, it is very poisonous. Duan Chengshi in his *You yang za zu* says: "*Que yu* 雀芋 is shaped like the head of a sparrow. When it is placed on a dry ground, [the ground] will be moistened. When it is placed on moist ground, it will dry. When flying birds come into contact with it, they fall to the ground. When running animals touch it, they are stiffened. It resembles *cao wu* [*tou*], but is even more extremely poisonous." It also says: "On Mount Wu gou shan in Jian ning jun an herb [named] *mu mi* 牧靡 is found. When crows or magpies are struck by the poison of *wu hui*, they immediately eat this herb to resolve it." It is unknown which pharmaceutical drug *mu mi* is.

【修治】【時珍曰】草烏頭或生用，或炮用，或以烏大豆同煮熟，去其毒用。

Pharmaceutical Preparation. [Li] Shizhen: *Cao wu tou* may be used fresh, or roasted, or is heat processed by boiling it together with black soybeans. This way its poison is eliminated and it can be used [for therapeutic purposes].

烏頭。*Wu tou.*

【氣味】辛，温，有大毒。【别録曰】甘，大熱，大毒。【普曰】神農、雷公、桐君、黄帝：甘，有毒。【權曰】苦、辛，大熱，有大毒。【大明曰】味蔹、辛，熱，有毒。【之才曰】莽草、遠志爲之使。反半夏、栝樓、貝母、白歛、白及。惡藜蘆。【時珍曰】伏丹砂、砒石。忌豉汁。畏飴糖、黑豆、冷水，能解其毒。

Qi and Flavor. Acrid, warm, very poisonous. *Bie lu*: Sweet, very hot, very poisonous. [Wu] Pu: Shen nong, Lei gong, Tong jun, Huang Di: Poisonous. [Zhen] Quan: Bitter, acrid, very hot, very poisonous. Da Ming: Flavor salty,[1108] acrid, hot, poisonous. [Xu] Zhicai: *Illiceum* [leaf] and *polygala* [root] serve as its guiding substances. [Ingested together,] it opposes *pinellia* [root], Japanese snake gourd, *fritillaria* [root], *ampelopsis* [root] and common *bletilla* [root]. It abhors *veratrum* [root]. [Li] Shizhen: It suppresses [the effects of] cinnabar and arsenic. [During a therapy with it] malt sugar, black soybeans and cold water are to be avoided. They can resolve its poison.

【主治】中風惡風，洗洗出汗，除寒濕痺，欬逆上氣，破積聚寒熱。其汁煎之名射罔，殺禽獸。本經。消胸上痰冷，食不下，心腹冷痰，臍間痛，不可俛仰，目中痛，不可久視。又墮胎。別録。主惡風憎寒，冷痰包心，腸腹㽲痛，痃癖氣塊，齒痛。益陽事，强志。甄權。治頭風喉痺，癰腫疔毒。時珍。

Control. Wind stroke, malign wind [intrusion], with shivering and sweating. It eliminates blockage related to the presence of cold and moisture, and cough with [qi] counterflow. It breaks through accumulations and concretions with alternating sensations of cold and heat. To obtain the juice and boil it [to a paste results in] *she wang*, aconite paste, "to cast a net." It kills fowl and animals. *Ben jing*. It dissolves phlegm and cold risen in the chest, with an inability to let food move down, phlegm[1109] related to cold in the central and abdominal region, pain in the navel region, inability to lower and raise the head, pain in the eyes, with an inability to see into the distance. Also, it stimulates abortion. *Bie lu*. It controls malign wind with an aversion to cold, cold phlegm enclosing the heart, flatulent pain[1110] in the intestines in the abdomen, qi lumps related to string-illness[1111] and aggregation-illness, and toothache. It boosts the yang affair (i. e., male sexual potency) and strengthens

---

1108 Instead of *xian* 薟, *Zheng lei* ch. 10, *wu tou* 烏頭, quoting *Rihua zi*, writes [疒僉]. The meaning is unclear; it may be a homophone use of *xian* 鹹, "salty."

1109 Instead of *tan* 痰, "phlegm," *Zheng lei* ch. 10, *wu tou* 烏頭, quoting *Bie lu*, writes *ji* 疾, "illness."

1110 *Jiao tong* 㽲痛, "flatulent pain," an illness sign of a pressing pain in the abdomen. BCGM Dict I, 249.

1111 *Xuan* 痃, "string-illness," a condition of acute pain located in the abdomen to the left and right of the umbilicus. BCGM Dict I, 591.

the mind. Zhen Quan. It serves to cure head wind[1112] with throat closure, swelling related to obstruction-illness[1113] and pin-illness[1114] poison. [Li] Shizhen.

17-21-01

烏喙 *Wu hui*

"A crow's beak." Alternative name *liang tou jian* 兩頭尖, "two pointed tips."

【氣味】辛，微温，有大毒。【普曰】神農、雷公、桐君、黄帝：有毒。【權曰】苦、辛，大熱。畏惡同烏頭。

Qi and Flavor. Acrid, slightly warm, very poisonous. [Wu] Pu: Shen nong, Lei gong, Tong jun, Huang Di: poisonous. [Zhen] Quan: Bitter, acrid, very hot. It fears and abhors [to be ingested] together with *wu tou* 烏頭.

【主治】風濕，丈夫腎濕陰囊癢，寒熱歴節，掣引腰痛，不能行步，癰腫膿結。又墮胎。别録。男子腎氣衰弱，陰汗，瘰癧歲月不消。甄權。主大風頑痺。時珍。

Control. Wind [intrusion] and the presence of moisture. Itching scrotum of husbands related to the presence of moisture in their kidneys. Alternating sensations of cold and heat with pervading joints [wind].[1115] Pain pulling on the lower back making it impossible to walk. Swelling and pus nodes related to an obstruction-illness. Also, it stimulates promotion. *Bie lu.* Weak kidney qi of males. Sweating in the yin [(i. e., genital) region]. Scrofula pervasion-illness[1116] failing to dissolve in the course of months and years. Zhen Quan. It controls massive wind[1117] and stubborn blockage. [Li] Shizhen.

1112 *Tou feng* 頭風, "head wind." Condition of wind evil attacking the head followed by pain, dizziness, itching. BCGM Dict I, 509.

1113 *Yong* 癰, "obstruction-illness," refers to an obstruction of vessels or other ducts inside the body. Qi rushing against the obstruction may cause a local swelling and eventually break through the surface to cause an abscess. BCGM Dict I, 641.

1114 *Ding* 丁, "pin[-illness]," also *ding* 疔, "pin-illness," refers to a deep-reaching and festering hardness in a tissue, eventually rising above the skin like a pinhead. BCGM Dict I, 127-129.

1115 *Li jie [feng]* 歴節[風], pervading joints [wind], a condition of *tong feng* 痛風, "pain wind," characterized by spontaneous sweating, shortness of qi/breath, aching joints, and difficulties in bending and stretching. BCGM Dict I, 314.

1116 *Luo li* 瘰癧, "scrofula pervasion-illness," when two or more connected swellings of the size of plum or date kernels appear either on the neck or in the armpits, or somewhere else on the body. BCGM Dict I. 329.

1117 *Da feng* 大風, "massive wind," may refer to sores caused by a massive intrusion of wind evil and also to conditions of leprosy. BCGM Dict I, 111.

17-21-02
射罔 *She wang*

Aconite paste "to cast a net."

【氣味】苦，有大毒。【之才曰】温。【大明曰】人中射罔毒，以甘草、藍汁、小豆葉、浮萍、冷水、薺苨，皆可一味禦之。

Qi and Flavor. Bitter, very poisonous. [Xu] Zhicai: Warm. Da Ming: When a human is struck by *she wang* poison, *glycyrrhiza* [root], indigo juice (16-43-02),[1118] mung bean leaves, ducksmeat, cold water and apricot-leaved *adenophora* [root] applied as single substance are able to rescue the [victim].

【主治】尸疰癥堅，及頭中風痺。別録。瘻瘡瘡根，結核瘰癧，毒腫及蛇咬。先取塗肉四畔，漸漸近瘡，習習逐病至骨。瘡有熟膿及黄水，塗之。若無膿水，有生血，及新傷破，即不可塗，立殺人。藏器。

Control. Corpse-qi attachment-illness[1119] with concretion-illness hardenings, and also blockage related to wind [intrusion] into the head. *Bie lu*. Scrofula sores; the base of sores. Nodular kernels with scrofula pervasion-illness,[1120] swelling caused by poison and snake bites. At first apply it to all four sides of the [affected] flesh. It gradually reaches the sore and slow by slow pursues the disease until it reaches the bones. When a sore is filled with pus and yellow water, apply [*she wang*] to it. If neither pus nor [yellow] water are present, and if [the sore] has fresh blood, or in the case of a fresh, open wound, do not apply it. It would kill that person instantly. [Chen] Cangqi.

【發明】【時珍曰】草烏頭、射罔，乃至毒之藥。非若川烏頭、附子，人所栽種，加以釀制殺其毒性之比。自非風頑急疾，不可輕投。甄權藥性論言其益陽事，治男子腎氣衰弱者，未可遽然也。此類止能搜風勝濕，開頑痰，治頑瘡，以毒攻毒而已，豈有川烏頭、附子補右腎命門之功哉？吾蘄郝知府自負知醫，因病風癬，服草烏頭、木鼈子藥過多，甫入腹而麻痺，遂至不救，可不慎乎。【機曰】烏喙形如烏嘴，其氣鋒鋭。宜其通經絡，利關節，尋蹊達徑，而直抵病所。煎爲射罔，能殺禽獸。非氣之鋒鋭捷利，能如是乎？【楊清叟曰】凡風寒濕痺，骨内冷痛，及損傷入骨，年久發痛，或一切陰疽腫毒。並宜草烏頭、南星等分，少加肉桂爲末，薑汁、

1118 Instead of *lan zhi* 藍汁, "indigo juice," *Zheng lei* ch. 10, *wu tou* 烏頭, writes *lan qing* 藍青.

1119 *Shi zhu* 尸疰, "corpse [qi] attachment-illness," a condition of a slowly developing infectious weakness. BCGM Dict I, 202.

1120 *Luo li* 瘰癧, "scrofula pervasion-illness," when two or more connected swellings of the size of plum or date kernels appear either on the neck or in the armpits, or somewhere else on the body. BCGM Dict I. 329.

熱酒調塗。未破者能内消，久潰者能去黑爛。二藥性味辛烈，能破惡塊，逐寒熱，遇冷即消，遇熱即潰。

Explication. [Li] Shizhen: *Cao wu tou* and *she wang* are extremely poisonous pharmaceutical drugs. They are not like *chuan wu tou* 川烏頭, *aconitum* [main tuber from Si] chuan, and *fu zi* 附子, *aconitum* [accessory tuber], that are cultivated by the people and processed to kill their poisonous nature. [*Cao wu tou* and *she wang*] should not be given lightly [to patients], except for stubborn, critical illnesses related to wind [stroke/intrusion]. Zhen Quan in his *Yao xing lun* says: "It boosts the yang affair," and "It serves to cure weak kidney qi of males." There is no evidence of this. [Substances of] this kind are only able to dispel wind and overcome moisture, to open [pathways blocked by] stubborn phlegm and to cure stubborn sores, because this is nothing more than their poison attacking [the patient's] poison. How could *chuan wu tou* 川烏頭, *aconitum* [main tuber from Si] chuan, and *fu zi* 附子, *aconitum* [accessory tuber], have a [therapeutic] potential of supplementing [the qi of] the right kidney, (i. e.,) the Gate of Life? Prefect Hao of my [home region] Qi [zhou] thought of himself to know medicine. Hence, when he suffered from wind [intrusion] with *xuan*-illness,[1121] he ingested excessive quantities of *cao wu tou* 草烏頭 and *mu bie zi* 木鼈子. They simply entered his abdomen whereupon he turned numb and eventually reached a status in which he could no longer be saved. [That example] must make one act cautiously! [Wang] Ji: *Wu hui* 烏喙 is shaped like a crow's, *wu* 烏, beak, *zui* 嘴. Its qi are very sharp. That makes it suitable [for use as a medication] to penetrate conduits and network [vessels], to free the movement of/through joints, and to find paths and access tracks leading [pharmaceutical drugs] directly to the location of a disease. Boiled to prepare *she wang*, it can kill fowl and animals. If it were not for the fast actions of its sharp qi, how could it have such [effects]? Yang Qingsou: For all conditions of blockage related to wind [intrusion] and the presence of cold and moisture, with painful cold in the bones, harm caused by injuries reaching into the bones, with a pain continuing for years, and also all types of swelling with poison related to an impediment-illness[1122] in the yin [(i. e., genital) region, the following recipe is applicable]. Grind equal amounts of *cao wu tou* and Indian turnip [root], with a little cinnamom bark added, into powder and apply it,

1121 *Xuan* 癬, "*xuan*-illness." Conditions of dermal lesions with initially erythema, papules, and itching gradually extending in all directions to form an irregular ring with clear boundaries. The skin is slightly elevated with small papules, blisters, and/or scales and scraps. The central lesion may appear to heal spontaneously, and it may reappear. Also, a designation of local lesions with itching, release of liquid and shedding of scabs. BCGM Dict I, 591.

1122 *Ju* 疽, "impediment-illness," refers to an obstruction of vessels or other ducts inside the body. Qi rushing against the impediment may cause a local swelling and eventually break through the surface to cause an abscess. BCGM Dict I, 277.

mixed with ginger juice and hot wine, [to the affected region]. If the [swelling] has not opened yet, it can dissolve its interior; if it has festered for a long time, it can eliminate the black, decayed [flesh]. The nature and the flavors of these two pharmaceutical drugs are acrid and violent; they can break through malign lumps and dispel cold and heat. When they encounter [a swelling related to] cold, they dissolve it. When they encounter [a swelling related to] heat, they stimulate excretion.

【附方】舊四，新四十八。
Added Recipes. Four of old. 48 newly [recorded].

陰毒傷寒。生草烏頭爲末，以葱頭蘸藥納穀道中，名提盆散。王海藏陰證略例。

Yin poison[1123] associated with harm caused by cold. [Grind] fresh *cao wu tou* into powder, dip the tip of an onion stalk into [the powder of] this pharmaceutical drug and insert it into the anus. [The recipe] is called "powder to lift a pot." Wang Haicang, *Yin zheng lue li.*

二便不通。即上方，名霹靂箭。

The two [minor (urination) and major, (defecation) kinds of] relief are blocked. The recipe is identical to the previous one. It is called "thunderbolt arrow."

中風癱瘓。手足顫掉，言語蹇澀。左經丸：用草烏頭炮去皮四兩，川烏頭炮去皮二兩，乳香、没藥各一兩，爲末。生烏豆一升，以斑蝥三七個，去頭翅，同煮，豆熟去蝥，取豆焙乾爲末。和匀，以醋麪糊丸梧子大。每服三十丸，温酒下。簡易方。

Wind stroke with paralysis, hands and feet tremble, language is impeded. The "pills to assist the conduits." [Grind] four *liang* of *cao wu tou*, roasted and with the skin removed, two *liang* of *chuan wu tou*, roasted and with the skin removed, as well as one *liang* each of frankincense and myrrh into powder. Boil one *sheng* of fresh black soybeans together with three times seven blister beetles, with their head and wings removed, and discard the beetles when the beans are done. Then dry the beans over a fire in a pan and [grind them into] powder. Evenly mix [this powder with the earlier powder] and with vinegar and wheat flour form a paste to make pills the size

1123 *Yin du* 陰毒, "yin poison," a condition of *shang han* 傷寒, "harm caused by cold," resulting in a flourishing of only yin qi and a diminution of yang qi, with cold extremities and a greenish facial complexion, pain in the abdomen and affecting the entire body, as well as a deep-lying and fine movement in the vessels. BCGM Dict I, 633 (where yang and yin are erroneously exchanged).

of *wu* seeds. Each time [let the patient] ingest 30 pills, to be sent down with warm wine. *Jian yi fang*.

癱瘓頑風，骨節疼痛，下元虛冷，諸風痔漏下血，一切風瘡。草烏頭、川烏頭、兩頭尖各三錢，硫黃、麝香、丁香各一錢，木鼈子五個，爲末。以熟蘄艾揉軟，合成一處，用鈔紙包裹，燒熏病處。名雷丸。孫天仁集效方。

Paralysis with stubborn wind [disease], painful bones and joints, depletion cold in the original [long-term depot (i. e., the kidneys)] in the lower [body part], all types of wind [disease] associated with leaking piles and blood discharge, and all types of sores related to wind [intrusion]. [Grind] three *qian* each of *cao wu tou*, *chuan wu tou* and *liang tou jian*, one *qian* each of sulphur, musk and cloves, as well as five pieces of *mu bie zi* (here: aconitum tuber, 17-20) into powder. Rub heat processed mugwort leaves from Qi [zhou] to a soft [powder], mix it with the earlier powder, wrap this in paper money and burn it to fumigate the location of the disease with the smoke. [This recipe] is called "thunder pills." Sun Tianren, *Ji xiao fang*.

諸風不遂。朱氏集驗方用生草烏頭、晚蠶沙等分，爲末。取生地龍搗和，入少醋糊丸梧子大。每服四五丸，白湯下，甚妙。勿多服，恐麻人。名鄂渚小金丹。

All types of wind [stroke with the limbs] failing to follow [one's will]. The *Zhu shi ji yan fang* [recommends to grind] equal amounts of fresh *cao wu tou* and late [generation] silkworm feces into powder. Then pound a living earth worm to pulp and mix it [with the powder], add a little vinegar and form [with wheat flour] a paste to make pills the size of *wu* seeds. Each time [let the patient] ingest four to five pills, to be sent down with clear, boiled water. Very wondrous. Do not let him ingest too many [pills]. They might numb that person. [This recipe] is called "little golden elixir from the islet in E."

經驗濟世方用草烏頭四兩去皮，大豆半升，鹽一兩，同以沙瓶煮三伏時，去豆，將烏頭入木臼搗三百杵，作餅焙乾爲末，酒糊丸梧子大，每空心鹽湯下十丸。名至寶丹。

The *Jing yan ji shi fang* [recommends to] boil four *liang* of *cao wu tou*, half a *sheng* of soybeans and one *liang* of salt in an earthenware jar for three full days. Then remove the soybeans and pound the *wu tou* in a wooden mortar 300 times. Prepare it to cakes, dry them over a fire in a pan and [grind them into] powder. With wine [and wheat flour] form a paste and make pills the size of *wu* seeds. Each time send down on an empty stomach with a salt decoction ten pills. [This recipe] is called the "highly precious elixir."

一切頑風。神應丹：用生草烏頭、生天麻各洗，等分，擂爛絞汁傾盆中。砌一小坑，其下燒火，將盆放坑上。每日用竹片攪一次，夜則露之。晒至成膏，作成小鋌子。每一鋌分作三服，用葱、薑自然汁和好酒熱服。乾坤秘韞。

All types of stubborn wind [diseases]. The "elixir with a divine response." Pound equal amounts of fresh *cao wu tou* and fresh *gastrodia* [root], all washed clean, to a pulp, squeeze it to obtain a juice and pour it into a pot. Dig a small pit in the ground and light a fire on its bottom. Place the pot on the pit. Every day stir [the juice] with a piece of bamboo once. During the night leave the pot in the open. Wait until [the juice] has dried in the sun into a paste. Form it to small sticks and each time divide one stick to be ingested in three portions. Ingest them with a hot mixture of the natural juice of onions, ginger and good wine. *Qian ku mi yun*.

一切風證。不問頭風痛風，黄鴉吊脚風痺。生淮烏頭一斤，生川烏頭一枚，生附子一枚，並爲末。葱一斤，薑一斤，擂如泥，和作餅子。以草鋪盤内，加楮葉於上，安餅於葉上，又鋪草葉蓋之。待出汗黄一日夜，乃晒之，舂爲末，以生薑取汁煮麪糊和丸梧子大。初服三十丸，日二服，服後身痺汗出即愈。避風。乾坤秘韞。

All types of wind [disease] conditions, including head wind, pain wind, yellow crow hoisting legs wind[1124] with blockage. [Grind] one *jin* of fresh *wu tou* from Huai, one fresh *wu tou* from [Si] chuan and one fresh *fu zi*, *aconitum* [accessory tuber], together into powder. Pound one *jin* of onions and one *jin* of ginger to a mud. Mix [it with the powder] and form cakes. Spread one layer of straw on a plate, add paper mulberry tree leaves on top of them, and place the cakes on top of these leaves. Then again spread straw on them to cover them. Leave it until it releases a yellow sweat for one day and one night, and [grind it] in a mortar into powder. Obtain the juice of fresh ginger, boil [the powder in it] and with wheat flour form a paste to make pills the size of *wu* seeds. In the beginning, ingest 30 pills; to be ingested twice a day. If the body experiences a blockage after ingestion, it is [a sign of] healing. [During this therapy] avoid wind. *Qian kun mi yu*.

破傷風病。壽域方用草烏頭爲末，每以一二分温酒服之，出汗。

Diseases of wind [intrusion] into an open wound. The *Shou yu fang* [recommends to grind] *cao wu tou* into powder. Each time ingest with warm wine one or two *fen* to cause sweating.

1124 *Huang ya diao jiao feng* 黄鴉吊脚風, lit.: "yellow crow hoisting legs [caused by] wind [intrusion]." *Diao jiao* 吊脚, "to hoist the legs," refers to contracted sinews, resulting from a blockage related to wind intrusion. To add *huang ya* 黄鴉, "yellow crow" to some disease terms was fashionable during the Song era and later; the conceptual origin and meaning of such designations remain unclear.

儒門事親方用草烏尖、白芷，并生研末。每服半錢，冷酒一盞，入葱白一根，同煎服。少頃以葱白熱粥投之，汗出立愈。

The *Ru men shi qin* has a recipe [recommending to grind] fresh *cao wu* pointed ends and fresh *angelica dahurica* [root] into powder. Each time ingest half a *qian*. Boil it with one cup of cold wine to which is added one onion root, and ingest this. After a short while eat a hot gruel made with onions. Once a sweating begins, a cure is achieved instantly.

年久麻痺，或歷節走氣，疼痛不仁，不拘男女。神授散：用草烏頭半斤，去皮爲末。以袋一個，盛豆腐半袋，入烏末在內，再將豆腐填滿壓乾，入鍋中煮一夜，其藥即堅如石，取出晒乾爲末，每服五分。冷風濕氣，以生薑湯下。麻木不仁，以葱白湯下之。活人心統。

Numbness lasting for years. Or pervading joints [wind][1125] with running qi, pain and numbness. Regardless of whether males or females are affected. The "powder conferred by spirits." Remove the skin of half a *jin* of *cao wu tou* and [grind it into] powder. Fill a pouch half with bean curd and add the [*cao*] *wu* [*tou*] powder to it. Then add further bean curd until [the pouch] is filled and squeeze it until it is dry. Give it into a cauldron and heat it for one night. The pharmaceutical drug will be as hard as a stone. Take it out, dry it in the sun and [grind it into] powder. Each time ingest five *fen*. In the case of wind [intrusion] with cold, send it down with a fresh ginger decoction. In the case of numbness, send it down with an onion decoction. *Huo ren xin tong*.

風濕痺木。黑神丸：草烏頭連皮生研、五靈脂等分，爲末，六月六日滴水丸彈子大。四十歲以下分六服，病甚一丸作二服，薄荷湯化下，覺微麻爲度。本事方。

Numbness related to wind [intrusion] and the presence of moisture. The "black spirit pills." [Grind] fresh *cao wu tou*, with its skin, and flying squirrel droppings into powder. On the sixth day of the sixth month drip water into it and prepare pills the size of a bullet. Patients 40 years of age or younger ingest this divided into six portions. In the case of a serious disease ingest one pill divided into two portions, to be sent down dissolved in a mint decoction, until there is a slight sensation of numbness. *Ben shi fang*.

1125 *Li jie* [*feng*] 歷節[風], pervading joints [wind], a condition of *tong feng* 痛風, "pain wind," characterized by spontaneous sweating, shortness of qi/breath, aching joints, and difficulties in bending and stretching. BCGM Dict I, 314.

風濕走痛。黑弩箭丸：用兩頭尖、五靈脂各一兩，乳香、没藥、當歸各三錢，爲末，醋糊丸梧子大。每服十丸至三十丸，臨卧温酒下。忌油膩、濕麪。孕婦勿服。瑞竹堂方。

Running pain related to wind [intrusion] and the presence of moisture. The "black crossbow arrow pills." [Grind] one *liang* each of *liang tou jian* and flying squirrel droppings, and three *qian* each of frankincense, myrrh and Chinese *angelica* [root] into powder. With vinegar [and wheat flour] paste form pills the size of *wu* seeds. Each time ingest from ten up to 30 pills, to be sent down at bedtime with warm wine. [During this therapy] oily and fat items, and moist noodles are to be avoided. Pregnant women must not ingest [these pills]. *Rui zhu tang fang*.

腰脚冷痛。烏頭三個，去皮臍，研末，醋調貼，須臾痛止。十便良方。

Painful cold in the lower back and legs. Grind three *wu tou* [tubers], with skin and navel[1126] removed, into powder. Mix it with vinegar and attach it [to the affected region]. After a short time, the pain ends. *Shi bian liang fang*.

膝風作痛。草烏、細辛、防風等分，爲末，摻靴襪中，及安護膝内，能除風濕健步。扶壽方。

Painful wind [intrusion] in the knees. [Grind] equal amounts of *cao wu* [*tou*], *asarum heteropoides* [root] and *saposhnikovia* [root] into powder. Give it into the boots or stockings, and also into the kneecap. It will be able to dispel wind and moisture and to strengthen one's ability to walk. *Fu shou fang*.

遠行脚腫。草烏、細辛、防風等分，爲末，摻鞋底内。如草鞋，以水微濕摻之。用之可行千里，甚妙。經驗方。

Legs swollen when walking for long distances. [Grind] equal amounts of *cao wu* [*tou*], *asarum heteropoides* [root] and *saphoshnikovia* [root] into powder and place it on the soles of the shoes. If the are shoes made of straw, moisten them with a little water. An application of this [method] lets one walk a thousand miles. Very wondrous. *Jing yan fang*.

脚氣掣痛，或胯間有核。生草烏頭、大黄、木鼈子作末，薑汁煎茶調貼之。又法：草烏一味爲末，以薑汁或酒糟同搗貼之。永類方。

Leg qi[1127] with tugging pain, sometimes with kernels developing in the hips. [grind fresh *cao wu tou*, rhubarb root and *momordica* seeds into powder. Boil a tea with ginger juice, mix this with the powder and apply it [to the affected region]. Another

1126 *Qi* 臍, "navel," is the indentation at the top of the tuber where it was connected with the stem of the plant. "To remove skin and navel" has the meaning of "to clean thoroughly."

1127 *Jiao qi* 脚氣, "leg qi." Painful, weak, swollen legs. BCGM Dict I, 248.

method: [Grind] *cao wu* [*tou*] alone into powder, pound it with ginger juice or distillers' grains [to a pulp] and apply this [to the affected region]. *Yong lei fang.*

濕滯足腫，早輕晚重。用草烏頭一兩，以生薑一兩同研，交感一宿。蒼术一兩，以葱白一兩同研，交感一宿。各焙乾爲末，酒糊丸梧子大。每服五十丸，酒下。艾元英如宜方。

Sluggish moisture in the feet causing swelling that is slight in the morning and severe at night. Grind one *liang* of *cao wu tou* together with one *liang* of fresh ginger, and let them interact for one night. Grind one *liang* of *atractylodes lancea* [rhizome] and one *liang* of onions and let them interact for one night. Dry both [mixtures] over a fire in a pan and [grind them into] powder. With wine and [wheat flour] form a paste and make pills the size of *wu* seeds. Each time ingest 50 pills, to be sent down with wine. Ai Yuanying, *Ru yi fang.*

除風去濕。治脾胃虛弱，久積冷氣，飲食減少。用草烏頭一斤，蒼术二斤，以去白陳皮半斤，生甘草四兩，黑豆三升，水一石，同煮乾，只揀烏、术晒焙爲末，酒糊丸梧子大，焙乾收之。每空心温酒下二三十丸，覺麻即漸減之。名烏术丸。集簡方。

To dispel wind and remove moisture, and to cure depletion and weakness of spleen and stomach, as well as long-time accumulations of cold qi, with decreased intake of beverages and food. Boil one *jin* of *cao wu tou*, two *jin* of *atractylodes lancea* [rhizome], half a *jin* of tangerine peels, with the white stuff discarded, four *liang* of fresh *glycyrrhiza* [roots] and three *sheng* of black soybeans in one *dan* of water until [the water] has dried. Then take out just the *wu* [*tou*] and the *atractylodes lancea* [rhizome], dry them in the sun and/or over a fire in a pan, and [grind them into] powder. With wine and [wheat flour] paste form pills the size of *wu* seeds, dry them over a fire in a pan and store them. Each time on an empty stomach send down with warm wine 20 to 30 pills. As soon as a feeling of numbness begins gradually reduce their number. [This recipe] is called "pills with *wu* [*tou*] and *atractylodes lancea* [rhizome]." *Ji jian fang.*

偏正頭風。草烏頭四兩，川芎藭四兩，蒼术半斤，生薑四兩，連鬚生葱一把，搗爛，同入瓷瓶，封固埋土中。春五、夏三、秋五、冬七日，取出晒乾。揀去葱、薑，爲末，醋麪糊和丸梧子大。每服九丸，臨卧温酒下，立效。戴古渝經驗方。

Unilateral and proper head wind.[1128] Pound four *liang* of *cao wu tou*, four *liang* of [Si] chuan *ligusticum* [root], half a *jin* of *atractylodes lancea* [rhizome], four *liang* of

1128 *Tou feng* 頭風, "head wind." Condition of wind evil attacking the head followed by pain, dizziness, itching. BCGM Dict I, 509.

fresh ginger and one handful of fresh onions with their hair to a pulp and fill it into a porcelain jar. Seal it tightly and bury it in the ground. In spring for five days. In summer for three days. In autumn for five days. In winter for seven days. Then take it out again, dry [the contents] in the sun and [grind them into] powder. Take out the onions and the ginger and grind [the remaining substances] into powder. With vinegar and wheat flour prepare a paste to make pills the size of *wu* seeds. Each time ingest nine pills, to be sent down with warm wine at bedtime. Immediately effective. Du Guyu, *Jing yan fang*.

久患頭風。草烏頭尖生用一分，赤小豆三十五粒，麝香一字，爲末。每服半錢，薄荷湯冷服。更隨左右嗜鼻。指南方。

Chronic suffering from head wind. [Grind] one *fen* of fresh *cao wu tou* pointed ends, 35 mung beans and one *zi* of musk into powder. Each time ingest half a *qian*, to be ingested cold with a mint decoction. Also, depending on whether [the pain is] on the left or right [side of the head] inhale [the powder into the respective] nostril. *Zhi nan fang*.

風痰頭痛。體虛傷風，停聚痰飲，上厥頭痛，或偏或正。草烏頭炮去皮尖半兩，川烏頭生去皮尖一兩，藿香半兩，乳香三皂子大，爲末。每服二錢，薄荷薑湯下，食後服。陳言三因方。

Headache related to wind [intrusion] and the presence of phlegm. Bodily weakness with harm caused by wind. Phlegm rheum collection. Rising ceasing [qi] causing headache, either unilateral or proper. [Grind] half a *liang* of *cao wu tou*, roasted, with the skin and the pointed ends removed, one *liang* of *chuan wu tou*, fresh, with skin and the pointed ends removed, half a *liang* of *agastache* [herb] and frankincense the size of three *gleditsia* pods into powder. Each time ingest two *qian*, to be sent down with a mint and ginger decoction. To be ingested after a meal. Chen Yan, *San yin fang*.

女人頭痛，血風證。草烏頭、巵子等分，爲末。自然葱汁，隨左右調塗太陽及額上，勿過眼，避風。濟生方。

Headache of women, with signs of a blood wind[1129] [condition]. [Grind] equal amounts of *cao wu tou* and *gardenia* [fruit] into powder, mix it with the natural juice of onions, and depending on whether [the pain is on the left or on the right] apply it to the left or right major yang [needle insertion hole at the temples], and also to

1129 *Xue feng* 血風, "blood wind," a condition introduced in *Zhu bing yuan hou lun* ch. 15 as brought about by an intrusion of wind evil qi into an unbalanced state of qi and blood, mostly in women. BCGM Dict I, 594.

the forehead. It must not be inflicted on the eyes. [During this therapy,] exposure to wind is to be avoided. *Ji sheng fang.*

腦洩臭穢。草烏去皮半兩，蒼术一兩，川芎二兩，並生研末，麪糊丸綠豆大。每服十丸，茶下。忌一切熱物。聖濟總録。

Malodorous, dirty brain outflow [from the nose]. Grind half a *liang* of *cao wu* [*tou*], with the skin removed, one *liang* of *atractylodes lancea* [rhizome] and two *liang* of [Si] chuan *ligusticum* [root], all fresh, into powder and form with a wheat flour paste pills the size of mung beans. Each time ingest ten pills, to be sent down with tea. [During this therapy] avoid all hot items. *Sheng ji zong lu.*

耳鳴耳癢，如流水及風聲，不治成聾。用生烏頭掘得，乘濕削如棗核大，塞之。日易二次。不過三日愈。千金方。

Sounds in the ears, and itching ears, as if there was flowing water or the sounds of wind. If this is not cured, it will end in deafness. Undig a fresh *wu tou* [tuber] and while it is still moist carve from it a piece the size of a Chinese date pit. Insert it [into the affected ear]. Replace it twice per day. A cure is achieved after no more than three days. *Qian jin fang.*

喉痺口噤不開，欲死。草烏頭、皂莢等分，爲末，入麝香少許。擦牙并嗃鼻内，牙關自開也。

Throat closure and clenched jaws that won't open and bring one close to dying. [Grind] equal amounts of *cao wu tou* and *gleditsia* pods/seeds into powder, add a little musk and rub this on the [patient's] teeth. At the same time, let him inhale it into his nose. The teeth will unlock as a result.

濟生方用草烏尖、石膽等分，爲末。每用一錢，醋煮皂莢汁調稀，掃入腫上，流涎數次，其毒即破也。

The *Ji sheng fang* [recommends to grind] equal amounts of *cao wu* [*tou*] pointed ends and chalanthite into powder. Each time use one *qian*. Mix a small amount with a decoction of *gleditsia* juice in vinegar and brush it on the swelling. There will be several streams of saliva, and they serve to crush the poison.

虚壅口瘡，滿口連舌者。草烏一個，南星一個，生薑一大塊，爲末，睡時以醋調塗手心足心。或以草烏頭、吴茱萸等分，爲末，蜜調塗足心。本事方。

A depletion with sores obstructing the mouth. They cover the entire mouth and also the tongue. [Grind] one *cao wu* [*tou* tuber], one Indian turnip [root] and one big piece of fresh ginger into powder, at bedtime mix it with vinegar and apply it to the palms of the hands and the soles of the feet. Or [grind] equal amounts of *cao wu tou* and *zanthoxylum* [fruit] into powder, mix it with honey and apply it to the soles of the feet. *Ben shi fang*.

疳蝕口鼻穿透者。草烏頭燒灰，入麝香等分，爲末貼之。

Gan-illness[1130] with an erosion of mouth and nose penetrating [the skin]. Burn *cao wu tou* to ashes, add an equal amount of musk, [grind this into] powder and attach it [to the affected region].

風蟲牙痛。草烏炒黑一兩，細辛一錢，爲末揩之，吐出涎。

Toothache related to wind [intrusion] and the presence of worms/bugs. [Grind] one liang of *cao wu* [*tou* tubers], roasted until they are black, and one *qian* of *asarum heteropoides* [root] into powder and apply it [to the affected teeth]. Spit out the saliva that forms.

一方：草烏、食鹽同炒黑，摻之。海上方。

Another recipe. Roast *cao wu* [*tou* tubers] and table salt together until [the tubers] are black and apply this [to the affected teeth]. *Hai shang fang*.

寒氣心疝三十年者。射罔、食茱萸等分，爲末，蜜丸麻子大。每酒下二丸，日三服。劉國英所秘之方。范汪東陽方。

Heart elevation-illness[1131] related to cold qi that has lasted for 30 years. [Grind] equal amounts of *she wang* and *zanthoxylum* [fruit] into powder and form with honey pills the size of hemp seeds. Each time send down with wine two pills, to be ingested three times a day. This is a recipe kept secret by Liu Guoying. Fan Wang, *Dong yang fang*.

寒瘧積瘧。巴豆一枚去心皮，射罔如巴豆大，大棗去皮一枚，搗成丸梧子大。清旦、先發時各服一丸，白湯下。肘後方。

Cold malaria, accumulation malaria.[1132] Pound one *croton* seed with the heart and the skin removed, a piece of *she wang* aconite paste the size of a *croton* seed, and one

1130 *Gan* 疳, "*gan*-illness," also: "sweets-illness," involves several complaints that affect children and adults, with causes and conditions too different to fall into a known disease category. BCGM Dict I, 180-188.

1131 *Xin shan* 心疝, "heart elevation-illness," a condition of heartache caused by cold qi, and accompanied by counterflow cold in the four extremities with the lips and mouth assuming a greenish-blue color. BCGM Dict I, 578.

1132 *Ji nue* 積瘧, "accumulation malaria," identical to *shi nüe* 食瘧, "food malaria." A condition of *nüe ji* 瘧疾, "malaria ailment," associated with food accumulation. The clinical appearance, in addition to regularly recurring alternating sensations of cold and heat, includes a feeling of distension and pain in the stomach tract and abdomen, sometimes with a tendency to avoid eating. BCGM Dict I, 240, 453.

Chinese date, with the skin removed, [to a pulp] and form pills the size of *wu* seeds. In the early morning, prior to an outbreak, ingest one pill, to be sent down with clear, boiled water. *Zhou hou fang*.

脾寒厥瘧。先寒後熱，名寒瘧。但寒不熱，面色黑者名厥瘧。寒多熱少，面黃腹痛，名脾瘧。三者並宜服此。賈耘老用之二十年，累試有效。不蛀草烏頭削去皮，沸湯泡二七度，以盞蓋良久，切焙研，稀糊丸梧子大。每服三十丸，薑十片，棗三枚，葱三根，煎湯清早服，以棗壓之。如人行十里許，再一服。絶勿飲湯，便不發也。蘇東坡良方。

Spleen [malaria], cold [malaria] and ceasing [yang qi] malaria. [Patients] sense cold first and heat afterwards. This is called "cold malaria." When they sense only cold and no heat at all, and if the facial complexion is black, this is called "ceasing [yang qi] malaria." If [patients] sense much cold and little heat, and if the face is yellow and the abdomen aches, this is "spleen malaria." For all three it is suitable to ingest the following [medication]. Old Jia Yun used it for 20 years; he repeatedly tested it and it proved to be effective. Cut off the skin from *cao wu tou* that is not moth infested and steep it in water boiled to bubbling two times seven times. Keep it covered in a bowl for a long time, then cut it into pieces, dry them over a fire in a pan, [grind them into] powder and form with a watery [wheat flour] paste pills the size of *wu* seeds. Each time ingest 30 pills. Boil them with ten ginger slices, three Chinese dates and three onion roots in clear water and ingest [the liquid] in the early morning. Press it down with Chinese dates. After the time it takes for someone to walk ten miles, ingest [the same dose] a second time. Do not drink boiled water. This will prevent an outbreak. Su Dongpo, *Liang fang*.

腹中癥結。害妨飲食，羸瘦。射罔二兩，椒三百粒，搗末，雞子白和丸麻子大。每服一丸，漸至三丸，以愈爲度。肘後方。

Nodular concretion in the abdomen blocking the consumption of beverages and food, and causing emaciation. Pound two *liang* of *she wang* and 300 pepper grains into powder. Mix it with chicken egg white and form pills the size of hemp seeds. Each time ingest one pill and gradually increase the dose to three pills until a cure is achieved. *Zhou hou fang*.

水泄寒痢。大草烏一兩，以一半生研，一半燒灰，醋糊和丸緑豆大。每服七丸，井華水下。忌生冷魚肉。十便良方。

Watery outflow and cold free-flux illness. Grind [to powder] one half of a big *cao wu* [*tou* tuber] weighing one *liang* fresh and the other half burned to ashes and form with a vinegar and [wheat flour] a paste to prepare pills the size of mung beans.

Each time ingest seven pills, to be sent down with well splendor water[1133]. [During this therapy] avoid fresh and cold items, fish and meat. *Shi bian liang fang*.

泄痢注下。三神丸：治清濁不分，泄瀉注下，或赤或白，腹臍刺痛，裹急後重。用台烏頭三個去皮尖，以一個火炮，一個醋煮，一個燒灰，爲末，醋糊丸綠豆大，每服二十丸。水瀉流水下，赤痢甘草湯下，白痢薑湯下。忌魚腥生冷。和劑局方。

A pouring discharge as outflow and free-flux illness. The "three spirits pills." They serve to cure a failure of clear and turbid [excretions] to separate with an outflow as pouring discharge, sometimes red, sometimes white, with a piercing pain in the abdominal region and at the navel, as well as internal tension and a feeling of heaviness. Remove the skin and the pointed ends from three *tai wu tou* [tubers].[1134] Roast one of them over a fire. Boil one of them in vinegar. Burn one of them to ashes, and [grind all of them together into] powder. With a vinegar and [wheat flour] paste form it to pills the size of mung beans. Each time ingest 20 pills. In the case of an outflow of water, send them down with running water. In the case of red free-flux illness, send them down with a *glycyrrhiza* [root] decoction. In the case of white free-flux illness, send them down with a ginger decoction. [During this therapy] fish, items with a smell of fish, fresh items and cold items are to be avoided. *He ji ju fang*.

結陰下血，腹痛。草烏頭，蛤粉炒，去皮臍切一兩，茴香炒三兩。每用三錢，水一盞，入鹽少許，煎八分，去滓，露一夜，五更冷服。聖濟錄。

Bound yin [qi] and blood discharge with abdominal pain. One *liang* of *cao wu tou* is fried with clam shell powder. Then the skin and the navel[1135] [of the tubers] are removed and they are cut into pieces. Add three *liang* of fried fennel. Each time boil three *qian* [of this mixture] down to 80% in one cup of water to which a little salt is added. Discard the dregs, leave [the decoction] in the open for one night, and ingest it cold in the early morning. *Sheng ji lu*.

老人遺尿不知出者。草烏頭一兩，童便浸七日，去皮，同鹽炒，爲末，酒糊丸綠豆大。每服二十丸，鹽湯下。普濟方。

Old people losing urine without noticing it. Soak one *liang* of *cao wu tou* in boys' urine for seven days, remove the skin, fry [the tubers] together with salt, grind them

1133 *Jing hua shui* 井華水, "well splendor water," i. e., the first water drawn from a well in the morning. BCGM Vol. II, 05-15-01.

1134 Instead of *tai wu tou* 台烏頭, *Ju fang* ch. 6, *zhi xie li* 治瀉痢, "to cure outflow and free-flux illness," *san shen wan* 三神丸, "three spirits pills," writes *cao wu* 草烏.

1135 *Qi* 臍, "navel," is the indentation at the top of the tuber where it was connected with the stem of the plant. "To remove skin and navel" has the meaning of "to clean thoroughly."

into powder and with wine [and wheat flour] prepare a paste to form pills the size of mung beans. Each time ingest 20 pills, to be sent down with a salt decoction. *Pu ji fang.*

内痔不出。草烏爲末，津調點肛門内，痔即反出，乃用枯痔藥點之。外科集驗方。

Internal piles that fail to appear. [Grind] *cao wu* [*tou into*] *powder*, mix it with saliva and apply it to the interior of the anus. When the piles appear, drip a "medication to let piles wither" on them. *Wai ke ji yan fang.*

疔毒初起。草烏頭七個，川烏頭三個，杏仁九個，飛羅麪一兩，爲末。無根水調搽，留口以紙蓋之，乾則以水潤之。唐瑶經驗方。

Pin-illness[1136] poison that has just begun to rise. [Grind] seven *cao wu tou* [tubers], three *chuan wu tou* [tubers], nine apricot kernels, and one *liang* of fine wheat flour into powder. Mix it with "water that has no root,"[1137] and apply [this to the affected region]. Cover [the affected region] with paper, leaving open one hole. When it has dried, moisten it with water. *Tang Yao jing yan fang.*

疔毒惡腫。生烏頭切片，醋熬成膏，攤貼。次日根出。又方：兩頭尖一兩，巴豆四個，搗貼。疔自拔出。普濟方。

Pin-illness poison with a malign swelling. Cut fresh *wu tou* to pieces, simmer them in vinegar to generate a paste, and apply it [to the affected region]. The root will come out the following day. Another recipe: Pound one *liang* of *liang tou jian* and four *croton* [seeds to a pulp] and apply it [to the affected region.] The pin-illness will be pulled out. *Pu ji fang.*

疔瘡發背。草烏頭去皮爲末，用葱白連鬚和搗，丸豌豆大，以雄黄爲衣。每服一丸，先將葱一根細嚼，以熱酒送下。或有惡心，嘔三四口，用冷水一口止之。即卧，以被厚蓋，汗出爲度。亦治頭風。乾坤秘韞。

Pin-illness sores effusing on the back. [Grind] *cao wu tou*, with the skin removed, into powder and pound it together with onions, with their hair retained, [to a pulp] to be formed to pills the size of garden peas. They are coated with realgar. Each time ingest one pill. First finely chew one onion root, then send [the pill] down with hot wine. It may be that [patients] feel nauseous and vomit three or four times. This can be stopped with one mouthful of cold water. Then they go to bed, warmly covered

1136 *Ding* 丁, "pin[-illness]," also *ding* 疔, "pin-illness," refers to a deep-reaching and festering hardness in a tissue, eventually rising above the skin like a pinhead. BCGM Dict I, 127-129.

1137 Water emerging from the brick wall of a well that has not been let free yet into the bottom of the well, is called "water without root." See also 05-15.

with a blanket until they sweat. [This recipe] also serves to cure head wind.[1138] *Qian kun mi yun.*

惡毒諸瘡，及發背、疔瘡、便毒等證。二烏膏：用草烏頭、川烏頭，于瓦上以井華水磨汁塗之。如有口，即塗四邊。乾再上。亦可單用草烏磨醋塗之。永類方。

All sores associated with malign poison, also: illness signs such as effusion on the back, pin-illness[1139] sores, and poison in the region of relief.[1140] The "ointment with two *wu* [*tou*]." Grind *cao wu tou* and *chuan wu tou* on a tile with the first water drawn from a well in the morning and apply the resulting juice [to the affected region]. If [the sores] have an opening, apply [the juice] on all four sides of it. When it has dried, apply [moist juice] again. It is also possible to grind just *cao wu* [*tou*] in vinegar and apply [the liquid to the affected region]. *Yong lei fang.*

大風癬瘡，遍身黑色，肌體麻木，痺痛不常。草烏頭一斤，刮洗去皮極净，攤乾。以清油四兩，鹽四兩，同入銚内，炒令深黄色。傾出剩油，只留鹽并藥再炒，令黑烟出爲度。取一枚擘破，心内如米一點白者始好，白多再炒。乘熱杵羅爲末，醋麪糊丸梧子大。每服三十丸，空心温酒下。草烏性毒難制，五七日間，以黑豆煮粥食解其毒。繼洪澹寮方。

Massive wind[1141] and *xuan*-illness[1142] sores. The entire body is black. Muscles and body are numb, with an unusually painful blockage. Scrape one *jin* of *cao wu tou* [tubers] to remove their skin and wash them very clean. Then spread them to let them dry. With four *liang* of clear oil and four *liang* of salt give them into a cauldron and fry them until they have assumed a deep yellow color. Turn [the cauldron] to let the remaining oil flow off, with only the salt and the pharmaceutical drug remaining.

1138 *Tou feng* 頭風, "head wind." Condition of wind evil attacking the head followed by pain, dizziness, itching. BCGM Dict I, 509.

1139 *Ding* 丁, "pin[-illness]," also *ding* 疔, "pin-illness," refers to a deep-reaching and festering hardness in a tissue, eventually rising above the skin like a pinhead. BCGM Dict I, 127-129.

1140 *Bian du* 便毒, "poison [in the region] of relief." A condition of swelling with poison developing in the body region associated with functions of 'minor relief', i.e. urination, and 'major relief', i.e. defecation. BCGM Dict I, 65.

1141 *Da feng* 大風, "massive wind," may refer to sores caused by a massive intrusion of wind evil and also to conditions of leprosy. BCGM Dict I, 111.

1142 *Xuan* 癬, "*xuan*-illness." Conditions of dermal lesions with initially erythema, papules, and itching gradually extending in all directions to form an irregular ring with clear boundaries. The skin is slightly elevated with small papules, blisters, and/or scales and scraps. The central lesion may appear to heal spontaneously, and it may reappear. Also, a designation of local lesions with itching, release of liquid and shedding of scabs. BCGM Dict I, 591.

They are fried again until a black smoke is emitted. Then take one [tuber] and open it. If inside there is one white content the size of a rice grain, it is beginning to be well done. If there are many such white [grains], fry [the remaining tubers] again. Eventually pound them as long as they are still hot and pass them through a sieve to obtain a powder. With vinegar and wheat flour prepare a paste to form pills the size of *wu* seeds. Each time ingest 30 pills, to be ingested with warm wine on an empty stomach. *Cao wu* has a poisonous nature that is difficult to check. Within three to five days prepare a rice gruel and eat it to resolve the poison. Ji Hong, *Dan liao fang*.

遍身生瘡，陰囊、兩脚尤甚者。草烏一兩，鹽一兩化水，浸一夜，炒赤爲末。猪腰子一具，去膜煨熟，竹刀切擣，醋糊丸緑豆大。每服三十丸，空心鹽湯下。澹寮方。

Sores that cover the entire body, especially severe on the scrotum and the two legs. Soak for one night one *liang* of *cao wu* [*tou*] in water in which one *liang* of salt was dissolved, then fry it until it turns red and [grind it into] powder. Remove the membrane of a pig's kidney, roast it until done, cut it with a bamboo knife to pieces and pound them [to powder]. With vinegar and [wheat flour] prepare a paste and form pills the size of mung beans. Each time ingest 30 pills, to be sent down on an empty stomach with a salt decoction. *Dan liao fang*.

一切諸瘡未破者。草烏頭爲末，入輕粉少許，臘猪油和搽。普濟方。

All kinds of sores that have not broken open yet. [Grind] *cao wu* [*tou*] into powder, add a little calomel, mix it with oil from a pig obtained in the 12th month, and apply this [to the affected region]. *Pu ji fang*.

瘰癧初作，未破，作寒熱。草烏頭半兩，木鼈子二個，以米醋磨細，入擣爛葱頭、蚯蚓糞少許，調勻傅上，以紙條貼，令通氣孔，妙。醫林正宗。

Scrofula pervasion-illness[1143] in its beginning. It has not broken open yet, with alternating sensations of cold and heat. Rub half a *liang* of *cao wu tou* and two pieces of *mu bie zi* (here presumably *aconitum carmichaeli* tuber, 17-20) with rice vinegar to a fine [powder], add onion tips, pounded to a pulp, and a small amount of earthworm feces. Mix this evenly, apply it [to the affected region] and cover it with a piece of paper, leaving a hole [in the paper] for the qi to pass through. Wondrous. *Yi lin zheng zong*.

馬汗入瘡，腫痛，急療之，遲則毒深。以生烏頭末傅瘡口，良久有黄水出，即愈。靈苑方。

1143 *Luo li* 瘰癧, "scrofula pervasion-illness," when two or more connected swellings of the size of plum or date kernels appear either on the neck or in the armpits, or somewhere else on the body. BCGM Dict I. 329.

Horse sweat has entered a wound causing painful swelling. This should be healed instantly. Otherwise, the poison will go deep. Apply fresh *wu tou* powder to the opening of the sore. After quite some time a yellow water will be emitted. This then is the cure. *Ling yuan fang*.

蛇蝎螫人。射罔傅之，頻易，血出愈。梅師方。

Someone bitten by a snake or stung by a scorpion. Apply *she wang* to [the affected region] and frequently replace it. When it bleeds, a cure is achieved. *Mei shi fang*.

中沙虱毒。射罔傅之佳。千金。

Struck by the poison of sand lice. To apply *she wang* is excellent. *Qian jin*.

17-22
白附子別録下品
Bai fu zi, FE *Bie lu*, lower rank.

***Aconitum coreanum* Lèvl., *Typhonium giganteum* Engl.**

【釋名】見後發明下。

Explanation of Names. See below under "Explication."

【集解】【別録曰】白附子生蜀郡。三月采。【弘景曰】此物久絶，無復真者。【恭曰】本出高麗，今出涼州以西，蜀郡不復有。生砂磧下濕地，獨莖似鼠尾草，細葉周匝，生於穗間，根形似天雄。【珣曰】徐表南州異物記云：生東海、新羅國及遼東。苗與附子相似。【時珍曰】根正如草烏頭之小者，長寸許，乾者皺文有節。

Collected Explanations. *Bie lu*: *Bai fu zi grows* in Shu jun. It is collected in the third month. [Tao] Hongjing: This item has vanished a long time ago. Genuine specimens have not been found again. [Su] Gong: Originally it came from Gao li. Today it comes from west of Liang zhou. In Shu jun it is no longer present. It grows in sandy deserts and on low-lying, moist ground. It has a single stem resembling that of Japanese *salvia* herbs. It is surrounded by numerous fine leaves growing between spikes. The root is shaped similar to carmichael's monkshood root. [Li] Xun: Xu Biao in his *Nan zhou yi wu ji* states: "It grows in Dong hai, Xin luo guo and Liao dong. The seedlings equal those of *aconitum carmichaeli*, *fu zi* 附子, plants." [Li] Shizhen: The root is truly similar to that of small *aconitum carmichaeli* [tubers], with a length of about one *cun*. Dried specimens have a wrinkled line design and knots.

【氣味】辛、甘，大温，有小毒。【保昇曰】甘、辛，温。【大明曰】無毒。【珣曰】小毒。入藥炮用。【杲曰】純陽，引藥勢上行。

Qi and Flavor. Acrid, sweet, very warm, slightly poisonous. [Han] Baosheng: Sweet, acrid, warm. Da Ming: Nonpoisonous. [Li] Xun: A little poisonous; it is roasted to be applied with pharmaceutical drugs. [Li] Gao: Pure yang. It guides the strength of pharmaceutical drugs to move upward.

【主治】心痛血痺，面上百病，行藥勢。別録。中風失音，一切冷風氣，面皯瘢疵。大明。諸風冷氣，足弱無力，疥癬風瘡，陰下濕癢，頭面痕，入面脂用。李珣。補肝風虚。好古。風痰。震亨。

Control. Heart pain and blood blockage. The hundreds of diseases affecting the face. It moves the strength of [other] pharmaceutical drugs. *Bie lu*. Wind stroke with a loss of voice. All cold and wind qi [disorders]. Facial gloom, scars and blemishes. Da Ming. All types of wind [intrusion] and cold qi, weak feet without strength. Sores related to *jie*-illness,[1144] *xuan*-illness[1145] and wind [intrusion]. Moisture and itching in the yin [(i. e., genital) region] below. Facial marks. It is used to prepare facial cremes. Li Xun. It supplements liver [qi] in the case of depletion with wind [intrusion]. [Wang] Haogu. Wind [intrusion] and phlegm. [Zhu] Zhenheng.

【發明】【時珍曰】白附子乃陽明經藥，因與附子相似，故得此名，實非附子類也。按楚國先賢傳云：孔休傷頰有瘢。王莽賜玉屑、白附子香，與之消瘢。

Explication. [Li] Shizhen: *Bai fu zi* is a pharmaceutical drug for the yang brilliance conduits. Because it is very similar to *fu zi* it was given the name ["white *fu zi*"]. The fact is, it is not related to *fu zi*, *aconitum carmichaeli*. According to the *Chu guo xian xian zhuan*, Kong Xiu was harmed at his cheek, resulting in a scar. Wang Mang gave him the "fragrant [crème made of] jade shard and *bai fu zi*." He applied it and it dissolved the scar.

【附方】新十二。

Added Recipes. 12 newly [recorded].

中風口喎，半身不遂。牽正散：用白附子、白僵蠶、全蝎並等分，生研爲末。每服二錢，熱酒調下。楊氏家藏方。

1144 *Jie*-illness 疥, vaguely identifiable skin ailment. BCGM Dict I, 249.

1145 *Xuan* 癬, "*xuan*-illness." Conditions of dermal lesions with initially erythema, papules, and itching gradually extending in all directions to form an irregular ring with clear boundaries. The skin is slightly elevated with small papules, blisters, and/or scales and scraps. The central lesion may appear to heal spontaneously, and it may reappear. Also, a designation of local lesions with itching, release of liquid and shedding of scabs. BCGM Dict I, 591.

Wind stroke with wryness of the mouth, and half the body no longer following one's will. The "powder to lead along proper [qi]." Grind equal amounts of fresh specimens of *bai fu zi*, white, stiff silkworms and complete scorpions into powder. Each time ingest two *qian*, to be sent down mixed with hot wine. *Yang shi jia cang fang.*

小兒暑風。暑毒入心，痰塞心孔，昏迷搐搦，此乃危急之證，非此丸生料瞑眩之劑不能伐之。三生丸：用白附子、天南星、半夏，並去皮，等分，生研，猪膽汁和丸黍米大。量兒大小，以薄荷湯下。令兒側卧，嘔出痰水即甦。全幼心鑑。

Children affected by summer heat and wind. When summer heat poison enters their heart, phlegm obstructs the heart orifices, with confusion and convulsions, this is a disease sign of a critical, tense condition. There is no way to attack it other than with these pills even though they are a preparation generating dizziness and nausea. The "pills with three fresh [items]." Remove the skin from equal amounts of fresh *bai fu zi*, fresh Indian turnip [root] and fresh *pinellia* [root]. Grind them and mix them with pig bile to form pills the size of millet. Let the child send them down a with mint decoction, with the number [of pills] corresponding to its age. Then let the child lie on its side. When it vomits phlegm and water it will regain consciousness. *Quan you xin jian.*

風痰眩運，頭痛氣鬱，胸膈不利。白附子炮去皮臍半斤，石膏煅紅半斤，朱砂二兩二錢半，龍腦一錢，爲末，粟米飯丸小豆大。每服三十丸，食後茶、酒任下。御藥院方。

Vertigo related to wind [intrusion] and the presence of phlegm. Headache with pent-up qi. Blocked passage through chest and diaphragm. [Grind] half a *jin* of *bai fu zi*, roasted, the skin and the navel[1146] removed, half a *jin* of gypsum, calcined until it has turned red, two and a half *liang* of cinnabar and one *qian* of borneol into powder and form with millet or cooked rice pills the size of mung beans. Each time ingest 30 pills, to be sent down after a meal with tea or wine, whichever is preferred. *Yu yao yuan fang.*

偏正頭風。白附子、白芷、猪牙皂角去皮，等分爲末。食後茶清服，仰卧少頃。普濟方。

Unilateral and proper headache. Remove the skin of equal amounts of *bai fu zi*, *angelica dahuria* [root] and small *gleditsia* pods/seeds and [grind them into] powder,

1146 *Qi* 臍, "navel," is the indentation at the top of the tuber where it was connected with the stem of the plant. "To remove skin and navel" has the meaning of "to clean thoroughly."

to be ingested after a meal with clear tea. Then lie down, the face showing upward, for a short time. *Pu ji fang.*

痰厥頭痛。白附子、天南星、半夏等分，生研爲末，生薑自然汁浸蒸餅丸緑豆大。每服四十丸，食後薑湯下。濟生方。

Headache related to phlegm and ceasing [qi]. Grind equal amounts of fresh *bai fu zi*, fresh Indian turnip [root] and fresh *pinellia* [root] into powder, soak it in the natural juice of fresh ginger, and with steamed cakes prepare pills the size of mung beans. *Ji sheng fang.*

赤白汗斑。白附子、硫黄等分，爲末，薑汁調稀，茄蒂蘸擦，日數次。簡便方。

Red and white sweat macules.[1147] [Grind] equal amounts of *bai fu zi* and sulphur into powder and prepare a thin mixture with ginger juice. Dip eggplant fruit base [into the liquid] and apply [the liquid on the affected region]. Several times a day. *Jian bian fang.*

面上皯黯。白附子爲末，卧時漿水洗面，以白蜜和塗紙上，貼之。久久自落。衛生易簡方。

Facial dark speckles. [Grind] *bai fu zi* into powder. At bedtime wash the face with water, mix [the powder] with honey and spread it on a piece of paper. Attach it [to the affected region]. After quite a long time [the speckles] will fall off. *Wei sheng yi jian fang.*

耳出膿水。白附子炮、羌活各一兩，爲末。猪、羊腎各一個，每個入末半錢，濕紙包，煨熟，五更食，温酒下。聖濟録。

Pus and water coming out of the ears. [Grind] one *liang* each of *bai fu zi*, roasted, and *notopterygium* [root] into powder. Fill half a *qian* of this powder separately into one pig kidney and one sheep kidney. Wrap them in moist paper, simmer them until done and eat them in the early morning hours, to be sent down with warm wine. *Sheng ji lu.*

喉痺腫痛。白附子末、枯礬等分，研末，塗舌上，有涎吐出。聖惠方。

Throat blockage with a painful swelling. Grind equal amounts of *bai fu zi* and processed alum into powder and apply it to the tongue. Spit out the saliva generated. *Sheng hui fang.*

1147 *Han ban* 汗斑, "sweat macule," identical to *li yang feng* 癧瘍風, "pervasion-illness with ulcers wind." A condition of white macules and dots appearing on the skin in the neck, on the chest, and below the armpits, without itching or pain. BCGM Dict I, 205, 315.

偏墜疝氣。白附子一個，爲末，津調填臍上，以艾灸三壯或五壯，即愈。楊起簡便方。

Unilateral descending [of scrotum] with elevation-illness qi.[1148] [Grind] one *bai fu zi* [root] into powder, mix it with saliva and place it on the navel. Cauterize it with mugwort [leaves] three or five times and this results in a cure. Yang Qi, *Jian bian fang*.

小兒吐逆不定，虛風喘急。白附子、藿香等分，爲末。每米飲下半錢。保幼大全方。

A child vomits with [qi] counterflow at irregular intervals, related to depletion wind[1149] and hectic panting. [Grind] equal amounts of *bai fu zi* and *agastache* [herb] into powder. Each time send down with a rice beverage half a *qian*. *Bao you da quan fang*.

慢脾驚風。白附子半兩，天南星半兩，黑附子一錢，並炮去皮，爲末。每服二錢，生薑五片，水煎服。亦治大人風虛，止吐化痰。宣和間，真州李博士用治吳內翰女孫甚效。康州陳侍郎病風虛極昏，吳內翰令服三四服，即愈。楊氏家藏。

Slow spleen fright wind.[1150] Roast together half a *liang* of *bai fu zi*, half a *liang* of Indian turnip [root] and one *liang* of black *aconitum* [accessory tuber], remove their skin and [grind them into] powder. Each time ingest two *qian*. To be ingested with a decoction of five fresh ginger slices in water. It also serves to cure depletion with wind [intrusion] of adults, ends vomiting and transforms phlegm. During the *xuan he* reign period (1119 – 1125), Doctor Li of Zhen zhou resorted to it to cure a granddaughter of Palace Writer Wu and it was very effective. In Kang zhou, Attendant Gentleman Chen suffered from depletion with wind [intrusion] and extreme dizziness. Palace Writer Wu let him ingest three to four doses, and he was cured. *Yang shi jia cang*.

1148 *Shan* 疝, "elevation-illness," a group of conditions characterized by violent abdominal pain, in some cases associated with constipation and anuria. BCGM Dict I, 417.

1149 *Xu feng* 虛風, "depletion wind," identical to *man jing feng* 慢驚風, slow fright wind." A condition of a *jing feng* 驚風, "fright wind," characterized by recurrent cramps in the presence or absence of fever. The cramps are slow and not very forceful. BCGM Dict I, 334, 584.

1150 *Man pi jing feng* 慢脾驚風, "slow spleen fright wind." A condition identical to *man jing feng* 慢驚風,"slow fright wind." BCGM Dict I, 335. See previous note.

17-23
虎掌本經下品
Hu zhang, FE *Ben jing*, lower rank.
天南星宋開寶
Tian nan xing, FE Song, *Kai bao*.

Arisaema thunbergii **Bl. Indian turnip.**

【釋名】虎膏綱目、鬼蒟蒻日華。【恭曰】其根四畔有圓牙，看如虎掌，故有此名。【頌曰】天南星即本草虎掌也，小者名由跋。古方多用虎掌，不言天南星。南星近出唐人中風痰毒方中用之，乃後人采用，别立此名爾。【時珍曰】虎掌因葉形似之，非根也。南星因根圓白，形如老人星狀，故名南星，即虎掌也。蘇頌説甚明白。宋開寶不當重出南星條，今併入。

Explanation of Names. *Hu gao* 虎膏, "tiger paste," *Gang mu*. *Gui ju ruo* 鬼蒟蒻, *Rihua*. [Su] Gong: The root on all four sides has round teeth, making it look like a "tiger paw," *hu zhang* 虎掌. Hence it has this name. [Su] Song: *Tian nan xing* 天南星, "the sky's southern star," is [the substance listed as] *hu zhang* 虎掌 in the *Ben cao*. Small ones are called *you ba* 由跋 (17-24). Ancient recipes often resorted to *hu zhang* 虎掌; they did not speak of *tian nan xing* 天南星. *Nan xing* appeared more recently when Tang people used it in recipes for wind stroke with phlegm and poison. From then on, people collected it for [therapeutic] use and this [second] name was established. [Li] Shizhen: *Hu zhang* 虎掌 [is called "tiger paw") because of a similarity of its leaves [with a tiger's paw], not because of [a similarity of] its root. [It is called] *nan xing* 南星, "southern star," because its root is round and white, with a shape similar to that of the [star] Canopus. Hence it is called "southern star," *nan xing* 南星. It is *hu zhang* 虎掌. Su Song says that it is very bright and white. The Song era *Kai bao* should not have listed *nan xing* 南星 in a separate entry. Here it is combined [with *hu zhang* in one entry].

【集解】【别録曰】虎掌生漢中山谷及冤句。二月、八月采，陰乾。【弘景曰】近道亦有。形似半夏，但大而四邊有子如虎掌。今用多破作三四片。方藥不甚用也。【恭曰】此是由跋宿根。其苗一莖，莖頭一葉，枝丫脥莖，根大者如拳，小者如雞卵，都似扁柿。四畔有圓牙，看如虎掌。由跋是新根，大如半夏二三倍，四畔無子牙。陶説似半夏，乃由跋也。【保昇曰】莖頭有八九葉，花生莖間。【藏器曰】天南星生安東山谷，葉如荷，獨莖，用根。【頌曰】虎掌今河北州郡有之。初生根如豆大，漸長大似半夏而扁，年久者根圓及寸，大者如雞卵。周匝生圓牙二三枚或五六枚。三四月生苗，高尺餘。獨莖上有葉如爪，五六出分布，尖而圓。一窠生七八莖，時出一莖，作穗直上如鼠尾。中生一葉如匙，裹莖作房，旁開一口，上下尖。中有花，微青褐色。結實如麻子大，熟即白色，自落布地，一子生一窠。九月苗殘取根。今冀州人菜圃中種之，呼爲天南星。又曰：天南星，處處平澤有之。二月生苗，似荷梗，其莖高一尺以來。葉如蒟蒻，兩枝相抱。五月開花似蛇頭，黃色。七月結子作穗似石榴子，紅色。二月、八月采根，似芋而圓扁，與蒟蒻相類，人多誤采，了不可辨。但蒟蒻莖斑花紫，南星根小，柔膩肌細，炮之易裂，爲可辨爾。南星即本經虎掌也。大者四邊皆有牙子，采時削去之。江州一種草，葉大如掌，面青背紫，四畔有牙如虎掌，生三四葉爲一本，冬青，不結花實，治心疼寒熱積氣，亦與虎掌同名，故附見之。【時珍曰】大者爲虎掌、南星，小者爲由跋，乃一種也。今俗又言大者爲鬼臼，小者爲南星，殊爲謬誤。

Collected Explanations. *Bie lu*: *Hu zhang* grows in the mountain valleys of Han zhong, and also in Yuan ju. It is collected in the second and eighth month; it is dried in the yin (i. e., shade). [Tao] Hongjing: It can also be found nearby. Its physical appearance resembles that of *pinellia* [root], but it is bigger and on its four sides it has "children" similar to a tiger's paw. When it is used today, it is mostly broken into three or four pieces. It is not often resorted to as a recipe pharmaceutical drug. [Su] Gong: This is the perennial root of *you ba* 由跋. Its seedling has one stem; at the tip of this stem is one leaf. Forked twigs grow close to the stem. Large roots have the size of fists; small ones that of chicken eggs. They always resemble a flat persimmon. On all four sides they have round teeth that make them look like a tiger's paw. *You ba* is the new root. It is two or three times bigger than a *pinellia* [root, and the latter] does not have seed-teeth on all four sides. When Tao [Hongjing] says that it resembles *pinellia* [root], then this is *you ba*. [Han] Baosheng: There are eight or nine leaves at the tip of the stem; the flowers grow from the stem. [Chen] Cangqi: Tian nan xing grows in the mountain valleys of An dong. The leaves resemble those of Indian lotus. It has a single stem. The root is used [for therapeutic purposes]. [Su] Song: Nowadays, *Hu zhang* is found in the *zhou* and prefectures of He bei. At the beginning of its growth the root has the size of a soybean. It slowly grows to the size of a *pinellia* [root], but is flat. Within one year it has a round root about one *cun* [in diameter], with the size of a chicken egg. It is surrounded by two or three, sometimes five or six round teeth. It grows a seedling in the third or fourth month, reaching a height of more than a *chi*. On its single stem leaves develop resembling claws. Five or six spread in all directions; they are pointed and round. From one "nest" seven or eight stems grow; sometimes one stem appears with spikes directed upward similar to the tail of mice/rats. In the center one leaf grows, shaped like a spoon. It encloses the stem and forms its "housing." On one side is an opening with pointed margins above and below and a flower in its center. They are of a weak greenish-brown color. They form fruits the size of hemp seeds. When they are ripe they are white. They fall down by themselves to cover the ground. Each seed forms one "nest." In the ninth month the seedling decays and the root is collected. Today, people in Ji zhou plant it in their vegetable gardens, and they call it *tian nan xing*. It is also said: *Tian nan xing* can be found everywhere in the marshlands of the plains. It grows a seedling in the second month, similar to Indian lotus roots. The stem is about one *chi* tall. The leaves are similar to those of devil's tongue. Two twigs are close to each other. In the fifth month flowers open resembling a snake head. They are yellow. In the seventh month seeds form with spikes resembling pomegranate seeds. They are red. The root is collected in the second and eighth month. It resembles taro [tubers], but is round and flat. It is related to devil's tongue. People often erroneously collect [the latter] because they are unable to distinguish them. However, the stem of devil's tongue has dots and its flowers are purple. [*Tian*] *nan xing* has a small root that is soft, oily and with fine flesh. When it is roasted it easily cracks. This is how they can be distinguished. [*Tian*] *nan xing* is the *hu zhang* recorded in the *Ben jing*. Large [roots] have teeths on all four sides; they are cut off to be discarded when [the root] is collected. In Jiang zhou a kind of an herb is found with leaves as big as a fist, a greenish front and a purple back. They have teeth on all four sides similar to a tiger's paw/*hu zhang*. Three or four leaves grow together, forming one base. In winter it is greenish; it does not form flowers and fruit. It serves to cure heart pain, alternating sensations of cold and heat, and qi accumulation. It has the same name as *hu zhang*. Hence it is presented here as an appendix. [Li] Shizhen: Large [roots] are *hu zhang* and [*tian*] *nan xing*; small ones are *you ba*. They are one kind. Today, is also commonly said that large [roots] are *gui jiu* 鬼臼, "demon's mortar," while small ones are [*tian*] *nan xing*. This is definitely wrong.

【修治】【頌曰】九月采虎掌根，去皮臍，入器中湯浸五七日，日換三四遍，洗去涎，暴乾用。或再火炮裂用。【時珍曰】凡天南星須用一兩以上者佳。治風痰有生用者，須以温湯洗净，仍以白礬湯，或入皂角汁，浸三日夜，日日換水，暴乾用。若熟用者，須於黄土地掘一小坑，深五六寸，以炭火燒赤，以好酒沃之。安南星於内，瓦盆覆定，灰泥固濟一夜取出用。急用即以濕紙包，於煻灰火中炮裂也。一法：治風熱痰以酒浸一宿，桑柴火蒸之，常洒酒入甑内，令氣猛。一伏時取出，竹刀切開，味不麻舌爲熟。未熟再蒸，至不麻乃止。脾虚多痰，則以生薑渣和黄泥包南星煨熟，去泥焙用。造南星麴法：以薑汁、礬湯，和南星末作小餅子，安籃内，楮葉包蓋，待上黄衣，乃取晒收之。造膽星法：以南星生研末，臘月取黄牯牛膽汁和劑，納入膽中，繫懸風處乾之。年久者彌佳。

Pharmaceutical Preparation. [Su] Song: The roots of *hu zhang* are collected in the ninth month. Remove their skin and the navel, give them into a vessel and soak them in hot water for five to seven days. Exchange [the water] three or four times a day. Then wash them to remove their saliva, dry them in the sun and use them [for therapeutic ends]. Or roast them over a fire until they crack and then use them. [Li] Shizhen: For all applications of *tian nan xing* [roots] weighing at least one *liang* are required to achieve excellent results. When fresh specimens are used to cure wind [intrusion] and phlegm, they must be washed clean with warm, boiled water. Then they are soaked in an alum decoction, sometimes with *gleditsia* fruit juice added, for three days and nights, with the water exchanged every day. Eventually they are dried in the sun and can be used. If they are to be used heat processed, dig a small pit in a yellow soil ground, about five to six *cun* deep. Heat it with a charcoal fire until it turns red and spray good wine into it. Then place the [*tian*] *nan xing* [roots] into [the pit], firmly cover it with an earthenware pot, seal [the edges of the pot] with ashes and mud, and remove [the root] again after one night for [therapeutic] use. In the case of an urgent need, wrap [the root] with moist paper and roast it over an ashes fire until it cracks. Another method. To cure wind [intrusion] with heat and phlegm, soak [the root] in wine for one night, steam it with a mulberry twig fire and repeatedly spray wine into the steamer to let its qi turn violent. After one full day and night remove it and cut it open with a bamboo knife. If it does not cause a numbing flavor on the tongue it is done. If it is not done yet, steam it again until it no longer causes numbing. Then stop. In the case of a spleen depletion with much phlegm, wrap a [*tian*] *nan xing* [root] with fresh ginger residue and yellow [soil] mud and simmer it until done. Remove the mud, bake [the root] over a slow fire, and use it [for therapeutic purposes]. The method to prepare [*tian*] *nan xing* [root] leaven. Form a small cake with ginger juice, alum decoction and [*tian*] *nan xing* powder. Place it into a basket and cover it with paper mulberry tree leaves. Wait until a yellow coating grows [on the root], remove it, dry it in the sun and store it. The method to prepare "bile [*tian nan*] *xing*." Grind a fresh [*tian*] *nan xing* [root] into powder, mix it with the bile of a yellow bull and insert it into the gall bladder. Fasten it and suspend it at a windy place to let it dry. When it is left there for years, it will be excellent.

【氣味】苦，温，有大毒。【别録曰】微寒。【普曰】虎掌：神農、雷公：苦，有毒。岐伯、桐君：辛，有毒。【大明曰】辛烈，平。【杲曰】苦、辛，有毒。陰中之陽，可升可降，乃肺經之本藥。【震亨曰】欲其下行，以黄蘗引之。【之才曰】蜀漆爲之使。惡莽草。【大明曰】畏附子、乾薑、生薑。【時珍曰】得防風則不麻，得牛膽則不燥，得火炮則不毒。生能伏雄黄、丹砂、焰硝。

Qi and Flavor. Bitter, warm, very poisonous. *Bie lu*: Slightly cold. [Wu] Pu: *Hu zhang*: Shen nong, Lei gong: Bitter, poisonous.[1151] Qi Bo, Tong jun: Acrid, poisonous. Da Ming: Violently acrid, balanced. [Li] Gao: Bitter, acrid, poisonous. A yang in yin [substance]. It can rise and it can descend. It is a basic pharmaceutical drug for the lung conduits. [Zhu] Zhenheng: If it is supposed to move downward, combine it with *phellodendron* bark to guide it. [Xu] Zhicai: Chinese quinine serves as its messenger; [ingested together,] it abhors *illiceum* [leaves]. Da Ming: It fears *aconitum* [accessory tuber], dried ginger and fresh ginger. [Li] Shizhen: Combined with *saposhnikovia* [root] it does not cause numbness. Combined with ox bile it does not cause dryness. Roasted over a fire it is no longer poisonous. As a fresh substance it can suppress [the effects of] realgar, cinnabar and nitrokalite.

【主治】心痛，寒熱結氣，積聚伏梁，傷筋痿拘緩，利水道。本經。除陰下濕，風眩。别録。主疝瘕腸痛，傷寒時疾，强陰。甄權。天南星：主中風麻痺，除痰下氣，利胸膈，攻堅積，消癰腫，散血墮胎。開寳。金瘡折傷瘀血，擣傅之。藏器。蛇蟲咬，疥癬惡瘡。大明。去上焦痰及眩運。元素。主破傷風，口噤身强。李杲。補肝風虚，治痰，功同半夏。好古。治驚癇，口眼喎斜，喉痺，口舌瘡糜，結核，解顱。時珍。

Control. Heart pain. Alternating sensations of cold and heat. Bound qi. Accumulations, concretions and hidden beams.[1152] Harm leading to sinew dysfunction and cramps. It frees the passage through the water pathways. *Ben jing*. It removes moisture from the yin [(i. e., genital) region] below, and wind [intrusion causing] dizziness. *Bie lu*. It controls elevation-illness with conglomeration-illness[1153] and intestinal pain, harm caused by cold and seasonal illness. It strengthens the yin [qi]. Zhen Quan. *Tian nan xing*: It controls wind stroke with numbness. It eliminates phlegm and discharges qi. It frees the passage through the chest and the diaphragm. It attacks hard accumulations, dissolves swelling related to obstruction-illness, disperses blood and aborts a fetus. *Kai bao*. Wounds caused by metal objects/weapons, fractures, stagnating blood. Pound [it to a pulp] and apply it [to the affected

1151 Instead of *you du* 有毒, "poisonous," *Yu lan* ch. 990, *hu zhang* 虎掌, quoting *Wu shi ben cao* 吴氏本草, writes *wu du* 無毒, "nonpoisonous."

1152 *Fu liang* 伏梁, "hidden beam," a condition of *ji* 積, "accumulation," associated with the heart. It is shaped like a lower arm. Below it rises from the navel; above it reaches to below the heart. It is accompanied by vexation. In serious cases patients spit blood. They cannot be cured for an extended period of time. BCGM Dict I, 175.

1153 *Shan jia* 疝瘕, "elevation-illness with conglomeration-illness." A lump-like swelling in the abdomen that alternately collects and then dissolves again. BCGM Dict I, 418.

region]. [Chen] Cangqi: Snake and worm/bug bites. *Jie*-illness,[1154] *xuan*-illness,[1155] malign sores. Da Ming. It removes phlegm from the upper [section of the Triple] Burner and dizziness with [brain] movement. [Zhang] Yuansu: It controls wind [intrusion] into an open wound, resulting in clenched jaw and a stiff body. Li Gao. It supplements liver [qi] with a wind [intrusion] into a state of depletion. It serves to cure phlegm. Its [therapeutic] potential is identical to that of *pinellia* [root]. [Wang] Haogu. It serves to cure fright epilepsy, with wry mouth and slanted eyes, throat blockage, sores in the mouth and on the tongue. Nodular kernels.[1156] Open skull.[1157] [Li] Shizhen.

【發明】【時珍曰】虎掌、天南星，乃手足太陰脾肺之藥。味辛而麻，故能治風散血；氣溫而燥，故能勝濕除涎；性緊而毒，故能攻積拔腫而治舌口喎糜。楊士瀛直指方云：諸風口噤，宜用南星，更以人參、石菖蒲佐之。

Explication. [Li] Shizhen: *Hu zhang*, [i. e.,] *tian nan xing*, is a pharmaceutical drug for the hand and foot major yin spleen and lung conduits. Hence it is able to cure wind [disorder] and to disperse blood. Its qi are warm and dry. Hence it can overcome moisture and dispel saliva. Its nature is hard and poisonous. Hence it is capable of attacking accumulations, pulling them out from a swelling, and of curing sores and wryness involving the tongue and the mouth. Yang Shiying in his *Zhi zhi fang* states: "For all kinds of wind [stroke] causing clenched jaw, it is advisable to use [*tian*] *nan xing*, and to assist it with ginseng [root] and *acorus* [root]."

【附方】舊十，新二十九。

Added Recipes. Ten of old. 29 newly [recorded].

中風口噤，目瞑，無門下藥者。開關散：用天南星爲末，入白龍腦等分，五月五日午時合之。每用中指點末，揩齒三二十遍，揩大牙左右，其口自開。又名破棺散。經驗方。

1154 *Jie*-illness 疥, vaguely identifiable skin ailment. BCGM Dict I, 249.

1155 *Xuan* 癬, "*xuan*-illness." Conditions of dermal lesions with initially erythema, papules, and itching gradually extending in all directions to form an irregular ring with clear boundaries. The skin is slightly elevated with small papules, blisters, and/or scales and scraps. The central lesion may appear to heal spontaneously, and it may reappear. Also, a designation of local lesions with itching, release of liquid and shedding of scabs. BCGM Dict I, 591.

1156 *Jie he* 結核, "nodular kernels," a condition identical to *luo li jie he* 瘰癧結核, nodular kernels of scrofula with pervasion-illness. BCGM Dict I, 250, 329

1157 *Jie lu* 解顱, "open skull," a condition of children whose fontanel fails to close until they have reached a certain age. 'BCGM Dict I, 251.

Clenched jaw caused by wind stroke. The eyes are darkened, and there is no entrance to [let the patient] send down a medication. The "powder to open barriers." Grind *tian nan xing* into powder and at noon on the fifth day of the fifth month add an equal amount of white borneol. Each time dip the middle finger into the powder and rub it on the [patient's] teeth 30, or at least 20 times. Rub the large teeth on the left and right, and his mouth opens as a result. [This recipe] is also called the "powder to break open coffins." *Jing yan fang*.

諸風口噤。天南星炮剉，大人三錢，小兒三字，生薑五片，蘇葉一錢，水煎减半，入雄猪膽汁少許，温服。仁齋直指方。

All types of clenched jaw caused by wind [intrusion]. Boil *tian nan xing*, roasted and cut into pieces, three *qian* if it is an adult [patient], three *zi* if it is a child, five slices of fresh ginger and one *qian* of *perilla* leaves in water down to one half. Add a little bile of a male pig and ingest this warm. *Ren zhai zhi zhi fang*.

小兒口噤，牙關不開。譚氏方：天南星一枚，煨熟，紙裹斜包，剪一小孔，透氣于口中，牙關自開也。

Clenched jaw of children, with an inability to open the tooth barrier. *Tan shi fang*: Simmer one *tian nan xing* [root] until done, wrap it in paper to make a package. Hold it tilted, cut a small hole and through [this hole] guide the qi [of the hot root] into the [patient's] mouth. This will open the tooth barrier.

一方：用生南星同薑汁擦之，自開。

Another recipe. Apply a mixture of fresh [*tian*] *nan xing* and ginger juice [to the patient's teeth]. They will open as a result.

小兒驚風。墜涎散：用天南星一兩重一個，換酒浸七伏時，取出安新瓦上，週迴炭火炙裂，合濕地出火毒，爲末，入硃砂一分。每服半錢，荆芥湯調下。每日空心一服，午時一服。經驗方。

Fright wind of children.[1158] The "powder to let saliva drop down." Soak one *tian nan xing* [root] weighing one *liang* in wine for seven full days, replacing the wine [with new wine regularly]. Then remove [the root] and place it on a new tile, and while turning it around roast it over a charcoal fire until it cracks. Then place it on moist ground to let the fire qi leave, and [grind it into] powder. Add one *fen* of cinnabar. Each time ingest half a *qian*, to be sent down mixed with *schizonepeta* [herb]. Ingest this on an empty stomach once every day, and ingest it once at noon. *Jing yan fang*.

1158 *Jing feng* 驚風, "fright wind," a condition of children characterised by jerking and arched back rigidity, eyeballs turned upward, and twitching hands and legs. BCGM Dict I, 261.

吐瀉慢驚。天王散：治小兒吐瀉，或誤服冷藥，脾虛生風痰慢驚。天南星一個，重八九錢者，去臍。黄土坑深三寸，炭火五斤，煅赤，入好酒半盞。安南星在内，仍架炭三條在上，候發裂取剉，再炒熟爲末，用五錢。天麻煨熟研末一錢，麝香一字，和匀。三歲小兒用半錢，以生薑、防風煎湯調下。亦治久嗽惡心。錢乙小兒方。

Vomiting and outflow with a chronic fright. The "celestial king's powder." It serves to cure children who vomit and have outflow, or who mistakenly ingested cold medication, and also chronic fright with wind phlegm[1159] related to spleen depletion. Take one *tian nan xing* [root] weighing eight or nine *qian* and remove the navel.[1160] Dig a pit in yellow soil three *cun* deep and calcine it with a fire of five *jin* of charcoal until its inside is red. First pour half a cup of good wine and then place the [*tian*] *nan xing* into [the pit] and put another three pieces of charcoal on top of it. Wait for the root to crack, remove it and file it to small pieces. Roast them another time, [grind them into] powder and mix five *qian* of it with one *qian* of *gastrodia* [root], cooked over a slow fire until done and [ground into] powder, and one *zi* of musk. For children three years of age use half a *qian*, to be sent down with a decoction of fresh ginger and *saposhnikovia* [root]. It also serves to cure long-lasting cough with nausea. Qian Yi, *Xiao er fang*.

風癇痰迷。墜痰丸：用天南星九蒸九晒，爲末，薑汁麵糊丸梧子大。每服二十丸，人參湯下。石菖蒲、麥門冬湯亦可。衛生寶鑑。

Wind epilepsy[1161] and phlegm confusion.[1162] Steam a *tian nan xing* [root] nine times, dry it in the sun nine times and [grind it into] powder. With ginger juice and wheat flour prepare a paste and form pills the size of *wu* seeds. Each time ingest 20 pills, to be sent down with a ginseng [root] decoction. An *acorus* [decoction] or an *ophiopogon* [tuber] decoction will do, too. *Wei sheng bao jian*.

1159 *Feng tan* 風痰, "wind phlegm," are pathogenic qi resulting from a combination of *feng* 風, "wind," and *tan* 痰, "phlegm," with the latter being brought about by the former. BCGM Dict I, 169.

1160 *Qi* 臍, "navel," is the indentation at the top of the tuber where it was connected with the stem of the plant. "To remove skin and navel" has the meaning of "to clean thoroughly."

1161 *Feng xian* 風癇, "wind epilepsy," a condition of *xian* 癇," epilepsy," resulting from the effects of wind evil. BCGM Dict I, 170

1162 *Tan mi* 痰迷, "phlegm confusion," a condition of mental disturbance with forgetfulness, loss of consciousness, and aphasia brought forth by an abundance of phlegm saliva diminishing the patient's mental capacities. BCGM Dict I, 493.

小兒癇瘖。癇後瘖不能言。以天南星濕紙包煨，爲末。雄猪膽汁調服二字。全幼心鑑。

Epilepsy and loss of voice of children. When following an epilepsy [children] have lost their voice, that is, they cannot speak. Wrap a *tian nan xing* [root] in moist paper , simmer it and [grind it into] powder. [Let the child] send down two *zi* mixed with the bile of a male pig. *Quan you xin jian.*

治癇利痰。天南星煨香一兩，朱砂一錢，爲末，猪心血丸梧子大。每防風湯化下一丸。普濟方。

To cure epilepsy and let phlegm flow off. [Grind] one *liang* of *tian nan xing*, simmered until it develops a fragrance, and one *qian* of cinnabar into powder and form with the blood from a pig's heart pills the size of *wu* seeds. Each time send down one pill dissolved in a *saposhnikovia* [root] decoction. *Pu ji fang.*

口眼喎斜。天南星生研末，自然薑汁調之。左貼右，右貼左。仁存方。

Wry mouth and slanted eyes. Grind a fresh *tian nan xing* [root] into powder, mix it with the natural juice of ginger and apply this on the right side [of the patient's face] if [the slanting is] on the left, and on the left side [of the patient's face] if it is on the right. *Rencun fang.*

角弓反張。南星、半夏等分，爲末。薑汁、竹瀝灌下一錢。仍灸印堂。摘玄方。

Arched reverse strain.[1163] [Grind] equal amounts of [*tian*] *nan xing* and *pinellia* [root] into powder, and force-feed one *qian* [to the patient mixed with either] ginger juice or bamboo stem juice. *Zhai xuan fang.*

破傷中風。胡氏奪命散，又名玉真散，治打撲金刃傷，及破傷風傷濕，發病强直如癇狀者。天南星、防風等分，爲末。水調敷瘡，出水爲妙。仍以温酒調服一錢。已死心尚温者，熱童便調灌二錢。鬬歐内傷墜壓者，酒和童便連灌三服即甦。亦可煎服。三因方。

An open wound struck by wind. "Mr. Hu's powder to seize fate." It is also called "powder with the true [strength of] jade." It serves to cure harm resulting from a blow, a fall or metal weapons, and also wound wind[1164] and [wounds] harmed by moisture, with [patients] suffering from a stiff posture similar to epilepsy. [Grind] equal amounts of *tian nan xing* and *saposhnikovia* [root] into powder, mix it with

1163 *Jiao gong fan zhang* 角弓反張, "arched reverse strain," arched back rigidity, opisthotonos, an illness sign of the body being bent backwards because of contracting muscles. BCGM Dict I, 247.

1164 *Po shang feng* 破傷風, "wound wind," a condition of lockjaw, arched back rigidity and convulsions, resulting from wounds struck by wind. BCGM Dict I, 379.

water and apply it to the sores. When water is emitted, this is the wondrous [effect of this therapy]. In addition, [let the patient] ingest mixed with warm wine one *qian*. [Patients] who have died already but are still warm are force-fed with two *qian* mixed with hot boys' urine. [Patients] hurt in a battle by falling or bruises are force-fed with [the powder mixed with] wine and boys' urine three times consecutively. [The powder] may also be ingested boiled [in water]. *San yin fang*.

破傷風瘡。生南星末，水調塗瘡四圍，水出有效。普濟方。
Sores related to wound wind. Mix fresh [*tian*] *nan xing* powder with water and apply it to all four sides of the sores. When [the sores] emit water, this is [evidence of the powder's] effects. *Pu ji fang*.

婦人頭風，攻目作痛。天南星一個，掘地坑燒赤，安藥於中，以醋一盞沃之，蓋定勿令透氣，候冷研末。每服一字，以酒調下。重者半錢。千金方。
Head wind[1165] of women, with [the wind] attacking the eyes and causing pain. Dig a pit in the ground and burn a fire to let it turn red. Then place of *tian nan xing* [root] into it, spray one cup of vinegar on it, and cover it tightly so that no qi can leave. Wait until the pharmaceutical drug has cooled and [grind it into] powder. Each time [let the woman] ingest one *zi*, to be sent down mixed with wine. For severe cases, [let her ingest] half a qian. *Qian jin fang*.

風痰頭痛不可忍。天南星一兩，荊芥葉一兩，爲末，薑汁糊丸梧子大。每食後薑湯下二十丸。
Wind phlegm[1166] with unbearable headache. [Grind] one *liang* of *tian nan xing* and one *liang* of *schizonepeta* leaves into powder. With ginger juice and [wheat flour] paste form pills the size of *wu* seeds. Each time send down with a ginger decoction 20 pills after a meal.

又上清丸：用天南星、茴香等分，生研末，鹽、醋煮麵糊丸。如上法服。並出經效濟世方。
Also, the "pills that let clear [qi] rise." Grind equal amounts of fresh *tian nan xing* and fresh fennel into powder, boil it with salt and vinegar, and with a wheat floor paste form pills to be ingested according to the method outlined above. Both [recipes] quoted from *Jing xiao ji shi fang*.

1165 *Tou feng* 頭風, "head wind." Condition of wind evil attacking the head followed by pain, dizziness, itching. BCGM Dict I, 509.

1166 *Feng tan* 風痰, "wind phlegm," are pathogenic qi resulting from a combination of *feng* 風, "wind," and *tan* 痰, "phlegm," with the latter being brought about by the former. BCGM Dict I, 169.

風痰頭運，目眩，吐逆，煩懣，飲食不下。玉壺丸：用生南星、生半夏各一兩，天麻半兩，白麵三兩，爲末，水丸梧子大。每服三十丸，以水先煎沸，入藥煮五七沸，漉出放温，以薑湯吞之。惠民和劑局方。

Wind phlegm and head movement.[1167] Dizziness, vexation and mental pressure, inability to eat and drink. The "jade kettle pills." [Grind] one *liang* each of fresh [*tian*] *nan xing*, and fresh *pinellia* [root], half a *liang* of *gastrodia* [root] and three *liang* of wheat flour into powder and with water form pills the size of *wu* seeds. Each time ingest 30 pills. First boil water to bubbling. Then add the medication and boil it to bubbling five to seven times. Filter the liquid, remove [the medication] and leave it until it is warm [instead of hot]. Swallow it with a ginger decoction. *Hui min ju he ji ju fang*.

腦風流涕。邪風入腦，鼻内結硬，遂流髓涕。大白南星切片，沸湯泡二次，焙乾。每用二錢，棗七個，甘草五分，同煎服。三四服，其硬物自出，腦氣流轉，髓涕自收。以大蒜、蓽茇末作餅，隔紗貼顖前，熨斗熨之。或以香附、畢茇末頻吹鼻中。直指方。

Brain wind[1168] with a flow of snivel. Evil wind has entered the brain, with hardened bound [qi] in the nose and an outflow of marrow and nasal mucus. Cut a big, white [*tian*] *nan xing* [root] into pieces. Steep them twice in water heated to bubbling and bake them over a slow fire until they are dry. Each time boil two *qian* together with seven Chinese dates and five *fen* of *glycyrrhiza* [root] and ingest this in three or four portions. The hard items will leave [the nose] as a result. The flow of qi in the brain revolves [as usual] and marrow and nasal mucus will be held back. With a powder made from garlic and long pepper prepare a cake, place it, separated by a thin piece of cloth, on the [patient's] forehead and press it with a hot flatiron. It is also possible to repeatedly blow a *cyperus* [root] and long pepper [powder] into the [patient's] nose. *Zhi zhi fang*.

小兒風痰，熱毒壅滯，凉心壓驚。抱龍丸：用牛膽南星一兩，入金錢薄荷十片，丹砂一錢半，龍腦、麝香各一字，研末，煉蜜丸芡子大。每服一丸，竹葉湯化下。全幼心鑑。

Wind phlegm of children. Heat poison is obstructed and remains at one place. The "pills that embrace dragons" cool the heart and press down fright. Add to one *liang*

1167 *Tou yun* 頭運, "head movement," identical to *tou xuan* 頭旋, "head spin." An illness sign of a feeling of vertigo as if one's own body and the scenery around were revolving. BCGM Dict I, 512.

1168 *Nao feng* 腦風, "brain wind," a condition of *tou feng* 頭風, "head wind," characterized by a simultaneous presence of cold evil, with headache, a feeling of cold in the neck and back, as well as running nose and tearflow. BCGM Dict I, 349.

of [*tian*] *nan xing*, [processed with] ox bile, ten pieces of mint, one and a half *qian* of cinnabar, and one *zi* each of borneol and musk, and grind them into powder. With heat refined honey form pills the size of *qian* seeds. Each time ingest one pill, to be sent down dissolved in a bamboo leaf decoction. *Quan you xin jian.*

壯人風痰及中風、中氣初起。星香飲：用南星四錢，木香一錢，水二盞，生薑十四片，煎六分，温服。王碩易簡方。

Strong persons with wind phlegm[1169] and wind stroke, with the qi causing the stroke just beginning to rise. The "beverage with [*tian nan*] *xing* and *costus* [root]." Boil four *qian* of [*tian*] *nan xing* and one *qian* of *costus* [root] in two cups of water with 14 fresh ginger slices down to 60% and ingest this warm. Wang Shuo, *Yi jian fang.*

痰迷心竅。壽星丸：治心膽被驚，神不守舍，或痰迷心竅，恍惚健忘，妄言妄見。天南星一斤，先掘土坑一尺，以炭火三十斤燒赤，入酒五升，滲乾。乃安南星在内，盆覆定，以灰塞之，勿令走氣。次日取出，爲末。琥珀一兩，朱砂二兩，爲末。生薑汁打麵糊丸梧子大。每服三十丸至五十丸，煎人參、石菖蒲湯下。一日三服。和劑局方。

Phlegm confusion with the orifices of the heart [obstructed]. The "pills of the Heavenly Body/God of Longevity." They serve to cure fright affecting heart and gallbladder, with their spirits no longer guarding their ordinary residence. Also, phlegm confusion with the orifices of the heart [obstructed] resulting in absent-mindedness and forgetfulness, absurd speaking and absurd visions. Prepare one *jin* of *tian nan xing*. First dig a pit, one *chi* deep, into the soil and with a fire lit by 30 *jin* of charcoal heat it until it turns red. Then pour five *sheng* of wine into it, and wait until it has seeped in and [the pit is] dry. Then place the *tian nan xing* into [the pit], cover it with an overturned bowl, and close the edges with ashes so that no qi will escape. The next day remove [the *tian nan xing*] and [grind it into] powder. [Grind] one *liang* of amber and two *liang* of cinnabar into powder, and with fresh ginger juice and wheat flour prepare a paste to form pills the size of *wu* seeds. Each time ingest 30 to 50 pills, to be sent down with a ginseng [root] and *acorus* decoction. To be ingested three times a day. *He ji ju fang.*

風痰注痛。方見羊躑躅下。

Wind phlegm and influx pain.[1170] For a recipe, see under the entry *yang zhi zhu* (17-35).

1169 *Feng tan* 風痰, "wind phlegm," are pathogenic qi resulting from a combination of *feng* 風, "wind," and *tan* 痰, "phlegm," with the latter being brought about by the former. BCGM Dict I, 169.

1170 *Zhu tong* 注痛, "influx pain," an illness sign of pain erratically changing its location. BCGM Dict I, 694.

痰濕臂痛右邊者。南星制、蒼术等分，生薑三片，水煎服之。摘玄方。

Pain in the arm on the right related to phlegm and the presence of moisture. Boil in water equal amounts of prepared [*tian*] *nan xing* and *atractylodes lancea* [rhizome], and three fresh ginger slices and ingest this. *Zhai xuan fang*.

風痰欬嗽。大天南星一枚，炮裂研末。每服一錢，水一盞，薑三片，煎五分，温服。每日早、午、晚各一服。十全博救方。

Wind phlegm and cough. Roast one big *tian nan xing* [root] until it cracks and grind it into powder. Each time ingest one *qian*, to be boiled in one cup of water, together with three ginger slices, down to 50%. To be ingested warm. Every day to be ingested once in the early morning, at noon and in the evening. *Shi quan bo jiu fang*.

氣痰欬嗽。玉粉丸：南星麴、半夏麴、陳橘皮各一兩，爲末，自然薑汁打糊丸如梧子大。每服四十丸，薑湯下。寒痰，去橘皮，加官桂。東垣蘭室秘藏。

Cough with qi [disorder and] phlegm. The "jade powder pills." [Grind] one *liang* each of [*tian*] *nan xing* leaven, *pinellia* [root] leaven and long-stored tangerine peels into powder, and with the natural juice of ginger and [wheat flour] prepare a paste to form pills the size of *wu* seeds. Each time ingest 40 pills, to be sent down with a ginger decoction. In the case of phlegm with the presence of cold remove the tangerine peels, and add *cassia* bark instead. [Li] Dongyuan, *Lan shi mi cang*.

清氣化痰。三仙丸：治中脘氣滯，痰涎煩悶，頭目不清。生南星去皮、半夏各五兩，並湯泡七次，爲末。自然薑汁和作餅，鋪竹篩內，以楮葉包覆，待生黄成麴，晒乾。每用二兩，入香附末一兩，糊丸梧子大。每服四十丸，食後薑湯下。王璆百一選方。

To clear up qi and transform phlegm. The "three hermits/immortals pills." They serve to cure qi stagnating in the central [stomach] duct, phlegm, saliva and vexing heart-pressure, unclear head and eyes. Steep five *liang* each of fresh [*tian*] *nan xing*, with the skin removed, and *pinellia* [root] together seven times in hot water and [grind them into] powder. With the natural juice of ginger form a cake and place it on a bamboo sieve. Cover it with paper mulberry tree leaves and wait for a yellow leaven to grow. Then dry [the cake] in the sun. Each time use two *liang*, add one *liang* of nutgrass [root] powder and prepare with a [wheat flour] paste pills the size of *wu* seeds. Each time ingest 49 pills, to be sent down after meals with a ginger decoction. Wang Qiu, *Bai yi xuan fang*.

温中散滯，消導飲食。天南星炮、高良薑炮各一兩，砂仁二錢半，爲末，薑汁糊丸梧子大。每薑湯下五十丸。和劑方。

To warm the center and to disperse sluggish [qi], to dissolve and guide beverages and food. [Grind] one *liang* each of *tian nan xing*, roasted, and lesser galangal [root] with two and a half *qian* of bastard cardamom [seeds] into powder, prepare with ginger juice and [a wheat flour] paste pills the size of *wu* seeds, and each time ingest with a ginger decoction 50 pills. *He ji ju fang*.

酒積酒毒。服此即解。天南星丸：用正端天南星一斤。土坑燒赤，沃酒一斗入坑，放南星，盆覆，泥固濟，一夜取出，酒和水洗净，切片，焙乾，爲末，入朱砂末一兩，薑汁麵糊丸梧子大。每服五十丸，薑湯下。蔡丞相、吕丞相嘗用有驗。楊氏家藏方。

Wine accumulation,[1171] wine poisoning. When this is ingested, the [poison] is resolved. The "pills with *tian nan xing*." Prepare one *jin* of best *tian nan xing* [roots]. Heat a pit in the soil until it turns red, spray one *dou* of wine into the pit. Place the [*tian*] *nan xing* [into the pit] and cover it with a turned-over bowl. Tightly seel it with mud. Remove [the roots] after one night, and wash them clean with a wine and water mixture. Cut them into pieces, bake them over a slow fire until they are dry, and [grind them into] powder. Add one *liang* of cinnabar powder, and with ginger juice and wheat flour prepare a paste to form pills the size of *wu* seeds. Each time ingest 50 pills, to be sent down with a ginger decoction. Prime Minster Cai and Prime Minister Lü once applied [this medication] and it proved to be effective. *Yang shi jia cang fang*.

吐泄不止，四肢厥逆，虚風不省人事，服此則陽回，名回陽散。天南星爲末，每服三錢，京棗三枚，水二鍾，煎八分，温服。未省再服。集效方

Unending vomiting and outflow. With ceasing [yang qi and qi] counterflow in the four limbs, depletion with wind [intrusion][1172] and an inability to recognize other persons or things. To ingest this lets the yang [qi] return. [The recipe] is called "powder to let yang [qi] return." Grind *tian nan xing* into powder. Each time ingest three *qian*, boiled together with three Chinese dates in two *zhong* of water down to 80%. If no effect shows, ingest this a second time. *Ji xiao fang*.

1171 *Jiu ji* 酒積, wine accumulation," a condition of *shi ji* 食積, "food accumulation," resulting from an excessive consumption of wine, often accompanied by a yellow facial complexion with depletion swelling, a distended, swollen abdomen, as well as vomiting and diarrhea. BCGM Dict I, 584

1172 *Xu feng* 虚風, "depletion wind," identical to *man jing feng* 慢驚風, slow fright wind." A condition of a *jing feng* 驚風, "fright wind," characterized by recurrent cramps in the presence or absence of fever. The cramps are slow and not very forceful. BCGM Dict I, 334, 584.

又方：醋調南星末，貼足心。普濟方。

Another recipe. Mix [*tian*] *nan xing* powder with vinegar and apply this to the soles of [the patient's] feet. *Pu ji fang.*

腸風瀉血，諸藥不效。天南星石灰炒焦黄色，爲末，酒糊丸梧子大，每酒下二十丸。普濟方。

Intestinal wind and blood outflow, with all medications having remained without effect. Roast *tian nan xing* with lime until it has assumed a yellow color, and [grind it into] powder. With wine and [wheat flour] prepare a paste to form pills the size of *wu* seeds. Each time send down with wine 20 pills. *Pu ji fang.*

吐血不止。天南星一兩，剉如豆大，以爐灰汁浸一宿，洗焙研末。每服一錢，以自然銅磨酒調下。勝金方。

Unending spitting/vomiting of blood. Cut a *tian nan xing* [root] weighing one *liang* to the size of a soybean, soak it in a furnace ashes liquid for one night, wash it, bake it over a slow fire and grind it into powder. Each time ingest one *qian*, to be send down mixed with wine in which natural copper was ground. *Sheng jin fang.*

初生貼顖。頭熱鼻塞者。天南星炮，爲末，水調貼顖上，炙手熨之。危氏得效方。

To be attached to the top of the head of a newborn. When the head is hot and the nose is blocked. Roast *tian nan xing*, [grind it into] powder and attach it mixed with water to the top of the [child's] head. Press it with a heated hand. *Wei shi de xiao fang.*

小兒解顱。顖開不合，鼻塞不通。天南星炮去皮，爲末，淡醋調緋帛上，貼顖門，炙手頻熨之，立效。錢乙小兒直訣。

Open skull of children.[1173] The top of the head is open and fails to close; the nose is stuffed, it passage is blocked. [Grind] *tian nan xing*, roasted and with the skin removed, into powder. Mix it with light vinegar and spread this on a piece of silk. Attach this to the [child's] fontanel and press it with a heated hand. Immediately effective. Qian Yi, *Xiao er zhi jue.*

解頤脱臼，不能收上。用南星末，薑汁調塗兩頰，一夜即上。醫説。

Dislocation of temporamandibular joints, unable to hold the chin. Mix [*tian*] *nan xing* powder with ginger juice and apply it to both cheeks. Within one night [the chin] is raised again. *Yi shuo.*

1173 *Jie lu* 解顱, "open skull," a condition of children whose fontanel fails to close until they have reached a certain age. BCGM Dict I, 251.

小兒口瘡。白屑如鵝口，不須服藥。以生天南星去皮臍，研末，醋調塗足心，男左女右。閻孝忠集效方。

Oral sores of children, with white flakes, resembling a goose-mouth.[1174] [To cure this] it is not necessary to let them ingest a medication. Grind *tian nan xing*, with the skin and the navel[1175] removed, into powder, mix it with vinegar and apply this to the sole of one of the [child's] feet; for males it is the left, and for females it is the right [sole]. Yan Xiaozhong, *Ji xiao fang.*

走馬疳蝕，透骨穿腮。生南星一個，當心剜空，入雄黃一塊，麵裹燒，候雄黃作汁，以盞子合定，出火毒，去麵爲末，入麝香少許，拂瘡數日，甚驗。經驗方。

Running horse *gan*-illness[1176] erosions penetrating the bones and passing through the cheeks. Cut out the heart from a fresh [*tian*] *nan xing* [root] and insert a lump of realgar into the hollow space. Enclose it with wheat flour and heat it until a juice is emitted from the realgar. Give it into a cup and seal it until the fire poison has left. Then remove the wheat flour and [grind the root] into powder. Add a little musk and apply this to the sores for several days. Very effective. *Jing yan fang.*

風蟲牙痛。南星末塞孔，以霜梅龕住，去涎。摘玄方。

Toothache related to wind [intrusion] and the presence of worms/bugs. Insert [*tian*] *nan xing* powder into the cavities, and fix it with white plums. Remove/spit out the saliva. *Zhai xuan fang.*

喉風喉痺。天南星一個，剜心，入白僵蠶七枚，紙包煨熟，研末。薑汁調服一錢，甚者灌之，吐涎愈。名如聖散。博濟方。

Throat wind,[1177] throat blockage. Carve out of one *tian nan xing* [root] the heart and insert seven white, stiff silkworms [into the hollow space], wrap it with paper and simmer it until done. Grind it into powder and ingest mixed with ginger juice one

1174 *E kou* 鵝口, "goose-mouth." A condition of *chuang* 瘡, "sores," with a white layer covering the mucous membranes and top of the tongue in a child's mouth making it resemble a goose-mouth. BCGM Dict I, 141.

1175 *Qi* 臍, "navel," is the indentation at the top of the tuber where it was connected with the stem of the plant. "To remove skin and navel" has the meaning of "to clean thoroughly."

1176 *Zou ma gan* 走馬疳, "running horse *gan*-illness," identical to *zou ma ya gan* 走馬牙疳, running horse dental *gan*-illness," a condittion of *ya gan* 牙疳, "dental *gan*-illness," that develops abruptly and turns into a serious condition, with festering decay beginning at the teeth and gums and eventually causing the teeth to erode and fall out. BCGM Dict I, 704.

1177 *Hou feng* 喉風, "throat wind," various conditions with mouth, tongue, and throat swelling and pain. BCGM Dict I, 217.

qian. In severe cases, [patients must be] force-fed. They spit out saliva and are cured. [This recipe] is named "sage-like powder." *Bo ji fang*.

痰瘤結核。南星膏：治人皮肌頭面上生瘤及結核，大者如拳，小者如栗，或軟或硬，不疼不痒，宜用此藥，不可輒用針灸。生天南星大者一枚，研爛，滴好醋五七點。如無生者，以乾者爲末，醋調。先用針刺令氣透，乃貼之。覺痒則頻貼，取效。嚴子禮濟生方。

Phlegm tumor[1178] with nodular kernels. The "[*tian*] *nan xing* ointment." It serves to cure persons developing tumors and nodular kernels on the skin, in the muscles, on the head and on the face, with big ones assuming the size of a fist, and small ones the size of Chinese chestnuts. They may be soft or hard, and they neither ache nor itch. For all these this medication is suitable; a generalized application of needling or cauterization is not advisable. Grind one large, fresh *tian nan xing* [root] to a pulpy [mass] and drip five to seven drops of good vinegar into it. If no fresh [root] is available, a dry [root] will do, too; it is [ground into] powder. Mix [the pulpy mass or the powder] with vinegar [to prepare an ointment]. First pierce a needle [into the tumor kernels] to allow the qi [of the ointment] to penetrate them. Then apply the [ointment]. When [the patient] feels an itch, repeat the application several times until an effect shows. Yan Zili, *Ji sheng fang*.

身面疣子。醋調南星末塗之。簡易方。

Warts on the body and the face. Mix [*tian*] *nan xing* powder with vinegar and apply this [to the affected region]. *Jian yi fang*.

17-24
由跋本經下品

You ba, FE *Ben jing*, lower rank.

Small, new root of **17-23: *Arisaema thunbergii* Bl., Indian turnip.**

【釋名】(missing)

【集解】【恭曰】由跋是虎掌新根，大于半夏一二倍，四畔未有子牙，其宿根即虎掌也。【藏器曰】由跋生林下，苗高一尺，似蒟蒻，根如雞卵。【保昇曰】春抽一莖，莖端有八九葉，根圓扁而肉白。【時珍曰】此即天南星之小者，其氣未足，不堪服食，故醫方罕用；惟重八九錢至一兩餘者，氣足乃佳。正如附子之側子不如附子之義也。

Collected Explanations. [Su] Gong: *You ba* are the new roots of *hu zhang* 虎掌. They are one or two times bigger than *pinellia* [roots], and they do not have tooth-

1178 *Tan liu* 痰瘤, "phlegm tumor," a condition identical to *luo li* 瘰癧, "scrofula with pervasion-illness." BCGM Dict I, 493, 329.

like seed outgrowths on all four sides. The perennial roots are *hu zhang*. [Chen] Cangqi: *You ba* grow under the trees in forests; the seedlings are one *chi* tall. They resemble those of devil's tongue. The roots are similar to chicken eggs. [Han] Baosheng: In spring one stem rises, with eight or nine leaves at the end of the stem. The root is round and flat and its meat is white. [Li] Shizhen: These are small *tian nan xing* [roots]. Their qi are insufficient, and they are not suitable to be ingested [as medication] or consumed as food. Therefore, phyisicians seldom use them. Only those weighing eight to nine *qian* up to more then one *liang* have sufficient qi and are excellent. This is exactly the same idea as that of the marginal seed-outgrowths, *ce zi* 側子, of *aconitum* accessory tubers, *fu zi* 附子, being not as good as *aconitum* accessory tubers, *fu zi* 附子, themselves.[1179]

【正誤】【弘景曰】由跋本出始興，今人亦種之。狀如烏翣而布地，花紫色，根似附子。苦酒摩塗腫，亦效。【恭曰】陶氏所說，乃鳶尾根，即鳶頭也。又言虎掌似半夏，是以鳶尾爲由跋，以由跋爲半夏，非惟不識半夏，亦不識鳶尾與由跋也。今南人猶以由跋爲半夏。【時珍曰】陳延之小品方亦以東海鳶頭爲由跋，則其訛誤久矣。

Correction of Errors. [Tao] Hongjing: *You ba* originally comes from Shi xing. Today, there are people who also plant it. It is shaped like crow feathers and covers the ground. Its flowers are purple; the root resembles *aconitum* accessory tubers. When it is rubbed in bitter wine and applied to swelling, it is effective, too. [Su] Gong: What Mr. Tao [Hongjing] says applies to the root of kite's tail iris, *yuan wei* 鳶尾, which is "kite's head," *yuan tou* 鳶頭. He also says Indian turnip, *hu zhang* 虎掌, resembles *you ba*, and this is because he considers kite's tail iris, *yuan wei* 鳶尾, to be *you ba* 由跋, and *you ba* 由跋 to be *pinellia* [root], *ban xia* 半夏. He not only is unfamiliar with *pinellia* [root], he also is not familiar with kite's tail iris and *you ba*. Today, southerners still identifiy *you ba* as *pinellia* [root]. [Li] Shizhen: Chen Yanzhi in his *Xiao pin fang*, too, identifies *yuan tou* 鳶頭, [i. e., the roots of kite's tail iris] from Dong hai as *you ba*. This error has survived for a long time.

【氣味】辛、苦，温，有毒。

Qi and Flavor. Acrid, bitter, warm, poisonous.

【主治】毒腫結熱。本經。

Control. Poison swelling and nodes with heat. *Ben jing*.

1179 See above, entries 17-17 and 17-19.

17-25
蒟蒻宋開寶
Ju ruo, FE Song, *Kai bao*.

Amorphallus revieri Durieu. Devil's tongue.

【釋名】蒻頭開寶、鬼芋圖經、鬼頭。

Explanation of Names. *Ruo tou* 蒻頭, *Kai bao*. *Gui yu* 鬼芋, "demon's taro," *Tu jing*. *Gui tou* 鬼頭, "demon's head."

【集解】【志曰】蒻頭出吴、蜀。葉似由跋、半夏，根大如盌，生陰地，雨滴葉下生子。又有斑杖，苗相似，至秋有花直出，生赤子，根如蒻頭，毒猛不堪食。亦名斑杖，與此不同。【頌曰】江南吴中出白蒟蒻，亦曰鬼芋，生平澤極多。人采以爲天南星，了不可辨，市中所收往往是此。但南星肌細膩，而蒟蒻莖斑花紫，南星莖無斑花黄爲異爾。【時珍曰】蒟蒻出蜀中，施州亦有之，呼爲鬼頭，閩中人亦種之。宜樹陰下掘坑積糞，春時生苗，至五月移之。長一二尺，與南星苗相似，但多斑點，宿根亦自生苗。其滴露之説，蓋不然。經二年者，根大如盌及芋魁，其外理白，味亦麻人。秋後采根，須净擦，或搗或片段，以釅灰汁煮十餘沸，以水淘洗，换水更煮五六遍，即成凍子，切片，以苦酒、五味淹食，不以灰汁則不成也。切作細絲，沸湯汋過，五味調食，狀如水母絲。馬志言其苗似半夏，楊慎丹鉛録言蒟醬即此者，皆誤也。王禎農書云：救荒之法，山有粉葛、蒟蒻、橡、栗之利。則此物亦有益于民者也。其斑杖，即天南星之類有斑者。

Collected Explanations. [Ma] Zhi: *Ruo tou* comes from Wu and Shu. The leaves resemble those of small Indian turnip [herbs] and *pinellia* [herbs]. The root has the size of a bowl. It grows on yin (i. e., shady) ground. Rain drops from its leaves and generates seeds. There is also a *ban zhang* 斑杖, "spotted cane," with a similar seedling. By autumn a flower comes out that is directed straight up and develops red seeds. The root is similar to *ruo tou* 蒻頭; it is violently poisonous and cannot be eaten. Bushy knotweed, *hu zhang* 虎杖, too, is named *ban zhang*; but it is different from the [item discussed] here. [Su] Song: White *ju ruo* coming from Wu zhong in Jiang nan is also called *gui yu* 鬼芋, "demon's taro." It grows in large numbers in the marshlands of the plains. People who collect it assume it is Indian turnip, *tian nan xing* 天南星. They are unable to distinguish the two. Those one gets on the market often are [Indian turnip]. However, the tissue of Indian turnip is fine and oily. While the stem of devil's tongue is spotted and its flowers are purple, the stem of Indian turnip has no spots and its flowers are yellow. That is the difference. [Li] Shizhen: Devil's tongue comes from Shu zhong; it can also be found in *Shi zhou*. It is [also] called "devil's head". People in Min zhong also plant it. For this purpose a pit is dug in the yin (i. e., shade) below trees and filled with manure. In spring a seedling grows which is relocated elsewhere at the latest in the fifth month. It has a length of one or two *chi*, and is similar to the seedlings of Indian turnip, except for its many spots. Its perennial root also grows a seedling by itself. What is said about rain drops [generating seeds], this is definitely not the case. After two years, the root has reached the size of a bowl or taro tuber. It is white outside and inside, and its flavor is numbing. The root is collected after autumn. It must be rubbed clean and is then either pounded or cut into pieces. It is boiled with a thick [furnace] ashes juice to bubbling, ten times or more, and then rinsed clean with water. Exchange the water and again boil it five or six times until it becomes a kind of jelly. Cut it into pieces and eat it with much bitter wine and the five flavors. If it is not [boiled] with the ashes juice, it will not form [a jelly]. It is cut into fine threads, and bubbling hot water is poured over them. Then they are mixed with the five flavors and eaten. They are shaped like the threads of jellyfish. Ma Zhi says that the seedling resembles that of *pinellia* [herbs]. Yang Shen in his *Dan qian lu* says "it is betel pepper." Both are wrong. Wang Zhen in his *Nong shu* states: "For being rescued in times of famine, the mountains hold *pueeraria* [root], devil's tongue, sawtooth oak and Chinese chestnuts for one's benefit." That is, this item is also good for the people. The *ban zhang* 斑杖, "spotted cane," is a kind of Indian turnip with spots.

17-25-01
根 *Gen*

Root [of *ju ruo*].

【氣味】辛，寒，有毒。【李廷飛曰】性冷，甚不益人，冷氣人少食之。生則戟人喉出血。

Qi and Flavor. Acrid, cold, poisonous. Li Tingfei: It is of cold nature, and very harmful to humans. When persons with cold qi eat it raw/fresh, it will pierce that person's throat and causes bleeding.

【主治】癰腫風毒，摩傅腫上。搗碎，以灰汁煮成餅，五味調食，主消渴。開寶。

Control. Obstruction-illness[1180] swelling with wind poison.[1181] Rub [the root] and apply it to a swelling. Pound it to pieces, boil it with a juice prepared from ashes

1180 *Yong* 癰, "obstruction-illness,"refers to an obstruction of vessels or other ducts inside the body. Qi rushing against the obstruction may cause a local swelling and eventually break through the surface to cause an abscess. BCGM Dict I, 641.

1181 *Feng du* 風毒, "wind poison," a condition caused by *feng* 風, "wind," and *du* 毒, "poison," resulting in a pathogenic evil qi including the characteristics of both. BCGM Dict I, 160.

[and water] and form a cake. Mix it with the five flavors and eat it. This controls melting with thirst.[1182] *Kai bao*.

【發明】【機曰】按三元延壽書云：有人患瘵，百物不忌，見鄰家修蒟蒻，求食之美，遂多食而瘵愈。又有病腮癰者數人，多食之，亦皆愈。

Explication. [Wang] Ji: According to the *San yuan yan shou shu*, once someone suffered from consumption, but failed to observe any [dietary and behavioral] restrictions. He witnessed how a neighbor prepared *ju ruo*, asked him [to let him have some] and when he ate it he was pleased by its flavor. Hence he ate a lot of it and his consumption was cured. Also, several persons suffering from cheek obstruction-illness ate a lot and they were all cured.

【附録】

Appendix.

17-25-A01

菩薩草宋圖經 ***Pu sa cao***, FE Song, *Tu jing*

Bodhisattva herb.

【頌曰】生江、浙州郡。凌冬不凋，秋冬有花直出，赤子如蒻頭。冬月采根用。味苦，無毒。主中諸毒食毒，酒研服之。又諸蟲傷，搗汁飲，并傅之。婦人妊娠欬嗽，搗篩蜜丸服，神效。

[Su] Song: It grows in the *zhou* and prefectures of Jiang and Zhe. It does not wither in winter. In autumn and winter flowers come out that are directed straight up. Their red seeds are similar to those of devil's tongue. In winter the root is collected for [therapeutic] application. Its flavor is bitter; it is nonpoisonous. To control being struck by all types of poison, and food poison, rub it in wine and ingest this. Also, for all types of harm caused by worms/bugs, pound it, drink the resulting juice and apply it [to the affected region]. For pregnant women with cough pound it, pass it through a sieve and with honey form pills to be ingested. Divinely effective.

1182 *Xiao ke* 消渴, "melting with thirst," most likely including cases of diabetes. BCGM Dict Vol I, 567.

17-26
半夏本經下品
Ban xia, FE *Ben jing*, lower rank.

***Pinellia ternata* (Thunb.) Breit.**

【釋名】守田本經、水玉本經、地文別録、和姑本經。【時珍曰】禮記月令：五月半夏生。蓋當夏之半也，故名。守田會意，水玉因形。

Explanation of Names. *Shou tian* 守田, "field guard," *Ben jing*. *Shui yu* 水玉, "water jade," *Ben jing*. *Di wen* 地文, "ground text/lines," *Bie lu*. *He gu* 和姑, "to harmonize an aunt," *Ben jing*.[1183] [Li] Shizhen: *Li ji*, Yue ling: "*Ban xia* 半夏 grows in the fifth month." The fact is, [the fifth month] is halfway, *ban* 半, through summer, *xia* 夏. Hence the name. "Field guard," refers to its purpose. "Water jade" is based on its physical appearance.

【集解】【別録曰】半夏生槐里川谷。五月、八月采根，暴乾。【普曰】生微丘或生野中，二月始生葉，三三相偶。白花圓上。【弘景曰】槐里屬扶風。今第一出青州，吴中亦有，以肉白者爲佳，不厭陳久。【恭曰】所在皆有。生平澤中者，名羊眼半夏，圓白爲勝。然江南者大乃徑寸，南人特重之。頃來互用，功狀殊異。其苗似是由跋，誤以爲半夏也。【頌曰】在處有之，以齊州者爲佳。二月生苗一莖，莖端三葉，淺緑色，頗似竹葉，而生江南者似芍藥葉。根下相重，上大下小，皮黄肉白。五月、八月采根，以灰裛二日，湯洗暴乾。蜀圖經云：五月采則虛小，八月采乃實大。其平澤生者甚小，名羊眼半夏。由跋絶類半夏，而苗不同。【斅曰】白傍𦰡子真似半夏，只是咬着微酸，不入藥用。

Collected Explanations. *Bie lu*: *Ban xia* grows in the river valleys of Huai li. The root is collected in the fifth and eighth month; it is dried in the sun. [Wu] Pu: It grows in low, hilly regions and in the wild. Its leaves begin to grow in the second month, with two or three of them forming a union. The flowers are white and round; they are on top [of the herb]. [Tao] Hongjing: Huai li belongs to Fu feng. Today, best quality [*ban xia*] comes from Qing zhou; it is also present in Wu zhong. That with white meat is excellent. If it is stored for a long time, it does not matter. [Su] Gong: It can be found everywhere. When it grows in the marshlands of the plains, it is called "sheep eye *ban xia*." [Roots that are] round and white are best. In Jiang nan, though, big specimens have a diameter of one *cun*, and southerners especially value them. They use the same fields [for them and for *ban xia*], but the [therapeutic] potentials and shapes [of both items] differ. The seedling [of "sheep eye *ban xia*"] resembles that of Indian turnip, *you ba* 由跋, and it is mistaken for *ban xia*. [Su] Gong: It can be found everywhere. Specimens from Qi zhou are excellent. In the

1183 Instead of *Ben jing* 本經, *Yu lan* ch. 992, *ban xia* 半夏, quotes *Wu shi ben cao* as its source.

second month it grows a seedling with one stem; at the tip of the stem are three leaves of a pale green color, somewhat resembling bamboo leaves. Those that grow in Jiang nan have leaves resembling those of *paeonia*. The root appears to double itself downward; with big [tubers] further up and small ones further down. The skin is yellow and the flesh is white. The root is collected in the fifth and eighth month. It is kept wrapped in ashes for two days. Then it is washed with hot water and dried in the sun. The *Shu tu jing* states: "Those collected in the fifth month are hollow and small; those collected in the eighth month are solid and big. Those from the marshlands in the plains are very small; they are named 'sheep eye *ban xia*.' *You ba* very much resembles *ban xia*, but the seedling differs." [Lei] Xiao: *Bai bang ji zi*[1184] is really similar to *ban xia*, except when you bite it it is has a slightly sour taste. It is not used as a medication.

【修治】【弘景曰】凡用，以湯洗十許過，令滑盡。不爾有毒，戟人咽喉。方中有半夏必須用生薑者，以制其毒故也。【斅曰】修事半夏四兩，用白芥子末二兩，釅醋二兩，攪濁，將半夏投中，洗三遍用之。若洗涎不盡，令人氣逆，肝氣怒滿。【時珍曰】今治半夏，惟洗去皮垢，以湯泡浸七日，逐日換湯，晾乾切片，薑汁拌焙入藥。或研爲末，以薑汁入湯浸澄三日，瀝去涎水，晒乾用，謂之半夏粉。或研末以薑汁和作餅子，日乾用，謂之半夏餅。或研末以薑汁、白礬湯和作餅，楮葉包置籃中，待生黄衣，日乾用，謂之半夏麴。白飛霞醫通云：痰分之病，半夏爲主，造而爲麴尤佳。治濕痰，以薑汁、白礬湯和之。治風痰，以薑汁及皂莢煮汁和之。治火痰，以薑汁、竹瀝，或荆瀝和之。治寒痰，以薑汁、礬湯入白芥子末和之，此皆造麴妙法也。

Pharmaceutical Preparation. [Tao] Hongjing: For all [medicinal] applications wash it with hot water more than ten times until [the surface of the roots] is no longer slippery. Otherwise [the root will remain to be] poisonous and pierces one's throat. When *ban xia* is used in a recipe, fresh ginger must also be used to check its poison. [Lei] Xiao: For its preparation, take four *liang* of *ban xia*. Add two *liang* of white mustard seed powder to two *liang* of thick vinegar, and stir this to obtain a turbid mixture. Then add the *ban xia* and wash it three times before using it [for medicinal purposes]. If the "saliva" [on the root] is not completely eliminated, it will cause a counterflow of one's qi, with liver qi causing anger and a feeling of fullness. [Li] Shizhen: When *ban xia* is processed today, they only wash it and remove its skin and dirt. Then it is soaked in hot water for seven days; with [the cooled water] replaced daily with hot water. Dry [the root] in the opening at a cool place and cut it into pieces. Mix them with ginger juice, dry them over a fire in a pan and add them

1184 *Bai bang ji zi* 白傍𦮼子, an herb of unknown identity.

to medication. Or grind [the root] into powder, give it with ginger juice into hot water and let it soak until the liquid is clear, after three days. Let the saliva/slime water trickle off, dry [the root] by basking it in the sun and then use [it for therapeutic purposes]. This is called "*ban xia* powder." Or mix the powder with ginger juice and prepare a cake. It is dried in the sun and then used. This is called "*ban xia* cake." Or mix the powder with ginger juice and alum in hot water and prepare a cake. Wrap it in paper mulberry tree leaves and place it into a basket until a yellow coating has formed. Then dry it in the sun and use this [for therapeutic purposes]. This is called *ban xia* leaven. Bai Feixia in his *Yi tong* states: "For diseases in the phlegm section, *ban xia* is the controlling [substance]; prepared to generate a leaven it is especially excellent. To cure phlegm with the presence of moisture, mix it with ginger juice and alum in hot water. To cure phlegm related to wind [intrusion] mix it with ginger juice and a *gleditsia* [pod/seed] decoction. To cure [diseases associated with] fire (i. e., heat) and phlegm mix it with ginger juice and bamboo stem juice, or *schizonepeta* juice. To cure [diseases associated with] cold and phlegm, mix it with ginger juice and alum in hot water, to which white mustard seeds are added. All these are the wondrous methods of a [*ban xia*] leaven preparation."

17-26-01
根 *Gen*

Root [of *ban xia*].

【氣味】辛，平，有毒。【別録曰】生微寒，熟温。生令人吐，熟令人下。湯洗盡滑用。【元素曰】味辛、苦，性温，氣味俱薄，沈而降，陰中陽也。【好古曰】辛厚苦輕，陽中陰也。入足陽明、太陰、少陽三經。【之才曰】射干爲之使。惡皂莢。畏雄黄、生薑、乾薑、秦皮、龜甲。反烏頭。【權曰】柴胡爲之使。忌羊血、海藻、飴糖。【元素曰】熱痰佐以黄芩，風痰佐以南星，寒痰佐以乾薑，痰痞佐以陳皮、白术。多用則瀉脾胃。諸血證及口渴者禁用，爲其燥津液也。孕婦忌之，用生薑則無害。

Qi and Flavor. Acrid, balanced, poisonous. *Bie lu*: Fresh it is slightly cold. Heat processed it is warm. Fresh it lets one vomit. Heat processed it causes discharge. To apply it it is washed with hot water and its slimy [saliva] surface is completely eliminated. [Zhang] Yuansu: Flavor acrid, bitter, nature warm. Qi and flavor are all weakly pronounced. It sinks and it ascends; it is a yang in yin [substance]. [Wang] Haogu: Its acrid [flavor] is strong; its bitter [flavor] is light. It is a yin in yang [substance]. It enters the three foot yang brilliance, [foot] major yin, and [foot] minor yang conduits. [Xu] Zhicai: Blackberry lily [root] serves as its guiding substance. [Ingested together,] it abhors *gleditsia* [pods/seeds]. It fears realgar, fresh ginger, dried ginger, *fraxinus* bark and tortoise carapaces. It is opposed to *aconitum* [main tuber]. [Zhen] Quan: *Bupleurum* [root] serves as its guiding substance. [During a therapy with *ban xia*,] sheep blood, *sargassum* herb and malt sugar are to be avoided. [Zhang] Yuansu: *Scutellaria* [root] helps it [in curing diseases associated with] heat and phlegm. Indian turnip [root] helps it [in curing diseases associated with] wind [intrusion] and phlegm. Dried ginger helps it [in curing diseases associated with] cold and phlegm. Tangerine peels and *atractylodes* [rhizome] help it [in curing] obstacle-illness[1185] associated with phlegm. Used often/in large amounts it causes spleen and stomach outflow. Its application is strictly forbidden for all signs of blood disease and thirst because it dries up body liquids. Pregnant women avoid it. An application [of *ban xia*] together with fresh ginger is not harmful.

【主治】傷寒寒熱，心下堅，胸脹欬逆，頭眩，咽喉腫痛，腸鳴，下氣止汗。本經。消心腹胸膈痰熱滿結，欬嗽上氣，心下急痛堅痞，時氣嘔逆，消癰腫，療痿黄，悦澤面目，墮胎。别録。消痰，下肺氣，開胃建脾，止嘔吐，去胸中痰滿。生者：摩癰腫，除瘤癭氣。甄權。治吐食反胃，霍亂轉筋，腸腹冷，痰瘧。大明。治寒痰及形寒飲冷傷肺而欬，消胸中痞，膈上痰，除胸寒，和胃氣，燥脾濕，治痰厥頭痛，消腫散結。元素。治眉稜骨痛。震亨。補肝風虚。好古。除腹脹，目不得瞑，白濁夢遺，帶下。時珍。

Control. Harm caused by cold; alternating sensations of cold and heat. Hardenings below the heart. Chest distension with cough and [qi] counterflow. Dizziness. Painful throat swelling. Intestinal sounds. [It serves to] discharge qi and end sweating. *Ben jing*. It serves to dissolve a feeling of fullness and bound [qi] in the central region and the abdomen, the chest and the diaphragm region. Cough with rising qi. Painful tension below the heart with hardening and obstacle-illness. Vomiting with [qi] counterflow related to seasonal qi. It dissolves obstruction-illness[1186] swelling. It heals dysfunction with yellow [complexion]. It provides the face and the eyes with a pleasant glossiness. It stimulates abortion. *Bie lu*. It dissolves phlegm, discharges lung qi, opens the stomach and strengthens the spleen. It ends vomiting, and eliminates a feeling of fullness related to the presence of phlegm in the chest. Fresh specimens are rubbed on obstruction-illness swelling. It removes tumorous goiter qi. Zhen Quan. It serves to cure vomiting of food with a turned over stomach, cholera with contorted sinews, cold in the intestines and the abdomen, phlegm malaria. Da Ming. It serves to cure [diseases associated with] cold and phlegm,

---

1185 *Pi* 痞, "obstacle-illness," a condition of an uncomfortable distension and fullness in the chest and abdominal region. When pressed there is no pain. BCGM Dict I. 371.

1186 *Yong* 癰, "obstruction-illness,"refers to an obstruction of vessels or other ducts inside the body. Qi rushing against the obstruction may cause a local swelling and eventually break through the surface to cause an abscess. BCGM Dict I, 641.

and cough related to a cold body, cold beverages and harm caused to the lung. It dissolves obstacle-illness[1187] in the chest and phlegm above the diaphragm. It eliminates cold from the chest, harmonizes stomach qi, and dries spleen moisture. It serves to cure headache related to the presence of phlegm and ceasing [yang qi]. It dissolves swelling and disperses bound [qi]. [Zhang] Yuansu. It serves to cure a painful bone ridge behind the eyebrows. [Zhu] Zhenheng. It supplements liver [qi] in the case of depletion and wind [intrusion]. [Wang] Haogu. It eliminates abdominal distension. [It serves to cure] inability of eyes to close to sleep. Uncontrolled loss of white, turbid [urine/sperm of males] during dreams. [Diseases] below the belt [of women]. [Li] Shizhen.

【發明】【權曰】半夏使也。虛而有痰氣，宜加用之。【頌曰】胃冷嘔噦，方藥之最要。【成無己曰】辛者散也，潤也。半夏之辛，以散逆氣結氣，除煩嘔，發音聲，行水氣而潤腎燥。【好古曰】經云，腎主五液，化爲五濕。自入爲唾，入肝爲泣，入心爲汗，入脾爲痰，入肺爲涕。有痰曰嗽，無痰曰欬。痰者，因欬而動脾之濕也。半夏能泄痰之標，不能泄痰之本。泄本者，泄腎也。欬無形，痰有形。無形則潤，有形則燥，所以爲流濕潤燥也。俗以半夏爲肺藥，非也。止嘔吐爲足陽明，除痰爲足太陰。柴胡爲之使，故小柴胡湯中用之，雖爲止嘔，亦助柴胡、黄芩主往來寒熱，是又爲足少陽、陽明也。【宗奭曰】今人惟知半夏去痰，不言益脾，蓋能分水故也。脾惡濕，濕則濡困，困則不能治水。經云：水勝則瀉。一男子夜數如厠，或教以生薑一兩，半夏、大棗各三十枚，水一升，瓷瓶中慢火燒爲熟水，時呷之，便已也。【趙繼宗曰】丹溪言二陳湯治一身之痰，世醫執之，凡有痰者皆用。夫二陳内有半夏，其性燥烈。若風痰、寒痰、濕痰、食痰則相宜。至于勞痰、失血諸痰，用之反能燥血液而加病，不可不知。【機曰】俗以半夏性燥有毒，多以貝母代之。貝母乃太陰肺經之藥，半夏乃太陰脾經、陽明胃經之藥，何可代也？夫欬嗽吐痰，虛勞吐血，或痰中見血，諸鬱，咽痛喉痺，肺癰肺痿，癰疽，婦人乳難，此皆貝母爲向導，半夏乃禁用之藥。若涎者脾之液，美味膏粱炙煿，皆能生脾胃濕熱，故涎化爲痰，久則痰火上攻，令人昏憒口噤，偏廢僵仆，蹇澁不語，生死旦夕，自非半夏、南星，曷可治乎？若以貝母代之，則翹首待斃矣。【時珍曰】脾無留濕不生痰，故脾爲生痰之源，肺爲貯痰之器。半夏能主痰飲及腹脹者，爲其體滑而味辛性温也。涎滑能潤，辛温能散亦能潤，故行濕而通大便，利竅而泄小便。所謂辛走氣，能化液，辛以潤之是矣。潔古張氏云：半夏、南星治其痰，而欬嗽自愈。丹溪朱氏云：二陳湯能使大便潤而小便長。聊攝成氏云：半夏辛而散，行水氣而潤腎燥。又和劑局方用半硫丸治老人虛秘，皆取其滑潤也。世俗皆以南星、半夏爲性燥，誤矣。濕

1187 *Pi* 痞, "obstacle-illness," a condition of an uncomfortable distension and fullness in the chest and abdominal region. When pressed there is no pain. BCGM Dict I. 371.

去則土燥，痰涎不生，非二物之性燥也。古方治咽痛喉痺，吐血下血，多用二物，非禁劑也。二物亦能散血，故破傷打撲皆主之。惟陰虛勞損，則非濕熱之邪，而用利竅行濕之藥，是乃重竭其津液，醫之罪也，豈藥之咎哉！甲乙經用治夜不眠，是果性燥者乎？岐伯云：衛氣行于陽，陽氣滿，不得入于陰，陰氣虛，故目不得瞑。治法：飲以半夏湯一劑，陰陽既通，其卧立至。方用流水千里者八升，揚之萬遍，取清五升，煮之，炊以葦薪，大沸，入秫米一升，半夏五合，煮一升半，飲汁一盃，日三，以知爲度。病新發者，覆盃則卧，汗出則已。久者三飲而已。

Explication. [Zhen] Quan: *Ban xia* is a guiding substance. For depletion with the presence of phlegm qi it should be resorted to as an additive. [Su] Song: For stomach cold and retching, it is a most important recipe drug. Cheng Wuji: Acrid [flavor] disperses and moistens. The acrid [flavor] of *ban xia* serves to disperse counter-flowing qi and bound qi. It eliminates vexing vomiting, helps to effuse voice sounds, stimulates the passage of water and qi and moistens dryness in the kidneys. [Wang] Haogu: The classic states: "The kidney controls the five liquids; it transform them to generate the five kinds of moisture." [Moisture] that enters [the kidneys] themselves becomes saliva. [Moisture] that enters the liver becomes tears. [Moisture] that enters the heart becomes sweat. [Moisture] that enters the spleen becomes phlegm. [Moisture] that enters the lung becomes snivel. With phlegm, that is to say: [silent] cough. Without phlegm, that is to say: [noisy] cough. Phlegm is the liquid of the spleen excited by cough. *Ban xia* is capable of draining phlegm as the tip [of a disease]; it is not able to drain the root [that is the cause] of phlegm. To drain the root is to drain the kidneys. Cough has no physical appearance. Phlegm has a physical appearance. That without physical appearance (i. e., the cough) is to be moistened; that with physical appearance (i. e., the phlegm) is to be dried. Hence what is at stake here is to make moisture flow off and to moisten what is dry. *Ban xia* is commonly held to be a pharmaceutical drug for the lung. That is not so. When it ends vomiting, that is an activity in the foot yang brilliance [conduits]; when it eliminates phlegm, that is an activity in the foot major yin [conduits]. *Bupleurum* [root] serves as its guidance substance. Hence [*ban xia*] is used as an ingredient of the "small decoction with *bupleurum* [root]."[1188] Although it serves to end vomiting, it also assists *bupleurum* [root] and *scutellaria* [root] in their control of alternating sensations of cold and heat, and these are activities in the foot minor yang and yang brilliance [conduits]. [Kou] Zongshi: Today, people only know that *ban xia* removes phlegm. No one says that it boosts spleen [qi]. The fact is, this is based on its ability

1188 *Xiao chai hu tang* 小柴胡湯, the "small decoction with *chai hu*," has the following ingredients: Bupleurum root, *scutellaria* root, ginseng root, *pinellia* root, dried *glycyrrhiza* root, fresh ginger, Chinese dates.

to separate waters. The spleen abhors moisture. When it is moist it has a problem of being immersed. With such a problem it is unable to govern the [body's] waters. The Classic states: "When water dominates, this results in outflow." When a male goes to the latrine several times during the night, he is taught to heat one *liang* of fresh ginger, 30 *ban xia* [roots] and 30 Chinese dates in a porcelain jar over a slow fire to prepare a "processed water," and to sip this over time. This will end [his problem]. Zhao Jizong: [Zhu] Danxi says: "The 'decoction with the two long-stored [ingredients]'[1189] serves to cure phlegm anywhere in the entire body." Throughout the times, physicians have accepted this, and whenever they encountered a phlegm [disease], they always used it. Now, one of the two long-stored [ingredients] is *ban xia*. By its nature it is violently drying. For wine phlegm, cold phlegm, moisture phlegm and food phlegm, it is a suitable [pharmaceutical drug]. However, when it comes to exhaustion phlegm or all types of phlegm related to blood loss, to use it would contrary [to one's intentions] dry the blood liquid and further add to the disease. That must be known! [Wang] Ji: Since *ban xia* by its nature is drying and poisonous, it is commonly replaced by *fritillaria* [root]. *Fritillaria* [root] is a pharmaceutical drug for the major yin lung conduits, while *ban xia* is a pharmaceutical drug for the major yin conduits of the spleen and the yang brilliance conduits of the stomach. How could it be possible to replace one by the other! Now, for cough with spitting of phlegm, depletion exhaustion with spitting of blood, or blood appearing in the phlegm, all [conditions of] pent-up qi, painful throat and throat blockage, lung obstruction-illness[1190] and lung dysfunction, obstruction-illness and impediment-illness,[1191] and women with difficult birth, for all these [disorders] *fritillaria* [root] is the appropriate guiding substance, while the use of *ban xia* as a pharmaceutical drug is to be avoided. Saliva is the liquid of the spleen. Delicacies of fat, rich and roasted food can generate moisture and heat in spleen and stomach. As a result, saliva is transformed to phlegm. When this continues for a long time, phlegm fire rises to attack above, causing confusion and lockjaw, hemilateral disablement and falls, speech disorder or speechlessness, with a transition from life to death between early morning and evening. How could these [conditions] be cured without resorting

1189 *Er chen tang* 二陳湯, the "decoction with two long-stored ingredients," has the following ingredients: *Ban xia*, tangerine peels, *poria*, dried *glycyrrhiza* root, fresh ginger, smoked plum.

1190 *Fei yong* 肺癰, "lung obstruction-illness," also: *fei yong* 肺壅, "lung obstruction," a condition of abscesses in the lung, with fever, chest pain, and vomiting of bad-smelling pus and blood. BCGM Dict I, 156.

1191 *Yong ju* 癰疽, "obstruction-illness, impediment-illness." refers to two vaguely distinguished obstructions/impediments of vessels or other ducts inside the body. Qi rushing against the obstruction may cause a local swelling and eventually break through the surface to cause an abscess. BCGM Dict I, 642.

to *ban xia* and Indian turnip [root]? When they are replaced by *fritillaria* [root, patients] might as well raise the head and wait for death. [Li] Shizhen: When moisture remains in the spleen, it does not generate phlegm. The reason is, the spleen is the source of phlegm; the lung is the vessel where phlegm is stored. *Ban xia* is capable of controlling phlegm rheum and abdominal distension because its physical body is smooth/slippery, its flavor is acrid and by its nature it is warm. The smoothness resulting from its saliva/slime can moisten; the acrid [flavor] and the warm [nature] can disperse and also moisten. Hence [*ban xia*] stimulates the passage of moisture and frees the passage of defecation. It opens the orifices and promotes an outflow of urine. This is an example of what it called "acrid [flavor] lets the qi run and can transform body liquid. Acrid [flavor] is used to moisten." Mr. Zhang Jiegu states: "When *ban xia* and Indian turnip [root] have cured phlegm, cough is healed as a result." Mr. Zhu Danxi states: "The 'decoction with two long-stored ingredients' can be engaged to moisten defecation and further urination." Mr. Cheng [Wuji] from Lao she states: "*Ban xia* is acrid and disperses. It stimulates the passage of water and qi, and moistens the dryness of the kidneys." Also, the *He ji ju fang* [recommends to] use the "pills with *ban* [*xia*] and sulphur"[1192] to cure depletion constipation of old people, always taking advantage of [*ban xia*'s ability to] smoothen and moisten. At all times it has been commonly held that Indian turnip [root] and *ban xia* by their nature are dry[ing]. That is a mistake. When the soil [i. e., the spleen] is devoid of moisture it is dry, and neither phlegm nor saliva are generated. But this is not caused by these two items because of their [alledged] dry[ing] nature. Ancient recipes often [recommend to] resort to these two items to cure throat pain and throat closure, blood spitting and blood discharge. Such preparations are not prohibited! Both these items also can disperse blood. Hence they are always resorted to for treating open wounds caused by blows. Only when for yin [qi] depletion with exhaustion and injury, that are not related to evil [qi] of moisture and heat, [*ban xia* and Indian turnip [root] are applied as pharmaceutical drugs to open the orifices and stimulate the passage of moisture, then this serves to further aggravate a deficit of body liquids, and this is a physician's crime! How could the pharmaceutical drugs be blamed! The *Jia yi jing* [recommends to] "use [*ban xia*] to cure insomnia." Is this so because of its dry nature? Qi Bo states: "The guardian qi pass through the yang [conduits]. When they are filled with yang qi, they cannot enter the yin [section], resulting in a yin qi depletion. Hence [such patients] cannot close their eyes and sleep. The method to cure this: [Let patients] drink one preparation of a '*ban xia* decoction.' Once the communication between yin and yang [qi] is reestab-

1192 The *ban liu wan* 半硫丸, "pills with *ban* [*xia*] and sulphur," has the following ingredients: *Ban xia*, sulphur, fresh ginger.

lished, [patients] will lie down and sleep instantly." The recipe [of the "*ban xia* decoction" is as follows.] Get eight *liang* of [river] water that has flowed a thousand *li*. Throw it up and make it splash 10 000 times. Let it turn clear, take five *sheng* of it and boil it. Then heat it with reed firewood until it massively bubbles, add one *sheng* of glutinous millet and five *ge* of *ban xia*, and boil it down to one and a half *sheng*. [Let patients] drink one cup of the juice, three times a day, until an effect shows. When the disease has just begun, [patients] will lie down and sleep once they have emptied one cup. They will sweat and [the disease] is cured. [When the disease] has lasted for a long time, they need to drink three [cups] to cure it.

【附方】舊十五，新五十三。

Added Recipes. 15 of old. 53 newly [recorded].

法制半夏。清痰化飲，壯脾順氣。用大半夏，湯洗七次，焙乾再洗，如此七轉，以濃米泔浸一日夜。每一兩用白礬一兩半，温水化，浸五日。焙乾，以鉛白霜一錢，温水化，又浸七日。以漿水慢火内煮沸，焙乾收之。每嚼一二粒，薑湯送化下。御藥院方。

The method to check [unwanted effects of] *ban xia*, [when it is used] to clear phlegm and to transform [phlegm] rheum. Wash a big *ban xia* [root] with hot water seven times. Dry it over a fire in a pan and wash it again. Do this seven times, then soak it for one day and one night in dense water that has been used to wash rice. For every *liang* [of *ban xia*] add one and a half *liang* of alum, dissolved in warm water, and let the [root] soak [in this water] for another five days. Then dry [the root] over a fire in a pan. Add one *qian* of lead acetate, dissolved in warm water, and soak [the root in this water] for another seven days. Then boil it in fermented water of foxtail millet over a slow fire to bubbling, dry it over a fire in a pan and store it. For each [application] chew one or two grains, to be sent down dissolved in a ginger decoction. *Yu yao yuan fang*.

紅半夏法。消風熱，清痰涎，降氣利咽。大半夏湯浸焙制如上法。每一兩入龍腦五分；朱砂爲衣染之。先鋪燈草一重，約一指厚，排半夏于上，再以燈草蓋一指厚。以炒豆焙之，候乾取出。每嚼一兩粒，温水送下。御藥院方。

The method [to prepare] "red *ban xia*" [when *ban xia* is used] to dissolve heat related to wind [intrusion], to clear phlegm-type saliva, to send down qi and to free the passage through the throat. Soak one big *ban xia* [root] in hot water, dry it over a fire in a pan and check [its unwanted effects] with the method described above. For every *liang* [of *ban xia*] add five *fen* of borneol and coat it with cinnabar. First spread a layer of common rush, about one finger thick, place the *ban xia* on top of it and cover it with another one finger-thick layer of common rush. Roast soybeans and bake [the *ban xia*] with them. Wait until they are dry and remove them. For each [application] chew one or two grains and send them down with warm water. *Yu yao yuan fang*.

化痰鎮心，袪風利膈。辰砂半夏丸：用半夏一斤，湯泡七次，爲末篩過，以水浸三日，生絹濾去滓，澄清去水，晒乾，一兩，入辰砂一錢，薑汁打糊丸梧子大。每薑湯下七十丸。此周府方也。袖珍方。

To transform/dissolve phlegm and calm the heart, to dispel wind and free the passage through the diaphragm. The "pills with cinnabar and *ban xia*." Steep one *jin* of *ban xia* in hot water seven times, [grind it into] powder and pass it through a sieve. Soak [the powder] in water for three days, strain it through thin, tough silk, wait for the liquid to clear and discard the water. Dry [the powder] in the sun. To one *liang* add one *qian* of cinnabar, and with ginger juice [and wheat flour] prepare a paste to form pills the size of *wu* seeds. Each time send down with a ginger decoction 70 pills. This is a recipe of the Zhou court. *Xiu zhen fang*.

化痰利氣。三仙丸，方見虎掌下。

To transform/dissolve phlegm and free the passage of qi. The "three hermits/immortals pills." For the recipe, see under [the entry] Indian turnip (17-23).

消痰開胃，去胸膈壅滯。斗門方用半夏洗泡，焙乾爲末，自然薑汁和作餅，濕紙裹，煨香。以熟水二盞，同餅二錢，入鹽五分，煎一盞，服之。大壓痰毒及酒食傷，極驗。

To transform/dissolve phlegm and open the stomach, to remove obstructions with sluggish [qi] from the chest and the diaphragm region. The *Dou men fang* [recommends to] wash and steep [in boiling water] *ban xia*, dry it over a fire in a pan and [grind it] into powder. Mix [the powder] with natural ginger juice and form a cake. Wrap it in moist paper, slowly roast it until it develops a fragrance, and form with two cups of boiled water a cake of two *qian*. Add five *fen* of salt, boil it down to one cup, and ingest it. This serves to vigorously suppress phlegm poison and any harm resulting from wine or food. Very effective.

經驗用半夏、天南星各二兩爲末，水五升，入壜内浸一宿，去清水，焙乾重研。每服二錢，水二盞，薑三片，煎服。

The *Jing yan*[1193] [recommends to grind] two *liang* each of *ban xia* and Indian turnip [root] into powder, soak them in a big earthen jug for one night, remove the clear

1193 Instead of *Jing yan* 經驗, *Zheng lei* ch. 10, *ban xia* 半夏, writes *Jing yan hou fang* 經驗後方.

water, dry them over a fire in a pan, repeat this, and then grind [them into powder]. Each time ingest two *qian* to be boiled in two cups of water with three slices of ginger. Ingest the decoction.

中焦痰涎。利咽，清頭目，進飲食。半夏泡七次四兩，枯礬一兩爲末，薑汁打糊，或煮棗肉，和丸梧子大。每薑湯下十五丸。寒痰加丁香五錢，熱痰加寒水石煅四兩。名玉液丸。和劑局方。

Phlegm-type saliva in the central [section of the Triple] Burner. [This recipe serves to] free the passage through the throat, clear head and eyes, and stimulate the intake of beverages and food. [Grind] four *liang* of *ban xia*, steeped [in hot water] seven times, and one *liang* of processed alum into powder, prepare with ginger juice [and wheat flour] a paste, or boil it with Chinese date meat, and form pills the size of *wu* seeds. Each time send down with a ginger decoction 15 pills. In the case of cold [qi] and phlegm, add five *qian* of clove. For heat [qi] and phlegm, add four *liang* of calcined calcite. [The recipe is] called "pills with jade liquid." *He ji ju fang*.

老人風痰。大腑熱，不識人，及肺熱痰實不利。半夏泡七次焙，硝石各半兩，爲末，入白麵一兩搗勻，水和丸緑豆大。每薑湯下五十丸。普濟。

Wind [intrusion] and phlegm of old people. Heat in the large repository,[1194] with an inability to recognize other persons. The lung is replete with heat [qi] and phlegm, and [the passage of qi through the lung] is blocked. [Grind] half a *liang* each of *ban xia*, steeped [in hot water] seven times and dried over a fire in a pan, and nitrokalite into powder. Add white wheat flour and pound this to an even mixture to be formed with water to pills the size of mung beans. Each time send down with a ginger decoction 50 pills. *Pu ji*.

膈壅風痰。半夏半斤，酸漿浸一宿，温湯洗五十遍，去惡氣，日乾爲末。漿水搜作餅，日乾，再研爲末。每五兩入生龍腦一錢，以漿水濃脚和丸雞頭子大。紗袋盛，避風處陰乾。每服一丸，好茶或薄荷湯嚼下。御藥院方。

Blocked diaphragm related to wind [intrusion] and phlegm. Soak half a *jin* of *ban xia* with Chinese lantern plant for one night, wash it with warm water 50[1195] times to remove its malign qi, dry it in the sun and [grind it into] powder. Add fermented water of foxtail millet to form a cake, dry it in the sun, and once again grind it into powder. For each five *liang* add one *qian* of fresh borneol, and with the dense dregs

1194 The term *da fu* 大腑, "big repository," is not well defined. It is sometimes identified as the Triple Burner, *san jiao* 三焦, as its upper, central and lower section are seen as the "largest" among all the depot and repository organs. It may also be simply a writing error of *da chang* 大腸, "large intestine."

1195 Instead of *wu shi* 五十, "50," *Zheng lei* ch. 10, *ban xia* 半夏, quoting *Yu yao yuan fang* writes *wu qi* 五七, "five times seven."

of fermented water of foxtail millet form pills the size of foxnut seeds. Fill them into a gauze bag and let them dry shielded from wind[1196] in a yin (i. e., shady) location. Each time ingest one pill, to be chewed and sent down with good tea or a mint decoction. *Yu yao yuan fang*.

搜風化痰，定志安神，利頭目。辰砂化痰丸：用半夏麴三兩，天南星炮一兩，辰砂、枯礬各半兩，爲末，薑汁打糊丸梧子大。每服三十丸，食後薑湯送下。和劑局方。

To search for wind [that has intruded and is to be dispelled] and transform phlegm, to stabilize the mind and pacify the spirit, and to benefit head and eyes. The "pills with cinnabar to transform phlegm." [Grind] three *liang* of *ban xia* leaven, one *liang* of Indian turnip [root] and half a *liang* each of cinnabar and processed alum into powder. With ginger juice [and wheat flour] prepare a paste to form pills the size of *wu* seeds. Each time ingest 30 pills, to be sent down with a ginger decoction following a meal. *He ji ju fang*.

痰厥中風。省風湯：用半夏湯泡八兩，甘草炙二兩，防風四兩。每服半兩，薑二十片，水二盞，煎服。奇效良方。

Phlegm and ceasing [yang qi] associated with wind stroke. The "decoction to reduce wind." Prepare eight *liang* of *ban xia*, soaked in hot water, two *liang* of *glycyrrhiza* [root], roasted, and four *liang* of *saposhnikovia* [root]. For each ingestion boil half a *liang* [of this mixture] with 20 slices of ginger in two cups of water and ingest the decoction. *Qi xiao liang fang*.

風痰頭運，嘔逆目眩，面色青黃，脉弦者。水煮金花丸：用生半夏、生天南星、寒水石煅各一兩、天麻半兩，雄黄二錢，小麥麵三兩爲末，水和成餅，水煮浮起，漉出，搗丸梧子大。每服五十丸，薑湯下，極效。亦治風痰咳嗽，二便不通，風痰頭痛。潔古活法機要方。

Movement in the head/vertigo related to wind [intrusion] and phlegm, vomiting with [qi] counterflow, dimmed vision, a greenish-yellow facial complexion, and a string-like [movement in the] vessels. The "pills with golden flowers boiled in water." [Grind] one *liang* each of fresh *ban xia*, fresh Indian turnip [root], and calcined calcite, half a *liang* of *gastrodia* [root], two *qian* of realgar, and three *liang* of wheat flour into powder, mix it with water and form cakes. Boil them in water until they have risen to float on the surface, strain [the liquid] to remove them and pound them to prepare pills the size of *wu* seeds. Each time ingest 50 pills, to be sent down with a ginger decoction. Extremely effective. They also serve to cure cough associat-

---

1196 Instead of *bi feng* 避風, "to avoid wind," "shielded from wind," *Zheng lei* ch. 10, *ban xia* 半夏, writes *tong feng* 通風, "passed through by wind."

ed with wind [intrusion] and phlegm, blockage of the two [major (i. e., defecation) and minor (i. e. urination) ways of] relief, and headache related to wind [intrusion] and phlegm. A recipe[recorded in Zhang] Jiegu's *Huo fa ji yao*.

風痰濕痰。清壺丸：半夏一斤，天南星半兩，各湯泡，晒乾爲末，薑汁和作餅，焙乾，入神麴半兩，白术末四兩，枳實末二兩，薑汁麵糊丸梧子大。每服五十丸，薑湯下。葉氏方。

Wind [intrusion] with phlegm; presence of moisture with phlegm. The "pills to clear the kettle." Soak half a *jin* of *ban xia* and half a *liang* of Indian turnip [root] separately in hot water, dry them in the sun and [grind them into] powder. Mix it with ginger juice and form cakes. Dry them over a fire in a pan, add half a *liang* of medicated leaven, four *liang* of *atractylodes* [rhizome] powder and two *liang* of immature and dried bitter orange fruits and form with a ginger juice and wheat flour paste pills the size of *wu* seeds. Each time ingest 50 pills, to be sent down with a ginger decoction. *Ye shi fang*.

風痰喘逆，兀兀欲吐，眩運欲倒。半夏一兩，雄黄三錢爲末。薑汁浸，蒸餅丸梧子大。每服三十丸，薑湯下。已吐者加檳榔。活法機要。

Panting with [qi] counterflow related to wind [intrusion] and phlegm. An extreme urge to vomit. Dizziness and a tendency to fall. [Grind] one *liang* of *ban xia* and three *qian* of realgar into powder. Soak it in ginger juice and with steamed cakes form pills the size of *wu* seeds. Each time ingest 30 pills, to be sent down with a ginger decoction. When vomiting has already started, add *areca* [nuts]. *Huo fa ji yao*.

風痰喘急。千緡湯：用半夏湯洗七個，甘草炙、皂莢炒各一寸，薑三片，水一盞，煎七分，温服。和劑局方。

Hectic panting related to wind [intrusion] and phlegm. The "decoction as effective as a thousand fishing lines." Wash seven *ban xia* [roots] in hot water, add roasted *glycyrrhiza* [roots] and fried *gleditsia* [pods/seeds], each of one *cun* length, and three slices of ginger and boil them in one cup of water down to 70%, to be ingested warm. *He ji ju fang*.

上焦熱痰，欬嗽。制過半夏一兩，片黄芩末二錢，薑汁打糊丸緑豆大。每服七十丸，淡薑湯食後服。此周憲王親製方也。袖珍方。

Heat [qi] and phlegm in the upper [section of the Triple] Burner. Prepare with one *liang* of processd *ban xia*, two *qian* of sliced *scutellaria* [root] powder and ginger juice a [wheat flour] paste to form pills the size of mung beans. Each time ingest 70 pills, to be ingested with a bland ginger decoction after a meal. This is a recipe designed by Zhou Xian wang in person. *Xiu zhen fang*.

肺熱痰嗽。制半夏、栝樓仁各一兩，爲末，薑汁打糊丸梧子大。每服二三十丸，白湯下。或以栝樓瓤煮熟丸。濟生方。

Lung heat with phlegm and cough. [Grind] one *liang* each of processed *ban xia* and Japanese gourd kernels into powder and form with a ginger juice and [wheat flour] paste pills the size of *wu* seeds. Each time ingest 20 to 30 pills, to be sent down with clear, boiled water. Or boil [the powder] with Japanese gourd pulp until done and form this to pills. *Ji sheng fang.*

熱痰欬嗽，煩熱面赤，口燥心痛，脉洪數者。小黄丸：用半夏、天南星各一兩，黄芩一兩半，爲末，薑汁浸蒸餅丸梧子大。每服五七十丸，食後薑湯下。潔古活法機要。

Heat, phlegm and cough. A vexing heat with a red face, a dry mouth, heart pain and a vast and accelerated [movement in the] vessels. The "little yellow pills." [Grind] one *liang* each of *ban xia* and Indian turnip [root], and one and a half *liang* of *scutellaria* [root] into powder. Soak it in ginger juice and with steamed cakes form pills the size of *wu* seeds. Each time ingest 50 to 70 pills, to be sent down with a ginger decoction after a meal. [Zhang] Jiegu, *Huo fa ji yao.*

小兒痰熱，欬嗽驚悸。半夏、南星等分，爲末。牛膽汁和，入膽内，懸風處待乾，蒸餅丸緑豆大。每薑湯下三五丸。摘玄方。

Phlegm and heat of children, with cough and fright palpitation. [Grind] equal amounts of *ban xia* and Indian turnip [root] into powder. Mix it with ox bile and fill it into the [gallbladder]. Suspend it at a windy location and wait until it has dried. With steamed cakes form pills the size of mung beans. Each time [let the child] send down with a ginger decoction three to five pills. *Zhai xuan fang.*

濕痰欬嗽，面黄體重，嗜卧，驚，兼食不消，脉緩者。白术丸：用半夏、南星各一兩，白术一兩半，爲末，薄糊丸梧子大。每服五七十丸，薑湯下。活法機要。

Cough with the presence of moisture and phlegm, the face is yellow and the body is heavy, with a desire to lie down. Fright and an inability to dissolve food. A slowed down [movement in the] vessels. The "pills with *atractylodes macrocephala* [rhizome]." [Grind] one *liang* each of *ban xia* and Indian turnip [root] with one and a half *liang* of *atractylodes macrocephala* [rhizome] into powder and with a water gruel form pills the size of *wu* seeds. Each time ingest 50 to 70 pills, to be sent down with a ginger decoction. *Huo fa ji yao.*

氣痰欬嗽，面白氣促，洒淅惡寒，愁憂不樂，脉濇者。玉粉丸：用半夏、南星各一兩，官桂半兩，爲末，糊丸梧子大。每服五十丸，薑湯下。活法機要。

Qi [disorder] with phlegm and cough, a white face and hectic [breath] qi, shivering and an aversion to cold, worries and unhappiness, and a rough [movement in the] vessels. The "jade powder pills." [Grind] one *liang* each of *ban xia* and Indian turnip [root] and half a *liang* of *cassia* bark into powder, and with [wheat flour] paste form pills the size of *wu* seeds. Each time ingest 50 pills, to be sent down with a ginger decoction. *Huo fa ji yao.*

小結胸痛，正在心下，按之則痛，脉浮滑者，小陷胸湯主之。半夏半升，黄連一兩，栝樓實大者一個，水六升，先煮栝樓取三升，去滓，内二味煮取二升，分三服。仲景傷寒論。

Painful minor bound chest,[1197] directly underneath the heart. When pressed it aches. The [movement in the] vessels is at the surface and smooth/slippery. This is controlled by the "minor decoction for a sunken chest." Prepare half a *sheng* of *ban xia*, one *liang* of *coptis* [rhizome], one large Japanese snake gourd and six *sheng* of water. First boil the Japanese snake gourd in the water down to three *sheng* and remove the dregs. Then add the remaining two substances and boil this down to two *sheng*, to be ingested divided into three portions. [Zhang] Zhongjing, *Shang han lun.*

濕痰心痛喘急者。半夏油炒爲末，粥糊丸緑豆大。每服二十丸，薑湯下。丹溪心法。

Moisture, phlegm, heart pain and hectic panting. Fry *ban xia* in oil, [grind it into] powder and with a rice congee paste form pills the size of mung beans. Each time ingest 20 pills, to be sent down with a ginger decoction. *Danxi xin fa.*

急傷寒病。半夏四錢，生薑七片，酒一盞，煎服。胡洽居士百病方。

Acute harm caused by cold disease. Boil four *qian* of *ban xia* with seven slices of fresh ginger in one cup of wine and ingest the decoction. Hu Qia jushi, *Bai bing fang.*

結痰不出，語音不清，年久者亦宜。玉粉丸：半夏半兩，桂心一字，草烏頭半字，爲末。薑汁浸蒸餅丸芡子大。每服一丸，夜卧含嚥。活法機要。

Bound phlegm that fails to come out, with blurred speech. [This recipe] is suitable even for cases having lasted for years. The "jade powder pills." [Grind] half a *liang*

1197 *Xiao jie xiong* 小結胸, "minor bound chest," a condition of *jie xiong* 結胸, "bound chest," brought forth by phlegm and heat, with the chest and abdomen experiencing distension, hardening and pain to a degree that one does not wish to have pressure applied there. BCGM Dict I, 252, 567.

of *ban xia*, one *zi* of shaved cinnamom bark and half a *zi* of *aconitum* [main tuber] into powder. Soak it in ginger juice and with steamed cakes form pills the size of *qian* seeds. Each time ingest one pill. At night at bedtime hold it in the mouth and swallow [the resulting saliva]. *Huo fa ji yao.*

停痰冷飲，嘔逆。橘皮半夏湯：用半夏水煮熟、陳橘皮各一兩。每服四錢，生薑七片，水二盞，煎一盞，温服。和劑局方。

Stagnating cold phlegm rheum, with vomiting and [qi] counterflow. The "decoction with tangerine peels and *ban xia.*" Prepare one *liang* each of *ban xia*, boiled in water until done, and long-stored tangerine peels. Each time ingest four *qian* [of this mixture] boiled with seven slices of fresh ginger in two cups of water down to one cup. To be ingested warm. *He ji ju fang.*

停痰留飲，胸膈滿悶，氣短惡心，飲食不下，或吐痰水。伏苓半夏湯：用半夏泡五兩，伏苓三兩。每服四錢，薑七片，水一鍾半，煎七分，甚捷徑。和劑局方。

Stagnating phlegm rheum, with a feeling of fullness in the chest and diaphragm region, and heart pressure, shortness of [breath] qi, nausea, and an inability to send down beverages and food. Sometimes accompanied by phlegm spitting. The "decoction with *poria* and *ban xia.*" Prepare five *liang* of *ban xia*, soaked in water, and three *liang* of *poria*. Each time ingest four *qian* [of this mixture] and boil them with seven slices of ginger in one and a half *zhong* of water down to 70%.[1198] A very fast shortcut [to healing]. *He ji ju fang.*

支飲作嘔。嘔家本渴，不渴者，心下有支飲也。或似喘不喘，似嘔不嘔，似噦不噦，心下憒憒，並宜小半夏湯。用半夏泡七次，一升，生薑半升，水七升，煮一升五合，分服。張仲景金匱要略。

A propping [phlegm] rheum causing vomiting. Patients who vomit should be thirsty, but here they are not thirsty and have a propping rheum below the heart. Or it seems as if they panted, but they do not pant, as if they vomited, but they do not vomit, as if they retched, but they do not retch. With a sensation of utter confusion below the heart. For all these conditions the "minor *ban xia* decoction" is suitable. Boil one *sheng* of *ban xia*, steeped [in hot water] seven times, and half a *sheng* of fresh ginger in seven *sheng* of water down to one *sheng* and five *ge*, and ingest this in several portions. Zhang Zhongjing, *Ji kui yao lüe.*

噦逆欲死。半夏生薑湯主之。即上方也。

1198 The amount to be ingested is missing here. *He ji ju fang* ch. 4, *zhi tan yin* 治痰飲, "to cure phlegm rheum," writes *qu ze kong xin fu* 去滓空心服, "remove the dregs and ingest [the liquid] on an empty stomach."

Retching with [qi] counterflow letting one wish to die. This is controlled by the "decoction with *ban xia* and *fresh ginger*." This is the recipe recorded above.

痘瘡噦氣。方同上。

Smallpox sores with retching of qi. Recipe identical to the one above.

嘔噦眩悸，穀不得下。半夏加伏苓湯：半夏一升，生薑半斤，伏苓三兩，切，以水七升，煎一升半，分温服之。金匱要略。

Vomiting and retching with dizziness and palpitation, and an inability to pass solid food [through the body] downward. The "decoction with *ban xia* extended with *poria*." Boil in seven *sheng* of water down to one and a half *sheng*: one *sheng* of *ban xia*, half a *jin* of fresh ginger and three *liang* of *poria*, cut, and ingest [the liquid] warm, divided into several portions. *Jin kui yao lüe*.

目不得眠。見發明下。

Inability to close the eyes and sleep. See under "Explication."

心下悸忪。半夏麻黄丸：半夏、麻黄等分，爲末，蜜丸小豆大。每服三十丸，日三。金匱要略。

Palpitation below the heart. The "pills with *ban xia* and *ephedra* [herb]." [Grind] equal amounts of *ban xia* and *ephedra* [herb] into powder, and form with honey pills the size of mung beans. Each time ingest 30 pills. Three times a day. *Jin kui yao lüe*.

傷寒乾啘。半夏熟洗，研末。生薑湯服一錢匕。深師方。

Harm caused by cold with dry retching. Boil *ban xia* until done, wash it and grind it into powder. Ingest with a fresh ginger decoction the amount held by a one *qian* spoon. *Shen shi fang*.

嘔逆厥逆，内有寒痰。半夏一升洗滑焙研，小麥麵一升，水和作彈丸，水煮熟。初呑四五枚，日三服。稍增至十五枚，旋煮旋呑。覺病減，再作。忌羊肉、餳糖。此乃許仁則方也。外臺秘要。

Vomiting with [qi] counterflow; ceasing [yang qi with qi] counterflow. Wash one *sheng* of *ban xia* to remove its slimy [exterior], bake it over a fire in a pan, grind it [to powder] and with one *sheng* of wheat flour and water form pills the size of a bullet. Boil them in water until done. At first swallow four or five pills, to be ingested three times a day. Gradually increase the dose up to 15 pills. Boil them and swallow them right away. If the disease feels like it is getting weaker, repeat the treatment. [During this therapy] mutton and malt sugar are forbidden. This is a recipe of Xu Renze. *Wai tai mi yao*.

嘔吐反胃。大半夏湯：半夏三升，人參三兩，白蜜一升，水一斗二升和，揚之一百二十遍。煮取三升半，温服一升，日再服。亦治膈間支飲。金匱要略。

Vomiting with a turned over stomach. The "major decoction with *ban xia*." Mix three *sheng* of *ban xia*, three *liang* of ginseng [root], and one *sheng* of white honey in one *dou* and two *sheng* of water, ladle it up and let it splash 120 times, boil it down to three and a half *sheng*, and ingest one *sheng* warm. To be ingested twice a day. It also serves to cure propping rheum in the diaphragm region. *Jin kui yao lüe*.

胃寒噦逆，停痰留飲。藿香半夏湯：用半夏湯泡炒黄二兩，藿香葉一兩，丁皮半兩，每服四錢，水一盞，薑七片，煎服。和劑局方。

Stomach cold with retching and [qi] counterflow. Stagnating phlegm rheum. The "decoction with *agastache* [leaves] and *ban xia*." Prepare two *liang* of *ban xia*, soaked in hot water and fried until it turns yellow, one *liang* of *agastache* leaves and half a *liang* of clove bark. Each time ingest four *qian*, to be boiled in one cup of water with seven slices of ginger. Ingest the decoction. *He ji ju fang*.

小兒吐瀉，脾胃虚寒。齊州半夏泡七次、陳粟米各一錢半，薑十片，水琖半，煎八分，温服。錢乙小兒。

Children with spitting/vomiting and outflow. Spleen and stomach depletion with cold. Boil in one and a half small cup down to 80%: one and a half *qian* each of *ban xia* from Qi zhou, steeped [in hot water] seven times, and long-stored millet, with ten slices of ginger, and [let the child] ingest [the liquid] warm. Qian Yi, *Xiao er*.

小兒痰吐，或風壅所致，或欬嗽發熱，飲食即嘔。半夏泡七次半兩，丁香一錢，以半夏末水和包丁香，用麵重包，煨熟，去麪爲末，生薑自然汁和丸麻子大。每服二三十丸，陳皮湯下。活幼口議。

Children spitting phlegm. This may be related to an obstruction caused by wind [intrusion]. They may cough with heat effusion, and vomit what they have drunk and eaten. Prepare half a *liang* of *ban xia*, steeped [in hot water] seven times, and one *qian* of cloves. Mix the *ban xia* with water and use this to wrap the clove. Wrap this in turn with wheat flour, and simmer it until done. Remove the wheat flour and [grind the rest into] powder. Mix [the powder] with fresh ginger juice and form pills the size of hemp seeds. Each time [let the child] ingest 20 to 30 pills, to be sent down with a tangerine peel decoction. *Huo you kou yi*.

妊娠嘔吐。半夏二兩，人參、乾薑各一兩，爲末。薑汁麪糊丸梧子大，每飲服十丸，日三服。仲景金匱要略。

Vomiting during pregnancy. ['Grind] two *liang* of *ban xia* and one *liang* each of ginseng [root] and dried ginger into powder, and form with a ginger juice wheat flour paste pills the size of *wu* seeds. Each time [the woman is to] ingest with a beverage ten pills, to be ingested three times a day. [Zhang] Zhongjing, *Jin kui yao lüe*.

霍亂腹脹。半夏、桂等分，爲末。水服方寸匕。肘後方。

Cholera with abdominal distension. [Grind] equal amounts of *ban xia* and *cassia* [bark] into powder and ingest with water the amount held by a square *cun* spoon. *Zhou hou fang*.

小兒腹脹。半夏末少許，酒和丸粟米大。每服二丸，薑湯下。不瘥，加之。或以火炮研末，薑汁調貼臍，亦佳。子母秘録。

Children with abdominal distension. Mix a small amount of *ban xia* powder with wine and form pills the size of millet. Each time [let the child] ingest two pills, to be sent down with a ginger decoction. If this remains without effect, increase the [dose]. Or roast it over fire in a pan, grind it into powder and apply it mixed with ginger juice to the [child's] navel. This, too, is excellent. *Zi mu mi lu*.

黄疸喘滿，小便自利，不可除熱。半夏、生薑各半斤，水七升，煮一升五合，分再服。有人氣結而死，心下暖，以此少許入口，遂活。張仲景方。

Yellow *dan*-illness/jaundice with panting, a feeling of fullness, and a free flow of urine. [In such a situation,] the heat must not be dispelled. Boil half a *jin* each of *ban xia* and fresh ginger in seven *sheng* of water down to one *sheng* and five *ge*, and ingest this divided into several portions. Once someone had bound qi and died. There was still warmth below his heart. A small amount of this [medication] was inserted into his mouth and he won his life back. A recipe of Zhang Zhongjing.

伏暑引飲，脾胃不利。消暑丸：用半夏醋煮一斤，伏苓半斤，生甘草半斤，爲末，薑汁麪糊丸梧子大。每服五十丸，熱湯下。和劑局方。

Latent summer heat with an urge to drink, and the passage through spleen and stomach blocked. The "pills to dissolve summer heat." [Grind] one *jin* of *ban xia*, boiled in vinegar, half a *jin* of *poria* and half a *jin* of fresh *glycyrrhiza* [root] into powder, and with a ginger juice wheat flour paste form pills the size of *wu* seeds. Each time ingest 50 pills, to be sent down with hot, boiled water. *He ji ju fang*.

老人虛秘，冷秘，及痃癖冷氣。半硫丸：半夏泡炒、生硫黄等分，爲末，自然薑汁煮糊丸如梧子大。每空心温酒下五十丸。和劑局方。

Old people with depletion and blocked [defecation], cold blockage, and string-illness[1199] and aggregation-illness with cold qi. The "pills with *ban* [*xia*] and sulphur." [Grind] equal amounts of *ban xia*, soaked in water and fried, and fresh sulphur into powder, boil it with natural ginger juice, and with [wheat flour] prepare a paste to form pills the size of *wu* seeds. *He ji ju fang*.

失血喘急。吐血下血，崩中帶下，喘急痰嘔，中滿宿瘀。用半夏搥扁，以薑汁和麪包煨黄，研末，米糊丸梧子大。每服三十丸，白湯下。直指方。

Loss of blood with hectic panting. Blood spitting and blood discharge. Collapsing center[1200] and [diseases] below the belt. Hectic panting and phlegm vomiting. A feeling of fullness in the center, and sluggish [food remaining in the body] overnight. Pound *ban xia* [roots] to flat pieces, mix them with ginger juice, wrap them with wheat flour, simmer them until they have turned yellow, grind them into powder and with a rice paste form pills the size of *wu* seeds. Each time ingest 30 pills, to be sent down with clear, boiled water. *Zhi zhi fang*.

白濁夢遺。半夏一兩，洗十次，切破，以木猪苓二兩，同炒黄，出火毒，去猪苓，入煅過牡蠣一兩，以山藥糊丸梧子大。每服三十丸，伏苓湯送下。腎氣閉而一身精氣無所管攝，妄行而遺者，宜用此方。蓋半夏有利性，猪苓導水，使腎氣通也。與下元虛憊者不同。許學士本事方。

Uncontrolled loss of white, turbid [urine/sperm] during dreams. Wash one *liang* of *ban xia* ten times and cut it to pieces. Roast them together with *polyporus sclerotium* until they have turned yellow. Let the fire poison leave, remove the *polyporus sclerotium*, add one *liang* of calcined oyster shells and with a Chinese yam paste form pills the size of *wu* seeds. Each time ingest 30 pills, to be sent down with a *poria* decoction. In the case of a kidney qi closure and if essence qi pass uncontrolled through the entire body and are lost, it is suitable to resort to this recipe. The fact is, *ban xia* by its nature frees passages, *polyporus sclerotium* guides water, and this serves to free the passage of kidney qi. This is a situation different from depletion and fatigue of the original [qi] in the lower [section of the Triple Burner, i. e., the kidney qi]. Xu xueshi, *Ben shi fang*.

1199 *Xuan* 痃, "string-illness," a condition of acute pain located in the abdomen to the left and right of the umbilicus. BCGM Dict I, 591.

1200 *Beng zhong* 崩中, "collapsing center," excessive vaginal bleeding outside of a menstruation period. BCGM Dict I, 58.

八般頭風。三次見效。半夏末，入百草霜少許，作紙撚燒烟，就鼻内嗃之。口中含水，有涎吐去，再含。衛生寶鑑。

The eight types of head wind. Applied three times it shows an effect. Add a little soot scratched from within a chimney of a furnace where all types of herbs had been burned to *ban xia* powder, [wrap it in] paper twirled to a stick, burn it to generate fumes and inhale them with the nose, while holding water in the mouth. When saliva is generated, spit it out and again hold water in the mouth. *Wei sheng bao jian.*

少陰咽痛，生瘡，不能言語，聲不出者，苦酒湯主之。半夏七枚打碎，雞子一枚，頭開一竅，去黄，納苦酒令小滿，入半夏在内，以鐶子坐于炭火上，煎三沸，去滓，置盃中，時時嚥之，極驗。未瘥更作。仲景傷寒論。

A minor yin [disorder] with a painful throat, a development of sores, an inability to speak, when no sound at all leaves [the throat]. The "decoction with bitter wine" controls it. Crush seven *ban xia* [roots] to pieces. Open the top of one chicken egg, remove the yoke and fill it a little with bitter wine. Then insert the *ban xia* [pieces] and place it with a metal ring with a handle on a charcoal fire. Boil it three times until bubbling, remove the dregs, give it into a cup and every now and then swallow it. Extremely effective. If no cure is achieved, repeat it. [Zhang] Zhongjing, *Shang han lun.*

喉痺腫塞。生半夏末嗃鼻内，涎出效。集簡方。

Throat blockage: closure because of a swelling. Inhale fresh *ban xia* powder into the nose. As soon as saliva is excreted, the effect becomes apparent. *Ji jian fang.*

骨哽在咽。半夏、白芷等分，爲末。水服方寸匕，當嘔出。忌羊肉。外臺秘要。

Choking on a bone in the throat. [Grind] equal amounts of *ban xia* and *angelica dahurica* [root] into powder and ingest with water the amount held by a square *cun* spoon. [The bone] is released by vomiting. [During this therapy,] mutton is to be avoided. *Wai tai mi yao.*

重舌木舌，脹大塞口。半夏煎醋，含漱之。

Doubled tongue,[1201] Wooden tongue.[1202] The distension [of the tongue] is big enough to block the mouth. Boil *ban xia* in vinegar, hold the decoction in the mouth and rinse [the tongue].

1201 *Chong she* 重舌, "doubled tongue," a condition with the growth underneath the tongue, mostly in children, of what appears like a second tongue. BCGM Dict I, 92.

1202 *Mu she* 木舌, "wooden tongue," a condition with the body of the tongue massively swollen to an extent that it fills the oral cavity and at the same time is as hard as wood. BCGM Dict I, 344.

又方：半夏二十枚，水煮過，再泡片時，乘熱以酒一升浸之，密封良久，熱漱冷吐之。

Another recipe. Boil 20 *ban xia* [roots] in water and let them soak for a while. [That is], steep them, while they are still hot, in one *sheng* of wine in a tightly sealed [vessel] for a long time. Rinse [the tongue] with the hot liquid and spit it out when it cools.

小兒顖陷。乃冷也。水調半夏末，塗足心。

Children with a sunken fontanel. This is [a condition related to] cold. Mix *ban xia* powder with water and apply this to the soles [of the child's feet].

面上黑氣。半夏焙研，米醋調敷。不可見風，不計遍數，從早至晚，如此三日，皂角湯洗下，面瑩如玉也。摘玄方。

Facial surface with black qi. Bake *ban xia* over a slow fire and grind it. Mix it with rice vinegar and apply it [to the affected region. The face] must not be exposed to wind. Do not count how often, [simply repeat the application] from early morning until night for three days. Then wash [the face] with a *gleditsia* [pod/seeds] decoction to remove [the medicinal application]. The face will be as lustrous as jade. *Zhai xuan fang.*

癩風眉落。生半夏、羊屎燒焦等分，爲末，自然薑汁日調塗。聖濟録。

Repudiation-illness, (i. e., massive) wind,[1203] with loss of eyebrows. [Grind] equal amounts of fresh *ban xia* and sheep dung, burned until scorched, into powder and apply it with the natural juice of ginger [to the affected region] every day. *Sheng ji lu.*

盤腸生產。產時子腸先出，產後不收者，名盤腸產。以半夏末頻嗜鼻中，則上也。婦人良方。

Birth with a twisted intestine.[1204] When in the course of a birth the intestine appears first, and after the birth is not drawn back again, this is called "birth with a twisted intestine." [Let the woman] repeatedly inhale *ban xia* powder into her nose, and [the intestine] will rise again. *Fu ren liang fang.*

產後運絶。半夏末，冷水和丸大豆大，納鼻中即愈，此扁鵲法也。肘後方。

1203 *Lai feng* 癩風, repudiation-illness (i. e., massive) wind," a condition of a chronic, infectious skin disease with insensitive skin, red macules, festering swelling, and, in severe cases, loss of eyebrows, harm to the eyes, and collapse of the patient's nose. BCGM Dict I, 111, 164.

1204 *Pan chang sheng chan* 盤腸生産, "birth with a twisted intestine," a condition at the time of birth with the vaginal wall or rectum appearing first and, after the child was born, being unable to retreat by themselves. BCGM Dict I, 369.

Vertigo with [qi movements threatened to be] cut off. Mix *ban xia* powder with cold water and form pills the size of soybeans. Insert them into the [woman's] nose and she will be cured. This is a method [applied] by Bian Que. *Zhou hou fang*.

小兒驚風。生半夏一錢，皂角半錢，爲末。吹少許入鼻，名嚏驚散，即甦。直指方。

Fright wind of children.[1205] [Grind] one *qian* of fresh *ban xia* and half a *qian* of *gleditsia* [pods/seeds] into powder and blow a small amount into the [child's] nose. [This recipe] is called "powder to sneeze out fright." [The child] will regain consciousness. *Zhi zhi fang*.

卒死不寤。半夏末吹鼻中，即活。南岳夫人紫靈魏元君方也。

Sudden death with unconsciousness. Blow *ban xia* powder into [the patient's] nose and he/she will return to life. This is a recipe of the Lady of Nan yue, the Original Sovereign Wei of the Purple Numinosity.[1206]

五絶急病。一曰自縊，二曰墻壓，三曰溺水，四曰魘魅，五曰産乳。並以半夏末，納大豆一丸入鼻中。心温者一日可活也。子母秘録。

Acute disease related to any of the five interruptions [of qi movements]. First: Suicidal hanging. Second: Fall from a wall. Third: Drowning in water. Fourth: Nightmare goblin [attachment]. Fifth: [Problems arising] during birth or nursing. For all of them insert one *ban xia* powder pill, the size of a soybean, into the [patient's] nose. [Patients] with warmth in their heart/central region can be brought back to life within one day [after the incident]. *Zi mu mi lu*.

疽發背及乳瘡。半夏末，雞子白調塗之。肘後方。

Impediment-illness[1207] effusing on the back and breast sores. Mix *ban xia* powder with egg white and apply this [to the affected region]. *Zhou hou fang*.

吹奶腫痛。半夏一個煨研，酒服立愈。

Inflated breast[1208] with painful swelling. Simmer one *ban xia* [root], grind it and [let the woman] ingest it with wine. This results in an instant cure.

1205 *Jing feng* 驚風, "fright wind," a condition of children characterised by jerking and arched back rigidity, eyeballs turned upward, and twitching hands and legs. BCGM Dict I, 261.

1206 See BCGM Dict III, 339.

1207 *Ju* 疽, "impediment-illness," refers to an obstruction of vessels or other ducts inside the body. Qi rushing against the impediment may cause a local swelling and eventually break through the surface to cause an abscess. BCGM Dict I, 277.

1208 *Chui ru* 吹乳, "inflated breast." Identical to *chui nai* 吹奶, "inflated breast." A condition with milk blocked after delivery and the breasts turning red and swelling. BCGM Dict I, 101.

一方：以末，隨左右嗃鼻，效。劉長春經驗方。

Another recipe. [The woman] inhales the powder into her left or right nostril depending on [which breast, on the left or right, is inflated]. Liu Changchun, *Jing yan fang.*

打撲瘀痕。水調半夏末塗之，一宿即没也。永類鈐方。

Stagnant [blood] and scars following a blow or fall. Mix *ban xia* powder with water and apply it [to the affected region]. After one night [stagnant blood and scars] will be eliminated. *Yong lei qian fang.*

遠行足趼。方同上。集簡方。

Callous feet after walking a long way. Recipe identical to the one above. *Ji jian fang.*

金刃不出，入骨脉中者。半夏、白歛等分，爲末。酒服方寸匕，日三服。至二十日自出。李筌太白經。

A metal blade is stuck in a bone or vessel and cannot be extracted. [Grind] equal amounts of *ban xia* and *ampelopsis* [root] into powder, and ingest with wine the amount held by a square *cun* spoon. To be ingested three times a day. [The blade] will come out within 20 days. Li Quan, *Tai bai jing.*

飛蟲入耳。生半夏末，麻油調，塗耳門外。本事方。

A flying bug has entered an ear. Mix fresh *ban xia* powder with sesame oil and apply this outside the entrance to the ear. *Ben shi fang.*

蝎蠆螫人。半夏末，水調塗之，立止。錢相公篋中方。

A person stung by a scorpion. Mix *ban xia* powder with water and apply this [to the affected region. The pain] ends immediately. Qian xiang gong, *Jia zhong fang.*

蝎瘻五孔相通者。半夏末，水調塗之，日二。聖惠方。

Fistula with five interconnected holes related to scorpion [stings]. Mix *ban xia* powder with water and apply this [to the affected region]. Twice a day. *Sheng hui fang.*

咽喉骨哽。半夏、白芷等分，爲末。水服方寸匕，當嘔出。忌羊肉。外臺秘要。

Choking on a bone in the throat. [Grind] equal amounts of *ban xia* and *angelica dahurica* [root] into powder and ingest with water the amount held by a square *cun* spoon. [The bone] is released by vomiting. [During this therapy,] mutton is to be avoided. *Wai tai mi yao.*[1209]

1209 As the 24 characters of this recipe text are identical to a passage further up, it is commonly omitted in modern BCGM editions.

17-26-02
莖涎 *Jing xian*

Saliva from the stem [of *ban xia*].

【主治】煉取塗髮眉，墮落者即生。雷斆。

Control. Process [the stem] with heat and remove [the saliva emitted]. Apply it to hair and eyebrows and where they have fallen off they will grow again. Lei Xiao.

17-27
蚤休本經下品

Zao xiu, FE *Ben jing*, lower rank.

***Paris polyphylla* Smith var. *chinensis* (Franch.) Hara. Love apple.**

【釋名】蚩休別録、螫休日華、紫河車圖經、重臺唐本、重樓金線唐本、三層草綱目、七葉一枝花蒙筌、草甘遂唐本、白甘遂。【時珍曰】蟲蛇之毒，得此治之即休，故有蚤休、螫休諸名。重臺、三層，因其葉狀也。金線重樓，因其花狀也。甘遂，因其根狀也。紫河車，因其功用也。

Explanation of Names. *Chi xiu* 蚩休, *Bie lu. Shi xiu* 螫休, *Rihua. Zi he che* 紫河車, *Tu jing. Chong tai* 重臺, *Tang ben. Chong lou jin xian* 重樓金線, *Tang ben.*[1210] *San ceng cao* 三層草, *Gang mu. Qi ye yi zhi hua* 七葉一枝花, "flower with seven leaves on one branch," *Meng quan. Cao gan sui* 草甘遂, *Tang ben. Bai gan sui* 白甘遂. [Li] Shizhen: When the poison of worms/bugs and snakes is cured with this [herb], it "rests," *xiu* 休. Hence all such names of *zao xiu* 蚤休, "letting fleas rest," and *shi xiu* 螫休, "letting scorpions rest," Names such as *chong tai* 重臺, "doubled platform," and *san ceng* 三層, "three layers," are based on the shape of the leaves. "Brocade/golden thread and double storied building," *jin xian chong lou* 金線重樓 is based on the shape of the flowers. ["Herbal and white] *gan sui*" 甘遂 is based on the shape of the root [that is similar to the *euphorbia* Kansui root]. The name "purple river cart," (i. e., placenta), *zi he che* 紫河車, is based on the therapeutic potential and usage [of this herb].

【集解】【別録曰】蚤休生山陽川谷及冤句。【恭曰】今謂重樓金線者是也。一名重臺，南人名草甘遂。一莖六七葉，似王孫、鬼臼、蓖麻輩，葉有二三層。根如肥大菖蒲，細肌脆白。【保昇曰】葉似鬼臼、牡蒙，年久者二三重。根如紫參，皮黃肉白。五月采根，日乾。【大明曰】根如尺二蜈蚣，大如肥紫菖蒲。【頌曰】即紫河車也。今河中、河陽、華、鳳、文州及江淮間亦有之。葉似王孫、鬼臼等，作二三層。六月開黃紫花，蕊赤黃色，上有金絲垂下。秋結紅子。根似肥薑，皮赤肉白。四月、五月采

1210 Instead of *Tang ben* 唐本, *Zheng lei* ch. 11, *zao xiu* 蚤休, names the *Tu jing* as earliest evidence of this alternative name.

之。【宗奭曰】蚤休無旁枝，止一莖挺生，高尺餘，顛有四五葉。葉有岐，似苦杖。中心又起莖，亦如是生葉。惟根入藥用。【時珍曰】重樓金線處處有之，生于深山陰濕之地。一莖獨上，莖當葉心。葉綠色似芍藥，凡二三層，每一層七葉。莖頭夏月開花，一花七瓣，有金絲蕊，長三四寸。王屋山產者至五七層。根如鬼臼、蒼朮狀，外紫中白，有粘、糯二種。外丹家采製三黃、砂、汞。入藥洗切焙用。俗諺云

七葉一枝花，深山是我家。
癰疽如遇者，一似手拈拏，
是也。

Collected Explanations. *Cao xiu* grows in the river valleys of Shan yang and in Yuan ju. [Su] Gong: [*Cao xiu*] is the item called *chong lou jin xian* 重樓金線 today. An alternative name is *chong tai* 重臺. The southerners call it "herbal *gan sui* 甘遂." It has one stem with six or seven leaves, resembling *paris bashanensis*, *dysosma versipellis*, and castor oil plants. The leaves have two or three layers, and the root resembles fat, big *acorus* [roots]. It has a fine texture, is white and crispy. [Han] Baosheng: The leaves resemble those of umbrella leaf [herbs] and *paris bashanensis* plants. Those older than a year have two or three layers. The root is similar to that of common bistort; it has a yellow skin and white meat. The root is collected in the fifth month; it is dried in the sun. Da Ming: The root is similar to a 1,2 *chi* long centipede, and it is as big as a fat, purple *acorus* [root]. [Su] Song: This is *zi he che* 紫河車. Today, it can also be found in He zhong, He yang, Hua, Feng and Wen zhou, and in the Jiang Huai region. The leaves resemble those of *paris* and umbrella leaf [herbs]. They appear with two or three layers. Yellow-purple flowers open in the sixth month; the anther bearing filaments are of red-yellow color. Golden threads hang down from above. Red seeds form in autumn. The root resembles fat ginger [roots]; the skin is red and the meat is white. They are collected in the fourth and fifth month. [Kou] Zongshi: *Cao xiu* has no branches. It has just one stem rising straight up, reaching a height of more than a *chi*. At its tip it has four or five leaves. These leaves are forked, resembling those of bushy knotweed. In their center yet another stem rises, and it grows leaves the same way. Only the root is used for pharmaceutical purposes. [Li] Shizhen: *Chong lou jin xian* can be found everywhere. It grows deep in the mountains at shady, moist places. A single stem rises, and this stem is situated in the center of the leaves. The green color of the leaves resembles that of *paeonia* [leaves]. In all, [the stem] has two or three layers, with each layer having seven leaves. During the summer months a flower opens at the top of the stem. One flower has seven petals with golden thread-like anther holding filaments that are three to four *cun* long. Those growing on Mount Wang wu shan have five to seven layers. The root is shaped like that of umbrella leaf [herbs] and *atractylodes lancea*. It is purple on the

outside and white inside. There are two kinds, one sticky, one glutinous. Experts of external elixirs collect them to check [the effects of] the three substances named *huang* 黄, "yellow,"[1211] cinnabar and mercury. For adding them to medication, they are washed, cut to pieces and baked over a slow fire, and are then used [for medicinal applications]. An appropriate common saying is:
"I am a flower with seven leaves on each branch.
My home is deep in the mountains.
When I encounter an obstruction- or impediment-illness,[1212]
they are nothing more than objects that can easily be picked up with your fingers."

17-27-01
根 ***Gen***

Root [of *zao xiu*].

【氣味】苦，微寒，有毒。【大明曰】冷，無毒。伏雄黄、丹砂、蓬砂及鹽。

Qi and Flavor. Bitter, slightly cold, poisonous. Da Ming: Cold, nonpoisonous. It suppresses [the effects of] realgar, cinnabar, borax and salt.

【主治】驚癇，摇頭弄舌，熱氣在腹中。本經。癲疾，癰瘡，除蝕，下三蟲，去蛇毒。别録。生食一升，利水。唐本。治胎風手足搐，能吐泄瘰癧。大明。去瘧疾寒熱。時珍。

Control. Fright epilepsy, with a swaying head and playful tongue. Heat qi are present in the abdomen. *Ben jing*. Peak-illness[1213] ailments. Obstruction-illness sores. [It] eliminates erosions, serves to discharge the three types of worms/bugs, and eliminates the poison of snakes. *Bie lu*. One *sheng* eaten fresh frees the passage of water. *Tang ben*. It serves to cure fetal wind[1214] with hands and feet pulled in. It is capable of [healing] scrofula pervasion-illness[1215] by causing vomiting and outflow.

1211 The three [items named "yellow",] *huang* 黄, are sulphur, *liu huang* 硫黄, realgar, *xiong huang* 雄黄, and orpiment, *ci huang* 雌黄.

1212 *Yong ju* 癰疽, "obstruction-illness, impediment-illness." refers to two vaguely distinguished obstructions/impediments of vessels or other ducts inside the body. Qi rushing against the obstruction may cause a local swelling and eventually break through the surface to cause an abscess. BCGM Dict I, 642.

1213 *Dian ji* 癲[疾], "peak ailment," a mental disturbance of depression and unhappiness, with a calm attitude and little incentive to speak. BCGM Dict I, 125.

1214 *Tai feng* 胎風, "fetal wind," a condition of *jing feng* 驚風, "fright wind," developed by children within 100 days following delivery. BCGM Dict I, 485.

1215 *Luo li* 瘰癧, "scrofula pervasion-illness," when two or more connected swellings of the size of plum or date kernels appear either on the neck or in the armpits, or somewhere else on the body. BCGM Dict I. 329.

Da Ming. It eliminates malaria ailments with alternating sensations of cold and heat. [Li] Shizhen.

【發明】【恭曰】摩醋，傅癰腫蛇毒，甚有效。【時珍曰】紫河車，足厥陰經藥也。凡本經驚癇、瘧疾、瘰癧、癰腫者宜之。而道家有服食法，不知果有益否也。

Explication. [Su] Gong: It is rubbed in vinegar to be applied to obstruction-illness swelling and snake poison [bites], and is very effective. [Li] Shizhen: *Zi he che* is a pharmaceutical substance for the foot ceasing yin conduits. For all conditions of fright epilepsy, malaria ailment, scrofula pervasion-illness and obstruction-illness swelling the *Ben jing* recommends it as suitable. The Daoists have included it in their approaches to ingesting [medicinal substances] for food. But it is not known whether it is beneficial or not.

【附方】新五。服食法。

Added Recipes. Five newly recorded. A method to ingest it as food.

紫河車根以竹刀刮去皮，切作骰子大塊，麪裹入瓷瓶中，水煮候浮漉出，凝冷，入新布袋中，懸風處待乾。每服三丸，五更初面東念呪，井水下，連進三服，即能休粮。若要飲食，先以黑豆煎湯飲之，次以藥丸煮稀粥，漸漸食之。呪曰："天朗氣清金雞鳴，吾今服藥欲長生。吾今不飢復不渴，賴得神仙草有靈。"

Use a bamboo knife to remove the skin of a *zi he che* root and cut it to pieces the size of a dice. Cover them with wheat flour, give them into a porcelain jar and boil them with water until they float on the surface. Filter [the liquid] to remove [the root] and let them harden while they cool. Then fill them into a new cloth bag and suspend them at a windy location until they have dried. Each time ingest three pills in that in the early morning hours at first you recite an exorcistic spell, and then send them down with well water. Ingest the three [pills] one after another. This enables you to end the consumption of food. If you feel a desire to drink and eat, drink a soybean decoction first. Then boil the medicinal pills in a watery gruel, and slowly eat it. The spell is: "Under a golden sky with clear qi the cocks crow. Today, I ingest this medication with the wish to have a long life. Today, to feel neither thirst nor hunger, I rely on a magic strength obtained with this divine herb of the immortals."

小兒胎風，手足搐搦。用蚤休即紫河車爲末。每服半錢，冷水下。衛生易簡方。

Fetal wind of children, with their hands and feet contracted. [Grind] *zao xiu*, that is, *zi he che*, into powder. Each time ingest half a *qian*, to be sent down with cold water. *Wei sheng yi jian fang.*

慢驚發搐，帶有陽證者。白甘遂末即蚤休一錢，栝樓根末二錢，同于慢火上炒焦黃，研勻。每服一字，煎射香、薄荷湯調下。錢乙小兒方。

Chronic fright effusing as contracted [limbs] and accompanied by signs of a yang [qi disorder]. Prepare one *qian* of white *gan sui* powder, that is *zao xiu*, and two *qian* of Japanese snake gourd root powder. Fry them together over a slow fire until they are scorched and turn yellow, and grind them to an evenly mixed [powder]. Each time ingest one *zi*, to be sent down mixed with a musk and mint decoction. Qian yi, *Xiao er fang.*

中鼠莽毒。金線重樓根，磨水服，即愈。集簡方。

Struck by the poison of *illiceum* [leaves]. Rub a *jin xian chong lou* root in water and ingest it. This results in a cure. *Ji jian fang.*

咽喉穀賊。腫痛。用重臺赤色者、川大黄炒、木鼈子仁、馬牙消各半兩，半夏泡一分，爲末，蜜丸芡子大，含之。聖惠方。

Grain intrusion in the throat,[1216] with a painful swelling. [Grind] half a *liang* each of *chong tai*, those of red color, rhubarb root from [Si] chuan, *momordica* seed kernels, and mirabilite, as well as one *fen* of *ban xia*, soaked, into powder and form with honey pills the size of *qian* seeds. [The patient] is to hold them in his mouth. *Sheng hui fang.*

17-28
鬼臼本經下品

Gui jiu. FE *Ben jing*, lower rank.

***Dysosma versipellis* (Hance) M. Cheng ex Ying. Umbrella leaf.**[1217]

【校正】併入圖經璚田草。

Editorial Correction. Inserted also here, from the *Tu jing*: *Qiong tian cao.*

【釋名】九臼本經、天臼別録、鬼藥綱目、解毒別録、爵犀本經、馬目毒公本經、害母草圖經、羞天花綱目、朮律草綱目、璚田草綱目、獨脚蓮土宿本草、獨荷草土宿、山荷葉綱目、旱荷綱目、八角盤綱目、唐婆鏡。【弘景曰】鬼臼根如射干，白而味甘，九臼相連，有毛者良，故名。【時

1216 *Gu zei* 穀賊, "grain intrusion," a condition of swelling and pain in the gullet resulting from an inadvertent ingestion of awns or spikes of cereals. BCGM Dict I, 196.

1217 *Gui jiu* 鬼臼, lit.: "a demon's mortars."

珍曰】此物有毒，而臼如馬眼，故名馬目毒公。殺蠱解毒，故有犀名。其葉如鏡、如盤、如荷，而新苗生則舊苗死，故有鏡、盤、荷、蓮、害母諸名。蘇東坡詩集云“璚田草俗號唐婆鏡”，即本草鬼臼也。歲生一臼，如黄精根而堅瘦，可以辟穀。宋祁劍南方物贊云：羞天花，蜀地處處有之。依莖綴花，蔽葉自隱，俗名羞天，予改爲羞寒花，即本草鬼臼也。贊云：“冒寒而茂，莖修葉廣。附莖作花，葉蔽其上。”以其自蔽，若有羞狀。〇别有羞天草，與此不同，即海芋也。

Explanation of Names. *Jiu jiu* 九臼, "nine mortars," *Ben jing*. *Tian jiu* 天臼, "heaven's mortars," *Bie lu*. *Gui yao* 鬼藥, "a demon's medication," *Gang mu*. *Jie du* 解毒, "resolves poison," *Bie lu*. *Jue xi* 爵犀, "venerated rhinoceros," *Ben jing*. *Ma mu du gong* 馬目毒公, "poison lord with horse eyes," *Ben jing*. *Hai mu cao* 害母草, "harm to the mother herb." *Tu jing*. *Xiu tian hua* 羞天花, "flowers shying away from heaven," *Gang mu*. *Shu lü cao* 术律草, *Gang mu*. *Qiong tian cao* 璚田草, "splendid field herb," *Gang mu*. *Du jiao lian* 獨脚蓮, "single leg lotus," *Tu su ben cao*. *Du he cao* 獨荷草, "single [leg] lotus herb," *Tu su*. *Shan he ye* 山荷葉, "mountain lotus leaves," *Gang mu*. *Han he* 旱荷, "parched lotus," *Gang mu*. *Ba jiao pan* 八角盤, "eight edges plate," *Gang mu*. *Tang po jing* 唐婆鏡, "aunt Tang's mirror." [Tao] Hongjing: The root of *gui jiu* resembles that of blackberry lily. It is white and has a sweet flavor. Nine "mortars," *jiu* 臼, cling together. When they have hair, they are good. Hence the name. [Li] Shizhen: This item is poisonous. Its "mortars" are similar to the eyes of horses. Hence the name "poison lord with horse eyes." It serves to kill *gu*[1218] and resolve poison. Hence the name [*jue*] *xi* [爵]犀, "venerable rhinoceros." The leaves are similar to mirrors, *jing* 盤, or plates, *pan* 鏡, or lotus, *he* 荷, and when a new seedling grows, the old seedlings die. Hence all the names such as *jing* 鏡, *pan* 盤, *he* 荷, *lian* 蓮 and "harming its mother," *hai mu* 害母. Su Dongpo in his *Shi ji* states: "Splendid field herb," *qiong tian cao* 璚田草, is commonly called " aunt Tang's mirror," *tang po jing* 唐婆鏡." This is the *gui jiu* 鬼臼 of the *Ben cao*. It grows one "mortar" per year. It is similar to Solomon's seal root, but harder and lean. It can be resorted to to avoid [the consumption of] grain/hard food. Song Qi in his *Jian nan fang wu zuan* states: "*Xiu tian hua* 羞天花 is present everywhere in Shu. The flowers cling to the stem; they are sheltered by the leaves and remain hidden. They are said to 'shy away from heaven,' *xiu tian* 羞天. I have changed this to *xiu tian hua* 羞寒花, 'flowers shying away from heaven.' This is the *gui jiu* 鬼臼 of the *Ben cao*. A eulogy reads:

'It resists cold and remains luxuriant.
The stem is embellished with broad leaves.

1218 *Gu du* 蠱毒, "*gu*-poison[ing]." (1) A poison emitted by certain worms/snakes with an ability to cause varying pathological changes in a person who has taken it in by means of wine or food. (2) Abdominal fullness, in some cases with blood spitting, and blood in the stool and urine. BCGM Dict I, 192 - 193. See BCGM 42-22.

Flowers are attached to the stem.
Leaves are above to shelter them.
[The flowers] hide themselves, as if they were shy'."

There is also a *xiu tian cao* 羞天草, "herb shying away from heaven." It is a different item; it is *alocasia* [root].

【集解】【別録曰】鬼臼生九真山谷及冤句。二月、八月采根。【弘景曰】鬼臼生山谷中。八月采，陰乾。似射干、术輩，又似鉤吻。有兩種：出錢塘、近道者，味甘，上有叢毛，最勝；出會稽、吴興者，大而味苦，無叢毛，力劣。今馬目毒公狀如黄精根，其臼處似馬眼而柔潤。今方家多用鬼臼而少用毒公，不知此那，復乖越如此。【恭曰】鬼臼生深山巖石之陰。葉如蓖麻、重樓輩。生一莖，莖端一葉，亦有兩岐者。年長一莖，莖枯則爲一臼。假令生來二十年，則有二十臼，豈惟九臼耶？根肉皮鬚並似射干，今俗用多是射干。而江南别送一物，非真者。今荆州當陽縣、硤州遠安縣、襄州荆山縣山中並貢之，亦極難得。【頌曰】今江寧府、滁、舒、商、齊、杭、襄、峽州、荆門軍亦有之，並如蘇恭所説。花生莖間，赤色，三月開後結實。又一説：鬼臼生深山陰地，葉六出或五出，如雁掌。莖端一葉如繖，旦時東向，及暮則西傾，蓋隨日出没也。花紅紫如荔枝，正在葉下，常爲葉所蔽，未常見日。一年生一莖，既枯則爲一臼，及八九年則八九臼矣。然一年一臼生而一臼腐，蓋陳新相易也，故俗名害母草。如芋魁、烏頭輩亦然，新苗生則舊苗死，前年之臼腐矣。而本草注謂全似射干，今射干體狀雖相似，然臼形淺薄，與鬼臼大異。鬼臼如八九個南星側比相疊，而色理正如射干。用者當使人求苗采之，市中不復有也。【時珍曰】鬼臼根如天南星相疊之狀，故市人道謂小者爲南星，大者爲鬼臼，殊爲謬誤。按黄山谷集云：唐婆鏡葉底開花，俗名羞天花，即鬼臼也。歲生一臼，滿十二歲，則可爲藥。今方家乃以鬼燈檠爲鬼臼，誤矣。又鄭樵通志云：鬼臼葉如小荷，形如鳥掌，年長一莖，莖枯則根爲一臼，亦名八角盤，以其葉似之也。據此二説，則似是今人所謂獨脚蓮者也。又名山荷葉、獨荷草、旱荷葉、八角鏡。南方處處深山陰密處有之，北方惟龍門山、王屋山有之。一莖獨上，莖生葉心而中空。一莖七葉，圓如初生小荷葉，面青背紫，揉其葉作瓜李香。開花在葉下，亦有無花者。其根全似蒼术、紫河車。丹爐家采根制三黄、砂、汞。或云其葉八角者更靈。或云其根與紫河車一樣，但以白色者爲河車，赤色者爲鬼臼，恐亦不然。而庚辛玉册謂蚤休陽草，旱荷陰草，亦有分别。陶弘景以馬目毒公與鬼臼爲二物，殊不知正是一物而有二種也。又唐獨孤滔丹房鏡源云：术律草有二種，根皆似南星，赤莖直上，莖端生葉。一種葉凡七瓣，一種葉作數層。葉似蓖麻，面青背紫而有細毛。葉下附莖開一花，狀如鈴鐸倒垂，青白色，黄蕊中空，結黄子。風吹不動，無風自摇。可制砂、汞。按此即鬼臼之二種也。其説形狀甚明。

Collected Explanations. *Bie lu*: *Gui jiu* grows in mountain valleys of Jiu zhen and in Yuan ju. The root is collected in the second and eighth month. [Tao] Hongjing: *Gui ju* grows in mountain valleys. It is collected in the eighth month, and dried in the yin (i. e., shade). It resembles blackberry lily [herbs] and *atractylodes lancea* [herbs]. It is also similar to *gelsemium* [herbs]. There are two kinds. Those coming from Qian tang and nearby have a sweet flavor. They are covered by clusters of hair and they are the very best. Those coming from Gui ji and Wu xing are big, have a bitter flavor and lack the clusters of hair. Their strength is inferior. Today's *ma mu du gong* is shaped similar to Solomon's seal root. The location of its "mortars" is reminiscent of the eyes of horses, but they are softer and moist. Today's recipe experts often use *gui jiu*; they seldom use [*ma mu*] *du gong*. It is unknown why they prefer the former over the latter. [Su] Gong: *Gui jiu* grows in the shade deep in the mountains and on cliff rocks. The leaves are similar to those of castor oil plants and love apple. It grows one stem, and there is one leaf at the end of the stem. There are also some with two separate leaves. When the stem has grown for a year, the stem withers and forms a "mortar." If it were left to live for 20 years, it might have 20 "mortars." Why does it have only nine "mortars"? The meat, the skin and the "whiskers" of the root, they all resemble those of blackberry lily [roots]. Today, they commonly use blackberry lily [roots]. Those sent from Jiang nan are a different item; they are not genuine [*gui jiu*]. Today Dang yang xian in Jing zhou, Yuan an xian in Jia zhou, and Jing shan xian in Xiang zhou send it as tribute to the Court; it is very difficult to obtain. [Su] Song: Today it is also present in Jiang ning fu, Chu, Shu, Shang, Qi, Hang, Xiang, Jia and Jing men jun. To all of them applies what Su Gong has said: Their flowers grow out of the stem. They are red and they form fruits after they have opened in the third month. It is also said: *Gui jiu* grows deep in the mountains on shady ground. Five or six leaves appear, similar to the claws of wild geese. At the end of the stem is a leaf similar to an umbrella. In the early morning it is directed toward the East. In the evening it is inclined toward the West. The fact is, its appearance and disappearance follow the sun. The flowers are red-purple, like lychee [flowers]. They are situated directly underneath the leaves. They are always covered by the leaves, and they never see the sun. When a stem has grown for one year, it withers and develops a "mortar." After eight and nine years, it has eight and nine "mortars." However, each year one "mortar" grows and one "mortair" perishes. The fact is, old and new replace each other. Hence [*gui jiu*] is commonly called "harming the mother herb." This is similar to items like taro tubers and [*aconitum*] main tubers. When a new seedling grows, the old seedling dies. The "mortar"[1219] of the

---

1219 Instead of *jiu* 臼, "mortar," *Zheng lei* ch. 11, *gui jiu* 鬼臼, quoting *Tu jing* writes *dou* 魁, "tuber."

previous year decays. A commentary on the *Ben cao* says that "[*gui jiu* roots] in all respects resembles blackberry lily [roots]." Today's blackberry lily [root] may have a similar physical appearance, but the shape of the "mortars" is quite insignificant while [those of] *gui jiu*, in contrast, are big. *Gui jiu* [roots] are similar to eight or nine Indian turnip [roots] clinging together; but their color and texture are completely similar to those of blackberry lily [roots]. For their [therapeutic] application, someone should be sent out to search for the seedlings and collect the [roots]. They are no longer offered on the market. [Li] Shizhen: The root of *gui jiu* is similar to several Indian turnip [roots] clinging together. Hence all[1220] the merchants on the markets claim that small specimens are Indian turnip [roots], and that big ones are *gui jiu*. That is a big mistake. According to the *Huang shan gu ji*, "*Tang po jing* 唐婆鏡 leaves at their base open flowers; they are commonly called *xiu tian hua* 羞天花. These are *gui jiu*. They grow one 'mortar' per year, and this is completed after 12 years. Then they can serve as a pharmaceutical drug. Today's recipe experts assume edible tulips (13-16) to be *gui jiu*, and they are wrong." Also, Zheng Qiao in his *Tong zhi* states: "*Gui jiu* leaves are similar to small lotus [leaves]; they are shaped similar to a bird's claw. [*Gui jiu*] grows one stem in a year; when the stem withers the root forms a 'mortar.' It is also called 'eight edges pan,' because this is what its leaves look like." Based on these two statements, it seems that [*gui jiu*] is [the item] called *du jiao lian* 獨脚蓮, "single leg lotus," by people today. It is also called *shan he ye* 山荷葉, "mountain lotus leaf," *du he cao* 獨荷草, "single [stem/leg] lotus herb," *han he ye* 旱荷葉, "parched lotus leaf," and *bai jiao jing* 八角鏡, "eight edge mirror." It can be found everywhere in the South deep in the mountains at shady, secluded locations. In the North it is present only on Mount Long men shan and Mount Wang wu shan. A single stem rises. The stem grows from the center of the leaves and is hollow. One stem has seven leaves. They are as round as small lotus leaves that have just begun to grow. They are greenish on their surface and purple on their back. When the leaves are rubbed, a fragrance of melons or plums develops. The flowers open below the leaves; some do not have flowers at all. The root in all respects resembles that of *atractylodes lancea* [rhizomes] and love apple. The experts for elixir [preparation in] furnaces collect the root to check [the effects of] the three substances named *huang* 黄, "yellow,"[1221] cinnabar and mercury. Some say that "those with eight edges leaves are of an even greater magic effect." Some say that "the root is identical to that of love apple, and that those of white color are love apple, while those of red color are *gui jiu*." This may not be so. The *Geng xin yu ce* says: "Love apple is a yang herb;

1220 Instead of *dao* 道, the Zhang edition of the BCGM writes *tong* 通, "throughout."

1221 The three [items named "yellow"], *huang* 黄, are sulphur, *liu huang* 硫黄, realgar, *xiong huang* 雄黄, and orpiment, *ci huang* 雌黄.

han he 旱荷 (i. e., *gui jiu*) is a yin herb." This, too, is a way to distinguish them. Tao Hongjing assumed *ma mu du gong* 馬目毒公 and *gui jiu* to be two different items; apparently he did not know that they are two kinds of one identical item. Also, the Tang era [author] Du Gutao in his *Dan fang jing yuan* states: "*Shu lü cao* 术律草 has two kinds. The roots of both kinds resemble those of arisaema lancea. A red stem rises straight up. The stem grows leaves at its ends. The leaves of one kind have seven petals, the leaves of the other kind form several layers. The leaves are similar to those of castor oil plants. They are greenish on their surface and purple on their back, and they have fine hair. Below the leaves and attached to the stem one flower opens. It is shaped like a bell and hangs upside down. It is of a greenish-white color. The anther bearing filaments are yellow and hollow. They form yellow seeds. When wind blows they do not move. When there is no wind, they sway spontaneously. They can serve to check [the effects of] cinnabar and mercury." Based on this, these may be the two kinds of gui jiu. The description of their physical shape is very clear.

17-28-01
根 *Gen*

Root [of *gui jiu*].

【氣味】辛，温，有毒。【別録曰】微温。【弘景曰】甘，温，有毒。【權曰】苦。【之才曰】畏垣衣。

Qi and Flavor. Acrid, warm, poisonous. *Bie lu*: Slightly warm. [Tao] Hongjing: Sweet, warm, poisonous. [Zhen] Quan: Bitter. [Xu] Zhicai: [Ingested together,] it fears wall moss.

【主治】殺蠱毒，鬼疰精物，辟惡氣不祥，逐邪，解百毒。本經。殺大毒，療欬嗽喉結，風邪煩惑，失魄妄見，去目中膚翳。不入湯。別録。主尸疰，殗殜勞疾，傳尸瘦疾。甄權。下死胎，治邪瘧癰疽，蛇毒，射工毒。時珍。

Control. It kills *gu* poison,[1222] demon attachment-illness and essence-spirit items. It repels malign qi and the inauspicious. It drives away evil and resolves the hundred poisons. *Ben jing*. It kills massive poison. It heals cough with [qi] nodes in the throat., vexing affection by wind evil, loss of *po*-soul and absurd visions. It removes skin membranes from the eyes. It is not prepared as decoction. *Bie lu*. It controls

1222 *Gu du* 蠱毒, "*gu*-poison[ing]." (1) A poison emitted by certain worms/snakes with an ability to cause varying pathological changes in a person who has taken it in by means of wine or food. (2) Abdominal fullness, in some cases with blood spitting, and blood in the stool and urine. BCGM Dict I, 192 - 193. See BCGM 42-22.

corpse [qi] attachment-illness[1223] with progressing calamity and exhaustion illness, corpse [qi] transmission with an emaciation-illness. Zhen Quan. It serves to discharge a dead fetus and to cure evil malaria, obstruction-illness and impediment-illness,[1224] snake poison and the archer's[1225] poison. [Li] Shizhen.

【發明】【頌曰】古方治五尸鬼疰、百毒惡氣多用之。又曰，今福州人三月采璚田草根葉，焙乾擣末，蜜丸服，治風疾。

Explication. [Su] Song: Ancient recipes often resort to it to cure the five types of corpse [qi][1226] and demon attachment-illness, the hundred poisonings and malign qi. It is also said that nowadays people in Fu zhou in the third month collect the root and leaves of umbrella leaf herb, bake them over a slow fire until they are dry, pound them into powder and with honey form pills to be ingested to cure wind illness.

【附方】新三。

Added Recipes. Three newly [recorded].

子死腹中，胞破不生，此方累效，救人歲萬數也。鬼臼不拘多少，黄色者，去毛爲細末，不用篩羅，只撚之如粉爲度。每服一錢，無灰酒一盞，同煎八分，通口服，立生如神。名一字神散。婦人良方。

A dead child in the abdomen. There is no birth despite a ruptured (amniotic) sac. This recipe is always effective. It has saved countless years of human life. Remove the hair of any amount of *gui jiu* of yellow color and [grind it] to fine powder. Do not pass it through a sieve. Just pinch it with your fingers and when it feels like a powder, this is it. Each time [let the woman] ingest one *qian*. Boil it in one cup of ash-free wine down to 80% and [let her] ingest it orally. A birth will happen immediately. [This recipe] is called "divine powder with one *zi* [of medication]." *Fu ren liang fang*.

1223 *Shi zhu* 尸疰, "corpse [qi] attachment-illness," a condition of a slowly developing infectious weakness. BCGM Dict I, 202.

1224 *Yong ju* 癰疽, "obstruction-illness, impediment-illness." refers to two vaguely distinguished obstructions/impediments of vessels or other ducts inside the body. Qi rushing against the obstruction may cause a local swelling and eventually break through the surface to cause an abscess. BCGM Dict I, 642.

1225 *She gong* 射工, "archer," 1.) a small bug in ancient times believed to live in water and be capable of "shooting" poison from its mouth at people, thereby causing disease; 2.) a condition caused by the archer's poison. BCGM Dict. I, 432. See 42-15.

1226 *Wu shi* 五屍," the five types of corpse [qi]." BCGM Dict I, 158.

射工中人，寒熱發瘡。鬼臼葉一把，苦酒漬，搗取汁。服一升，日二次。千金方。

Someone struck by the [poison of the] archer, with an effusion of [the poison through] sores and alternating sensations of cold and heat. One handful of *gui jiu* leaves are soaked in bitter wine first and then pounded to obtain a juice. Ingest one *sheng*, twice a day. *Qian jin fang*.

黑黄急病。黑黄，面黑黄，身如土色，不妨食，脉沉，若青脉入口者死。宜烙口中黑脉、百會、玉泉、章門、心俞。用生鬼臼搗汁一小盞服。乾者爲末，水服。三十六黄方。

An acute disease of black and yellow. "Black and yellow" [is to say:] the facial complexion is black-yellow; the body has the color of soil. [Patients] do not mind to eat; the [movement in their] vessels is in the depth. When greenish vessels enter their mouth, they die. For this it is advisable to brand/cauterize the black vessels in the mouth, and the needle insertion holes *bai hui* (GV-20), *yu quan* (CV-3), *zhang men* (LV-13) and *xin shu* (BL-15), and to ingest a small cup of juice obtained by pounding fresh *gui ju*. [When only] dry [*gui ju* is available, grind it into] powder and ingest it with water. *San shi liu huang fang*.

17-29
射干本經下品

She gan. FE *Ben jing*, lower rank.

***Belamcanda chinensis* (L.) DC. Blackberry lily.**

【釋名】烏扇本經、烏翣別録、烏吹別録、烏蒲本經、鳳翼拾遺、鬼扇土宿、扁竹綱目、仙人掌土宿、紫金牛土宿、野萱花綱目、草薑別録、黄遠吴普。【弘景曰】射干方書多音夜。【頌曰】射干之形，莖梗疏長，正如射之長竿之狀，得名由此爾。而陶氏以夜音爲疑，蓋古字音多通呼，若漢官僕射，主射事，而亦音夜，非有別義也。【時珍曰】其葉叢生，横鋪一面，如烏翅及扇之狀，故有烏扇、烏翣、鳳翼、鬼扇、仙人掌諸名。俗呼扁竹，謂其葉扁生而根如竹也。根葉又如蠻薑，故曰草薑。翣音所甲切，扇也。

Explanation of Names. *Wu shan* 烏扇, *Ben jing*. *Wu sha* 烏翣, *Bie lu*. *Wu chui* 烏吹, *Bie lu*. *Wu pu* 烏蒲, *Ben jing*. *Feng yi* 鳳翼, *Shi yi*. *Gui shan* 鬼扇, *Tu su*. *Bian zhu* 扁竹, *Gang mu*. *Xian ren zhang* 仙人掌, *Tu su*. *Zi jin niu* 紫金牛, "purple gold ox," *Tu su*. *Ye xuan hua* 野萱花, *Gang mu*. *Cao jiang* 草薑, *Bie lu*. *Huang yuan* 黄遠, Wu Pu. [Tao] Hongjing: [The *she* of] *she gan* 射干 in recipe texts is mostly read *ye* 夜. [Su] Song: The physical appearance of *she gan* 射干 is a long-stretched thin stem, looking exactly like the long rod, *gan* 竿, [required for a bow] to shoot, *she*

射, [an arrow].[1227] This is the origin of its name. Mr. Tao [Hongjing] was not sure about the reading [of *she* 射] as *ye* 夜. The fact is, the readings of ancient characters often overlapped. For example, during the Han dynasty the official *pu she* 僕射 was responsible for all affairs related to shooting, *she* 射. But [his title] was also read [*pu* 僕] *ye* 夜. The meaning remained the same. [Li] Shizhen: The leaves grow as clusters; they spread horizontally like the wings of crows, *wu chi* 烏翅, or a fan, *shan* 扇. Hence it was given names such as "black fan," *wu shan* 烏扇 and *wu sha* 烏翣, "a phoenix's wings," *feng yi* 鳳翼, "a demon's fan," *gui shan* 鬼扇, and "an immortal/hermit's palm," *xian ren zhang* 仙人掌. A common name is "flat bamboo," *bian zhu* 扁竹. That is to say, its leaves grow flat and the root is similar to that of bamboo. Root and leaves also are similar to those of lesser galangal, *man jiang* 蠻薑. Hence the name "herbal *jiang*," *cao jiang* 草薑. *Sha* 翣 is split read *suo* 所 *jia* 甲. It means "fan," *shan* 扇也。

【集解】【别録曰】射干生南陽山谷田野。三月三日采根，陰乾。【弘景曰】此是烏翣根，黄色，庭臺多種之。人言其葉是鳶尾，而復有鳶頭，此若相似爾，恐非烏翣也。又别有射干相似而花白莖長，似射人之執竿者，故阮公詩云射干臨層城。此不入藥用。【恭曰】鳶尾葉都似射干，而花紫碧色，不抽高莖，根似高良薑而肉白，名鳶頭。【保昇曰】射干高二三尺，花黄實黑。根多鬚，皮黄黑，肉黄赤。所在皆有，二月、八月采根，去皮日乾。【藏器曰】射干、鳶尾二物相似，人多不分。射干即人間所種爲花草名鳳翼者，葉如烏翅，秋生紅花、赤點。鳶尾亦人間所種，苗低下於射干，狀如鳶尾，夏生紫碧花者是也。【大明曰】射干根潤，形似高良薑大小，赤黄色淡硬，五、六、七、八月采。【頌曰】今在處有之，人家種之。春生苗，高一二尺。葉大類蠻薑而狹長横張，疏如翅羽狀，故名烏翣。葉中抽莖，似萱草莖而强硬。六月開花，黄紅色，瓣上有細文。秋結實作房，中子黑色。一説射干多生山崖之間，其莖雖細小，亦類木。故荀子云西方有木，名曰射干，莖長四寸，生於高山之上是也。陶弘景所説花白者，自是射干之類。【震亨曰】根爲射干，葉爲烏翣，紫花者是，紅花者非。【機曰】按諸注則射干非一種，有花白者，花黄者，花紫者，花紅者。丹溪獨取紫花者，必曾試有驗也。【時珍曰】射干即今扁竹也。今人所種，多是紫花者，呼爲紫蝴蝶。其花三四月開，六出，大如萱花。結房大如拇指，頗似泡桐子，一房四隔，一隔十餘子。子大如胡椒而色紫，極硬，咬之不破。七月始枯。陶弘景謂射干、鳶尾是一種。蘇恭、陳藏器謂

1227 Instead of *she zhi chang gan zhi Zhuang* 射之長竿之狀, *Zheng lei* ch. 10, *she gan* 射干, quoting the *Tu jing*'s describes this item's lengthy stem, *jing chang* 莖長, as *si she ren zhi chi gan zhe* 似射人之執竿者. "resembling the rod held by an archer." Also describing the lengthy stem as *zheng ru chang gan zhuang* 正如長竿狀, "shaped exactly like a long rod." In the BCGM these two phrases were combined and *she ren* 射人, "archer," was erroneously changed to *she zhi* 射之.

紫碧花者是鳶尾，紅花者是射干。韓保昇謂黄花者是射干。蘇頌謂花紅黄者是射干，白花者亦其類。朱震亨謂紫花者是射干，紅花者非。各執一説，何以憑依？謹按張揖廣雅云：鳶尾，射干也。易通卦驗云：冬至射干生。土宿真君本草云：射干即扁竹，葉扁生，如側手掌形，莖亦如之，青緑色。一種紫花，一種黄花，一種碧花。多生江南、湖、廣、川、浙平陸間。八月取汁，煮雄黄，伏雌黄，制丹砂，能拒火。據此則鳶尾、射干本是一類，但花色不同。正如牡丹、芍藥、菊花之類，其色各異，皆是同屬也。大抵入藥功不相遠。【藏器曰】射干之名有三：佛經云射干貂獄，此是惡獸，似青黄狗，食人，能緣木；阮公云"射干臨層城"者，是樹，殊有高大者；本草射干是草，即今人所種者也。

Collected Explanations. *Bie lu*: *She gan* grows in the mountain valleys of Nan yang and in the open country. The root is collected on the third day of the third month; it is dried in the yin (i. e., shade). [Tao] Hongjing: This is the root of *wu sha* 烏翣. It is yellow. It is often planted on garden terraces. People say that its leaves are those of kite's tail iris, and that it also has [a root resembling] kite's [tail iris'] head. If they resemble each other indeed, it may not be *wu sha* 烏翣. There is yet another plant resembling *she gan*. It has white flowers and a long stem, looking like the rod held by an archer. Hence Ruan gong in a poem states: "*She gan* look down on the city walls from above." This item is not used as medication. [Su] Gong: All the leaves of kite's tail iris resemble those of *she gan*, but its flowers are of a purple-jade-bluish color, and [*she gan*] does not rise as a tall stem. The root is similar to that of lesser galangal, with white meat. It is named kite's head, *yuan tou* 鳶頭. [Han] Baosheng: *She gan* is two to three *chi* tall. Its flowers are yellow and the fruits are black. The root has many "whiskers." Its skin is yellow-black; the meat is yellow-red. It can be found everywhere. The root is collected in the second and eighth month. Its skin is removed and [the naked root] is dried in the sun. [Chen] Cangqi: *She gan* and kite's tail iris are two similar items. People often cannot distinguish them. The *she gan* planted by people is a blossoming herb called *feng yi* 鳳翼, "phoenix wings." Its leaves are similar to a bird's wings. In autumn it grows a red flower, with fire-red dots. Kite's tail iris, too, is planted by people. Its seedling is shorter than that of *she gan*, and it is shaped like a kite's tail. In summer it grows purple-jade-bluish flowers. Da Ming: The root of *she gan* is moist. Its size is about that of lesser galangal [roots]. It is of bland red-yellow color, and it is hard. It is collected in the fifth, sixth, seventh and eighth month. [Su] Song: Today it is present everywhere, and households plant it. In spring it grows a stem, reaching a height of one to two *chi*. The leaves are as big as those of lesser galangal, but they are narrow, lengthy and spread horizontally. They are similar to the wing feathers [of birds]. Hence the name *wu sha* 烏翣, "crow's feather." From the midst of the leaves a stem rises; it resembles the stem of a yellow day lily, but is more robust and harder. It opens flowers of a yellow-red color in the sixth month, with a fine line design on the petals. In autumn fruit "housing"/capsules form with black seeds inside. It is also said that *she gan* often grows on cliffs, with a stem that maybe fine and small but is related to trees, nevertheless. Hence this is the one of which *Xun zi* states: "There is a tree in the West that is named *she gan*. Its stem has a length of four *cun*, and it grows on high mountains." Those said by Tao Hongjing to have white flowers, they are definitely related to *she gan*. [Zhu] Zhenheng: The root is *she gan*; the leaves are *wu sha* 烏翣. When the flowers are puple, it is [*she gan*]. When the flowers are red, it is something else. [Wang] Ji: According to all comments, there is not only one kind of *she gan*. There are [*she gan* herbs] with white flowers, yellow flowers, purple flowers, and red flowers. As [Zhu] Danxi only accepted those with purple flowers, he must have successfully tested them [to be aware of their effects]. [Li] Shizhen: *She gan* is today's *bian zhu* 扁竹, "flat bamboo." Those planted by people today are mostly those with purple flowers. They call them *zi hu jie* 紫蝴蝶, "purple butterfly." The flowers open in the third and fourth month; with six anthers. They have the size of blackberry lily [flowers]. They form [fruit] "housing"/capsules the size of a thumb; somewhat resembling soaked dragon tree seeds. One "housing"/capsule has four divisions, and each division has more than ten seeds. The seeds have the size of black pepper, with a purple color. They are extremely hard and cannot be bitten to pieces. In the seventh month, [the flowers] begin to wither. Tao Hongjing says: "*She gan* and kite's tail iris are one kind." Su Gong and Chen Cangqi say: "Those with flowers of purple-jade-bluish color are kite's tail iris, and those of flowers of red color are *she gan*." Han Baosheng says: "Those with yellow flowers are *she gan*." Su Song says: "Those with red-yellow color flowers are *she gan*; those with white flowers are related to them." Zhu Zhenheng says: "Those with purple flowers are *she gan*, those with red color are not." As each of them has made a specific statement, how can one find the one to depend on? Now, Zhang Qi in his *Guang ya* states: "Kite's tail iris is *she gan*." The *Yi tong gua yan* states: "*She gan* grows at Winter Solstice." The *Tu su zhen jun ben cao* states: "*She gan* is *bian zhu* 扁竹. The leaves grow flat, similar to the palm of a hand lying on its side. The stem is similar; it is of greenish-green color. One kind has purple flowers. One kind has yellow flowers. One kind has jade-bluish flowers. Many grow in the flat land of Jiang nan, Hu, Guang, Chuan and Zhe. The juice is obtained in the eighth month. It is boiled with realgar, checks [the effects of] cinnabar and can limit the [strength/duration of] fire." Based on this, kite's tail iris and *she gan* basically are of one group, but the colors of their flowers are not identical. This is truly the same as with items such as *paeonia* root bark, [white and red] *paeonia* bark, and *chrysanthemum* flowers. Their colors differ, but they all belong to the same group. Generally speaking, their therapeutic potentials do not lie far apart. [Chen] Cangqi: In all, there are three [kinds of] *she gan*. In Buddhist books a *she gan diao jiu* 射干貂獄 is referred to. This is a malign, wild animal resembling greenish-yellow dogs. It eats humans and is capable of letting wood turn green. When Ruan gong states: "*She gan* look down on the city walls from above," these are trees, with some of them being quite tall. The *she gan* of the *Ben cao* is an herb. It is the one planted by people today.

17-29-01
根 *Gen*

Root [of *she gan*].

【修治】【斅曰】凡采根，先以米泔水浸一宿，漉出，然後以篁竹葉煮之，從午至亥，日乾用。

Pharmaceutical Preparation. [Lei] Xiao: Whenever the root is collected it is first soaked for one night in water that has been used to wash rice. Strain the liquid to remove [the root]. Next boil it together with the leaves of the *jin* 篁 variety of bamboo, from *wu* 午 hrs. (11 – 13) to *hai* 亥 hrs. (21 – 23), dry it in the sun and use [it for therapeutic purposes].

【氣味】苦，平，有毒。【別録曰】微温。久服令人虛。【保昇曰】微寒。【權曰】有小毒。【元素曰】苦，陽中陰也。【時珍曰】寒。多服瀉人。

Qi and Flavor. Bitter, balanced, poisonous. *Bie lu*: Slightly warm. Ingested over a long time it causes depletion. [Han] Baosheng: Slightly cold. [Zhen] Quan: A little poisonous. [Zhang] Yuansu: Bitter. It is a yin in yang [substance]. [Li] Shizhen: Cold. If ingested in large quantities it lets one have outflow.

【主治】欬逆上氣，喉痺咽痛，不得消息，散結氣，腹中邪逆，食飲大熱。本經。療老血在心脾間，欬唾，言語氣臭，散胸中熱氣。別録。苦酒摩塗毒腫。弘景。治疰氣，消瘀血，通女人月閉。甄權。消痰，破癥結，胸膈滿，腹脹氣喘，痃癖，開胃下食，鎮肝明目。大明。治肺氣喉痺爲佳。宗奭。去胃中癰瘡。元素。利積痰疝毒，消結核。震亨。降實火，利大腸，治瘧母。時珍。

Control. Cough with rising qi. Throat blockage and painful throat making it impossible to breathe. [This item serves to] disperse bound qi, and evil [qi] in the abdomen with [qi] counterflow. Massive heat related to [the consumption of] food and beverages. *Ben jing*. It heals old blood stagnating in the region of heart and spleen, coughing up of spittle, and malodorous qi emitted when speaking. It disperses heat in the chest. *Bie lu*. Rub it in bitter wine and apply this to poison swelling. [Tao]

Hongjing. It serves to cure attachment-illness qi,[1228] It dissolves stagnant blood and opens the passage of blocked female menstruation. Zhen Quan. It dissolves phlegm and breaks through conglomeration-illness nodes. [It serves to cure a feeling of] fullness in the chest and diaphragm region, abdominal distension and qi panting, as well as string-illness[1229] and aggregation-illness. It opens the skin and allows food to move down. It presses down liver [qi] and clears the eyes. Da Ming. It is an excellent substance to cure a blocked passage of lung qi through the throat. [Kou] Zongshi. It removes obstruction-illness[1230] sores inside the stomach. [Zhang] Yuansu. It frees the passage of accumulated phlegm and [heals] elevation-illness with poison.[1231] It dissolves node kernels. [Zhu] Zhenheng. It lets repletion fire descend, frees the passage through the large intestine, and serves to cure malaria mother [of lumps].[1232] [Li] Shizhen.

【發明】【震亨曰】射干屬金，有木與火，行太陰、厥陰之積痰，使結核自消甚捷。又治便毒，此足厥陰濕氣，因疲勞而發。取射干三寸，與生薑同煎，食前服，利三兩行，甚效。【時珍曰】射干能降火，故古方治喉痺咽痛爲要藥。孫真人千金方治喉痺有烏翣膏。張仲景金匱玉函方治欬而上氣，喉中作水雞聲，有射干麻黄湯。又治瘧母鼈甲煎丸，亦用烏扇燒過。皆取其降厥陽相火也。火降則血散腫消，而痰結自解，癥瘕自除矣。

Explication. [Zhu] Zhenheng: *She gan* is associated with [the phase] metal; it has [the faculties of the phases] wood and fire. It stimulates the passage of phlegm accumulated in the major yin and ceasing yin [conduits], and lets node kernels dissolve very fast. Also, it serves to cure poison in the [region of urination/defecation] relief, that is, moisture qi in the foot ceasing yin [conduits] that have effused as a result of consumption and exhaustion. Boil a three *cun* long *she gan* [root] together with

1228 *Zhu qi* 疰氣, "attachment-illness qi," 1.) a condition identical to *gui zhu* 鬼疰, "demon attachment-illness." 2.) An etiological agent of turbid qi issued by demonic beings or encountered on burial grounds and in mountain forests that is capable of bringing forth demon attachment-illness. BCGM Dict I, 693.

1229 *Xuan* 痃, "string-illness," a condition of acute pain located in the abdomen to the left and right of the umbilicus. BCGM Dict I, 591.

1230 *Yong* 癰, "obstruction-illness,"refers to an obstruction of vessels or other ducts inside the body. Qi rushing against the obstruction may cause a local swelling and eventually break through the surface to cause an abscess. BCGM Dict I, 641.

1231 *Shan* du 疝毒, "elevation-illness with poison." Documented in the BCGM only twice. Presumably a writing error of à *bian du* 便毒, "poison [in the region] of relief." BCGM Dict I, 418.

1232 *Nüe mu* 瘧母, "malaria-mother [of lumps]." A condition of a long-lasting sequence of malaria outbreaks where over time hard lumps develop below the flanks. BCGM Dict I, 365.

fresh ginger and ingest this prior to a meal. This will free three, or at least two, [bowel] movements. Very effective. [Li] Shizhen: *She gan* can send fire down. Hence in ancient recipes it is considered it to be an important pharmaceutical drug to cure throat blockage and painful throat. Sun zhenren in his *Qian jin fang* [recommends to] cure throat blockage with a "*wu sha* 烏翣 ointment." Zhang Zhongjing in his *Jin kui yu han fang* [recommends] a "decoction with *she gan* and *ephedra* [herb]" to cure cough with rising qi, and the croaking sound of greenish frogs in the throat. Also, to cure malaria mother [of lumps] with the "pills with boiled tortoise shells," he resorted to burned *wu shan* 烏扇. All [these recipes] make use [of *she gan*'s ability to] send down the ceasing yang[1233] minister fire. Once the fire is moved down, the blood disperses and the swelling dissolves, with the result that phlegm nodes are resolved and any concretion-illness and conglomeration-illness is eliminated.

【附方】舊二，新八。

Added Recipes. Two of old. Eight newly [recorded].

咽喉腫痛。射干花根、山豆根，陰乾爲末，吹之如神。袖珍方。

Painful throat swelling. Dry *she gan* flowers and root, and bushy *sophora* in the yin (i. e., shade) and [grind them into] powder. Blown [into the patient's throat, the powder] is divinely [effective]. *Xiu zhen fang*.

傷寒咽閉，腫痛。用生射干、猪脂各四兩，合煎令焦，去滓，每噙棗許，取瘥。龐安常傷寒論。

Harm caused by cold resulting in throat closure and painful swelling. Boil four *liang* each of fresh *she gan* and lard until they are scorched. Remove the dregs. Each time hold as much as the size of a Chinese date in the mouth until a cure is reached. Pan Anchang, *Shang han lun*.

喉痺不通，漿水不入。外臺秘要用射干一片，含嚥汁，良。

Complete throat blockage, when even fermented water of foxtail millet will not enter it. The *Wai tai mi yao* [recommends to] hold one piece of *she gan* in the mouth and to swallow the resulting juice. Good.

醫方大成用扁竹新根擂汁嚥之，大腑動即解。或醋研汁噙，引涎出亦妙。

The *Yi fang da cheng* [recommends to] pound a fresh *bian zhu* root to obtain a juice and to swallow it. [The problem] is resolved with a massive bowel movement. Or

1233 According to Zhu Zhenheng, *she gan* is able to stimulate a movement of accumulated phlegm in the ceasing yin section. Hence the character yang 陽 here may be an erroneous writing of yin 陰.

grind [the root] with vinegar and hold the juice in the mouth. It will stimulate salivation with a wondrous effect.

便民方用紫蝴蝶根一錢，黄芩、生甘草、桔梗各五分，爲末，水調頓服，立愈。名奪命散。

The *Bian min fang* [recommends to grind] one *qian* of *zi hu jie* root and five *fen* each of *scutellaria* [root], fresh *glycyrrhiza* [root] and *platycodon* [root] into powder and ingest it mixed with water all at once. A cure is achieved immediately. [The recipe] is called "powder to snatch life from fate."

二便不通，諸藥不效。紫花扁竹根生水邊者佳，研汁一盞服，即通。普濟方。

The two reliefs (defecation and urination) blocked, with all medications remaining without effect. *Bian zhu* root of a plant with purple flowers growing at the side of waters is excellent. Grind it to obtain a juice and ingest one cup. This will open [the passage of urination and defecation]. *Pu ji fang*.

水蠱腹大，動摇水聲，皮膚黑。用鬼扇根擣汁，服一盃，水即下。肘後方。

Massive abdominal water *gu* distension,[1234] with sounds of water when moving and swaying and a black skin. Pound *gui shan* root to obtain a juice and ingest one cup of it. The water will be discharged. *Zhou hou fang*.

陰疝腫刺。發時腫痛如刺。用生射干擣汁與服，取利。亦可丸服。肘後方。

Swelling and yin [(i. e., genital) region] elevation-illness[1235] with a piercing [pain]. When [the elevation-illness] develops, a swelling occurs with a piercing pain. Pound fresh *she gan* to obtain a juice and ingest it. Immediately effective. It is also possible to ingest it as pills. *Zhou hou fang*.

乳癰初腫。扁竹根如僵蠶者，同萱草根爲末，蜜調傅之，神效。永類方。

Breast obstruction-illness[1236] swelling in its early stage. [Grind] *bian zhu* roots, resembling stiff silkworms, together with yellow day lily roots into powder, mix it with honey and apply this [to the affected region]. Divinely effective. *Yong lei fang*.

1234 *Shui gu fu da* 水蠱腹大, "massive abdominal water *gu* distension," identical to *gu zhang* 鼓脹, "drum[-like] distension." A condition of an abdominal distension and big upswell brought forth by stagnant water qi accumulating in the abdomen. BCGM Dict I, 196, 469.

1235 *Shan* 疝, "elevation-illness," a group of conditions characterized by violent abdominal pain, in some cases associated with constipation and anuria. BCGM Dict I, 417.

1236 *Ru yong* 乳癰, "breast obstruction-illness," a condition of acute putrefication of a woman's breast. Often encountered if a woman, following delivery, experiences *chui nai* 吹奶, "inflated breast," or *du ru* 妒乳, "jealousy breast." BCGM Dict I, 412.

中射工毒，生瘡者。烏翣、升麻各二兩，水三升，煎二升，温服。以滓敷瘡上。姚僧坦集驗方。

Struck by the archer's poison,[1237] resulting in a growth of sores. Boil two *liang* each of *wu sha* and *cimicifuga* [rhizome] in three *sheng* of water down to two *sheng*, and ingest this warm. Apply the dregs to the sores. Yao Sengtan, *Ji yan fang*.

17-30
鳶尾本經下品

Yuan wei. FE *Ben jing*, lower rank.

***Iris tectorum* Maxim. Kite's tail iris.**

【釋名】烏園本經。根名鳶頭。【時珍曰】並以形命名。烏園當作烏鳶。

Explanation of Names. *Wu yuan* 烏園, *Ben jing*. The root is called *yuan tou* 鳶頭, "a kite's head." [Li] Shizhen: Both names refer to the physical appearance [of this substance]. *Wu yuan* 烏園 should be written *wu yuan* 烏鳶, "black kite."

【集解】【別録曰】烏鳶生九疑山谷。五月采。【弘景曰】方家言是射干苗，而主療亦異，當別是一種。方用鳶頭，當是其根，療體相似，而本草不題。【恭曰】此草所在有之，人家亦種。葉似射干而闊短，不抽長莖，花紫碧色。根似高良薑，皮黄肉白，嚼之戟人咽喉，與射干全別。射干花紅，抽莖長，根黄有臼。【保昇曰】草名鳶尾，根名鳶頭，亦謂之鳶根。葉似射干，布地生。黑根似高良薑而節大，數個相連。九月、十月采根，日乾。【時珍曰】此即射干之苗，非別一種也。肥地者莖長根粗，瘠地者莖短根瘦。其花自有數色。諸家皆是强分。陳延之小品方言，東海鳶頭即由跋者，亦訛也。東海出之故耳。

Collected Explanations. *Bie lu*: *Wu yuan* grows in the valleys of Mount Jiu yi shan. It is collected in the fifth month. [Tao] Hongjing: Recipe experts say that this is the seedling of blackberry lily, but their control and therapeutic [usages] differ. It must be a different kind. When recipes [recommend to] use *yuan tou* 鳶頭, this must be its root. Their therapeutic functions are similar, but the *Ben cao* does not mention it. [Su] Gong: This herb is present everywhere, and people also plant it. The leaves resemble those of blackberry lily, but are broad and short. [The plant] does not rise up as a long stem. Its flowers are of a purple-jade-bluish color. The root resembles that of lesser galangal, with a yellow skin and white meat. When chewed it pierces through one's throat. This is entirely different from blackberry lily. Blackberry lily has red flowers and rises up as a long stem. The root is yellow and forms "mortars."

1237 *She gong* 射工, "archer," 1.) a small bug in ancient times believed to live in water and be capable of "shooting" poison from its mouth at people, thereby causing disease; 2.) a condition caused by the archer's poison. BCGM Dict. I, 432. See 42-15.

[Han] Baosheng: The herb is named "kite's tail." The root is named "kite's head." It is also referred to as "kite root." The leaves resemble those of blackberry lily; their growth covers the ground. The black root resembles that of lesser galangal, but has large nodes several of which are linked together. The root is collected in the ninth and tenth month; it is dried in the sun. [Li] Shizhen: This is nothing but the seedling of blackberry lily; it is not a different kind of its own. On fat earth the stem is long and the root is crude. On poor ground, the stem is short and the root is lean. The flowers may have several colors; and the distinctions made by all experts are forced. When Chen Yanzhi in his *Xiao pin fang* states: "*Yuan tou* from Dong hai is the root of Indian turnip," this is wrong, too, because this is [simply *yuan wei*] coming from Dong hai."

【氣味】苦，平，有毒。【恭曰】有小毒。

Qi and Flavor. Bitter, balanced, poisonous. [Su] Gong: Slightly poisonous.

【主治】蠱毒邪氣，鬼疰諸毒，破癥瘕積聚，去水，下三蟲。本經。殺鬼魅，療頭眩。别録。

Control. *Gu* poison[1238] and evil qi. All types of poison related to demon attachment-illness. It breaks through concretion-illness and conglomeration-illness,[1239] accumulations and collections, removes water, and serves to discharge the three types of worms/bugs. *Ben jing*. It kills demonic seduction-specters[1240] and heals dizziness in the head. *Bie lu*.

1238 *Gu du* 蠱毒, "*gu*-poison[ing]." (1) A poison emitted by certain worms/snakes with an ability to cause varying pathological changes in a person who has taken it in by means of wine or food. (2) Abdominal fullness, in some cases with blood spitting, and blood in the stool and urine. BCGM Dict I, 192 - 193. See BCGM 42-22.

1239 *Zheng jia* 癥瘕, "concretion-illness and conglomeration-illness." The two terms are often used interchangeably and do not signify two distinctly different conditions. Concretion-illness and conglomeration-illness result from a disharmony of cold and warmth resulting in a failure to transform beverages and food. Nodes form when the clash with the qi of the long-term depots. BCGM Dict I, 677.

1240 *Gui mei* 鬼魅, "demonic seduction-specters." 1.) An etiological agent capable of bringing forth sudden violent diseases, strange diseases and recurring diseases believed to be associated with the activity of demons by people since antiquity. 2.) A condition of sudden violent or unusual or recurrent natures that are difficult to explain. Hence since antiquity there is a belief that such conditions are caused by demonic intrusion. BCGM Dict I, 200.

【附方】舊一，新一。

Added Recipes. One of old. One newly [recorded].

飛尸遊蠱着喉中，氣欲絶者。鳶尾根削去皮，納喉中，摩病處，令血出爲佳。陳藏器本草拾遺。

Flying corpse [qi][1241] and roaming *gu* [poison] attached inside the throat and threatening to interrupt the qi [flow]. Insert a *yuan wei* root, with the skin removed, into the affected throat and rub the location of the disease until it bleeds [to achieve a result this is] excellent. Chen Cangqi, *Ben cao shi yi.*

鬼魅邪氣。四物鳶頭散：東海鳶頭、黄牙即金牙、莨菪子、防葵各一分，爲末，酒服方寸匕。欲令病人見鬼，增防葵一分。欲令知鬼，又增一分，立驗。不可多服。陳延之小品方。

Demonic seduction-specters and evil qi. The "powder with four items, including *yuan tou*." [Grind] one *fen* each of *yuan tou* from Dong hai, native gold (referred to here as "yellow tooth, i. e., gold tooth"), henbane seeds and *peucedanum* [root] into powder and ingest with wind the amount held by a square *cun* spoon. If it is intended to let the patient have visions of demons, add an additional fen of *peucedanum* [root]. If he is supposed to meet a demon, again add one more *fen*. Immediately effective. An overdose is to be avoided. Chen Yanzhi, *Xiao pin fang*.

17-31
鳳簪綱目
***Yu zan*.** FE *Gang mu.*

***Hosta plantaginea* (Lam.) Ascherson. Assumption lily.**[1242]

【釋名】白鶴仙。【時珍曰】並以花象命名。

Explanation of Names. *Bai he xian* 白鶴仙, "white crane immortal." [Li] Shizhen: The names reflect the image of the flowers.

【集解】【時珍曰】玉簪處處人家栽爲花草。二月生苗成叢，高尺許，柔莖如白菘。其葉大如掌，團而有尖，葉上紋如車前葉，青白色，頗嬌瑩。六七月抽莖，莖上有細葉。中出花朶十數枚，長二三寸，本小末大。未開時，正如白玉搔頭簪形，又如羊肚蘑菇之狀；開時微綻四出，中吐黄蕊，

1241 *Fei shi* 飛屍, "flying corpse [qi]." A condition with sudden outbreaks and frequently changing appearances that do not show a regular pattern. BCGM Dict I, 156.

1242 *Yu zan* 玉簪, lit.: "a hairpin made of jade."

頗香，不結子。其根連生，如鬼臼、射干、生薑輩，有鬚毛。舊莖死則根有一臼，新根生則舊根腐。亦有紫花者，葉微狹。皆鬼臼、射干之屬。

Collected Explanations. [Li] Shizhen: *Yu zan* is planted as a flower herb by people everywhere. In the second month it grows a cluster of stems, reaching a height of more than a *chi*. The soft stems are similar to those of celery cabbage. Its leaves have the size of a palm; they are round with a pointed end. On the surface of the leaves is a line design similar to the leaves of Asiatic plantain. They are of greenish-white color, quite charming and lustrous. A stem rises up in the sixth and seventh month. Fine leaves grow on the stem. In their center a cluster of more than ten flowers appears. They are two to three *cun* long, small at their base and big at the end. Before they open, they truly look like the tips of hairpins made of white jade, or like sheep belly mushrooms. When they open they break up with four anthers, with yellow filaments emerging from the center that are quite fragrant. [The flowers] do not form seeds. The roots grow linked to each other, similar to those of umbrella leaf herbs, blackberry lily and fresh ginger. They are covered with "whisker" hair. When the old stem dies the roots form a "mortar," and when a new root grows, the old root rots. There are also specimens with purple flowers, and slightly narrow leaves. They all are related to umbrella leaf herbs and blackberry lily.

17-31-01
根 *Gen*

Root [of *yu zan*].

【氣味】甘、辛，寒，有毒。

Qi and Flavor. Sweet, acrid, cold, poisonous.

【主治】搗汁服，解一切毒，下骨哽，塗癰腫。時珍。

Control. Pound it to obtain a juice and ingest it to resolve all types of poison and to discharge a bone that is stuck in the throat. It is applied to obstruction-illness[1243] swelling. [Li] Shizhen.

1243 *Yong* 癰, "obstruction-illness,"refers to an obstruction of vessels or other ducts inside the body. Qi rushing against the obstruction may cause a local swelling and eventually break through the surface to cause an abscess. BCGM Dict I, 641.

【附方】新五。

Added Recipes. Five newly [recorded].

乳癰初起。内消花，即玉簪花，取根擂酒服，以渣傅之。海上方。

Breast obstruction-illness[1244] that has just begun to rise. Pound the root of *nei xiao hua* 内消花,[1245] that is, *yu zan hua*, with wine and [let the woman] ingest this. Apply the dregs [to the affected region]. *Hai shang fang.*

婦人斷產。白鶴仙根、白鳳仙子各一錢半，紫葳二錢半，辰砂二錢，搗末，蜜和丸梧子大。產内三十日，以酒半盞服之。不可着牙齒，能損牙齒也。摘玄方。

To end the reproductive faculties of a woman. Pound one and a half *qian* of *bai he xian* root and white touch-me-not seeds, two and a half *qian* of trumpet flower and two *qian* of cinnabar into powder and form with honey pills the size of *wu* seeds. Ingest them with half a cup of wine within 30 days after a birth. They must not touch the teeth. They could injure the teeth. *Zhai xuan fang.*

解斑蝥毒。玉簪根擂水服之，即解。趙真人濟急方。

To resolve blister beetle poison. Grind a *yu zan* root in water and ingest this. This resolves [the poison]. Zhao zhenren, *Ji ji fang.*

下魚骨哽。玉簪花根、山裏紅果根，同搗自然汁，以竹筒灌入咽中，其骨自下。不可着牙齒。臞仙乾坤生意。

To discharge a fish bone stuck in the throat. Pound *yu zan hua* root and hawthorne root to obtain a natural juice and force-feed it by means of a bamboo tube into the [patient's] throat. The bone will be discharged. Do not touch the teeth. Quxian, *Qian kun sheng yi.*

刮骨取牙。玉簪根乾者一錢，白砒三分，白硇七分，蓬砂二分，威靈仙三分，草烏頭一分半，爲末。以少許點疼處，即自落也。余居士選奇方。

To smear something on a bone to extract a tooth. [Grind] one *qian* of *yu zan* root, dried, three *fen* of arsenic, seven *fen* of white sal ammoniac, two *fen* of borax, three *fen* of Chinese *clematis* [root] and one and a half *fen* of *aconitum* [main tuber] into powder and drip a small amount on the painful location. The [tooth] falls off as a result. Yu Jushi, *Xuan qi fang.*

1244 *Ru yong* 乳癰, "breast obstruction-illness," a condition of acute putrefication of a woman's breast. Often encountered if a woman, following delivery, experiences *chui nai* 吹奶, "inflated breast," or *du ru* 妒乳, "jealousy breast." BCGM Dict I, 412.

1245 *Nei xiao hua* 内消花, lit.: the "flower to dissolve internally."

17-31-02
葉 *Ye*

Leaf [of *yu zan*].

【氣味】同根。

Qi and Flavor. Identical to the root.

【主治】蛇虺螫傷，搗汁和酒服，以渣傅之，中心留孔洩氣。時珍。

Control. Harm caused by the bite of a snake or venomous viper. Pound [the leaves] and ingest the resulting juice mixed with wine. Apply the dregs to [the affected region] and leave an opening in the middle for the qi to flow off. [Li] Shizhen.

17-32
鳳仙綱目
Feng xian, FE *Gang mu*

***Impatiens balsamina* L. Touch-me-not.**

【釋名】急性子救荒、旱珍珠綱目、金鳳花綱目、小桃紅救荒、夾竹桃救荒、海蒳音納、染指甲草救荒、菊婢。【時珍曰】其花頭翅尾足俱具，翹然如鳳狀，故以名之。女人采其花及葉包染指甲。其實狀如小桃，老則迸裂，故有指甲、急性、小桃諸名。宋光宗李后諱鳳，宮中呼爲好女兒花。張宛丘呼爲菊婢。韋居呼爲羽客。

Explanation of Names. *Ji xing zi* 急性子, "one with a hurried nature," *Jiu huang*. *Han zhen zhu* 旱珍珠, "parched pearls," *Gang mu*. *Jin feng hua* 金鳳花, "golden phoenix flower," *Gang mu*. *Xiao tao hong* 小桃紅, "redness of a small peach," *Jiu huang*. *Jia zhu tao* 夾竹桃, "peaches clinging to bamboo," *Jiu huang*. *Hai na* 海蒳, read *na* 納, *za zhi jia cao* 染指甲草, "herb to dye fingernails," *Jiu huang*. *Ju bei* 菊婢, "*chrysanthemum* servant-girl." [Li] Shizhen: This flower has a head, wings, a tail and feet, all turned up like those of a phoenix. Hence the name. Females collect the flowers and the leaves to paint their fingernails. The fruits are shaped like small peaches; when they are old they crack. Hence all the names such as *zhi jia* 指甲, "fingernail," *ji xing* 急性, "hurried nature," and *xiao tao* 小桃, "small peach." The Song [Emperor] Guang zong's [wife] Empress Li's [personal] tabooed name was *feng* 鳳, "phoenix." Hence those in the palace called [*feng xian*] *hao nü er hua* 好女兒花, "good girls' flower," instead. Zhang Wanqiu called it *ju bei* 菊婢, "*chrysanthemum* servant-girl." Wei Jun called it *yu ke* 羽客, "feathered visitor."

【集解】【時珍曰】鳳仙人家多種之，極易生。二月下子，五月可再種。苗高二三尺，莖有紅白二色，其大如指，中空而脆。葉長而尖，似桃、柳葉而有鋸齒。椏間開花，或黃或白，或紅或紫，或碧或雜色，亦自變易，狀如飛禽，自夏初至秋盡，開謝相續。結實纍然，大如櫻桃，其形微長，色如毛桃，生青熟黃，犯之即自裂。皮卷如拳，苞中有子似蘿蔔子而小，褐色。人采其肥莖汋醃，以充萵筍。嫩葉渫，浸一宿，亦可食。但此草不生蟲蠹，蜂蝶亦不近，恐亦不能無毒也。

Collected Explanations. [Li] Shizhen: *Feng xian* is often planted by households; it grows very easily. Put the seeds down in the second month; in the fifth month they can be replanted. The seedling is one to two *chi* tall; the stem has two colors: red and white. It has the size of a finger; it is hollow and brittle. The leaves are long and pointed; they resemble peach and willow leaves with teeth. Flowers open in the forks; they may be yellow, white, red, purple, jade-bluish or of mixed color. They also may undergo changes. They are shaped like flying birds. From early summer to the end of autumn flowers open continuously, forming fruits one linked to another. They have the size of cherrys but with a somewhat lengthy shape. The color is that of hairy peaches; it is greenish as long as they are fresh and yellow when they are ripe. When knocked against, they crack open and the skin curls up like a fist. The seeds in an "envelop" resemble radish seeds, but they are smaller and of brown color. People collect the fat stems, preserve them in brine and pass them off as lattuce shoots. When the scattered tender leaves are soaked overnight, they, too, are edible. However, as this herb does not generate worms/bugs and as neither bees/wasps nor butterflies approach it, one wonders how it can be that it is nonpoisonous.

17-32-01
子 *Zi*

Seeds [of *feng xian*].

【氣味】微苦，温，有小毒。

Qi and Flavor. Slightly bitter, warm, slightly poisonous.

【主治】産難，積塊噎膈，下骨哽，透骨通竅。時珍。

Control. Difficult births. Accumulation lumps and gullet occlusion. They send down a bone stuck in the throat. They pass through bones and open orifices. [Li] Shizhen.

【發明】【時珍曰】鳳仙子其性急速，故能透骨軟堅。庖人烹魚肉硬者，投數粒即易軟爛，是其驗也。緣其透骨，最能損齒，與玉簪根同，凡服者不可着齒也。多用亦戟人咽。

Explication. [Li] Shizhen: *Feng xian* seeds by their nature are hurried and fast. Hence they can pass through bones and soften what is hard. When cooks boil hard fish and meat, they just add several [*feng xian*] seeds and [the fish and the meat] easily soften and become pulpy. This is the evidence. As they penetrate bones, they are very capable of destroying teeth, similar to the root of assumption lily. Whenever they are ingested they must not touch the teeth. Used often they also pierce one's throat.

【附方】新五。

Added Recipes. Five newly [recorded].

產難催生。鳳仙子二錢，研末。水服，勿近牙。外以蓖麻子隨年數搗塗足心。集簡方。

To hasten birth in cases of difficult delivery. Grind two *qian* of *feng xian* seeds into powder and [let the woman] ingest it with water. It must not come close to her teeth. For an external application, pound a number of castor beans corresponding to her age and apply [the resulting pulp] to the soles of her feet. *Ji jian fang.*

噎食不下。鳳仙花子酒浸三宿，晒乾爲末，酒丸綠豆大。每服八粒，温酒下。不可多用，即急性子也。摘玄方。

Gullet occluding food that fails to move down. Soak *feng xian* flower seeds in wine for three nights, dry them in the sun and [grind them into] powder. With wine form pills the size of mung beans. Each time ingest eight pills, to be sent down with warm wine. They must not be resorted to in large quantities; after all, these are the "seeds with a hurried nature." *Zhai xuan fang.*

咽中骨哽欲死者。白鳳仙子研水一大呷，以竹筒灌入咽，其物即軟。不可近牙。或爲末吹之。普濟方。

Choking on a bone stuck in the throat, and death is imminent. Grind white *feng xian* seeds in one large mouthful of water and force-feed it with a bamboo tube into the [patient's] throat. The item [stuck there] softens as a result. [The water-seeds mixture] must not come close to [the patient's] teeth. It is also possible [to [grind the seeds] into powder and blow it [into the throat]. *Pu ji fang.*

牙齒欲取。金鳳花子研末，入砒少許，點疼牙根，取之。摘玄方。

To extract a tooth. Grind *jin feng hua* seeds into powder, add a little arsenic and drip this on the root of the aching tooth. Then extract it. *Zhai xuan fang.*

小兒痞積。急性子、水葒花子、大黄各一兩，俱生研末。每味取五錢，外用皮硝一兩拌勻。將白鵓鴿一個，或白鴨亦可，去毛屎，剖腹，勿犯水，以布拭净，將末裝入内，用線紥定，沙鍋内入水三盌，重重紙封，以小火煮乾，將鴿、鴨翻調焙黄色，冷定。早辰食之，日西時疾軟，三日大便下血，病去矣。忌冷物百日。孫天仁集效方。

Children with an obstacle-illness accumulation. Grind one *liang* each of *ji xing* seeds, prince's feather seeds and rhubarb root, all fresh, into powder. For each application take five *qian* of [the powder] and additionally mix it evenly with one *liang* of mirabilite. Then take one white rock pigeon, a white duck will do, too, remove its feathers and excrements, cut open its abdomen - it must not come into contact with water, wipe it clean with a piece of cloth, and fill the powder into it. Tightly fasten it with a thread and give it, wrapped in several layers of paper, into an earthen pot filled with three bowls of water. Boil it over a small fire until the water has dried. Turn the pigeon, or the duck, while it is baked until it has turned yellow, and let it cool. [The child] is to eat it early the next morning, and by the time the sun is in the West, its [obstacle-]illness will have softened. On the third day [the child] will defecate blood, and the disease is gone. [During this therapy,] cold items are to be avoided for 100 days. Sun Tianren, *Ji xiao fang*.

17-32-02

花 *Hua*

Flower [of *feng xian*].

【氣味】甘，滑，温，無毒。

Qi and Flavor. Sweet, soft, warm, nonpoisonous.

【主治】蛇傷，擂酒服即解。又治腰脇引痛不可忍者，研餅晒乾爲末，空心每酒服三錢，活血消積。時珍。

Control. For harm caused by a snake, pound it in wine, ingest this and [the poison] is resolved. Also, to cure unbearable pain pulling on the lower back and flanks, grind [the flowers], prepare a cake, dry it in the sun and [grind it into] powder. Each time ingest on an empty stomach with wine three *qian*. This serves to quicken the blood and dissolve accumulations. [Li] Shizhen.

【附方】新一。

Added Recipes. One newly [recorded].

風濕卧牀不起。用金鳳花、柏子仁、朴硝、木瓜煎湯洗浴，每日二三次。内服獨活寄生湯。吴旻扶壽精方。

Wind [intrusion] and the presence of moisture making one lie down and not want to get up. Boil *jin feng hua*, arborvitae seed kernels, mirabilite and qince and wash [the patient] with the decoction two or three times a day. He is also to ingest the "decoction with *angelica biserrata* conveying life." Wu Min, *Fu shou jing fang*.

17-32-03
根、葉 *Gen, Ye*

Root, leaf [of *feng xian*].

【氣味】苦、甘、辛，有小毒。

Qi and Flavor. Bitter, sweet, acrid, slightly poisonous.

【主治】雞魚骨哽，誤吞銅鐵，杖撲腫痛，散血通經，軟堅透骨。時珍。

Control. Choking on a chicken and fish bone. If a copper or iron item is swallowed accidentally. Painful swelling resulting from flogging or a fall. It disperses blood and opens the passage through the conduits; it softens what is hard and penetrates bones. [Li] Shizhen.

【附方】新三。

Added Recipes. Three newly [recorded].

咽喉物哽。金鳳花根嚼爛噙嚥，骨自下，雞骨尤效。即以温水漱口，免損齒也。亦治誤吞銅鐵。危氏得效方。

Choking on an item stuck in the throat. Chew a *jin lan hua* root until it has turned pulpy, hold it in the mouth, swallow [the resulting liquid] and the bone moves down. It is especially effective for chicken bones. Then rinse the mouth with warm water to avoid injuring the teeth. It also serves to heal if a copper or iron item is accidentally swallowed. *Wei shi de xiao fang.*

打杖腫痛。鳳仙花葉搗如泥，塗腫破處，乾則又上，一夜血散即愈。冬月收取乾者，研末水和塗之。葉廷器通變要法。

Painful swelling caused by flogging. Pound *feng xian* flowers and leaves to a pulpy, muddy mass and apply it on the swelling and where [the skin] has broken open. When it has dried, apply it again. Within one night the blood is dispersed, and this is the cure. When during winter [only] dried [flowers and leaves] are available, grind them into powder, mix them with water and apply this [to the affected region]. Ye Tingqi, *Tong bian yao fa.*

馬患諸病。白鳳仙花連根葉熬膏，遇馬有病，抹其眼四角上，即汗出而愈。衛生易簡方。

All types of horse diseases. Simmer white *feng xian* flowers with the root and the leaves to a paste. When you encounter a horse with a disease, apply it on the four corners of its eyes. This will let it sweat, and this is the cure. *Wei sheng yi jian fang.*

17-33
坐拏草宋圖經
Zuo na cao, FE Song, *Tu jing*.

Unidentified.

【集解】【頌曰】生江西及滁州。六月開紫花結實。采其苗入藥，江西甚易得。後因人用有效，今頗貴重。【時珍曰】按一統志云：出吉安永豐縣。

Collected Explanations.. [Su] Song: It grows in Jiang xi and in Chu zhou. It opens flowers and forms fruits in the sixth month. They collect the seedling and add it to medication; in Jiang xi it is obtained most easily. Because its application was effective, later on and to this day, it is greatly valued. [Li] Shizhen: According to the *Yi tong zhi*, it comes from Yong feng xian in Ji an.

【氣味】辛，熱，有毒。

Qi and Flavor. Acrid, hot, poisonous.

【主治】風痺，壯筋骨，兼治打撲傷損。蘇頌。

Control. Blockage related to wind [intrusion]. It strengthens sinews and bones, and at the same time it serves to cure injuries caused by blows and falls. Su Song.

【發明】【頌曰】神醫普救方治風藥中已有用者。【時珍曰】危氏得效方麻藥煮酒方中用之。聖濟録治膈上虛熱，咽喉噎塞，小便赤濇，神困多睡，有坐拏丸。用坐拏草、大黄、赤芍藥、木香、升麻、麥門冬、黄芪、木通、酸棗仁、薏苡仁、枳殼等分，爲末。蜜丸梧子大。每服二十丸，麥門冬湯下。

Explication. [Su] Song: It is already recorded in the *Shen yi pu jiu fang* as one of the pharmaceutical drugs used for curing wind [intrusion]. [Li] Shizhen: The *Wei shi de xiao fang* [recommends its] use in a recipe for numbing (anesthesizing) medication boiled in wine. The *Sheng ji lu* has the "pills with *zuo na*" for depletion heat above the diaphragm, blocked throat, red and rough urination, and spirit taxation with severe sleepiness. It uses equal amounts of *zhu na cao*, rhubarb root, red *paeonia* [root], *costus* [root], *cimicifuga* [rhizome], *ophiopogon* [tuber], *astragalus* [root], *akebia* [herb], jujube kernels, Job's tears kernels, and unripe oranges, ground into powder and formed with honey to pills the size of *wu* seeds. Each time ingest 20 pills, to be sent down with an *ophiopogon* [tuber] decoction.

【附録】
Appendix

17-33-A01
押不蘆 *Yabulu*

【時珍曰】按周密癸辛雜志云：漠北回回地方有草名押不蘆。土人以少許磨酒飲，即通身麻痺而死，加以刀斧亦不知。至三日則以少藥投之即活。御藥院中亦儲之。貪官污吏罪甚者，則服百日丹，皆用此也。昔華陀能刳腸滌胃，豈不有此等藥耶？

[Li] Shizhen: According to Zhou Mi's *Gui xin za zhi*, "north of the desert in the region of the muslims there is an herb named *yabulu*. The locals rub a small amount in wine and drink it. This numbs/anesthesizes the body and that person dies. He will not even notice whether he was cut by a knife or axe. Three days later he is given a small dose of a medication and will come back to life." The Imperial Pharmaceutical Office stores it, too. Officials who have committed a severe crime ingest the "one hundred days elixir" [to withstand the pain inflicted during their punishment]. They all resort to this [recipe]. In ancient times Hua Tuo was able to cut open the intestines and rinse the stomach. Why should he not have possessed such medication?

17-34
曼陀羅花綱目
Mantuoluo hua, FE *Gang mu.*

***Datura metel* L. Downy thorn apple.**

【釋名】風茄兒綱目、山茄子。【時珍曰】法華經言佛説法時，天雨曼陀羅花。又道家北斗有陀羅星使者，手執此花，故後人因以名花。曼陀羅，梵言雜色也。茄乃因葉形爾。姚伯聲花品呼爲惡客。

Explanation of Names. *Feng qie er* 風茄兒, "wind eggplant," *Gang mu*. *Shen qie zi* 山茄子, "mountain eggplant." [Li] Shizhen: The *Fa hua jing* says that when Buddha recited his sutras, *mantuoluo* 曼陀羅 flowers rained from heaven. The Daoists hold that the Big Dipper has sent a *tuoluo* 陀羅 star emissary, holding this plant in his hand. Hence, later on, people named this flower after him. *Mantuoluo* 曼陀羅 in Sanskrit means "multi-colored." [The name] *qie* 茄, "eggplant," refers to the shape of the leaves. In Yao Bosheng's "categories/ranks of flowers," it is called *e ke* 惡客, "malicious visitor."[1246]

【集解】【時珍曰】曼陀羅生北土，人家亦栽之。春生夏長，獨莖直上，高四五尺，生不旁引，綠莖碧葉，葉如茄葉。八月開白花，凡六瓣，狀如

1246 See BCGM Dict III, 581, 582.

牽牛花而大，攢花中折，駢葉外包，而朝開夜合。結實圓而有丁拐，中有小子。八月采花，九月采實。

Collected Explanations. [Li] Shizhen: *Mantuoluo* grows in the North; households also plant it. It grows in spring and reaches maturity in summer. One single stem rises straight up, reaching a height of four to five *chi*. When it grows it never diverges to the side. The stem is green; the leaves are jade-bluish. The leaves are similar to eggplant leaves. A white flower opens in the eighth month, with six petals. It is shaped like *pharbitis* flowers, but is bigger. The [petals] cluster in the center of the flower and are split. Always two are enclosed by a leaf. They open in the morning and close at night. The [flower] forms round fruit with a handle stick, and small seeds inside. The flower is collected in the eighth month; the fruits are collected in the ninth month.

17-34-01
花、子 *Hua, Zi*

Flower, seeds [of *mantuoluo hua*].

【氣味】辛，温，有毒。

Qi and Flavor. Acrid, warm, poisonous.

【主治】諸風及寒濕脚氣，煎湯洗之。又主驚癇及脱肛，并入麻藥。時珍。

Control. For all types of wind [intrusion] and leg qi[1247] with the presence of cold and moisture, boil [*mantuoluo*] and with the decoction wash the [affected region]. Also, it controls fright epilepsy and prolapsed anus, and is added to numbing/anesthesizing medication. [Li] Shizhen.

【發明】【時珍曰】相傳此花笑采釀酒飲，令人笑；舞采釀酒飲，令人舞。予常試之，飲須半酣，更令一人或笑或舞引之，乃驗也。八月采此花，七月采火麻子花，陰乾，等分爲末。熱酒調服三錢，少頃昏昏如醉。割瘡灸火，宜先服此，則不覺苦也。

Explication: [Li] Shizhen: According to tradition, if [the person] who collects this flower laughs, and if it is then used to brew wine, [the wine] will make people laugh. If [the person] who collects this flower dances, and if it is then used to brew wine, [the wine] will make people dance. I have tested this several times. When it is drunk to at least half of one's heart's content, it will let others, too, either laugh or dance. This was the proof. In the eighth month this flower is collected; hemp flowers are collected in the seventh month. They are dried in the yin (i. e., shade) and equal amounts are [ground into] powder. Ingest mixed with hot wine three *qian*. Within

1247 *Jiao qi* 脚氣, "leg qi." Painful, weak, swollen legs. BCGM Dict I, 248.

a short time you will feel dizzy as if drunk. This should be ingested prior to surgery and cauterization. Then you cannot feel the pain.

【附方】新三。

Added Recipes. Three newly [recorded].

面上生瘡。曼陀羅花晒乾研末，少許貼之。衛生易簡方。

Facial sores. Dry *mantuoluo hua* in the sun, grind it into powder and apply a little [to the affected region]. *Wei sheng yi jian fang*.

小兒慢驚。曼陀羅花七朵，重一字，天麻二錢半，全蝎炒十枚，天南星炮、丹砂、乳香各二錢半，爲末。每服半錢，薄荷湯調下。御藥院方。

Children with chronic fright. [Grind] seven *mantuoluo hua*, weighing on *zi*, two and a half *qian* of *gastrodia* [root], ten complete scorpions, fried, and two and a half *qian* of Indian turnip, roasted in a pan, cinnabar and frankincense into powder. Each time [let the child] ingest half a *qian*, to be sent down mixed with a mint decoction. *Yu yao yuan fang*.

大腸脱肛。曼陀羅子連殼一對，橡斗十六個，同剉，水煎三五沸，入朴硝少許，洗之。儒門事親。

Anal prolapse of the large intestine. File together to pieces one pair of *mantuoluo* seeds with their shell, and 16 sawtooth oak fruits, and boil them in water to bubbling, three to five times. Add a little mirabilite and [use the liquid to] wash [the affected region]. *Ru men shi qin*.

17-35
羊躑躅本經下品

Yang zhi zhu, FE *Ben jing*, lower rank.

***Rhododendron molle* (Bl.) G. Don. Azalea.**

【釋名】黄躑躅綱目、黄杜鵑蒙筌、羊不食草拾遺、鬧羊花綱目、驚羊花綱目、老虎花綱目、玉枝別録。【弘景曰】羊食其葉，躑躅而死，故名。鬧，當作惱。惱，亂也。

Explanation of Names. *Huang zhi zhu* 黄躑躅, *Gang mu*. *Huang du juan* 黄杜鵑, *Meng quan*. *Yang bu shi cao* 羊不食草, "an herb that sheep won't eat," *Shi yi*. *Nao yang hua* 鬧羊花, "the flower that troubles sheep," *Gang mu*. *Jing yang hua* 驚羊花, "the flower that frightens sheep," *Gang mu*. *Lao hu hua* 老虎花, "tiger flower," *Gang mu*. *Yu zhi* 玉枝, "jade branch," *Bie lu*. [Tao] Hongjing: When sheep, *yang* 羊, eat its leaves, they stagger, *zhi zhu* 躑躅, and die. Hence the name. *Nao* 鬧, "to trouble," should be written *nao* 惱. *Nao* 惱 is *luan* 亂, "to confuse."

【集解】【別録曰】羊躑躅生太行山川谷及淮南山。三月采花，陰乾。【弘景曰】近道諸山皆有之。花黄似鹿葱，不可近眼。【恭曰】花亦不似鹿葱，正似旋花色黄者也。【保昇曰】小樹高二尺，葉似桃葉，花黄似瓜花。三月、四月采花，日乾。【頌曰】所在有之。春生苗似鹿葱，葉似紅花，莖高三四尺。夏開花似凌霄花、山石榴輩，正黄色，羊食之則死。今嶺南、蜀道山谷遍生，皆深紅色如錦綉。然或云此種不入藥。【時珍曰】韓保昇所説似桃葉者最的。其花五出，蕊瓣皆黄，氣味皆惡。蘇頌所謂深紅色者，即山石榴名紅躑躅者，無毒，與此別類。張揖廣雅謂躑躅一名决光者，誤矣。决光，决明也。按唐李紳文集言：駱谷多山枇杷，毒能殺人，其花明艷，與杜鵑花相似，樵者識之。其説似羊躑躅，未知是否？要亦其類耳。

Collected Explanations. *Yang zhi zhu* grows in the river valleys of Mount Tai xing shan and on the mountains in Huai nan. The flowers are collected in the third month; they are dried in the yin (i. e., shade). [Tao] Hongjing: Today it can be found in all the mountain regions nearby. The flowers are yellow[1248] and resemble those of yellow day lily. They must not come into contact with the eyes. [Su] Gong: The flowers do not resemble those of yellow day lily; they certainly resemble the yellow flowers of hedge bindweed. [Han] Baosheng: These are small trees, two *chi* tall. The leaves resemble the leaves of peach trees; the flowers are yellow and resemble melon flowers. The flowers are collected in the third and fourth month; they are dried in the sun. [Su] Song: They can be found everywhere. In spring they grow a stem similar to that of yellow day lily. The leaves resemble those of safflower. The stem is three to four *chi* tall. In summer it opens a flower similar to trumpet flowers and those of Chinese azalea. They are of an ordinary yellow color. When sheep eat them, they die. Today, they grow everywhere in Ling nan and Shu dao, and they all are of a deep red color similar to embroidered brocade. Still, there are some who state that this kind is not added to medication. [Li] Shizhen: When Han Baosheng says that [its leaves] resemble the leaves of peach trees, he is entirely right. Each flower has five anthers. The anther holding filaments and the petals are all yellow. Qi and flavor are all malign. Those said by Su Song to be of a deep red color, they are Chinese azalea, named *hong zhi zhu* 紅躑躅, and they are nonpoisonous. They are of a different group as [the item discussed] here. When Zhang Qi in his *Guang ya* says that *zhi zhu* 躑躅 is also called *jue guang* 决光, he is mistaken. *Jue guang* 决光 is *jue ming* 决明, fetid *cassia* (16-23). According to the Tang era's *Li Shen wen ji*, "in

1248 Instead of *huang* 黄, "yellow," *Zheng lei* ch. 10, *yang zhi zhu* 羊躑躅, quoting Tao Yinju writes *miao* 苗, "seedling."

Luo gu much mountain loquat can be found; its poison can kill humans. Its flowers are bright and beautiful; similar to azalea flowers. Those who gather firewood are familiar with them." They say that they resemble *yang zhi zhu*, but it is not know whether this is really so. But they are probably related.

17-35-01
花 *Hua*

Flower [of azalea].

【氣味】辛，温，有大毒。【權曰】惡諸石及麵，不入湯使。伏丹砂、硇砂、雌黄。畏巵子。

Qi and Flavor. Acrid, warm, very poisonous. [Zhen] Quan: [Ingested together,] it abhors all types of mineral [drugs] and wheat flour; it must not be added to substances prepared as decoction. It suppresses [the effects of] cinnabar, sal ammoniac, and orpiment. It fears *gardenia* seeds.

【主治】賊風在皮膚中淫淫痛，温瘧惡毒，諸痺。本經。邪氣鬼疰蠱毒。別録。

Control. Robber wind[1249] with a pain as if there was something in the skin. Malign poison associated with warmth malaria. All types of blockage. *Ben jing*. Evil qi, demon attachment-illness, *gu* poison.[1250] *Bie lu*.

【發明】【頌曰】古之大方多用躑躅。如胡洽治時行赤散，及治五嗽四滿丸之類，并治風諸酒方皆雜用之。又治百病風濕等，魯王酒中亦用躑躅花。今醫方捋脚湯中多用之。南方治蠱毒下血，有躑躅花散，云甚勝。【時珍曰】此物有大毒，曾有人以其根入酒飲，遂至于斃也。和劑局方治中風癱瘓伏虎丹中亦用之，不多服耳。

Explication. [Su] Song: Ancient complex recipes often use *zhi zhu*. For example, Hu Qia in his "red powder" to cure epidemic [diseases], and also in the "pills for a fourfold fullness" to cure cough, and also in all types of [medicinal] wine recipes to cure wind [intrusion], it was always resorted to. Also, to cure the hundreds of diseases with wind [intrustion] and the presence of moisture, *zhi zhu* flower was used as an ingredient in "King Lu's wine." Today's physicians often use it as an ingredient of the "decoction to stroke the legs." In the South a "*zhi zhu* flower powder" exists

1249 *Zei feng* 賊風, "robber wind," a condition caused by qi that appear in a season they do not belong to. More at BCGM Dict I, 667.

1250 *Gu du* 蠱毒, "*gu*-poison[ing]." (1) A poison emitted by certain worms/snakes with an ability to cause varying pathological changes in a person who has taken it in by means of wine or food. (2) Abdominal fullness, in some cases with blood spitting, and blood in the stool and urine. BCGM Dict I, 192 - 193. See BCGM 42-22.

to cure *gu* poisoning with blood discharge. It is said to be of superior effectiveness. [Li] Shizhen: This item is very poisonous. There have been people who put its root into wine and drank it, resulting in their death. The *He ji ju fang* also recommends it as an ingredient of the "elixir to make a tiger crouch" to cure wind-stroke with paralysis. It is not ingested in large quantities.

【附方】新四。

Added Recipes. Four newly [recorded].

風痰注痛。躑躅花、天南星，並生時同擣作餅，甑上蒸四五遍，以稀葛囊盛之。臨時取焙爲末，蒸餅丸梧子大。每服三丸，温酒下。腰脚骨痛，空心服。手臂痛，食後服。大良。續傳信方。

Influx pain[1251] related to wind [intrusion] and phlegm. Pound *zhi zhu* flowers and Indian turnip as long as they are fresh [to pulp] and prepare a cake. Steam it on a steam pot four or five times and fill it into a pouch made of thin *pueraria* [fibers]. When the time [of an application] is close, take it out [of the pouch], dry it over a fire in a pan, [grind it into] powder and prepare it with a steamed cake to pills the size of *wu* seeds. Each time ingest three pills, to be sent down with warm wine. In the case of leg qi with aching bones, ingest them on an empty stomach. In the case of painful hands and arms, ingest them after a meal. Very good. *Xu chuan xin fang.*

痛風走注。黄躑躅根一把，糯米一盞，黑豆半盞，酒、水各一盌，徐徐服。大吐大泄，一服便能動也。醫學集成。

Wind pain,[1252] always on the move. [Boil] a handful of yellow *zhi zhu* flowers, one cup of glutinous rice, half a cup of black soybeans in one bowl each of wine and water, and ingest this in small amounts. One ingestion will stimulate massive vomiting and massive outflow. *Yi xue ji cheng.*

風濕痺痛，手足身體收攝不遂，肢節疼痛，言語蹇澀。躑躅花酒拌蒸一炊久，晒乾爲末。每以牛乳一合，酒二合，調服五分。聖惠方。

Painful blockage related to wind [intrusion] and the presence of moisture. Hands, feet, the entire body are paralyzed and do not follow one's will, the joints of the extremities ache, and language is impeded. Mix *zhi zhu* flowers with wine and steam this for as long as it takes to cook a meal. Then dry this and [grind it into] powder.

1251 *Zhu tong* 注痛, "influx pain," an illness sign of pain erratically changing its location. BCGM Dict I, 694.

1252 *Tong feng* 痛風, "pain wind," a condition of *bi* 痹, "blockage," with rheumatic pain in the limb joints following an intrusion of evil qi such as wind, cold, moisture, and/or heat. BCGM Dict I, 507.

Each time ingest five *fen* of a mixture with one *ge* of cow milk and two *ge* of wine. *Sheng hui fang.*

風蟲牙痛。躑躅一錢，草烏頭二錢半，爲末，化蠟丸豆大。綿包一丸咬之，追涎。海上仙方。

Toothache related to wind [intrusion] and the presence of worms/bugs. [Grind] one *qian* of *zhi zhu* and two and a half *qian* of *aconitum* [main tuber] into powder, dissolve it in honey and form pills the size of soybeans. Wrap one pill in silk floss and bite on it to stimulate salivation. *Hai shang xian fang.*

【附録】

Appendix

17-35-A01

山躑躅 ***Shan zhi zhu***

***Rhododendron simsii* Planch. Chinese azalea.**

【時珍曰】處處山谷有之。高者四五尺，低者一二尺。春生苗葉，淺緑色。枝少而花繁，一枝數萼，二月始開花如羊躑躅，而蒂如石榴花，有紅者、紫者、五出者、千葉者。小兒食其花，味酸無毒。一名紅躑躅，一名山石榴，一名映山紅，一名杜鵑花。其黄色者，即有毒羊躑躅也。

[Li] Shizhen: It is found everywhere in mountain valleys. Tall ones reach a height of four to five *chi*, short ones a height of one to two *chi*. In spring it grows a seedling and leaves of a pale green color. It has few branches but a profuse growth of flowers. One branch has several calyxes. Beginning with the second month flowers open resembling those of azalea, while its fruit base is similar to that of pomegranate flowers. Some are red, some are purple. Some have five petals, some have a thousand leaves. Children eat its flowers. They are sour and nonpoisonous. Other names are "red *zhi zhu*," "mountain *zhi zhu*," "shining mountain red," and "cuckoo flower." Those of yellow color are poisonous azalea.

17-35-A02

羊不喫草拾遺 ***Yang bu chi cao***, FE *Shi yi.*

Unidentified.[1253]

【藏器曰】生蜀川山谷，葉細長，在諸草中羊不喫者是也。味苦、辛，温，無毒。主一切風血，補益，攻諸病。煮之，亦浸酒服。【時珍曰】此草似羊躑躅而云無毒，蓋别有此也。

1253 *Yang bu chi cao* 羊不喫草, lit.: "the herb that sheep won't eat."

[Chen] Cangqi: It grows in the mountain valleys of Shu chuan. Its leaves are fine and long. Among all the herbs it is the only one sheep won't eat. Flavor bitter, acrid, warm, nonpoisonous. It controls all types of wind [intrusion] and blood [disorder], it supplements and boosts [the qi] and it attacks all types of disease. It is ingested either boiled [as decoction] or soaked in wine. [Li] Shizhen: This herb resembles azalea, but is said to be nonpoisonous. The fact is, it is something different.

17-36
芫花本經下品
***Yuan hua*, FE *Ben jing*, lower rank.**

***Daphne Genkwa* Sieb. et Zucc. Daphne flower.**

【校正】自木部移入此。

Editorial Correction. Moved here from the section "woods."

【釋名】杜芫別録、赤芫吴普、去水本經、毒魚別録、頭痛花綱目、兒草吴普、敗華吴普。根名黄大戟吴普、蜀桑別録。【時珍曰】芫或作杬，其義未詳。去水言其功，毒魚言其性，大戟言其似也。俗人因其氣惡，呼爲頭痛花。山海經云首山其草多芫是也。

Explanation of Names. *Du yuan* 杜芫, *Bie lu. Chi yuan* 赤芫, Wu Pu. *Qu shui* 去水, *Ben jing. Du yu* 毒魚, *Bielu. Tou tong hua* 頭痛花, *Gang mu. Er cao* 兒草, Wu Pu. *Bai hua* 敗華, Wu Pu. The root is named *huang da ji* 黄大戟, Wu Pu. *Shu sang* 蜀桑, *Bie lu.* [Li] Shizhen: *Yuan* 芫 is also written *yuan* 杬; the meaning is unclear. *Qu shui* 去水, "removes water," refers to its [therapeutic] potential. *Du yu* 毒魚, "poisonous fish/to poison fish," refers to its nature. *Da ji* 大戟, "large lance," refers to a similarity in their appearance. Because of its malign qi common people call it *tou tong hua* 頭痛花, "headache flower." The *Shang hai jing* states: "Among the flowers of Mount Shou shan are many *yuan* 芫." This is [the item discussed here].

【集解】【別録曰】芫花生淮源川谷。三月三日采花，陰乾。【普曰】芫根生邯鄲。二月生葉，青色，加厚則黑。華有紫、赤、白者。三月實落盡，葉乃生。三月采花，五月采葉，八月、九月采根，陰乾。【保昇曰】近道處處有之。苗高二三尺，葉似白前及柳葉，根皮黄似桑根。正月、二月花發，紫碧色，葉未生時收采，日乾。葉生花落，即不堪用也。【頌曰】在處有之。宿根舊枝莖紫，長一二尺。根入土深三五寸，白色，似榆根。春生苗葉，小而尖，似楊柳枝葉。二月開紫花，頗似紫荆而作穗，又似藤花而細。今絳州出者花黄，謂之黄芫花。【時珍曰】顧野王玉篇云：杬木出豫章，煎汁藏果及卵不壞。洪邁容齋隨筆云：今饒州處處有之。莖幹不純是木。小人争鬬者，取葉挼擦皮膚，輒作赤腫如被傷以誣人。至和鹽擦卵，則又染其外若赭色也。

Collected Explanations. Bie lu: *Yuan hua* grows in the river valleys of Huai yuan. The flower is collected on the third day of the third month; it is dried in the yin (i. e., shade). [Wu] Pu: The root grows in Han dan. It grows a leaf in the second month. It is of greenish color and turns black when [the leaf] grows thicker. The flower may be purple, red and white. All fruits fall down in the third month, and a new leaf grows. The flower is collected in the third month; the leaf is collected in the fifth month. The root is collected in the eighth and ninth month. They are dried in the yin (i. e., shade). [Han] Baosheng: It is found everywhere nearby. The seedling is two to three *chi* tall. The leaves resemble those of *cynanchum stauntonii* and willow leaves. The root has a yellow skin; it resembles a mulberry tree root. The flower blossoms in the first and second month; it is of purple-jade-bluish color. It is collected and stored before the leaf grows. It is dried in the sun. When the leaves grow the flowers fall down and are no longer suitable for [medicinal] use. [Su] Song: It is found everywhere. The perennial root has old branches from which a purple stem [rises], reaching a height of one or two *chi*. The root enters the soil three to five *cun* deep. It is white, similar to the roots of Siberian elms. In spring it grows a seedling with small, pointed leaves, similar to the leaves on willow branches. A purple flower opens in the second month; it is quite similar to Chinese redbud flowers, but has spikes. It also resembles gamboge flowers, but is finer. Those nowadays coming from Jiang zhou with yellow flowers are called "yellow *yuan hua*." [Li] Shizhen: Gu Yewang in his *Yu pian* states: "*Yuan mu* 杬木 comes from Yu zhang. Fruits and eggs do not decay when processed with the juice obtained by boiling it in water." Hong Mai in his *Rong zhai sui bi* states: "Today it can be found everywhere in Rao zhou. Its leaves and trunk are not pure wood. When someone of lower status has fought in a brawl, he rubs his skin with the leaves. Then his skin swells and turns red and he falsely accuses [his opponent] of having injured him. If you apply it to an egg with salt, its exterior appears brown in color."

【修治】【弘景曰】用當微熬。不可近眼。【時珍曰】芫花留數年陳久者良，用時以好醋煮十數沸，去醋，以水浸一宿，晒乾用，則毒滅也。或以醋炒者次之。

Pharmaceutical Preparation. [Tao] Hongjing: For a [therapeutic application] it should be slightly simmered. It must not come into contact with the eyes. [Li] Shizhen: *Yuan hua* that has been stored for quite a long time over several years is good. For an application boil it in good vinegar ten or more times to bubbling, remove the vinegar, soak it in water for one night, dry it in the sun and then make use of it. This way, the poison is eliminated. It may also be fried in vinegar, which is the second best [method of preparation].

【氣味】根同。辛，温，有小毒。【别録曰】苦，微温。【普曰】神農、黄帝、雷公：苦，有毒。扁鵲、岐伯：苦。李當之：有大毒，多服令人洩。【之才曰】决明爲之使。反甘草。

Qi and Flavor. Identical to the root. Acrid, warm, slightly poisonous. *Bie lu*: Bitter, slightly warm. [Wu] Pu: Shen nong, Huang Di, Lei gong: Bitter, poisonous. Bian Que, Qi Bo: Bitter. Li Dangzhi: Very poisonous. Ingested in large amounts it causes outflow. [Xu] Zhicai: Fetid *cassia* [seeds] serve as its guiding substance. [Ingested] together,] it is opposed to *glycyrrhiza* [root].

【主治】欬逆上氣，喉鳴喘，咽腫短氣，蠱毒鬼瘧，疝瘕癰腫，殺蟲魚。本經。消胸中痰水，喜唾，水腫，五水在五臟皮膚及腰痛，下寒毒肉毒。根療疥瘡。可用毒魚。别録。治心腹脹滿，去水氣寒痰，涕唾如膠，通利血脉，治惡瘡風痺濕，一切毒風，四肢攣急，不能行步。甄權。療欬嗽，瘴瘧。大明。治水飲痰澼，脇下痛。時珍。

Control. Cough with rising qi counterflow. Panting with noise in the throat. Throat swelling with shortness of [breath] qi. [It serves to cure] the poison of worms/bugs, demon malaria, elevation-illness with conglomeration-illness,[1254] and obstruction-illness[1255] swelling. It kills worms/bugs and fish. *Ben jing*. It dissolves phlegm and water [accumulation] in the chest, with a tendency to spit, water swelling, the five types of water [accumulation] in the five long-term depots and the skin, as well as lower back pain. It serves to discharge cold poison and meat poison. The root heals *jie*-illness[1256] sores. It can be used to poison fish. *Bie lu*. It serves to cure distension of the central and abdominal region with a feeling of fullness. It removes water qi with cold and phlegm, and a snivel with the consistency of glue. It frees the passage of blood through the vessels. It serves to cure malign sores, blockage related to wind [intrusion] and the presence of moisture, all types of poisonous wind [intrusion], contraction and cramps of the four limbs making it impossible to walk even for a few steps. Zhen Quan. It heals cough and miasmatic malaria.

1254 *Shan jia* 疝瘕, "elevation-illness with conglomeration-illness." A lump-like swelling in the abdomen that alternately collects and then dissolves again. BCGM Dict I, 418.

1255 *Yong* 癰, "obstruction-illness,"refers to an obstruction of vessels or other ducts inside the body. Qi rushing against the obstruction may cause a local swelling and eventually break through the surface to cause an abscess. BCGM Dict I, 641.

1256 *Jie*-illness 疥, vaguely identifiable skin ailment. BCGM Dict I, 249.

Da Ming. It serves to cure water accumulation, phlegm flush[1257] and pain below the flanks. [Li] Shizhen.

【發明】【時珍曰】張仲景治傷寒太陽證，表不解，心下有水氣，乾嘔發熱而欬，或喘或利者，小青龍湯主之。若表已解，有時頭痛出汗，不惡寒，心下有水氣，乾嘔，痛引兩脇，或喘或欬者，十棗湯主之。蓋小青龍治未發散表邪，使水氣自毛竅而出，乃内經所謂開鬼門法也。十棗湯驅逐裏邪，使水氣自大小便而洩，乃内經所謂潔净府、去陳莝法也。夫飲有五，皆由内啜水漿，外受濕氣，鬱蓄而爲留飲。流于肺則爲支飲，令人喘欬寒熱，吐沫背寒。流于肺則爲懸飲，令人欬唾，痛引缺盆兩脇。流于心下則爲伏飲，令人胸滿嘔吐，寒熱眩運。流于腸胃則爲痰飲，令人腹鳴吐水，胸脇支滿，或作泄瀉，忽肥忽瘦。流于經絡則爲溢飲，令人沉重注痛，或作水氣胕腫。芫花、大戟、甘遂之性，逐水洩濕，能直達水飲窠囊隱僻之處。但可徐徐用之，取效甚捷。不可過劑，洩人真元也。陳言三因方以十棗湯藥爲末，用棗肉和丸，以治水氣喘急浮腫之證，蓋善變通者也。楊士瀛直指方云：破癖須用芫花，行水後便養胃可也。【好古曰】水者，肺、腎、脾三經所主，有五臟六腑十二經之部分。上而頭，中而四肢，下而腰脚。外而皮毛，中而肌肉，内而筋骨。脉有尺寸之殊，浮沉之别，不可輕瀉。當知病在何經何臟，方可用之。若誤投之，則害深矣。芫花與甘草相反，而胡洽居士方治痰癖飲癖，以甘遂、大戟、芫花、大黄、甘草同用。蓋欲其大吐以泄濕，相反而相激也。

Explication. [Li] Shizhen: To control harm caused by cold associated with major yang illness signs, when the exterior fails to open and water qi stay below the heart, with dry retching, heat effusion and cough, sometimes with panting, sometimes with free-flow, Zhang Zhongjing [recommends the] "minor greenish dragon decoction."[1258] When the exterior has opened, with occasional headache and sweating, no aversion to cold, and water qi staying below the heart, with dry retching and pain pulling on the two flanks, sometimes associated with panting, sometimes with cough, this is controlled with the "ten Chinese dates decoction."[1259] The fact is, when the evil [qi] have not been dispersed and effused from the exterior yet, the "minor greenish dragon decoction" lets the water qi leave [the body] through the hair pores. This is the method called

1257 *Tan pi* 痰澼, "phlegm flush," a condition identical to *tan pi* 痰癖, "phlegm aggregation-illness." A disease brought forth by stagnant phlegm rheum. BCGM Dict I, 494-495.

1258 The ingredients of *Xiao qing long tang* 小青龍湯, "minor greenish dragon decoction" include *ephedra* herb, *paeonia* root, *asarum heteropoides* herb, dried ginger, *glycyrrhiza* root, *cassia* twig, *schisandra* seed, and *pinellia* tuber

1259 *Shi zao tang* 十棗湯, "ten Chinese dates decoction," with the following ingredients: Chinese dates, wikstroemea flower, kansui root, *da ji*.

in the *Nei jing* "opening of demon gates."[1260] The "ten Chinese dates decoction" lets water qi flow out together with the major (i. e., defecation) or minor (i. e., urination) relief. This is what is called in the *Nei jing* the method "to cleanse the palace,"[1261] and "to remove old straw."[1262] Now, there are five kinds of rheum. All of them result from an intake of water or soup inside, or from the absorption of moisture qi from outside. They are stored pent-up and become stagnant rheums. When they flow into the lung, this is a "propping rheum." It lets one pant or cough with alternating sensations of cold and heat. [Patients] spit foam and feel cold in the back. When they flow into the lung,[1263] this results in a "suspended rheum."[1264] It lets one cough with spitting, with a pain pulling on the "empty basin" (needle insertion hole ST-12). When they flow into the area below the heart, this results in a "hidden rheum." It lets one vomit with a feeling of fullness in the chest, alternating sensations of cold and heat, dizziness and [blood induced brain] movement. When they flow into the intestines and the stomach, this results in "phlegm rheum." It lets one have abdominal sounds and spit water, with a propping fullness in the chest and the flanks, and occasionally with outflow, or a sudden gain of weight or sudden emaciation. When they flow into the conduits and network [vessels], this results in a "spilling rheum." It lets one have a feeling of extreme heaviness and influx pain,[1265] sometimes with a surface swelling caused by water qi. *Yuan hua*, Peking spurge and kansai [root] by their nature drive out water and let moisture flow off. They are able to directly proceed to the location of a hidden pouch of water rheum. When they are used in moderate amounts, their effects show very fast. They must not be overdosed, lest they drain one's original qi. In his *San yin fang*, Chen Yan [recommends to] grind the pharmaceutical drug ingredients of the "ten Chinese dates decoction" into powder, mix it with Chinese date meat and form pills because in cases of surface swelling with hectic panting caused by water qi they will transform [the swelling] and free the flow [of the stagnant water]. Yang Shiying

1260 *Su wen* ch. 14. Paul U. Unschuld and Hermann Tessenow, *Huang Di Nei Jing Su Wen. An Annotated Translation of Huang Di's Inner Classic*, 2 vols. University of California Press, Berkeley and Los Angeles, 2011. Vol. 1, 244.

1261 Ibid. 245.

1262 Ibi. 243.

1263 Instead of *liu yu fei* 流于肺, "flows into the lung," *Jin kui* 2nd ch., *tan yin ke sou bing mai zheng bing zhi* 痰飲欬嗽病脉證并治, "cures for [movements in] the vessels and disease signs of phlegm rheum and cough, discussing *xuan yin* 懸飲, "suspended rheum," writes *shui liu yu xie xia* 水流于脇下, "water flows into the region below the flanks."

1264 *Xuan yin* 懸飲, "suspended rheum," a condition of *yin* 飲, rheum, disease brought forth by rheum flowing into the region below the flanks with cough and vomiting causing pain. BCGM Dict I, 593.

1265 *Zhu tong* 注痛, "influx pain," an illness sign of pain erratically changing its location. BCGM Dict I, 694.

in his *Zhi zhi fang* states: "To break through an aggregation-illness the application of *yuan hua* is a must. After the passage of the water has been stimulated, the stomach should be nourished." [Wang] Haogu: "Water is controlled by the three conduits associated with the lung, the kidneys, and the spleen. It is present in the five long-term depots, the six short-term repositories and the 12 conduits. Above it is in the head. In the middle it is present in the four limbs. Below it is in the lower back and the legs. In the exterior it is in the skin and the hair. In the middle it is in the muscles and the flesh. In the interior it is in the sinews and the bones. The [movement in the] vessels appears at the different [locations of] *chi* and *cun* [at the writs], and with different manifestations at the surface or in the depth. One must not drain them carelessly. It is essential to know in which of the conduits and in which of the long-term depots a disease is situated, and only then [the afore-mentioned substances *yuan hua*, Peking spurge and kansai root] can be used. If they are mistakenly 'tossed' [into a patient], the damage that results is profound." *Yuan hua* and *glycyrrhiza* [root] oppose each other. Still, Hu Qia jushi in a recipe to cure phlegm aggregation-illness and rheum aggregation-illness [recommends to] use kansai [root], Peking spurge [root], *yuan hua* and *glycyrrhiza* [root] together. The fact is, when it is intended to cause massive vomiting to reach an outflow, their mutual opposition is a mutual incentive to being effective.

【正誤】【慎微曰】三國志云：魏初平中，有青牛先生，常服芫花，年百餘歲，常如五六十人。【時珍曰】芫花乃下品毒物，豈堪久服？此方外迂怪之言，不足信也。

Correction of Errors. [Tang] Shenwei states: "During the *chu ping* reign period (190 - 193) of the Wei dynasty, a [Daoist] Mister of the Black Ox regularly ingested *yuan hua*. Even at his age of more than 100 years he always seemed to be like someone aged 50 or 60 years." [Li] Shizhen: *Yuan hua* is a poisonous item of "lower rank." How could it be suitable for a long time ingestion? This recipe is based on weird sayings; they are not based on sufficient evidence to be believed.

【附方】舊五，新一十九。

Added Recipes. Five of old. 19 newly [recorded].

卒得欬嗽。芫花一升，水三升，煮汁一升，以棗十四枚，煮汁乾。日食五枚，必愈。肘後方。

Sudden cough. Boil one *sheng* of *yuan hua* in three *sheng* of water down to one *sheng*. Boil it with 14 Chinese dates until the liquid has dried. Eat five [of these Chinese dates] per day and a cure will definitely by achieved. *Zhou hou fang*.

卒嗽有痰。芫花一兩，炒，水一升，煮四沸，去滓，白糖入半斤。每服棗許。勿食酸鹹物。張文仲備急方。

Sudden cough with phlegm. Boil one *liang* of *yuan hua*, fried, in one *sheng* of water four times to bubbling. Remove the dregs, add half a *jin* of white sugar to them, and each time ingest as much as the size of a Chinese date. [During the treatment] do not eat sour and salty items. Zhang Wenzhong, *Bei ji fang*.

喘嗽失音。暴傷寒冷，喘嗽失音。取芫花連根一虎口，切，暴乾。令病人以薦自裹，舂令灰飛揚，入其七孔中。當眼淚出，口鼻皆辣，待芫根盡乃止。病即愈。古今録驗。

Panting, cough and loss of voice. Sudden damage caused by cold, with panting, cough and loss of voice. Cut a handful of *yuan hua* flowers with their roots to pieces and dry them in the sun. Let the patient wrap himself with a straw mat,[1266] [pound the *yuan hua*] in a mortar so that the dust flies around and enters the [patient's] seven orifices. This will cause tearflow from his eyes, and his mouth and nose will feel a biting as if by pepper. Continue this until the *yuan* [*hua*] root is all used up. This cures the disease. *Gu jin lu yan*.

乾嘔脇痛。傷寒有時頭痛，心下痞滿，痛引兩脇，乾嘔短氣，汗出不惡寒者，表解裏未和也，十棗湯主之。芫花熬、甘遂、大戟各等分，爲散。以大棗十枚，水一升半，煮取八合，去滓納藥。强人服一錢，羸人半錢，平旦服之，當下利病除。如不除，明旦更服。仲景傷寒論。

Dry vomiting with painful flanks. Harm caused by cold with an occasional headache, obstruction-illness[1267] and a feeling of fullness below the heart, with the pain pulling on the two flanks, dry vomiting and shortness of [breath] qi, sweating and no aversion to cold. This is a condition where internal harmony is not achieved yet after an exterior [issue] has been resolved. It is controlled by the "ten Chinese dates decoction."[1268] [Grind] equal amounts of *yuan hua*, simmered, kansai [root] and Peking spurge [root] into powder. Boil, together with ten Chinese dates, one and a half *sheng* of water down to eight *ge*. Remove the dregs and enter the pharmaceutical substances. A strong person ingests one *qian*, a lean person half a *qian*. To be ingested during the day. This will cause a free-flow discharge, and the disease is

1266 *Yi jian zi guo* 以薦自裹 is an abbreviated version of *yi jian zi ying jiu li* 以薦自縈就裹, "wrap himself with a straw mat," a phrase found in *Wai tai* ch. 9, *ke shi sheng fang* 欬失聲方, "recipes for cough with loss of voice, quoting the *Gu jin lu yan*.

1267 *Yong* 癰, "obstruction-illness,"refers to an obstruction of vessels or other ducts inside the body. Qi rushing against the obstruction may cause a local swelling and eventually break through the surface to cause an abscess. BCGM Dict I, 641.

1268 *Shi zao tang* 十棗湯, "ten Chinese dates decoction," with the following ingredients: Chinese dates, *wikstroemea* flower, kansai root, *da ji*. Here without the *wikstroemea* flowers.

eliminated. If this is not the case, ingest [the same medication] the next day again. [Zhang] Zhongjing, *Shang han lun*.

水腫支飲及癖飲。用十棗湯加大黃、甘草，五物各一兩，大棗十枚同煮，如法服。一方加芒硝一兩。胡洽百病方。

Water swelling, propping rheum and aggregation-illness with rheum. Boil one *liang* each of the following five items: [the three ingredients of] the "ten Chinese dates decoction"], expanded by rhubarb [root] and *glycyrrhiza* [root], together with ten Chinese dates in water and ingest this as usual. Another recipe [recommends to] add one *liang* of mirabilite. Hu Qia, *Bai bing fang*.

天行煩亂。凝雪湯：治天行毒病七八日，熱積胸中，煩亂欲死。用芫花一斤，水三升，煮取一升半，漬故布薄胸上。不過再三薄，熱則除。當温四肢，護厥逆也。千金方。

Epidemic, vexing disorder. The "coagulated snow decoction." It serves to cure an epidemic poison disease lasting seven or eight days, with a heat accumulation in the chest and a vexing disorder bringing one close to dying. Boil one *jin* of *yuan hua* in three *sheng* of water down to one and a half *jin*. Soak on old piece of cloth [in the liquid] and apply it on the chest. The heat will have vanished after no more than two or three such applications. The four limbs must kept warm to prevent a ceasing [yang qi] counterflow. *Qian jin fang*.

久瘧結癖在腹脇，堅痛者。芫花炒二兩，朱砂五錢，爲末，蜜丸梧子大。每服十丸，棗湯下。直指方。

In the case of a long-lasting malaria with a bound [qi] aggregation-illness in the abdomen and the flanks, and a painful hardening, [grind] two *liang* of *yuan hua* and five *qian* of cinnabar into powder and form with honey pills the size of *wu* seeds. Each time ingest ten pills, to be sent down with a Chinese dates decoction. *Zhi zhi fang*.

水蠱脹滿。芫花、枳殼等分，以醋煮芫花至爛，乃下枳殼煮爛，搗丸梧子大。每服三十丸，白湯下。普濟方。

Water *gu* with distension[1269] and a feeling of fullness. Prepare equal amounts of *yuan hua* and unripe oranges. In vinegar boil the *yuan hua* until it has become a pulpy mass. Then add the unripe oranges and boil them until they have become a pulpy mass. Pound it to prepare pills the size of *wu* seeds. Each time ingest 30 pills, to be sent down with clear, boiled water. *Pu ji fang*.

1269 *Shui gu fu da* 水蠱腹大, "massive abdominal water *gu* distension," identical to *gu zhang* 鼓脹, "drum[-like] distension." A condition of an abdominal distension and big upswell brought forth by stagnant water qi accumulating in the abdomen. BCGM Dict I, 196, 469.

酒疸尿黄。發黄，心懊痛，足脛滿。芫花、椒目等分，燒末。水服半錢，日二服。肘後方。

Dan-illness caused by wine,[1270] with yellow urine. Heart annoyance with pain and a feeling of fullness in the feet and shinbones. Burn equal amounts of *yuan hua* and Chinese pepper to obtain a powder and ingest with water half a *qian*. To be ingested twice a day. *Zhou hou fang*.

背腿間痛。一點痛，不可忍者。芫花根末，米醋調傅之。如不住，以帛束之。婦人産後有此，尤宜。袖珍方。

Painful region from the back to the thighs. An unbearable pain at one point. Mix *yuan hua* root powder with rice vinegar and apply this [to the affected region]. If [the pain] fails to end, fasten [the medication] with a piece of cloth. When a woman has this following delivery, it is especially suitable. *Xiu zhen fang*.

諸般氣痛。芫花醋煮半兩，玄胡索炒一兩半，爲末。每服一錢。男子元臟痛，葱酒下。瘧疾，烏梅湯下。婦人血氣痛，當歸酒下。諸氣痛，香附湯下。小腸氣痛，茴香湯下。仁存方。

All types of painful qi [disorder]. [Grind] half a *liang* of *yuan hua*, boiled in wine, and one and a half *liang* of *corydalis* [tuber] into powder. Each time ingest one *qian*. When males have a painful [external] original long-term depot (i. e., the testicles), they send it down with onion wine.[1271] In the case of a malaria illness, send it down with a smoked plum decoction. Women with a painful blood or qi [disorder] send it down with a Chinese *angelica* [root] wine. For all types of painful qi [disorder] send it down with a nutgrass [root] decoction. In the case of painful qi [disorder] in the small intestine, send it down with a fennel decoction. *Rencun fang*.

鬼胎癥瘕，經候不通。芫花根三兩剉，炒黄爲末。每服一錢，桃仁煎湯調下。當利惡物而愈。聖惠方。

Demon fetus,[1272] that is a concretion-illness and/or conglomeration-illness, with blocked menstruation. File three *liang* of *yuan hua* roots to pieces, fry them until they have turned yellow, and [grind them into] powder. Each time [let the woman] ingest one *qian*, to be sent down mixed with a peach kernel decoction. *Sheng hui fang*.

1270 *Jiu dan* 酒疸, "*dan*-illness [caused by] wine." A condition of *huang dan* 黄疸, "yellow *dan*-illness," resulting from an excessive consumption of wine/alcoholic beverages. BCGM Dict I, 271.

1271 *Cong jiu* 葱酒, an alcoholic beverage made from husked rice, ginger and spring onions.

1272 *Gui tai* 鬼胎, "demon fetus," a condition of *zheng jia* 癥瘕, "concretion-illness and conglomeration-illness," assuming an appearance of pregnancy, with blocked menses and abdominal distension. BCGM Dict I

催生去胎。芫花根剥皮，以綿裹，點麝香，套入陰穴三寸，即下。攝生妙用方。

To speed up birth and remove a [dead] fetus. Cut the skin from a *yuan hua* root, wrap it in silk fabric, dip it in musk and insert it three *cun* deep into [the woman's] yin opening (i. e., vagina). This serves to discharge [the baby/fetus]. *She sheng miao yong fang.*

產後惡物不下。芫花、當歸等分，炒，爲末。調一錢服。保命集。

When following delivery the malign items (i. e., lochia) are not discharged. Fry equal amounts of *yuan hua* and Chinese *angelica* [root] and [grind them into] powder, to be ingested in a dose of one *qian* mixed [with water]. *Bao ming ji.*

心痛有蟲。芫花一兩醋炒，雄黃一錢，爲末。每服一字，溫醋湯下。乾坤生意。

Heart/stomach pain related to the presence of worms/bugs. [Grind] one liang of *yuan hua*, fried in vinegar, and one *qian* of realgar into powder. Each time ingest one *zi*, to be sent down with a warm vinegar decoction. *Qian kun sheng yi.*

牙痛難忍。諸藥不效。芫花末擦之，令熱痛定，以溫水漱之。永類方。

Toothache hard to bear. When all types of medication have remained without an effect. Rub [the teeth] with *yuan hua* powder until they are hot. This will settle the pain. Rinse [the teeth] with warm water. *Yong lei fang.*

白禿頭瘡。芫花末，猪脂和傅之。集效方。

White baldness sores on a head. Mix *yuan hua* powder with lard and apply this [to the affected region]. *Ji xiao fang.*

癰腫初起。芫花末，和膠塗之。千金方。

Obstruction-illness[1273] swelling that has just begun to rise. Mix *yuan hua* powder with glue and apply it [to the affected region]. *Qian jin fang.*

癰癤已潰。芫花根皮搓作撚，插入，則不生合，令膿易竭也。集簡方。

Obstruction-illness pimples that have begun to fester. Roll the skin of a *yuan hua root* to a stick and insert it into [the open pimple]. This way a closing growth is prevented and all the pus flows out easily. *Ji jian fang.*

1273 *Yong* 癰, "obstruction-illness,"refers to an obstruction of vessels or other ducts inside the body. Qi rushing against the obstruction may cause a local swelling and eventually break through the surface to cause an abscess. BCGM Dict I, 641.

痔瘡乳核。芫根一握，洗净，入木臼搗爛，入少水絞汁，於石器中慢火煎成膏。將絲線於膏内度過，以線繫痔，當微痛。候痔乾落，以紙撚蘸膏納竅内，去根，當永除根也。一方，只搗汁浸線一夜用，不得使水。經驗方。

Piles with teat-like kernels. Wash one handful of *yuan* [*hua*] roots clean and pound them in a wooden mortar to a pulpy mass. Add a little water and squeeze it to obtain a juice. Boil this in a stone vessel over a slow fire to generate a paste. Pull a silk thread several times through the paste and use it to tie off the piles. This will cause some pain. Wait until the piles have dried and fall off. Then dip a paper stick into the paste and insert it into the opening to remove the root [of the piles]. This serves to eliminate the root forever. Another recipe. Simply pound [the roots], soak the silk [thread] in the resulting juice for one night, and then apply it. This does not require water. *Jing yan fang*.

瘰癧初起。氣壯人用芫根擂水一盞服，大吐利，即平。黄州陳大用所傳。瀕湖集簡方。

Scrofula pervasion-illness[1274] that has just begun to rise. Persons with robust qi ingest one cup of water in which a *yuan* [*hua*] root was ground. This results in massive vomiting and free-flow, flattening [the swelling]. [A recipe] handed over by Chen Dayong of Huang zhou. *Binhu ji jian fang*.

便毒初起。芫根擂水服，以渣傅之，得下即消。黄州熊珍所傳。瀕湖集簡方。

Poison in the [region of urination/defecation] relief that has just begun to rise. Grind *yuan* [*hua*] root in water and ingest [the resulting juice]. Apply the dregs [to the affected region]. With a discharge [the poison] is dissolved. [A recipe] handed over by Xiong Zhen of Huang zhou. *Binhu ji jian fang*.

贅瘤焦法。甘草煎膏，筆粧瘤之四圍，上三次。乃用芫花、大戟、甘遂等分，爲末，醋調。别以筆粧其中，勿近甘草。次日縮小，又以甘草膏粧小暈三次如前，仍上此藥，自然焦縮。危氏得效方。

The method to scorch a redundancy tumor. Fry *glycyrrhiza* [root] to generate a paste. Apply [this paste] with a brush on all four sides of the tumor. Do this three times. Then [grind] equal amounts of *yuan hua*, Peking spurge and kansai [root] into powder, mix it with vinegar and apply it with a brush to the center [of the tumor]. It must not touch the *glycyrrhiza* [root paste surrounding it]. The next day [the tumor] will have shrunk. Again apply the *glycyrrhiza* [root] paste as a thin layer [around the

1274 *Luo li* 瘰癧, "scrofula pervasion-illness," when two or more connected swellings of the size of plum or date kernels appear either on the neck or in the armpits, or somewhere else on the body. BCGM Dict I. 329.

tumor], three times as before. And then apply the medicinal [powder to the center] once more. [The tumor] will be scorched and shrinks. *Wei shi de xiao fang.*

一切菌毒。因蛇蟲毒氣，熏蒸所致。用芫花生研，新汲水服一錢，以利爲度。危氏得效方。

All types of fungi poison. The poison qi of snakes and worms/bugs that have been transmitted [to a patient] via steam fumes. Grind fresh *yuan hua* and ingest with newly drawn water one *qian* until a free-flow is reached.

17-37
蕘花音饒本經下品

***Rao hua*, 蕘** read *rao* 饒. FE *Ben jing*, lower rank.

***Wikstroemia canescens* (Wall.) Meissn.**

【釋名】【時珍曰】蕘者，饒也。其花繁饒也。

Explanation of Names. [Li] Shizhen: *Rao* 蕘 is 饒, "plentiful." Its flowers are "numerous," "plentiful," *fan rao* 繁饒也.

【集解】【時珍曰】蕘花生咸陽川谷及河南中牟。六月采花，陰乾。【弘景曰】中牟者，時從河上來，形似芫花而極細，白色。【恭曰】苗似胡荽，莖無刺。花細，黄色，四月、五月收，與芫花全不相似也。【保昇曰】所在有之，以雍州者爲好。生岡原上，苗高二尺許。【宗奭曰】今京洛間甚多。【時珍曰】按蘇頌圖經言：絳州所出芫花黄色，謂之黄芫花。其圖小株，花成簇生，恐即此蕘花也。生時色黄，乾則如白，故陶氏言細白也。或言無蕘花，以桃花代之，取其利耳。

Collected Explanations. [Li] Shizhen: *Rao hua* grows in river valleys of Xian yang and in Zhong mu in Hen nan. The flowers are collected in the sixth month. They are dried in the yin (i. e., shade). [Tao] Hongjing: Specimens [said to be] from Hong mu often arrive there by river transport. Their physical appearance is similar to that of daphne flowers, but they are extremely fine and of white color. [Su] Gong: The seedling resembles that of coriander; the stem has no thorns. The flowers are fine and yellow. They are gathered in the fourth and fifth month, and they are not at all similar to daphne flowers. [Han] Baosheng: [*Rao hua*] can be found everywhere. Specimens from Yong zhou are considered to be good. It grows on hills and on the plains; the seedling is about two *chi* tall. [Kou] Zongshi: Today much of it can be found in the Jing luo region. [Li] Shizhen: According to Su Song's *Tu jing*, "daphne flowers coming from Jiang zhou are yellow; they are called 'yellow daphne flowers'." The illustration [in the *Tu jing*] shows a small plant with flowers growing as clusters. I wonder if that is *rao hua*. As long as [the flowers are] fresh, they are yellow; when they are dried they are white. Hence Mr. Tao [Hongjing] says "fine and white." Some say that when *rao hua* is not at hand, it is substituted with peach flowers, resorting to the latter's ability to free [a stagnating flow].

【氣味】苦，寒，有毒。【别録曰】辛，微寒，有毒。

Qi and Flavor. Bitter, cold, poisonous. *Bie lu*: Acrid, slightly cold, poisonous.

【主治】傷寒温瘧，下十二水，破積聚大堅癥瘕，蕩滌腸中留癖、飲食、寒熱邪氣，利水道。本經。療痰飲欬嗽。别録。治欬逆上氣，喉中腫滿，疰氣蠱毒，痃癖氣塊。甄權。

Control. Harm caused by cold and warmth malaria. It serves to discharge the twelve kinds of water [retention], breaks through accumulations and collections, massive hardenings, concretion-illness and conglomeration-illness.[1275] It cleanses the intestines of stagnating conglomeration-illness, beverages and food, and evil qi with alternating sensations of cold and heat. It frees the passage through the water pathways. *Ben jing*. It heals phlegm rheum with cough. *Bie lu*. It serves to cure cough with rising qi, a swelling in the throat with a feeling of fullness, attachment-illness qi,[1276] *gu* poisoning,[1277] string-illness[1278] and aggregation-illness with qi lumps. Zhen Quan.

【發明】【宗奭曰】張仲景傷寒論以蕘花治利者，取其行水也。水去則利止，其意如此。今用之當斟酌，不可過使與不及也，須有是證乃用之。【好古曰】仲景小青龍湯云：若微利，去麻黄，加蕘花如雞子大，熬令赤色。用之蓋利水也。【時珍曰】蕘花蓋亦芫花之類，氣味主治大略相近。

Explication. [Kou] Zongshi: When Zhang Zhongjing in his *Shang han lun* resorts to *rao hua* to cure free-flow, he uses its ability to stimulate the movement of water.

1275 *Zheng jia* 癥瘕, "concretion-illness and conglomeration-illness." The two terms are often used interchangeably and do not signify two distinctly different conditions. Concretion-illness and conglomeration-illness result from a disharmony of cold and warmth resulting in a failure to transform beverages and food. Nodes form when the clash with the qi of the long-term depots. BCGM Dict I, 677.

1276 *Zhu qi* 疰氣, "attachment-illness qi," 1.) a condition identical to *gui zhu* 鬼疰, "demon attachment-illness." 2.) An etiological agent of turbid qi issued by demonic beings or encountered on burial grounds and in mountain forests that is capable of bringing forth demon attachment-illness. BCGM Dict I, 693.

1277 *Gu du* 蠱毒, "*gu*-poison[ing]." (1) A poison emitted by certain worms/snakes with an ability to cause varying pathological changes in a person who has taken it in by means of wine or food. (2) Abdominal fullness, in some cases with blood spitting, and blood in the stool and urine. BCGM Dict I, 192 - 193. See BCGM 42-22.

1278 *Xuan* 痃, "string-illness," a condition of acute pain located in the abdomen to the left and right of the umbilicus. BCGM Dict I, 591.

When the water is eliminated, the free-flow ends. That is the meaning underlying its usage. Today's usage should be based on careful deliberations; it must not be applied in too large or too small amounts. [Wang] Haogu: [Zhang] Zongjing in the context of his "minor greenish dragon decoction"[1279] states: "If it is a case of minor free-flow, omit the *ephedra* [herb], and add a lump of *rao hua* the size of a chicken egg. Simmer it until it has turned red." The fact is, its application will free the flow of water." [Li] Shizhen: The fact is, *rao hua* belongs to a group with daphne. Their qi, flavor and therapeutic control are quite similar.

17-38
醉魚草綱目
Cui yu cao, FE *Gang mu.*

Buddleya lindleyana Fort. Dr. Lindley's *buddleya*.

【釋名】鬧魚花綱目、魚尾草綱目、槐木。

Explanation of Names. *Nao yu hua* 鬧魚花, "noisy fish flower," *Gang mu. Yu wei cao* 魚尾草, "fish tail herb," *Gang mu. Lu mu* 槐木, "pulley wood."

【集解】【時珍曰】醉魚草南方處處有之。多在塹岸邊，作小株生，高者三四尺。根狀如枸杞。莖似黃荆，有微稜，外有薄黃皮。枝易繁衍，葉似水楊，對節而生，經冬不凋。七八月開花成穗，紅紫色，儼如芫花一樣。結細子。漁人采花及葉以毒魚，盡圉圉而死，呼爲醉魚兒草。池沼邊不可種之。此花色狀氣味並如芫花，毒魚亦同，但花開不同時爲異爾。按中山經云：熊耳山有草焉，其狀如蘇而赤華，名曰葶薴，可以毒魚。其此草之類與？

Collected Explanations. [Li] Shizhen: *Cui yu cao* is present everywhere in the South. It is often found at the side of moats and at river banks. It grows as a small trunk, with tall ones reaching a height of three to four *chi*. The root is shaped like that of *lyceum* herbs. The stem resembles that of *vitex* herbs. It has slight edges, and on the outside a thin, yellow skin. The branches easily multiply. The leaves resemble those of water willows. They grow facing each other at the nodes. Throughout winter they do not wither. Flowers forming spikes open in the seventh and eighth month. They are red-purple in color, very much like daphne flowers. They form fine seeds. Fishermen collect the flowers and the leaves to poison fish. The entire [fish pond] enclosure is filled with dead [fish. Hence this herb] is called "herb to intoxicate fish." It cannot be planted near ponds. The flower, color, shape, qi and flavor, they all

1279 The ingredients of *Xiao qing long tang* 小青龍湯, "minor greenish dragon decoction" include *ephedra* herb, *paeonia* root, *asarum heteropoides* herb, dried ginger, *glycyrrhiza* root, *cassia* twig, *schisandra* seed, and *pinellia* tuber

are similar to those of daphne flowers, and their ability to poison fish is the same, too. The only difference is that the times when they open flowers are not the same. According to the *Zhong shan jing*, "On Mount Xiong er shan is an herb shaped like *perilla* herbs but with red flowers. It is called *ting ning* 葶苧 and serves to poison fish." Maybe it is related to the herb discussed here?

17-38-01

花、葉 *Hua, Ye*

【氣味】辛、苦，温，有小毒。

Qi and Flavor. Acrid, bitter, warm, slightly poisonous.

【主治】痰飲成齁，遇寒便發，取花研末，和米粉作粿，炙熟食之，即效。又治誤食石斑魚子中毒，吐不止，及諸魚骨鯁者，搗汁，和冷水少許嚥之，吐即止，骨即化也。久瘧成癖者，以花填鯽魚腹中，濕紙裹煨熟，空心食之，仍以花和海粉搗貼，便消。時珍。

Control. Roaring [panting] caused by phlegm rheum, with an aggravation-illness when it meets cold. Grind *zui yu cao* into powder, mix it with rice flour and form rice cakes. Roast them until done and eat them. This is effective. It also serves to cure persons who are poisoned and vomit without end because they mistakenly have eaten bass roe, and all cases of choking on a bone. Pound [the herb] to obtain a juice, mix it with cold water and [let the patient] sip it in small amounts. This ends the vomiting and dissolves a bone [stuck in the throat]. In the case of an aggregation-illness generated in the course of malaria, stuff the flowers into the abdomen of a golden carp, wrap [the fish] in moist paper, simmer it until done and eat it on an empty stomach. Also, mix the flowers with clam shell powder [1280] and apply this [to the affected region].

17-39

莽草本經下品

Mang cao, FE *Ben jing*, lower rank.

***Illiceum lanceolatum* A. C. Smith.**

【校正】自木部移入此。

Editorial Correction. Moved here from the section "trees."

【釋名】𦵗草音罔、芒草山海經、鼠莽。【弘景曰】莽本作𦵗字，俗訛呼爾。【時珍曰】此物有毒，食之令人迷罔，故名。山人以毒鼠，謂之鼠莽。

1280 For *hai fen* 海粉, clam shell powder, see BCGM 46-10-02.

Explanation of Names. *Wang cao* 菵草, [菵] read *wang* 罔, *mang cao* 芒草, *Shan hai jing*. *Shu mang* 鼠莽, "mouse/rat grass." [Tao] Hongjing: The character *mang* 莽 originally was written *wang* 菵, but it is commonly misread [*mang* 莽]. [Li] Shizhen: This item is poisonous. Those who eat it will be confused, *mi wang* 迷罔. Hence the name. The mountain people use it to poison mice/rats. They call it *shu mang* 鼠莽, "mouse/rat grass."

【正誤】【別録曰】一名葞，一名春草。【禹錫曰】按爾雅云：葞，春草。孫炎注云：藥草也，俗呼爲菵草。郭璞注云：一名芒草。所見異也。【時珍曰】葞，音尾，白薇也。薇、葞字音相近爾。别録白薇下云：一名春草。而此又以爲菵草，蓋因孫炎之誤也。今正之。

Correction of Errors. *Bie lu*: Alternative names *mi* 葞 and *chun cao* 春草, "spring herb." [Zhang] Yuxi: According to the *Er ya*, "Mi 葞 is *chun cao* 春草." Sun Yan in a comment states: "This is a pharmaceutical herb. It is commonly called *wang cao* 菵草." Guo Pu in his comment states: "Alternative name: *mang cao* 芒草." Apparently, this is a different [item]. [Li] Shizhen: 葞 is read *wei* 尾; it is *bai wei* 白薇, *cynanchum atratum*. The reading of the characters 薇 and 葞 is quite similar. The entry *bai wei* 白薇 in the *Bie lu* says: "Alternative name *chun cao* 春草." This, in turn, is considered to be *wang cao* 菵草. The fact is, this is based on the erroneous statement by Sun Yan. It is corrected here.

【集解】【別録曰】莽草生上谷山谷及冤句。五月采葉，陰乾。【弘景曰】今東間處處皆有，葉青辛烈者良。人用搗以和陳粟米粉，納水中，魚吞即死浮出，人取食之無妨。【頌曰】今南中州郡及蜀川皆有之。木若石南而葉稀，無花實。五月、七月采葉，陰乾。一説藤生，繞木石間。既謂之草，乃蔓生者是也。【宗奭曰】莽草諸家皆謂之草，而本草居木部。今世所用，皆木葉如石南葉，枝梗乾則皺，揉之其臭如椒。【斅曰】凡用葉，勿用尖及攣生者。【時珍曰】范子計然云：莽草出三輔，青色者善。

Collected Explanations. *Bie lu*: *Mang cao* grows in the mountain valleys of Shang gu and in Yuan ju. The leaves are collected in the fifth month; they are dried in the yin (i. e., shade). [Tao] Hongjing: Today it is present everywhere in the East. Greenish leaves with a violent, acrid [flavor] are good. People pound it, mix it with long-stored millet flour and give it into waters. The fish swallow it and come dead to the surface. Humans can eat them without problem. [Su] Song: Today it can be found everywhere in the *zhou* and prefectures in the South and also in Shu chuan. The tree is similar to that of *plotinia*, but it has fewer leaves, and no flowers or fruits. The leaves are collected in the fifth and seventh month; they are dried in the yin (i. e., shade). It is also said that "it grows as a vine, winding around trees and rocks." But it is called "herb," *cao* 草, hence it is a creeper. [Kou] Zongshi: All the experts call *mang cao* 莽草 an "herb," but the *Ben cao* lists it in the section *mu* 木, "woods/trees." [The items] used today are tree leaves similar to *plotinia* leaves. When the branches are dry and have hardened, they are wrinkled, and when they are rubbed they release a bad smell similar to Chinese pepper. [Lei] Xiao: For all [medicinal] applications of the leaves, do not use those that are pointed and rolled up. [Li] Shizhen: The *Fan zi Jiran* states: "*Mang cao* comes from San fu. Specimens that are greenish in color are good."

17-39-01
葉 *Ye*
Leaf [of *mang cao*].

【修治】【斅曰】凡使，取葉細剉，以生甘草、水蓼二味，同盛入生稀絹袋中，甑中蒸一日，去二件，曬乾用。

Pharmaceutical Preparation. [Lei] Xiao: For all [medicinal] applications, cut the leaves to fine pieces, fill them together with fresh *glycyrrhiza* [root] and water pepper into a pouch made of thin, tough silk and steam it in a steaming pot for one day. Then remove both items [from the pouch], dry [the *mang cao*] in the sun and use it [for medicinal purposes].

【氣味】辛，温，有毒。【普曰】神農：辛。雷公、桐君：苦，有毒。【時珍曰】莽草制雌黄、雄黄而有毒，誤食害人。惟紫河車磨水服，及黑豆煮汁服，可解。豆汁澆其根即爛，性相制也。

Qi and Flavor. Acrid, warm, poisonous. [Wu] Pu: Shen nong: Acrid. Lei gong: Bitter, poisonous. [Li] Shizhen: *Mang cao* controls [the effects of] orpiment and realgar, but is poisonous itself. If eaten by mistake it is harmful. [Such poison] can be resolved only by ingesting water in which love apple [leaves] have been rubbed, and also by ingesting a black soybean decoction. When soybean juice is poured on a [*mang cao*] root, it rots. Their natures check each other.

【主治】風頭，癰腫乳癰，疝瘕，除結氣疥瘙。殺蟲魚。本經。療喉痺不通，乳難。頭風癢，可用沐，勿令入眼。别録。治風疽，疝氣，腫墜凝血，治瘰癧，除濕風，不入湯服。主頭瘡白秃殺蟲。與白歛、赤小豆爲末，雞子白調如糊，熁毒腫，乾更易上。甄權。治皮膚麻痺，煎濃湯淋。風蟲牙痛。大明。

Control. Wind head.[1281] Swelling related to obstruction-illness,[1282] breast obstruction-illness.[1283] Elevation-illness with conglomeration-illness.[1284] *Jie*-illness with itch. It kills worms/bugs and fish. *Ben jing*. Complete throat blockage. Difficulties to let nursing milk. Head wind with itch. It can be used to wash [the affected region], but must not enter the eyes. *Bie lu*. It serves to cure wind [intrusion] and impediment-illness,[1285] elevation-illness[1286] qi, dropped, swollen [testicles] and coagulated blood. It serves to cure scrofula pervasion-illness,[1287] and removes moisture and wind. It is not given into hot water/decoctions to be ingested. It controls sores on the head associated with white baldness, and kills worms/bugs. [Grind] it together with *ampelopsis* [root] and red mung beans into powder, mix it with egg white to form a paste and apply this to the poison swelling to let it melt. When [the paste] has dried, replace it [with a moist paste]. Zhen Quan. To cure numbness of the skin boil it to a thick decoction and pour it [on the affected region]. [It serves to cure] toothache associated with wind [intrusion] and worms/bugs. Da Ming.

【發明】【頌曰】古方治風毒痺厥諸酒，皆用菵草。今醫家取葉煎湯，熱含少頃吐之，治牙齒風蟲及喉痺甚效。【宗奭曰】濃煎湯，淋渫皮膚麻痺。周禮翦氏掌除蠹物，以莾草熏之則死。【時珍曰】古方治小兒傷寒，有莾草湯。又瑣碎録云：思村王氏之子，生七日而兩腎縮入。一醫云：此受寒氣而然也。以硫黄、茱萸、大蒜研塗其腹，以菵草、蛇牀子燒烟，熏其下部而愈也。

Explication. [Su] Song: For all [medicinal] wines [recommended in] ancient recipes to cure wind poison causing blockage/numbness and ceasing [yang] qi they used

1281 *Feng tou* 風頭, "wind head," a condition wind evil attacking the head followed by pain, or dizziness, or itching. BCGM Dict I, 509.

1282 *Yong* 癰, "obstruction-illness,"refers to an obstruction of vessels or other ducts inside the body. Qi rushing against the obstruction may cause a local swelling and eventually break through the surface to cause an abscess. BCGM Dict I, 641.

1283 *Ru yong* 乳癰, "breast obstruction-illness," a condition of acute putrefication of a woman's breast. Often encountered if a woman, following delivery, experiences *chui nai* 吹奶, "inflated breast," or *du ru* 妒乳, "jealousy breast." BCGM Dict I, 412.

1284 *Shan jia* 疝瘕, "elevation-illness with conglomeration-illness." A lump-like swelling in the abdomen that alternately collects and then dissolves again. BCGM Dict I, 418.

1285 *Ju* 疽, "impediment-illness," refers to an obstruction of vessels or other ducts inside the body. Qi rushing against the impediment may cause a local swelling and eventually break through the surface to cause an abscess. BCGM Dict I, 277.

1286 *Shan* 疝, "elevation-illness," a group of conditions characterized by violent abdominal pain, in some cases associated with constipation and anuria. BCGM Dict I, 417.

1287 *Luo li* 瘰癧, "scrofula pervasion-illness," when two or more connected swellings of the size of plum or date kernels appear either on the neck or in the armpits, or somewhere else on the body. BCGM Dict I. 329.

mang cao. Today's physicians use the leaves to prepare a decoction. [Patients] are to hold it in the mouth for a short while and than to spit it out. This serves to cure teeth affected by wind [intrusion] and worms/bugs, and throat blockage, and is very effective. [Kou] Zongshi: Prepare a thick decoction and pour it on the skin [to cure] numbness. According to the *Zhou li*, Mr. Jian was in charge of repelling moths. He steamed them with *mang cao* and they died. [Li] Shizhen: Ancient recipes included a *mang cao* decoction to cure children with harm caused by cold. Also, the *Suo sui lu* states: "In the village Si, the two testicles of a seven day old child of Mr. Wang were withdrawn [into the abdomen]. A physician said: 'This has happened because they were exposed to cold qi.' Grind sulphur, *evodia* [root][1288] and garlic [to a paste] and apply this to [the child's] abdomen. Burn *wang cao* and *cnidium* [herb] and with the fumes steam its lower body parts. This cures [its disease]."

【附方】舊四，新五。

Added Recipes. Four of old. Five newly [recorded].

賊風腫痺。風入五臟恍惚，宜莽草膏主之。莽草一斤，烏頭、附子、躑躅各二兩，切，以水和醋一升，漬一宿。猪脂一斤，煎三上三下，絞去滓。向火，以手摩病上三百度，應手即瘥。若耳鼻疾，可以綿裹塞之。疥癬雜瘡，並宜摩之。肘後方。

Robber wind[1289] with swelling and blockage/numbness. Absent-mindedness resulting from wind intrusion into the five long-term depots. The "paste with *mang cao*" is suitable to control this. Cut one *jin* of *mang cao* and two *liang* each of *aconitum* [main tuber], *aconitum* [accessory tuber] and azalea to pieces, and soak them in one *sheng* of a mixture of water and vinegar for one night. Then boil this with one *jin* of lard added three times until bubbling, let it cool three times and squeeze it to remove the dregs. [Let the patient] be close to a fire and with your hands rub the location of the disease [with the liquid] 300 times. This results in a cure. In the case of an illness in the ears or the nose, wrap [the medication] in a silk fabric and stuff it into [the affected ear or nose]. For *jie*-illness[1290] and *xuan*-illness[1291] it is suitable to rub [the liquid into the affected regions]. *Zhou hou fang*.

1288 *Zhu yu* 茱萸 is ambiguous. It could also refer to *zanthoxylum* [fruit] and Asiatic cornelian cherry

1289 *Zei feng* 賊風, "robber wind," a condition caused by qi that appear in a season they do not belong to. More at BCGM Dict I, 667.

1290 *Jie*-illness 疥, vaguely identifiable skin ailment. BCGM Dict I, 249.

1291 *Xuan* 癬, "*xuan*-illness." Conditions of dermal lesions with initially erythema, papules, and itching gradually extending in all directions to form an irregular ring with clear boundaries. The skin is slightly elevated with small papules, blisters, and/or scales and

小兒風癎，掣瘲戴眼，極者日數十發，又治大人賊風。莽草、雷丸各一雞子黄大，化猪脂一斤，煎七沸，去滓，摩痛處，勿近目及陰，日凡三四次。外臺秘要。

Wind epilepsy[1292] of children, with clonic convulsions affecting the eyes; in severe cases there are tens of fits each day. It also serves to cure adults affected by robber wind. Dissolve *mang cao* and thunderball fungus, each of an amount the size of egg yolk, in one *jin* of lard by boiling this to bubbling seven times. Then remove the dregs, and rub [the liquid] into the location of the pain. It must not come into contact with the eyes and the yin [(i. e. genital) region]. Three to four times a day. *Wai tai mi yao*.

頭風久痛。莽草煎湯沐之，勿令入目。聖惠方。

Head wind[1293] with long-lasting pain. Boil *mang cao* and wash [the affected region] with the decoction. It must not enter the eyes. *Sheng hui fang*.

風蟲牙痛。肘後方用莽草煎湯，熱漱冷吐。一加山椒皮。一加獨活。一加郁李仁。一加芫花。一加川椒、細辛各等分。煎湯熱漱冷吐。

Toothache related to wind [intrusion] and the presence of worms/bugs. The *Zhou hou fang* [recommends to] boil *mang cao* and to rinse [the teeth] with the hot decoction. When it is cold, spit it out. Another [recipe] adds the skin of mountain pepper. Another [recipe] adds *angelica biserrata* [root]. Another [recipe] adds Chinese dwarf cherry kernels. Another [recipe] adds daphne flowers. Another [recipe] adds equal amounts of Chinese pepper and *asarum heteropoides* [roots]. Boil [the mixtures] and with the hot decoction rinse [the teeth]. When it has cooled, spit it out.

聖惠用莽草半兩，皂角三挺去皮子，漢椒七粒，爲末，棗肉丸芥子大。每以一丸塞孔中，吐涎取效。

The *Sheng hui* [recommends to grind] half a *liang* of *mang cao*, three *gleditsia* pods, with skin and seeds discarded, and seven Chinese pepper grains into powder. Mix it with Chinese date meat and form pills the size of mustard seeds. Each time insert one pill into the hole [in the affected tooth] and spit out the resulting saliva until an effect shows.

---

scraps. The central lesion may appear to heal spontaneously, and it may reappear. Also, a designation of local lesions with itching, release of liquid and shedding of scabs. BCGM Dict I, 591.

1292 *Feng xian* 風癎, "wind epilepsy," a condition of *xian* 癎," epilepsy," resulting from the effects of wind evil. BCGM Dict I, 170

1293 *Tou feng* 頭風, "head wind." Condition of wind evil attacking the head followed by pain, dizziness, itching. BCGM Dict I, 509.

瘰癧結核。莾草一兩爲末，雞子白調塗帛上，貼之。日二易，取效止。聖惠方。

Scrofula pervasion-illness[1294] with nodular kernels. [Grind] one *liang* of *mang cao* into powder, mix it with egg white, smear it on a piece of cloth and apply this [to the affected region] until an effect shows. Then end [the application]. *Sheng hui fang.*

癰瘡未潰。方同上，得痛爲良。肘後方。

An obstruction-illness sore that has not yet started to fester. Recipe identical to the one above. When a pain is felt, this is good. *Zhou hou fang.*

乳腫不消。莽草、小豆等分，爲末，苦酒和，傅之。衛生易簡方。

Breast swelling that fails to dissolve. [Grind] equal amounts of *mang cao* and mung beans into powder, mix it with bitter wine and apply this [to the affected region]. *Wei sheng yi jian fang.*

狗咬昏悶。浸椒水調莽草末，傅之。便民圖纂。

Dizziness and heart-pressure following a dog bite. Mix *mang cao* powder with water in which Chinese pepper was soaked and apply this [to the affected region]. *Bian min tu zuan.*

17-40
茵芋本經下品
Yin yu, FE *Ben jing*, lower rank.

***Skimmia reevesiana* Fort.**

【釋名】莞草別録、卑共別録。【時珍曰】茵芋本作因預，未詳其義。莞草與莆莞名同。

Explanation of Names. *Guan cao* 莞草, *Bie lu*. *Bei gong* 卑共, *Bie lu*. [Li] Shizhen: *Yin yu* 茵芋 originally was written *yin yu* 因預. The meaning is not clear. The name *guan cao* 莞草 is identical to that of *pu guan* 莆莞.

【集解】【別録曰】茵蕷生太山川谷。三月三日采葉，陰乾。【弘景曰】好者出彭城，今近道亦有。莖葉狀似莽草而細軟，連細莖采之。方用甚稀，惟合療風酒。【大明曰】出自海鹽。形似石南，樹生，葉厚，五、六、七月采。【頌曰】今雍州、絳州、華州、杭州亦有之。春生苗，高三四尺，莖赤。葉似石榴而短厚，又似石南葉。四月開細白花，五月結實。二月、四月、七月采莖葉，日乾。

1294 *Luo li* 瘰癧, "scrofula pervasion-illness," when two or more connected swellings of the size of plum or date kernels appear either on the neck or in the armpits, or somewhere else on the body. BCGM Dict I. 329.

Collected Explanations. *Bie lu*: *Yin yu* grows in the river valleys of Mount Tai shan. The leaves are collected on the third day of the third month; they are dried in the yin (i. e., shade). [Tao] Hongjing: Good specimens come from Peng cheng. Today it can also be found everywhere else. The stem and the leaves are shaped similar to *illiceum* [stem and leaves], but they are fine and soft. They are collected together with the fine stem. They are very seldom resorted to in recipes. They only occur in [recipes for medicinal] wines to heal wind [intrusion]. Da Ming: [*Yin yu*] comes from Hai yan. With its physical appearance it resembles *photinia* [plants]. It grows as a tree with thick leaves that are collected in the fifth, sixth and seventh month. [Su] Song: Today it is present in Yong zhou, Jiang zhou, Hua zhou and also in Hang zhou. In spring it grows a seedling reaching a height of three to four *chi*; its stem is red. The leaves resemble those of pomegranade [plants], but they are short and thick. They also resemble the leaves of *photinia* [plants]. In the fourth month [*yin yu*] opens fine, white flowers; in the fifth month they form fruits. Stem and leaves are collected in the second,[1295] fourth, and seventh month. They are dried in the sun.

17-40-01

莖、葉 *Jing, Ye*

Stem, leaf [of *yin yu*].

【氣味】苦，温，有毒。【别録曰】微温，有毒。【權曰】苦辛，有小毒。

Qi and Flavor. Bitter, warm, poisonous. *Bie lu*: Slightly warm, poisonous. [Zhen] Quan: Bitter, acrid, slightly poisonous.

【主治】五臟邪氣，心腹寒熱，羸瘦，如瘧狀，發作有時，諸關節風濕痺痛。本經。療久風濕走四肢，脚弱。别録。治男子女人軟脚毒風，拘急攣痛。甄權。一切冷風，筋骨怯弱羸顫。入藥炙用。大明。

Control. Evil qi affecting the five long-term depots. Alternating sensations of cold and heat in the central and abdominal region with emaciation and occasional outbreaks similar to malaria. Painful blockage related to wind [intrusion] and the presence of moisture in all the joints. *Ben jing*. It heals long-lasting wind and moisture entering the four limbs, with weakness of the legs. *Bie lu*. It serves to cure soft legs of males and females related to poison wind, with painful contraction and cramps. Zhen Quan. All types of cold and wind [intrusion]. Sinews and bones affected by timidity and weakness, with emaciation and shivering. To be added to medicines, it is fried. Da Ming.

1295 Instead of *er* 二, "second [month]," *Zheng lei* ch. 10, *yin yu* 茵芋, quoting the *Tu jing* writes *san* 三, "third."

【發明】【時珍曰】千金、外臺諸古方，治風癇有茵蕷丸，治風痺有茵蕷酒，治婦人産後中風有茵蕷膏，風濕諸方多用之。茵蕷、石南、莽草皆古人治風妙品，而近世罕知，亦醫家疏缺也。

Explication. [Li] Shizhen: All the ancient recipes in the *Qian jin* and the *Wai tai* [recommend to use] the "pills with *yin yu*" to cure wind epilepsy, the "wine with *yin yu*" to cure blockage caused by wind [intrusion], and the "*yin yu* paste/ointment" to cure women struck by wind following delivery. [The ancients] often resorted to [*yin yu*] in all the recipes for wind [intrusion] and the presence of moisture. *Yin yu*, *photinia* [leaves] and *illiceum* [leaves] are wondrous items used by the ancients to cure wind [intrusion], but they are little known today. Even physicians neglect and omit them.

【附方】舊一，新二。

Added Recipes. One of old. Two newly [recorded].

茵蕷酒。治賊風，手足枯痺拘攣。用茵蕷、附子、天雄、烏頭、秦艽、女萎、防風、防已、石南葉、躑躅花、細辛、桂心各一兩，十二味切，以絹袋盛，清酒一斗漬之。冬七、夏三、春秋五日，藥成。每服一合，日二服，以微痺爲度。方出胡洽居士百病方。圖經本草。

The "wine with *yin yu*." It serves to cure robber wind,[1296] with hands and feet dried up, numb and cramped/contracted. Cut to pieces one *liang* each of the following 12 substances: *yin yu*, *aconitum* [accessory tuber], carmichael's monkshood [root], *aconitum* [main tuber], large *gentiana* [root], clematis creeper, *saposhnikovia* [root], *stephania tetandra* [root], *photinia* leaves, azalea flowers, *asarum heteropoides* [root] and shaved cinnamom bark. Fill them into a tough silk pouch and soak it in one *dou* of clear wine, in winter for seven, in summer for three and in spring and autumn for five days, to generate a medication. Each time ingest one *ge*, to be ingested twice a day until a slight numbness develops. This recipe is quoted from Hu Qia jushi's *Bai bing fang*. *Tu jing ben cao*.

茵芋丸。治風氣積滯成脚氣，發則痛者。茵芋葉、炒薏苡仁各半兩，郁李仁一兩，牽牛子三兩，朱砂末半兩。右爲末，煉蜜丸如梧子大。每服二十丸，五更薑棗湯下，取利。未利再服，取快。本事方。

The "pills with *yin yu*." They serve to cure stagnating wind qi accumulation resulting in leg qi,[1297] [a disease] that is painful when it is active. [Prepare] half a *liang* each of

1296 *Zei feng* 賊風, "robber wind," a condition caused by qi that appear in a season they do not belong to. More at BCGM Dict I, 667.

1297 *Jiao qi* 脚氣, "leg qi." Painful, weak, swollen legs. BCGM Dict I, 248.

yin yu leaves and fried Job's tears kernels, one *liang* of Chinese dwarf cherries, three *liang* of *pharbitis* seeds and half a *liang* of cinnabar powder. [Grind] these substances into powder and form with heat refined honey pills the size of *wu* seeds. Each time ingest 20 pills, to be sent down in the early morning hours with a ginger and Chinese dates decoction. This results in a free-flow. If no free-flow follows, ingest [the pills] again. *Ben shi fang.*

產後中風。茵芋五兩，木防己半斤，苦酒九升，漬一宿。猪脂四升，煎三上三下，膏成。每炙，熱摩千遍。千金方。

Struck by wind following delivery. Soak for one night five *liang* of *yin yu* and half a *jin* of queen coralbead [vine] in nine *sheng* of bitter wine. Then boil [the liquid] with four *sheng* of lard three times until bubbling and let it cool three times until a paste has formed. Each time roast [the paste] and rub [the woman] with the hot [paste] a thousand times. *Qian jin fang.*

17-41
石龍芮本經中品

Shi long rui, FE *Ben jing*, middle rank.

***Ranunculus sceleratus* L. Cursed crow foot.**

【校正】併入菜部水堇。

Editorial Correction. *Shui jin* 水堇 from the section "vegetables" is included here.

【釋名】地椹本經、天豆別録、石能別録、魯果能別録、水堇吴普、音謹，又音芹。苦堇爾雅、堇葵郭璞、胡椒菜救荒、彭根別録。【弘景曰】生于石上，其葉芮芮短小，故名。【恭曰】實如桑椹，故名地椹。【禹錫曰】爾雅云：齧，苦堇也。郭璞云：即堇葵也。本草言味甘，而此云苦者，古人語倒，猶甘草謂之大苦也。【時珍曰】芮芮，細皃。其椹之子細芮，故名。地椹以下，皆子名也。水堇以下，皆苗名也。苗作蔬食，味辛而滑，故有椒、葵之名。唐本草菜部“水堇”係重出，今依吴普本草合併爲一。

Explanation of Names. *Di shen* 地椹, *Ben jing*. *Tian dou* 天豆, *Bie lu*. *Shi neng* 石能, *Bie lu*. *Lu guo neng* 魯果能, *Bie lu*. *Shui jin* 水堇, Wu Pu, [with 堇] read *jin* 謹, also read *qin* 芹. *Ku jin* 苦堇, *Er ya*. *Jin kui* 堇葵, Guo Pu. *Hu jiao cai* 胡椒菜, *Jiu huang*. *Peng gen* 彭根, *Bie lu*. [Tao] Hongjing: It grows on rocks, *shi* 石. The leaves are fragile, *rui rui* 芮芮, short and small. Hence the name. [Su] Gong: The fruits are similar to mulberry fruits, *shen* 椹,. Hence the name *di shen* 地椹, "ground mulberry fruits." [Zhang] Yuxi: The *Er ya* states: "*Nie* 齧 is *ku jin* 苦堇." Guo Pu states: "This is *jin kui* 堇葵. The *Ben cao* says: 'Flavor sweet,' but here [in the *Er ya*] it is stated to be bitter. The language of the ancients tended to reverse [the facts]. For example, they said of *glycyrrhiza* [root, the 'sweet herb' (*gan cao* 甘草) root,] that it is 'very bitter'." [Li] Shizhen: *Rui rui* 芮芮 is "fine," *xi* 細. Mulberry fruits, *shen* 椹. are fine and fragile, *xi rui* 細芮. Hence the names. The names [in the list given above] following *di shen* 地椹 are names of the seeds. The names [in the list given above] following *shui jin* 水堇 are names of the seedling. The seedling can be prepared as an edible vegetable with an acrid, smoothing flavor. Hence names such as *jiao* 椒, "pepper," and *kui* 葵, "Chinese mallow." The *Tang ben cao* with its *shu jin* 水堇 entry in the section "vegetables" lists [*shi long rui*] twice. Here now following the *Wu Pu ben cao* both are combined in one entry.

【集解】【别録曰】石龍芮生太山川澤石邊。五月五日采子，二月、八月采皮，陰乾。【弘景曰】今出近道。子形粗，似蛇牀子而扁，非真好者，人言是蓄菜子也。東山石上所生者，其葉芮芮短小，其子狀如葶藶，黄色而味小辛，此乃是真也。【恭曰】今用者，俗名水堇。苗似附子，實如桑椹，生下濕地，五月熟，葉、子皆味辛。山南者粒大如葵子。關中、河北者細如葶藶，氣力劣於山南者。陶以細者爲真，未爲通論。又曰：堇菜野生，非人所種。葉似蕺，花紫色。【藏器曰】爾雅云：芨，堇草。注云：烏頭苗也。蘇恭注天雄亦云：石龍芮葉似堇草，故名水堇。據此，則堇草是烏頭苗，水堇定是石龍芮，更非别草也。【頌曰】今惟出兖州。一叢數莖，莖青紫色，每莖三葉，其葉短小多刻缺，子如葶藶而色黄。蘇恭所説乃水堇，非石龍芮也。兖州所上者，正與本經及陶氏説合，爲得其真。【宗奭曰】石龍芮有兩種：水中生者，葉光而末圓；陸地生者，葉毛而末鋭。入藥須水生者。陸生者又謂之天灸，而補不足，莖冷失精。【時珍曰】蘇恭言水堇即石龍芮，蘇頌非之，非矣。按漢吴普本草石龍芮一名水堇，其説甚明。唐本草菜部所出水堇，言其苗也。本經石龍芮，言其子也。寇宗奭所言陸生者，乃是毛堇，有大毒，不可食。水堇即俗稱胡椒菜者，處處有之，多生近水下濕地。高者尺許，其根如薺。二月生苗，叢生。圓莖分枝，一枝三葉。葉青而光滑，有三尖，多細缺。江淮人三四月采苗，瀹過，晒蒸黑色爲蔬。四五月開細黄花，結小實，大如豆，狀如初生桑椹，青緑色。搓散則子甚細，如葶藶子，即石龍芮也。宜半老時采之。范子計然云：石龍芮出三輔，色黄者善。

Collected Explanations. *Bie lu*: *Shi long rui grows* on the rocks at the side of rivers and marshlands on Mount Tai shan. The seeds are collected on the fifth day of the fifth month. The skin is collected in the second and eighth month. They are dried in the yin (i. e., shade). [Tao] Hongjing: Today it comes from nearby. The seeds have a crude shape, similar to those of *cnidium* [herbs], but they are flat. People say that these are not the real and good specimens; they call them "stored vegetables." Those growing on the rocks of the mountains in the East have fragile, short and small leaves. Their seeds are shaped like those of wood whitlow grass. They are yellow in color, and of a slightly acrid flavor. These are the real [*shi long rui*] specimens. [Su] Gong: That used today is commonly called *shui jin* 水堇. Its seedling resembles that of *aconitum* [accessory tuber]. Its fruits are similar to mulberry fruits. It grows in low-lying marshlands. [The fruits] ripen in the fifth month. The leaves and the seeds are of acrid flavor. Those from Shan nan have kernels the size of Chinese mallow seeds. Those from Guan zhong and He bei have [seeds] as fine as those of wood whitlow grass. The strength of their qi is less than that of specimens from Shan nan. Tao [Hongjing] considers those with fine [seeds] to be real/genuine [*shi long rui*], but this is not accepted in all discourses. It is also said: *Jin cai* 堇菜 is a vegetable growing in the wild; it is not planted by people. The leaves resemble those of shepherd's purse; the flowers are purple in color. [Chen] Cangqi: The *Er ya* states: "*Ji* 芨 is *qin cao* 堇草."[1298] A comment states: "This is the seedling of *aconitum* [main tuber]." Su Gong commenting on carmichael's monkshood [root] states: "The leaves of *shi long rui* resemble those of *qin cao* 堇草; hence the name *shui qin* 水堇." Based on this, *qin cao* 堇草 is the seedling of *aconitum* [main tuber]. *Shui qin* 水堇, for sure, is *shi long rui* 石龍芮. It cannot be another herb. [Su] Song: Today it only comes from Yan zhou. It forms clusters with several stems. The stems are greenish-purple in color. Each stem has three leaves. The leaves are short and small, with many notches. The seeds resemble those of wood whitlow grass, but they are yellow in color. What Su Gong describes is *shui jin* 水堇, not *shi long rui* 石龍芮. Those grown in Yan zhou perfectly agree with the statements made in the *Ben jing* and by Mr. Tao [Hongjing]. They refer to the real [*shi long rui*]. [Kou] Zongshi: There are two kinds of *shi long rui*. Those growing in waters have shiny leaves with round tips. Those growing on land have hair and pointed tips. For medicinal applications those growing in waters are chosen. Those growing on land are also called *tian jiu* 天灸, "heavenly cauterization." They serve to supplement insufficient [qi], in cases of a sensation of cold in the "stalk," (i. e., penis) and uncontrolled loss of essence/sperm. [Li] Shizhen: Su Gong says that *shui jin* 水堇 is *shi long rui* 石龍芮. Su Song denies it. He is wrong. According to the Han era[1299] *Wu Pu ben cao*, an alternative name of *shi long rui* is *shui jin*. This is very clear. The *shui jin* recorded in the section "vegetables" of the *Tang ben cao* is a reference to its seedling. The *shi long rui* in the *Ben jing* is a reference to its seeds. When [Kou] Zongshi speaks of those growing on land, these are "hair *jin* 堇." They are very poisonous, and not edible. The

1298 For an identification of *qin/jin cao* as Chinese elder, *shuo diao* 蒴藋, *sambucus chinensis* Lindl., see 16-41.

1299 Instead of Han 漢 (dynasty), ch. 1 of the *Li dai zhu jia ben cao* 歷代諸家本草, *Wu shi ben cao*, quoting [Han] Baosheng writes: Wei 魏 (dynasty).

shui jin that is commonly called *hu jiao cai* 胡椒菜, "black pepper vegetable," can be found everywhere. Much of it grows near waters in low-lying marshland. Tall ones reach a height of more than a *chi*. The root is similar to that of shepherd's purse. It grows seedlings in the second month; they grow as clusters. The stem is round and separates into branches. Each branch has three leaves. The leaves are greenish, shiny and smooth, with three pointed ends and many fine notches. The people in the Jiang Huai region collect the seedlings in the third and fourth month. Having cleansed/boiled them, they dry them in the sun, steam them until they have turned black and prepare them as vegetables. Fine, yellow flowers open in the fourth and fifth month, forming small fruits the size of soybeans. They are shaped like mulberry fruits that have just grown and are greenish-green in color. When they are rubbed very fine seeds appear similar to seeds of wood whitlow grass. They are the *shi long rui* 石龍芮. It is advisable to collect them when they are half ripe. The *Fan zi ji ran* states: "*Shi long rui* that comes from San fu and is yellow in color is good."

17-41-01
子 *Zi*

Seeds [of *shi long rui*].

根皮同。

Root and skin are of identical [qi and flavor].

【氣味】苦，平，無毒。【普曰】神農：苦，平。岐伯：酸。扁鵲：大寒。雷公：鹹，無毒。【之才曰】大戟爲之使，畏茱萸、蛇蛻皮。

Qi and Flavor. Bitter, balanced, nonpoisonous. [Wu] Pu: Shen nong: Bitter, balanced. Qi Bo: Sour. Bian Que: Very cold. Lei gong: Salty, nonpoisonous. [Xu] Zhicai: Peking spurge serves as its guiding substance. [Ingested together,] it fears *evodia* [fruit] and snake sloughs.

【主治】風寒濕痺，心腹邪氣，利關節，止煩滿。久服輕身，明目不老。本經。平腎胃氣，補陰氣不足，失精莖冷。令人皮膚光澤，有子。別録。逐諸風，除心熱燥。大明。

Control. Blockage related to wind [intrusion] and the presence of cold and moisture, evil qi in the central and abdominal region. It frees the passage through the joints and ends vexing sensations of fullness. Ingested over a long time, it relieves the body of its weight, clears the eyes and prevents aging. *Ben jing*. It balances kidney and stomach qi and supplements insufficient yin qi with an uncontrolled loss of essence/sperm and a sensation of cold in the "stalk," (i. e., penis). It makes one's skin shiny and moist, and lets one have children. *Bie lu*. It eliminates all types of wind and removes heat and dryness from the heart. Da Ming.

【發明】【時珍曰】石龍芮乃平補之藥，古方多用之。其功與枸杞、覆盆子相埒，而世人不知用，何哉？

Explication. [Li] Shizhen: *Shi long rui* is a pharmaceutical drug that balances and supplements [qi]. It is often used in ancient recipes. Its [therapeutic] potential is comparable to that of *lycium* [fruits] and *rubus* seeds but our contemporaries do not know how to use it. How can this be!

17-41-02

水堇 *Shui jin*

【氣味】甘，寒，無毒。【時珍曰】微辛、苦，濇。

Qi and Flavor. Sweet, cold, nonpoisonous. [Li] Shizhen: Slightly acrid, bitter, astringent.

【主治】擣汁，洗馬毒瘡，并服之。又塗蛇蝎毒及癰腫。唐本。久食除心下煩熱。主寒熱鼠瘻，瘰癧生瘡，結核聚氣，下瘀血，止霍亂。又生擣汁半升服，能殺鬼毒，即吐出。孟詵。

Control. Pound it and use the resulting juice to wash [regions affected by] horse [sweat] poison, and in addition ingest it. It is also applied to poison [bites] by snakes and scorpions and obstruction-illness[1300] swelling. *Tang ben*. Ingested over a long time it removes vexing heat from below the heart. It controls alternating sensations of cold and heat associated with mouse fistula,[1301] scrofula pervasion-illness[1302] with a growth of sores, and nodular kernels with qi collections. It discharges stagnating blood and ends cholera. Also to pound fresh [*shui jin*] and ingest half a *sheng* of its juice can kill demon poison that is then spat out.

【發明】【詵曰】堇葉止霍亂，與香茙同功。香茙即香葇也。

Explication. [Meng] Shen: *Jin* 堇 leaves end cholera. Their [therapeutic] potential is identical to that of *elsholtzia* [herbs]. *Xiang mu* 香茙 is *xiang ru* 香葇.[1303]

1300 *Yong* 癰, "obstruction-illness,"refers to an obstruction of vessels or other ducts inside the body. Qi rushing against the obstruction may cause a local swelling and eventually break through the surface to cause an abscess. BCGM Dict I, 641.

1301 *Shu lou* 鼠瘻, "mouse fistula," BCGM Dict I, 466, identical to *luo li* 瘰癧, "scrofula pervasion-illnes."

1302 *Luo li* 瘰癧, "scrofula pervasion-illness," when two or more connected swellings of the size of plum or date kernels appear either on the neck or in the armpits, or somewhere else on the body. BCGM Dict I. 329.

1303 For a suggestion to read 香葇 as *xiang rou* rather than *xiang ru*, see BDGM 16-47.

【附方】舊二，新一。

Added Recipes. Two of old. One newly [recorded].

結核氣。堇菜日乾爲末，油煎成膏。摩之，日三五度便瘥。孟詵食療。

Bound kernel qi. Dry *jin* vegetable in the sun and [grind it into] powder. Boil it with oil to generate a paste. Rub it [into the affected regions], three to five times a day. This will result in a cure. Meng Shen, *Shi liao*.

蛇咬傷瘡。生堇杵汁塗之。萬畢術。

Sores resulting from harm caused by snakebites. Pound fresh *jin* 堇 to obtain a juice and apply it [to the affected region]. *Wan bi shu*.

血疝初起。胡椒菜葉挼按揉之。集簡方。

Elevation-illness[1304] related to blood [accumulation] that has just begun to rise. Rub the leaves of *hu jiao cai* 胡椒菜 and massage them [into the affected region]. *Ji jian fang*.

17-42
毛茛音艮拾遺

Mao gen, read *gen*, FE *Shi yi*.

***Ranunculus japonicus* Thunb. Japanese buttercup.**

【校正】併入毛建草。

Editorial Correction. *Mao jian cao* 毛建草 is included here.

【釋名】毛建草拾遺、水茛綱目、毛堇音芹、天灸衍義、自灸綱目、猴蒜。【時珍曰】茛乃草烏頭之苗，此草形狀及毒皆似之，故名。肘後方謂之水茛，又名毛建，亦茛字音訛也。俗名毛堇，似水堇而有毛也。山人截瘧，采葉挼貼寸口，一夜作泡如火燎，故呼爲天灸、自灸。

Explanation of Names. *Mao jian cao* 毛建草, *Shi yi*. *Shui gen* 水茛, *Gang mu*. *Mao qin* 毛堇, read *qin* 芹; *tian jiu* 天灸, *Yan yi*. *Zi jiu* 自灸, *Gang mu*. *Hou suan* 猴蒜, "monkey's garlic." [Li] Shizhen: *Gen* 茛 is the seedling of *aconitum* [main tuber]. This herb is similar [to that of *aconitum* main tuber] in view of both its physical appearance and toxicity. Hence the name. The *Zhou hou fang* names it *shui gen* 水茛; it is also named *mao jian* 毛建, which is a misreading of the character 茛. The commonly used name is *mao jin* 毛堇. It resembles *shui jin* 水堇 (17-41-02) but has hair. When the mountain people have malaria they collect the leaves, rub them and apply this to the "inch opening." In the course of one night blisters form as if

1304 *Shan* 疝, "elevation-illness," a group of conditions characterized by violent abdominal pain, in some cases associated with constipation and anuria. BCGM Dict I, 417.

burned by fire. Hence they call it *tian jiu* 天灸, "heaven's cauterization" and *zi jiu* 自灸, "natural cauterization."

【集解】【藏器曰】陶注鉤吻云：或是毛莨。蘇恭云：毛莨是有毛石龍芮也，有毒，與鉤吻無干。葛洪百一方云：菜中有水莨，葉圓而光，生水旁，有毒，蟹多食之。人誤食之，狂亂如中風狀，或吐血，以甘草汁解之。又曰：毛建草，生江東地，田野澤畔。葉如芥而大，上有毛。花黃色。子如蒺藜。【時珍曰】毛建、毛莨即今毛堇也，下濕處即多。春生苗，高者尺餘，一枝三葉，葉有三尖及細缺。與石龍芮莖葉一樣，但有細毛爲别。四五月開小黃花，五出，甚光艷。結實狀如欲綻青桑椹而有尖峭，與石龍芮子不同。人以爲鵝草者，大誤也。方士取汁煮砂伏硫。沈存中筆談所謂石龍芮"有兩種：水生者葉光而末圓，陸生者葉毛而末鋭"，此即葉毛者，宜辨之。

Collected Explanations. [Chen] Cangqi: In his comment on *gelsemium* [herb], *gou wen* 鉤吻 (17-47), Tao [Hongjing] states: "It may be *mao gen* 毛莨." Su Gong states: "*Mao gen* 毛莨 is cursed crow foot (17-41) with hair. It is poisonous. It is not related to *gelsemium* [herb], *gou wen* 鉤吻." Ge Hong in his *Bai yi fang* states: "Among vegetables is a *shui gen* 水莨. Its leaves are round and shiny. It grows at the side of waters and is poisonous. Crabs eat lots of it. When humans mistakenly eat it, they are mad and confused as if struck by wind; sometimes they spit blood. This is resolved with *glycyrrhiza* [root] juice." It is also said: *Mao gen* herbs grow in Jiang dong; in the open land in the wild adjacent to marshlands. The leaves are similar to mustard leaves, but they are bigger. They have hair on their surface. The flowers are yellow in color. The seeds are similar to those of wood whitlow grass. [Li] Shizhen: *Mao jian* 毛建 and *mao gen* 毛莨 are today's *mao jin* 毛堇. Much of it grows in low-lying marshland. In spring it grows a seedling; it is about a *chi* tall. One branch has three leaves. Each leaf has three pointed ends and fine notches. It is identical to the stem and the leaves of cursed crow foot, *shi long rui* 石龍芮, but differs in that it has fine hair. Small, yellow flowers open in the fourth and fifth month, with five petals each. They are very shiny. They form fruits shaped like greenish mulberry fruits that are about to split open, and they have sharply pointed ends, which is different from the seeds of cursed crow foot, *shi long rui* 石龍芮. When people identify it as sneezeweed, this is a grave mistake. Recipe masters use the juice to boil cinnabar and to suppress [the effects of] sulphur. Shen Cunzhong in his *Bi tan* says: "Cursed crow foot, *shi long rui*, has two kinds. Those growing in waters have shiny leaves and round tips. Those growing on land have hairy leaves and pointed ends." [The item discussed] here is [the cursed crow foot] with hair; they must be distinguished.

【附録】
Appendix

17-42-A01
海薑 *Hai jiang*
陰[1305]命 *Yin ming*

Unidentified.

【藏器曰】陶注鉤吻云：海薑生海中，赤色，狀如石龍芮，有大毒。又曰：陰命生海中，赤色，着木懸其子，有大毒。今無的識者。

[Chen] Cangqi: In his comment on *gou wen* 鉤吻, Tao [Hongjing] states: "*Hai jiang* grows in the sea, it is red in color and shaped like cursed crow foot. It is very poisonous." It is also said: *Yin ming* grows in the sea; it is red in color. Its seeds hang down attached to trees. It is very poisonous. Today, both are unknown.

17-42-01
葉及子 *Ye and Zi*

Leaf and seeds [of *mao gen*].

【氣味】辛，温，有毒。

Qi and Flavor. Acrid, warm, poisonous.

【主治】惡瘡癰腫，疼痛未潰，搗葉傅之，不得入瘡令肉爛。又患瘧人，以一握微碎，縛於臂上，男左女右，勿令近肉，即便成瘡。和薑搗塗腹，破冷氣。藏器。

Control. Malign sores and obstruction-illness[1306] swelling that are painful and have not yet started to fester. Pound the leaves and apply the [resulting pulp to the affected region]. It must not enter the sores lest it cause the flesh to rot. Also, for persons suffering from malaria, cut a handful to pieces, [fill them into a silk pouch] and fasten it to the [patient's] arm, for males to the left and for females to the right [arm]. It must not come into contact with the flesh. Mix [the leaf pieces] with ginger, pound this [mixture] and apply [the resulting pulp] to the [patient's] abdomen. This will break through cold qi [accumulations]. [Chen] Canqi.

1305 Instead of yin 陰, *Zheng lei* ch. 11, writes *yin* 蔭.

1306 *Yong* 癰, "obstruction-illness," refers to an obstruction of vessels or other ducts inside the body. Qi rushing against the obstruction may cause a local swelling and eventually break through the surface to cause an abscess. BCGM Dict I, 641.

17-43
牛扁本經下品

Niu bian. FE *Ben jing*, lower rank.

***Aconitum barbatum* Pers. var. *puberulum* Ledeb.**

【釋名】扁特唐本、扁毒唐本。

Explanation of Names. *Bian te* 扁特, *Tang ben*. *Bian du* 扁毒, *Tang ben*.

【集解】【別録曰】牛扁生桂陽川谷。【弘景曰】今人不復識此。【恭曰】此藥似堇草、石龍芮輩，根如秦艽而細，生平澤下濕地。田野人名爲牛扁，療牛虱甚效。太常名扁特，或名扁毒。【保昇曰】今出寧州。葉似石龍芮、附子等。二月、八月采根，日乾。【頌曰】今潞州一種名便特，六月有花，八月結實。采其根苗，搗末油調，殺蟣虱。主療大都相似，疑即扁特也，但聲近而字訛耳。

Collected Explanations. *Bie lu*: *Niu bian* grows in the river valleys of Gui yang. [Tao] Hongjing: Today, people no longer know of it. [Su] Gong: This pharmaceutical drug resembles [plants] such as Chinese elder and cursed crow foot. The root is similar to that of large gentiana, but it is finer. It grows in marshlands of the plains, and in low-lying marshland. People in the open country call it niu bian 牛扁. It very effectively heals oxen infested with lice. It is often called *bian te* 扁特 and also *bian du* 扁毒. [Han] Baosheng: Today it comes from Ning zhou. The leaves resemble those of cursed crow foot and *aconitum*. The root is collected in the second and eighth month; it is dried in the sun. [Su] Song: Today in Lu zhou is a kind named *bian te* 便特. It opens flowers in the sixth month and forms fruits in the eighth month. [People] collect its roots and seedlings, pound them into powder and mix it with oil to kill lice and their nymphs/eggs. Its [potential to] control and heal [disease] is quite similar [to that of *niu bian*]. Maybe [*bian te* 便特] is *bian te* 扁特. The pronunciation is similar, just one character is mistaken.

【氣味】苦，微寒。無毒。

Qi and Flavor. Bitter, slightly cold. Nonpoisonous.

【主治】身皮瘡熱氣，可作浴湯。殺牛虱小蟲，又療牛病。本經。

Control. For body skin sores associated with heat qi, it can be prepared to a hot bathing liquid. It kills ox lice and small worms/bugs. It also heals the diseases of oxen. *Ben jing*.

【附録】
Appendix.

17-43-A01
虱建草拾遺 *Shijiancao*, FE*Shiyi*

Unidentified.

【藏器曰】苦，無毒。主蟣虱。挼汁沐頭，虱盡死。人有誤吞虱成病者，擣汁服一小合。亦主諸蟲瘡。生山足濕地，發葉似山丹，微赤，高一二尺。又有水竹葉，生水中。葉如竹葉而短小，可生食，亦去蟣虱。

[Chen] Cangqi: Bitter, nonpoisonous. It controls lice and their nymphs/eggs. Press it to obtain a juice and wash the head with it. All lice die. When someone has mistakenly swallowed lice and falls ill, pound it to obtain a juice and let him ingest one modest *ge*. It also controls all types of sores related to worms/bugs. The leaves it develops[1307] resemble those of wild scarlet lily. They are slightly red. [The herb] is one or two *chi* tall. There is also [a kind called] *shui zhu ye* 水竹葉, "water bamboo leaf." It grows in water. Its leaves are similar to bamboo leaves, but are short and small. They can be eaten raw. They, too, eliminate lice and their nymphs/eggs.

17-44
蕁麻蕁音燖宋圖經
***Xun ma*, 蕁 read *xun* 燖, FE Song, *Tu jing*.**

***Urtica laetevirens* Maxim. Nettle.**

【釋名】毛藙。【時珍曰】蕁字本作藙。杜子美有除藙草詩，是也。

Explanation of Names. *Mao qian* 毛藙. [Li] Shizhen: The character *xun* 蕁 was originally written *qian* 藙. Du Zimei has a poem about "Getting rid of the *qian* herb." This is the one [discussed here].

【集解】【頌曰】蕁麻生江寧府山野中。【時珍曰】川、黔諸處甚多。其莖有刺，高二三尺。葉似花桑，或青或紫，背紫者入藥。上有毛芒可畏，觸人如蜂蠆螫蠚，以人溺濯之即解。有花無實，冒冬不凋。挼投水中，能毒魚。

Collected Explanations. [Su] Song: *Xun ma* grows in the wild in the mountains of Jiang ning fu. [Li] Shizhen: Today, very much of it is present everywhere in Chuan and Qian. Its stem has thorns and reaches a height of two to three *chi*. The leaves resemble those of mulberry; they may be greenish or purple. Those with a purple back are added to medication. They have hairy awns on their surface one should watch

1307 Instead of *fa* 發葉, "the leaves it develops," *Zheng lei* ch. 9, *shi jian cao* 虱建草, writes *jing ye* 莖葉, "stem and leaves."

for. When they sting one this is similar to being stung by bees/wasps or scorpions. This is resolved by pouring human urine [on the affected region]. Its flowers have no fruits. In winter they do not wither. Rubbed and tossed into water, they can kill fish.

【氣味】辛、苦，寒，有大毒。吐利人不止。

Qi and Flavor. Acrid, bitter, cold, very poisonous. It lets one vomit and have free-flow without end.

【主治】蛇毒，搗塗之。蘇頌。風瘮初起，以此點之，一夜皆失。時珍。

Control. For snake [bite] poison, pound it and apply [the pulp to the affected region]. [Su] Song. Wind papules that have just begun to rise. Drip this on them and in the course of one night they all vanish. [Li] Shizhen.

17-45
格注草唐本草
Ge zhu cao, FE *Tang ben cao.*

Unidentified.

【集解】【恭曰】出齊魯山澤間，葉似蕨。根紫色，若紫草根，一株有二寸許。二月、八月采根，五月、六月采苗，日乾用。

Collected Explanations. [Su] Gong: It comes from the mountains and marshlands of the region of Qi and Lu. The leaves resemble those of *pteridium* vegetables. The root is purple, similar to the root of *arnebia* [herbs]. The trunk/plant is about two *cun* tall. The root is collected in the second and eighth month. The seedlings are collected in the fifth and sixth month. They are dried in the sun and used [for therapeutic purposes].

【氣味】辛、苦，温，有大毒。

Qi and Flavor. Acrid, bitter, warm, very poisonous.

【主治】蠱疰諸毒疼痛等。唐本。

Control. *Gu* attachment-illness[1308] and all types of painful poisoning. *Tang ben.*

1308 *Gu zhu* 蠱疰, "*gu*-attachment-illness," a condition of abdominal fullness with accumulations, pain and emaciation brought forth by *gu* poison, in some cases with blood spitting, and blood in the stool and urine. The illness takes many different forms. BCGM Dict I, 193.

17-46
海芋綱目
Hai yu. FE *Gang mu*.

***Alocasia macrorhiza* (L.) Schott.**[1309]

【釋名】觀音蓮綱目、羞天草玉册、天荷綱目、隔河仙見下。

Explanation of Names. *Guan yin lian* 觀音蓮, "Guanyin's lotus," *Gang mu*. *Xiu tian cao* 羞天草, "the herb that is ashamed to show itself to heaven," *Yu ce*. *Tian he* 天荷, "heaven's lotus," *Gang mu*. *Ge he xian* 隔河仙, see below.

【集解】【時珍曰】海芋生蜀中，今亦處處有之。春生苗，高四五尺。大葉如芋葉而有幹。夏秋間抽莖開花，如一瓣蓮花，碧色。花中有蕊，長作穗，如觀音像在圓光之狀，故俗呼爲觀音蓮。方士號爲隔河仙，云可變金。其根似芋魁，大者如升盌，長六七寸，蓋野芋之類也。庚辛玉册云：羞天草，陰草也。生江廣深谷澗邊。其葉極大，可以禦雨，葉背紫色。花如蓮花。根葉皆有大毒。可煅粉霜、硃砂。小者名野芋。宋祁海芋贊云：
木幹芋葉，擁腫盤戾。
農經弗載，可以治癘。

Collected Explanations. [Li] Shizhen: *Hai yu* grows in Shu; today it is also present everywhere else. In spring it grows a seedling, reaching a height of four to five *chi*. It has big leaves similar to taro leaves, but they have a stem. In summer and autumn, a stem rises and opens a flower similar to a single petal lotus flower. It is jade-bluish in color. In the center of the flower are the filaments; they are long and form spikes, and this looks like Guanyin surrounded by her halo. Hence the common name "Guanyin lotus." The recipe masters call it *ge he xian* 隔河仙, "hermit/immortal beyond the river," stating that it can change [things to] gold. Its root resembles a taro tuber; large ones are as big as a bowl of one *sheng*, and they reach a length of six to seven *cun*. The fact is, they belong to a group with wild taro. The *Geng xin yu ce* states: "*Xiu tian cao* is a yin herb. It grows at the side of deep valley ravines in Jiang guang. Its leaves are extremely big; they can protect one from rain. The back of the leaves is purple. The flowers are similar to those of lotus. Root and leaves are very poisonous. They can serve to calcine calomel and cinnabar. Small ones are called "wild taro." Song Qi in his "*hai yu* eulogy" states:
"A wooden stem and taro leaves. Big as if swollen.
Not recorded in agriculture classics. It can be used to cure epidemics."

【氣味】辛，有大毒。

Qi and Flavor. Acrid, very poisonous.

1309 *Hai yu* 海芋, lit.: "sea taro."

【主治】瘧瘴毒腫風癩。伏硇砂。時珍。

Control. Malaria, miasmatic poison swelling, wind [intrusion] repudiation-illness.[1310] It suppresses [the effects of] sal ammoniac. [Li] Shizhen.

【附録】
Appendix.

17-46-A01
透山根 *Tou shan gen*

Unidentified.

【時珍曰】按岣嶁神書云：透山根生蜀中山谷。草類蘼蕪，可以點鐵成金。昔有人采藥，誤斫此草，刀忽黄軟成金也。又庚辛玉册云：透山根出武都。取汁點鐵，立成黄金。有大毒，人誤食之，化爲紫水。又有金英草，亦生蜀中。狀如馬齒莧而色紅，摸鐵成金。亦有大毒，入口殺人，須臾爲紫水也。又何薳春渚紀聞云：劉均父吏部罷官歸成都。有水銀一篋，過峽篋漏，急取渡旁叢草塞之。久而開視，盡成黄金矣。宋初有軍士在澤州澤中割馬草歸，鐮皆成金。以草燃釜，亦成黄金。又臨安僧法堅言：有客過於潛山中，見一蛇腹脹，齧一草以腹磨之而消。念此草必能消脹，取置篋中。夜宿旅館，聞鄰房有人病腹脹呻吟，以釜煎藥一盃與服。頃之不復聞聲，念已安矣。至旦視之，其人血肉俱化爲水，獨骸骨在牀爾。視其釜，則通體成金矣。觀何氏所載，即是透山根乃金英草之類。如此毒草，不可不知，故備載之耳。

[Li] Shizhen: According to the *Gou lou shen shu*, "*tou shan gen* grows in the mountain valleys of Shu zhong. The herb is related to *ligusticum*. It can be dripped on iron to generate gold. In ancient times someone collected pharmaceutical drugs. He mistakenly cut this herb. Suddenly his knife turned yellow and soft and transformed to gold." Also, the *Geng xin yu ce* states: "*Tou shan gen* comes from Wu du. When the juice is dripped on iron it immediately turns into gold. It is very poisonous. When humans mistakenly consume it, they transform to purple water. There is also a 'golden splendor herb,' It, too, grows in Shu zhong. It is shaped like purslane, but is red in color. When it is rubbed on iron, [the iron] turns into gold. It, too, is very poisonous. Once it has entered the mouth, that person dies and within a short moment turns into purple water." Also, as He Yuan in his *Chun zhu ji wen* states: "Liu Xunfu was dismissed from office in the Ministry of Personnel and returned to Cheng du.
He carried with him a box with mercury. When he crossed a gorge, the box leaked. He quickly collected a bunch of herbs from the side of the ferry to stop the hole.

1310 *Da feng lai* 大風癩, "massive wind [i. e.,] repudiation-illness," most likely including cases of leprosy/Aussatz. BCGM Dict I, 111, 293

After quite some time he opened [the box] to inspect [its contents], and everything had turned into yellow gold." At the beginning of the Song era, a soldier in the marshland of Ze zhou cut grass to feed his horse. When he returned, his sickle had turned into gold. The pot he had heated the herbs with had also turned into yellow gold. Also, Monk Fa jian from Lin an says: "Once a visitor while passing through the Qian shan mountains saw a snake with a bloated abdomen. It broke down an herb, rubbed its abdomen on it, and [the bloating] melted away. So he thought that this herb is certainly able to dissolve swelling and he took some of it with him. The night he spent in an inn, When he heard someone in an adjacent room groaning because of abdominal bloating, he boiled some of the [herb] in a cauldron to prepare a medication and gave it to him to ingest it. After a short while he no longer heard anything and assumed that [the other man's problem] had been solved. The next morning he looked after him, but that man's blood and flesh had all turned into water; only the skeleton remained on the bed. Then he looked at the cauldron, it, too, had entirely turned into gold." In view of the monk's record, this [herb] was of one group with *tou shan gen* and[1311] *jin ying cao*. Such a poisonous herb must be known. Therefore it is recorded here for [everybody to] be prepared!

17-47
鉤吻本經下品
Gou wen, FE *Ben jing*, lower rank.

***Gelsemium elegans* (Gardn.et Champ.) Benth.**

【釋名】野葛本經、毒根吴普、胡蔓草圖經、斷腸草綱目、黄藤綱目、火把花。【弘景曰】言其入口則鉤人喉吻也。或言"吻"當作"挽"字，牽挽人腸而絶之也。【時珍曰】此草雖名野葛，非葛根之野者也，或作冶葛。王充論衡云：冶，地名也，在東南。其説甚通。廣人謂之胡蔓草，亦曰斷腸草。入人畜腹内，即粘腸上，半日則黑爛，又名爛腸草。滇人謂之火把花，因其花紅而性熱如火也。岳州謂之黄藤。

Explanation of Names. *Ye ge* 野葛, *Ben jing*. *Du gen* 毒根, "poison root," Wu Pu. *Hu man cao* 胡蔓草, "creeper herb of the Hu," *Tu jing*. *Duan chang cao* 斷腸草, "the herb that severs intestines," *Gang mu*. *Huang teng* 黄藤, "yellow vine," *Gang mu*. *Huo ba hua* 火把花, "torch flower." [Tao] Hongjing: It is said that when it has entered the mouth, it "hooks," *gou* 鉤, that person's throat. Others say: "*Gou* 吻 should be written wan 挽, 'to pull,' as it pulls, *qian wan* 牽挽, that person's intestines and sev-

1311 The Jiang xi edition, the Qian edition and the Zhang edition of BCGM all have *nai* 乃, "this is." However, in view of the earlier Gen xin yu ce quote 又有金英草, "there is also a 'golden splendor herb'," the character *nai* 乃 appears to be an erroneous writing of *ji* 及, "and."

ers them." [Li] Shizhen: Even though this herb is called *ye ge* 野葛, it is definitely not a wild kind of *ge gen* 葛根, *pueraria* [root]. Still others write [*ye ge* 野葛] as *ye ge* 冶葛. Wang Chong in his *Lun heng* states: "*Ye* 冶 is the name of a place in the South-East." This is quite to the point. People in Guang call it *hu man cao* 胡蔓草, "herb of the Hu and Man people;" it is also called *duan chang cao* 斷腸草, "the herb that severs the intestines." When it enters and collects in one's abdomen, it clings to the intestines. Within half a day they turn black and rot. It is also called *lan chang cao* 爛腸草, "the herb that lets the intestines rot." People in Dian call it *huo ba cao* 火把花, "handheld fire/torch flower," because its flowers are red, and by its nature it is hot like fire. In Yue zhou they call it *huang teng* 黃藤, "yellow vine."

【集解】【別録曰】鉤吻生傅高山谷及會稽東野，折之青烟出者名固活。二月、八月采。【普曰】秦鉤吻一名除辛，生南越山及寒石山，或益州。葉如葛，赤莖大如箭而方，根黃色，正月采之。【恭曰】野葛生桂州以南，村墟閭巷間皆有。彼人通名鉤吻，亦謂苗爲鉤吻，根名野葛。蔓生，其葉如柿。其根新采者，皮白骨黃。宿根似地骨，嫩根如漢防己，皮節斷者良。正與白花藤相類，不深別者，頗亦惑之。新者折之無塵氣。經年以後則有塵起，從骨之細孔中出。今折枸杞根亦然。本草言折之青烟起者名固活爲良，亦不達之言也。人誤食其葉者致死，而羊食其苗大肥，物有相伏如此。博物志云"鉤吻蔓生，葉似鳧葵"是也。【時珍曰】嵇含南方草木狀云：野葛蔓生，葉如羅勒，光而厚，一名胡蔓草。人以雜生蔬中毒人，半日輒死。段成式酉陽雜俎云：胡蔓草生邕州、容州之間。叢生。花扁如巵子而稍大，不成朶，色黃白。其葉稍黑。又按嶺南衛生方云：胡蔓草葉如茶，其花黃而小。一葉入口，百竅潰血，人無復生也。時珍又訪之南人云：鉤吻即胡蔓草，今人謂之斷腸草是也。蔓生，葉圓而光。春夏嫩苗毒甚，秋冬枯老稍緩。五六月開花似欅柳花，數十朶作穗。生嶺南者花黃，生滇南者花紅，呼爲火把花。此數説皆與吴普、蘇恭説相合。陶弘景等別生分辨，並正于下。

Collected Explanations. *Gou wen* grows in the mountain valleys of Fu gao, and in the wild east of Gui ji. Those that when broken release a greenish smoke are called *gu huo* 固活. They are collected in the second and eighth month. [Wu] Pu: *Gou wen* from Qin is also called *chu xin* 除辛. It grows in the Nan yue shan and Han shi shan mountains, and also in Yi zhou. The leaves are similar to *pueraria* [leaves]. The red stem is square and has the size of an arrow. The root is yellow; it is collected in the first month. [Su] Gong: *Ye ge* 野葛 grows south of Gui zhou. It can be found everywhere in deserted villages and along lanes. All the people there call it *gou wen* 鉤吻. It is also said that the seedling is called *gou wen* 鉤吻, while the root is called *ye ge* 野葛. It grows as a creeper; its leaves are similar to persimmon [leaves]. The skin of a freshly collected root is white; the "bone" is yellow. The perennial root resembles *lycium* roots. Tender roots are similar to *stephania tetandra* [roots]. Those with the skin broken at the nodes are good. They are closely related to Chinese star jasmine. If they are not carefully distinguished, one may be misled. When fresh specimens are broken, they do not release dust qi. Only after a year has passed the dust [in them] rises and comes out of the fine holes of the "bone." When today *lycium* roots are broken, this is so, too. When the *Ben cao* says that those are good that release a greenish fume when broken and are called *gu huo* 固活, this is not a sufficiently detailed record. When humans mistakenly eat its leaves, they die. When sheep eat the seedlings, they become fat. This is how things suppress others. The *Bo wu zhi* states: "*Gou wen* grows as a creeper. The leaves resemble those of *nymphoides* [herbs]." That is correct. [Li] Shizhen: Ji Han in his *Nan fang cao mu zhuang* states: "*Ye ge* 野葛 grows as a creeper. The leaves are similar to those of sweet basil. They are shiny and thick. Another name is *hu man cao* 胡蔓草. People mix it with fresh vegetables to poison others. They die within half a day." Duan Chengshi in his *You yang za zu* states: "*Hu man cao* grows as clusters in the region of Yong zhou and Rong zhou. The flowers are flat like those of mountain *gardenia*, just a little bigger. [The flowers] do not form clusters; they are yellow-white. The leaves are somewhat black." Also, according to the *Ling nan wei sheng fang*, "the leaves of *hu man cao* are similar to tea [leaves]. The flowers are yellow and small. When only one leaf enters the mouth, blood will spill out of one hundred orifices. Such a person will not be brought back to life." [I, Li] Shizhen, visited people in the South to ask them [about this herb]. They stated: "*Gou wen* is *hu man cao*. It is the one called by people *duan chang cao*, 'the herb that severs intestines,' today. It grows as a creeper. The leaves are round and shiny. In spring and summer the tender seedling is extremely poisonous. In autumn and winter it has dried, is old and [the poison] is a bit slower. In the fifth and the sixth month it opens flowers similar to the flowers of Schneider's *zelkova* and willows. Tens of them appear as clusters forming spikes. Those that grow in Ling nan have yellow flowers; those growing in Dian nan have red flowers. They are called 'torch flower'." All these records agree with those of Wu Pu and Su Gong. Tao Hongjing and others go into more detail. They are quoted below.

【正誤】【弘景曰】五符經亦言鉤吻是野葛。覈事而言，似是兩物。野葛是根，狀如牡丹，所生處亦有毒，飛鳥不得集，今人用合膏服之無嫌。鉤吻別是一物，葉似黃精而莖紫，當心抽花，黄色，初生極類黃精，故人采多惑之，遂致死生之反。或云鉤吻是毛茛，參錯不同，未詳云何？【斅曰】凡使黄精勿用鉤吻，真似黃精，只是葉有毛鉤子二個。黃精葉似竹葉。又曰：凡使鉤吻，勿用地精，莖苗相同。鉤吻治人身上惡毒瘡，其地精殺人也。【恭曰】鉤吻蔓生，葉如柿。陶言飛鳥不集者，妄也。黃精直生，葉似柳及龍膽草，殊非比類。毛茛乃有毛石龍芮，與鉤吻何干？【頌曰】江南人說黃精莖苗稍類鉤吻。但鉤吻葉頭極尖而根細，與蘇恭所說不同，恐南北之產異也。【禹錫曰】陶說鉤吻似黃精者，當是。蘇說似柿葉者，別是一物也。又言苗名鉤吻，根名野葛者，亦非通論。【時珍曰】神農本草鉤吻一名野葛，一句已明。草木狀又名胡蔓草，顯是藤生。吳普、蘇恭所說正合本文。陶氏以藤生爲野葛，又指小草爲鉤吻，復疑是毛茛，乃祖雷斆之說。諸家遂無定見，不辨其蔓生、小草，相去遠也。然陶、雷所說亦是一種有毒小草，但不得指爲鉤吻爾。昔天姥對黃帝言：黃精益壽，鉤吻殺人。乃是以二草善惡比對而言。陶氏不審，疑是相似，遂有此說也。餘見"黃精"下。

Correction of Errors. [Tao] Hongjing: The *Wu fu jing* says: "*Gou wen* 鉤吻 is *ye ge* 野葛." A close examination leads one to say that they appear to be two different items. *Ye ge* is the root. It is shaped like *paeonia* [root]. The places where [*ye ge*] grows are poisonous; birds do not gather there. Today, people use [*ye ge*] to prepare a paste that is ingested without any problem. *Gou wen* is something different. The leaves resemble those of Solomon's seal; the stem is purple. A yellow flower rises from its center. In the beginning it is very much like Solomon's seal. When the ancients went out to collect [Solomon's seal] they often were misled [and took *gou wen*. Its application] ended in death rather than life. Some say: "*Gou wen* is Japanese buttercup, *mao gen* 毛茛 (17-42)." This mixes up different items. Why was it not clearly stated? [Lei] Xiao: Whenever it is intended to apply Solomon's seal [root], do not use *gou wen*! It is really similar to Solomon's seal except for that the leaves [of *gou wen*] have two hairy hooks, while the leaves of Solomon's seal resemble the leaves of bamboo. It is also said: Whenever it is intended to apply *gou wen*, do not use *di jing* 地精. The stem and the seedling [of *gou wen* and *di jing*] are identical. But, *gou wen* serves to cure malign poison sores on the human body, while *di jing* kills one.[1312] [Su] Gong: *Gou wen* grows as a creeper; the leaves are similar to those of persimmon. When Tao [Hongjing] says that birds do not collect [where *gou wen* grows], this is nonsense. Solomon's seal grows straight up; the leaves resemble willow [leaves] and Korean *gentiana* [leaves]. They are definitely not related. Japanese buttercup, *mao gen* 毛茛, is hairy cursed crow foot, *shi long rui* 石龍芮. What does it have in common with *gou wen*? [Su] Song: People in Jiang nan say that Solomon's seal stem and seedlings are somewhat related to *gou wen*. However, the tip of *gou wen* leaves is pointed, and the root is fine. This is different from what Su Gong says. Perhaps the products of the South and the North differ. [Zhang] Yuxi: When Tao [Hongjing] says that "*gou*

1312 *Di jing* 地精 is an alternative name of ginseng root, *ren shen* 人参, and *polygonum multiflorum*, *he shou wu* 何首烏, both of which are described as "nonpoisonous." The *di jing* referred to here may be another herb.

wen resembles Solomon's seal," he is right. When Su [Gong] says that "[its leaves] are similar to persimmon leaves," then this is another item. It is also said that the seedling is called *gou wen* 鉤吻 while the root is called *ye ge* 野葛. This was not accepted in all discourses. [Li] Shizhen: The *Shen nong ben cao* [states] of *gou wen* that "its alternative name is *ye ge.*" This one sentence makes everything clear. In the *Cao mu zhuang* it is also called *hu man cao* 胡蔓草. Obviously it grows as a creeper. The statements by Wu Pu and Su Gong perfectly agree with the original text. Mr. Tao [Hongjing] identifies the creeper as *ye ge*, and the small herb as *gou wen*, and he was not sure if it could be Japanese buttercup. Following Lei Xiao's statement, all the experts failed to arrive at a definite view; they failed to distinguish between creeper and small herb, which are quite distant from each other. Now, Tao [Hongjing] and Lei [Xiao], too, refer to a small poisonous herb, but this should not be identified as *gou wen*. In ancient times, Tian Lao said to Huang Di: "Solomon's seal boosts longevity. *Gou wen* kills one." This is a comparision of the good and malign qualities of these two items. Mr. Tao [Hongjing] failed to examine [this statement]; he assumed they might be related to each other, and hence made his statement. For further details, see under the entry "*huang jing* 黄精," Solomon's seal (12-08).

【氣味】辛，温，大有毒。【普曰】神農：辛。雷公：有毒殺人。【時珍曰】其性大熱。本草毒藥止云有大毒，此獨變文曰大有毒，可見其毒之異常也。【之才曰】半夏爲之使，惡黄芩。

Qi and Flavor. Acrid, warm, very poisonous.[1313] [Wu] Pu: Shen nong: Acrid. Lei gong: It is poisonous and kills humans. [Li] Shizhen: Its nature is very hot. The *Ben cao* says of poisonous pharmaceutical substances "has much poison." Only for the present [substance] this wording is changed to "is very poisonous." From this it can be seen that its poison is extraordinarily strong. [Xu] Zhicai: *Pinellia* [root] serves as its guiding substance. [Ingested together,] it abhors *scutellaria* [root].

【主治】金瘡乳痓，中惡風，欬逆上氣，水腫，殺鬼疰蠱毒。本經。破癥積，除脚膝痺痛，四肢拘攣，惡瘡疥蟲，殺鳥獸。擣汁入膏中，不入湯飲。别録。主喉痺咽塞，聲音變。吴普。

Control. Wounds caused by metal objects/weapons, and disorders affecting the female breast. Being struck by malign wind. Cough with counterflow of rising qi. Water swelling. It kills demons associated with an attachment-illness and *gu* poi-

1313 Instead of *da you* 大有, both the *da guan* 大觀 and the *zheng he* 政和 edition of the *Zheng lei* write *you da* 有大. Beginning with the Ming editions of the *Zheng lei* this was changed to *da you* 大有, an error followed by the *Ben cao gang mu*.

son.[1314] *Ben jing*. It breaks through concretion-illness and accumulations. It removes painful blockage from the legs and knees, as well as cramp and contraction of the four limbs. Malign sores and *jie*-illness[1315] with the presence of worms/bugs. It kills fowls and animals. It is pounded and the resulting juice is made into pastes, not decoctions that are drunk. *Bie lu*. It controls blocked throat with an altered sound of the voice. Wu Pu.

【發明】【藏器曰】鉤吻食葉，飲冷水即死，冷水發其毒也。彼土毒死人懸尸樹上，汁滴地上生菌子，收之名菌藥，烈於野葛也。蕹菜搗汁，解野葛毒。取汁滴野葛苗即萎死。南人先食蕹菜，後食野葛，二物相伏，自然無苦。魏武帝噉野葛至尺，先食此菜也。【時珍曰】按李石續博物志云：胡蔓草出二廣。廣人負債急，每食此草而死，以誣人。以急水吞即死急，慢水吞死稍緩。或取毒蛇殺之，覆以此草，澆水生菌，爲毒藥害人。葛洪肘後方云：凡中野葛毒口不可開者，取大竹筒洞節，以頭拄其兩脇及臍中。灌冷水入筒中，數易水。須臾口開，乃可下藥解之。惟多飲甘草汁、人屎汁，白鴨或白鵝斷頭，瀝血入口中，或羊血灌之。嶺南衛生方云：即時取雞卵抱未成雛者，研爛和麻油灌之。吐出毒物乃生，稍遲即死也。

Explication. [Chen] Cangqi: If after eating *gou wen* leaves one drinks cold water, he dies. Cold water effuses its poison. When a person has died of [*gou wen*] poison, the locals hang his corpse on a tree. The juice that drips on the ground creates mushrooms. They are stored as "mushroom medication." They are even more violently [poisonous] than *ye ge* 野葛. [People] pound swamp morning glory, *weng cai* 蕹菜 (27-02), to obtain a juice. It serves to resolve the poison of *ye ge*. When this juice is dripped on a *ye ge* seedling, it withers. People in the South first eat swamp morning glory and then they eat *ye ge*. The two items suppress each other's [effects], and [*ye ge* is eaten] without problem. Emperor Wu di of the Wei once ate a *chi*-long *ye ge* [root]. He had eaten this vegetable first. [Li] Shizhen: According to Li Shi's *Xu bo wu zhi*, "*hu man cao* comes from the two Guang [regions]. When Guang people are deeply in debt, they always eat this herb and die. This is to blame the person [for whom they are in debt]. If [the herb] is swallowed with fast running water, they die right away. If it is swallowed with slow flowing water, the dying is slowed down. Some take a poisonous snake and kill it. Then they cover it with this herb. They pour water on it and mushrooms grow from it. They are prepared as a poisonous medication to harm people." Ge Hong in his

1314 *Gu du* 蠱毒, "*gu*-poison[ing]." (1) A poison emitted by certain worms/snakes with an ability to cause varying pathological changes in a person who has taken it in by means of wine or food. (2) Abdominal fullness, in some cases with blood spitting, and blood in the stool and urine. BCGM Dict I, 192 - 193. See BCGM 42-22.

1315 *Jie*-illness 疥, vaguely identifiable skin ailment. BCGM Dict I, 249.

Appendix

5. Weights and measures

5.1 Measures of capacity

1 *zhong* 鍾, 663 liters, equal to 64 *dou* 斗
Also: size of a wine cup, or small jug.
1 *hu* 斛, "bushel," 107. 37 liters, equal to 10 *dou* 斗
1 *dan* 石, "bushel," also written *shuo* 碩, equal to 1 *hu* 斛
1 *dou* 斗, "peck," 10.74 liters, equal to 10 *sheng* 升
1 *sheng* 升, "pint," 1.07 liters, equal to 10 *ge* 合
1 *ge* 合, equal to 0.11 liters

5.2 Measures of weight

1 *cheng* 秤, 7.5 kg, equal to 15 *jin* 斤
1 *jin* 斤, "catty," 500 grams, equal to 16 *liang* 兩,
1 *liang* 兩, "ounce," 31.25 grams, equal to 10 *qian* 錢
1 *qian* 錢, 3.13 grams, equal to 10 *fen* 分
1 *fen* 分, 0.31 grams, equal to 10 *li*
1 *li* 厘, 0.031 grams, the thousandth part of a *liang* 兩
1 *yi* 鎰, equal to 20 or 24 *liang* 兩
1 *dan* 石, "picul," 60 kg, equal to 120 *jin* 斤

1 *zhu* 銖, "scruple," 1.3 grams, one 24th part of a *liang* 兩,
equal to 100 grains of millet
1 *zi* 字, the weight of a quarter of a copper coin covered with the powder of a
pharmaceutical substance
1 *wen* 文, the weight of one coin.

5.3 Measures of length

1 *li* 里, equal to 1800 *chi*
1 *zhang* 丈, "stave," equal to 10 *chi* 尺
1 *li* 厘, the thousandth part of a *chi* 尺
1 *chi* 尺, "foot," equal to 10 *cun* 寸
1 *cun* 寸, "inch," varying over time between 0.9 and 1.2 Western inches
1 ren 仞, equivalent to seven or eight *chi* 尺

5.4 Measures of the size of pills

zao seed, *zao zi* 皂子, the size of *gleditsia* seeds
soybean, *dou* 豆, the size of a soybeans
qian seed, *qian zi* 芡子, the size of *Euryale ferox* Salisb. seeds
mung bean, *lü dou* 緑豆, the size of *vigna radiata* L. Wilczek beans
red mung bean, *chi xiao dou* 赤小豆, the size of *vigna umbellata* (Thunb.) Ohwi
et Ohashi
wu [*tong*] seed, *wu* [*tong*] *zi* 梧桐子, the size of *Firmiana platanifolia* (L.f.)
Marsili seeds
bullet, *dan zi* 彈子, the size of a firearm bullet
hemp seed, *ma zi* 麻子, the size of *Cannabis sativa* L. seeds
white soybean, *bai dou* 白豆, *Vigna unguiculata* (L.) Walp. var. *cylindrica* (L.)
Ohashi seeds
rice bean, *xiao dou* 小豆, the size of *vigna umbellata* (Thunb.) Ohwi et Ohashi
dragon eyes, *long yan* 龍眼, the size of longan seeds
mustard seeds, *jie zi* 芥子, the size of seeds of *brassica juncea* (L.) Czern.et Coss.
jujube kernels, *suan zao* 酸棗, of *zizyphus jujuba* Mill. var. *spinosa* (Bunge) Hu ex
H. F. Chow

6. Lists of Substances

6.1 Pharmaceutical substances of plant origin mentioned in BCGM ch. 15 - 17 in passing. Herbs with an entry of their own are marked with their entry number.

By Ulrike Unschuld

Note 1. The earlier a text has been written, the less certain can be today's botanical identification of a substance. 2. The botanical species given in the following list may not include all species possibly covered by a Chinese plant name. Here only the most common identifications are provided as a first hint at the nature of a pharmaceutical substance referred to in a recipe or elsewhere. 3. Wherever available, the *Zhong hua ben cao's* 中华本草, Shanghai 1999, identification of botanical substances was adopted as authoritative. 4. All recipes requiring an ingestion of medication with wine relate to low alcohol rice wine.

A

Acanthopanax [root-bark/stem]. *Wu jia* [*pi*] 五加[皮], *mu gu* 木骨
  Acanthopanax gracilistylus W.W. Smith

Achyranthes [leaf]. *Niu xi* [*ye*] 牛膝[葉], 16-02
  Achyranthes bidentata Bl.

Aconite paste. *She wang* 射罔
  Made from the tubers of *aconitum carmichaeli* Debx.

Aconitum [accessory tuber]. *Fu zi* 附子, *she wang* 射罔, *cao wu* 草烏, 17-17
  Aconitum carmichaeli Debx.

Aconitum [main tuber]. *Wu tou* 烏頭, 17-21
  Aconitum carmichaeli Debx.

Acorus [root]. *Chang pu* 菖蒲
  Acorus gramineus Ait. (M. Br.)

Adenophora, apricot-leaved, [root], *Ji ni* 薺苨
  Adenophora trachelioides Maxim.

Adenophora [root]. *Sha shen* 沙參
Adenophora stricta Miq.
Agastache [herb]. *Huo xiang* 藿[香]
Agastache rugosa (Fisch. et Mey.) O. Kuntze
Agrimonia herb. *Lang ya* 狼牙, 17-05
Agrimonia pilosa Ledeb.
Ailanthus [tree/herb]. *Chun chu* 椿樗, *feng yan cao* 鳳眼草
Ailanthus altissima (Mill.) Swingle
Akebia [herb]. *Mu tong* 木通
Akebia quinata (Thunb.) Decne.
Alfalfa. *Mu xu* 苜蓿
Medicago hispida Gaertn.
Alisma [root]. *Ze xie* 澤瀉
Alisma orientalis [Sam.] Juzep.
Alocasia [root]. *Hai yu* 海芋, 17-46
Alocasia macrorhiza (L.) Schott.
Aloes wood. *Chen xiang* 沉香
Aquilaria agallocha (Lour.) Roxb.
Amaranth [herb], *Xian* 莧
Amaranthus tricolor L.
Ampelopsis [root]. *Bai lian* 白斂
Ampelopsis japonica (Thunb.) Makino
Anemarrhena [root]. *Zhi mu* 知母
Anemarrhena asphodeloides Bunge.
Angelica biserrata [root]. *Du huo* 獨活
Angelica biserrata, Shan et Yuan.
Angelica dahurica [root]. *Bai zhi* 白芷, *guan* 莞
Angelica dahurica (Fisch. ex Hoffm.) Benth. et Hook f. ex Franch. et Sav. cv.
Apricot [kernel/seed]. *Xing* [*ren*] 杏[仁/人]
Armeniaca vulgaris Lam.
Arborvitae [tree/leaf/seed kernels]. *Bai* [*zi ren*] 柏[子仁], *ce bai ye* 側柏葉
Platycladus orientalis (L.) Franco
Areca [nut]. *Bin lang* 檳榔
Areca catechu L.
Aristolochia [fruit]. *Du lin teng* 都淋藤, *ma dou ling* 馬兜鈴藤
Aristolochia contorta Bunge

Arnebia [herb, root]. *Zi cao* 紫草, *di xue* 地血
Arnebia euchroma (Royle) Johnst.
Artemisia anomala [herb]. *Liu ji nu* 劉寄奴, 15-21
Artemisia anomala S.Moore
Artemisia scoparia [herb]. *Yin chen* [*hao*] 茵蔯[蒿], 15-07
Artemisia scoparia Waldst. et Kit.
Asafetida. *E wei* 阿魏
Resin of *Ferula assa foetida* L.
Asarum caulescens [root]. *Du heng* 杜衡
Asarum caulescens Maxim.
Asarum heteropoides [root]. *Xi xin* 細辛
Asarum heteropoides Fr. Schmidt var. *manshuricum* (Maxim.) Kitag.
Asiatic cornelian cherry. *Shan zhu yu* 山茱萸
Cornus officinalis Sieb. et Zucc.
Asiatic elder. *Jie gu* [*mu*], 接骨[木]
Sambucus williamsii Hance
Asiatic plantain [herb/root/seed]. *Che qian* [*cao/zi*] 車前[草/子], 16-30
Plantago asiatica L.
Asparagus [root], *Tian men dong* 天門冬
Asparagus cochinchinensis (Lour.) Merr.
Astragalus [root]. [*Huang*] *qi* [黃]芪, *huang qi* 黄耆
Astragalus membranaceus Bunge var. *mongolicus* (Bunge) P. K. Hsiao
Atractylodes lancea [rhizome]. *Cang zhu* 蒼朮
Atractylodes lancea Thunb.
Atractylodes macrocephala [rhizome]. *Bai zhu* 白朮
Atractylodes macrocephala Koidz.
Auricularia fungus. *Mu er* 木耳
Auricularia auricula (L. ex Hook.) Underw.
Azalea [flower]. *Yang zhi zhu* 羊躑躅, 17-35
Rhododendron molle (Bl.) G. Don

B

Banana. *Gan jiao* 甘蕉, 15-47
Musa sapientum L
Barnyard grass. *Bai* 稗
Echinochloa crusgalli (L.) Beauv.
Bastard cardamon. *Sha ren* 砂仁, *suo sha mi* 縮砂蔤
Amomum villosum Lour.

Betel pepper. *Ju jiang* 蒟醬
Piper betle, L.

Bitter bamboo. *Ku zhu* 苦竹
Pleiobastus amarus (Keng) f.

Bitter orange fruit, immature and dried. *Zhi shi* 枳實
Poncirus trifoliata (L.) Raf.

Bitter orange fruit, cut in half and dried. *Zhi ke* 枳殼
Poncirus trifoliata. (L.) Raf.

Black cardamom. *Yi zhi ren/zi* 益智仁/子
Alpinia oxyphylla Miq.

Black mustard. *Jie* 芥
Brassica juncea (L.) Czern.et Coss.

Black pepper. *Hu jiao* 胡椒
Piper nigrum L.

Blackberry lily [root]. *Wu sha* 烏翣, *xuan hua* 萱花, *she gan* 射干, 17-29
Belamcanda chinensis (L.) DC.

Bland bamboo leaves. *Dan zhu ye* 淡竹葉, 16-08
Lopatherum gracile Brongn.

Box myrtle. *Yang mei* 楊梅
Myrica rubra (Lour.) Sieb. et Zucc.

Broom plant. *Du zhou* 獨帚, *di fu* 地膚, 16-24
Kochia scoparia (L.) Schrad.

Brown's lily [bulb]. *Bai he* 百合
Lilium brownii F.E. Brown ex Miellez var. *viridulum* Baker

Buckwheat [rhizome]. *Qiao mai* 蕎麥
Fagopyrum esculentum Moench

Bupleurum [root]. *Chai hu* 柴胡
Bupleurum chinense D.C.

Bushy knotweed [root]. *Ku zhang* 苦杖, *hu zhang* 虎杖
Polygonum cuspidatum Sieb. et Zucc.

Bushy *sophora*. *Shan dou gen* 山豆根
Sophora tonkinensis Gagnep.

C

Calabash. *Ku hu lu* 苦壺蘆, *ku hu* 苦瓠
Lagenaria siceraria (Molina) Standl. var. *microcarpa* (Naud.) Hara.

Calthrop [fruit]. *Ji li* 蒺藜, 16-61
Tribulus terrestris L.

Camphor mint. *Shui su* 水蘇, *ji su* 雞蘇
Stachys japonica Miq

Caper spurge. *Qian jin zi* 千金子, *xu sui* 續隨, 17-10
Euphorbia lathyris L

Carmichael's monkshood [root]. *Tian xiong* 天雄, 17-18
Aconitum carmichaeli Debx.

Carpesium [leaf/root]. *Tian ming jing* 天名精, *he shi* 鶴虱, *di song* 地菘, *du niu xi* 杜牛膝, 15-43
Carpesium abrotanoides L.

Carrot. *Hu luo bo* 胡蘿蔔
Daucus carota L. var. *sativa* Hoffm.

Cassia, cinnamomum cassia bark. *Gui* 桂, *la gui* 辣桂
Unscraped bark from smaller, younger branches of Cinnamom-tree
Cinnamomum cassia Presl.

Castor bean, castor oil plant. *Bi ma* 蓖麻, *pi ma* 蜱麻, 17-13
Ricinus communis L.

Cat thistle. *Xiao ji* 小薊, *mao ji* 猫薊,
Cirsium setosum (Willd.) MB.

Catalpa [tree]. *Qiu* 楸
Catalpa bungei C.A. Mey.

Cattail [pollen]. *Pu* [*huang*] 蒲[黄]
Typha spp.

Celery. *Qin* 芹
Apium graveolans L.

Celery cabbage. [*Shan*] *bai cai* [山]白菜, *song* 菘, *yun tai* 芸薹
Brassica campestris L.

Chaulmoogra. *Da feng zi* 大風子
Hydnocarpus anthelmintica Pierre

Chinese *angelica* [root]. *Dang gui* 當歸
Angelica sinensis (Oliv.) Diels

Chinese artichoke. *Gan lu zi* 甘露子
Stachys sieboldii Miq.

Chinese *azalea*. *Ying shan hong* 映山紅, 17-35-A01
Rhododendron simsii Planch.

Chinese cedar wood. *Shan* 杉
Cunninghamia lanceoloata (Lambt.) Hook.

Chinese celery. *Shui qin* 水芹
Oenanthe javanica (Bl.) DC.
Chinese chestnut. *Li* 栗
Castanea molissima L.
Chinese chive. *Xie bai* 薤白
Allium macrostemon Bge.
Chinese *clematis* [root]. *Wei ling xian* 威靈仙
Clematis chinensis Osbeck.
Chinese coffee tree [fruit]. *Fei zao [jia]* 肥皂[莢]
Gymnocladus chinensis Baill.
Chinese creeping fern. *Wu jiu* 烏韭
Odontosoria chinensis (L.) J. Sm
Chinese date. [*Da*] *zao* [大]棗, *jiao zao* 膠棗.
Zizyphus jujuba Mill.
Chinese dwarf cherries. *Yu li* 郁李
Cerasus japonica (Thunb.) Lois
Chinese elder. *Shuo diao* 蒴藋, *lu ying* 陸英, *jin cao* 堇草, 16-40, 16-41
Sambucus chinensis Lindl.
Chinese foxglove [root/rhizome]. *Di huang* 地黃, *hu* 苄, 16-01
Rehmannia glutinosa (Gaertn.) Libosch. ex Fisch et Mey.
Chinese indigo plant [leaf]. *Lan* [*ye*] 藍[葉], *da qing* 大青
1. *Liao lan* 蓼藍, *Polygonum tinctorium* Lour.
2. *Song lan* 菘藍, *Isatis indigofera* L.
3. *Ma lan* 馬藍, *Baphicacanthus cusia* (Nees) Bremek
4. *Mu lan* 木藍, *Indigofera tinctoria* L.
Chinese iris. *Ma lin zi* 馬藺子, 15-40
Iris lactea Pall. var. *chinensis* (Fisch.) Koidz.
Chinese lantern plant. *Suan jiang* 酸漿, *deng long cao* 燈籠草, 16-16
Physalis alkekengi L. var. *franchetii* (Mast.) Makino
Chinese leek. *Jiu* 韭
Allium tuberosum Rottl. ex Spreng.
Chinese *ligusticum*. *Gao ben* 藁本
Ligusticum sinense Oliv.
Chinese mallow. *Kui* 葵, 16-10
Malva verticillata L.
Chinese pepper. [*Hua*] *jiao* [花]椒, *jiao hong* 椒紅, *jiao mu* 椒目
Xanthoxylum amatum DC.

Chinese quinine. *Shu qi* 蜀漆, *chang shan* 常山; *heng shan* 恒山 17-14
Dichroa febrifuga Lour.

Chinese redbud. *Zi jing* 紫荆
Cercis chinensis Bge.

Chinese sage. *Dan shen* 丹參
Salvia miltiorrhiza Bunge

Chinese Sarsaparilla. *Ba qi* 菝葜
Smilax china L.

Chinese star jasmine. *Bai hua teng* 白花藤
Trachelospermum jasminoides (Lindl.) Lem.

Chinese sumac gallnut. *Wu bei zi* 五倍子
Galls produced by *Schlechtendalia chinensis* on leaves of *Rhus javanica* L. and other spec.

Chinese sweet gum. *Feng* [*xiang zhi*] 楓[香脂]
Liquidambar formosana Hance.

Chinese yam. *Shan yao* 山藥, *shu yu* 薯蕷
Dioscorea opposita Thunb.

Chrysanthemum flower. *Ju hua* 菊花
Dendranthema morifolium (Ramat) Tzvel.

Cimicifuga [rhizome]. *Sheng ma* 升麻
Cimicifuga foetida L.

Cinnamom tree, unscraped bark. *Rou gui* 肉桂
Cinnamomum cassia Presl.

Clematis creeper. *Nü wei* 女萎
Clematis apiifolia DC.

Climbing nightshade. *Pai feng teng* 排風藤
Solanum lyratum Thunb.

Cloves. *Ding xiang* 丁香, *ji she xiang* 雞舌香
Flower buds of *Syzygium aromaticum* (L.) Merr. et Perry

Cnidium [herb]. *She chuang* 蛇牀, *zao ji* 棗肌
Cnidium monnieri (L.) Cusson

Cocklebur. *Cang er* [*ye*] 蒼耳[葉], *xi er* 枲耳, *yang fu lai* 羊負來, 15-42
Xanthium sibiricum Patrin ex Widder

Cockscomb [seed]. *Ji guan* [*zi*] 鷄冠[子], 15-26
Celosia cristata L.

Coconut. *Ye zi* 椰子
Cocos nucifera L.

Cowpea. *Jiang dou* 豇豆, 江豆
Vigna unguiculata (L.) Walp.
Croton seed. *Ba dou* 巴豆, *gang zi* 剛子
Croton tiglium L.
Cudweed. *Shu er cao* 鼠耳草, *fo er cao* 佛耳草, 16-22
Gnaphalium affine D.Don
Cursed crow foot. *Shi long rui* 龍芮, 17-41
Ranunculus sceleratus L.
Cuscuta [seed]. *Tu si zi* 兔絲子
Cuscuta chinensis Lam.
Cynanchum atratum [root]. *Bai wei* 白薇
Cynanchum atratum Bunge
Cynanchum paniculatum [root]. *Xu chang qing* 徐長卿
Cynanchum paniculatum (Bunge) Kitag.
Cynanchum stauntonii [root]. *Bai qian* 白前
Cynanchum stauntonii (Decne.) Schltr. ex Lèvl.

D

Dahurian *patrinia*. *Bai jiang* 敗醬, 16-19
Patrinia scabiosaefolia Fisch. exTrev.
Dandelion. *Pu gong ying* 蒲公英
Taraxacum mongolicum Hand-Mazz.
Daphne [flower]. *Yuan hua* 芫花, 17-36
Daphne genkwa Sieb. et Zucc.
Dark plum. *Mei* 梅
Armeniaca mume Sieb.
Demon needle [herb]. *Gui zhen* [*cao*] 鬼針[草]
Bidens bipinnata L.
Desert broomrape. [*Rou*] *cong rong* [肉]蓯蓉
Cistanche deserticola Y. C. Ma.
Devil's tongue. *Ju ruo* 蒟蒻, 17-25
Amorphallus revieri Durieu
Diarrhena herb. *Zong xin cao* 粽心草, *long chang cao* 龍常草, 15-52
Diarrhena manshurica Maxim.
Dictamnus [root bark]. *Bai xian* [*pi*] 白鮮[皮]
Dictamnus angustifolius G. Don ex Sweet.
Dioscorea [root]. *Bi xie* 萆薢
Dioscorea collettii Hook f. var. *hypoglauca* (Palibin) Péi et Ting

Dragon tree. *Tong* 桐
Paulownia fortunei (Seem.) Hemsl.
Dryopteris [root]. *Guan zhong* 貫衆, *feng wei cao* 鳳尾草
Dryopteris crassirhizoma Nakai
Ducksmeat. *Fu ping* 浮萍
Spirodela polyrhiza (L.) Schleid.

E

Edible tulip. *Shan ci gu* 山慈姑, 17-15-A01
Tulipa edulis (Miq.) Baker
Eggplant. *Qie* 茄, *luo su* 落蘇
Solanum melogena L.
Eleocharis [fruit]. *Fu ci* 鳧茈
Eleocharis dulcis (Burm. f.) Trin. ex Henschel
Elsholtzia [herb]. *Xiang ru* 香薷, *xiang ru* 香葇
Elsholtzia ciliata (Thunb.) Hyland
Ephedra [herb]. *Ma huang* 麻黄, 15-49
Ephedra sinica Stapf
Eriocaulon [scape and flower]. *Gu jing cao* 穀精草, 16-62
Eriocaulon buergerianum Koern.
Eucommia [bark]. *Du zhong* 杜仲
Eucommia ulmoides Oliv.
Eupatorium [herb/leaf]. *Lan* [*cao*] 蘭[草]
Eupatorium fortunei Turcz.
Evodia [fruit]. [*Wu*] *zhu yu* [吴]茱萸
Evodia rutaecarpa (Juss.) Benth.

F

Fennel [fruit]. *Hui xiang* 茴香, *huai xiang* 懷香
Foeniculum vulgare Mill.
Fetid *cassia* [seeds]. *Jue ming* [*zi*] 决明[子], 16-23
Cassia tora L.
Five-leaves herb. *Wu ye cao* 五葉草
Erodium stephanianum Willd.
Floss grass. *Mao hua* 茅花; *bai mao* 白茅
Imperata cylindrica (L.) Beauv. var. *major*

Forsythia [fruit]. *Lian qiao* 連翹, 16-39
Forsythia suspensa (Thunb.) Vahl.
Foxnut [fruit/seeds]. *Ji tou* [*shi*] 雞頭[實], *qian zi* 芡子.
Euryale ferox Salisb.
Fraxinus bark. *Qin pi* 秦皮
Fraxinus rhynchophylla Hance
Fringed pink. *Qu mai* 瞿麦, *shi zhu* 石竹, 16-25
Dianthus superbus S.;
Fritillaria [root]. *Bei mu* 貝母
Fritillaria unibracteata Hsiao et K.C. Hsia

G

Galgant. *Shan nai* 山柰
Kaempferia galanga L.
Gamboge. *Teng huang* 藤黄
Garcinia morella Desv.(M.J.)
Garden daisy [seed]. *Peng hao* 蓬蒿, *tong hao* [*zi*] 茼蒿[子], 同蒿[子]
Chrysanthemum carinatum Schousb.
Garden lettuce. *Wo ju* 萵苣
Lactuca sativa L.
Garden sorrel. *Tu da huang* 土大黄.
Rumex acetosa L.
[Mountain] *gardenia* [fruit]. [*Shan*] *zhi zi* [山]卮子
Gardenia jasminoides Ellis.
Gastrodia [root/seedling]. *Chi jian* 赤箭, *tian ma* [*miao*] 天麻[苗]
Gastrodia elata BL
Gelsemium [herb]. *Huang teng* 黄藤, *ye ge* 野葛, *gou wen* 鈎吻, 17-47
Gelsemium elegans (Gardn.et Champ.) Benth.
Gingko [seed]. *Bai guo* 白果
Ginkgo biloba L.
Ginseng [root]. *Ren shen* 人參
Panax ginseng C. A. Meyer
Gleditsia [pod/seed], [bark]. *Zao jiao* 皂角, *zao jia* 皂莢
Gleditsia sinensis Lam.
Glycyrrhiza [root]. *Gan cao* 甘草, *fen cao* 粉草
Glycyrrhiza uralensis Fisch.
Golden eye grass. *Xian mao* 仙茅
Curculigo orchioides Baertn.

Great burdock [seeds]. *Niu bang* 牛蒡, *e shi* 惡實, *shu nian zi* 鼠粘子, 15-41
Arctium lappa L.

H

Hawthorne. *Shan zha* 山楂, *shan li hong guo* 山裏紅果
Crataegus pinnatifada Bunge var. major N.F. Br.
Hedge bindweed [flower/root]. *Gu zi hua* 鼓子花, *xuan hua* 旋花[根]
Calystegia sepium (L.) R. Br.
Hemp [herb]. *Qing ma* 青麻, *huo ma* 火麻, *xi ma* 菒麻
Cannabis sativa L.
Hemp seeds. *Da ma zi* 大麻子, *da ma ren* 大麻仁
Cannabis sativa L.
Henbane [seed]. *Lang dang* 莨菪, *tian xian* [*zi*] 天仙[子], 17-11
Hyoscyamus niger F. W. Schmidt
Hibiscus [root bark]. *Mu jin* 木槿
Hibiscus syriacus L.
Himalayan teasel herb [root]. *Xu duan* 續斷, 15-31
Dipsacus asperoides C. Y. Cheng et T. M. Ai.
Honeysuckle [stem]. *Ren dong* [*teng*] 忍冬[藤], *jin yin teng* 金银藤, *lu si teng* 鷺鷥藤
Lonicera japonica Thunb.
Horse thistle. *Ma ji* 馬薊, 15-30
Cirsium japonicum Fisch. ex DC.
Horseheal [flower/leaf/root]. *Xuan fu hua* 旋覆花, *di di jin* [*gen*] 滴滴金[根], 15-24
Inula japonica Thunb.

I

Illiceum [leaf]. *Mang cao* 莽草, *shu mang* 鼠莽, 17-39
Illiceum lanceolatum A. C. Smith
Indian lotus seed germs. *Lian rou* 蓮肉
The green germs of the mature seeds of *Nelumbo nucifera* Gaertn.
Indian lotus flower. *Lian hua* 蓮花, *han dan* 菡萏, *fu rong* 芙蓉
Indian lotus rhizome node. *Ou jie* 藕節
Indian lotus stalk with leaves. *He* 荷
Nelumbo nucifera Gaertn.
Indian mallow. *Qing ma* 苘麻, 15-36
Abutilon theophrasti Medic.

Indian pokewee [root]. *Shang lu* 商陸[根], 17-02
Phytolacca acinosa Roxb.
Indian strawberry. *She mei* 蛇莓, *she mei* 蛇苺
Duchesnea indica (Andr.) Focke
Indian turnip [root]. [*Tian*] *nan xing* [天]南星, *hu zhang* 虎掌, 虎杖, 17-23, 17-24
Arisaema thunbergii Bl.
Indigo. [*Qing*] *dai* [青]黛
Prepared from --> Chinese Indigo plants
Indocalamus [leaf]. *Ruo* 箬
Indocalamus tesselatus (Munro) Keng
Ink plant. *Han lian cao* 旱蓮草, 16-38
Eclipta prostrata (L.) L.

J

Japanese *artemisia*. *Mu hao* 牡蒿, 15-15
Artemisia japonica Thunb.
Japanese brome. *Yan mai* 燕麦
Bromus japonicus Thunb.
Japanese buttercup. *Mao gen* 毛茛, 17-42
Ranunculus japonicus Thunb.
Japanese *cayratia*. *Wu zhao long* 五爪龍
Cayratia japonica (Thunb.) Gagnep.
Japanese dock. *Yang ti* 羊蹄
Rumex crispus L. var. japonicus (Houtt.) Makino
Japanese ginger [root/herb]. *Rang he* 蘘荷, *su pu* 宿蒪, 15-48
Zingiber mioga (Thunb.) Rosc.
Japanese musk maple. *Fu bei* 腐婢.
Premna microphylla Wall. ex Schauer
Japanese *salvia*. *Shu wei cao* 鼠尾草, 16-35
Salvia japonica Th.
Japanese snake gourd. *Tu gua* 土瓜, *gua lou* 瓜蔞
Trichosanthes cucumeroides (Ser.) Maxim.
Japanese thistle. *Da ji* 薊, *xiao ji* 小薊, *mao ji* 猫薊 15-30
encompassing:
Tiger thistle: *da ji* 薊
Cirsium japonicum Fisch. ex DC.

Cat thistle: *xiao ji* 小薊, *mao ji* 猫薊,
Cirsium setosum (Willd.) MB.

Job's tears. *Yi yi ren* 薏苡仁
Seeds of *coix lacryma* L.

Jujube, *suan zao* 酸棗
Zizyphus jujuba Mill. var. *spinosa* (Bunge) Hu ex H.F.Chow

K

Kansui [root]. *Gan sui* 甘遂, 17-09
Euphorbia kansui T. N. Liou ex T.P. Wang

Keiske *artemisia*. *Yan lü* 菴藺, 15-03
Artemisia keiskeana Miq.

Kite's tail iris. *Yuan wei* 鳶尾, 17-30
Iris tectorum Maxim.

Kleinian cinquefoil. *She han* 蛇含, 16-33
Potentilla kleiniana Wight et Arn.

Korean gentian. *Long dan cao* 龍膽草
Gentiana scabra Bunge

Korean lawngrass. *Jie lü cao* 結縷草
Zoysia japonica Steud.

L

Lady's thumb. *Ma liao* 馬蓼, 16-49
Polygonum persicaria L.

Lamb's quarters. *Li* 藜
Chenopodium album L.

Large *gentiana* [root]. *Qin jiao* 秦艽
Gentiana macrophylla Pall.

Large-leaved senna. *Jiang mang* 茳芒, 16-23-A01
Cassia sophora L.

Lesser galangal [root]. *Gao liang jiang* 高良薑, *man jiang* 蠻薑
Alpinia officinarum Hance

Libanotis [herb]. *Xie hao* 邪蒿, 斜蒿
Libanotis seseloides (Fisch. et Mey. ex Turcz.) Turcz.

Ligusticum [root]. *Xiong qiong* 芎藭, *chuan xiong* 川芎, *mi wu* 蘼蕪, *fu xiong* 撫芎, *que niao xiong* 雀腦芎
Ligusticum chuanxiong Hort.

Lindera [root]. *Wu yao* 烏藥
Lindera aggregata (Sims.) Kosterm.
Linear leaf thistle. *Ku ao* 苦芙, 15-32
Cirsium chinense Gardn. et Champ.
Long pepper. *Bi ba* 華茇
Piper longum L.
Longan [seed]. *Long yan* 龍眼
Dimocarpus longan Lour.
Loofah. *Si gua* 絲瓜
Luffa cylindrica (L.) Roem.
Loquat. *Pi pa* 枇杷
Eriobotrya japonica L.
Love apple [root]. *Zao xiu* 蚤休, *chong tai* 重臺, *zi he che* 紫河車, 17-27
Paris polyphylla Smith var. *chinensis* (Franch.) Hara
Lychee [fruit]. *Li zhi* 荔枝
Litchi chinensis Sonn.
Lycium root bark. *Di gu pi* 地骨皮
Lycium barbarum L.
Lycium [seed]. *Gou qi* [*zi*] 枸杞[子]
Lycium chinense Mill.

M

Madder. *Qian* 蒨, 茜
Rubia cordifolia L.
Maesa [leaf]. *Tu chang shan* 土常山, 17-14-A01
Maesa japonica (Thunb.) Moritzi
Magnolia flower bud. *Xin yi* 辛夷
Magnolia biondii Pamp.
Magnolia bark. *Hou po* 厚朴
Magnolia officinalis Rehd. et Wils.
Malabar nightshade. *Luo kui* 落葵
Basella alba L.
Mayflower glorybower. *Da qing* 大青, 15-37
Clerodendrum cyrtophyllum Turcz.
Metaplexis [leaf]. *Luo mo* 蘿藦, *wan lan* 芄蘭, *bai huan teng* 白環藤
Metaplexis japonica (Thunb.) Makino
Mimosa [bark]. *He huan* 合歡
Albizzia julibrissin Durazz.

Mint. *Bo he* 薄荷, *jin qian bo he* 金錢薄荷
Mentha canadensis L.
Momordica seed. *Mu bie zi* 木鼈子
Momordica cochinchinensis (Lour.) Spreng.
Morinda [root]. *Ba ji* [*tian*] 巴戟[天]
Morinda officinalis How.
Mulberry tree bark. *Sang bai pi* 桑白皮
Morus alba L.
Musk melon fruit base. *Gua di* 瓜蒂
Cucumis melo L.
Mysore thorn. *Yun shi* 雲實, 17-12
Cesalpinia decapetala (Roth) Alston

N

Naked barley. *Kuang mai* 穬麥
Hordeum vulgare var. *nudum* Hook. f.
Nanmu [tree]. *Nan* 楠
Phoebe zhennan S.Lee et F.N.Wei
Natural indigo. *Qing dai* 青黛
Prepared from → Chinese indigo plants
Nettle. *Qian ma* 蕁麻, 17-44
Urtica laetevirens Maxim.
Notopterygium [root]. *Qiang huo* 羌活
Notopterygium incisum Ting ex H. T. Chang
Nutgrass. *Suo cao* 莎草, *xiang fu* [*zi*] 香附[子]
Cyperus rotundus L.
Nutmeg. *Rou dou kou* 肉豆蔻
Myristica fragrans Houtt.
Nymphoides [herb]. *Jin lian zi* 金蓮子, *shui xing* 水荇, *fu kui* 鳧葵
Nymphoides peltatum (Gmel.) O. Ktze.

O

Okra. *Huang shu kui* 黄蜀葵, 16-13
Abelmoschus manihot (L.) Medic.
Onion [white]. *Cong* 葱. *Cong bai* 葱白.
Onion seed. *Cong shi* 葱實
Allium fistulosum L.

Ophiopogon [tuber]. *Mai men dong* 麥門冬, 16-05
Ophiopogon japonicus (L. f.) Ker-Gawl.
Orange, unripe. *Zhi qiao* 枳殼
Citrus aurantium L.

P

Paeonia [root], white/red. [*Bai/chi*] *shao yao* [白/赤]芍藥
Paeonia veitchii Lynch.
Paeonia root bark. *Mu dan* [*pi*] 牡丹[皮], *bai mu dan gen* [*pi*] 白牡丹根[皮]
Paeonia suffruticosa Andr.
Pak choi. *Song cai* 菘菜
Brassica rapa subsp. *chinensis*
Paper mulberry tree. *Chu* 楮
Broussonetia papyrifera (L.) Vent.
Paris [root]. *Mu meng* 牡蒙, *wang sun* 王孫
Paris bashanensis Wang et Tang
Pea. *Bi dou* 畢豆, *hu dou* 胡豆
Pisum sativum L.
Peach [seed]. *Tao* [*ren*] 桃[仁]
Amygdalus persica L.
Peking spurge [root]. *Da ji* 大戟, 17-07
Euphorbia pekinensis Rupr.
Pennycress. *Xi ming* 菥蓂
Thlaspi arvense L.
Perilla [stem/leaf]. *Zi su* 紫蘇, *bai su* 白蘇
Perilla frutescens (L.) Britt. var.*arguta* (Benth.) Hand.-Mazz.
Perilla herb. *Ren* 荏.
Perilla frutescens (L.) Britt.
Persian lilac fruit. *Shan lian zi* 山楝子
Melia azedarach L.
Persimmon fruit calyx. *Shi di* 柿蒂
Diospyros kaki Thunb.
Peucedanum [root]. *Fang kui* 防葵, 17-04
Peucedanum japonicum Thunb.
Pharbitis [seed]. [*Hei*] *qian niu* [*zi*] [黑]牽牛子, [*bai*] *qian niu* [白]牽牛
Pharbitis nil (L.) Choisy
Phellodendron bark. *Huang bo* 黃蘗, 黃檗, 黃柏
Phellodendron amurense Ruppr.

Photinia [leaf]. *Shi nan* 石南
Photinia serrulata Lindl.
Pinellia [root]. *Ban xia* 半夏, 17-26
Pinellia ternata (Thunb.) Breit.
Platycodon [root]. *Jie geng* 桔梗
Platycodon grandiflorus (Jacq.) A. DC.
Polygala [root]. *Yuan zhi* 遠志
Polygala tenuifolia Willd.
Polygonatum odoratum [root]. *Wei rui* 萎蕤
Polygonatum odoratum (Mill.) Druce
Polygonum multiflorum [root]. *He shou wu* 何首烏
Polygonum multiflorum Thunb.
Polypody. *Gu sui bu* 骨碎補
Drynaria fortunei (Kunze) J.Smith
Polyporus sclerotium. *Zhu ling* 猪苓
Polyporus umbellatus (Pers.) Fr.
Pomegranate [flower/seeds]. *Shi liu* [*hua*/zi] 石榴[花/子]
Punica granatum L.
Poplar. *Bai yang* 白楊
Populus davidiana Dode
Poppy. *Yu mi* 御米
Papaver somniferum L.
Poria. *Fu ling* 茯苓, *fu shen* 伏神
Sclerotium of *Poria cocos* (Schw.) Wolf
Prince's feather. *Qing xiang* 青葙, 15-25
Celosia argentea L.
Prunus plum. *Li* 李
Prunus salicina Lindl. Plum.
Pteridium vegetable. *Jue* 蕨
Pteridium aquilinum (L.) Kuhn var. *latiusculum* (Desv.) Underw.
Pueraria [root]. *Ge* [*gen*] 葛[根]
Pueraria lobata (Willd.) Ohwi
Pulsatilla herb. *Bai tou weng cao* 白頭翁草
Pulsatilla chinensis (Bunge) Regel
Purple aster [root]. *Zi wan* 紫菀, 16-03
Aster tataricus L. f. .Purple aster.

Purple *chrysanthemum*. *Ma lan* 馬蘭
Kalimeris indica (L.) Sch.-Bip.
Purslane. *Ma chi* [*xian*] 馬齒[莧]
Portulaca oleracea L.
Pyrrosia [leaf]. *Shi wei* 石韋
Pyrrosia lingua (Thunb.) Farw.

Q

Queen coralbead. *Mu fang ji* 木防己
Cocculus orbiculatus (L.) DC.
Quince. *Mu gua* 木瓜
Chaenomeles speciosa (Sweet) Nakai

R

Radish [seed]. *Luo bo* 蘿蔔, *lai fu* [*zi*] 萊菔[子]
Raphanus sativus L.
Ramie plant. *Zhu* [*ma*] 苧[麻], 15-35
Boehmeria nivea (L.) Gaud.
Rape turnip. *Wu jing* 蕪菁, *man jing* 蔓菁
Brassica rapa L.
Red cardamom. *Cao guo* 草果
Amomum tsao-ko Crevost et Lemaire
Red knotweed. [*Shui*] *hong* [*cao*] [水]葒[草], *liao hong* 蓼洪, 16-50
Polygonum orientale L.
Red mung bean. *Chi xiao dou* 赤小豆, *hong dou* 紅豆
Vigna umbellata (Thunb.) Ohwi et Ohashi
Rhubarb root. *Da huang* 大黃, 17-01
Rheum palmatum L.
Roof pine. *Wa song* 瓦松
Orostachys fimbriata (Turcz.) Breger
Rubus seed. *Fu pen zi* 覆盆子
Rubus chingii Hu

S

Safflower. *Hong hua* 紅花, *hong lan* 紅藍, 15-27
Carthamus tinctorius L.

Sanguisorba [root]. *Di yu* 地榆
Sanguisorba officinalis L.
Saposhnikovia [root]. *Fang feng* 防風
Saposhnikovia divaricata (Turcz.)
Sargassum herb. *Hai zao* 海藻
Sargassum fusiforme (Harv.) Setch.
Sawtooth oak. *Xiang shi* 橡實, *xiang dou* 橡斗
Quercus acutissima Carr.
Schisandra seed. *Wu wei zi/he* 五味子/核
Schisandra chinensis Turcz. Baill.
Schizonepeta [spike, fruit]. *Jing jie* 荆芥
Schizonepeta multifida (L.) Briq.
Schneider's zelkova. *Ju* 櫸
Zelkova schneideriana Hand.-Mazz.
Scrophularia [root]. *Xuan shen* 玄參, *chong tai* 重臺
Scrophularia ningpoensis Hemsl.
Scurfy pea. *Po gu zhi* 破故紙
Psoralea corylifolia L.
Scutellaria [root]. *Huang qin* 黃芩
Scutellaria baicalensis Georgi
Sesame [seed]. *Ju sheng* [*zi*] 巨勝[子], *zhi ma* 脂麻
Sesamum indicum L.
Shaved cinnamom bark. *Gui xin* 桂心
Cinnamomum cassia Presl.
Shepherd's purse. *Ji cai* 蕺菜
Capsella bursa-pastoris (L.) Medic.
Siberian elm. *Yu* 榆
Ulmus pumila L.
Siberian milfoil. *Shi* 蓍
Achillea alpina L.
Siberian motherwort. *Yi mu* [*cao*] 益母[草], *chong wei* 茺蔚, 15-17
Leonurus japonicus Houtt.
Sievers wormwood. *Bai hao* 白蒿, *lou hao* 蔞蒿, 15-10
Artemisia sieversiana Ehrhart ex Willd
Silkwormthorn. *Zhe* 柘
Maclura tricuspidata Carr.

Sim's azalea. *Shan shi liu* 山石榴, *shan zhi zhu* 山躑躅, 17-35-A01
Rhododendron simsii Planch.
Simpleleaf chastetree [seeds]. *Man jing* 蔓荆[子]
Vitex trifolia L. var. *simplicifolia* Cham.
Skimmia [stem/leaf]. *Yin yu* 茵蕷, 17-40
Skimmia reevesiana Fort.
Sow thistle. *Ku ju* 苦苣,
Ixeris chinensis (Thunb.) Nakai subsp. *versicolor* (Fisch. ex Link) Kitam. and *ku mai* 苦蕒, *Ixeris denticulata* (Houtt.) Stebb
Soft rush. [*Shi*] *long chu* [石]龍芻, 15-51
Juncus setchuensis L.
Seven-leaf nightshade. *Qi gu cao* 漆姑草, 16-17
Solanum septenlobum Bunge
Sneezeweed. *E* [*bu shi*] *cao* 鵝[不食]草
Centipeda minima (L.) A.Br. et Ascher.
Solomon's seal [root]. *Huang jing* 黄精
Polygonatum sibiricum Delar. ex Redoute
Sophora japonica [tree leaves]. *Huai* [*ye*] 槐[葉]
Sophora japonica L.
Sophora [root]. *Ku shen* 苦參
Sophora flavescens Ait.
Spiked millet. *Qing liang mi* 青粱米
Setaria italica (L.) Beauv.
Spurge. [*Cao*] lü ru [草]藺茹, 17-06
Euphorbia ebracteolata Hayata
St. Paulswort. *Nian hu cai* 粘糊菜, 15-44
Siegesbeckia orientalis L.
Stemona [root]. *Bai bu* 百部
Stemona sessilifolia Miq.
Stephania tetrandra [root]. *Fang ji* 防己
Stephania tetrandra Moore
Stonecrop. *Jing tian* 景天
Hylotelephium erythrostictum (Miq.) H. Ohba
Storax. *Su he xiang* 蘇合香
Liquidambar orientalis Mill.
Strong fragrant loosestrife. *Hui cao* 蕙草
Lysimachia foenum-graecum Hance

Sugar cane. *Gan zhe* 甘蔗
Saccharum sinensis Roxb.
Swamp morning glory. *Weng cai* 蕹菜
Ipomea aquatica Forsk.
Sweet basil. *Lan xiang* 蘭香, *luo le* 羅勒, *xiang cai* 香菜
Ocimum basilicum L.
Sweet wormwood. *Liu ji nu cao* 劉寄奴草, 15-21
Artemisia anomala S. Moore, 15-21

T

Tangerine peel. *Chen pi* 陳皮, *ju pi* 橘皮, *ju hong* 橘紅
Citrus reticulata Blanco
Taro [seeds/tuber]. [*Ye*] *yu* [野]芋, *yu zi* 芋子, *yu kui* 芋魁
Colocasia esculenta L. Schott
Taxillus mistletoe. *Zhan si* 占斯
Taxillus nigrans (Hance) Danser
Terminalia fruit. *He li le* 訶黎勒, *he zi* 訶子
Terminalia chebula Retz.
Thunderball fungus. *Lei wan* 雷丸
Polyporus mylittae Cook at Mass.
Thyme-leaf spurge. *Di jin* 地锦
Euphorbia humifusa Willd. *E. maculata* L.
Tiger thistle. *Hu ji* 虎薊, 15-30
Cirsium japonicum Fisch. ex DC.
Touch-me-not. *Feng xian* 鳳仙, 17-32
Impatiens balsamina L.
Trachycarpus [palm]. *Zong lü* 椶櫚
Trachycarpus fortunei (Hook) H.Endl.
Trichosanthes [root]. *Tian hua fen* 天花粉, *gua lou* [*gen*] 栝樓[根]
Trichosanthes kirilowii Maxim.
Trumpet flower. *Ling xiao* 凌霄, *zi wei* 紫葳
Campsis grandiflora (Thunb.) Loisel ex K. Schum.
Turczaninowia [root]. *Nü wan* 女菀, 16-04
Turczaninowia fastigiata (Fisch.) DC.

U

Ulmus [fruit]. *Wu yi* 蕪荑
Ulmus macrocarpa Hance
Umbrella leaf herb [root]. *Gui jiu* 鬼臼, *qiong tian cao* 璚田草, 17-28
Dysosma versipellis (Hance) M. Cheng ex Ying
Uniflower Swiss centaury. *Lou lu* 漏蘆, 15-33
Stemmacantha uniflorum (L.) Dittrich

V

Veratrum [root]. *Li lu* 藜蘆, 17-15
Veratrum nigrum L.
Vervain. *Ma bian cao* 馬鞭草, 16-32
Verbena officinalis L.
Vitex [herb]. *Huang jing* 黄荆, *mu jing* 牡荆
Vitex negundo L. var. *cannabifolia* (Sieb.et Zucc.) Hand.-Mazz.

W

Wall moss. *Yuan yi* 垣衣
Weissia controversa Hedw.
Walnut. *Hu tao* 胡桃
Juglans regia L.
Wartweed. *Ze qi* 澤漆, 17-08
Euphorbia helioscopia L.
Water pepper. *Liao* 蓼, 16-47, 16-48
Polygonum hydropiper L.
Wax gourd. *Dong gua* 冬瓜
Benincasa hispida (Thunb.) Cogn.
Welted thistle. *Fei lian* 飛廉, 15-34
Carduus crispus L.
Wheat [bran]. *Fou mai* 浮麥, *fu* 麩
Triticum aestivum L.
Wikstroemea [herb]. *Rao hua* 蕘花, 17-37
Wikstroemia canescens (Wall.) Meissn.
Wild hop. *Lü cao* 葎草
Humulus scandens (Lour.) Merr.
Wild turmeric. *Yu jin* 鬱金
Curcuma longa L.

Wild scarlet lily. *Shan dan* 山丹
Lilium concolor Salisb.
[Weeping] willow. [*Yang*] *liu* [楊]柳
Salix babylonica L.
Winter aster. *Ye ju* [*hua*] 野菊[花], *ku yi* 苦薏, 15-02
Dendranthema indicum (L.) des Moul.
Winter daphne [root]. *Rui xiang* 瑞香
Daphne acutiloba Rehd.
Winter horsetail. *Mu zei* 木賊, 15-50
Hippochaete hiemale (L.) Borher
Wolfsbane. *Lang du* 狼毒, 17-03
Stellaria chamaejasme L.
Wood whitlow grass. *Ting li* 葶藶, 16-29
Lepidium apetalum Willd.
Wormwood herb. *Qing hao* 青蒿, 15-08
Artemisia carvifolia Buch.-Ham. ex Roxb.

Y

Yellow day lily. *Xuan cao* 萱草, *lu cong* 鹿葱, 16-06
Hemerocallis citrina Baroni

Z

Zanthoxylum [fruit]. *Dang* [*zi*] 欓[子], *shi zhu yu* 食茱萸, *wu zhu yu* 吴茱萸
Zanthoxylum ailanthoides Sieb. et Zucc.

6.2. Substances discussed in chapters 15 – 17 in a separate entry. Listed in alphabetical order of their proper pin yin names with their popular English names where available and references to their entry.

A

Ai 艾, common mugwort. 15-05

B

Bai fu zi 白附子, *aconitum coreanum* Lèvl. 17-22
Bai hao 白蒿, sievers wormwood. 15-10
Bai jiang 敗醬, dahurian *patrinia*. 16-19
Ban bian lian 半邊蓮, *lobelia*. 16-67
Ban xia 半夏, *pinellia ternata*. 17-26
Bi ma 蓖麻, castor oil plant. 17-13
Bi se le 必似勒, unidentified. 15-40-A01
Bian xu 萹蓄, common knotgrass. 16-59
Bo luo hui 博落迴, unidentified. 17-13-A01

C

Can cai 蠶菜, *leonurus pseudomacranthus*. 15-18
Can wang cao 蠶繭草, Japanese knotweed. 16-55
Ce zi 側子, *aconitum* [marginal "child" tuber]. 17-19
Chang shan 常山, *shu qi* 蜀漆, Chinese quinine. 17-14
Che qian 車前, asiatic plantain. 16-30
Chong wei 茺蔚, Siberian motherwort. 15-17
Chui hu gen 槌胡根, unidentified. 16-07
Cui yu cao 醉魚草, Dr. Lindley's *buddleya*. 17-38

D

Da huang 大黄, rhubarb. 17-01
Da ji 大戟, Peking purge. 17-07
Da ji 大薊, *xiao ji* 小薊, *cirsium japonicum*. 15-30
Da qing 大青, mayflower glorybower. 15-37
Dan zhu ye 淡竹葉, bland bamboo leaves. 16-08

Deng xin cao 燈心草, common rush. 15-53
Di fu 地膚, broom plant. 16-24
Di huang 地黃, Chinese foxglove. 16-01
Di wu gong 地蜈蚣, golden hair starviolet. 16-66
Di yang mei 地楊梅, woodrush. 16-64
Dong kui 冬葵, Chinese mallow. 16-10
Du jing shan 杜莖山, Japanese maesa. 17-14-A01
Du yong jian jun 獨用將軍, *triosteum sinuatum*. 16-70
Dui lu 對廬, unidentified. 15-03-A01

E

E shi 惡實, great burdock. 15-41

F

Fan hong hua 番紅花, saffron. 15-28
Fang kui 防葵, *peucedanum japonicum*. 17-04
Fei lian 飛廉, welted thistle. 15-34
Feng xian 鳳仙, touch-me-not. 17-32
Fu zi 附子, *aconitum* [accessory tuber]. 17-17

G

Gan jiao 甘蕉, banana. 15-47
Gan lan 甘藍, cabbage varieties. 16-46
Gan sui 甘遂, Kansui. 17-09
Ge zhu cao 格注草, unidentified. 17-45
Gou she cao 狗舌草, dog's tongue herb. 16-31
Gou wei cao 狗尾草, green bristlegrass. 16-37
Gou wen 鉤吻, *Gelsemium elegans*. 17-47
Gu jing cao 穀精草, pipewort. 16-62
Gui jiu 鬼臼, umbrella leaf. 17-28
Gui zhen cao 鬼針草, beggar tick. 16-69

H

Hai gen 海根, *polygonum virginicum*. 16-52
Hai jiang 每薑, unidentified. 17-42-A01
Hai jin sha 海金沙, climbing fern. 16-63
Hai yu 海芋, *alocasia macrorhiza*. 17-46

Hong cao 葒草, red knotweed. 16-50
Hong lan hua 紅藍花, safflower. 15-27
Hu lu ba 胡盧巴, fenugreek. 15-39
Hu mian mang 胡面莽, unidentified. 16-01-A01
Hu zhang 虎杖, bushy knotweed. 16-57
Hu zhang, tian nan xing 虎掌天南星, Indian turnip. 17-23
Huang hua hao 黃花蒿, yellow flower wormwood. 15-09
Huang shu kui 黃蜀葵, okra. 16-13
Huo tan mu cao 火炭母草, Chinese knotweed. 16-53

J

Ji guan hua 雞冠花, cockscomb. 15-26
Ji li 蒺藜, calthrop. 16-61
Jian chun luo 剪春羅, mullein pink. 16-27
Jian zhong xiao 見腫消, *gynura segetum*. 16-71
Jiao hao 角蒿, Chinese *incarvillea*. 15-11
Jin cao 藎草, small carpetgrass. 16-60
Jin zhan cao 金盞草, marigold. 16-28
Jiu niu cao 九牛草, *chrysanthemum decaisneanum*. 15-16
Ju ruo 蒟蒻, devil's tongue. 17-25
Ju 菊, *chrysanthemum*. 15-01
Jue ming 決明, fetid *cassia*. 16-23

K

Ku ao 苦芺, linear leaf thistle. 15-32
Kuan dong hua 款冬花, coltsfoot. 16-21

L

Lan dian 藍澱, indigo. 16-44
Lan 藍, indigo plant. 16-43
Lang ba cao 狼把草, threelobe beggarticks. 16-36
Lang dang 莨菪, henbane. 17-11
lang du 狼毒, wolfsbane. 17-03
Lang ya 狼牙, hairy agrimony. 17-05
Li chang 鱧腸, ink plant. 16-38
Li lu 藜蘆, false hellebore. 17-15
Li shi 蠡實, Chinese iris. 15-40

M

N

Nü wan 女菀, *turczaninowia fastigiata*. 16-04

P

Pan dao zeng 攀倒甑, unidentified. 16-72
Pu sa cao 菩薩草, Bodhisattva herb. 17-25-A01

Q

Qian nian ai 千年艾, 1000 year old common mugwort. 15-06
Qing dai 青黛, natural indigo. 16-45
Qing hao 青蒿, wormwood. 15-08
Qing ma 苘麻, Indian mallow. 15-36
Qing xiang zi 青葙子, Prince's feather. 15-25
Qu jie cao 曲節草, Japanese *peristrophe*. 15-22
Qu mai 瞿麥, fringed pink. 16-25
Que qiao 雀翹, unidentified. 16-45-A01

R

Rang he 蘘荷, Japanese ginger. 15-48
Rao hua 蕘花, *wikstroemia canescens*. 17-37
Ruo 箬, unidentified. 15-45

S

San bai cao 三白草, Chinese lizard's tail. 16-54
Shan ci shi 山慈石, edible tulip. 17-15-A01
Shan zhi zhu 山躑躅, Chinese azalea. 17-35-A01
Shang lu 商陸, Indian pokeweed. 17-02
She gan 射干, blackberry lily. 17-29
She han 蛇含, kleinian cinquefoil. 16-33
She wang cao 蛇网草, hill-buckwheat. 16-56
Shen guo gen 參果根, unidentified. 17-15-A02
Shi jian cao 虱建草, unidentified. 17-43-A01
Shi long chu 石龍芻, soft rush. 15-51
Shi long rui 石龍芮, cursed crow foot. 17-41
Shi 蓍, Siberian milfoil. 15-04
Shu kui 蜀葵, common hollyhock. 16-11
Shu qu cao 鼠麴草, cudweed. 16-22
Shu wei cao 鼠尾草, Japanese *salvia*. 16-35

T

W

X

Y

Ya bu lu 押不蘆, *yabulu*. 17-33-A01
Ya zhi cao 鴨跖草, day flower. 16-09
Yan lai hong 雁來紅, redness derived from wild geese. 15-25-A02
Yan lü 菴藺, Keiske *artemisia*. 15-03
Yan zhi 燕脂, rouge. 15-29
Yang bu chi cao 羊不喫草, unidentified. 17-35-A02
Yang zhi zhu 羊躑躅, azalea. 17-35
Ye ju 野菊, winter aster. 15-02
Yin chen hao 茵蔯蒿, virgate wormwood. 15-07
Yin di jue 陰地厥, moonwort. 15-14
Yin yu 茵蕷, *skimmia reevesiana*. 17-40
Ying chun hua 迎春花, winter jasmine. 16-20
You ba 由跋, small root of Indian turnip. 17-24
You cao 蕕草, crabgrass. 16-58
Yu zan 玉簪, assumption lily. 17-31
Yuan hua cao 雲花草, unidentified. 15-49-A01
Yuan hua 芫花, daphne flower. 17-36
Yuan wei 鳶尾, kite's tail iris. 17-30
Yun shi 雲實, Mysore thorn. 17-12

Z

Zao xiu 蚤休, love apple. 17-27
Ze qi 澤漆, wartweed. 17-08
Zhu ma 苧麻, ramie plant. 15-35
Zi hua di ding 紫花地丁, purpleflower violet. 16-68
Zi wan 紫菀, purple aster. 16-03
Zuo na cao 坐拏草, unidentified. 17-33

6.3 Substances discussed in chapters 15 – 17 in a separate entry. Listed in alphabetical order of their currently accepted scientific identification with reference to their entry.

A

B

Belamcanda chinensis (L.) DC. 17-29
Bidens pilosa L. 16-69
Bidens tripartite L. 16-36
Boehmeria nivea (L.) Gaud. 15-35
Brassica oleracea L. var. *capitata* L. 16-44
Buddleya lindleyana Fort. 17-38

C

Calendula arvensis L. 16-28
Carduus crispus L. 15-34
Carpesium abrotanoides L. 15-43
Carthamus tinctorius L. 15-27
Cassia sophora L. 16-23-A01
Cassia tora L. 16-23
Celosia argentea L. 15-25
Celosia cristata L. 15-26
Cesalpinia decapetala (Roth) Alston. 17-12
Chrysanthemum decaisneanum Matsum. 15-16
Cirsium chinense Gardn. et Champ. 15-32
Cirsium japonicum DC. 15-30
Clerodendrum cyrtophyllum Turcz. 15-37
Commelina communis L. 16-09
Crocus sativus L. 15-28
Cynanchum thesinides (Freyn) K. Schum. 16-34

D

Daphne Genkwa Sieb. et Zucc. 17-36
Datura metel L. 17-34
Dendranthema indicum (L.) des Moul. 15-02
Dendranthema morifolium (Ramat) Tzvel. 15-10
Dianthus superbus S. 16-25
Diarrhena manshurica Maxim. 15-52
Dichroa febrifuga Lour. 17-14
Digitaria sanguinalis (L.) Scop. 16-58
Dipsacus asperoides C. Y. Cheng et T. M. Ai. 15-31
Dysosma versipellis (Hance) M. Cheng ex Ying. 17-28

E

F

G

H

I

J

R

S

Stellaria chamaejasme L. 17-03
Stemmacantha uniflorum (L.) Dittrich. 15-33

T

Tribulus terrestris R. 16-61
Trigonella foenum-graecum L. 15-39
Triosteum sinuatum Maxim. 16-70
Tubocapsicum anomalum (Franch. et Sav.) Makino. 16-15
Turczaninowia fastigiata (Fisch.) DC. 16-04
Tussilago farfara L. 16-21

U

Urtica laetevirens Maxim. 17-44

V

Vaccaria segetalis (Neck.) Garcke. 16-26
Veratrum nigrum L. 17-15
Verbena officinalis L. 16-32
Viola philipica Cav. 16-68

W

Wikstroemia canescens (Wall.) Meissn. 17-37

X

Xanthium sibiricum Patrin ex Widder. 15-42

Z

Zingiber mioga (Thunb.) Rosc. 15-48